# Health Promotion Strategies Through the Lifespan

## SECOND CANADIAN EDITION

# Health Promotion Strategies Through the Lifespan

## SECOND CANADIAN EDITION

### RUTH BECKMANN MURRAY
St. Louis University

### JUDITH PROCTOR ZENTNER
Director of Health Services, Hickory Hill Furniture Corporation

### VERNA PANGMAN
University of Manitoba

### CLARE PANGMAN
University of Manitoba

With contributions to Chapter 1 by
### JOANNE LOUIS
University of Toronto

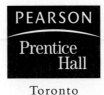

PEARSON

Prentice
Hall

Toronto

**Library and Archives Canada Cataloguing in Publication**

Health promotion strategies through the lifespan / Ruth Beckmann Murray . . . [et al.].—2nd
   Canadian ed.

   Includes index.
   ISBN-13: 978-0-13-615601-7

   1. Health promotion—Textbooks.   2. Life cycle, Human—Textbooks.   3. Nursing assessment—
Textbooks.   4. Developmental psychology—Textbooks.   I. Murray, Ruth Beckmann
II. Series: Prentice Hall health (Toronto, Ont.)

RT48.H44 2009          613          C2008-901644-0

ISBN-13: 978-0-13-615601-7
ISBN-10: 0-13-615601-0

Vice-President, Editorial Director: Gary Bennett
Acquisitions Editor: Michelle Sartor
Marketing Manager: Colleen Gauthier
Developmental Editor: Helen Smith/Catherine Belshaw
Production Editor: Jennifer Parks/Cheryl Jackson
Copy Editor: Susan Broadhurst
Proofreader: Anne Borden
Production Coordinator: Andrea Falkenberg/Sarah Lukaweski
Compositor: Integra
Permissions Researcher: Sandy Cooke
Art Director: Julia Hall
Cover and Interior Designer: Anthony Leung
Cover Image: Rick Gomez/Masterfile

2 3 4 5   12 11 10

Printed and bound in the United States of America.

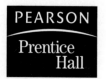

# Dedication

*This book is dedicated to*

*Students—for their inspiration*

*Friends—for their assistance*

*Our families—for their patience*

Ruth Beckmann Murray

Judith Proctor Zentner

*We dedicate this book to our loving parents,*

*Rose and William, and Essie and Harvey, whose spirits inspired us*

*in our journey to create and complete the first and second*

*Canadian editions with care and consideration.*

Verna Pangman

Clare Pangman

# Contents

# Preface

**Prepared by Verna C. Pangman and Clare Pangman**

Welcome to *Health Promotion Strategies through the Lifespan*, Second Canadian Edition. This new text serves to fulfill the need for a uniquely Canadian perspective of health promotion in nursing programs across the country. In preparing this second Canadian edition of the Murray and Zentner text, we endeavoured throughout to present a current and enriching Canadian orientation to the topics presented in the previous work, which will allow instructors and students to identify with these topics in a context that is most relevant for them.

The health of individuals and families is of paramount importance in our society today. Health promotion and wellness activities have exerted a profound influence on the complex decisions made by health professionals in widely varied health care settings across Canada. Nursing professionals work in collaboration with individuals and families to pursue optimum health practices that enhance the quality of life. Based on this premise, our main priority was to focus on a health promotion and preventative frame of reference throughout the lifespan, while remaining mindful of cultural differences.

We began by writing a prelude to the textbook. This prelude focuses first on the Canadian historical perspective of health promotion and secondly on the importance of the principles of health promotion in the delivery of care. In each subsequent chapter, emphasis has been placed on Canadian data and Canadian research findings relevant to each lifespan stage. The importance of evidence-based practice has been highlighted to promote wellness in individuals and families. In addition, the wellness diagnosis is presented to assist the reader in focusing on the strengths of the individual and family. The importance of the *Canadian Multiculturalism Act* is emphasized because it affects all Canadians in every province and territory. Therefore, the cultural aspect in the context of the health beliefs, attitudes, and behaviours of the individual and the family are incorporated into planning, implementing, and evaluating health care.

## APPROACH AND ORGANIZATION

The general organization followed in the first Canadian edition has been retained in the second Canadian edition. That is, each chapter follows a common sequence. Family development and relationships, physiological concepts, nutrition, rest and sleep, leisure, and health promotion are followed by psychosocial, cognitive, emotional, and moral/spiritual development. Finally, health care and family-centred nursing applications complete each chapter, with emphasis on common health issues. A Canadian perspective on Aboriginal populations is prevalent throughout this edition.

We have outlined some of the many changes and additions made for this edition. Over the next 25 years, the aging of the Canadian population will increase dramatically as baby-boomers enter late life. The proportion of the population over the age of 65 is expected to grow from the current 13 percent to 21 percent by the year 2026. This demographic transformation of Canadian society has profound consequences for all aspects of individual life, community, and the general public. We hope that you enjoy this second Canadian edition of *Health Promotion Strategies through the Lifespan*.

## NEW TO THIS EDITION

This second Canadian edition continues to be an important text for nursing students at both the undergraduate and graduate levels. As well, this text will be of value to practising nurses, because it brings updated Canadian research applications to a variety of settings. As in the previous Canadian edition, the purpose of the text is to promote the health of clients and their families through careful assessment, implementations, and evaluation—each of which is important for nurses in the twenty-first century.

For example, the "Canadian Guidelines for Water Quality" are presented in Chapter 2, as well as the "Canadian Nurses' Position Statement on Food Safety and Security as Determinants of Health." Some of the recent disease outbreaks in Canada and the world are taken into account, including SARS, West Nile Virus, and Mad Cow Disease. Census Canada 2001 figures on such topics as family structures, roles, and functions, and divorce rates are again incorporated into the second Canadian edition. Information on Canadian single parent families, as well as on step-families, is included. Of particular interest in Chapter 8 is the treatment of *Canada's Food Guide*, as it has been adapted for children. In Chapter 9, the relationship between grandparenting and the three main types of child care available in Canada are also introduced. The effects of poverty on Canadian children are discussed. The issues of obesity and eating disorders are newly addressed in Chapter 11, along with Canadian teenage pregnancy, STI (Sexually Transmitted Infections), and Canadian data on AIDS. Unique to this new edition is the Canadian research findings on the positive aspects of the caregiver's role. New Canadian data is employed in Chapter 14 to identify pertinent issues relating to the elderly; issues considered here cover everything from elder abuse to retirement. Finally, discussions of the place of one's death discussed in Chapter 15 have been based on important Canadian research findings, including the Canadian definition of "brain death," and the position of the CACCN (Canadian Association of Critical Care Nurses) on life support. Canadian data on organ and tissue transplantation, and the CNA (Canadian Nurses Association) statement on how nurses can support organ donation are now included here, as well. No less interesting is the information added to the second Canadian edition on stem cell research and cloning policies in Canada, along with the concept of euthanasia and the "right to die" movement, Compassionate Care Initiative, advance directives, and assisted suicide—all from a Canadian perspective.

It is important that nurses continually update their knowledge of health promotion, because complex societal changes and uncertainties occur each day in the health care delivery system throughout Canada. Because of Canada's geographical and cultural diversity, health professionals—including nurses—are continually faced with the necessity of being able to recognize and address health promotion challenges to ensure the provision of adequate health service for their clients and their families. The knowledgeable application of the current, relevant, and important research findings, as presented in this edition, will help the nurse engage with confidence in evidence-based practice. Delivering the best health promotion and prevention agendas appropriately aimed at the precise level of the health of Canadians is a never-ending challenge to health providers. The ultimate goal with all clients (individual or family) is to empower them to achieve optimal well-being.

## KEY FEATURES

A new paradigm of teaching/learning skills continues to be the basis for this edition. Each of these processes is based upon well-developed principles of adult learning.

**Objectives** and **Introductions** clearly summarize the core concepts explored in each chapter.

**Narrative Vignette** boxes, introduced in the first Canadian edition, include reflective questions. Here students can apply their knowledge to plausible scenarios that require them to make informed decisions.

An **Evidence-Based Practice** box, also introduced in the first Canadian edition is again included in each chapter, using recent findings from Canadian research studies.

**Nursing Care and Nursing Application** descriptions provide at-a-glance reference material that can be applied in the nursing environment.

**Case Situations** are designed to guide the student to apply knowledge in a practical setting.

The **Controversy Debate** feature engages the student with important points of contention and debate that all nursing professionals encounter. These exercises provide a valuable forum for discussion.

New **Figures** and **Tables** throughout the second Canadian edition add explanation, accessibility, and visual appeal to the concepts presented.

**Key Terms** are **bolded** and *definitions* are italicized in the text.

**Critical Thinking Questions** continue to appear throughout each chapter and serve to keep the student thinking about how the topics discussed apply to their own experiences.

**Chapter Summary** and **Interesting Websites** sections enhance the student's learning, appreciation, and understanding of the topics discussed.

## INSTRUCTOR SUPPLEMENT

**Instructor's Manual.** This manual includes a rich compilation of teaching-learning strategies, tips, group and individual activities, and additional resources to assist instructors with implementing the text into the course curriculum. It also includes sample test questions for each chapter (matching, multiple choice, true-false, and short answer), as well as a sample final exam. The Instructor's Manual is available for downloading from a password-protected section of Pearson Education Canada's online catalogue (www.pearsoned.ca/highered). Navigate to your book's catalogue page to view a list of those supplements that are available. See your local sales representative for details and access.

## COURSESMART eTEXTBOOK

CourseSmart is a new way for instructors and students to access textbooks online anytime from anywhere. With thousands of titles across hundreds of courses, CourseSmart helps instructors choose the best textbook for their class and give their students a new option for buying the assigned textbook as a lower-cost eTextbook. For more information, visit www.coursesmart.com.

# Acknowledgments

We wish to acknowledge and graciously thank all of those dedicated individuals who gave freely of their precious time to assist us in the completion of this second Canadian adaptation.

In particular, we wish to acknowledge and to express our thanks to the following:

Administration and colleagues at the Faculty of Nursing, University of Manitoba, for their unending support and encouragement. We would not have been able to complete this work without their significant encouragement and contributions.

Research assistants for their enthusiasm and unending work in assisting us to collect data from various scholarly books and journals.

Library administration and staff, who many times pointed us in the right direction in our literature searches and provided us with many creative ideas and suggestions.

We are grateful to the following reviewers who provided valuable feedback on all or part of the manuscript:

- Sheryl Boblin, McMaster University
- Susan Brajtman, University of Ottawa
- Gail Bremer, Langara College
- Nancy Carter, McMaster University
- Rose Doyle, Kwantlen University College
- Shantha George, Grant MacEwan College
- Lynda Johnston, Douglas College
- Claudette Kelly, Thompson Rivers University
- Judith MacDonnell, University of Toronto
- Sue McLeod, Seneca College of Applied Arts and Technology
- Lucia New, Saskatchewan Institute of Applied Arts and Sciences
- Robin Scobie, University of Victoria
- Jacqueline C. Gahagan, Dalhousie University
- Kristin Knibbs, University of Saskatchewan
- Virginia Vandall-Walker, Athabasca University
- Catherine Sheffer, Dalhousie University

The entire editorial and production staff at Pearson Education Canada and, in particular, Michelle Sartor, Helen Smith, Cheryl Jackson, Andrea Falkenberg, and Sarah Lukaweski, for their talents and patience.

# Prelude to the Textbook

## HEALTH PROMOTION IN CANADA

Health promotion is the continuous process of enabling people to improve and to increase control over their well-being and health. According to Maville and Huerta, Canada is recognized as having launched health promotion in the global community.[1] In fact, other countries have adopted several of the Canadian theoretical frameworks for health promotion in order to instigate their own health promotion programs.[2] The most significant challenge in implementing health promotion strategies is the ongoing paradigm shift from a medical model of treatment to a primary health care model.

## DEVELOPMENTAL PERSPECTIVES

In 1974, the publication of the report of the then minister of National Health and Welfare, the Honourable Marc Lalonde entitled *A New Perspective on the Health of Canadians* outlined a framework for health comprised of four main elements: lifestyle, environment, human biology, and health care organization.[3] This report was received favourably by Canadians, and it continues to receive national and international acclaim. The report led to the development of successful health promotion programs associated with personal behaviours and lifestyles.[4] The Lalonde Report marked the first stage of health promotion in Canada.[5]

One important global initiative related to health promotion was the World Health Organization (WHO) Conference in 1978. This conference identified primary health care as the route to achieve "Health for All" by the year 2000.[6] Member states of the WHO, including Canada, decided to act towards the principles of "Health for All."[7] Canada hosted the first International Conference on Health Promotion in 1986. Two key documents released at that time, *The Ottawa Charter for Health Promotion* and *Achieving Health for All: A Framework for Health Promotion*,[8] alerted Canadians to the underlying conditions within society that determine health.

*The Ottawa Charter* called for action in five areas: (1) to build healthy public policy to ensure that policies contribute to health promoting conditions; (2) to create supportive environments; (3) to strengthen community action so that communities have the capacity to set priorities and take action on issues affecting their health; (4) to develop personal skills to meet life challenges, and (5) to reorient health services to focus on the needs of the entire person and invite a collaboration among providers and users of services.[9] *The Ottawa Charter* has been translated into over 40 languages, and it serves as a guide for health promotion around the world.

The second document, *Achieving Health for All*, focused attention on three key health promotion challenges for Canadians: (1) reducing inequities in health, (2) increasing the emphasis on prevention of disease, and (3) increasing people skills to cope with chronic disease and disability.[10] The framework put forward three mechanisms to meet these challenges: self-care, mutual aid, and health environments. It also suggested three strategies: community participation, strengthening community health services, and health public policy.[11]

To continue the journey of Canada's involvement in health promotion, it is important to note that, in 1989, the members of the Population Health Program at the Canadian Institute for Advanced Research (CIAR) began to increase the understanding of multiple and interactive factors that influence health status and function, including social, economic, genetic, and health care, as well as the complex interrelationships among them. Taking into account the work of CIAR, in 1994 the federal, provincial, and territorial health ministers released their report—*Strategies for Population Health: Investing in the Health of Canadians*.[12] The contents of this report included timely and relevant information on the determinants of health. Most importantly, it proposed a population health conceptual framework based on five categories of determinants which underpin the health of a population: (1) personal health practices, (2) individual capacity and coping skills, (3) the social and economic environment, (4) the physical environment, and (5) health services.[13]

The Canadian government established the National Forum on Health in October 1994.[14] The mandate of the National Forum on Health was to ensure that Canada's health care system was equipped for the challenges of the future. The National Forum recommended transforming knowledge about health into action, mainly through a broader awareness of the determinants of health.[15] In 1997, the National Forum on Health delivered its report and made recommendations that support the following four principles of primary health care: (1) public participation, (2) accessibility, (3) health promotion and disease prevention, and (4) intersectorial collaboration. The one principle not supported by the National Forum is the principle of appropriate technology.[16] The National Forum on Health officially ended its operations in June 1997.[17]

Since the late 1980s, the term "population health" has been used to explain an approach that focuses on the range of individual and collective elements and conditions, and the interactions among them, that determine the health and well-being of Canadians.[18] The goals of a population approach are intended not only to maintain, but to improve, the health and well-being of an entire population and to decrease inequities in health status among various population groups.[19] Further deliberations at Health Canada have led to the following list of determinants for future population health policy and research directions: income and social status; social support networks; education, employment, and working conditions, social and physical environments; biology and genetic endowment; personal health practices and coping skills; healthy child development; and health services. As a result of recent discussions within Health Canada, gender and culture have been added to this list of determinants.[20]

In the mid-1990s, Hamilton and Bhatti of the Health Promotion Development Division of Health Canada constructed a population health promotion model, which explains the relationship between population health and health promotion. Hamilton and Bhatti's model emphasizes that to improve people's health we must take action on the full range of health determinants.[21] That is, the model illustrates how a population health approach can be implemented through comprehensive health promotion strategies to influence the factors and conditions that determine health. This model also stresses the need for evidence-based decision-making procedures to ensure the development of population health promotion activities.[22]

In 1999, the Canadian Population Health Initiative (CPHI) was launched to expand the public's knowledge of population health. The CPHI mission is twofold: first to facilitate a better understanding of factors that affect the health of individuals and communities, and second, to contribute to the development of health policies that decrease inequities and promote the health and well-being of Canadians.[23] The Canadian Population Health Initiative Action Plan 2007–2010 was released to guide CPHI's strategic direction over those three years. The key areas of focus include mental health and resilience, reducing gaps in health, place and health, and promoting healthy weights.[24]

Reforming primary health care has been a constant message since the early 1980s. Now that we've reached the new millennium, what is the status of health promotion in the lives of Canadians? According to the Canadian Institute for Health Information, health and health care continue to be top priorities for Canadians.[25] As part of the Action Plan for Health System Renewal in September 2000, federal, provincial, and territorial first ministers agreed that improvements to primary health care are critical to the renewal of health services that touch Canadians in all facets of their lives.[26] The federal government established an $800 million primary health care transition fund in September 2000 to support the efforts of provinces and territories and to develop and implement transitional primary health care reform initiatives. The suggested changes to the structure of primary health care were intended to help achieve the

following: (1) better health for citizens by placing the focus on preventing illness and promoting health, (2) better access to, and integration of, primary health care services, and (3) greater job satisfaction for health care providers, by encouraging them to use their skills to full potential and by improving working conditions.[27]

Evidence was accumulating that social and economic health disparities were growing in Canada; and these disparities were contributing to increased health costs and other social burdens. Consequently, an important conference was held in Toronto, in 2002, which was attended by concerned social and health policy experts, community representatives, and health researchers.[28] This conference examined the ten key social determinants of health to explore the implications of these conditions for the health of Canadians and to outline policy directions to improve the health of Canadians. Those determinants identified as paramount to the health of Canadians and relevant to policy were early childhood development, employment and working conditions, education, food security, housing shortages, health care services, income and its equitable distribution, social exclusion, social safety nets, and unemployment and employment security.[29] The conference resulted in the Toronto Charter on the Social Determinants of Health. The Charter itself is, and will continue to be, a significant tool for promoting health and social justice, both within and outside Canada.[30]

In 2002, the federal, provincial, and territorial health ministers agreed to work together on an integrated Pan-Canadian Healthy Living Strategy. The goals of this strategy were to improve overall health outcomes and to decrease health disparities by addressing the common preventable risk factors—namely physical inactivity and unhealthy eating. Health promoting strategies aimed at targeting all Canadians, while focusing on children and youth, Aboriginal peoples, and all other vulnerable groups.[31]

The First Ministers' Health Accord of 2003 and the 10-Year Plan to Strengthen Health Care in Canada in 2004 moved from debating health care renewal to emphasizing the delivery of care.[32] The Health Accord of 2003 identifies primary health care as the cornerstone of tomorrow's health care system. The First Ministers agreed to make the timely access to quality care a reality for all Canadians.[33]

The combined results of the Romanow Commission on the Future of Health Care in Canada, the Kirby Senate Committee Final Report on the State of the Health Care System in Canada, and several provincial reports (including those of Clair, Fyke, and Mazankowski) indicated specifically that Canadians not only want, but expect, improved access to quality services from the health care system.[34] Specifically, Roy Romanow recommended the creation of a Health Council of Canada, which would help foster collaboration and cooperation among provinces, territories, and the federal government. The council would play a key role in establishing common indicators to measure the performance of the health care system and reporting the results to Canadians on a regular basis. In fact, after the 2003 and 2004 Health Care Accords, the Health Council of Canada was uniquely charged with tracking health care renewal and reporting its progress to Canadians.[35]

Recently, there has been a revitalization of the vision of primary health care. In 2005, governments across the Americas (including Canada) reaffirmed their commitments to the principles and strategies of primary health care by signing the Declaration of Montevideo.[36] The focus on the reorientation of health care systems towards primary health care requires the adjustment and adaptation of health promotion and disease prevention strategies by all involved—from governments to clients, families, and communities.[37]

It is interesting to note that some concerns are reported in the literature regarding meaningful health promotion, or disease prevention aspects, within the health care system. It has been stated, for example, that in order for health promotion to flourish in Canada, a great deal of community involvement is necessary.[38] Certain difficulties appear to be inherent in federally driven programs that emphasize the community participation of disadvantaged groups. Other difficulties in implementing health promotion projects stem from limited funding and understaffing.[39] Given these issues, to what extent can we as Canadians expect answers from the health ministers as they continue to meet, deliberate and make decisions regarding the state of our health?

## THE ROLE OF HEALTH PRACTITIONERS

For the past two decades, the Canadian Nurses Association (CNA) has been promoting primary health care as a helpful strategy to guide the reform of the health care system.[40] The influence of the CNA has been clear because it was the only national health association to advocate primary health care. In fact, nursing response to health promotion occurred within the context of primary health care.[41] In 2000, the *Nursing Strategy for Canada* was made public by the federal, provincial, and territorial health ministers, after significant consultation with nurses and other health care stakeholders. The goal of the strategy was to put mechanisms in place and to maintain an adequate supply of nursing personnel who were well-educated, well-distributed, and deployed to meet the health needs of Canadians. The final report of the *Nursing Strategy for Canada*, released in September 2003, indicated that the collaborative approach had resulted in significant progress towards the objective that nurses play a vital and effective role in the delivery of health care in Canada.[42] An important aspect in the delivery of health care is the emphasis placed first on health promotion practice to include strategies directed at clients, families, and communities and second, on promoting social and environmental change at the societal level.[43]

In 2004, the Canadian Nurses Association (CNA) actively participated at a meeting with the First Ministers in a 10-year Plan to Strengthen Health Care. CNA collaborated and partnered with other health care organizations on joint policy and media relations initiatives. Consequently, this collaborative effort produced a document called *Common Vision for the Canadian Health System*, which was delivered widely through the media with interviews, statements, and news releases. CNA undertook a particularly relevant study called *Toward 2020: Visions for Nursing*, in a strong endeavour to lay the groundwork for the role of nursing in planning health care for the twenty-first century. Funded by Health Canada through the Office of Nursing Policy, one of the goals of the study was to propose scenarios for the nursing profession in the year 2020 that would maximize the contributions of nursing in the promotion of the health of Canadians.[44] Villeneuve and MacDonald, the principal investigators in the study, stress that one critical underlying premise of primary health care is collaboration between health care practitioners and consumers of care.[45] In fact, collaborative, client-centred practice urges the active participation of each discipline to promote the health of clients by encouraging respect for the contribution of all health care professionals. In 2006, the Canadian Nurses Association (CNA) published a position paper entitled *Interprofessional Collaboration*.[46] Here it is emphasized that interdisciplinary collaboration requires effective teamwork and that in order for teams to function efficiently, the team must be supported by a strong team leader.[47] Nurse leaders need to learn as much as possible about collaboration as a process and about the roles of other health professionals to work effectively in the promotion of the health of clients and their families in various health care settings. Nursing has the potential to contribute in significant and varied ways to the interdisciplinary development of health promotion.[48]

Exerting influence on the implementation of primary health care will require concerted action on the part of nurses throughout the country.[49] Nurses can take many measures to ensure that the changes taking place in the health care system reflect the primary health care model with emphasis on health promotion practice.

Fortunately, nurses are becoming more politically active and some have begun to lobby their local politicians to ensure that health care plans reflect the current health concerns of their communities.[50] One notable example of a politically active nurse is that of "Street Nurse" Cathy Crowe whose achievements and endeavours, which are worthy of wide public attention, may be monitored on her own website: www.tdrc.net/CathyCrowe.htm. Nurses generally need to play an even broader role in health promotion in today's society by being visible and making certain that the nursing voice is heard at the decision-making table as the health system moves toward primary health care.

As you read and reflect upon how the Canadian concepts of health promotion interact and connect with the material retained from earlier editions of this work, you will note that the theme of health promotion is indeed directed toward individuals and families throughout the lifespan. Think carefully about the health promotion strategies presented in the text. At the same time, consider alternate strategies that you, as an individual, might devise and implement under various circumstances you encounter as a health care professional. We hope you will seek to help clients and their families deal with day-to-day health issues as they strive to lead healthy lives.

## ENDNOTES

1. Maville, J.A., and C.G. Huerta, Health Promotion in Nursing. Albany, NY: Delmar Thompson Learning, Inc., 2002.
2. Maville, and Huerta, Health Promotion in Nursing.
3. Lalonde, M., A New Perspective on the Health of Canadians: A Working Paper. Ottawa: Government of Canada. Quoted in M.J. Stewart, Community Nursing: Promoting Canadians' Health (2nd ed.). Toronto: W.B. Saunders, 2000. Vollman, A. R., E. T. Anderson, and J. McFarlane, Canadian Community as Partner: Theory and Practice in Nursing. Philadelphia: Lippincott Williams & Wilkins, 2004.
4. Public Health Agency of Canada (PHAC), Appendix A: The Evolution of the Population Health Paradigm, Website: www.phac-aspc.gc.ca/phsp/phdd/docs/common/appendix_a.html.
5. Glouberman, S., and J. Millar, Evolution of the Determinants of Health Policy, and Health Information Systems in Canada, American Journal of Public Health, 93, no. 3, (2003), 388–392.
6. World Health Organization, Primary Health Care: Report on the International Conference on Primary Health Care, Alma Alta, USSR, 6–12 September 1978. Quoted in M.J. Stewart, Community Nursing: Promoting Canadians' Health (2nd ed., p. 34). Toronto: W.B. Saunders, 2000.
7. Lemire Rodger, G., and S.M. Gallagher, The Move Toward Primary Health Care in Canada: Community Health Nursing from1985 to 2000, in M.J. Stewart, ed., Community Nursing: Promoting Canadians' Health (2nd ed., pp. 37–38). Toronto: W.B. Saunders, 2000.
8. Public Health Agency of Canada (PHAC), Population Health Promotion: An Integrated Model of Population Health and Health Promotion, Website: www.phac-aspc.gc.ca/ph-sp/phdd/php/php.htm April 2007.
9. PHAC, Population Health Promotion: An Integrated Model of Population Health and Health Promotion, Website: www.phac-aspc.gc.ca/ph-sp/phdd/php/php.htm April 2007.
10. PHAC, Population Health Promotion: An Integrated Model of Population Health and Health Promotion, Website: www.phac-aspc.gc.ca/ph-sp/phdd/php/php.htm April 2007.
11. West, L., Trends and Issues in Health Care. Toronto: McGraw-Hill Ryerson Ltd., 2003.
12. PHAC, Appendix A: The Evolution of the Population Health Paradigm, Public Health Agency of Canada, Appendix B: Population Health Framework, Website: www.phac-aspc.gc.ca/ph-sp/phdd/docs/common/appendix_b.html April 2007
13. Noseworthy, T.W., Continuing to Build on our Legacy: National Forum on Health, 1994–1997, in M.J. Stewart, ed., Community Nursing: Promoting Canadians' Health (2nd ed., pp. 33–37). Toronto: W.B. Saunders, 2000.
14. Noseworthy, Continuing to Build on our Legacy: National Forum on Health, 1994–1997, in M.J. Stewart, ed., Community Nursing: Promoting Canadians' Health (2nd ed., pp. 33–37). Toronto: W.B. Saunders, 2000.
15. Lemire Rodger, and Gallagher, The Move Toward Primary Health Care in Canada: Community Health Nursing from 1985 to 2000.
16. Stewart, M.J., Framework Based on Primary Health Care Principles, in M.J. Stewart, ed., Community Nursing: Promoting Canadians' Health (2nd ed., pp. 58–59). Toronto: W.B. Saunders, 2000.
17. Health Canada, Health Care—National Forum on Health, Website: www.hc-sc.gc.ca/ April 2007 Site navigation: Home>health care system>commissions & inquiries>national forum on health.
18. Public Health Agency of Canada, Towards a Common Understanding: Clarifying the Core Concepts of Population Health: Introduction, Website: www.phac-aspc.gc.ca/ph-sp/phdd/docs/common/intro.html April 2007.
19. Public Health Agency of Canada, The Statistical Report on the Health of Canadians 1999: An Overview. Website: www.phac-aspc.gc.ca/ph-sp/phdd/report/stat/over.html April 2007.
20. PHAC, Towards a Common Understanding: Clarifying the Core Concepts of Population Health: Introduction, Website: www.phac-aspc.gc.ca/ph-sp/phdd/docs/common/intro.html April 2007.
21. Public Health Agency of Canada, Population Health Promotion: An Integrated Model of Population Health and Health Promotion, Website: www.phac-aspc.gc.ca/ph-sp/phdd/php/php.htm April 2007.
22. PHAC, Population Health Promotion: An Integrated Model of Population Health and Health Promotion.
23. Canadian Population Health Initiative, The Canadian Population Health Initiative (CIPHI). Website: http://secure.cihi.ca/ April 2007.
24. Canadian Population Health Initiative, About the Canadian Population Health Initiative (CPHI): Mission. Website: http://secure.cihi.ca/ April 2007. Canadian Institute for Health Information, The Canadian Population Health Initiative Action Plan 2007–2010, Ottawa: Author, 2006.
25. Canadian Institute of Health Information, Health Care in Canada, 2002, Ottawa: Author. Website: http://secure.cihi.ca/cihiweb/splash.html April 2007.
26. Health Canada, Primary Health Care, Website: www.hc-sc.gc.ca/hcs sss/prim/index_e.html April 2007.
27. Health Canada, Primary Health Care, Website: www.hc-sc.gc.ca/hcs-sss/prim/index_e.html April 2007.
28. Raphael, D., T. Bryant, and A. Curry-Stevens, Toronto Charter Outlines Future Health Policy Directions for Canada and Elsewhere, Health Promotion International, 19, no. 2, (2004), 269–273.
29. Reutter, L. Health and Health Care in Canada, in Canadian Fundamentals of Nursing 1, 7 (P. A. Potter, A. G. Perry, J. C. Ross-Kerr, and M. J. Wood eds., 2006).
30. Raphael, D., T. Bryant, and A. Curry-Stevens, Toronto Charter Outlines Future Health Policy Directions for Canada and Elsewhere, Health Promotion International, 19, no. 2, (2004), 269–273
31. Public Health Agency of Canada, Health Promotion, Healthy Living, The Integrated Pan-Canadian Healthy Living Strategy, Website: www.phac-aspc.gc.ca/ April 2007.
32. Health Council of Canada, Health Care Renewal in Canada: Clearing the Road to Quality – Annual Report to Canadians 2005. Toronto: Author, 2006.
33. Health Canada, Ten Year Plan to Strengthen Health Care, Website: www.hc-sc.gc.ca/index_e.html April 2007.
34. West, Trends and Issues in Health Care.
35. Health Council of Canada, Health Care Renewal in Canada: Clearing the Road to Quality.

36. Health Council of Canada, Health Care Renewal in Canada: Clearing the Road to Quality.

37. Martin, C. M., Towards a Framework for Primary Health Care Transition in Canada: A Discussion Document. Ottawa: Canadian Alliance of Community Health Centre Associations, 2006. Website: www.cachca.ca/main>useful resources>documents> towards April 2007.

38. Segall, A., and N.L. Chappell, Health and Health Care in Canada. Toronto: Pearson Education Canada Inc., 2000.

39. Boyce, W.F., Influence of Health Promotion Bureaucracy on Community Participation: A Canadian Case Study. Health Promotion International, 17 no. 1 (2002), 61–68.

40. Lemire Rodger, G., Canadian Nurses Association, in M. McIntyre and E. Thomlinson, eds., Realities of Canadian Nursing: Professional, Practice, and Power Issues (pp. 124–137). Philadelphia: Lippincott, 2003.

41. MacDonald, M. A., Health Promotion: Historical, Philosophical, and Theoretical Perspectives in Transforming Health Promotion Practice: Concepts, Issues, and Applications 22, 34 (L. Young and V. Hayes eds., 2002).

42. Health Canada, Nursing Strategy for Canada, October 2000 Website: www.hc-sc.gc.ca/ahc-asc/activit/strateg/nurs-infirm-eng.php August 2008

43. MacDonald, M. A., Health Promotion: Historical, Philosophical, and Theoretical Perspectives in Transforming Health Promotion Practice: Concepts, Issues, and Applications 22, 34 (L. Young and V. Hayes eds., 2002).

44. Canadian Nurses Association. Operational Report of the Chief Executive Officer: June 2004 to June 2006. Ottawa: Athor, 2006.

45. Villeneuve, M., and J. MacDonald, Toward 2020: Visions for Nursing. Ottawa: Canadian Nurses Association.

46. Canadian Nurses Association, Position Statement: Interprofessional Collaboration. Author, 2006.

47. Enhancing Interdisciplinary Collaboration in Primary Health Care (EICP) Initiative. Enhancing Interdisciplinary Collaboration in Primary Health Care in Canada, (2005) Ottawa: The Conference Board of Canada.

48. MacDonald, M. A., Health Promotion: Historical, Philosophical, and Theoretical Perspectives in Transforming Health Promotion Practice: Concepts, Issues, and Applications 22, 34 (L. Young and V. Hayes eds., 2002).

49. Canadian Nurses Association, Primary Health Care—The Time Has Come, Nursing Now: Issues and Tends in Canadian Nursing, 16 (September 2003), 1–4.

50. CNA Primary Health Care—The Time Has Come, Nursing Now: Issues and Tends in Canadian Nursing, 16 (September 2003), 1–4.

# Part I
## Influences on the Developing Person and Family Unit

# Chapter 1

## Sociocultural Influences on the Person and Family

*The culture and subcultures into which we are born encompass us and direct us for life. We learn an identity, values, beliefs, norms and habits of life, language, relationships, time, space, work, play, right, wrong, and physical and mental health practices.*

Ruth Beckmann Murray

*Caring relationships based on respect are central to a multicultural environment.*

P. Moffitt and J. Wuest, Spirit of the Drum: The Development of Cultural Nursing Praxis, Canadian Journal of Nursing Research, 34(4) (2002), 115.

## Objectives

*Study of this chapter will enable you to:*

1 Define *culture* and *subculture*, and describe various types of subcultures.

2 Examine characteristics of a culture, and determine how they affect the people under your care.

3 Evaluate values, and discuss how they influence clients, families, and health care workers.

4 Consider ways to identify diverse groups within Canada.

5 Defend the importance of nurses providing cultural care to Canadians.

6 Examine several health trends occurring in Canada.

7 Compare and contrast attitudes toward health and illness.

8 Analyze the influences of socioeconomic levels on the health status of persons and groups.

9 Identify key concepts of health promotion.

10 Determine how knowledge of cultural and socioeconomic levels can contribute to the effectiveness of health promotion.

11 Evaluate ways to meet the needs of a person with cultural values and a socioeconomic level different from your own.

12 Apply knowledge about the teaching–learning process to a health promotion education program.

# SOCIOCULTURAL INFLUENCES

When people talk or act differently from you, consider that to them you may also seem to talk or act differently. Many such differences are cultural and should be understood rather than laughed at or ignored.

*J. Zentner*

All humans have the same needs, but these needs vary in their individual natures because of culture.[1] Culture includes using language, art forms, and games to communicate with others; establishing birth and death practices; rearing children; developing unique interpretations about the world; forming organizations; and making, saving, using, and changing tools. Humans are heirs to the accumulation of the wisdom and folly of preceding generations, and, in turn, they teach others their beliefs, feelings, and practices. People (your clients, their families, and you) are deeply affected by the culture they learn during their early years, often more so than by the cultural knowledge they acquire later.

Culture plays a critical role in health care delivery. Clients and their families must understand the care given, as well as how to navigate the maze of the health care system.[2] Nurses must understand their individual values and unique cultures before working with others. Nurses must deal with these issues not only in a culturally sensitive way, but also in a humanly responsive way to meet the needs of individuals.[3] An understanding of cultural and socioeconomic class systems and their influences on the development of behaviour is essential to understanding yourself and the person under your care.

---

## CRITICAL THINKING

*Take a moment to reflect on your own understanding of the meaning of culture.*

---

# CULTURE

Srivastava states that culture is a difficult term to define simply and without ambiguity.[4] The Canadian Nurses Association (CNA) describes culture as shared patterns of values and learned behaviours transmitted socially over time that distinguish the members of one group from another.[5] Culture involves the full range of accepted and common beliefs, values, attitudes, patterns of meanings, and behaviours held by a group of people. It is complex and significant because it enables people to navigate and make sense of their world through shared meanings and patterns of behaviour.[6] These ways of being are transmitted from one generation to the next and also from a dominant society to immigrants who become members of that society. Culture is a complex integrated system that also includes knowledge, skills, art, law, customs, and any other acquired habits and capabilities of a human being. Aspects of culture are shared, learned, and perpetuated by members of that culture.[7] All these aspects provide a pattern for living together.

## Subculture

A **subculture** is *a group of persons within a larger culture of the same age, socioeconomic level, ethnic origin, education, or occupation, or with the same goals who have a unique identity but are related to the total culture in certain ways.*

Within society there are a number of subcultures. A description of a few subcultures—ethnic, family, religious, regional, and socioeconomic—follows.

**Ethnic** The term **ethnic** pertains to *a group of people distinguished from other people by race or nationality that possesses common physical and mental traits as a result of heredity, cultural traditions, language or speech, customs, and common history.* Cultural background is a fundamental component of one's ethnic background.[8] In Canada, there are many European ethnic subcultures, such as Slovakian (German, Italian, Polish, or Slavic), Scandinavian (Danish, Norwegian, Icelandic, Finnish, or Swedish), Swiss, French, Dutch, and Russian. There are also ethnic subcultures from the United Kingdom: English, Irish, Welsh, and Scottish. Markers of racial or ethnic identity comprise every conceivable skin colour hue, and sometimes the markers are as much a matter of socialization, ideology, and attitude as of pigmentation.

According to the 2006 Canadian Census, ethnic origin refers to the ethnic or cultural group(s) to which an individual's ancestors belonged.[9] In that census, more than 200 different ethnic origins were reported. The list includes cultural groups associated with Canada's first peoples: North American Indian, Métis, and Inuit. (Note: For statistical and other purposes, the Government of Canada usually divides the Aboriginal population into four categories: (1) North American Indians registered under the *Indian Act*, (2) North American Indians not registered under the *Indian Act*, (3) Métis, and (4) Inuit.[10]) Other cultural groups included in this census were the French, English, Scottish, and Irish. The list also reflects the history of immigration to Canada in the past 100 years, with such groups as German, Italian, Chinese, Ukrainian, Dutch, Polish, and others. A host of new ethnic origins has emerged as a result of changing sources of immigrants to Canada, including Kosovars from Yugoslavia; Azerbaijani and Georgians from Central Asia; Pashtun from Afghanistan; Yemeni and Saudi Arabians from the Middle

East; Khmer from Southeast Asia; Nepali and Kashmiri from South Asia; Congolese, Yoruba, and Ashanti from Africa; and Bolivians, Maya, and Caribbean Indians from Central and South America.[11] How far back can you trace your own ethnic or cultural group in Canada?

In both the 1996 and 2006 censuses, an increased number of people reported being either Canadian or Canadien as part of their ethnic heritage. It is important to note that those people had English or French as a mother tongue, were born in Canada, and had both parents born in Canada.[12] English and French are Canada's official languages and are also the two languages most likely to be spoken in the country.[13] The *Official Languages Act*, adopted in 1969, gave these languages equal status, rights, and privileges in federal institutions. Other languages are recognized as non-official or heritage languages. In parts of Canada where Aboriginal groups are prevalent, a small portion of the population speaks neither English nor French. Furthermore, in large ethnic communities, this same phenomenon occurs because many immigrants have never learned either official language.[14]

In Canadian society, generally English and French predominate; however, more than 100 other languages are also spoken.[15] The rapid cultural shift has affected health care, especially in the area of medical communication. For example, Canadians who have a relatively low level of literacy in either official language cannot use the printed health information available to them.

**Family**  **Family culture** *refers to family life, which is part of the cultural system.* The family is the medium through which the larger cultural heritage is transmitted to the child. Family culture consists of ways of living and thinking that constitute the familial and sexual aspects of group life. These include courtship and marriage patterns, sexual mores, intimate partnerships, status and relationships of men and women, parent–child relationships, childrearing, responsibilities to parents, and attitudes toward unmarried people, children, divorce, homosexuality, and various health problems.[16]

Family rituals are the collective way of working out household routines and using time within the family culture. These rituals are indicators of family values. **Ritual** is *a system of definitely prescribed behaviours and procedures.* Ritual provides exactness in daily tasks of living and has a sense of rightness about it. The more often the behaviour is repeated, the more it comes to be approved and therefore habitual. Thus, rituals inevitably develop in family life as a result of the intimacy of relationships and the repetition or continuity of certain interactions. Rituals change from one life cycle to another. Examples include rituals of marriage, of childbirth, as well as when children go to school and when they leave the home. Rituals are important in child development because they

- Are group habits that communicate ways of doing things. Rituals are attitudes related to events, including family etiquette, affectionate responses between family members, organization of leisure time, and education for group adjustment.

- Promote solidarity and continuity by promoting unconsciously performed habitual behaviour that brings harmony to family life. Many rituals continue into the next generation, increasing the person's sense of worth, security, and family continuity or identity.

- Aid in maintaining self-control through disciplinary measures.

- Promote feelings of euphoria, sentimentality, or well-being; for example, through celebrations on special occasions.

- Dictate reactions to threats; for example, during times of loss, illness, or death.[17]

---

## CRITICAL THINKING

*In what ways have the rituals with which you grew up come to affect you in your adult life?*

---

Family influences are discussed more extensively in Chapter 4.

**Religious**  All cultures, subcultures, and ethnic groups possess certain values, customs, and practices common to every culture. They share certain values, customs, and practices with some other cultures, and they have certain values, customs, and practices unique to their group. **Religious culture** also *influences a person, because a religion constitutes a way of living, behaving, and thinking, and therefore is a kind of culture.* Religious influences on values, attitudes, and behaviours are discussed in Chapter 3.

---

## CRITICAL THINKING

*What types of cultural services have you seen implemented in urban hospitals?*

---

**Regional**  The population in Canada's small towns and rural areas grew by 1 percent between 2001 and 2006. In 2006, just less than 20 percent of Canadians were living in rural areas—that is, in areas located outside urban centres with a population of at least 10 000.[18]

Based on defined rules regarding total population and population density, Statistics Canada categorizes all land in Canada as either urban or rural. An urban area has a minimum population concentration of 1000 persons and a population density of at least 400 persons per square kilometre. By default, all territory outside urban areas is classified as rural.[19]

There are two types of rural areas: those close to urban centres and those that are more remote. In rural areas close to urban centres, more than 30 percent of the labour force commutes to work in the nearby urban centre. In remote rural areas, the population has remained nearly the same as in 2001. The lack of growth in these rural areas is often due to the migration of young adults to metropolitan areas to pursue their educations or find jobs.[20]

Rural dwellers use the same adaptive strategies and products as urban dwellers, and their value systems may be similar. Differences between rural and urban dwellers may depend more on the geography, climate, and history of the area than on socioeconomic status, race, ethnicity, or religion.

Population density, population size, and distance from health care facilities are criteria frequently used in defining rural areas. *Ruralness* is a matter of perspective; to some people, it means "smaller than here." Differences within rural populations and among rural areas are substantial. Among rural people, age, income, race, ethnicity, and occupation all contribute to different values, customs, and definitions of health. To consider health resources in rural communities, a Canadian provincial regional health authority conducted a study to explore and analyze mental health services and other resources used by rural consumers. Interestingly, it revealed that access to mental health services was challenging for residents of many rural communities. It also discovered that a number of programs and services available for the rural people in some communities were not available in other communities.[21]

**Socioeconomic** **Socioeconomic level** is *a cultural grouping of persons who, through group consensus and similarity of financial position or wealth, occupation, and education, have come to have a similar status, lifestyle, and language, as well as similar interests, feelings, attitudes, and overt behaviours.*

# THREE CHARACTERISTICS OF CULTURE

Understanding the characteristics of culture will help you understand and work with people from various cultures. Take a moment to reflect on the cultural differences that you recall seeing in your childhood friends and in your neighbourhood. What stands out to you?

## Culture Is Learned

The first of the three basic characteristics of culture is that it is learned. People function physiologically in much the same way throughout the world, but their behaviours are learned and are therefore relatively diverse. Because of culture, a child is ascribed or acquires a certain **status** or *position of prestige*. The child learns or assumes certain **roles**, *patterns or related behaviours expected first by others and later by oneself that define the behaviours and adjustment for a given group.* The behaviours, values, attitudes, and beliefs are learned through cultural transmission as one generation passes culture to the next.[22] This learned culture becomes a matter of tradition, even though the culture allows choices within certain limits. What a person learns during development is of great significance.

## Culture Is Stable but Changing

The second basic characteristic of culture is that it is subject to, and capable of, change in order to remain viable and adaptive, although it is basically a stable entity. The stabilizing features are traditions, group pressure, and the ready-made solutions to life's problems that are provided for the group, enabling individuals to anticipate the behaviour of others, predict future events, and regulate their lives within the culture.[23]

Another stabilizing aspect of culture is the use of language, even though the meanings of words change over time. Although language forms vary from culture to culture, the terms for *mother* and *father* sound alike across some cultural lines, perhaps because certain vocalizations are easy for children to learn and articulate. Even though Canada is officially bilingual, French-speaking majorities predominate mainly in Quebec and northern New Brunswick, and Engish-speaking majorities tend to occupy the rest of Canada.[24]

Aboriginal cultures, being oral in nature, are transmitted through speech rather than written text. Aboriginal languages, which are symbols of Aboriginal cultural and group identity, are many and diverse. Language serves not only as a means of interacting but also as a way of connecting people with their past and of grounding their emotional, social, and spiritual selves. Despite the efforts of Canadian Aboriginal peoples to preserve their languages, these languages are endangered. If they are lost, the consequences will have a profound effect on the Aboriginal peoples' cultural survival.[25]

Language emphasizes the particular values of a culture. For example, neither the language of the Nootka Indians on Vancouver Island nor that of the Hopi in the American southwest has a separate subject and predicate as English does. These languages describe an event as a whole using a single term. The Indo-European languages, including English, emphasize *time* while the Natives in Alaska have numerous concepts to describe the varieties of *space*. Inuktitut, the language of the Inuit, is widely used throughout the North, and thus the Inuit across the Arctic can understand one another. Even though dialects and accents vary from region to region, Inuktitut is considered a single language.[26] One thing a person new to the language might notice is that a single word may be spelled in many different ways.

## CRITICAL THINKING

*What factors may contribute to the potential loss of Aboriginal languages?*

The meeting ground between cultures is in language and **dialect**, *a variety of a language spoken by a distinct group of people in a definite place.* Dialects are related to racial and ethnic backgrounds, geographic regions, and neighbourhoods. If words are not understood in relation to the culture, a breakdown of communication and relationships occurs. Choice of words, syntax, intonation, and level of emotion in speech all convey meaning.[27] As Chinese Canadians have made gains in education and employment, they have also made conscious efforts to develop a sense of community and to increase the awareness of Chinese culture.[28] Although Chinese people read and write with the same script characters, they can employ any of several dozen different dialects when they speak. The "official" dialect taught in schools in China is Mandarin, which is the dialect of Beijing, the capital of China.[29]

Because of the increasing variety of languages that we now encounter in Canada, such as the many Chinese dialects, it is important for health professionals to listen carefully to the language spoken, be accepting of the dialect, and validate meanings of words when necessary during the assessment and intervention phases of health care delivery. Cultural and language differences can have a significant impact on miscommunication, misdiagnoses, and inappropriate treatments.[30]

A culture makes change possible through its inventions, discoveries, and diffusion. The process of invention is constant in our society. For example, scientists make strides in medical research that enhance our quality of life. Another aspect of cultural change is discovery. Technological advancements, such as the Canadian-made BlackBerry, have resulted from scientific discovery. Diffusion is the spread of cultural traits from one society to the next. The ability to electronically send information around the globe has been a powerful tool in cultural transmission.[31]

Many industrial societies, including Canada, are moving into a **postindustrial or postmodern society**. In 1973, Daniel Bell, a sociologist, coined the term *post-industrialism* to refer to technology that supports an information-based economy.[32] Production in postindustrial societies focuses on computers and other electronic devices that not only create but also process as well as store and apply information. Individuals in postindustrial societies concentrate on learning skills for jobs in high-tech communication. The following are some of the problem areas of postmodern society:

- Need for more professional knowledge
- Greater expectations of the public
- More goods considered to be public goods
- Lack of measurements to show what is actually needed and thus where money and resources should be directed
- A changing demography with more urban concentration
- Increased life expectancy
- Changing values, with little understanding of the historical roots of a culture
- Power struggles between groups.[33]

## CRITICAL THINKING

*In what ways do events of the postindustrial era affect the practice of health care professionals?*

## Culture Has Components and Patterns

The third basic characteristic of culture is that every culture has certain components or patterns. Components and patterns influence, and are influenced by, adaptation to climate, use of natural resources, geography, sanitation facilities, diet, group biological and genetic factors, and disease conditions and health practices. Knowledge of cultural values is essential for providing culturally sensitive care as you interact with, assess, teach, and intervene with people of various cultures.

Table 1-1 describes the various components of cultures, with examples.[34]

## CULTURAL CARE

Did you know that Canada was the first nation in the world to make multiculturalism an official policy? In 1971, the multicultural policy focused on the fact that Canada had no official culture but recognized those of all ethnic backgrounds. The *Canadian Multiculturalism Act* was passed in 1988 to preserve Canada's multicultural heritage. Both racial and cultural equalities are now protected by law due to the passage of this Act.[35] In other words, multiculturalism, a fundamental feature of Canadian society, focuses on the equal participation of individuals and communities of all origins and on the preservation of multicultural heritage.[36]

## Table 1-1 Components of All Cultures

| Component of the Culture | Purpose or Meaning | Examples |
|---|---|---|
| Provision of physical welfare; feeding, clothing, and shelter patterns | Survival and maintenance of population. Health promotion. | Production and processing of food, shelter, clothing. Personal and health care patterns. Production and use of tools. Manufacturing, industrialization. Change of land terrain for home building, farming, industry. Health care services. |
| Communication systems | Basis for interaction and cohesion. Vehicle for transmission and preservation of the culture. Distinguishes groups from each other. | Language and dialects. Vocabulary and word taboos. Nonverbal behaviour. Voice tone, rhythm, speed, pronunciation. Facial expressions, gestures, symbols. Mass media. Computers. Music. Art. Satellites. |
| Exchange of goods and services | Production and distribution of goods and services. Work roles. Payment. Obtain at least necessities or luxury, depending on culture. | Barter. Trade. Commerce. Financial institutions. Economic policies. Regulatory mechanisms. Health care institutions and services. |
| Travel and transportation | Provision for obtaining goods and services. Mobility within and across cultures, societies, nations. | Walk. Use of animals, such as dog, llama, horse, oxen. System of car, truck, railway, air travel transport. |
| Social controls; institutions of government | Maintenance of order. Organization of people, society, government. Regulation of time and activity. Power systems. | **Mores**, *morally binding attitudes*. **Customs**, *long-established practices having force of unwritten laws*. Value systems. Laws. Policies. Regulations. Public or group opinion. Political offices; kingships; dictators. |
| Forms of property | Necessities to maintain survival. May contribute to person's worth, status, social position. | Personal belongings. Personal property. Real estate. Financial institutions and systems. |
| Human response patterns | Family relationships structure other relationships and "taken-for-granted" activities to maintain the group. Values, beliefs, attitudes taught for socialization of person into culture. Ready-made solutions to life problems and goal achievements. Relationships structured by age, sex, status, wealth, power, number of kin, wisdom. | Rules for all social interaction, handling competition, conflict, cooperation, and games. Intimate habits of daily living personally and in groups. Manner in which one's body, home, property perceived. Daily "taken-for-granted" activities and interactions. Use of time and space. Health care roles and practices. |
| Family and sexual patterns | Maintain structure for care and support of others. Regulate relationships for survival, harmony, generational longevity. | Wedding ceremonies. Birth, childbearing practices. Family division of labour. Roles assigned to men, women, children. Inheritance rights. Care of elderly. Guardianship. Forms of kinship. Divorce proceedings, or removal of undesired member, such as infanticide, burial of woman with husband, or elders leaving tribe to die. Use of time and space. |

*(continued)*

Table 1-1 (continued)

| Component of the Culture | Purpose or Meaning | Examples |
|---|---|---|
| Knowledge | Survival and expansion of group and desired practices. Contributes to improved living standards through inventions, products, practices, services. Technologic innovation, mobility to higher social status. | Reasoning process. Education system, informal and local, formal and national. Skills. Values. **Science**, *systematized knowledge based on observation, study, experimentation*. Traditions. Folklore. Folk and scientific medical, nursing, and health care practices. |
| Belief system | Guides behaviour of individuals and group during daily life, at special events, occasions, celebrations. Provides meaning to life and death. Indicates priorities. Guides health and illness behaviour. | Religion. Ethical codes. Magical ideas and practices. Taboos. Rituals. Methodology. Philosophy. Organized institution of the church. Values and norms. |
| Artistic and aesthetic expression | Expression of meaning in life and death, feelings ranging from joy to sorrow, depending on situation. Spiritual expression. Expression of individual talents. Health promotion. Therapy and rehabilitation in illness. | Painting. Music. Dance. Architecture. Sculpture. Literature. Aesthetic expressions also in body adornment. Use and decoration of space and surrounding environment, such as floral gardens. |
| Recreation and leisure activities | Socialization. Use of leisure time. Travel to other cultures. | Play activities and tools. Games. Organized sports. Leisure activities depend on climate, terrain, available time, resources. |

Canada is a nation, both diverse and cohesive, united by a set of shared values that includes the respect of an individual's dignity and rule of law, freedom, equality, compassion, and fairness. Canada's framework for diversity recognizes that respect for cultural distinctiveness is intrinsic to an individual's sense of self-worth, which, in turn, encourages participation, achievement, and eventually attachment to the nation.[37]

## CRITICAL THINKING

*What criticisms can you think of regarding multiculturalism in Canada?*

## Importance of Cultural Concepts

In the mid-1960s, Leininger, the founder and pioneering leader of transcultural nursing, came to Canada to promote the ideas, definitions, and functional concepts of transcultural nursing.[38] She assisted health care providers to recognize the important and growing need of establishing a body of research-based knowledge and skills for providing informed cultural care to Aboriginal people and immigrants. **Transcultural nursing** is *the humanistic and scientific study and comparative analysis of different cultures and subcultures throughout the world in relation to differences and similarities in caring, health, illness, beliefs, values, life ways, and practices so that this knowledge can be used to provide culture-specific and cultural-universal nursing care to people.* The goal is to develop a body of knowledge so that transcultural nursing concepts, theories, and practices are an integral part of nursing education, service, and research. Leininger has developed *general principles* to guide transcultural practice, education, and research. These principles emphasize human rights and ethical considerations related to cultural care. Leininger describes the importance of a nurse being prepared for worldwide nursing and argues that transcultural nursing education should occur worldwide.[39]

## Transcultural Nursing

According to Andrews and Boyle, a thorough transcultural nursing assessment guide[40] would inform nurses of how to assess and work with clients who differ in the following ways:

- Biocultural variations and cultural aspects of the incidence of disease
- Communication

- Cultural affiliations
- Cultural sanctions and restrictions
- Developmental considerations
- Educational background
- Health-related beliefs and practices
- Kinship and social networks
- Nutrition
- Religious affiliation
- Values orientation

## Cultural Competence

Although multiculturalism and the theory of transcultural nursing paved the way for a discussion of culture within society and health care, these approaches have been critiqued. In particular, multicultural perspectives tend to stereotype and collapse ethnicities into categories. This oversimplification of "other" cultures then generates harmful stereotypes.[41] This perspective also implies that ethnic groups have homogenous cultures, without acknowledging the differences within the groups.[42] For example, even though there are physical similarities between Caucasian people from England and from Ireland, there is considerable difference in the worldviews between people from these groups. The concentration on ethnicity in transcultural nursing is a limitation because the perspective does not acknowledge the influence that other social factors have on health and health care.

While research has demonstrated that racial and ethnic disparities exist—for example, minority groups suffer disproportionately from cardiovascular disease, diabetes, asthma, and cancer—social factors are the greatest contributors to poor health.[43] These social factors are multifactorial, but members of racial and ethnic communities tend to be more socially disadvantaged, have lower levels of education, live in areas with greater environmental hazards, and work in jobs with higher rates of occupational hazards than the majority population.[44] It is these socioeconomic factors, such as poverty, employment, housing, and violence, that have a great influence on health, *not* race and ethnicity.

The 1998 Mental Health Plan, *Revitalizing and Rebalancing BC's Mental Health System*, identified strategies for mental health care reform in British Columbia. Within the plan, services were designed for individuals with serious mental illness, such as schizophrenia, bipolar, and other affective disorders. Yet, those with serious mental illnesses represent only 3 percent of the individuals with mental health issues in British Columbia. As well, within the Aboriginal community, mental health problems are rooted in the unique cultural identities, histories, and sociopolitical contexts of Aboriginal peoples. By focusing on a medical model for mental health care reform, the poverty, homelessness, and despair that influences the mental health of some Aboriginal people were inadequately addressed.[45]

Within nursing, considerations of not only culture, but also the socioeconomic influences on health are essential. As health care workers, it is important to recognize that every person, including oneself, has culture. Inherent to every culture are values, and these values influence how nurses give and receive health care. Attitude patterns make up a culture's **value system**, *its concept of how people should behave in various situations as well as which goals they should pursue and how.*[46] The value system of one culture may conflict with those of another at times.

All people have some prejudice. **Prejudice** has been described as a set of *unfavourable, intolerant, injurious, preconceived ideas formed before important facts are known.* Cultural safety requires nurses to examine their own cultural identity and beliefs and to explore how these may impact on the nurse–patient relationship.[47] The box entitled "Self-Assessment of Cultural Attitudes" contains

### Self-Assessment of Cultural Attitudes

To become more aware of your own attitudes and feelings about people of other racial and ethnic backgrounds, ask yourself the following questions:

1. What is your cultural or subcultural background?
2. What is your earliest memory of racial or ethnic differences?
3. What messages have you received in your life regarding people of various nationalities?
4. How much experience did you have with people from a socioeconomic group different from your own while you were growing up?
5. Describe an experience with a person from another sexual orientation with whom you have felt comfortable or uncomfortable.
6. In what way have these experiences with people affected your behaviour toward people from the group(s)?
7. What have you observed in the media about the portrayal of people from different religious groups?
8. Have you had interactions with people with disabilities within your own community?
9. What have you observed about the interaction of people from diverse cultural backgrounds in your school, church, workplace, or other organizations to which you belong?
10. What do you plan to do to increase your understanding of a person who is different from you?

a questionnaire that can help you assess your own cultural attitudes and perceptions.

**Cultural competence** is *the ability of a health care provider, agency, or system to respond to the unique trends of a population whose cultures are different from that of the mainstream or dominant society.* The importance of culture at all levels—client, provider, administration, and policy—is acknowledged and incorporated into health care. Basic beliefs about the nature of health and disease vary widely among cultures. It is not necessary to know everything about a person's culture to treat or give care competently. Cultural competence is an educational process that includes self-awareness, cultural knowledge, and the ability to develop working relationships across lines of difference, to be flexible, and to use intercultural communication skills.

Cultural care congruence will explain and predict outcomes. Three principles for client therapy goals are (1) cultural care preservation or maintenance, (2) cultural care accommodation or negotiation, and (3) cultural care repatterning or restructuring. These principles are defined as follows:

- **Cultural care preservation** refers to *assistive, facilitative, or enabling acts that preserve cultural values and ways of life viewed as beneficial to the client.*

- **Cultural care accommodation** refers to *assistive, facilitative, or enabling acts that reflect ways to adapt or adjust health care services to fit clients' needs, values, beliefs, and practices.*

- **Cultural care repatterning** refers to *altered designs to help clients change health or life patterns that are meaningful; the cognitive way in which one recognizes different attributes and features of a culture for new patterns of care to become evident and for retention or preservation of selected values, beliefs, or practices of the culture.*

## CULTURAL POPULATIONS IN CANADA

According to the 2006 Census of Population, in 2006 there were 31.6 million people in Canada.[48] This population reflects a cultural, ethnic, and linguistic profile that has become a permanent aspect of Canadian society.

## Aboriginal People

Canada's Aboriginal population is composed of three groups—the North American Indian, the Inuit, and the Métis—each of which is linguistically and culturally distinct.[49] The 2001 Aboriginal Peoples Survey presents a statistical portrait of the well-being of the Aboriginal population living in non-reserve areas across Canada. People who did not identify themselves as Aboriginal were also included in the survey if they were registered under the *Indian Act* and/or were members of a band or First Nation. The results indicate that, overall, the Aboriginal non-reserve population rated its health status as lower than that of the total Canadian population.[50]

According to the Report of the Royal Commission on Aboriginal Peoples, "the term Aboriginal obscures the distinctiveness of the First Peoples of Canada, namely Inuit, Métis and First Nations."[51] Among the First Nations alone, there are more than 50 distinct groupings, and among Inuit, several dialects exist within Inuktitut. The Métis people speak a variety of First Nations languages, such as Cree, Ojibwa, or Chipewyan, as well as Michif, a language that evolved from the Métis people's varied ancestry. The cultural and linguistic variations among these particular groups are greater than the variations among the European nations.[52] It is interesting that in the 2001 Canadian Census, nearly one million people reported having an Aboriginal identity.[53]

**Health Status of Aboriginal People** Type 2 diabetes is extremely common in the Aboriginal population. Even Aboriginal children are now being diagnosed with type 2 diabetes, a condition that once occurred mainly in older adults.[54] In fact, numerous recent publications attest to a significant disparity between the health of Aboriginal people and that of the Canadian population in general.[55]

According to Young, health research may answer why such disparities exist as well as provide solutions for eliminating them.[56] Type 2 diabetes has become a more serious health problem within the non-reserve Aboriginal population than within the total Canadian population.[57] Furthermore, according to Health Canada, evidence exists that the prevalence of diabetes is even higher among the Aboriginal population living on reserves.[58] Five other chronic conditions known to be more prevalent within the non-reserve Aboriginal population are high blood pressure, arthritis or rheumatism, asthma, stomach problems or intestinal ulcers, and heart problems. It is interesting to note, however, that about 69 percent of Aboriginal people aged 15 to 24 in non-reserve areas rated their health as very good or excellent compared with 71 percent of the total population in the same age group (see Table 1-2). While Aboriginal young people report levels of health status similar to those reported by the general Canadian youth population, with each successive age group the perceived health status of Aboriginal people declines more rapidly than it does in the total Canadian population.[59]

**Table 1-2** Self-Rated Health Status by Age Group for the Aboriginal Identity Non-Reserve Population 15 Years and Over, Canada, 2001 Aboriginal Peoples Survey[1,2,3]

| | Total self-rated health status[4] | | Excellent or very good | | Good | | Fair or poor | | Invalid or not stated | |
|---|---|---|---|---|---|---|---|---|---|---|
| | Number | percent | Number | percent | Number | percent | Number | percent | Number | percent |
| **Total Aboriginal identity non-reserve population aged 15+** | 547 870 | 100.0 | 308 530 | 56.3 | 144 830 | 26.4 | 94 220 | 17.1 | 300E | 0.0E |
| 15–24 | 136 750 | 100.0 | 94 640 | 69.2 | 33 640 | 24.5 | 8400 | 6.1 | 80E | 0.0E |
| 25–34 | 120 060 | 100.0 | 77 500 | 64.5 | 30 800 | 25.6 | 11 660 | 9.7 | 100E | 0.0E |
| 35–44 | 131 440 | 100.0 | 72 970 | 55.5 | 36 440 | 27.7 | 21 990 | 16.7 | x | x |
| 45–54 | 86 670 | 100.0 | 39 880 | 46.0 | 23 990 | 27.6 | 22 780 | 26.2 | x | x |
| 55 and over | 72 940 | 100.0 | 23 540 | 32.2 | 19 960 | 27.3 | 29 390 | 40.2 | x | x |

Source: Statistics Canada, Catalogue No. 89–589 of Aboriginal Peoples Survey 2001—Initial Findings: Well-Being of the Non-Reserve Aboriginal Population. Chart 1: Excellent or Very Good Self-Rated Health Status, Page 12. Used with permission.

[1] Excludes the population that did not answer the Health Section of the APS questionnaire and those with invalid or unstated ages.

[2] Aboriginal Identity population includes those people who reported on the APS at least one of the following: (1) Identification as North American Indian, Métis and/or Inuit; (2) Registered Indian status; and/or (3) Band membership.

[3] Non-reserve population includes Aboriginal people that do not live on Indian reserves, with the exception of the Northwest Territories, in which case the total (reserve and non-reserve) Aboriginal population is included.

[4] The sum of the values of each category may differ from the total due to rounding.

## CRITICAL THINKING

*What do you think causes type 2 diabetes among Aboriginal people? What health promotion strategies might benefit these people who live in northern communities?*

Tester and McNicoll make an exceptional point regarding Aboriginal youth.[60] They claim that the Government of Nunavut faces one of the highest suicide rates in the world, particularly among young Inuit males.[61]

Jenkins and his colleagues at the Department of Epidemiology and Biostatistics at McGill University examined the health status of Inuit infants and focused on Canadian Inuit communities with reference to other circumpolar regions.[62] Their results indicated that a wide range of interrelated factors affect the health of Inuit infants. These include their demographic, social, economic, and physical environments as well as their culture's personal health practices and the availability of quality, culturally appropriate health services. In addition, throughout the Arctic, Inuit infants experience higher mortality and poorer health than their non-Inuit counterparts. They also suffer disproportionately from bacterial and viral infections.[63]

To address the growing health concerns, a proposal was made in September 1999 to create a research institute devoted to Aboriginal health.[64] A group of leading Aboriginal and non-Aboriginal Canadian health researchers urged the federal government to consider funding dedicated to Aboriginal health research. This group strongly believed that such an approach would contribute significantly to the overall health and well-being of Aboriginal people. The Canadian Institute of Health Research (CIHR) was presented with the group's recommendations and launched the Institute of Aboriginal Peoples' Health (IAPH) in early 2000.[65] One of IAPH's goals is to present the results of accessible, appropriate, and easily understood health research to Aboriginal people.[66]

In Canada, the Aboriginal cultural revival is beginning to have an effect on mainstream society.[67] It is important that health care professionals taking care of Aboriginal people and their families are aware of culturally appropriate health care that takes into account the health beliefs, practices, and traditional healing systems that their clients and families may prefer. Within the Canadian health care delivery system, nurses provide the majority of health services to Aboriginal people in various settings.[68]

## Immigration

Over the past 100 years, immigration has shaped Canada, adding not only to the nation's ethnic composition but also to its cultural makeup. Canada had a higher rate of

## EVIDENCE-BASED PRACTICE

# Cross-Cultural Relationships between Nurses and Filipino-Canadian Patients

The purpose of this study was to describe culturally embedded values that implicitly guide Filipino-Canadian patients' interactions with Canadian nurses and that are integral to nurse–patient relationships. A focused ethnography was conducted with a purposive sample of 23 Filipino Canadians who received care in Canadian hospitals. Data consisted of interviews, field notes, and diary.

### Practice Implications

The findings revealed the following:

When receiving care, patients delineated *hindi ibang tao* (one of us) and *ibang tao* (not one of us) and this determined their preference for who performed personal and private tasks or received information.

The urgency of the patients' conditions, the intimacy required for most nursing procedures, and the short hospitalizations meant that patients often interacted without progressing through the cultural levels of *pakikitungo* (formality), *pakikibagay* (adjustability), and *pakikisama* (acceptance).

Consequently, the crisis of being hospitalized forced patients to move immediately toward the cultural levels of *pakikipagpalagayangloob* (mutual comfort) or *pakikiisa* (oneness).

Patients' willingness to trust and to share their *kapwa*-oriented (culturally-oriented) worldview in relating with fellow human beings, and their use of the languages of words, gazes, touch, and food, allowed nurses to become *hindi ibang tao* (one of us).

Caregiving roles and establishing relationships also distinguished that *hindi ibang tao* (one of us) was to *bantay* (watch over) the patient, whereas *ibang tao* (not one of us) was expected to *alaga* (care for) them (i.e., provide professional care).

### Implications for Nurses

Communicating and caring effectively for Filipino Canadians requires an understanding of Filipino Canadians' languages of words, gazes, touch, and food and their levels of interaction. Culturally safe nurse–patient relationships can then develop.

Source: Pasco, A.C., J.M. Morse, and J.K. Olsen, Cross-Cultural Relationships between Nurses and Filipino Canadian Patients, *Journal of Nursing Scholarship*, Third Quarter (2004), 239–246. Adapted courtesy of Blackwell Publishing.

population growth than any other G8 country between 2001 and 2006.[69] An increase in international immigration was primarily responsible for the acceleration of Canada's growth rate over the last five years. In fact, roughly two-thirds of Canada's population growth now comes from international migration. Meanwhile, the remaining one-third comes from natural increase—that is, growth resulting from more births than deaths.

The growth of the visible minority population in Canada during the last several decades is the result of immigration patterns. While earlier immigrants were mainly of European descent, new arrivals are more likely to have been born in non-European countries. It is important to note that the visible minority population (those other than Aboriginal peoples who are non-Caucasian in race or non-white in colour, as defined by the *Employment Equity Act*) is growing faster than the total population.[70]

In 2001, about one-eighth of Canada's population was from visible minorities. Canada's visible minority population is predominantly urban and dominated by a few large groups. At present, almost three-quarters of Canada's visible minorities reside in its three largest cities: Montreal, Toronto, and Vancouver. By 2017, two ethnic groups—South Asian and Chinese—are expected to account for half of the visible minority population, with each group numbering approximately two million.[71]

Immigration continues to influence the cultural composition of the population of Canada. Immigrants from other lands choose to come to a specific location, with the intention of taking up permanent residence, reuniting with family, and finding employment. Various events in the country of origin may cause the shift:

1. Political upheavals
2. Religious strife
3. Failure of national economic policies
4. Ethnic conflict and humanitarian crises
5. Wars, warlords vying for power, and separatist movements
6. Warring criminal factions, such as drug cartel conflicts
7. Multiple natural disasters and famines

**Health Status of Immigrants** McDonald states that it is now accepted that new immigrants to Canada, Australia, and the United States enjoy significant health advantages relative to comparable native-born populations in these countries. One obvious reason for this is that individuals in good health are more inclined and better able to emigrate than those in poor health. Another reason is that employability, which is a factor in granting permission to immigrate to Canada, includes a certain health status. Finally, before potential immigrants are admitted, they must undergo medical screening to ensure that that they do not suffer from serious medical conditions.[72]

Factors contributing to variations in the health status of immigrants include length of residence in Canada, country of origin or ethnicity, gender, age, level of education, and economic position. Ali and Perez studied the Canadian immigrant's health status (mental and physical health) using data from Statistics Canada Cross-sectional 2000/2001 Canadian Community Health Survey.[73] After analyzing the data, they found that immigrants who had arrived in Canada in recent years had the lowest rates of depression and alcohol dependence compared with immigrants who had been in Canada for 30 years or longer. Alcoholism and depression rates among immigrants from Asia, Africa, South and Central America, and the Caribbean were significantly lower than among the Canadian-born average. The results for chronic disorders generally indicated a gradient, wherein the health of immigrants becomes progressively worse as their length of stay in Canada increases. These results for chronic conditions in general corroborate other previous Canadian findings.[74] This indicates that the health status of immigrants who have resided in Canada for decades deteriorates over time and tends, eventually, to match the health status of the Canadian-born population.

## Influence of Groups and Media on Cultural Values

**Social Value Groups** Sociologist and pollster Michael Adams examined Canadian social values in his book *Sex in the Snow*, published in January 1997.[75] According to Adams, when Canadians are divided by their social values, 12 distinct psychographic "tribes," or social value groups, emerge. These can be organized under three categories: (1) the elders category (over age 60) comprises three subgroups; (2) the baby boomers category (at present roughly ages 39 to 49) comprises four subgroups; and (3) the Generation X category (at present roughly ages 25 to 49) comprises five subgroups. The fact that the greatest number of social value groups exists among Generation Xers reflects a trend toward increasingly diverse Canadian values. Adams has attributed this trend to the effects of technological advances, such as the Internet, that allow Canadians to cross cultural boundaries, and in doing so to explore a host of diverse values.[76] Canada's own techno-evangelist Don

Tapscott believes that the Net Generation, also called Generation Y, has grown up with computers and is wired for cyberspace.[77] Computers are no longer seen as "technology," but as tools and devices that are vital to everyday life. In addition, individuals of the Net Generation prefer the Internet to television because it provides abundant information as well as email and chat rooms.[78]

Adams states that in 1997 to 1999, some untoward reactions occurred in terms of how Canadians perceive their own lives on the one hand and the changing context of the Canadian society on the other. Overwhelming economic and technological forces appear to be going beyond the control of Canadians, leaving them with a growing sense of insecurity.[79]

---

### CRITICAL THINKING
*What is your understanding of a global community?*

---

**Influence on Health of Social Value Groups** The media exerts a profound influence on the psychosocial development of children.[80] The average Canadian child watches nearly 14 hours of television each week.[81] By the time he or she graduates from high school, the average teenager will have spent more time viewing television than being in the classroom.[82] Viewing television has the potential to generate both positive and negative effects on children and adolescents. A number of television programs for children can have positive effects. For example, by watching *Pinky Dinky Doo*, children will possibly be inspired to invent their own games, sharpen their listening skills, expand their vocabulary, and, most importantly, have a good time.[83] On the negative side, the Canadian Paediatric Society and the College of Family Physicians of Canada are concerned that too many children are sitting inside watching television instead of playing outdoors. This realization is alarming because most children already sit in school for five to seven hours per day. Other concerns are the increased reliance on television, video games, and computer technology as pastimes for children as well as the decreasing priority of physical education in Canadian schools. All these factors are cited by experts as major reasons for the growing numbers of sedentary children and teenagers. In fact, the Canadian Paediatric Society, the College of Family Physicians of Canada, and the Canadian Teachers' Federation have issued a joint call for action urging parents, educators, policy-makers, and politicians to act immediately to address the rise in child and youth physical inactivity and obesity.[84] A study by Ozmert, Yoran, and Yurdakok was the first to use the Child Behavior Checklist (CBCL) to examine the effects of television viewing on child behaviour. The findings revealed that children who watched television excessively were more withdrawn, exhibited more social problems, and displayed delinquent and aggressive behaviours. These same children also demonstrated less effective social behaviour and had lower school achievement scores.[85] The instances of violence shown on television are increasing. The average child sees 12 000 depictions of violent acts on television yearly, including many depictions of rape and murder. More than 1000 studies confirm that lengthy exposure to viewing violence increases the occurrences of aggressive behaviour.[86]

The Internet has a significant potential for providing children and youth with access to valuable educational information; however, in many instances, the lack of editorial standards limits the credibility of the Internet as a quality source of information.[87] The detrimental effects of sitting for long periods at a computer can contribute to obesity, underdeveloped social skills, and various forms of addictive behaviour.[88]

## HEALTH TRENDS IN SOCIETY

In the past decade, a review of polls, surveys, and reports indicates that Canadians cherish a number of values related to health care. Measurements of support for the principles of the *1984 Canada Health Act* are undertaken frequently in order to determine whether Canadians support the fundamental values of their health care system. Results have indicated that out of the five principles (universality, accessibility, portability, comprehensiveness, and public administration), the highest support is for universality, while the lowest support is for public administration. These findings indicate clearly that Canadians still believe in universality and that Medicare is highly valued.[89]

Mendelsohn examined the evolution of Canadian public opinion on the health care system over the previous 20 years. He states that Canadians are very supportive and proud of their health care system as well as supportive of the principles of the *Canada Health Act*; however, Canadians have also perceived deterioration in the quality of the system during the past decade, particularly with regards to waiting times for specialists, waiting times at emergency rooms, availability of the best technology, and adequate numbers of available doctors and nurses.[90] Mendelsohn also says that Canadians continue to resist privatization (payment for private health care services by patients) but they are seeking proposals to protect and improve the public health care system. It is interesting to note that several years after Mendelsohn's report to the Romanow Commission, health care remains a top concern for Canadians. The new trend, however, is that an increasing proportion of Canadians is giving serious consideration to private health care possibilities.[91]

In the past two decades, Canadians' values have gradually shifted toward greater personal autonomy, empowerment, and the desire to make choices on their own in a wide range of areas. There has been a dramatic rise in the use of professional services such as chiropractors, physiotherapists, and dentists—professionals other than physicians.[92]

Several trends are important to health care: the emphasis on an information society, the use of high technology, the long-term perspective, the decentralization of services, the use of self-help practices, the use of networking, the seeking of multiple options, the rise of more women in leadership positions, and the decline of the welfare state. The numbers of instances of aggression and violence vary from one culture to another, but any violence is disruptive to the health of Canadians. People react differently to frequent exposures to violence. They may tolerate it, develop disease symptoms, project their own aggression onto others, develop a neurotic preoccupation with it, or act violently themselves to discharge rage. We see examples in society of each reaction in the form of physical, emotional, and social illnesses.

In 2001, the anthrax cases reported in the United States heightened public awareness of bioterrorism. While the probability of such an attack in Canada is low, the consequences would be severe should one occur. It is therefore important to have emergency plans in place. These plans are critical if the health care system is to respond effectively. Note that, in 2003, the outbreak of severe acute respiratory syndrome (SARS) in several Canadian cities stressed the importance of coordinated efforts at all levels of government, as well as at international agencies.[93]

## SOCIAL DETERMINANTS OF HEALTH

The previous discussion regarding the influence of culture highlights a number of different ways to conceptualize health. At a 2002 Toronto conference, a special group of social and health policy experts, community representatives, and health researchers considered the state of 11 key social or societal determinants of health. The social determinants identified as relevant and important to the health of Canadians were early childhood development, education, employment and working conditions, food security, health care services, housing shortages, income and equitable distribution, social exclusion, social safety nets, unemployment, and employment security. These social determinants reflected an increasing concern that the social safety nets were eroding. As a result of the conference, the Toronto Charter on the Social Determinants of Health was developed to outline action for government at all levels, the media, public health, and health agencies and associations. This charter is, and will continue to be, a valuable tool for the promotion of health and social justice.[94]

## Poverty in Canada

Sociologists use the concept of poverty in two different ways. **Relative poverty**, which by definition is inevitable and universal, refers to the *deprivation of some individuals in relation to those who have more*. The richest and most egalitarian societies have within their number some people who reside in relative poverty. More critical is **absolute poverty**, *a deprivation of resources that is life-threatening*. Macionis and Gerber state that even in affluent Canada, which has a social safety net, families go hungry, reside in inadequate housing, and endure poor health because of critical states of poverty.[95]

## Who Is Poor?

A disproportionate number of children, elderly people, homeless people, refugees, and new immigrants are poor. Further, chronically ill and unemployed persons may become poor. Poor people may be of any race or ethnic group.

*Vulnerable populations* are social groups, often poor, but they may be in the middle or even upper economic levels. They are people who are often subordinated or discriminated against, marginalized, or disenfranchised. They have low social status and lack power in social and political

relationships and experience relatively more illness, premature death, and lower quality of life overall than comparable groups. These misfortunes are related to a lack of resources and increased exposure to risk.

Child poverty rates are disproportionately high among vulnerable social groups. Such children are more likely to drop out of school and become unemployed. Approximately half (52 percent) of low-income children in Canada live in female lone-parent families.[96] An increasing body of research indicates that lone mothers and their children are at a higher-than-average risk of health problems.[97] Based partly on the increase in the Aboriginal population, the plight of First Nations children in their rural communities, as well as the condition of urban Aboriginal children, requires sustained action to ensure that these children will thrive, not merely survive.[98] Infant mortality is higher among the poor, in isolated communities, and among Aboriginal peoples.[99]

The 2006 Report Card on Child and Family Poverty in Canada states that close to 1.2 million children—almost one out of six children in Canada—still live in poverty.[100] Campaign 2000 continues to be a non-partisan, cross-country coalition of more than 120 national, provincial, and community organizations committed to working together to end child and family poverty in Canada. Campaign 2000 challenges the leaders of each of Canada's political parties to develop a Poverty Reduction Strategy with targets, time-tables, and funding commitments. Furthermore, it contends that this strategy should be developed through substantive consultation with Canadians, including those with lived experience of poverty.[101]

In Canada, the economic status of seniors is important to their quality of life in a number of ways. For example, income plays an important role in determining seniors' physical and mental health, their life expectancy, the quality of their housing, and many other aspects of well-being.[102] In fact, personal income and wealth likely influence how a senior participates in society. The financial situation of seniors in Canada has improved significantly over the last 25 years.[103] Although poverty rates among seniors have declined, large disparities across groups remain. Immigrated seniors are more likely than Canadian-born seniors to have low incomes, and the income gap between genders is still highly evident.[104] Elderly women are far more likely than men to depend on Old Age Security (OAS) and Guaranteed Income Supplement (GIS), rather than private pension plans, as important sources of income. For the most part, private pension plans remain a benefit of non-immigrants. Among unattached elderly women, the incidence of low income is particularly high for the separated and the divorced, followed by the widowed. Never-married elderly women fare better but are still less well off relative to women who live common-law or are married.[105]

People of all ages and from all walks of life are among the homeless. Becoming a single parent or working at low-paying jobs adds to the risk of living on the street, especially if living with family members is not an alternative. The duration of homelessness varies from a short time to many years, depending on the cause and on the type of social services and assistance available to the person. In recent years, the homeless population has become younger and better educated. An increasing number of women with children and even entire family units live on the street. The homeless are represented by all racial groups and are found in all geographic areas. In Canada, ill health among homeless people is a major and growing concern. Homelessness is associated with both increased hospital costs and length of stay. Also associated with homeless clients are medical and surgical conditions that become complicated by secondary diagnoses of substance abuse or mental illness.[106] Canada remains one of the few countries in the world without a comprehensive affordable housing strategy and permanent funding for this issue.[107] This situation requires attention by all governmental levels. The reader is encouraged to consider the housing work of Cathy Crowe, a Toronto street nurse. Visit her at http://trdc.net/index.php?page=cathy-crowe, or search for her name on the Internet.

Refugees who are suddenly displaced because of war may be forced to live in a country that is not of their choosing with only the meagre goods they can carry. Because of their life experiences as refugees, a variety of physical health problems may arise after arrival. Mental health problems may begin because of losses suffered in the country of origin, refugee camp living, torture, and culture shock on arrival in Canada. Post-traumatic stress disorder (PTSD) is to be expected.[108] Many immigrants may have economic problems, but they are less likely to be in poverty than refugees.

One concern that arises in examining the issue of cultural minorities and health is that of various conflicting explanations. In Canada, many members of cultural minorities are economically deprived.[109] This fact makes it not only complicated, but also difficult to determine how much cultural uniqueness or economic disadvantage, or some combination of both, is responsible for health status. Canadians who experience inadequate income, dependency on welfare, stresses, substandard living conditions, physical violence, sexual abuse, and substance abuse understandably suffer worse health than other Canadians do.[110]

---

## CRITICAL THINKING

*What is your perception of the socioeconomic class system in Canada?*

## Health Status and Socioeconomic Class

What can be said about Canada's socioeconomic classes and the health of Canadians? Most Canadians enjoy a relatively high level of health.[111] This overall high standard of health, however, is not shared equally by all Canadians. For example, life expectancy, which is an important indicator of population health, varies both from region to region and with one's socioeconomic level. Regarding regions, life expectancy is generally higher in southern urban areas in, or west of, Ontario. Meanwhile, life expectancy is generally lower in remote regions, or in the northern parts of certain provinces. Many of these regions have significant populations of Aboriginal people. Interestingly, low life expectancies are not linked with any one specific cause. The mortality rates in regions with low life expectancies are higher for most causes of death.[112]

Roos and Mustard claim that health varies with socioeconomic status.[113] One example is that those who are better educated and have higher incomes can expect to have better health. According to these researchers, the general health status of the lower and middle socioeconomic groups will depend primarily on changes in social policy, such as the improvement of educational opportunities. Another study, conducted by Kosteniuk and Dickinson (Department of Sociology, University of Saskatchewan), found that having a higher household income, being retired, and growing older are all significantly associated with lower stress levels.[114] Higher-income Canadians experience greater levels of control and social support, while older Canadians experience lower rates of social support but higher rates of social involvement. When the effects of low income on infant health were studied, the researchers concluded that less-than-sufficient household incomes were associated with poorer health and higher hospital admissions in the first five months of life. This occurred even after adjusting for factors known to affect infant health, including the mother's level of education.[115] Similar results were found by another group of Canadian researchers, who concluded that children from poor families have more health problems than do children from better-off families. Furthermore, children of single mothers have more health problems than do children from two-parent families.[116] Another Canadian study of 6748 women aged 20 to 64 found that women in the lowest income group are about five times more likely to report poor or marginal health. Not surprisingly, those with higher incomes are more likely to report better health.[117]

## Where Are the Poor People?

Poverty has been examined thoroughly in Canada, in both rural and urban areas. The chair of the Rural Ontario Municipal Association (ROMA) states that poverty is a municipal issue in rural areas. Poor people who reside in rural areas are generally unemployed, with limited access to opportunity, child care, or transportation. These tend to be people who are underhoused or seniors who are becoming isolated as families move away. Municipal governments have an important role to play in terms of economic development to respond to dynamic local needs.[118] Meanwhile, the *Report on Reflections on Rural and Northern Poverty* indicates that the best solution to address poverty in rural and northern communities is to cultivate vibrant communities. Suggested approaches include creating local employment opportunities, including access to jobs as well as job training, retraining, and pre-employment supports. At the same time, community workers need to recognize the need to respect cultural and physical diversity and to recognize barriers such as inadequate housing, transportation, health and well-being services, child care, and educational and training opportunities that inhibit individuals from escaping from poverty. Finally, federal, provincial, and municipal governments must work collaboratively rather than in isolation or against one another.[119]

Regarding urban poverty, a report entitled *Urban Poverty in Canada: A Statistical Profile* examined poverty in Canada at the local level and compared the situation in cities across the country. The findings indicated that poverty increased throughout Canada in the early 1990s, but more so in the metropolitan areas. Cities in Quebec tended to have the highest poverty rates, while cities in southern Ontario tended to have the lowest poverty rates. In the Atlantic provinces, the Prairies, and British Columbia, cities reported poverty rates that ranged widely.[120]

## HEALTH PROMOTION

The sociocultural influences, trends in society, poverty, and social determinants of health are important considerations for the conditions that create, maintain, and support health. Health is desired universally, and in most societies health is linked with goals of human development, satisfaction of basic needs, work, quality of life, and social well-being. These associations not only have enlarged the scope of social objectives but also have improved Canadians' understanding of what makes them healthy and well. How health is identified, both physically and emotionally, varies from culture to culture, as do ideas about the factors related to health and illness.

Health promotion refers to behaviours that are directed to increasing the well-being and self-actualization of an individual or group. Health promotion focuses on efforts to approach or move toward a high level of health and well-being.[121] Along with new definitions of health, health promotion strategies have evolved. The biomedical approach to health promotion sees health as the absence of disease. The behavioural (lifestyle) approach focuses on physical functioning, ability, and well-being, both physical and emotional. The behavioural approach has led to a focus on developing interventions linked to disease prevention and health promotion such as the following:[122]

1. Health history and physical assessment
2. Health-promoting behaviours, including nutritional practices, physical activity, and stress management
3. Health-protecting behaviours, including avoiding abuse of tobacco, alcohol, and chemical substances, and exposure to environmental hazards and injuries

The socioenvironmental approach to health promotion considers social well-being at the individual and community level. This approach addresses key psychosocial risk factors as the social determinants of health. Based on the Ottawa Charter, this approach uses five key actions: strengthen community action, create supportive environments, develop healthy public policy, develop personal skills, and reorient health systems.[123]

When considering the health of populations, primary health care (PHC), which has been adopted by the World Health Organization (WHO) and by Canada, has been internationally accepted as the most effective way to meet health needs in communities around the globe.[124] PHC is usually equated with five principles that emphasize promotion, prevention, and an investment in sustainability. These principles include public participation, health promotion and disease prevention, the use of appropriate skills and technology, accessibility (an equal distribution of care), and intersectorial collaboration (the integration of social and health services, education, and links between hospitals and community services).[125]

### Influence of Health Promotion
By international standards, Canadians are healthy. The general population rates its own health as excellent or very good. In fact,

Canada can boast of having one of the highest life expectancies in the world: 77 years for men and 82 years for women.[126] So where are the health concerns?

In Canada, a high burden of chronic illness exists along with a growing level of health inequality among different groups in Canadian society. The key factors in health inequalities are income, Aboriginal identity, gender, and disability.[127] Regarding activity levels, more than half of Canadians (51 percent) aged 12 and older in 2005 said they were active or moderately active, an increase from 43 percent in 2000–2001. More males (53 percent) than females (49 percent) said they were active or moderately active in 2005. However, almost one-third (32 percent) of Canadians aged 18 years and older said their height and weight corresponded to a body mass index (BMI) in the overweight category. In addition, 15 percent said their height and weight corresponded to a BMI in the obese category, an increase from 14 percent in 2000–2001.[128] In Canada, obesity places a substantial burden on public health, and individuals with more extreme levels of obesity place themselves at an increased risk or face premature death.[129]

The Integrated Pan-Canadian Healthy Living Strategy is a conceptual framework based on a population health approach that strives to focus on some of the root causes that lead to poor health outcomes.[130] The strategy, approved by the federal, provincial, and territorial Ministers of Health, was launched in October 2005.[131] This approach addresses the working and living environments that affect an individual's health, the conditions that enable and support people in making healthy choices, and the health services required to promote and maintain health.[132] Nurses have the skills and knowledge to make primary health care the way of the future for all Canadians.[133]

Canada on the Move (COTM) is a national initiative aimed at increasing the Canadian population's awareness of and participation in regular physical activity using pedometers through a Web-based platform.[134] COTM began when Canadian Institutes of Health Research (CIHR) collaborated with Kellogg Canada and several other partners to promote activity. Use of the website (www.canadaonthemove.ca) was encouraged on Kellogg's cereal boxes. Meanwhile, separate press releases from CIHR and Kellogg Canada publicized the initiative and stressed the importance of increased walking.[135] The results of a study conducted by Plotnikoff and his researchers, who assessed the characteristics of participants visiting the websites, indicated that the COTM website presents a viable approach to reaching a diverse demographic group. That is, the study suggested that website assessment and intervention systems have the potential to reach large, albeit self-selected, samples of Canadians.[136]

## Health Promotion in Nursing Practice

Care and caring are basic to health, health promotion, and illness prevention. For more information, see the box entitled "Key Definitions Related to Health and Health Promotion." **Caring** is understood to be *assistive, supportive, or facilitative actions directed toward another person or group with evident or anticipated needs to ameliorate or improve a human condition or way of life.*[137]

In Canada, the need for effective nursing and health care leadership has been recognized as being critical for client and family care in all settings, including the development of policies and health promotion strategies. Nursing leadership encompasses a wide range of challenges and competencies to ensure quality client outcomes. What are these competencies? They include caring, modelling, and mentoring, as well as envisioning and decision making. At the 2003 Conference on Leadership in Ottawa, three areas of focus for nursing leaders were identified: (1) building practice environments; (2) developing primary health care; and (3) promoting evidence-based practice.[138] It is clear, then, that today's effective nurse must not only plan nursing care for the client and families but also collaborate, in a co-operative manner, with members of the health care team to reach the common goal of quality care for all.

Economic, political, and environmental factors that contribute to poor health must be addressed in health planning and policy formation.[139] Community participation increases access to health care. It provides for greater efficiency, effectiveness, and coordination of services and leads to equity in, and self-reliance of, a population. It requires time, energy, cultural knowledge, trust and respect, common goals, and constant dialogues. Nurses are in a key position to foster this model of health promotion and to conduct themselves accordingly within the consequent empowerment.[140]

## Culturally Competent Care

The CNA has been examining ways to incorporate cultural practices into health promotion activities.[141] The four key responsibilities set out by the CNA for nurses who wish to provide culturally appropriate care are as follows:

- Self-assessment—nurses need to spend time exploring their own personal attitudes and values about health in order to appreciate not only their own experiences but others' understanding of health as well.
- Cultural knowledge—involves the true understanding of others' health beliefs and values that can affect their responses to such personal events as birth practices,

- **Health:** State of well-being in which a person is able to use purposeful, adaptive responses and processes physically, mentally, emotionally, spiritually, and socially in response to internal and external stimuli (stressors) to maintain relative stability and comfort and to strive for personal objectives and cultural goals.

- **Wellness:** Ability to adapt, to relate effectively, and to function at near-maximum capacity; includes self-responsibility, nutritional awareness, physical fitness, stress management, environmental sensitivity, productivity, expression of emotions, self-expression in a variety of ways, creativity, personal care, and home and automobile safety.

- **Bio-psychosocial or holistic health:** High level and total view of health; unity of body, mind (feelings, beliefs, attitudes), and spirit, and person's interrelatedness with others and the environment.

- **Health promotion:** Activities that increase the levels of health and well-being and actualize or maximize the health potential of individuals, families, groups, communities, and society.

- **Health-protective behaviour:** Any behaviour performed by a person, regardless of the perceived or actual health status, to protect, promote, or maintain health, whether or not that behaviour is actually effective.

- **Primary prevention:** Activities that decrease the probability of occurrence of specific illness or dysfunction in an individual, family, group, or community and reduce incidence of new cases of disorder in a population by combating harmful forces that operate in the community and by strengthening the capacity of people to withstand these forces.

- **Secondary prevention:** Early diagnosis and treatment of the pathological process, thereby shortening disease duration and severity and enabling a person to return to normal function as quickly as possible.

- **Tertiary prevention:** Restoring a person to optimum function through rehabilitation and within the constraints of the problem when a defect or disability is fixed, stable, or irreversible.

- **Risk:** Exposure to possible loss, injury, or danger; the *probability* of the occurrence of a particular event.

- **Risk factor:** Factors or characteristics *associated* with an increased probability of experiencing a particular event. Association means that the risk factor and the condition often occur together, but that the risk factor may or may not be a cause.

death and dying, spirituality, and alternative or traditional therapies.

- Verbal and non-verbal communication—both are essential for clients and families to access the services they require. Facilitative techniques, such as listening, respecting, empathizing, and, in particular, being open, are helpful.

- Partnerships among clients, providers, and funding agencies—essential for quality care. Frequently, it becomes necessary to develop ways that incorporate culturally diverse practices into health care services to optimize health outcomes for the client. The development of partnership (intersectorial collaboration) is an important principle of health promotion.

All health professionals, not only nurses, can contribute to achieving the goal of health promotion to clients and their families in different communities. In essence, collaborative teamwork among health care professionals is the key to providing cultural connections. Health care professionals need to understand each discipline's knowledge base, practice styles and philosophies, and practice goals if mutual respect in an interdisciplinary

environment is to occur.[142] As part of this effort, cross-cultural services are becoming a growing need in the health care system in both urban and rural communities.

Learning about another's cultural background can promote feelings of respect and humility. It can enhance one's understanding of the person and the family: their needs, likes and dislikes, behaviours, attitudes, care and treatment approaches, and whether they might be influenced by sociocultural causes of disease.

Assessment involves observing, listening, and talking with the client and, frequently, the family. Some people communicate best in their first (or native) language when they are ill. Further, an elderly person may speak only his or her native language at home, having never learned English. Currently there is an emphasis of support for any group endeavouring to maintain its language because language provides strength and connectedness within a community. What can you do to help?

Because of the diversity of cultures found in Canada, there are a considerable number of people for whom English is not their first language. Hence, you may need to use an interpreter to assist you with assessment, care planning, and intervention. Become acquainted with

| Table 1-3 | Five Steps to Working Effectively with Interpreters |
|---|---|
| Step 1 | Recognize the need for an interpreter. |
| Step 2 | Seek out the appropriate type of interpreter. |
| Step 3 | Clarify the role of the interpreter and that of the health care provider. |
| Step 4 | Maintain control and engage in direct conversation with the client. |
| Step 5 | Be vigilant for errors in interpretation. |

Source: Srivastava, R., Working with Interpreters in Healthcare Settings. In R. Srivastava (ed.), *The Healthcare Professional's Guide to Clinical Cultural Competence* (p. 127, Table 6-1). Toronto: Elsevier, 2007.

people in the community who speak other languages fluently and can be interpreters or translators for health care professionals. Table 1-3 provides guidelines for working with an interpreter.

# HEALTH PROMOTION STRATEGIES
## Health Teaching

Health teaching is one way to have a lasting effect on the health practices of a different cultural group. Health education specifically transmits information, mobilizes the inner resources of the person, and helps people adopt and maintain healthful practices and lifestyles. Others cannot make decisions for a person, but the person should be provided with sufficient information concerning choices so that he or she can make intelligent decisions. Table 1-4 lists some good teaching principles and methods.

Various pressures interfere with attempts at health teaching. Behind poor health habits lies more than ignorance, economic pressure, or desires. Misdirected motivation plays a strong part in continuing certain non-preferential practices, in spite of your efforts at education. Motivation, moreover, is influenced by a person's culture and his or her status and role in that culture, and by social pressures for conformity. Starting programs of health promotion can be difficult when people place a low value on health, cannot recognize cause-and-effect relationships in disease, lack future-time orientation, or are confused about the existence of preventive measures in their culture. Thus, preventive programs or innovations in health promotion must be shaped to fit the cultural and health profiles of the population. Long-range health promotion and disease prevention goals stand a better chance of implementation if they are combined with measures to meet immediate needs. A mother is more likely to heed your

| Table 1-4 | Principles and Methods of Teaching |
|---|---|

**General Approach**

1. Convey respect; be genuine.
2. Reduce social distance between self and others as much as possible.
3. Promote sense of trust and an open interaction; a trusting relationship fosters self-understanding and motivation to follow a teaching plan.
4. Elicit description of feelings from the client about the subject matter or situation to relieve tension and meet the learner's needs.
5. Be organized.
6. Use a comfortable setting and audiovisual aids as necessary.
7. Encourage questions, disagreement, and comments to ensure that your presentation stays focused on client needs and meets teaching goals.
8. Encourage, support, and reinforce as you present content.

**Teaching Specific Content**

1. Begin at knowledge level of client; consider client's readiness to learn.
2. Determine what client wants to know and already knows.
3. Answer the client's questions first; the client will then be more receptive to the information presented.
4. Build on what the client knows. Gently refute myths or misunderstandings.
5. Relate information to behaviour patterns, lifestyle, and sociocultural background to increase likelihood of it being followed by the client.
6. Assist client in reworking your ideas to fit cultural, religious, or family values and customs to ensure that the material to be learned will be practised.
7. Present the content in a logical sequence.
8. Present more basic or simpler content before more advanced or complex information.
9. Present one idea, or a group of related ideas, at a time, rather than presenting many diverse ideas at once.
10. Demonstrate as you describe directions, suggestions, or ideas, if possible.
11. Break content into units and a series of sessions, if necessary. Do not present too many ideas at one time.
12. Teach the family as thoroughly as the client to ensure that suggestions about interpersonal relationships and other concerns will be followed.
13. Present the same information to friends, the employer, the occupational health nurse, the schoolteacher, the clergyman, or the significant community leader, if possible and relevant.
14. Provide written instructions in addition to oral presentations.
15. Provide feedback and reinforcement to the client as you provide opportunities for practice and review.

advice on how to prevent her sick child's condition from getting worse if you give the child immediate care and attention.

## Individual Teaching

**Programmed Learning** Material is presented in carefully planned sequential steps through program instruction books or a computer program. One frame of information is presented at a time. The learner then tests his or her grasp of the information in the frame by writing or, in the case of a computer program, keying in a response to a question, which is usually in a multiple-choice format. The book or computer then gives the correct response. If the learner's response was incorrect, the program presents a repetition of the information, or it might provide a more detailed explanation.

**Literature** *Pamphlets and brochures* describe preventive measures, signs and symptoms of disease, and major steps of intervention. These are published by many health care organizations and agencies, often for specific diseases or groups.

*Autobiographies* of persons with certain disease processes and "how-to" books by persons who have experienced certain health problems directly or indirectly pass along suggestions to others.

**Audiovisual Material** *Videotapes or DVDs* that explain preventive measures, disease processes, or specific instructions can be loaned to the client. He or she can stop the player at any point and replay certain sections until satisfied with the learning. "Talking Books" is a program that records information for the visually impaired. Closed-circuit television or videotape setups allow the person to hear and view material.

Note that these methods of individual instruction are individual only to a certain point. Only when the client can check learning with a *resource person*, ask further questions as necessary, and receive help in making personal applications will learning become significant. That process involves you. The client will not learn from a machine alone.

**Computer/Internet** Instructions for prevention and health care for any condition, as well as other information related to growth, development, and care of children, adolescents, or adults of any age, are available through computer-based instruction formats. Computer programs for client teaching are available to home care and health care agencies. For example, a diagram along with instructions can teach a patient about bypass surgery. Or, a parent can be shown exactly how tubes will be placed in a child's ear.

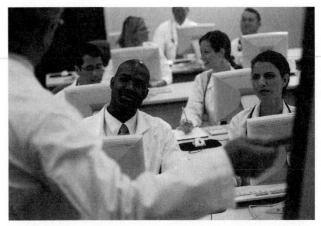

Group teaching provides an opportunity to provide health teaching to individuals with similar health concerns and problems.

## Group Teaching

Client groups provide a channel through which feelings and needs can be expressed and met, especially if the clients have similar concerns, such as colostomy or diabetes. Thus, you can use the group process either to enhance health teaching or as therapy to aid clients in coping with their problems. You may work with a group that has formed to accomplish some specific goal, such as losing weight, promoting research to find a cure for cancer, or providing guidance to parents with mentally retarded children. In some cases, information is not enough. Social support is also necessary, especially when clients are engaging in a lesser-valued activity, such as avoiding excessive consumption of sweet foods.

## Evaluation of Teaching

1. Check frequently to determine whether the content is of interest and is being understood.

2. Have the client repeat some content, or give examples of application of the content.

3. Have the client review previously covered content and its application at each teaching session.

4. Determine the amount of learning that has occurred.

## Advocacy

With your knowledge of cultures, you can be a client's advocate to ensure accessibility and appropriateness of services. Moreover, you can help the health care system care for clients in a culturally sensitive way, or you can work with several agencies toward that goal.

What does good health mean to you and your family? According to Health Canada, it is a major resource for personal, social, and economic development and an important aspect of quality of life. Health promotion strategies aim to make these conditions favourable through advocacy.[143] Health professionals should be visible and accessible, and they need to speak for health in its broadest sense. It is the essence of caring.

What is essential to practice is not only awareness of cultural values and sensitivity to different beliefs and practices, but also a response to human needs.[144] In their case analysis of Latin American refugees who had immigrated to Canada, Hrycak and Jakubec recommend a social advocacy approach with interventions focusing on three areas: the client, the health professional, and public policy. In regards to the client, listening to his or her history and context is valuable. For the health professional, inter-disciplinary workshops could provide venues for issues affecting refugees. Finally, public policy interventions can advocate for the needs of refugees.[145] For example, in an article on exploring perinatal health in Indo-Canadian women, Lynam, Gurm, and Dhari cite that an important strategy to improve pregnancy outcomes among these women is providing resources within the health care system as well as in the community.[146]

Changes in society may cause a variety of problems for individuals and families. Be a supportive listener; validate realistic ideas; prepare the client to adapt to a new or changing environment; and be aware of community agencies or resources that can provide additional help. See Table 1-5 for guidelines on making referrals. You may be able to provide your client with significant support. Develop a better awareness of your own personal philosophy for promoting a feeling of stability in your life so that you, in turn, can assist the client and the family to explore their feelings and formulate a philosophy for coping with change.

## Telehealth

**Telehealth**—*electronically transmitted clinician consultation*— has improved access to care for people in rural or underserved areas, and it is also increasingly used in health promotion education, illness prevention, and prevention of unnecessary hospitalizations. Telehealth can reduce the number of home care visits through computer monitoring made possible by audiovisual transmission over phone lines, which enable the client and care provider to see and hear each other. The client controls the video monitor, which prevents intrusions into privacy. You can also use this modern technology yourself to continue learning about cultural care and to help contribute to improved care.

In Canada, some jurisdictions—particularly in the North—are investing significantly in telehealth technology

**Table 1-5 Guidelines for Making a Referral**

1. Know the available community resources and the services offered.
2. Recognize when you are unable to further assist or work with the client; be honest about your own limits and your perceived need for a referral. Avoid implying rejection of the client.
3. Explore client readiness for referral. The client may also have ideas about referrals and sources of help or may be unwilling to use community agencies.
4. Determine which other professionals had contact with the client and confer with them about the possibility of referral. Various ethnic and racial groups prefer using extended family or the church.
5. Discuss the possibility of referral with a specific person at the selected agency before referral.
6. Inform parents of your recommendations and obtain their consent and co-operation if the client is a minor.
7. Be honest in explaining the services offered by the referral agency. Do not make false promises about another agency's services or roles.
8. Describe specifics about location, how to get to the referral place or person, where to park and enter, and what to expect on arrival.
9. Have the client (or parent) make the initial appointment for the new service if he or she is willing to do so; some people may prefer that you make the initial contact. Tell the person that you have called the agency and that he or she is expected.
10. Do not release information to the referral agency, or person, without written permission from the client (or parent).
11. Ask the client to give you feedback about the referral agency, or person, to help you evaluate your decision and to help you make a satisfactory referral selection for future individuals or families who are in need of help.

and activities to improve service delivery in rural and remote areas.[147] In Manitoba, the Telehealth Network has extensively increased rural access to health care. A satellite, or ground link, connects health care providers with clients, or with each other. Participants at each end can talk with, hear, and see each other. Additional specialized equipment, such as digital cameras, digital otoscopes, and document cameras, improve assessment and information sharing.[148] In Halifax, the establishment of the Izaak Walton Killam (IWK) Telehealth Program, by Chris-Anne Ingram, has been not only challenging but also rewarding in bringing health care to clients and their families. Furthermore, Telehealth is able to bring continuing education to clinicians regardless of distance.[149]

The National Initiative for Telehealth Framework of Guidelines was developed over a 20-month period and involved many steps and activities. Its focus is related to the rendering of clinical services (e.g., teletriage, telecare, and teleconsultation). The guidelines will serve as a useful point of reference; and they will undoubtedly contribute to the general development of the Telehealth field in Canada.[150]

The CNA, in a statement on telepractice, acknowledges the growing importance of Telehealth and the roles that nurses can play in this area. The organization's position underlines the importance of safe, competent, and ethical involvement in Telehealth. The CNA implies that nurses must provide nursing telepractice services consistent with the Codes of Ethics for Registered Nurses.[151]

The use of health informatics, including such innovations as Telehealth, decision-support systems, virtual education, and workload measurement through electronic charting, is increasingly widespread in nursing practice throughout the health care system.[152]

---

**CRITICAL THINKING**

*Arrange to meet with a Telehealth contact for an observational experience. What questions will you ask to become more informed about Telehealth?*

---

## Community Health Protection

Community health protection involves risk reduction behaviours and endeavours to change harmful environmental and social conditions. Harm reduction, in spite of its controversy, has become a widely adopted strategy, primarily because of the devastating harm and cost associated with substance use. The harm reduction approach aims to do the following:

- Offer a practical alternative that focuses on the consequences of harmful behaviours rather than on judging whether the behaviours are morally right or wrong.

- Accept alternatives to abstinence such as needle exchange programs and methadone maintenance.

- Base itself on consumer input and demand, rather than on a top-down policy.

- Support "low-threshold" access to treatment and a friendly approach in order to facilitate treatment options.

- Base itself on compassion, rather than judgment.[153]

This particular nonjudgmental approach treats the drug user as an individual with dignity and rights. It neither condones nor condemns drug use, but respects it as a choice.[154]

In many Canadian cities, HIV and hepatitis C (HCV) have become endemic among injection drug users (IDUs)

and, in turn, these diseases bring about numerous health problems, such as endocarditis. In September 2003, the City of Vancouver opened a medically supervised safer injecting facility (SIF) as a pilot operation. There, injection drug users can inject preobtained illicit drugs under the supervision of medical staff. Wood and his associates report that preliminary observations suggest that the site has been successful in attracting IDUs into its program, and it has helped to decrease public drug use. Due to the complex evaluation process, however, it will be several years before researchers can completely assess the SIF's impacts.[155]

## Sites for Health Promotion and Wellness Programs

Today, industries and some hospitals and other work settings are adding programs for their employees that target topics such as stress reduction, exercise, smoking cessation, and nutritional and weight guidance, particularly with reference to obesity and sodium and cholesterol dietary reduction. Some industries have also established employee assistance programs to help any employee with substance abuse problems so that he or she can be a safe, dependable worker. Some settings offer daycare services to workers with young children to reduce stress related to child care. Others provide stress management programs for their employees and their clients. Some companies have near-24-hour facilities that offer fully equipped exercise rooms, gyms, handball courts, whirlpool baths, and other features.

Health promotion sites could also be established in retirement centres, on campuses, in daycare centres, stores, housing projects, neighbourhood community centres, schools, churches, laundry facilities, and senior nutrition centres. Such sites would be more acceptable to many cultural populations than the hospital or traditional outpatient setting for health screening, well-child checkups, immunizations, and counselling.

---

**CRITICAL THINKING**

*What do you know about traditional healing practices?*

---

## Holistic Nursing

**Holistic nursing** is *nursing practice that has as its goal the healing of the whole person.* **Holism** involves *understanding the relationships among the biological, psychological, social, and spiritual dimensions of a person, that the whole is greater than the sum of the parts, and that a person is an integrated being who is interacting with internal and external environments.*[156]

## Non-traditional, Complementary, and Alternative Methods to Health Care

The use of Complementary Therapies and Alternative Health Care (CAHC) is becoming increasingly widespread in Canada, with significant implications for health delivery.[157] It is estimated that approximately 50 percent of Canadians use some form of natural health products or "complementary" or "alternative" medicine.[158]

Your knowledge of cultures will enable you to practise **holistic care** that *promotes the retention of cultural values and norms as part of the nursing process.* Holistic healing practices

---

### CASE SITUATION

You are a Nurse Unit Manager in the health services unit in a rural hospital in northern Alberta. Over the past year, you have noticed that the rate of admission for First Nations people with diabetes, from all neighbouring communities (some 4000 residents), has increased by 15 percent overall, with a range of 11 to 18 percent, with the highest increase found in the most remote community. When you reported the results of your survey at an interdisciplinary health team meeting, the members decided to form a specific task force group that will include yourself. The mandate of the task force, referred to as the Down with Diabetes Operation Task Force Group (DDO-TFG), is to develop a set of health-promoting strategies within a month's time. The health team unit agreed to implement the strategies as soon as they were developed. It was agreed that the strategies should be developed in co-operation with the communities; in fact, where possible, they should be developed on-site within the communities to promote as much joint commitment as possible.

1. At the first meeting (tomorrow), what guidelines will you suggest that the DDO-TFG follow as it begins to build a valuable community health program with the First Nations people?

2. At the first meeting of the DDO-TFG, after you were resoundingly commended for the excellent set of guidelines you presented, you were urged by the members to provide the preliminary design of an initial assessment/evaluation tool for use in the communities when DDO becomes fully operational.
   a. What will be your first steps in creating such an instrument? What help will you need? Who, or what agencies, might provide assistance to you?
   b. What procedural steps will you propose to the DDO-TFG to test and refine the instrument in time for the expected opening of the DDO a few weeks from now?

---

combine the best of two worlds: the wisdom and sensitivity of cultures and the technology and precision of the modern world. Although holistic practitioners use conventional therapies in many cases, the emphasis on the whole person—his or her physical, emotional, intellectual, spiritual, and sociocultural dimensions—remains. The focus is on disease prevention and health promotion as the individual takes responsibility for his or her own health and well-being. The nurse–client relationship is the key to holistic nursing care because the person has come to expect a caring interaction with the healer.

As part of the Health Products and Food Branch of Health Canada, the Natural Health Products Directorate (NHPD) is the regulating authority for natural products for sale in Canada. Its role is to ensure that Canadians have ready access to natural health products that are safe, effective, and of high quality while respecting freedom of choice and philosophical and cultural diversity. Under the Natural Health Products Regulations, which came into effect on January 1, 2004, natural health products (NHPs) are defined as:

- Vitamins and minerals
- Herbal remedies
- Homeopathic medicines
- Probiotics
- Other products such as amino acids and essential fatty acids[159]

What processes may be used to integrate complementary and alternative health practices into mainstream health care? Reflect on the following critical thinking question for a few minutes before responding.

---

### CRITICAL THINKING

*What are some ethical issues that accompany the use of CAHC?*

---

## Alternative Therapies

To be able to comprehend the meaning of alternative therapies, one may be drawn to the definition provided by Montbriand for her research project. She notes that alternative therapies entail a wide scope of health-related products or healing practices initiated or prescribed by self, family, network of friends, or an alternative health care practitioner who does not have the recognized authority to prescribe, as authorized by the provincial Colleges of Physicians and Surgeons or by the Canadian Medical Association.[160] Montbriand's results are most informative for health professionals. For example, one of her findings indicates that all three groups of professionals (doctors, nurses, and pharmacists) have recognized the need for evidence-based information about alternative therapies.

Today, many nurses are involved in the debate on complementary and alternative therapies. Mulkins, Morse, and Best state that complementary therapy is congruent with health promotion and disease prevention.[161] Thorne and a group of researchers studied a geographically diverse Canadian population with inflammatory bowel disease (IBD) and found that the use of complementary/alternative medicine (CAM) is common among them, and that it is generally perceived by the users to be beneficial and safe.[162] In a study by a Harvard University team, the folk remedy of drinking cranberry juice for urinary tract infections has been found to be effective in preventing recurring infection.

---

### CRITICAL THINKING

*What do you know about herbal remedies?*

---

While some controversy may remain about CAM therapies, it is imperative that nurses know the position of their provincial/territorial regulatory body on the provision of alternative therapies.

## Role of Nurses

Each province in Canada differs in the legal authority, reimbursement practices, and prescription authority assigned to nurses in advanced practice. These factors greatly influence the extent to which a nurse can be an entrepreneur.

**Clinical Nurse Specialist** The CNA's position statement on the Clinical Nurse Specialist (CNS) indicates that the CNS contributes significantly to the health of Canadians within a primary health care framework. Did you know that, historically speaking, the role of the CNS was introduced into the Canadian health care system in the 1960s? As health care became more complex, the trend toward specialization intensified and the result was the development of advanced nursing practice roles. The CNS, as a practitioner, provides expert client care based on in-depth knowledge of a wide scope of nursing and other relevant sciences. Most importantly, the regulation of CNS practice is within the current scope of nursing practice and existing regulatory approaches.[163]

**Nurse Practitioner** The Canadian Nurse Practitioner Initiative (CNPI), led by the CNA, is a pan-Canadian framework for the sustained integration of nurse practitioners as essential providers of quality health care. The goal of CNPI is to facilitate the integration of the nurse practitioner role in the health system to improve Canadians' access to health services in all communities.[164]

**Certification** The CNA Certification Program continues to grow in the number of nursing specialities, examinations given, and nurses certified by the program. By achieving CNA certification, nurses commit to a national standard of professional competence that demonstrates a broad scope of understanding within their specialty.[165]

The future belongs to nurses who are able to respond effectively to new demands and who have the courage to follow their convictions. In turn, people from diverse backgrounds will have more options in terms of selecting the type of health care service that best meets their needs. Then, culturally based primary health care can become a reality.

## SUMMARY

1. You will encounter diverse value systems and customs in your care of clients and families.

2. Understanding cultural and subcultural backgrounds will enhance your care of the client, family, group, and community.

3. People from the *same* culture are uniquely different from each other, but they also share similarities.

4. People from *different* cultural backgrounds share similarities as well as differences in various life patterns and values.

5. Cultural background has a major influence on development and health.

6. You will practise principles of cultural care in every health care setting that are based on concepts learned in this chapter.

7. Our hope is that you engage in lifelong learning about your own and others' cultures. Doing so will enable you to interact with, relate to, assess, intervene with, and care for your client as effectively as possible.

## Interesting Websites

## Key Terms

absolute poverty (15)

bio-psychosocial or holistic health (19)

caring (18)

cultural care accommodation (10)

cultural care preservation (10)

cultural care repatterning (10)

cultural competence (10)

customs (7)

dialect (6)

ethnic (3)

family culture (4)

health (19)

health promotion (19)

health-protective behaviour (19)

holism (23)

holistic care (24)

holistic nursing (23)

mores (7)

postindustrial or postmodern society (6)

prejudice (9)

primary prevention (19)

relative poverty (15)

religious culture (4)

risk (19)

risk factor (19)

ritual (4)

roles (5)

science (8)

secondary prevention (19)

socioeconomic level (5)

status (5)

subculture (3)

Telehealth (22)

tertiary prevention (19)

transcultural nursing (8)

value system (9)

wellness (19)

# Chapter 2

## Environmental Influences on the Person and Family

*Preventing pollutants and toxins from entering our air, water and food would have a profound effect on public health in Canada.*

Dr. David Suzuki, Canadian scientist, activist, and broadcaster

## Objectives

*Study of this chapter will enable you to:*

1 Examine the scope of environmental pollution, both outdoors and indoors.

2 Describe the benefits of including human health as a component of environmental assessment.

3 Describe the importance of greenhouse gas emissions.

4 Identify sources of air pollution in your community and specify resulting hazards to human health.

5 List types of water pollution and describe resultant health problems.

6 Determine substances that cause soil pollution and specify their effects on health.

7 Examine types of food pollution and consider their effects on health.

8 Identify sources of noise pollution in various settings.

9 Contrast different types of surface pollution and resultant health problems.

10 Describe health hazards encountered in the home and on the job and the major effects of these contaminants.

11 Analyze ways that you can prevent or reduce environmental, food, and noise pollution.

12 Determine measures of environmental sustainability that you can take as a nurse.

13 Evaluate your professional responsibility, in the practice area, in assessing for illness caused by environmental pollutants.

Although ecology is a well-publicized subject, the physical environment in which we live is often taken for granted and overlooked as a direct influence on people and their health. You may wonder why a book discussing major influences on the developing person, family unit, and their health contains a chapter about humans and their environment. Yet where we live and the condition of that area—its air, water, and soil—determine to a great extent how we live, what we eat, the disease agents to which we are exposed, our state of health, and our ability to adapt. This chapter focuses primarily on noxious agents to which many people in Canada are exposed in the external environment. Because of the interdependence of people, only those living in isolated rural areas escape the unpleasant effects of our urban, technologically advanced society. Yet even the isolated few may encounter some kind of environmental pollution, whether through groundwater contaminated from afar, food shipped into the area, smog blown from a nearby city, or contaminated rain or snow. Further, the pollutants discussed in this chapter are observed worldwide.

Nursing in the past was concerned primarily with the client's immediate environment in the hospital or home. Today nursing and health care are extended to include assessment of the family and community as well as the individual. Interventions are directed toward promoting a healthy, sustainable environment for individuals and families and maintaining public health standards and federal regulations. Understanding specific environmental health problems, their sources, and their effects will enable you to function effectively, both as a citizen and as a health care professional in working with clients and their families in the hospital or community.

## HISTORICAL PERSPECTIVE

The entire environment has been, and continues to be, a vital part of our existence. Human skill in manipulating the environment has produced tremendous benefits, but none has been without a price—the high price of pollution. Pollution of our environment, in addition to being a health threat, offends aesthetic, spiritual, social, and philosophic values. Environmental pollution is a complex, significant problem requiring multiple solutions (see Figure 2-1).

The world appears to be shrinking in size due mainly to rapidly occurring advances in technology, either in communication or transportation. Global attention has been directed to the effects of acid rain on forests, the depletion of the ozone layer, and global warming. People certainly learn more about other countries when news of disease outbreaks elsewhere appears in the media. One example is that of severe acute respiratory syndrome (SARS). The health of the planet and the health of its people are becoming more inseparable. Today, the public faces the challenge and the need to become highly aware of the connection between environmental hazards and human health.[1]

The official recognition of the status of the earth's environmental problems and the impact of these problems on human health was perhaps first stated by governments at the 1992 Rio Earth Summit.[2] At the Rio Summit, it was acknowledged that a clearer understanding and a precise identification of these global environmental health issues were required. It was also evident that a collective stance

**Figure 2-1** Human interrelationship with the environment

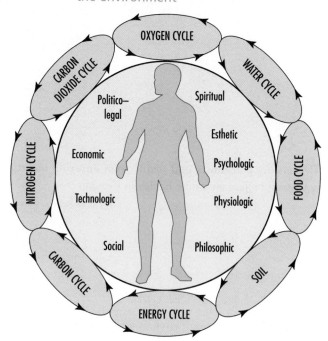

was needed among communities and countries to act on these issues.[3] Environmental health may be defined as the study of those aspects that influence both human health and the well-being of the population.[4] Such aspects may include exposure to environmental contamination, hazards, or pollutants that are detrimental to health. Governments and individuals are recognizing the urgent need to study and provide education on the impact of the environment upon human health. This is imperative if we are to achieve the goal of health for all.

Health Canada is committed to making Canada's population among the healthiest in the world. It works closely with other federal agencies, departments, and health stakeholders to reduce health and safety risks in Canada.[5] It is also responsible for ensuring that human health is included as a component of environmental assessment. Environmental assessment (EA) is a planning tool used to identify the potential effects of projects and activities on the environment.[6] With the broadening of EA to include related health and other social considerations, more reason exists to give health greater priority in all aspects of decision making.[7] EA provides decision-makers with the information they need to approve projects that are compatible with a healthy, sustainable environment.[8] EA requires a team effort, involving both health professionals and specialists in a variety of environmental, economic, social, and technical areas that can have an impact on health. An up-to-date review of important publications on EA can be found on the Canadian Environmental Assessment Agency website (www.ceaa.gc.ca/).[9] The *Canadian Environmental*

Assessment Act, passed in 1992 and proclaimed in June 1995, is a federal statute that requires federal departments to conduct environmental assessments for prescribed projects and activities before providing federal approval or financial support.[10]

More recently, human health and well-being were recognized as the ultimate goal of sustainable development. The World Commission on Environment and Development (WCED) has published a report that has come to be known as the Brundtland Report. It developed the guiding principles for sustainable development, which is defined as development that meets the needs of the present without compromising the ability of future generations to meet their own needs.[11]

Health for all and sustainable development will require a broad range of cross-sectoral strategies that go beyond the traditional domain of the health sector and include other policy sectors such as environment and natural resource management, economic development, education, housing, and agriculture. It is widely recognized that further improvements in health will also require significant efforts from many different sectors of society. With its emphasis on health and the environment and its multi-disciplinarity, EA is an important means of contributing to *health for all* and *sustainable development*.[12]

In October 2000, the Quebec City Consensus Conference on Environmental Health Indicators convened to examine the challenges facing environmental health monitoring and surveillance and to discuss the possibility of developing consensus on many of these issues.[13] The May 2003 National Round Table on the Environment and the Economy recommended that the federal government establish a small set of easily understood environmental and sustainable development indicators to track factors of importance to Canadians.[14]

Recognizing that both the health of Canadians and the country's social and economic progress are fundamentally linked to the quality of the environment, in the October 2004 Speech from the Throne the Government of Canada announced its commitment to working with provincial and territorial partners to build sustainable development systematically into its decision making. To accomplish this, more reliable and more accessible information is needed to guide the actions of Canadians and their governments.[15] In essence, Canadians need clearly defined environmental indicators—measuring sticks that can track the results that have been achieved through the efforts of governments, industries, and individuals to protect and improve the environment. Following expert advice, three environmental indicators were selected by which the federal government and its partners can track progress and be held accountable for taking steps to have cleaner air, lower greenhouse gas emissions, and cleaner water. The indicators are *air quality*, *greenhouse gas emissions*, and *fresh water quality*.

These Canadian Environmental Sustainability Indicators supplement traditional health and economic measures such as gross domestic product, so that Canadians can better understand the interrelationship between the economy, the environment, and human health and well-being.[16]

*What other indicators can you think of that might effectively measure the health status of a community?*

The *Canadian Environmental Protection Act* (CEPA) is Canada's principal piece of federal environmental protection legislation. It addresses issues that include controlling toxic substances, public participation, biotechnology, nutrients, hazardous wastes, fuel standards and vehicle emissions, international air and water pollution, disposal of materials at sea, and other measures.[17] In 1994, the House of Commons Standing Committee on Environment and Sustainable Development was handed the task of conducting a five-year review of CEPA. The committee recommended a new approach whereby the emphasis in CEPA would shift from the *management* of pollution to its *prevention*.[18] As a result, the cornerstone of CEPA (1999) is pollution prevention. Adequate prevention of pollution and harmful waste production helps to decrease risks to the environment and to human health.[19] Other methods of protecting the environment focus mainly on managing waste and pollution after they have been detected. Adhering to a preventive approach helps us manage risks to human health by protecting the quality of air, land, ecosystems, and nature (see Figure 2-2).[20] The National Pollutant

**Figure 2-2** The pollution paradigm shift

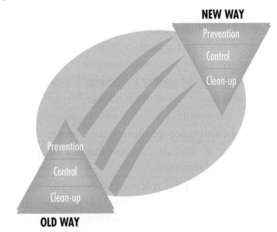

Source: *Informing Canadians on Pollution, 2003*, ISBN: 0-662-36412-0, Catalogue No. En40-7771 2003E, URL: www.ec.gc.ca/npri/communities
Figure 3—The Pollution Prevention Paradigm Shift. Year of Publication 2003.

Release Inventory (NPRI) is a database of information on annual releases to air, water, and land. The same database maintains records of off-site transfers for disposal or recycling.[21] The NPRI is the only nationally legislated, publicly accessible inventory of its kind in Canada. It was established in 1992 and mandated under CEPA. It requires companies to report specific information on the release and transfer of pollutants to the federal government on an annual basis.[22] Other federal legislation regarding protection of the environment includes the following:

- The *Arctic Waters Pollution Prevention Act*, which prohibits depositing waste of any type in the Arctic.

- The *Fisheries Act*, which prohibits depositing harmful substances in water that is frequented by fish.

- The *Canada Shipping Act*, which monitors the discharge of garbage and oil, or oily substances, from ships.

- The *Motor Vehicle Safety Act*, which establishes standards on emissions from gasoline- and diesel-powered motor vehicles.[23]

## CRITICAL THINKING

*In what ways can municipal governments collaborate with the provincial and federal governments in dealing with environmental issues?*

The recognition of the interdependence of human health and the health of the global ecosystems is growing.[24] A serious concern exists over the condition of the environment and the effects of chemical and biological contamination. Interestingly, this concern includes not only contamination effects on human health, but also the viability of ecosystems and numerous species. Public attention has been drawn to the many reports linking environmental exposure to unfavourable human health responses in our industrialized society.[25] For example, the literature which examines the effects of chemicals on the hormone systems of humans and animals is growing steadily. Due to a newly identified illness pattern—the "sick building" syndrome—indoor air quality in modern buildings has also been investigated.[26] Even though there is debate in the scientific community about environmental health problems, health care professionals remain the most credible source of information regarding the health effects of environmental exposures.[27]

Nature plays a vital role in human health and well-being, and parks and nature preserves play a significant role by providing access to nature for individuals and communities. Studies suggest that contact with nature can be an effective strategy in the prevention of mental illness. Clearly, collaborative strategies between research, primary

health, social services, urban planning, and environmental management sectors can have an impact on improving public health.[28]

Before leaving this section, it is important to understand that a new way of managing the environment has emerged over the last few years. Environmental agencies are establishing mechanisms for ensuring that information is easily accessible and readily understood. These efforts have been aided by recent advances in information and communication technology. According to the Task Force on a Canadian Information System for the Environment to the Minister of the Environment, Canada is one of the most connected countries in the world. It is the world leader in the use of geographic information systems and satellite-based remote sensing technology for data collection on the environment.[29] The three Canadian Environmental Sustainability Indicators—air quality, greenhouse gas emissions, and fresh water quality—provide important information, not only about Canada's environmental sustainability, but also about the health and well-being of the people of Canada and our economic growth and lifestyle choices.[30]

The following sections focus on health issues related to air quality (including greenhouse gas emissions), fresh water quality, soil pollution, food safety, noise pollution, surface pollution, and occupational hazards. A brief discussion of the sustainability of health promotion interventions is also provided.

## AIR QUALITY

In various settings, you will care for clients and their families who have diseases caused by air pollution. Strong evidence exists that air pollution is the most harmful environmental problem in Canada. In terms of human health effects, it causes thousands of deaths, millions of illnesses, billions of dollars in health care expense, and tens of billions of dollars in lost productivity every year.[31]

In Canada, and in most countries in the world, the effects of air pollution and global warming are contributing to a general anxiety in the population about the environment. The reason for this anxiety is that a potential exists for extensive adverse health effects and devastating climate change.[32] Air pollution levels tend to increase with higher temperatures. This relationship reflects the fact that the causes of global warming and air pollution are similar.[33] Edwards has found that almost two out of three Canadians claim that pollution has made their health worse (see Figure 2-3). In fact, more than half of Canada's population expresses concern about air quality.[34]

Asthma is increasingly prevalent in many industrialized countries, including Canada.[35] Asthma is a disease that

**Figure 2-3** The health effects of air pollution

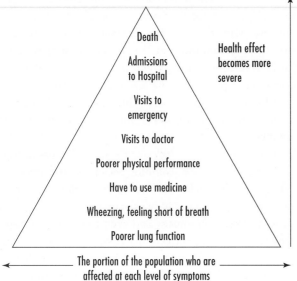

The health effects of air pollution may vary from subtle problems, to troubling symptoms, to hospital visits and early deaths.

Source: Reproduced with permission of the Canadian Public Health Association. Originally published in *Canadian Journal of Public Health, 92*(3) (May/June 2001).

causes breathing problems. The most common factors affecting the asthmatic client are allergens, respiratory irritants, and viral infections.[36] Examples of outdoor pollutants that can exacerbate asthma include ground-level ozone and sulphur dioxide. Meanwhile, the indoor irritant of tobacco smoke represents an even greater risk.[37] Manfreda and his co-researchers examined the variability of asthma-related manifestations and medication use in six sites across Canada (Vancouver, Winnipeg, Hamilton, Montreal, Halifax, and Prince Edward Island). Their findings were then compared to those from sites that had participated in a recent European survey. They concluded that the significant variation in the prevalence of asthma symptoms and attacks and in the use of asthma medication between Canada and international sites suggests a correlation between asthma and environmental conditions.[38] In the management of asthma, environmental control and education should be instituted for all asthma clients and their families.[39] For both mothers and fathers of young children with asthma, the most time-consuming caregiving task is to provide emotional and developmental support for their children.[40]

Health Care Without Harm is an international coalition working to transform the health care industry that has developed a guide called *Risks to Asthma Posed by Indoor Health Care Environments: A Guide to Identifying and Reducing Problematic Exposures.* This guide aims to inspire action by health professionals to attend to environmental factors and maximize opportunities for health promotion and disease prevention.[41]

McCarthy and her researchers conducted a pilot study to compare outcomes for parents who participated in empowerment compared to traditional approaches to asthma education. The findings indicated that both approaches resulted in increased knowledge. These findings have implications for asthma education and for the education of health professionals.[42]

## Sources of Air Pollution

Air quality influences our lives in a variety of ways. Air pollution has significant effects on both human health and the natural environment.

The eight most important pollutants found in the air are carbon monoxide, sulphur oxides, nitrogen oxides, heavy metals, volatile organic compounds (VOCs), gaseous ammonia, ground-level ozone, and fine particulate matter.[43] The latter two pollutants are the main components of smog and are the focus of air quality indicators. It is important to note that ground-level ozone and fine particulate matter have been linked to health impacts ranging from minor respiratory problems to hospitalizations and premature deaths.[44] Air pollution is most harmful to the very young, the very old, and persons with respiratory and cardiac disease. According to Frank, children are especially vulnerable to the health effects of air pollution for a number of reasons: they have a smaller body size, they generally spend more time than adults being active outdoors, and their

---

### CASE SITUATION

Jean-Paul is a ten-year-old boy admitted to the emergency unit of the large urban hospital where you work. Jean-Paul's mother has informed you that he is highly allergic to cats and smoke and that anxiety appears to exacerbate his asthma attacks. The doctor has discussed Jean-Paul's asthmatic management with the mother and has discharged him with several prescriptions for asthma drugs. As Jean-Paul's nurse, you decide to conduct some discharge teaching.

#### Questions

1. What issues will you address in your discharge teaching with Jean-Paul and his mother?
2. List the relevant health promotion strategies in this case.
3. The mother's main question for you is: "How likely is Jean-Paul to have another asthmatic attack?" How do you answer her?

lungs are still developing.[45] It is important to note that evidence for the effects of air pollution on children has increased significantly in recent years. Essentially, pollution exposure is implicated in the development of chronic disease or impairment.[46]

Ground-level ozone, which causes adverse health effects, must be distinguished from stratospheric ozone, which provides that vital service of blocking the sun's ultraviolet radiation. Ground-level ozone is a key component of smog. It is formed by atmospheric reactions involving nitrogen oxides, VOCs, and sunlight. Higher temperatures and sunlight intensity tend to exacerbate the formation of ground-level ozone.[47]

Fine particulate matter poses a powerful threat to human health because the particles travel deep into the lungs. The formation of fine particulate matter is complex and its sources are varied. Transportation and industrial emissions are the main contributors, while wood-burning stoves or fireplaces for home heating are also significant sources. Other sources include dust from wind erosion and ash from forest fires.[48]

Human exposure to ground-level ozone and fine particulate matter is of particular concern because there is no established threshold of concentration below which these pollutants are safe and no longer pose a risk to human health.[49]

In 2006, Canada and the United States developed an agreement that has guided both countries in successfully continuing to reduce their emissions of sulphur dioxide and nitrogen oxides—the major contributors to acid rain. The Air Quality Agreement has provided important opportunities for collaboration between Canada and the United States in environmental improvements as well as in diplomacy and working relationships. Both countries rely on the Agreement as a mechanism to address air pollution issues, and both countries are committed to its continuing viability and relevance as new bilateral issues occur.[50]

Canada's National Ambient Air Quality Objectives (NAAQOs) are national goals for outdoor air quality. They protect not only public health but also the environment and certain aesthetic properties of the environment.[51] The establishment of NAAQOs is a dynamic and continuous process. Air quality objectives are developed to reflect the current state of understanding about an air pollutant, to establish a national indicator for assessing the quality of air in all parts of Canada, and to provide guidance to governments in implementing risk management decisions such as planning control strategies and setting local standards.[52] Air quality is monitored by both the federal and the provincial governments. The Air Quality Index (AQI), also referred to as the Index of the Quality of Air (IQUA), is an indicator of overall air quality developed to inform the public about the general or prevailing air quality in their communities.[53] The lower the AQI, the better the air quality. AQI values for Ontario can be obtained from the Ontario Ministry of the Environment's website at www.airqualityontario.com.[54] It is important to note that the NAAQOs do not provide a measure of overall air quality. They provide only a means of evaluating the levels of individual pollutants. In Ontario, an AQI network provides the public with air quality information across the province.[55]

*Large sport utility vehicles*, with their poor gas mileage, are exacerbating global warming because of the amount of carbon dioxide produced. The *car driven daily to work*, in contrast to mass transit systems, can also be considered an enemy to the environment and even to society. Transport Canada is working to protect the environment and develop a more sustainable transportation system. In fact, its Advanced Technology Vehicle Program tests new, more environmentally friendly vehicles, such as new diesel and hybrid cars, with a view to adapting them to meet Canada's high safety standards and incorporating them into the Canadian market. The program travels across the country showcasing these vehicles to raise public awareness of advanced technology vehicles and developments in engines, power trains, construction material and methods, as well as fuel.[56]

In Canada, the federal government is developing an integrated strategy for: (1) clean air for vehicles and the fuels that power them; (2) trans-boundary air pollution with the United States and other countries; (3) industrial pollution; and (4) encouraging Canadians to develop solutions to clean air issues.[57]

**Greenhouse Gas Emissions** Emissions of greenhouse gases have been closely studied by scientists and governments since the early 1990s. Naturally occurring greenhouse gases—mainly carbon dioxide, nitrous oxide, methane, and water vapour—help regulate the earth's climate by trapping heat in the atmosphere and reflecting it back to the surface.[58] However, the earth's climate is changing. Some of this change is due to natural variations that have taken place over millions of years, but increasingly, human activities such as the use of fossil fuels in transportation, manufacturing, heating, cooling, and electricity generation are the greatest sources of greenhouse gas emissions.[59] Canada has seen a rise in average temperature of about 1°C since 1950, with six of the warmest years on record occurring in Canada between 1995 and 2005.[60] The greenhouse gas emissions indicator tracks the annual release of greenhouse gases, which are the major contributors to climate change.[61]

Addressing climate change requires two complementary actions: reducing greenhouse gas emissions and adapting to climate change. Canadians are already adjusting to a variable climate. However, climate change places new stresses on health throughout the population.[62] Higher temperatures are expected to increase the occurrence of heat-related illnesses such as heat exhaustion and heat stroke, and to exacerbate existing conditions related to circulatory, respiratory, and nervous system problems. Table 2-1 outlines the potential health impacts from climate change and variability.[63] Nurses need to be aware of current health outcomes of climate change and plan health promotion strategies to assist individuals and their family members to prevent illness and adapt accordingly in their environment.

## Indoor Air Pollution

Some significant indoor pollutants are carbon monoxide, asbestos particles, nitrogen oxides, formaldehyde, and radon.

### Table 2-1 Potential Health Impacts from Climate Change and Variability

| Health Concerns | Examples of Health Vulnerabilities |
|---|---|
| Temperature-related morbidity and morality | • Cold- and heat-related illnesses<br>• Respiratory and cardiovascular illnesses<br>• Increased occupational health risks |
| Health effects of extreme weather events | • Damaged public health infrastructure<br>• Injuries and illnesses<br>• Social and mental health stress due to disasters<br>• Occupational health hazards<br>• Population displacement |
| Health problems related to air pollution | • Changed exposure to outdoor and indoor air pollutants and allergens<br>• Asthma and other respiratory diseases<br>• Heart attacks, strokes, and other cardiovascular diseases<br>• Cancer |
| Health effects of water- and food-borne contamination | • Enteric diseases and poisoning caused by chemical and biological contaminants |
| Vector-borne and zoonotic diseases | • Changed patterns of diseases caused by bacteria, viruses, and other pathogens carried by mosquitoes, ticks and other vectors |
| Health effects of exposure to ultraviolet rays | • Skin damages and skin cancer<br>• Cataracts<br>• Disturbed immune function |
| Population vulnerabilities in rural and urban communities | • Seniors<br>• Children<br>• Chronically ill people<br>• Low income and homeless people<br>• Northern residents<br>• Disabled people<br>• People living off the land |
| Socioeconomic impacts on community health and well-being | • Loss of income and productivity<br>• Social distribution<br>• Diminished quality of life<br>• Increased costs to health care<br>• Health effects of mitigation technologies<br>• Lack of institutional capacity to deal with disasters |

Source: Government of Canada. *Climate Change Impacts and Adaptation: A Canadian Perspective.* Ottawa: Natural Resources Canada, 2004. Copied with permission of Her Majesty the Queen in Right of Canada.

Office workers and others in North America and Europe who work in buildings with inadequate ventilation systems that create poor mechanical airflow regularly report a *variety of non-specific but illness-producing symptoms*. The buildings have been referred to as "sick buildings," giving rise to "**sick building syndrome.**" Symptoms include the following:

- Irritation of the skin, eyes, nose, and throat
- Mental and physical fatigue
- Headache; difficulty concentrating
- Dizziness
- Eye, nose, and throat irritation
- Frequent respiratory infections
- Hypersensitivity reactions

Exposure to other indoor pollutants, such as cigarette smoke and inhalants, increases these symptoms.[64]

It is somewhat disconcerting to note that only minimal attention has been paid to indoor pollutant issues in schools. Poor indoor air quality affects the capacity to concentrate and learn. Further, it increases the likelihood of bacterial and viral infections, and allows mould growth to occur. A multidisciplinary research team from Dalhousie University in Halifax, with sponsorship from Health Canada, has begun a three-year exploration of the issue of indoor air quality in schools. The aim of the project is to develop standard guidelines and recommendations that will be pilot-tested in various schools across Canada.[65]

**Tobacco Smoke** Tobacco smoke is linked to an increase in asthma and respiratory infections, especially in children. It appears that passive smoking produces elevated risks for coronary heart disease that are similar to low-level active smoking (about one cigarette per day).[66] In Canada, de Groh and Morrison state that the rates of home exposure to environmental tobacco smoke vary dramatically by province.

### CRITICAL THINKING

*What health program could you develop in your area of work to promote smoke-free homes?*

**Household Products** Cleaning and home maintenance products are a multibillion-dollar industry in Canada. The huge selection of products on the retail shelf often makes it difficult for consumers to know what is safe to buy. Some ingredients may be carcinogens or reproductive toxins. Many can produce fumes that cause respiratory irritation on contact. Some are carcinogenic when fumes or particles are inhaled over time. Other ingredients, such as bleach and phosphates, raise environmental concerns. As

an example, individuals have been using methylene chloride, or products containing methylene chloride, as a paint stripper. Methylene chloride is listed as a possible human carcinogen (Group 2B) by the International Agency for Research on Cancer (IARC). There are no warning label requirements in Canada for methylene chloride, which is sold in hardware and home improvement outlets both as a pure product and as an ingredient in a wide range of paint strippers and similar products.[67]

Hospitals have a unique form of indoor air pollution. Fumes from disinfectants, such as glutaraldehyde, a sterilizing agent for instruments; surgical smoke or laser plume from tissue being cut, vaporized, or coagulated; and waste gases from anaesthetic agents affect health care workers and patients. A small amount of glutaraldehyde fumes can cause respiratory and dermatologic problems. Surgical smoke or laser plume can cause respiratory symptoms, burning and watery eyes, nausea, and viral contamination and regrowth. Nurses who work in recovery rooms are likely to feel fatigue from breathing the patients' exhaled anaesthesia gases.[68]

## Health Promotion Strategies

Indoor air pollution can be controlled by several measures: proper venting of gas stoves, heaters, and wood stoves; painting over materials that emit radon and formaldehyde; and daily airing of the house. Houseplants, especially spider plants, can be used to absorb air pollutants in the home.

Only in becoming aware of these factors as personal health threats will we seriously consider alternatives to using two or three cars, seek to know the serious hazards in our jobs, become concerned about houses downwind from an industrial site or the amount of ultraviolet light we receive, and use less dangerous products for many household tasks.

## FRESH WATER QUALITY

Good-quality water in adequate quantities is fundamental to human health, ecosystems, and economic performance. In Canada, water is used mostly by households and in industries such as electricity generation, manufacturing, agriculture, mining, and petroleum extraction.[69]

Pollution of water from the natural processes of aquatic animal and plant life, combined with human-made waste, constitutes another hazard to the delicate state of human health. Human-made water pollution has two major origins: *point sources* and *non-point sources*. Point sources are those that discharge pollutants from a well-defined place (e.g., outlet pipes of sewage treatment plants and factories). Non-point sources consist of runoff from city streets, construction sites, farms, and mines.

## Types of Water Pollution

Water pollution is a global problem, as is air pollution. As our environment changes, can we believe that all of our water sources will remain pristine? The fact is that preserving clean and safe drinking water sources is becoming a priority because of global pollution.[70] There is a critical link between human health and a fresh, clean water supply. McQuigge has shown that human, industrial, and agricultural waste productions are escalating. Unfortunately, these wastes find their way into the groundwater, which increases the risk of pathogens such as bacteria and viruses. These same waste production sources are also largely responsible for the presence of dangerous chemicals in the water.[71] In Ontario, and elsewhere in Canada, the standards for potability of 30 to 40 percent of private wells are below standard.[72] In addition, the quality of surface water can change due to inputs of human waste, nutrients, and chemicals, resulting in greater risks associated with drinking water.[73]

The fresh water quality indicator reports the status of surface fresh water quality at selected monitoring sites across the country, including the Great Lakes and northern Canada.[74]

In 2007, Health Canada, in co-operation with the Federal-Provincial-Territorial Committee on Drinking Water of the Federal-Provincial-Territorial Committee on Health and the Environment, published the *Summary of Guidelines for Canadian Drinking Water Quality*, which supersedes all previous versions.[75] The Summary provides microbiological, chemical, physical, and radiological parameters for drinking water quality. For example, the microbiological parameter regarding public drinking water systems states that water samples should show no *Escherichia coli* (E. coli). E. coli denotes fecal contamination as well as the chance of enteric pathogens being present. Both may unfavourably affect human health. If E. coli is detected, municipal officials may issue a boil-water advisory, which advocates a rolling boil for one minute to ensure safety for drinking purposes. Corrective actions directed toward a detected source of contaminated water supply should be taken. For all semi-public and private drinking water supply systems, water samples are expected to contain no E. coli, and no water sample should contain total coliform bacteria. Testing for E. coli and total coliforms should be carried out in all drinking water systems.[76] For more information on the requirements for Canadian drinking water, visit www.hc-sc.gc.ca/ewh-semt/water-eau/drink-potab/index_e.html.

Pip conducted a survey of bottled drinking water available in Manitoba. She claims that the bottled water samples studied indicated great variation in quality. Some even exceeded the Canadian quality guidelines for drinking water for total dissolved solids (TDSs), chloride, and lead.[77]

---

### CRITICAL THINKING

*Why is it important for a health professional to know the difference between total coliform bacteria and fecal coliform bacteria?*

---

### CONTROVERSY DEBATE

## Drinking Well Water: What Is the Risk?

While enjoying some well-earned time alone in a quiet restaurant, you find yourself seated next to a family of four (two children under 12 years of age). This family is joined by an older couple who have obviously known them from a common rural community some distance away. From their animated conversations you realize they have all been evacuated to your community from a region you heard about on the radio. This region had experienced a rapid spring thaw and heavy rains causing both small rivers in the area to overflow their banks and cause some flooding. Flooding, it seems, has never been experienced in this community in living memory. The two families have just received word that transportation is available the next day to return them to their homes after a two-week absence. The women mention their eagerness to be home again do their own cooking. Although home damage has been moderate in their neighbourhood, considerable ground flooding has occurred—especially near the hog-producing ranch and the beef cattle operation located in their community. Both operations, you learn, are close to where they live.

As a health care professional, you wonder about the water supply for the home community of these folks seated next to you.

1. What do you feel is your responsibility to these six people regarding your concerns about their water supply?

2. If you decide to introduce yourself to discuss the matter with them, how do you start?

3. If you learn from them that no official contact person has been made available to them regarding their safety on returning home, what will you say to them?

4. What health-promoting options are open to you to assist these people?

5. Is it possible that there is no issue here and that you could be considered a "busybody" for interfering?

## Issues Regarding Water Purification

The outbreak of E. coli in the water supply of Walkerton, Ontario, and *Cryptosporidium* species found in the water in North Battleford, Saskatchewan, were events that compromised public health.[78] Manure from cattle farms in the area together with inadequate water treatment processes are the suspected causes of these outbreaks. The disease outbreaks that resulted from the public drinking water systems drew the attention of several levels of government, and the public, to the critical need to examine water safety and have a supply of safe drinking water available in communities.

In April 2005, a community of about 1900 Cree people 10 kilometres upstream from James Bay was evacuated due to sewage-contaminated drinking water. The same community was evacuated again after flooding in April 2006.[79] As these incidents illustrate, Aboriginal, local, provincial, and federal governments must co-operate to provide safe drinking water and to take action in the event of floods and other disasters.[80]

Polluted water cannot be used for recreational purposes. Backpackers, campers, swimmers, windsurfers, and water skiers have all felt the impact of water pollution. In addition to the health risks associated with bad water, the odour and unsightliness of polluted water destroy the beauty of any natural setting. Lake Winnipeg, the world's tenth largest freshwater lake, is in ecological peril. The lake's health and sustainability has been seriously eroded from increasingly dangerous levels of algae blooms. Numerous forums have been held and the participants have made many recommendations, including the reconstruction of wetland detoxification sites deemed to be essential in controlling nutrient loading from rivers and streams that flow into Lake Winnipeg.[81]

### CRITICAL THINKING

*What do you need to know to better understand the quality of drinking water?*

Proper legislation can help prevent some health problems associated with contaminated water. For example, in Manitoba, the *Water Protection Act* sets water quality standards, objectives, and guidelines.[82]

A community health needs and resources assessment study was conducted in Newfoundland and Labrador between 1997 and 2004. The purpose of the study was to assess health beliefs and practices, satisfaction with health and community services, and concerns in relation to community health. The results indicated that the quality of drinking water was a serious concern.[83]

Nurses and other health professionals need to be aware of the challenge of ensuring that drinking water is safe. They need to work with individuals and families in communities to strengthen communication strategies related to risks associated with drinking contaminated water, and they need to increase public awareness of the importance of safe drinking water. Nurses also need to become politically active by lobbying and writing letters to government officials urging them to protect and improve drinking water sources.[84] Further, but not finally, they need to collaborate with other members of the health care team to promote the health of the population.

The health of future generations and their chance to enjoy the beauty, taste, and power of our country's water depend on those of us who are so carelessly polluting it. Water, like oxygen, is essential to life, development, and health.

### CRITICAL THINKING

*What other health promotion strategies can nurses implement in the community to make certain that drinking water is safe for use?*

## SOIL POLLUTION

Health problems from soil pollution are on the rise. Knowledge is essential for the recognition, treatment, and prevention of soil contamination issues. Soil contamination can cause long-term health problems because certain crops and vegetables can absorb soil contaminants.

Canada has become one of the world's foremost agricultural nations due to its abundance of rich farmland. Canada's soils must be kept free from bacterial, fungal, and insect pests in order to produce high yields of quality crops. The federal government has developed the Pest Management Regulatory Agency (PMRA), which is responsible for the protection of human health and the environment by decreasing the risks associated with pest-control products.[85] All pesticides sold, used, or imported into Canada and intended to manage, attract, destroy, or repel pests are regulated by the PMRA. These products include chemicals, devices, and organisms. The use of pesticides is regulated by the *Pest Control Products Act* as well as provincial/territorial legislation. The new *Pest Control Products Act* (2002) has initiated somewhat more rigorous requirements for manufacturers by requiring them to provide safety data on their products and to conduct post-registration surveillance.[86]

Dioxins are unwanted byproducts produced by both industrial processes and natural events, such as forest fires and incomplete combustion.[87] Dioxin, a known human carcinogen and a possible endocrine disrupter, can be formed during the incineration or burning of polyvinyl chloride (PVC) products. That is, dioxin is released into the environment, drains into the soil and water sources, and is absorbed by plants. Animals, as well as people, then consume of these altered plants.[88]

PVC, a firm and fragile plastic, is used in a wide range of health products such as bedding covers, blood bags, intravenous tubing, catheters, gloves, and respiratory products.[89] To make it pliable, DEHP—di(2-ethylhexyl)phthalate—is added.[90] DEHP can leach from the PVC and into clients.

In 1998, Health Canada issued an advisory for the disposal of soft vinyl teethers and rattles, designed for sucking and mouthing by very young children who have high oral contact (three or more hours a day on a daily basis). Health Canada is monitoring other products such as toys from manufacturers, importers, and distributors.[91]

All of the possible additional sites of dioxin contamination are not yet known, but dioxin is being found in many areas of the United States and Canada, including the Canadian Arctic.[92] In the Arctic, concern is being expressed as dioxins bio-accumulate in the marine food web and in animals that are hunted and eaten by Inuit.[93]

It is of utmost importance that nurses promote and implement environmentally safe health care. Nurses have a responsibility to advocate for the environment and should strive to be environmentally responsible.[94]

## CRITICAL THINKING

*How can you lobby industries for the reduction of dioxin?*

# FOOD SAFETY

Safe food and good nutrition are both important to the health and welfare of Canadians. Maintaining the safety of Canada's food supply is a shared responsibility among government, industry, and consumers. One of the best ways to promote and protect good health is to eat a nutritious and balanced diet. Some of Health Canada's most important responsibilities are to establish policies, set standards, and provide advice and information on the safety and nutritional value of food. Another is to administer the provisions of the *Food and Drug Act* that relate to public health, safety, and nutrition.[95]

The Canadian Food Inspection Agency provides all federal inspection services related to food. It enforces the food safety and nutritional quality standards established by Health Canada.[96]

The globalization of the food supply, the demand for more food sources worldwide, and rapid advances in food science and technology have collectively resulted in new foods, often known as novel foods. Health Canada assesses the safety of all genetically modified and novel foods proposed for sale in Canada.[97]

Botulism is rare in Canada—only 18 cases were reported in 1997—but the spores of *C. botulinum* are claimed to be the most lethal substance known.[98] Three main clinical forms of botulism exist: food borne, intestinal, and wound related. Food-borne botulism results when food contaminated by a preformed neurotoxin is eaten. The most frequent source of botulism in Canada is home-prepared products such as canned foods, fermented Inuit food, and improperly stored marine meat.[99] Suspect botulism in a client with acute onset of gastrointestinal, autonomic, and cranial nerve dysfunction. The earliest and most frequently observed symptom of infant botulism is constipation, followed by lethargy, poor feeding, ptosis, difficulty swallowing, hypotonia, and generalized weakness ("floppy baby").[100] When botulism is suspected, a member of the Botulism Reference Service (BRS) of Canada should be called immediately—day or night.[101]

## CRITICAL THINKING

*In conversing with a mother at the clinic, you learn that she intends to feed her infant canned fruit and vegetables. What will you say to this woman and what do you want her to realize?*

Food additives are subject to review and safety testing before they are considered for approval by the Health Products and Food Branch, Bureau of Chemical Safety of Health Canada.[102] Foods containing additives are continuously monitored for adverse reactions and hazards. If at any time a food additive is considered harmful, the food containing that additive is removed from the market. It is important to note that aspartame (known as NutraSweet or Equal) does not cause cancer. However, it is advisable to use artificial sweeteners in moderation.[103]

The CNA's position statement—"Food safety and security are determinants of health"—addresses several food-related health hazards. One such health hazard is obesity in Canadian adults and children. Another stems from the public concern about food products developed through genetic engineering. The concern points to the transparency and scientific evaluation of environmental and human health outcomes.[104] The CNA recommends that governments increase the monitoring of processes for production, storage, and preparation of food products.[105]

In January 2003, Health Canada proposed the Nutritional Labelling Regulations, making nutrition labelling mandatory on most food labels. The new Nutrition Facts Table usually appears in a standard format to help consumers make informed choices about the foods they buy and eat.[106] The new labelling requirements apply only to

## Food Additives

You have been diagnosed recently with type 2 diabetes. Your doctor is quite insistent that you reduce the sugar intake in your diet and develop a plan of exercise. You have always enjoyed your morning coffee (and, come to think of it, your desserts!) sweetened. Now, with diabetes on your mind, your thoughts turn to artificial sweeteners. However, you recall some media articles that claimed that artificial sweeteners cause cancer. You live alone and do your own cooking and meal preparation. It now seems that you must readjust some of your living habits.

1. What is an artificial sweetener? Which one has been removed from the market? Why was it removed?

2. What other health-promoting strategies might you implement to decrease your sugar levels?

3. What do you plan to do now about your physical activity?

4. What measures will you implement to help yourself maintain your plans?

---

pre-packaged foods. Foods that are exempt include fresh fruits and vegetables, for example.

In Canada's north, the Inuit are discovering that much of their food source is slowly being contaminated by pollutants. On average, Inuit women have levels of polychlorinated biphenyls (PCBs) in their breast milk that are five to ten times higher than those of women in southern Canada.[107] The Northern Contaminants Program (NCP) has provided an avenue to assist the Inuit in eliminating pollutants harmful to their health and the health of their environment.[108]

### CRITICAL THINKING

*What are some health-promoting strategies to address food supplies for the Inuit in the Arctic?*

---

**Biopesticides**, or **biological pesticides,** are *pesticides derived from natural materials such as animals, plants, bacteria, and certain minerals.* For example, canola oil and baking soda are biopesticides.[109] There are three main types of biopesticides:[110]

1. *Microbial pesticides* contain a bacterium, fungus, virus, or protozoan that controls bugs, weeds, or plant diseases.

2. *Biopesticides* are substances that plants produce from genetic material that has been added to the plant. Then the plant manufactures the substance that destroys the pest.

3. *Biochemical pesticides* are naturally occurring substances that control pests by non-toxic mechanisms, in contrast to conventional pesticides, which are synthetic and kill or inactivate the pest. For example, pheromones interfere with the growth or mating of a pest.

In Canada, pesticides are strictly regulated by federal and provincial laws. Pesticides cannot be sold without approved testing and subsequent registration by Health Canada's PMRA.[111]

## NOISE POLLUTION

As a nurse, you will care for people of all ages, in many different settings, who have a hearing deficit sometimes caused by noise pollution. Noise pollution can be defined as any unwanted sound. Sources of noise pollution include aircraft, road vehicles, rail cars, construction and landscaping equipment, home and car stereo systems, household appliances, and power tools.[112] Motorcycles and motor scooters can also be added to the list. Sensory stimulation plays a major role in psychological and physiologic development and is therefore directly related to physical, mental, and social well-being. Sound is but one form of sensory stimulation. One means of determining the potential hazard of any sound is to measure its loudness. The *measurement of sound loudness* is stated in **decibels**. Table 2-2 lists examples of common sound pollutants and their decibel readings.

## Effects of Noise Pollution

Sound overload affects everyone at some time by intruding on privacy and shattering serenity. In addition to hearing loss, it can impair communication and interfere with social relationships as well as causing irritability, chronic headache, tinnitus, insomnia, depression, fatigue, and tension. Although noise pollution is not directly related to mental illness, it can induce latent mental disorders.[113] Noise has also been associated with elevated blood cholesterol levels, atherosclerosis, and accident proneness. It can also cause hearing damage.[114] In addition, research

## Table 2-2 Common Sound Pollutants and Their Decibel Readings

| Sound | Decibels | Sound | Decibels |
|---|---|---|---|
| Rustle of leaves | 10 | Air compressor | 95 |
| Library whisper | 30 | Power lawnmower | 80–95 |
| Normal conversation | 60 | Dirt bike | 95 |
| Electric shaver | 60–86 | Farm tractor | 98 |
| Car | 60–90 | Power drill | 100 |
| Office (busy) | 70–85 | Street sweeper | 100 |
| Vacuum cleaner | 72–75 | Chain saw | 100–110 |
| Dishwasher | 76–96 | Outboard motor | 102 |
| Minibike | 76 | Jet flying at 300 metres | 103 |
| Shop tools | 80–95 | Ambulance siren | 105 |
| Loud street noise | 80–100 | Stereo headset | 110 |
| Alarm clock | 80 | Riveting gun | 110 |
| Washing machine | 80 | Jackhammer | 115–130 |
| Video arcade | 80–105 | Motorcycle | 115 |
| Subway | 80–114 | Live rock music | 120 |
| Snowmobile | 85–120 | Gunshot | 130–140 |
| Heavy city traffic | 90–95 | Jet plane at takeoff | 150 |
| Food blender in home | 93 | Rocket engine | 180 |
| Pneumatic hammer | 95 | | |

indicates that less obvious physiologic changes in the digestive, cardiovascular, endocrine, and nervous systems can occur from noise. Humans do not adapt well to excessive sound, as was once thought; but they do learn to tolerate it. Even when a person is asleep, noise cannot be shut out completely. He or she may frequently awaken, exhausted by the efforts to sleep in the midst of excessive external stimuli. What, for you, are examples of excessive noise levels?

Health Canada plays a significant role in reducing noise levels. Examples of its activities in this area include the following:

■ Advising government departments and agencies, industry, and the public of any health-related issues.

■ Providing information, guidelines, voluntary standards, and compliance and regulation programs for the protection of workers and general public.

■ Tracking and reviewing scientific papers by experts in the field.

■ Conducting research concerning the possible health effects of community, recreational, work-related, and aircraft noise.[115]

## Health Promotion Strategies

Although not every harmful form of sound can be avoided, certain measures can decrease the risk of hearing loss:

■ Wear protective ear coverings.

■ Shorten exposure time.

■ Have regular hearing examinations.

■ Seek immediate medical attention for any ear injury or infection.

■ Wear earplugs when exposed to loud noise for a long time or to intense sound even for a short time.

■ Use sound-absorbing materials to reduce noise at home and at work.

■ Do not use several noisy machines at one time.

■ Do not drown out unwanted noise with other noise.

You can educate the public about the hazards of excess noise and ways to reduce noise in the home environment:

■ Hang heavy drapes over windows closest to outside noise sources.

■ Use foam pads under mixers and blenders.

- Use carpeting in areas of heavy foot traffic.
- Use upholstered instead of hard-surfaced furniture.
- Install sound-absorbing ceiling tile in the kitchen.

Some surprising sources—hospitals, long-term care facilities, and personal care homes—may actually contribute to symptoms because of high noise levels.

## SURFACE POLLUTION

The management of waste has become one of the most pressing issues throughout the world. Waste management is seen as the disposal, removal, or storage of solid waste and sewage (including industrial discharges and nuclear waste).[116]

In Canada, three main approaches to solid waste disposal prevail.[117] One is burial—in up-to-date sanitary landfills that satisfy guidelines related to aesthetics, health, and the monitoring and prevention of leaching. Leaching is the diffusion of materials into groundwater from the landfill site. The second approach to solid waste disposal is incineration, which is sometimes used, under controlled conditions, to burn solid waste. Incineration has been the main method for disposing of the wide range of combustible materials that constitute biomedical wastes because it can significantly reduce the volume of waste material and can destroy organic material.[118] The third approach to waste management is transformation. An example of this process is anaerobic digestion by microorganisms or pyrolysis (chemical decomposition caused by combustion in an oxygen-deprived environment). This process can reduce waste volume by up to 91 percent.[119]

Waste management is everyone's responsibility—not only in Canada but worldwide. For society, the best way to manage waste is to incorporate the 4Rs, which are listed in order of preference: reduce, reuse, recycle, and recover.[120] Reducing the amount of waste is the most effective way to fight the flow of garbage into a landfill. Reusing material and products is the next best option. The process of recycling involves using material from old products to develop new products. Finally, recovery involves harvesting energy or worthwhile products from waste materials. The fourth R is difficult for individuals to put into practice. Consequently, it is geared towards industry.[121]

### CRITICAL THINKING

*What products could you reuse in your own home rather than disposing of them?*

In Canada, Waste Reduction Week is organized by a coalition of non-governmental, not-for-profit environment groups from each of the provincial and territorial jurisdictions. It informs and engages Canadians by providing them with "themed" specific facts and statistics on current wasteful practices. Individuals and families are then provided with practical strategies that encourage them to contribute to the solutions and successes of waste-free living.[122] (Visit www.wrwcanada.com for more information on this topic.)

## Hazardous Waste Disposal

Canadians produce more than 30 million tons of solid waste per year, of which 8 million are considered hazardous waste.[123] Put another way, more than one-quarter of our waste is hazardous!

Hazardous waste handling and disposal practices fall under the combined jurisdictions of federal, provincial, and territorial agencies. In 1980, the federal *Transportation of Dangerous Goods Act* (TDGA) was established. This Act and its pursuant Regulations (1985) present a blueprint of co-operation for all levels of government responding to public concerns on the need for the safe transportation of dangerous goods and hazardous wastes.[124] Most provinces are willing to use the TDGA classification system, but they tend to cling to their own provincial transport regulations and manifest systems. The Canada–U.S. Bilateral Agreement, signed in 1986, sets out specific conditions for the export and import of hazardous waste between the two countries. In 1989, a Waste Management Branch was created within Environment Canada to coordinate the growing involvement of the federal government in waste management activities. Through the Green Plan (1990) consultations, Canadians strongly supported the need to increase controls over toxic chemicals. The federal government, under the Green Plan, made a concentrated commitment to regulate and control the export and import of hazardous wastes at border ports.[125]

Although most hazardous wastes are generated by manufacturing industries, the military contributes significantly to the total volume. Hospitals, medical research laboratories, mining operations, service stations, retailers, and householders also contribute to the problem of hazardous-waste production.[126] Only a small percentage of the hazardous waste currently generated is disposed of in an environmentally sound manner. The rest threatens our water and air quality as well as our water and land ecosystems.

Hazardous waste can become a threat to human health in various ways: direct exposure of persons at or near the disposal site; direct exposure of persons as a result of accidents during transport of the waste; exposure to polluted air during improperly controlled incineration; and the contamination of groundwater and food.

**Nuclear Waste** The use of nuclear energy—power produced by fission reactors—has caused much concern and debate among the people of both Canada and the United States. The concerns centre around two major issues: the long-term disposal of radioactive waste and the safety of the reactors.

When a utility shuts down a reactor at the end of its period of usefulness, it is faced with the problem of what to do with intensely radioactive materials. At present, only three means of disposal exist: dismantlement of the reactor, with the debris shipped to a burial site; entombment of the reactor in a concrete structure; and protective storage that would prevent public access for 30 to 100 years. Even though nuclear power is more than 30 years old, the problem of safe disposal of radioactive waste has not yet been solved.

The seriousness of problems associated with the safety of nuclear reactors for generating electricity is well illustrated by a highly publicized event in 1986. At a nuclear power plant at Chernobyl, in the former Soviet Union, a fire in the plant's nuclear reactor sent a cloud of deadly radiation into the air. Some people in the plant died immediately, and hundreds of people in the vicinity developed radiation sickness. Contamination was so severe that the escaped radiation was detected by monitoring devices around the world.[127] The management of, and protection against, such life-threatening events of radiation exposure are both difficult and challenging.

Because of these concerns, and the fact that non-renewable resources such as oil are diminishing, alternative energy sources such as solar and wind power are now being explored.

**Hospital Waste** In Canada, incineration has been the main disposal method of the broad range of combustible materials that constitute biomedical waste in hospitals. This method can significantly reduce the volume of waste material, and it can destroy unwanted organic matter. The Canadian Council of Ministers of the Environment has recently proposed new incinerator standards that will reduce current dioxin and mercury emissions by 80 percent.[128] However, driven by rising waste-disposal costs and public disfavour toward incineration, several Canadian hospitals have implemented programs recently to downsize the amount of misclassified biomedical waste entering the waste system. Over 18 months, a Toronto hospital reduced the volume of biomedical waste produced each month from 14 800 kg to 6300 kg. The resulting monthly saving amounted to $5599.[129]

---

**CRITICAL THINKING**

*Through what methods did the Toronto hospital reduce the volume of biomedical waste?*

---

In its position statement *Medical Waste: Role of Nurses and Nursing*, the International Council of Nurses (ICN) states that each nurse has a duty to reduce or eliminate the negative impact of medical waste on the environment.[130] In fact, the ICN supports a number of initiatives to reduce the harmful impact of medical wastes:

- Client and family education on the impact of environmental pollution
- Waste disposal choices that reduce incineration to a maximum
- Waste treatment choices that minimize toxic disinfectants and sterilants
- Limiting the use of pesticides
- Use of the marketplace to develop low-toxicity products—for example, replacing chlorinated plastics (PVC), latex, and mercury[131]

As professionals, nurses need to be aware of the consequences of the medical waste produced by the health sector. Nursing organizations must:

- Define and regulate nursing competencies in environmental health
- Develop coalitions with other professionals for safe waste disposals
- Advocate for safe waste disposal mechanisms
- Advocate for the involvement of direct care nurses in decision making regarding environmental care
- Facilitate nurses' access to continuing education programs on the topic of medical waste
- Apply a precautionary approach to product evaluation and selection that protects the environment[132]

Nurses, both in clinical settings and in management positions, should collaborate with other health care professionals to develop policies that deal with the thoughtful and considerate purchase of supplies, as well as with the production and elimination of medical waste. In fact, nurses can play an active role from the inside through advocacy, education, and the implementation of effective strategies to reduce medical waste.

---

**CRITICAL THINKING**

*What strategies can you, as a nurse, implement to reduce medical wastes on your clinical unit?*

---

**Lead Poisoning** According to Sanborn, Abelsohn, Campbell, and Weir, lead levels in North American children and adults have decreased in the past three decades.[133] However, lead persists in the environment in lead paint, old plumbing, and contaminated soil.[134] Blood lead levels, once considered safe, are now known to cause subtle but chronic health problems. Lead-related health problems include developmental neurotoxicity; reproductive dysfunction; and toxicity to the blood, kidneys, and endocrine system. Most lead exposure is preventable. Diagnosing lead poisoning is a fairly simple process compared to diagnosing the health effects of exposures to other environmental toxins. The accurate assessment of lead poisoning, however, requires specific knowledge of its possible sources, such as lead smelters or battery recycling plants. In addition, the accurate assessment of lead poisoning is improved by knowing about possible high-risk groups, such as people who live in pre-1950s homes with lead-based paint. Finally, using appropriate laboratory tests to detect lead poisoning is very important.[135]

The effect of a child's exposure to environmental hazards is likely to be greater than, or different from, the effects shown by adults. Children have immature immune and detoxification systems and are less able to cope with environmental exposures. Children absorb more lead and other substances through the gastrointestinal tract than adults.[136] By implementing effective health-promoting strategies, case finding, and treatment interventions for lead exposure, the child, the family, and the larger community all reap the benefits of better health.

The National Pollutant Release Inventory (NPRI) provides Canadians with access to information on industrial and commercial pollution in their communities.[137] The NPRI is an important document that Environment Canada makes available to Canadians as an annual public report on pollutant releases. The NPRI may be accessed through an online database.

## OCCUPATIONAL HAZARDS

Increasingly, we learn of the health hazards that many workers face daily at their jobs. Monotony, paced work, and performance pressures are major sources of stress in many jobs, and they can contribute to disease pathology. Muscle strains, backaches, fractures, burns, eye injuries, effects of excess heat or cold, and other accidental emergencies are frequently taken for granted by the public. But workers may not experience the consequences of the hidden environmental hazards—the chemicals or radiation they work with directly or indirectly—until years later. In the past, the causes of many physical illnesses remained unsolved. But there is a greater understanding today of occupational hazards. Not only do miners and factory workers become ill because of their work environment, hospital and other health care workers may also suffer due to conditions encountered at work.

Health care workers provide services that expose them to serious short- and long-term health problems. Non-fatal occupational injuries and diseases are more common in hospital establishments and nursing care facilities than in private industry. There are five categories of hazard exposure:

1. *Biological or infectious:* Exposure to HIV and hepatitis viruses is most common.
2. *Chemical:* Exposure to germicidal sterilizing agents, chemotherapy agents, and latex (see Table 2-3).
3. *Environmental and mechanical:* Lifting, use of poorly designed equipment or workstations, lack of assistive devices, and inadequate staffing cause back and musculoskeletal injuries.
4. *Physical:* Shift work causing biologic rhythm disturbance and sleep-wake cycle disruptions (cause gastrointestinal problems, chronic fatigue, accidents); physical injury from violent patients; exposure to heat, cold, vibration, radiation, natural rubber latex, laser non-ionizing radiation (see Table 2-3), and noise (causes high blood pressure, headaches); and computers (cause muscle and eye strain).
5. *Psychosocial:* Shift work causing biologic rhythm disturbance and sleep-wake cycle disruptions (cause depression, interpersonal conflicts); noise (causes irritability, lowered concentration); job stress from work overload, shift work, inadequate staffing and resources, organizational politics, dealing with dying and death, and various illnesses, injuries, and accidents.[138]

In Canada, the enforcement of health and safety legislation in the workplace lies primarily with the provinces and territories. Although variations in legislation and regulations governing occupational health may exist, both the employer and the employee have obligations to maintain high quality standards under the health and safety legislation.[139] Although the provinces and territories carry most of the responsibility for occupational health, the federal government assumes jurisdiction for its own employees as well as for employees at certain types of work sites, such as nuclear power workstations, banks, and transportation businesses.[140]

A comprehensive federally legislated system to ensure the safe use of hazardous material in the Canadian workplace is the Workplace Hazardous Materials Information System (WHMIS). The WHMIS's purpose is to decrease illness and injury through workplace hazard communication.[141] Many of the requirements and exemptions of WHMIS legislation have been incorporated into the *Hazardous Products Act* and the *Hazardous Materials Information Review Act*.[142] Suppliers, employers, and workers all have responsibilities under the *Hazardous Products Act*. The supplier must label the product or container, and must provide a material safety data sheet (MSDS) to its customers. Employers must provide education and training sessions to employees who are exposed to hazardous products. Employers must also make certain that all controlled products are correctly labelled and that an MSDS is present for each controlled product. The MSDS must provide accurate details on the product's identification, chemical and toxicological properties, hazardous ingredients, and effects on health. The MSDS is also expected to specify measures for personal protection, first aid, and prevention.

The *Workers' Compensation Act* was introduced to protect both employers and employees from work-related injuries and the occurrence of illnesses. Compensation legislation, related to work injury and disease, is in place in all provinces and territories.[143] The agency that deals with compensation in most provinces is the Workers' Compensation Board, which is governed by the *Workers' Compensation Act*.[144] The thrust of the Workers' Compensation Board is threefold: it is autonomous, employers pay for the costs, and it determines the benefits allotted to the worker.[145] In making decisions, the Workers' Compensation Board must take into account all relevant facts and circumstances relating to the case before it.

---

## CRITICAL THINKING

*What health-related cases should be submitted to the Workers' Compensation Board for consideration?*

---

The Canadian Centre for Occupational Health and Safety (CCOHS) is a federal government agency whose purpose is to support the mission of abolishing Canadian work-related illnesses and injuries. Established in 1978, the CCOHS is governed by a council that represents three key stakeholder groups: the government (federal, provincial, and territorial), employers, and employees. The council mandates the CCOHS's unbiased approach to information dissemination relating to occupational health and safety.[146]

In addition, other policies and standards are applicable to the safety and health of workers. For example, the Canadian Standards Association (CSA) supports standards development in organizations, trade and industry, government departments in Canada, and the global marketplace. The CSA has earned an international reputation for both integrity and technical credibility.[147]

Canada's human rights legislation protects workers and provides for workers' freedom in the workplace. It requires employers to consider individual differences. Workers in both the public and the private sectors have the right to

organize and bargain in a collective manner. While the law protects collective bargaining, limitations exist that vary from province to province, such as for some public-sector workers who provide essential services.[148]

---

## CRITICAL THINKING

*Besides nurses, who else in the public sector provides essential services?*

---

Frequently, organizations ensure that certain special policies are in place for the health and safety of the worker. One such policy is the sexual harassment policy. Such policies should be clearly written and should include a definition of sexual harassment with examples of unacceptable behaviours. Organizational policies should be clearly indicated by ensuring that procedures exist to allow victims to register complaints and that such complaints will be considered immediately. The prime consideration is to indicate clearly that sexual harassment is not to be tolerated at any level in the organization.[149]

According to Statistics Canada, nurses' work-related injuries cost more than those of firefighters or police officers who are engaged in high-risk occupations. Factors such as poor workplace maintenance, inadequate equipment, and supply shortages increase nurses' risk for injury.[150] One of the thrusts of the CNA's *Position Statement on Quality Professional Practice Environments for Registered Nurses* is that developing and supporting quality professional practice is a responsibility shared by practitioners, employers, governments, regulatory bodies, professional associations, educational institutions, unions, and the public.[151] Other investigators have also described work-related health hazards for nurses.[152]

Often, occupational hazards are taken for granted. They are seen as part of the job. Employees in laundry and dry-cleaning establishments, for example, suffer hazards of excess heat, humidity, and noise. They encounter falls and accidents from slipping on wet floors, back injury and muscle strain from lifting, and circulatory problems from standing. Janitorial workers may have contact with dangerous chemicals in cleaning agents. Asthma is an occupational hazard for animal workers, veterinarians, farmers, bakers, carpenters, welders, and many other workers.

Industrial nurses and safety engineers emphasize wearing protective clothing and using protective equipment. Yet there are problems. The employee may not want to be bothered with cumbersome protective clothing; or the protective clothing and equipment given to a female worker may be too large and heavy and thus be ill-fitting and not protective, because they are designed for the male employee. (A few companies do specialize in protective clothing designed for women.) Oversized hardhats, safety shoes and gloves, and ear protectors that fit improperly can actually contribute to an accidental injury.

Length of exposure to an industrial substance often determines whether it will cause disease or death. The amount of exposure to the worker often depends on the production phase involved, and certain substances may cause diseases in certain areas of the body (such as specific forms of cancer). Gender is also a factor. Some substances affect the reproductive organs of women (or the fetus), but do not affect men. Some substances do not affect the male reproductive organs, but the exposed father's genes may contribute to fetal damage. Unfortunately, such information often becomes available only after the damage has been done.

Various pollutants and agents are health hazards. However, accidental injury, gun-related homicide, fire, and explosions are occupational hazards to many workers, including police officers, firefighters, emergency medical workers, and workers in any service establishment, particularly those that are open during late night or early morning hours. School teachers, staff, and students are also at risk for death from homicide (shootings) or fire.

Farming, whether corporate farming or on a smaller scale, or being employed as a farm labourer or migrant worker, is one of the most dangerous occupations. Some of the reasons are as follows:

1. Use of hazardous equipment or machinery can cause traumatic injury or death if it is not well maintained, if it is incorrectly or hurriedly operated, or in cases of rollover or turnover accidents. The high cost of parts may result in farm owners not buying protective devices. An accident involving farm machinery may not be detected for many hours, in contrast to an accident in a factory.

2. Exposure to environmental changes or temperature extremes (often drastic, harsh, or sudden) may contribute to cardiac, respiratory, and vascular diseases.

3. Exposure to herbicides, insecticides, anhydrous ammonia fertilizer (82 percent ammonia), and other agricultural chemicals may cause a variety of health problems.

4. Exposure to dust, silage, and manure gases; mould, fungi, and inhaled chemicals; and exposure to carbon monoxide gas from faulty exhaust systems or from working in enclosed areas may cause a variety of health problems.

5. Complications may arise from wounds that are contaminated by soil, manure, or chemicals and from traumatic injuries causing severe blood loss.

6. The effects of consistently long hours of hard work with insufficient sleep can have an impact (especially during busy seasons of planting and harvest) as well as stress related to uncertainties that accompany farming as an occupation and dependence on weather conditions.

7. Exposure to excessive machinery noise can cause hearing loss.

8. Not taking time for safety practices and a denial of the need for safety habits or protective shields or clothing can cause health problems, and are often the result of heavy workload, sense of pressure and hurry, and cost factors.

Children and the elderly may be especially vulnerable to the above hazards as they help with chores and farm work beyond their physical capacity.

The hazards of the factory or mine can extend beyond the workplace and endanger the workers' families and other residents of the community. Even if workers shower before leaving work, the total removal of all dust particles of some chemicals or elements is difficult. As a result, some communities become known for a high incidence of certain types of cancer, or skin or respiratory disease.

Table 2-3 summarizes common industrial agents (various substances, elements, or chemicals) and their major known effects. Refer to the endnotes for more information.[153]

Many occupational hazards exist for women and men. Clerical and other workers who regularly use video display terminals and computers have higher stress-related illnesses; more eye strain, neck and back strain, and headaches; and suffer greater emotional burnout.

Remember that the worker may have come into contact with a variety of harmful substances and that presenting symptoms may often seem unrelated to the occupation. Learn to become attuned to significant cues that can assist you in being particularly thorough and careful in your assessment.

## HEALTH PROMOTION IN NURSING PRACTICE

### Global Responsibility

The environment and people are interdependent. What we do to the environment and how we live affects everyone, eventually worldwide. One relevant example is the destruction of rain forests to obtain their products. What is destroyed cannot be regained, and synthetic development may not be adequate.[154]

The size, concentration, and mobility of populations have greatly increased. The spread of diseases, such as HIV/AIDS, Ebola virus hemorrhagic disease, pulmonary syndrome virus, hepatitis C virus, tuberculosis, cholera,

Table 2-3 Effects of Some Common Industrial Agents on the Worker

| Agent | Type of Industry or Occupation | Body Area Affected |
|---|---|---|
| Acetaldehyde | Chemical; paint | All body cells, especially brain and respiratory tract |
| Acetic anhydride | Textile | Exposed tissue damage, especially eyes and respiratory tract (ulceration, irritation) |
| Acetylene | Welding; plastic; dry cleaning | Respiratory tract asphyxiant; explosive, especially when combined with certain substances |
| Acrolein | Chemical | Skin. Eyes. Respiratory tract |
| Allyl chloride | Plastic | Skin. Respiratory tract. Kidney |
| Ammonia | Chemical; leather; wool; farmers; refrigeration workers | Eyes. Skin. Respiratory tract (ulceration, irritation) |
| Anaesthetic gases (leakage from equipment, exhalation of patients) | Surgical nurses; medical, hospital, dental, veterinary workers | Reproductive organs (spontaneous abortions, infertility, congenital abnormalities and cancer, whether male or female exposure) Neurological system (drowsy, irritable, headache) Respiratory tract (infections, cancer) Leucopenia Lymphoma |
| Aniline | Paint; rubber; dye manufacture | Skin. Hematopoietic system. Respiratory system |
| Arsenic | Mines; smelters; leather; chemical; oil refinery; ship builders; insecticide and pesticide makers and sprayers; pottery workers; agriculture; brass and bronze makers | Skin (ulcerations, cancer) Lungs. Liver (cancer) Neurological damage. Gastrointestinal symptoms Reproductive system (birth defects, chromosome alterations); if acute exposure, death in 1 to 7 days |
| Asbestos | Brake mechanics; mines; textiles; insulation; paint; sheet metal workers; shipyard workers; construction; plastics; pipe fitters; maintenance workers; millers; present on city streets | Respiratory tract (cancer, asbestosis, bronchitis, emphysema). Laryngeal cancer. Gastrointestinal tract (cancer) More harmful to people who smoke |
| Benzene | Rubber; chemicals; explosives; paints and paint strippers; shoemakers; dye users; office workers; chemists; hospital workers; solvent cleaner users; coke oven workers; furniture finishers; artists; degreasers | Skin. Liver. Brain (carcinogenic). Respiratory system Hematopoietic system (anemia, leukemia). Reproductive system (chromosome mutations in males, menstrual irregularities, stillbirths) |
| Beryllium | Foundry; metallurgic; aerospace; nuclear; household appliance; production, metal cans; shipbuilding | Skin and eyes (inflammation, ulcers). Respiratory tract (acute inflammation and berylliosis, chronic lung infection). Systemic effects on heart, liver, spleen, kidneys |

(continued)

Table 2-3 (continued)

| Agent | Type of Industry or Occupation | Body Area Affected |
|---|---|---|
| Butyl alcohol | Lacquer; paint | Eyes. Skin. Respiratory tract |
| Cadmium | Smelters; storage battery workers; silver industry; plastics; dental; pigment makers; artists; electrical workers; households (silver cleaner, ice cube trays); plating; alloys | Gastrointestinal tract (irritation, cancer). Reproductive system (decreased sperm count, impotence). Kidneys Respiratory tract. Hematopoietic system |
| Carbon disulphide | Rubber; viscose rayon workers; plastics; soil treaters; wax, glue, or resin makers; medical; laboratory workers; agriculture | Gastrointestinal tract. Cardiovascular. Liver. Kidneys. Brain Reproductive system (decreased sperm count, decreased libido, impotence, infertility, menstrual changes, stillbirth, spontaneous abortion) |
| Carbon tetrachloride | Solvent; dry cleaning; paint; chemical laboratory; household (fire extinguishers) | Skin. Gastrointestinal tract. Liver. Kidneys. Bladder Brain. Respiratory tract (irritation and carcinogen) |
| Chemotherapy (antineoplastic) medications | Medical; nurses | Skin and cornea (irritation, ulcers). Hair loss. Leucopenia. Reproductive system (fetal damage, miscarriage, cancer). Liver and other organs (may be carcinogenic) (some need special handling; effects vary with specific agent) |
| Chlorine | Industrial bleaching; laundry; chemical industries; swimming pool maintenance | Eyes. Respiratory tract. Skin (irritation, ulcerations, infections, cancer) Skin discolouration (orange) |
| Chloroform (chlorinated hydrocarbons) | Chemical; plastics; dry cleaners; drug workers; electronic equipment workers; insect control | Heart degeneration. Liver. Kidneys. Reproductive system (infertility, male and female). Brain. Skin |
| Chromium | Chrome plating; chemical; industrial bleaching; glass and pottery; linoleum makers; battery makers; metal cans and coatings | Irritating to all body cells, skin, eyes, respiratory tract (cancer, ulcerations), liver, kidneys |
| Cleaning agents, solvents | Maintenance workers; painters; households | Respiratory tract (irritation, allergy, asthma, cancer) Eyes (irritation, ulcers) Skin (ulcers, dermatosis, cancer) |
| Coal combustion products (soot, tar, coal tar products) | Gashouse workers; asphalt, coal tar, or pitch workers; coke oven workers; mines; plastics; roofers; waterproofers; metal coating workers; ship building | Skin. Respiratory tract. Larynx. Gastrointestinal tract Scrotum. Urinary tract. Bladder (carcinogenic to all areas) Hyperpigmentation of skin |
| Cotton, flax, hemp, lint | Textile Cigarette smokers especially affected | Respiratory tract (byssinosis–chest tightness, dyspnoea, cough, wheezing; chronic bronchitis) |
| Creosol | Chemical; oil refining | Denatures and precipitates all cellular protein Skin. Eyes. Respiratory Tract. Liver. Kidneys. Brain |
| Dichloroethyl ether | Insecticide; oil refining | Respiratory tract |
| Dimethyl sulphate | Chemical; pharmaceutical | Eyes. Respiratory tract. Liver. Kidneys. Brain |

(continued)

Table 2-3 (continued)

| Agent | Type of Industry or Occupation | Body Area Affected |
|---|---|---|
| Dyes | Dye workers | Urinary bladder (cancer) |
| Ethylene oxide | Hospital workers (sterilization); workers using epoxyresins | Skin. Eyes (infection, ulcers, burns) Neurological system (drowsy, weak). Leukemia; lymphoma Respiratory tract (dyspnoea, cyanosis, pulmonary edema, cancer) Gastrointestinal tract (vomiting, cancer) Reproductive organs (chromosome damage, spontaneous abortion, fetal damage, infertility in male and female) |
| Exhaust fumes | Mechanics; gas station and garage workers | Respiratory tract. Urinary bladder (cancer) |
| Formaldehyde | Laboratory workers; medical (cold sterilization); mechanics; textile workers; home insulators; mobile home owners; households (wet-strength paper towels, permanent-press clothing, foam insulation) | Reproductive tract (gene mutation) Liver. Lungs. Skin (infection, ulcers, cancer) Eyes, nose, throat (irritation) Neurological system (headache, fatigue, memory loss, nausea) |
| Freon | Refrigeration; aerosol propellants | Respiratory tract. Cardiovascular system |
| Fungus, parasites, microorganisms | Food; animal; outdoor workers; clinical laboratory workers | Skin. Respiratory tract (infection, including hepatitis B) |
| Germicidal agents | Health care providers; maintenance and cleaning workers | Skin (contact allergy, dermatosis) |
| Hydrogen chloride | Meat wrappers | Respiratory tract (irritation and asthma) |
| Hydrogen sulphide | Mines; oil wells; refineries; sewers | Respiratory tract (respiratory paralysis in high concentrations). Eyes |
| Iron oxide | Mines, iron foundries; metal polishers and finishers | Respiratory tract (cancer). Larynx |
| Laser, non-ionizing radiation | Health care providers | Eye and skin injury at the point of contact |
| Latex (natural rubber products) | Health care providers; patients with multiple hospitalizations; maintenance/cleaning workers; workers in industries that manufacture or use latex products; anyone with history of allergy | Skin hives, contact allergy, when touched by latex Respiratory tract (rhinorrhea, asthma, chronic sinus infection) Potential for anaphylactic shock |
| Lead | Auto; smelters; plumbing; paint; metallurgic; battery workers; plumbers; plastics; pottery; ceramics; gasoline station attendants; electronics; manufacture; shipbuilding; shoemakers; households; exposure in 120 industries | Hematopoietic. Cardiovascular (hypertension) Liver. Kidneys. Central nervous system and brain (behavioural change). Muscles; bone. Gastrointestinal tract. Reproductive system (decreased sperm count, chromosome mutation, causes fetal damage or spontaneous abortion during first trimester of pregnancy, infertility in male and female, stillbirth, impotency, menstrual irregularities) |

(continued)

Table 2-3 (continued)

| Agent | Type of Industry or Occupation | Body Area Affected |
|---|---|---|
| Leather | Leather; shoe | Nasal cavity and sinuses. Urinary bladder (carcinogenic). Larynx |
| Lye | Households (drain openers, oven and other cleaners) | Eyes (corneal ulceration) Skin (ulcerations) Respiratory tract (irritation) |
| Manganese | Mine; metallurgic; welders; shipbuilding | Respiratory tract. Liver. Brain |
| Mercury | Electrical and laboratory workers; dye makers; explosives; drug workers; plastics; paint; pesticide workers; households; exposure in 80 different types of industries | Toxic to all cells. Skin (ulcers, dermatosis, hyperpigmentation) Respiratory tract. Liver Brain damage. Reproductive system (infertility in male and female, spontaneous abortions, birth defects). Reduced vision. Psychic changes Exposure of pregnant women causes congenital defects and retardation in child |
| Methylene chloride | Paint removers | Respiratory tract (irritant, carcinogen). Skin. Eyes. Liver. Brain. Heart. Gastrointestinal tract |
| Mica | Rubber; insulation | Respiratory tract |
| Naphthalene | Textile cleaners | Larynx (cancer). Eyes. Lungs |
| Nickel | Metallurgic; smelter; electrolysis workers | Skin. Respiratory tract (infection and cancer). Reproductive tract |
| Nitric acid | Chemical industries; electroplaters; jewellers; lithographers | Skin (ulcerations, orange discoloration) Eyes (ulcerations) |
| Nitrobenzene | Synthetic dyes | Skin. Hematopoietic system. Brain |
| Nitrogen dioxide | Chemical; metal; arc welding; explosives; silos | Eyes. Respiratory tract. Hematopoietic system |
| Organophosphates (pesticides; insecticides) | Agriculture; pesticide manufacturers and sprayers; exterminators | Reproductive system (congenital anomalies) Brain dysfunction and neurological damage (memory loss, disorientation, ataxia, liver and convulsions). Kidneys (cancer) Respiratory tract (infections, cancer). Cardiovascular system |
| Pentachlorophenol | Wood preservative industry | Liver. Kidneys. Nervous system. Reproductive system. Carcinogenic to all systems |
| Petroleum products | Rubber; textile; aerospace; workers in contact with fuel oil, coke, paraffin, lubricants Dry cleaning; diesel jet testers | Skin. Respiratory tract. Larynx. Scrotum. Carcinogenic to all systems. Dermatosis. Hyperpigmentation of skin |
| Phenol | Plastics | Corrosive to all tissue, liver, kidneys, brain Skin (ulceration) |

*(continued)*

Table 2-3 (continued)

| Agent | Type of Industry or Occupation | Body Area Affected |
|---|---|---|
| Polyurethane | Plastics and most other industries | Respiratory tract (asthma, cancer). Dermatosis |
| Printing ink | Printers | Respiratory tract (irritation). Larynx (cancer). Urinary bladder (cancer) |
| Radiation | Health care providers: doctors, nurses, dentists, radiologists, and x-ray technicians (diagnostic, fluoroscopy, treatment, isotopes), physical therapists (diathermy), microbiologists and laboratory technicians (electron microscope); office workers (some types of computers and office machines); radar systems (police, weather, airport workers); nuclear generating stations; AM, FM, TV broadcasting stations; atomic workers; food workers; fibre workers; households (microwave ovens, some computers) | Reproductive system (chromosome irritation, sterility in men and women, birth defects, impotence, cancer). Hematopoietic system (leukemia). Thyroid (cancer). Other body systems bone and skin (cancer) |
| Rubber dust | Rubber | Respiratory tract (chronic disease, cancer). Dermatosis |
| Silica | Mines; foundries, ceramic or glass production | Respiratory tract (silicosis, pneumoconiosis, emphysema) |
| Sulphur dioxide | Oil refineries; ore smelting; brewery workers; flour bleachers; paper; sulphuric acid workers | Respiratory tract (acute exposure causes laryngospasm, circulatory arrest, death) |
| Talc dust | Mines | Respiratory tract (cancer). Calcification of pericardium |
| Tetraethyl lead | Chemical | Hematopoietic system. Brain |
| Thallium | Pesticide; fireworks or explosives | Skin. Eyes. Respiratory and gastrointestinal tracts. Kidneys. Brain |
| Toluene | Metal coatings; rubber; paint; clerical workers; printers; cosmetologists; plastics | Skin. Respiratory tract. Liver. Hematopoietic system. Brain (may cause drunken state and accidents). Reproductive system (infertility, birth defects, chromosome damage in male). Kidneys |
| Trichloroethylene | Chemical-metal degreasing; contact cement; paint; plastics; upholstery cleaners | Skin. Liver. Kidneys. Brain (carcinogen). Cardiac system |
| Vinyl chloride | Plastic; rubber; insulation; organic-chemical synthesizers; polyvinyl-resin makers | Skin. Respiratory tract (asthma). Cancer in the liver, kidney, spleen, and brain. Reproductive system (chromosome mutation, stillbirth, spontaneous abortion); exposure of pregnant woman to polyvinyl chloride causes defective fetus |
| Wood products | Furniture | Respiratory tract (asthma). Larynx (cancer) |
| Zinc | Plating; in brass, bronze, other alloys | Respiratory tract. Neurological system. Hematopoietic system |

dengue fever, diphtheria, Lyme disease, bubonic plague, and yellow fever has increased dramatically, according to the World Health Organization (WHO). New diseases have emerged in the past 20 years and are a threat to all countries. There are several reasons for new and re-emerging diseases:[155]

■ Changes in lifestyle, including overcrowded cities where population growth has outpaced supplies of clean water and adequate housing

■ Dramatic increases in national and international travel, whereby a traveller may spread the disease from one country to another before falling ill

■ Deterioration of traditional public health activities, such as surveillance and diagnostic laboratories, needed to recognize emerging problems quickly

■ Antibiotic resistance, so that effective treatment of gonorrhea, staphylococcal infections, dysentery, malaria, and even the simplest infection is difficult

■ Existence of unrecognized microorganisms in nature that are as deadly as the Ebola virus and will be distributed as people go into remote areas

Canada has experienced some serious health-related outbreaks in recent years, which we'll now consider briefly.

Severe acute respiratory syndrome (SARS) is thought to have arisen in southern China in November 2002.[156] The outbreak of SARS in Canada, especially in Toronto in 2003, was dramatic and devastating. The findings of a survey conducted in a large Toronto tertiary-care institution reported that the SARS outbreak had significant psychosocial effects on hospital staff, as well as on their families and their lifestyles. However, these effects differed depending on one's occupation and perceived risk. The results also indicated the need for strategies to address psychosocial distress and concern and to provide assistance for employees during times of crisis.[157] A second phase of the outbreak (SARS II) was declared in Toronto in the same year. Fortunately, a multidisciplinary approach to manage this second phase of the outbreak was undertaken at North York General Hospital. This successful approach was made possible through the collaboration and hard work of many individuals, as well as through open and active interaction among all departments, employees, and clients.[158]

Bauman and her colleagues conducted an exploratory investigation with nurse administrators who held key positions during the epidemic. Based on relevant literature and interviews, the nurse administrators confirmed the lack of space capacity in the health care system and indicated that the community and long-term care sectors had less capacity than acute care facilities did. The findings indicate that capacity issues should be addressed as part of larger human resource initiatives to create a more flexible workforce. Since SARS, a number of government and organizational initiatives have been developed to increase nursing capacity.[159]

Since its arrival in North America in 1999, West Nile virus (WNV) has spread rapidly across the United States and into Canada.[160] The prevention of WNV transmission relies on the elimination of breeding sites for mosquitoes and the use of personal protection.[161] Sayao and her team of researchers reviewed clinical and laboratory information that was obtained from a retrospective review of client hospital and clinical charts. Clients were included in the study if they showed serological evidence of WNV infection. Inclusion criteria also included clinical evidence of aseptic meningitis, encephalomyelitis, cerebellar syndrome, or motor neuronopathy.[162] Three clients received a treatment course of 3 million units IFN alpha-2b, administered by subcutaneous injection once per day for 14 days. The researchers found marked improvement in two patients who received IFN alpha-2b. This finding raised preliminary optimism toward this potential treatment.[163]

A survey was conducted in the Five Hills Health Region situated in the south-central area of Saskatchewan. This region reported the highest WNV case rates in the 2003 outbreak. The findings indicated that this was the highest seroprevalence rate of WNV recorded in North America thus far. Many factors could have influenced the outbreak, such as early prolonged hot weather, eco-region, level of mosquito control programs, personal protective behaviours, and urban and rural community differences.[164]

Bovine spongiform encephalopathy (BSE), or "mad cow disease," is a progressive fatal disease of the nervous system of cattle.[165] Only two cases of BSE have ever been diagnosed in Canada. The first was found in 1993 in a beef cow that had been imported from Britain in 1987. The animal carcass and the herd were destroyed and additional measures were taken immediately by the federal government to deal with any risk that Canadian cattle might have been affected. The second case of BSE was reported in May 2003. The animal was condemned to slaughter, so no meat from the carcass entered the food system. The Canadian Food Inspection Agency (CFIA) responded with a comprehensive investigation that tested some 2000 animals. All test results were negative for BSE. Canada, as well as many other countries, has taken precautions to prevent the introduction and spread of BSE.[166]

The Norwalk virus, a common cause of vomiting and diarrheal illness each winter, has often been referred to as "stomach flu." Infections have been linked to outbreaks of vomiting and/or diarrhea in institutions such as child care centres and long-term facilities as well as on cruise ships, camps, schools, and households. Immunity to the Norwalk virus is strain-specific and temporary, so everyone should take precautions to prevent its spread to others. Frequent handwashing with soap and running water is important, especially after visits to the washroom and before handling food.[167]

The first human case of avian influenza, or "bird flu," was diagnosed in 1997 in Hong Kong. The avian flu virus is found in nasal secretions and droppings of wild and domestic fowl. In humans, avian flu causes manifestations similar to other influenza infections. Clients who die succumb to pneumonia and respiratory distress symptoms. To prevent the spread of infection, it is necessary to observe standard precautions and use good hand hygiene practices.[168]

The CNA's position statement *Global Health and Equity* states that health is a global issue and that global health—the optimal well-being of all humans from an individual and global perspective—is a fundamental human right that should be accessible to all. All health professionals, including nurses, have the right and responsibility to raise awareness of the root cause of inequity in global health and to participate in finding solutions. Strategies such as collaboration, co-operation, and communication among all health professionals are imperative to improving the quality of global health.[169]

Canada is continually assessing international scientific information as it becomes available and modifying policies as required, based on new information.

## Personal Responsibility

Consider the environment, the various social institutions, and the population as a complex of interacting, interdependent systems. Environmental problems are a concern to everyone and are of equal consequence to every part of the world. Each of us shares the earth, so we are all responsible for its well-being. Environmental pollution is our collective responsibility and requires our collective solutions. A fourfold environmental protection system is useful for continuously identifying, analyzing, and controlling environmental hazards:

1. Surveillance: maintaining awareness of what people and industries are doing to the air, water, and land and of the effect of these actions on health; monitoring exposure
2. Development of criteria for the detection of pollution; detection
3. Research: including data from various records
4. Compliance: getting local government and industry to accept and implement new standards

**Citizen Role** An informed public can certainly help to establish such a system, but the financial support and legislative and administrative guidance of federal, provincial, and local governments provide the most feasible solutions. Lobby your governments to pass legislation that protects the environment. Support the production of biodegradable products from potato scraps, corn, molasses, beets, and castor oil. These non-petroleum ingredients can be transformed into a strong, flexible plastic that will degrade completely.

---

### CRITICAL THINKING

*What interventions are important to you regarding the environment in promoting the health of individuals and their families?*

---

**Lifestyle Changes** The box entitled "Conservation Solutions" summarizes individual and community activities to conserve resources, reduce pollution, and make lifestyle changes. For some people, following the suggestions means major changes—in shopping differently, in carefully disposing of articles, or in transportation—or it could mean planting a patio or rooftop garden or limiting the number of pets.

Quiet surroundings are a natural resource, too. Make your own life quieter through personal habits. Help to preserve local recreation sites that offer natural surroundings. Lobby the government for adequate acoustical standards in homes, apartments, hospitals, and industrial buildings and for noiseless kitchen equipment. Participate in local government planning to decrease town and city noise in relation to transportation routes, zoning, and industrial sites.

**Support for Conservation** In Canada, Greenpeace, founded in 1971, is an independently funded organization that works to protect the environment. It now has offices in more than 30 countries worldwide. Its mission is to protect biodiversity in all its forms, and prevent the pollution of oceans, land, air, and fresh water. It seeks to end all nuclear threats, and promotes peace, world disarmament, and nonviolence. Public education is an important element of Greenpeace's mandate.[170]

## Professional Responsibility

Although health care and nursing responsibilities have been interwoven throughout this chapter, consider that your primary responsibilities are detection through thorough assessment, making suggestions for intervention based on health promotion and prevention of illness, health teaching, and advocacy related to policy development and legislation.

The CNA's *Policy Statement on a Joint CNA/CMA Position Statement on Environmentally Responsible Activity in the Health Sector* states that its purpose is to express the commitment of both the CNA and the Canadian Medical Association (CMA) to accelerate responsible activity toward the environment within the health sector.[171] The CNA argues that nurses and physicians, as decision-makers, caregivers, and role models for health behaviour, should not only encourage but also implement measures to achieve environmentally responsible activity.[172] These professionals have the responsibility to encourage international professional bodies and their members to lobby their governments to promote healthy environments. One example of such a cause is the problem of toxic waste disposal in the developing world.

Nurses, physicians, and other health professionals have the prime responsibility to provide leadership in implementing the 4R principle to reduce, reuse, recycle, and recover. All health professionals should feel obligated to educate Canadians about maintaining a healthy environment in the workplace and in their communities.

*The Canadian Handbook on Health Impact Assessment, Volume 2: Decision Making in Environmental Health Impact Assessment* was written by a group of doctors and other professionals, for health professionals—doctors, nurses, and environmental health inspectors. While some of these professionals might lack expertise in the area of environmental assessment, they are asked frequently to provide their perspectives on issues such as the community health impacts of mining developments, landfill sites, or high-voltage lines. This handbook has been prepared for use by other stakeholders who plan and conduct environmental assessments and impact studies in Canada. Examples of such stakeholders include consulting firms in the fields of social science and engineering.[173]

Fraser states that nurses need to have a basic knowledge of environmental threats and their effects on various communities.[174] Nurses must be aware that environmental contaminants may affect the quality of life throughout the lifespan. People with kidney disease, compromised immune systems, or genetic predispositions to slow chemical metabolism react differently to environmental contaminants. In fact, the most vulnerable are children and pregnant women because of their relatively high metabolic rate and caloric demands.[175] The CNA's position statement *The Environment Is a Determinant of Health* notes that acute and chronic diseases, as well as death, are frequently triggered by the contamination of water.[176] In fact, environmental contaminants and health concerns are particularly relevant in cases of asthma, impaired capacity to learn, reduced fertility, and cancers. The CNA firmly believes that the quality of health, and thus life, can be improved by minimizing the use of products containing contaminants.[177]

Nurses at each level of instruction need to confront their own attitudes toward the environment and health, and determine ways in which they will help to educate and inform their clients about such matters. Curricula need to reflect health protection, health promotion, and the prevention of illness in rural, northern, and urban communities.

---

## CRITICAL THINKING

*What types of health-promotion courses dealing with the environment would you develop in your own program of studies? State your rationale.*

---

## Assessment

Screening for occupational diseases resulting from exposure to contaminants is most accurately done by occupational health nurses and physicians rather than by employees in corporate medical groups. Increasingly, there are improved radiological and blood chemistry diagnostic tests to detect diseases that are related to occupations, including a blood test to detect pesticide contamination. It is important to reinforce the knowledge of workers and the protective strategies they employ on the job. Keep abreast of medical advances.[178]

## Conservation Solutions

### Energy Solutions

- Use **public transportation**; carpool; bike, or walk rather than drive a car if feasible.
- Invest in **ample insulation**, weather stripping, and caulking for the home and workplace.
- **Use electricity and hot water efficiently**. Buy energy-saving household appliances.

- **Reduce demand for energy** by turning off the lights, radio, and television when no one is using them; run dishwasher and washer and dryer only when they have full loads.
- **Make the most of oven heat**—bake foods in batches; turn oven off shortly before baking is finished and use remaining heat to complete the job.
- **Dry clothes outdoors** on a line.

>

- **Use the clothes dryer efficiently**; separate loads into heavy and lightweight items as lighter ones take less time.

- **In winter, turn down the thermostat a few degrees**, especially at night and when house is empty. In **summer**, if using **air conditioning, turn thermostat up a few degrees**. Regularly service the furnace and air conditioner.

- **Close off** and do not heat or cool **unused rooms**; use insulating shades and curtains on cold winter nights and hot summer days.

## Food Solutions

- **Eat foods lower on the food chain**—fruits, vegetables, and grains; decrease consumption of meat and animal products.

- **Read the labels on food**; buy foods that have not been heavily processed. Learn which additives are harmful.

- **Support laws that ban harmful pesticides**, drugs, and other chemicals used in food production. Support markets that offer pesticide-free food.

- **Avoid food from endangered environments**, such as rain forests.

## Water Solutions

- **Fix leaks** promptly.

- Install sink faucet aerators and **water-efficient shower-heads**, which use two to five times less water with no noticeable decrease in performance.

- Take showers, not baths, to **reduce water consumption**.

- **Do not let water run** when it is not actually being used while showering, shaving, brushing teeth, or handwashing clothes.

- **Use ultra-low-flush or air-assisted toilets**, saving 60 to 90 percent water. Composting toilets use no water and recycle organic waste.

- **Buy phosphate-free, biodegradable soaps and detergents**; ask your supermarket to carry them if it does not.

- Do not run the tap until the water is cold to get a drink. Instead, **keep water in a refrigerator bottle**.

- **Economize water** when washing the car, sprinkling the lawn, and removing debris from surfaces. Repair leaks.

## Toxins and Pollutants Solutions

- Read labels; **buy the least toxic products** available; find out the best disposal methods for toxic products.

- Avoid purchasing clothes that require dry cleaning, which uses toxic chlorinated solvents. **Dry clean clothes only when necessary**.

- **Avoid contact with pesticides** by thoroughly scrubbing or peeling foodstuffs; if possible, maintain your own garden without use of pesticides.

- **Test your home for radon**, especially if you live on the east coast.

- **Ask your service station to use CFC recovery equipment** when repairing auto air conditioners.

- **Use more energy-efficient cars**.

- **Keep your automobile in top working condition** with a regular tune-up; make sure that anti-pollution controls are working properly.

- **Operate your vehicle properly**; do not idle or rev engine; drive at a steady pace; obey speed limits.

- **Support legislative initiatives that encourage industry to modify manufacturing processes** to eliminate the production of hazardous wastes and to reuse and recycle wastes when possible.

## Waste Reduction and Recycling Solutions

- **Buy products in bulk or with the least amount of packaging**. (A major contributor to acid rain is sulphur dioxide, one of the chemicals used to process virgin paper. In the very low-oxygen environment of the trash dump, paper or plastic may take 40 or more years to degrade.)

- **Buy products that are recyclable**, repairable, reusable, and biodegradable; avoid disposables. (Every three months, enough aluminium cans are thrown away to rebuild an entire commercial fleet.)

- **Separate your recyclable garbage** such as newspaper, glass, paper, aluminium, and organic waste.

- **Recycle newspapers**. Each weekend thousands of trees are made into newspapers that are not recycled.

- **Use recycled products**. Landfills are rapidly being exhausted, and the cost of recycling must be recovered.

- **Buy recycled paper for all uses**. It takes nearly 18 000 kilowatt-hours of electricity to produce 1 tonne of paper from virgin wood pulp. It takes 64 percent fewer kilowatt-hours (approximately 6500) to produce 1 tonne of recycled paper from waste paper.

- **Recycle used** oil to be re-refined for lubricants.

- Urge your area to use **Glasphalt** from recycled glass for parking areas and roadways.

## Housekeeping Solutions

- **Use simple substances for cleaning**. An all-purpose cleaner, safe for all surfaces, is 4 litres of hot water, 60 mL sudsy ammonia, 60 mL vinegar, and 15 mL baking soda. After use, wipe surface with water to rinse.

- **Keep drains open by using the following mix** once weekly: 250 mL baking soda, 250 mL salt, 60 mL cream of tartar. Pour 60 mL of the mixture weekly into the drain; follow with a pot of boiling water. If drain is clogged, pour in 60 mL baking soda followed by 120 mL vinegar. Close drain until fizzing stops. Then flush with boiling water.

- **Use low-phosphate or phosphate-free detergents** to wash clothes and dishes.

>

- **Use natural furniture- and floor-polish products**; such products use lemon oil or beeswax in a mineral oil base.

- **Use non-toxic products to control pests**. Control ants by sprinkling barriers of talcum powder, chalk, bone meal, or boric acid across their trails. Control cockroaches by dusting lightly with borax. Control ticks and fleas on pets by applying an herbal rinse. Boil 60 mL of fresh or dried rosemary in a litre of water: Steep for 20 minutes, strain, and cool. Then sponge on pet. Air-dry.

- **Maintain air circulation and clean ventilation systems** and ducts to remove fungi, mould, pollen, toxic residues, sprays, and other contaminants. Avoid hair spray and cleaning sprays.

- **Manage household hazardous waste**: buy only what is needed; do not store waste with household products; give unused product to someone else that may be able to use them rather than disposing of them. Do not pour oil, grease, or hazardous chemicals down the drain.

### Tree-Saver Solutions

- **Plant trees**; as trees grow, they remove carbon dioxide from the atmosphere through photosynthesis, slowing buildup of carbon dioxide. (Carbon dioxide causes more than 50 percent of the greenhouse effect.)

- **Plant fast-growing poplar tree hybrids** that suck contamination from soil and groundwater through **phytoremediation**, *a process that stores or metabolizes chemical and releases volatile compounds through leaves.*

- Join efforts to **save forests** from being cleared or burned. When forests are burned, carbon is released, adding to carbon dioxide buildup and global warming.

### Preservation of Life and Environment Solutions

- **Do not burn leaves or garbage**; instead, compost organic materials.

- **Do not buy endangered plants**, animals, or products made from overexploited species (furs, ivory, reptile skin, or tortoise shell).

- **Avoid buying wood from the tropical rain forests** unless it was propagated by sustainable tree farming methods.

- **Buy products from companies that do not pollute** or damage the environment.

- **Join, support, and volunteer your time to organizations working on environmental causes**.

- **Contact your elected representatives** through letters, emails, calls, or visits to communicate your concerns about conservation and environmental issues.

- **Advocate saving the wetlands**, which help filter pollution out of waterways, protect communities from floods, and sustain fish and wildlife.

---

An example of questions usually not asked on standard health history forms that you could use in assessment of the employed client is presented in Figure 2-4. Be sure to consider the client's issues, strengths, and healthy responses, such as knowledge capacity, empowerment, and social network.

## Nursing Strategies

Health teaching and advocacy can increase client and community awareness and contribute to the prevention of illness from pollutants or hazards. Encourage people to read labels and current literature on products. Natural or human-made chemical pollution in soil, water, and food products can produce various adverse effects, ranging from slight health impairments to death.

You may have an opportunity to teach people who earn a living as pesticide applicators and handlers. They should follow these precautions:

- Wear rubber or neoprene gloves while handling pesticides to avoid skin contact.

- Keep pesticide-soiled clothing separate from other family laundry.

- Empty all cuffs and pockets before doing laundry so trapped pesticide granules do not dissolve in wash water.

- Wash all clothing daily that is worn while applying pesticides. The longer the garments are stored before laundering, the more difficult it is to remove the pesticide.

- Pre-rinsing is an effective way to dislodge pesticide residue.

- Wash only a few items at a time, and wash for a 12- to 14-minute cycle. Use the recommended amount of heavy-duty detergent. Liquid detergents are more effective than powders in removing oil-based pesticides.

- The hotter the water—preferably 60 degrees C (140 degrees F)—the more effectively pesticide is removed.

- It may be necessary to discard heavily contaminated clothing.

**Figure 2-4** Occupational history form

---

1. Occupational history (start with last job first).

| | COMPANY | DATE EMPLOYED | JOB |
|---|---|---|---|
| (a) | _____ | _____ | _____ |
| (b) | _____ | _____ | _____ |
| (c) | _____ | _____ | _____ |
| (d) | _____ | _____ | _____ |

2. In these jobs, have you ever been exposed to:
   Excessive radiation or radioactive material? _____
   Excessive noise? _____    Excessive heat or light? _____

3. Have you worked in dusty trades? _____
   With any specific chemicals? _____
   In any vapours or fumes?_____
   If your answer is yes to any questions in (2) and (3), please elaborate. _____
   _____
   _____

4. Has a job ever made you "sick"? _____    If so, which job? _____
   Explain how you were sick. _____

5. Have you ever worn any protective equipment or a specific support? _____
   If so, what? _____

6. Have you ever had a serious work injury? _____    If so, please describe. _____
   _____

7. Have you ever had several minor work injuries? _____    If so, please describe. _____
   _____

8. Have you ever applied for, or received, workers' compensation? _____

9. Have you ever had a pension for disability? _____
   _____

---

- To remove possible pesticide residues from the washing machine tub, run the washer through a complete cycle using detergent and a full level of hot water.

Another dangerous problem associated with chemical pollution is its possible carcinogenic effect. Incidence of specific forms of cancer can vary depending on exposure to specific compounds, a common example being the high incidence of lung cancer in Canada because of heavy tobacco use. Be aware and knowledgeable about the incidence of chemically produced cancer in your region. Health teaching can then be directed at trying to eliminate or control the responsible carcinogenic chemical.

A research study was conducted to explore the determinants of support for and reported smoke-free policies in restaurants and bars across four countries (United States, Canada, United Kingdom, and Australia). In the study, the International Tobacco Control (ITC) Four Country Survey found that smokers adjust, accept, and comply with smoke-free laws. Further, support and compliance are remarkably similar across countries given the notably different levels of smoke-free policies.[179]

In their article *Making Canadian Healthcare Facilities 100 Percent Smoke-Free: A National Trend Emerges*, the authors state it is inevitable that all Canadian health care facilities will eventually ban tobacco products in their buildings and on their grounds. That is, they look forward to a time when no one expects to smoke on Canadian health care properties.[180]

Encourage people to use protective clothing and sunscreen lotions to prevent overexposure to the sun and potential skin cancer or melanoma (see the "Evidence-Based Practice" box). Prevent overexposure to ionizing radiation by making certain that unnecessary x-ray studies are not taken, by keeping a record of the frequency of such studies, and by carefully using a lead shield when x-ray examinations are given.

The biochemical response to chemical pollution or radiation can influence the cells in various ways. **Teratogenic** (*producing fetal malformations*) and **mutagenic** (*producing hereditary changes*) are two such changes in cells. Be aware that these changes can occur in both the client and the health care provider when they are exposed to radiation. Remember, radiation can also be carcinogenic. Genetic counselling is indicated for individuals who have been exposed to radiation. Citizens should know of the possibility of dealing effectively and therapeutically with biochemical changes, whether prenatal or in any other stage of growth and development. As a professional, you can encourage officials and consumers in your community to develop innovative technologies to cope with the hazardous effects of our current lifestyle.

Educate the public about current issues influencing health and the environment, including environmental toxins and pollutants, nuclear energy and energy alternatives, resource recovery and recycling, chemical and biologic warfare, and occupational hazards.

In the past 100 years, disease and death have been reduced because of preventive public health measures in the form of environmental control, such as water and waste management, rodent and insect control, and the development of housing codes. Now we are again faced with problems and diseases that have an environmental impact. Prevention can begin with informed consumer groups that have educational and work projects as their goals. It can begin with your responsibility for the client's environment.

## Client's Immediate Environment

Besides a feeling of responsibility for the community and physical environment in which the client lives, you also have a responsibility for that individual's immediate environment

---

### EVIDENCE-BASED PRACTICE
# Predictors of Sun Protection in Canadian Adults

Data from light-skinned respondents of the 1996 *National Survey on Sun Exposure & Protective Behaviours* who spent more than $N$ minutes per day of their leisure time in the sun ($N = 1027$) were analyzed. Multivariable logistic regression models were developed to identify four types of sun protection behaviour (avoiding the sun between 11 a.m. and 4 p.m., seeking shade, wearing protective clothing, applying sunscreen to the body). The analysis also included data of reports of the use of these four practices in combination.

The results showed the following:

1. At least one protective behaviour was performed by 81 percent of respondents.

2. Each protective behaviour was practised by between 40 and 48 percent of individuals.

3. Respondents more likely to perform the behaviours in combination were:

   (a) older individuals,

   (b) women,

   (c) those who wanted a tan,

   (d) those who found sun protection practices inconvenient, or

   (e) those forgetful about protection from the sun.

4. Women were less likely than men to wear protective clothing.

5. Older individuals were less likely to report sunscreen use.

6. Individuals with a higher education level were more likely to report wearing protective clothing and applying sunscreen.

7. Respondents reporting a higher income level reported sunscreen use more often.

8. Only 30 percent of respondents reported always/often employing three or four of the behaviours.

9. Younger adults were less likely to report the following: avoiding the sun during peak hours, seeking shade, and wearing protective clothing.

10. Men, who have a higher incidence of skin cancer, were less likely than women to engage in sun protection.

11. Men tended to report finding sun protection practices inconvenient; and they tended to report a lack of concern about the health effects of excessive sun exposure.

### Health Promotion Implications

Canadians need to adopt the use of a greater number of sun protection strategies, especially during peak hours. The results of poor sun protection practices among younger individuals is particularly perilous because sun exposure early in life has been found to be associated with high-risk melanoma and other skin cancers later in adulthood. Therefore, as a health care professional, you are challenged to devise effective means to educate all clients—young people and men, in particular—regarding the risks of sun exposure.

Source: Purdue, M.P., "Predictors of Sun Protection in Canadian Adults," *Canadian Journal of Public Health, 93*(6) (2002), 470–474. Used with permission.

while receiving health care. The client's surroundings should constitute a **therapeutic milieu** *free of hazards and conducive to recovery, physically and emotionally.*

The client's surroundings should be clean and adequately lit, ventilated, heated, and safe. Precautions should always be taken to prevent injury. Falls should be prevented by removing obstacles and electric cords from walking areas and having the person wear well-fitted shoes. The use of adequate support while walking should be encouraged. Lock the bed or wheelchair while the client is moving to and from them. In the home, be sure that electric cords and scatter rugs are not placed so that the person could fall. Wipe up spilled liquids immediately. Use sterile technique and proper handwashing methods to ensure that you bring no pathogenic organisms to the client. Avoid excessive noise from personnel and equipment to the degree possible. Various pieces of equipment used in client care must be monitored for safe function.

The *aesthetic environment* is also important for rest. Arrange articles on the bedside table in a pleasing manner if the client is unable to do so. Keep unattractive equipment and supplies out of sight as much as possible. Electric equipment should be in proper repair and function. Minimize offensive odours and noise. Place the person's bed or chair by a window or door so that the person can watch normal activity rather than stare at the ceiling or walls. As a nurse, involve yourself in making the entire ward, as well as the clients' rooms, look pleasing. Consider colour combinations and the use of drapes, furniture, clocks, calendars, pictures, and various artefacts to create a more homelike atmosphere. The committee in charge of decorating and building should include at least one nurse. You may need to volunteer to ensure that nursing and, indirectly, clients are represented in such programs.

The client's surroundings should be safe and attractive, but the *emotional climate of the unit and entire institution affects clients and staff as well.* The client and family are quick to respond and react to the attitudes and manner of the staff. Here are some questions you might ask yourself:

■ How do I treat delivery workers who bring gifts and flowers to clients?

■ Do I participate in the joy that remembrances bring to the client?

■ Do I treat visitors as welcome guests or as foreign intruders?

The emotional climate should radiate security and acceptance. Warmth should prevail and promote a sense and feeling of trust, confidence, and motivation within the client as he or she and the staff work together to cope with problems. The emotional relationship between the client and the health care staff should help the client reach the goal of maximum health.

In a truly therapeutic milieu, the *staff members also feel a sense of harmony among themselves.* There is mutual trust and acceptance between staff and supervisors, and supervisors recognize work well done by the staff. As a result, staff feel motivated to continue to learn and to improve the quality of client care. Staff are not likely to give individualized, comprehensive, compassionate care in an agency where they are not treated like individuals or where their basic professional needs are not met.

*Be aware of environmental pollution* in the health care environment. "No smoking" should be the rule. Sometimes there are designated smoking areas outside the building so that employees or visitors who smoke must go outdoors. It is difficult to teach a client the adverse effects of smoking and nicotine when an odour of cigarette smoke hangs on the clothing of the health care worker. Moreover, health care providers benefit from practising what they teach others. Health care providers and clients may also come in contact with agents listed in Table 2-3. Constant vigilance is necessary to detect harmful agents and prevent or reduce their use. Early assessment of harmful effects to reduce the symptoms and proper interventions for dermatosis, allergens, or other symptoms is essential.

There are times when the treatment for the client's infection or the therapy modalities may affect the health care provider—for example, radiotherapy and chemotherapy. Proper precautions should be taken to protect the provider from excess exposure and to protect the client. Carefully follow guidelines for handling chemotherapeutic and radioactive materials.

Measures to reduce work-related hazards in health care environments include:

1. Provide safer needle-stick devices and needle disposal containers.
2. Substitute less toxic sterilizing or cleaning substances.
3. Design work and computer systems space with high-efficiency ventilation and high-quality ergonomics to avoid muscle and vision strain.
4. Use work practice controls, such as handwashing, good hygiene, housekeeping measures, and immunization.
5. Use assistive devices for lifting.
6. Provide adequate staffing; create permanent shifts to avoid shift rotation.
7. Use personal protective equipment, such as gloves and equipment that are latex-free, low protein, and powder-free. Wear gowns and respiratory masks. Use lead shields.
8. Provide occupational health and safety training programs.

Joan Petruck, a health and safety coordinator with the East Central Regional Health Authority in Camrose, Alberta, formed a sharp-injury prevention task team from various health care settings. The team's mandate was to investigate how and why sharp injuries were occurring, and then to develop a realistic strategy for preventing future injuries. The team worked together from the premise that injuries are both predictable and preventable.[181] One of the changes introduced by the task team was to replace penlets with retractable, disposable lancets. Petruck claims that since retractable lancets were introduced, injuries have been eliminated in the facilities.[182] The team is currently investigating the cost of retractable syringes. They believe these syringes will eliminate both the risk posed by recapping and the danger from needles encountered in the laundry or garbage.

If you are caring for persons in the home, you are limited in the amount of change you can make. You can point out such hazards as electric cords in the walking area, however. You can suggest furniture rearrangement if you think that the person could function more easily with the change. You can put a clock in sight, pull the drapes, or place needed materials within the client's reach, if feasible.

Health Canada, the Centers for Disease Control and Prevention (CDC), and the World Health Organization (WHO) have developed infection control guidance for health care workers at risk.[183] One such recommendation is that handwashing is the most important hygiene measure in preventing the spread of infection. The College of Registered Nurses in Manitoba launched a public awareness campaign on handwashing aimed at helping Manitobans stay healthier.[184] The campaign targets handwashing, an easy way to stop the spread of illness and disease in the home, in the workplace, at school, and in public places. Manitoba's registered nurses encourage everyone to make frequent handwashing a habit.[185]

Specific ways of meeting the client's environmental needs differ at various developmental stages. The components of a therapeutic milieu are different for the baby than for the middle-aged client. However, a safe, secure environment, both physically and psychologically, must be present for both. An accurate determination of the factors that make up the environment and making appropriate changes may be the first steps in promoting health.

It is past time for all of us to ask ourselves certain basic questions. How much energy and natural resources do we need to sustain life, to maintain the high standard of living in Canada? How much are we willing to pay for benefits that will not poison us with side effects? How does population growth affect the use and abuse of natural resources? Will strictly controlled energy allocation be necessary because people refuse to abide by suggested limits? Must children continue to grow up exposed to all types of hazards in the environment? What more can each of us do personally and professionally to maintain a health-fostering environment?

## SUMMARY

1. Health and development are adversely affected by air, water, soil, food, noise, and surface pollution.

2. Sources of air pollution are carbon monoxide; sulphur and nitrogen oxide; suspended particles such as dust, ash, aerosols, and asbestos; tobacco smoke; hydrocarbons; ozone; photochemical smog; acid rain; radioactive substances; formaldehyde; and radon.

3. Sources of water pollution are sewage and pathogenic organisms; plant nutrients; synthetic and inorganic chemicals; sediment; radioactive material; oil spills; and heat from industrial processes.

4. Sources of food pollution include pesticides and food additives such as antibiotics and hormones administered to animals that are produced for food; contaminated water and soil used in food production; and contamination from pathogens during food processing or handling.

5. Noise pollution in the home and workplace produces numerous adverse health and safety effects.

6. Sources of surface pollution include open dumps; landfills; incineration of waste; salvage operations; unsafe disposal of hazardous, pathogenic, or radioactive wastes in the home or workplace; and lead found in soil, the home, and the workplace.

7. Health workers must be aware of various health hazards in the workplace—for the clients and their families as well as themselves.

8. Health care workers have global, local, personal, and professional responsibilities for promoting health and controlling pollution effects and preventing further hazards to health and development populations.

9. Health care workers must engage in legislative advocacy, public education, public policy changes, and the creation of societal resources to foster a healthy environment.

## Interesting Websites

### Air Quality

**www.hc-sc.gc.ca/air/**

Visit Health Canada's Air Quality website to learn more about how air pollution affects us and what you can do to help reduce it. Just follow the links that interest you.

### Natural Resources Canada (NRCan)

**www.nrcan.gc.ca/**

NRCan plays a pivotal role in helping shape the important contributions of the natural resources sector to the Canadian economy, society, and environment. This sector—forests, energy, minerals and metals, and landmass, as well as related industries—is one of the most productive, high-tech sectors in the global economy.

### Climate Change

**www.ec.gc.ca/climate/**

This site provides information on the effects of climate change, what we can do, and opportunities for community group work. Climate change is one of the most significant environmental challenges the world has ever faced. Visit this site and learn more.

### Canadian Medical Association Journal

**www.cmaj.ca/**

This online journal provides daily updates on such topics as clinical guidelines, health alerts, and drug advisories, as well as general information.

### BioRegulations: Rules and Guidelines

**http://bioregulations.gc.ca/**

Visit this site to find out about various Canadian federal and provincial regulations and guidelines concerning biotechnology in the sectors of agriculture, aquaculture, energy, environment, forestry, health, and mining.

### The Canadian Nurses Association

**www.cna-nurses.ca/cna/**

The CNA's site provides information on various position statements and articles regarding the environment.

## Key Terms

| | | | |
|---|---|---|---|
| **biological pesticides** (38) | **decibels** (38) | **phytoremediation** (54) | **teratogenic** (56) |
| **biopesticides** (38) | **mutagenic** (56) | **sick building syndrome** (34) | **therapeutic milieu** (57) |

# Chapter 3

## Spiritual and Religious Influences on the Person and Family

*Faith is the soul riding at anchor.*

H.W. Shaw

## Objectives

*Study of this chapter will enable you to:*

1  Define the terms *religious* and *spiritual* and determine your personal meaning of each.

2  Compare and contrast the major tenets of the Hindu, Sikh, Buddhist, Jainist, Shinto, Confucian, Taoist, Islamic, Jewish, Christian, and North American Indian religions.

3  Differentiate the major tenets of the various branches of Christianity: Roman Catholicism, Eastern Orthodoxy, various Protestant denominations, and other Christian sects.

4  Gain an overview of the variety of religions in Canada.

5  Discuss how religious beliefs influence the lifestyle and health status of individuals and families.

6  Identify more clearly your religious or spiritual beliefs and explore how they might influence your practice.

7  Discuss your role in helping to meet the spiritual needs of clients and their families.

8  Describe specific nursing measures that can be used to meet the needs of persons with different religious and spiritual backgrounds.

Until an illness occurs, the person may give no thought to the meaning of his or her life or spiritual beliefs. But when he or she feels vulnerable and fearful of the future, solace is sought. Religion and spiritual beliefs can provide that solace.

The attitude that medical science is superior to the spiritual dimension or to religion has affected us all. Yet the spiritual dimension and religion are there as they always have been. Each culture has had some organization to sustain the important rituals and myths of its people. Primitive peoples combined the roles of physician, psychiatrist, and priest.

> I had the cancer patient visualize an army of white blood cells attacking and overcoming the cancer cells.

> Within two weeks the cancer had diminished and he was rapidly gaining weight. He is alive and well today.

Is this a priest or a faith healer talking? Actually, it is a prominent tumour specialist. An internationally known neurosurgeon says, "In a very real sense, medicine is now—as it has always been—faith healing." Other health providers have seen life return after death. Thus, some health workers are trying to reunite the biopsychospiritual being.

History reveals that in the 5th century A.D., society began to change, and religion and scientific theory began to separate. Through a long process, the two theories are now sharing dialogue. In her manuscript "Suggestion for Thought," Florence Nightingale attempted to integrate science and mysticism. She felt the universe was an incarnation of a divine intelligence that regulated all things through law. She recognized that humans have spiritual needs; spiritual care enables the person to be conscious of the presence of God, the creator and sustainer of the universe.[1]

*Spiritual care has continued to be part of the nursing tradition.* The inclusion of nursing responsibility for spiritual care is cited by the CNA's Code of Ethics for Registered Nurses, the International Council of Nurses' Code of Ethics, and the American Holistic Nurses Association's standards for holistic nursing practice.[2]

There has been an increased awareness of the link between health and religion, and today the subject is being discussed and researched more openly.[3] Pangman states that research on the family has confirmed the importance of spirituality, particularly in families that have demonstrated the tenacity and ability to cope effectively with stress.[4] Studies show that people who practise religion have a lower incidence of hypertension, depression, and suicide.[5] One study indicates that a higher power supports these people and that having a relationship with God forms a foundation for their psychological well-being.[6] Furthermore, persons with high levels of spiritual well-being can cope more effectively with AIDS or chronic illness, and they can care better for clients with AIDS.[7]

An interpretive phenomenological study investigated the meaning of the experience of feeling healthy among people living with chronic illness and/or disability. The study was conducted with eight participants living with a variety of different chronic conditions.[8] The results provided a valuable mosaic of themes to express the participant's health experience. One of the themes included acquiring a state of grace whereby the participants attributed their experience of feeling healthy to an awareness of their spirituality and a sense of connectedness, wholeness, harmony, and peacefulness.[9] Another study interviewed 88 adult patients (50 percent men) about their religious beliefs and practices. These patients had been admitted to a Canadian tertiary care psychiatry inpatient unit. The results indicated that certain religious practices may protect against the severity of symptoms. It seems certain that these practices increase life satisfaction among psychiatric inpatients.[10]

Several articles in medical and nursing journals have discussed physicians and nurses who pray with their patients. The authors claim that prayer has added to the effectiveness of therapy.[11] Recently, several articles on the importance of prayer in nursing practice have appeared in scholarly journals.[12] These articles stress that prayer, as well as being a significant practice in most religions, results in comfort, and it sustains coping ability among individuals and their families.

---

## CRITICAL THINKING

*What is your personal understanding of the meaning of a sense of connectedness?*

---

# DEFINITIONS

**Religion** is defined on various levels: *a belief in a supernatural or divine force that has power over the universe and commands worship and obedience; a personal and institutional system of beliefs; a comprehensive code of ethics or philosophy; a set of practices that are followed; a church affiliation; the conscious pursuit of any object the person holds as supreme. In short, religion signifies that a group of people have established and organized practices that are related to spiritual concerns.*

This definition, however, does not portray the constancy and fervency that can at times underlie religious belief. In every human there seems to be a **spiritual dimension**, *a quality that goes beyond religious affiliation, which strives for inspiration, reverence, awe, meaning, and purpose, even in those who do not believe in any God. The spiritual dimension tries to be in harmony with the universe, strives for answers about the infinite, and especially comes into focus as a sustaining power when the person faces emotional stress, physical illness, or death. It goes outside a person's own power.*[13]

Spirituality is the umbrella for religion. It is the framework for beliefs, values, and rituals. Spirituality, however, is broad and need not include religious practice. **Spirituality**, according to Chilton,[14] *is an inner strength related to a belief in, and sense of, interconnection with a greater power.* Native spiritual life is founded on a belief in the fundamental interconnectedness of all natural aspects, all forms of life where primary importance is attached to Mother Earth. The symbol of a circle is significant in Native beliefs, and is often referred to as the Medicine Wheel.[15] The Medicine Wheel is a powerful and sacred symbol of the universe depicting the circularity of life and the four components of the self: body, mind, emotion, and spirit. The Medicine Wheel incorporates the values, beliefs, and social mores of the traditional Aboriginal culture. Common Native healing practices include shamanism, herbal remedies, and various purification rituals such as smudging and sweat lodges.[16] Some authors subsume spirituality or spiritual needs under cultural traditions or philosophic beliefs, or they describe spirituality as including all positive human qualities.

Culture, philosophy, love, and reverence for another human being are all *humanizing influences*. In the midst of our specialized health care, you have an opportunity to go beyond the dogma to bring together the biopsychospiritual being through the study of the religions, religious symbols, and spiritual values of your clients and their families.

---
CRITICAL THINKING

*How would you define or describe your own spirituality?*
---

## WORLD RELIGIONS

Use the following information about world religions in your assessments and intervention and in teaching clients and family members. Understanding these beliefs will help you work in a more complete manner with your co-workers. When exploring the spiritual heritage of health care, a fundamental need exists to become aware of the religious influences that have shaped and guided health care throughout history. This point is critical in contemporary society where there is a vast ethnic, racial, and cultural diversity.[17]

*Religions have several characteristics in common:*

■ A worldview, a way of perceiving reality; a description of existence and life meaning; assumptions about the universe and life

■ Basis of authority or source(s) of power

■ A portion of scripture or sacred word

■ An ethical code that defines right and wrong

■ A psychology and identity so that its adherents fit into a group and the world is defined by the religion

■ Aspirations or expectations

■ Certain notions and beliefs about what follows death

See Figure 3-1, "The Golden Rule," for the similarities in this phrase reflected in each religion.[18]

Religion influences worldviews with respect to living and dying. For instance, the Quran, the holy book of Islam, teaches that death is an inevitable part of life. Meanwhile, in the Greek culture, which is influenced by the Eastern Orthodox Church, death is usually viewed as a great tragedy. Similarly, at the time of death, the Hindu client may want to repeat verses from the Bhagavad-Gita. It becomes critical for health workers such as nurses to be able to provide access to prayer beads, prayer books, and other religious items.[19]

The following discussion presents a more detailed insight into each major world religion through personality sketches. *Each person has a fictitious name and represents not a single person but a composite of knowledge gained from the authors' interviews, reading, and personal experiences.* Although these personalities are presented as acting and thinking in a certain way, remember that the person's culture, family background, and personality all affect how that person lives out a religious experience.

 Hinduism and Sikhism

Rama tells us that nothing is typically **Hindu** and that anyone who puts religion in neat packages will have difficulty comprehending his outlook. Rama is named after **Ramakrishna**, *the greatest saint of Hinduism of the 19th century.* The history of Rama's religion goes back to approximately 1500 B.C., when the **Vedas**—*divine revelations*—were written. His main religious texts are the **Upanishads**, or *scriptures*, and the **Bhagavad-Gita**, a *summary of the former with additions. The most expressive and universal word of God is* **Om**, *or* **Aum**. This word provides the most important auditory and visual symbol in Rama's religion.*

Rama speaks of some of the worship practices popular in India today: of the family and local deities and of the trinity—**Brahma**, *the creator*, **Vishnu**, *the preserver and god of love*, and **Shiva**, *the destroyer*.

Rama tells of his own shrine in his home where, in the presence of various pictures of **incarnations** (*human forms of God*) and with incense burning, he meditates. He also thinks of Buddha, Mohammed, and Jesus as incarnations and sometimes reads from the scriptures being inspired by their teachings, although they represent other major religions.

Despite this vast array of deities and the recognition that all religions are valid, Rama believes in one universal concept: **Brahman**, the *Divine Intelligence*, the *Supreme Reality*. Rama believes that all paths lead to the understanding that this "reality" exists as part of all physical beings, especially humans. Rama's entire spiritual quest is directed toward uniting his *inner and real self*, the **atman**, with the concept of Brahman. So, although Rama has gone through several stages of desire—for pleasure, power, wealth, fame, and humanitarianism—the last stage, his desire for freedom, for touching the infinite, is his main goal. Figure 3-2 expresses that journey.

---
*See the symbol at the beginning of this section. A transliteration of the script is *a, u, m*. It is written in English as *Om*, or *Aum*. *Om*, *God*, and *Brahman* are synonymous and mean a *consciousness* or *awareness* rather than a personified being.

**Figure 3-1** The Golden Rule

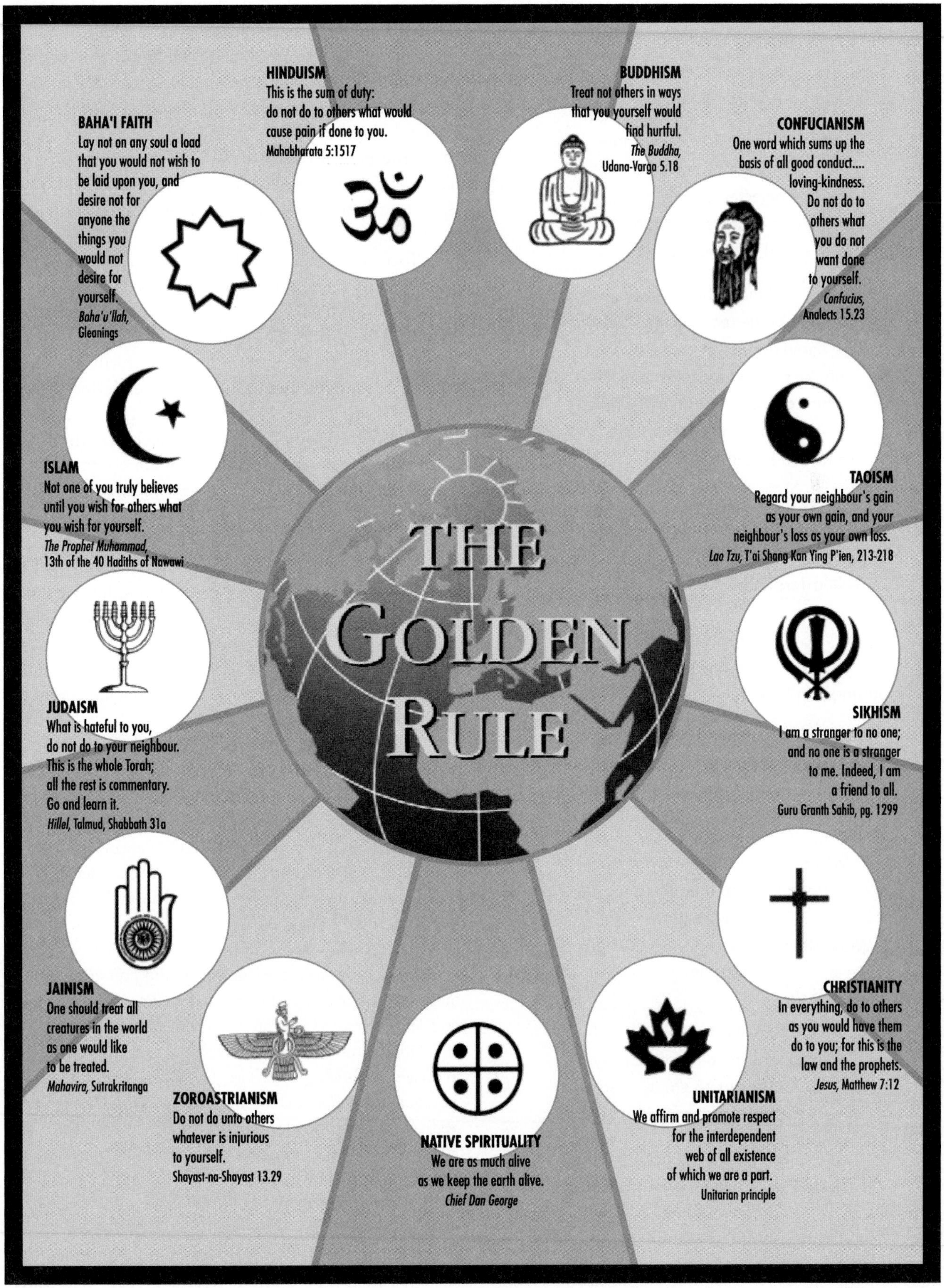

**BAHA'I FAITH**
Lay not on any soul a load that you would not wish to be laid upon you, and desire not for anyone the things you would not desire for yourself.
*Baha'u'llah,* Gleanings

**HINDUISM**
This is the sum of duty: do not do to others what would cause pain if done to you.
Mahabharata 5:1517

**BUDDHISM**
Treat not others in ways that you yourself would find hurtful.
*The Buddha,* Udana-Varga 5.18

**CONFUCIANISM**
One word which sums up the basis of all good conduct.... loving-kindness. Do not do to others what you do not want done to yourself.
*Confucius,* Analects 15.23

**ISLAM**
Not one of you truly believes until you wish for others what you wish for yourself.
*The Prophet Muhammad,* 13th of the 40 Hadiths of Nawawi

**TAOISM**
Regard your neighbour's gain as your own gain, and your neighbour's loss as your own loss.
*Lao Tzu,* T'ai Shang Kan Ying P'ien, 213-218

**JUDAISM**
What is hateful to you, do not do to your neighbour. This is the whole Torah; all the rest is commentary. Go and learn it.
*Hillel,* Talmud, Shabbath 31a

**THE GOLDEN RULE**

**SIKHISM**
I am a stranger to no one; and no one is a stranger to me. Indeed, I am a friend to all.
Guru Granth Sahib, pg. 1299

**JAINISM**
One should treat all creatures in the world as one would like to be treated.
*Mahavira,* Sutrakritanga

**ZOROASTRIANISM**
Do not do unto others whatever is injurious to yourself.
Shayast-na-Shayast 13.29

**NATIVE SPIRITUALITY**
We are as much alive as we keep the earth alive.
*Chief Dan George*

**UNITARIANISM**
We affirm and promote respect for the interdependent web of all existence of which we are a part.
Unitarian principle

**CHRISTIANITY**
In everything, do to others as you would have them do to you; for this is the law and the prophets.
*Jesus,* Matthew 7:12

Note: This is a reduced version of a 56 x 74 cm four-colour poster available in Canada from Broughton Books, sales@bbroughton.com, and in USA from Pflaum Publishing, service@pflaum.com. Used with permission.

**Figure 3-2** Gita is a way of life. (Written by A.D. Desai, Boulder, Co.)

**GITA IS A WAY OF LIFE**
a way of karma—
a way to Moksha

Like a lamp of a steady flame
Not overjoyed by achievements.
Nor dejected by calamities.
One observes the light
and darkness evenly.

Reigning the senses,
Within the reasonable limits
knowing that atma is eternal
unlike physical existence of self—
which changes from time to time,
bound by one's karmas and
controlled by the "treacherous" mind

But the wise one
bows to the Lord in humility
in the "wake" of humble surrender
offers karma without desire
For this can only be led by
"Gyana" the light
That enlightens by the practice of
uniting mind and body to a peaceful Omkar.

Unyielding to one's pride & passion
Persisting destructive thoughts,
Undisillusioned by the illusions
of this world as "Maya."

Where—what is there is not there
But what doesn't seem to be there (atma) is very
much present
When the veil is unfurled by the light of
"Gyana"

One reaches the Lord even by the feel of
His existence—
One opens the path of eternity
—a journey to an empty road
Where the tripti of the desired senses
Have evaporated in the air as the water takes
the form of vapour
It's then that one realizes . . . the blissful
state of atma
Vibrating OM! OM!! OM!! chanting
"Om Namo Bhagawate Vasudevaya. Om!!"

Rama is interested in health and illness only as a guide to this goal. He feels that the human love for the body is a cause for illness. He says, for example, that if we overeat we get a stomach ache. He views the pain as a warning—in this case, to stop overeating. He does not oppose medical treatment if absolutely necessary, but he believes that medicine can sometimes dull the pain and then the person overeats again, thus perpetuating the cause of the problem. Medical or psychiatric help, Rama says, is at best transitory. The cause of the pain must be rooted out.

To avoid dwelling on physical concerns, Rama strives for moderation in eating and in other body functions. He considers only the atman as real and eternal and the body as unreal and finite. The body is a temple, a vehicle, no more. He tries to take care of it so that it will not scream at him because of overindulgence or underindulgence. Rama is a vegetarian. He believes that meat and intoxicants would excite his senses too much. Yet the Hindu diet pattern is flexible; definite rules are not set. If Rama is sick, he tries to bear his illness with resignation, knowing its temporary nature. He believes that the prayer of supplication for body cure is the lowest form of prayer, whereas the highest form is devotion to God. To him, death and rebirth are nearly synonymous, for the atman never changes and always remains pure. He compares the atman to the ocean: as ocean water can be put into various containers without changing its nature, so can the atman be put into various physical and human containers without changing its nature.

Thus, if death is imminent, Rama believes that the body, mind, and senses weaken and become lifeless but that the never-changing atman is ready to enter into a new form of life, depending on the person's knowledge, deeds, and past experiences. Full acceptance of death is encouraged. Death is a friend to be faced bravely, calmly, and confidently.

Rama says that as a devotee of God he is following a *training course* called **yoga**. As a preliminary, however, he must establish certain moral qualifications. He must strive for self-control, self-discipline, cleanliness, and contentment. He must avoid injury, deceitfulness, and stealing. His overwhelming desire to reach God can be implemented through one or a combination of the four yoga paths: (1) **inana yoga** through *reading and absorbing knowledge*; (2) **bhakti yoga** through the *devotion of emotion and love*; (3) **karma yoga** through *work dedicated to God*; and (4) **raja yoga** through *psychological experiments on oneself*. Rama combines the first three by reading and memorizing portions of the ancient scriptures, by meditating daily at his shrine, and by dedicating the results of his professional work to God.

Rama mentions that various forms of yoga have spread around the world to form hybrid groups with varied purposes. One branch that has appeared in medical centres is **hatha yoga**, meaning *sun and moon, symbolizing an inner balance that is achieved through muscle and breathing exercises*. Ultimately, the body is prepared for meditation through these exercises.

From the bhakti emphasis comes **Sikhism**, founded by Nanak, who was born in 1469. The Sikhs had nine other gurus, or spiritual mentors, who sequentially taught that God was the one and only reality. The fifth guru compiled the scripture. Starting as a pacifist group, the Sikhs evolved to warriors.

For Rama, religion is not something to be picked up and put down according to a schedule or one's mood. It is a constant and all-pervading part of his life, every value and action, and the life of his country. India's literature and art are witness to this fact. Religion also influences family life and structure. Basically, marriage is for life, and people usually marry someone at the same social level. The husband is treated with respect, and the mother is thought of as ideal. The family is patrifocal; the father usually has final authority. All family members are close. Elders are respected, cared for when they are ill, and considered as experienced models; children and grandchildren seek their wisdom. Children have reverence for both father and mother, and backtalk is unthinkable. Friends are to be treated as brothers and sisters, and visitors are always treated congenially.

Rama will be married soon and gives us some insight into the ceremony and meaning. The traditional Indian wedding customs were formulated more than 5000 years ago. Each ceremony, each occasion, and each ritual has a deep philosophical meaning and purpose. The ceremony is performed in Sanskrit, the most ancient surviving language in the world. It is meant to unite two souls so firmly that after they are married, although their bodies remain separate, their souls merge and become spiritually one. Thus, divorce is unacceptable.[20]

First, eight sacred blessings are given. Then the groom is welcomed amid recitations including the five elements. The bride follows the bridesmaids and grooms-men and is welcomed following an exchange of garlands between bride and groom. The couple declares their union and ties together the ends of scarves that each is wearing. The bride and groom then walk around a fire (purifier), taking seven sacred steps, each signifying vows and promises made to each other. Finally, the rings are exchanged.[21]

---

## CRITICAL THINKING

*How effectively do you see yourself being able to relate to a client who lives by the teachings of Sikhism?*

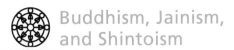

# Buddhism, Jainism, and Shintoism

Umeko Sato is a member of the sect of **Buddhism** called **Soka Gakkai**. This sect is a powerful religion in Japan, with a government party, a university, and a grand temple representing it. This organization, which includes about 10 percent of Japan's population, known previously as a militant proselytizing group, has toned down this phase and is living more graciously with other sects and creeds. Based on the **Lotus Sutra**, *part of the Buddhist scriptures*, its doctrine advocates the three values of happiness: profit, goodness, and beauty. Sato is attracted by the practicality of the teaching, the mottoes that she can live by, the emphasis on small group study, and present world benefits, especially healing.

Although Sato's beliefs at some points seem in direct contrast to the original Buddhist teachings, she is happy to explain the rich multi-religious tradition that her family has had for generations. She emphasizes that she is affected by the **Confucian** emphasis on the family unit, by Christianity's healing emphasis, by **Shintoism**, the state religion of Japan until 1945, and by **Buddhism**, which originated about 600 B.C. in India with a Hindu named Siddhartha Gautama.

Currently, approximately 90 percent of Japan's people adhere to both Buddhism and Shintoism, although the nation has never been known as devout. Less than 1 percent is Christian. Another small religion is **Jainism**. The "Jains" hark back to the 6th century B.C., about the same time as Buddha. Their fundamental tenet is **ahimsa**, *a refusal to injure any living thing*. Jains believe that every living thing has a soul. Although the Jains are found in Japan and other countries, they probably are known best for their bird hospital in Old Delhi, India, which treats 20 000 birds each year.

Gautama, shortly after a historic enlightenment experience during which he became the Buddha, preached a sermon to his followers and drew on the earth a wheel representing the continuous round of life and death and rebirth. Later, eight spokes were added to illustrate the sermon and to provide the most explicit visual symbol of Buddhism today.* Sato repeats Buddha's four noble truths: (1) life is disjointed or out of balance, especially in birth, old age, illness, and death; (2) the cause of this imbalance is ignorance of one's own true nature; (3) removal of this ignorance is attained by reaching **Nirvana**, *the divine state of release*, the *ultimate reality*, the *perfect knowledge* via (4) the eightfold path.

The eight spokes of the wheel represent the eightfold path used to reach Nirvana. Sato says that followers subscribe to right knowledge, right intentions, right speech, right conduct, right means of livelihood, right effort, right

---

*See the symbol at the beginning of this section.

mindfulness, and concentration. From these concepts has arisen a moral code that, among other things, prohibits intoxicants, lying, and killing of any kind (which explains why Buddhists are often vegetarians).

Sato explains that she cannot omit mention of the *one austere movement within the Mahayana branch*, the **Zen sect**. Taking this example from Gautama's extended contemplation of a flower, Zen followers care little for discourse, books, or other symbolic interpretations and explanations of reality. Hours and years are devoted to meditation, contemplation of word puzzles, and consultation with a Zen master. In seeking absolute honesty and truthfulness through such simple acts as drinking tea or gardening, the Zen student hopes to experience enlightenment. In North America, a version of Buddhism called *Buddhaharma* is emerging. Women and men are considered equal. This group provides meditations for the public on a CD-ROM disk.

Sato next turns to her former state religion, **Shintoism**. Whereas Buddhism produced a solemnizing effect on her country, Shintoism had an affirmative and joyous effect. Emperor, ancestor, ancient hero, and nature worship form its core. Those who follow Shintoism, she says, feel an intense loyalty and devotion to every lake, tree, and blossom in Japan and to the ancestral spirits abiding there. They also have a great concern for cleanliness, a carryover from early ideas surrounding dread of pollution in the dead.

Sato says that her parents have two god shelves in their home. One contains wooden tablets inscribed with the name of the household's patron deity and a symbolic form of the goddess of rice and other texts and objects of family significance. There her family performs simple rites such as offering a prayer or a food gift each day. In a family crisis, perhaps an illness, the family conducts more elaborate rites, such as lighting tapers or offering rice brandy. The other god shelf, in another room, is the Buddha shelf; if a family member dies, a Buddhist priest, the spiritual leader, performs specified rituals there.

Shintoism and Buddhism perceive death as a "natural" process that marks the finality of the body inhabited by the person in this life, not the end of life itself.[22]

Buddhism teaches the living how to die well. The elderly, or feeble, are to prepare themselves mentally for a state that would be conducive for a good rebirth. The person is to remain watchful and alert in the face of death, to resist distraction and confusion, to be lucid and calm. Distinct instructions are given as to what to expect as life leaves the body, as the person enters an intermediary state, and as Nirvana is about to occur.

So, although Sato has grasped a new religious path for herself, her respect for tradition remains.

In giving care to a person with Umeko Sato's background, be aware of the varied religious influences on her life.

The sect's emphasis on the here and now, rather than on the long road to Nirvana, may place a high value on physical health so that the person can benefit from the joys and beauty of this life. The person may readily voice impatience with the body's dysfunction. You, too, can respond to the great concern for cleanliness, the desire to have family nearby, and the need for family rites that are offered for the sick member. Should a family member be dying, you may see some ambivalence. The family member may want to prepare him- or herself in the traditional way, but someone with Sato's background, with emphasis on present world benefits and healing, may deny that there is a valid preparation for death.

 Confucianism and Taoism

Wong Huieng is a young teacher in Taiwan simultaneously influenced by **Taoism**, the *romantic and mystical*, and **Confucianism**, the *practical and pragmatic*. To provide insights into these Chinese modes of thinking, although it is more representative of Taoism, Wong Huieng uses the **yin–yang symbol**.* The symbol is a circle, representing **Tao** or the *absolute*, in which two tear shapes fit perfectly into one another, each containing a small dot from the other. Generally **yang** is *light or red*, and **yin** is *dark*. Ancient Chinese tradition says that everything exists in these two interacting forces. Each represents a group of qualities. **Yang** is *positive or masculine—dry, hot, active, moving, and light*. **Yin** is *feminine or negative—wet, cold, passive, restful, and empty*. For example, fire is almost pure yang and water almost pure yin, but not quite. The *combination of yin and yang constitutes all the dualisms a person can imagine*: day–night, summer–winter, beauty–ugliness, illness–health, life–death. Both qualities are necessary for life in the universe; they are complementary and, if in harmony, good. Yang and yin energy forces are embodied in the body parts and affect food preferences and eating habits.

Huieng translates this symbol into a relaxed philosophy of life: "If I am sick, I will get better. Life is like going up and down a mountain; sometimes I feel good and sometimes I feel bad. That's the way it is." Although educated, she is not interested in climbing the job ladder, accumulating wealth, or conquering nature. Her goal is to help provide money to build an orphanage in a natural wooded setting.

Huieng thinks of death as a natural part of life, as the peace that comes when the body is worn out. She admits, however, that when her father died, human grief took hold of her. Before his death, her mother went to the Taoist temple priest and got some incense that was to help cast the sickness from his body. After death, they kept his body in

---

*See the symbol at the beginning of this section.

the house for the required time, 49 days. The priest executed a special ceremony every seven days. Her mother could cry only one hour daily, from 2:00 until 3:00 in the morning. Now her mother talks through the priest to her father's ghost. Although Huieng regards this practice as superstitious and thinks that painting a picture of a lake and mountain is a more fitting way to erase her grief, she looks at the little yellow bag, containing a blessing from the priest, hanging around her neck, and finds it comforting if not intellectually acceptable.

Now Huieng turns to her practical side and talks about **Confucius**, the *first saint of the nation*. Although **Lao-tzu**, the *founder of Taoism*, is a semi-legendary figure said to have vanished after he wrote the *bible of Taoism*, **Tao-te-ching**, Confucius has a well-documented existence.

Confucius, born in 551 B.C., wrote little. His disciples wrote the **Analects**, *short proverbs, embodying his teachings*. He is revered as a teacher, not as a god. Huieng does not ask him to bless her but tries to emulate him and his teachings, which she has heard since birth. The temple in his memory is a place for studying, not for praying. And on his birthday, a national holiday, people pay respect to their teachers in his memory.

Five important terms in Confucius' teaching are **Jen**, *a striving for goodness within*; **Chun-sui**, *establishing a gentlemanly or womanly approach with others*; **Li**, *knowing how relationships should be conducted and having respect for age*; **Te**, *leading by virtuous character rather than by force*; and **Wen**, *pursuing the arts as an adjunct to moral character*. Huieng stresses that the directives for family relationships are found in Li. So strongly did Confucius feel about the family that he gave directives on proper attitudes between father and son, elder brother and junior brother, and husband and wife. Also, Huieng believes she cannot harm her body because it was given to her by her parents. Her concept of immediate family includes grandparents, uncles, aunts, and cousins. Her language has more words for relationships between relatives than the English language does.

Huieng believes that in caring for her body, she cares for her family, the country, and the universe. Essentially, to her, all people are family.

Important in your understanding of a person with Wong Huieng's background is the dualism that exists in such thinking. Acceptance of the particular version of mysticism and practicality and of the yin and yang forces that are seen as operating within self will help in building a foundation of personalized care.

The person may have more respect for older than younger staff members and may respond well to teaching. There may be a strong desire to attain and maintain wellness. These factors are directly related to the religious teaching, and you can use them to enhance care. Additionally, talk slowly to the person if language is an issue. Rely on family members to help you understand the person's feelings. Permit familiar foods. Remember that foods are divided into appropriate groups for types of illness. Address the person by the proper name. Do not use excessive touch signals unless they are invited. Remember, this person may be in awe of health care authority and may be intimidated.

 Islam

Omar Ali is *Muslim*, a member of **Islam**, the youngest of the major world religions.* "There is no God but Allah; Muhammad is His Prophet"† provides the key to Omar's beliefs. He must say this but once in his life as a requirement, but he will repeat it many times as an affirmation. Muslims believe in a final judgment day when everyone will be judged and sent either to Paradise or to the fire of hell, depending on how justly he or she lived life according to God's laws. They believe that everyone, except children before the age of puberty, are responsible for their own good and bad actions and deeds and that no one can intercede on behalf of another.

Omar has also been influenced by 3000-year-old **Zoroastrianism**, which is *a religion of pre-Islamic Iran* that flourishes in Bombay today. Likewise, it was a monotheistic religion even though dualism was also espoused.

Omar is an Egyptian physician whose religious tradition was revealed through Muhammad, born approximately A.D. 571 in Mecca, then a trading point between India and Syria on the Arabian Peninsula. Hating polytheism and paganism in any form, Muhammad recited God's revelation to him as is documented in the **Quran**,‡ *scriptures*. Omar believes in the biblical prophets, but he calls Muhammad the greatest—the seal of Prophets.

Through the Quran and the **Hadith**, *the traditions*, Omar has guidelines for his thinking, devotional life, and social obligations. He believes that he is a unique individual with an eternal soul. He believes in a heaven and hell, and while on earth he wants to walk the straight path.

To keep on this path, Omar prays five times a day: generally on rising, at midday, in the afternoon, in the early evening, and before retiring. Articles needed are water and a prayer rug. Because the Quran emphasizes cleanliness of body, Omar performs a ritual washing with running water over the face, arms, top of head, and feet before each prayer. Omar explains that for the bedridden client this

---

*A portion of this section was contributed by Caroline Samiezadé-Yazd, RN, MSN, PNP.

†These words are a translation of the sacred calligraphy in the symbol shown at the beginning of this section. The prophet's name is sometimes spelled Mohammad.

‡Sometimes spelled *Koran*.

requirement can be accomplished by pouring water out of some sort of receptacle. If a Muslim's entire body is considered ritually unclean, he or she must wash the entire body. If water is unavailable or the person cannot bathe, clean soil may be used in place of the ritual washing. After this washing, the Muslim needs either a ritually clean cloth or a prayer rug and a clean place to pray. He or she may not face a dirty area such as the bathroom when praying, even if this area is in the line toward Mecca. The Muslim must physically readjust in this case to comply with Islamic regulations. Then, facing Mecca, the Muslim goes through a series of prescribed bodily motions and repeats various passages in praise and supplication.

Omar observes **Ramadan**, *a fast month*,* during which time he eats or drinks nothing from sunrise to sunset; after sunset he takes nourishment only in moderation. He explains **fasting** (*abstinence from eating*) as a discipline that aids him in understanding those with little food and, more importantly, as a submission to Allah. At the end of Ramadan, he enters a festive period with feelings of goodwill and gift exchanges. The sick, the very old, pregnant and lactating mothers, children, and Muslims who require the ingestion or injection of substances throughout the day hours are exempt without penalty from practice of this belief.

Omar has made one pilgrimage to Mecca, another requirement for all healthy and financially able Muslims. He believes that the experience created a great sense of brotherhood, for all of the pilgrims wore similar modest clothing, exchanged news of followers in various lands, and reviewed their mutual faith. The twelfth day of the pilgrimage month is the **Feast of Sacrifice (Eida-Fita)**, when all Muslim families kill a lamb in honour of Abraham's offering of his son to God.

In line with the Quran's teaching, Omar does not eat pork (including such items as bologna, which may contain partial pork products). He does not gamble, drink intoxicants, use illicit drugs, or engage in religiously unlawful sexual practices such as premarital sex, homosexuality, and infidelity. The emphasis on strict moral upbringing includes dating, dancing, drinking, and sex outside marriage, and all are forbidden. This emphasis puts the Muslim on a common ground with conservative Christians. Abstinence from drug use also helps to eliminate many potential health and social problems.

Omar worships no images or pictures of Muhammad because the prophet is not deified. Nor does he hang or display pictures of any prophet or any god or worship statues or religious symbols. He gives a portion of his money to the poor, because Islam advocates a responsibility to society.

Omar points out that not all Arabs are Muslims, and not all Muslims are Arabs. Arabs come from a number of nations stretching from Morocco to the Persian Gulf. Persons who are Arab Muslims speak Arabic and uphold the tenets of Islam. Omar emphasizes the importance of gaining specific knowledge about their complex social structure. The centrality of religion and the family are closely related, and this centrality reflects many aspects of health care.

Omar mentions that parts of the basic Islam faith are used by an American-based group commonly known as the **Black Muslims (Nation of Islam)**. Known to have stringent, seclusionist rules, the Black Muslims are rapidly increasing in number and power. They seem to be moving away from orthodox Islam. Members may not become politically involved. Membership is especially appealing to young black men who are attracted to the masculine focus, the structure, and the emphasis on self-help and self-esteem.

Omar outlines the ideas of his religion as it applies to his profession. He believes that he can make a significant contribution to health care, but also believes that what happens is essentially God's will. Submission to God is the very meaning of Islam. This belief produces a very fluid feeling of time, and it promotes a sense of fatalism. Planning ahead for a Muslim is not as strong a value as it is in Western culture. It is believed that if God's will is defied, the evil eye will appear.

Muslim clients who are ill are excused from many, but not all, religious rules, but many will still want to follow them as closely as possible. Even though in a body cast and unable to get out of bed, a client may want to go through prayers symbolically. The person might recite the first chapters of the Quran, centred on praise to Allah, which are often used in times of crises. Family is a great comfort in illness, and praying with a group is strengthening, but the Muslim has no priest; the relationship is directly with God. Some clients may seem fatalistic, completely resigned to death, whereas others, hoping it is God's will that they live, co-operate vigorously with the medical program. Muslims do not discuss death openly, because if they did, the client and family may lose all hope and the client could die as a result. Instead, Muslims tend to communicate grief in gradual stages rather than immediately and all at once. Further, they make it a point never to let the affected person lose hope. Even in the gravest of situations, the family will not attempt to prepare for the death even when it is imminent. After death, a body must be washed with running water by a Muslim and the hands folded in prayer. Muslims do not perform autopsies, embalm, or use caskets for burials. Instead, they wrap a white linen cloth around the dead person and place the body into the ground facing Mecca. Knowledge of these attitudes and traditions can greatly enhance your care.

*Coming during the ninth month of the Muslim year, always at a different time each year by the Western calendar, and sometimes spelled *Ramazan*.

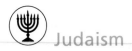

# Judaism

Seth Lieberman, strongly influenced by the emphasis on social concern in **Judaism**, is a psychiatrist. In the Jewish community, each member is expected to contribute to others' needs according to his or her ability. Jews have traditionally considered their community as a whole responsible for feeding the hungry, helping the widowed and orphaned, rescuing the captured, and even burying the dead. Jewish retirement homes, senior citizens' centres, and medical centres are witnesses to this philosophy.

Seth cannot remember when his religious instruction began—it was always there. He went through the motions and felt the emotion of the Sabbath eve with its candles and cup of sanctification long before he could comprehend his father's explanations. Book learning followed, however, and he came to understand the fervency with which his people study and live the law as given in the **Torah**, *the first five books of the Bible*, and in the **Talmud**, *a commentary and enlargement of the Torah*. His spiritual leader is the *rabbi*. His *spiritual symbol* is the **menorah**.*

His own *entrance into a responsible religious life and manhood* was through the **bar mitzvah**, a ceremony that took place in the synagogue when he was 13. Girls are also educated to live responsible religious lives, and congregations now have a ceremony similar to the bar mitzvah, called the **bat mitzvah**, for girls.

Although he was raised in an Orthodox home, Seth and his family are now members of the Reform sect. He mentions another group, the Conservatives. The **Orthodox** followers *believe that God gave the law*. It was written exactly as He gave it; and *it should be followed precisely*. **Reform Jews** *believe that the law was written by inspired men* at various times and therefore is *subject to reinterpretation*. Seth says he follows the traditions because he values traditions, rather than because God demands it. **Conservatives** *are in the middle, taking some practices from both groups*. Overriding any differences in interpretation of ritual and tradition is the fundamental concept expressed in the prayer "Hear, O Israel, the Lord our God, the Lord is One." Not only is He one, He loves His creation, wants His people to live justly, and wants to bless their food, drink, and celebration. Judaism's double theme might be expressed as "Enjoy life now, and share it with God." Understandably then, Seth's religious emphasis is not on an afterlife, although some Jewish people believe in one. Jews have had a history of

suffering, but the inherent value of suffering or illness is not stressed. Through their observance of the law, the belief of their historical role as God's chosen people, and their hope for better days, Jews have survived seemingly insurmountable persecution.

Seth offers guidelines for working with a Jewish person in a hospital or nursing home. Although Jewish law can be suspended when a person is ill, the client will be most comfortable following as many practices as possible.

Every Jew observes the **Sabbath**, *a time for spiritual refreshment, from sundown on Friday to shortly after sundown on Saturday*. During this period, Orthodox Jews may refuse freshly cooked food, medicine, treatment, surgery, and use of radio, television, and writing equipment lest the direction of their thinking be diverted on this special day. An Orthodox male may want to wear a **yarmulke** or *skullcap* continuously, use a *prayer book* called **Siddur**, and use **phylacteries**, *leather strips with boxes containing scriptures*, at weekday morning prayer. Also, the ultra-Orthodox male may refuse to use a razor because of the Levitical ban on shaving.

Some Orthodox Jewish women observe the rite of **mikvah**, *an ancient ritual of family purity*. From marriage to menopause (except when pregnant) these women have no physical or sexual relations with their husbands from 24 hours before menstruation until 12 days later when a ritual immersion in water renders them ready to meet their husbands again.

Jewish dietary laws have been considered by some scholars as health measures: to enjoy life is to eat properly and in moderation. The Orthodox, however, obey them because God so commanded. Food is called **treyfe** (or *treyfah*) if it is *unfit*; and **kosher** if it is *ritually correct*.

Forbidden food sources include pig, horse, shrimp, lobster, crab, oyster, and fowl that are birds of prey. Meats approved are from those animals that are ruminants and have divided hooves. Approved fish must have both fins and scales. Also, kosher animals must be healthy and slaughtered in a prescribed manner. Because of the Biblical passage that says not to soak a young goat in its mother's milk, Jews do not eat meat products and milk products together. Neither the utensils used to cook these products, nor the dishes from which these products are eaten are ever intermixed.

*Guidelines for a satisfactory diet* for the Orthodox are as follows:

- Serve milk products first, meat second. Meat can be eaten a few minutes after milk, but milk cannot be taken for six hours after meat.

- If a person completely refuses meat because of incorrect slaughter, encourage a vegetarian diet with protein supplements, such as fish and eggs, which are considered neutral unless prepared with milk or meat fat.

---

*See the symbol at beginning of this section. The seven-branched candelabrum stands for the creation of the universe in seven days, the centre light symbolizes the Sabbath, and the candlelight symbolizes the presence of God in the Temple.

- Buy frozen kosher products marked *U*, *K*, or *pareve*.
- Heat and serve food in the original container and use plastic utensils.

Two important holy days are Rosh Hashanah and Yom Kippur. **Rosh Hashanah**, *the Jewish New Year*, is a time to meet with the family, give thanks to God for good health, and renew traditions. **Yom Kippur**, the *Day of Atonement*, is a time for asking forgiveness of family members for wrongs done, and it occurs ten days later. On Yom Kippur, Jews fast for 24 hours, a symbolic act of self-denial, mourning, and petition. **Tisha B'av**, the *day of lamentation*, recalling the destruction of both Temples of Jerusalem, is another 24-hour fast period. **Pesach** or **Passover** (eight days for Orthodox and Conservative, seven days for Reform) *celebrates the ancient Jews' deliverance from Egyptian bondage*. **Matzo**, *unleavened bread*, replaces leavened bread during this period.

Some say that the Jewish person is preoccupied with health. Jews are future-oriented and want to know diagnosis and how a disease will affect business, family life, and social life. The Jewish people as a whole are highly educated, and although they respect the doctor, they may obtain several medical opinions before carrying out a treatment plan.

Although family, friends, and a rabbi may visit the ill, especially on or near holidays, they will also come at other times. Visiting the sick is a religious duty. And although death is final to many Jews, except for living on in the memories of others, guidelines exist for this time. When a Jewish person has suffered irreversible brain damage and can no longer say a **bracha**, *a blessing to praise God*, or perform a **mitzvah**, *an act to help a fellow*, he or she is considered a "vegetable" with nothing to save. Prolonging the life by artificial means may not be recommended. But until then, the dying client must be treated as the complete person he or she always was, capable of conducting his or her own affairs and entering into relationships.

Jewish tradition says never to leave the bedside of the dying person. Knowledge of this tradition can be of value to the dying and the mourners. The dying soul should leave in the presence of people, and the mourner is shielded from the guilt of thinking that the client was alone at death or that more could have been done. The bedside vigil also serves as a time to encourage a personal confession by the dying, which is a *rite of passage* to another phase of existence (even though unknown). This type of confessional is said throughout the Jewish life cycle whenever one stage has been completed. Confessional on the deathbed is a recognition that one cycle is ending and another cycle is beginning. Recitation of the *Shema* in the last moments before death helps the dying to affirm faith in God and focus on the most familiar rituals of life.

Immediate burial and specified mourning also move the remaining loved ones through the crisis period. (Note, however, that if a Jew dies on the Sabbath, he or she cannot be moved, except by a non-Jew, until sundown.) After the burial, the mourners are fed a meal of replenishment called *se'udat havra'ah*. This step symbolizes the rallying of the community and the sustenance of life for the remaining. Also, Jews follow the custom of **sitting shiva** or *visiting with remaining relatives for one week after the death*.

Judaism identifies a *year of mourning*. The first three days are of deep grief; clothes may be torn to symbolize the tearing of a life from others. Seven days of lesser mourning follow, leading to 30 days of gradual readjustment. The remainder of the year calls for remembrance and healing. During that year, a prayer called the mourner's *Kaddish* is recited in religious services. It helps convey the feeling of support for the mourner. At the annual anniversary of death, a candle is burned and special prayers are said.

So from circumcision of the male infant on the eighth day after birth to his deathbed, and from the days of the original menorah in the sanctuary in the wilderness until the present day, the followers of Judaism re-enact their traditions. Because many of these traditions remain an intrinsic part of the Jew, even when striving to maintain or regain wellness, the preceding guidelines offer a foundation for knowledgeable care.

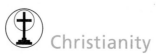

## Christianity

Beth Meyer, a *Roman Catholic*, Demetrius Callas, an *Eastern Orthodox*, and Jean Taylor, a *Protestant*, are Christian nurses representing the three major branches of **Christianity**. Although Christianity divided into Eastern Orthodox and Roman Catholicism in A.D. 1054, and the Protestant Reformation provided a third division in the 16th century, these nurses share some basic beliefs, most importantly that Jesus Christ, as described in the Bible, is God's son. When Jesus was born in Palestine, "B.C." changed to "A.D." The details of His 33 years are few, but His deeds and words recorded in the Bible's New Testament show quiet authority, loving humility, and an ability to perform miracles and to visit easily with people in varied social positions.

The main symbol of Christianity is the cross,* but it signifies more than a wooden structure on which Jesus was crucified. It also symbolizes the finished redemption—Christ rising from the dead and ascending to the Father to rule with Him and continuously pervade the personal lives of His followers.

Christians observe **Christmas** as *Christ's birthday*; **Lent** as a *season of penitence and self-examination preceding*

---

*See the symbol at the beginning of this section.

**Good Friday,** *Christ's crucifixion day,* and **Easter,** *His Resurrection day.*

Beth, Demetrius, and Jean rely on the New Testament as a guideline for their lives. They believe that Jesus was fully God and fully man at the same time, that their original sin (which they accept as a basic part of themselves) can be forgiven, and that they are acceptable to God because of Jesus Christ's life and death. They believe that God is three persons: the Father, the Son, and the Holy Spirit (Holy Ghost), the last providing a spirit of love and truth.

Beth, Demetrius, and Jean differ in some worship practices and theology, but all highly regard their individuality as children of God, and they hope for life with God after death. They feel responsible for their own souls, the *spiritual dimension of themselves,* and for aiding the spiritual needs of their patients.

**Roman Catholic Church** Roman Catholicism, according to Beth, is a religion based on the dignity of the person as a social, intellectual, and spiritual being made in the image of God. She traces the teaching authority of the church through the scriptures: God sent His Son to provide salvation and redemption from sin. He established the Church to continue His work after ascension into heaven. Jesus chose apostles to preach, teach, and guide. He appointed Saint Peter as the Church's head to preserve unity and to have authority over the apostles. The mission given by Jesus to Saint Peter and the apostles is the same that continues to the present through the Pope and his bishops. Beth notes that in the last several years, women in the Roman Catholic Church—both nuns and laywomen—are speaking out more on issues and are asking for more recognition and respect as God's spokespeople.

Beth believes that the seven **Sacraments** are *grace-giving rites that give her a share in Christ's own life and help sustain her in her efforts to follow His example.* The Sacraments that are received once in life are Baptism, Confirmation, Holy Orders, and usually Matrimony.

Through **baptism,** Catholics believe that the *soul is incorporated into the life of Christ and shares His divinity.* Any infant in danger of death should be baptized, even an aborted fetus. If a priest is not available, you can perform the sacrament by pouring water on the forehead and saying, "I baptize thee in the name of the Father, of the Son, and of the Holy Spirit." The healthy baby is baptized some time during the first weeks of life. Adults are also baptized when they convert to Catholicism and join the church.

**Confirmation** *is the sacrament in which the Holy Spirit is imparted in a fuller measure to help strengthen the individual in his or her spiritual life.* **Matrimony** *acknowledges the love and lifelong commitment, usually between a man and a woman.* **Holy Orders** *ordain deacons and priests.*

The Sacraments that may be received more than once are **Penance** (*confession*), the **Eucharist** (*Holy Communion*), and the **Anointing of the Sick** (*sacrament of the Sick*). Beth believes that **Penance,** *an acknowledgment and forgiveness of her sins in the presence of a priest,* should be received according to individual need even though it is required only once a year by church law. The **Mass,** often called the **Eucharist,** is the *liturgical celebration whose core is the sacrament of the Holy Eucharist.* Bread and wine are consecrated and become the body and blood of Christ. The body and blood are then received in Holy Communion.

The Eucharist is celebrated daily, and all Roman Catholics are encouraged to participate as often as possible. They are required by church law to attend on Sundays (or late Saturdays) and on specified holy days throughout the year, unless prevented by illness or some other serious reason.

Beth is glad that the Anointing of the Sick has been modified and broadened, and she explains the rite to client and family to allay anxiety. Formerly known as Extreme Unction, or the last rites, this sacrament was reserved for those near death. Now **Anointing of the Sick,** *symbolic of Christ's healing love and the concern of the Christian community,* can provide spiritual strength to those less gravely ill. After anointing with oil, the priest offers prayers for the forgiveness of sin and for the restoration of health. Whenever possible, the family should be present to join in the prayers.

If the client is dying, extraordinary artificial measures to maintain life may be unnecessary. At the hour of death, the priest offers Communion to the dying person by means of a special formula. This final Communion is called *Viaticum.* In sudden deaths, the priest should be called and the anointing and Viaticum should be administered if possible. If the person is dead when the priest arrives, there is no anointing, but the priest leads the family in prayer for the person who just died.

Beth divides the Roman Catholic funeral into three phases: the **wake,** *a period of waiting or vigil during which the body is viewed and the family is sustained through visiting;* the **funeral mass,** *a prayer service incorporated into the celebration of the Mass;* and the **burial,** *the final act of placing the person in the ground.* (This procedure may vary somewhat, in that some Catholics are now choosing cremation.) The mourners retain the memory of the dead through a Month's Mind Mass, celebrated a month after death, and anniversary masses. Finally, the priest integrates the liturgy for the dead with the whole parish liturgical life.

Beth is convinced that her religious practice contributes to her health. She believes that the body, mind, and spirit work together and that a spirit free of guilt and grievances and fortified with the strength of Christ's life has positive effects on the body. She believes that suffering and illness are allowed by God because of our disobedience (original sin) but that they are not necessarily willed by God or given as punishment for personal sin.

While in the hospital, a Roman Catholic may want to attend Mass, have the priest visit, or receive the Eucharist at bedside. (Fasting an hour before the sacrament is traditional, but in the case of physical illness, fasting is not necessary.) Other symbols that might be comforting are a Bible, prayer book, holy water, lighted candle, crucifix, and rosary.

**Eastern Orthodox Church** The Eastern Orthodox Church, the main denomination, is divided into groups by nationality. The **Greek Eastern Orthodox faith** is discussed by Demetrius. Each group has the **Divine Liturgy**, the *Eucharistic service*, in the native language and sometimes in English also. Although similar in many respects to the Roman Catholic faith, the Eastern Orthodox faith has no pope. The seven sacraments are followed with slight variations. Baptism is by triple immersion: the priest places the infant in a basin of water and pours water on the forehead three times. He then immediately confirms the infant by anointing with holy oil.

If death is imminent for a hospitalized infant and the parents or priest cannot be reached, you can baptize the infant by placing a small amount of water on the forehead three times. Even a symbolic baptism is acceptable, but only a living being should receive the sacrament. Adults who join the church are also baptized and confirmed.

The **Unction of the Sick** has never been practised as a last rite by the Eastern Orthodox; it is a *blessing for the sick*. Confession at least once a year is a prerequisite to participation in the Eucharist, which is taken at least four times a year: at Christmas, at Easter, on the Feast Day of Saint Peter and Saint Paul (June 30), and on the day celebrating the Sleeping of the Virgin Mary (August 15).

Fasting from the last meal in the evening until after **Communion**, another term for the Eucharist, is the general rule. Other fast periods include each Wednesday, representing the seizure of Jesus; each Friday, representing His death; and two 40-day periods, the first before Christmas and the second before Easter.

Fasting, to Demetrius, means that he must avoid meat, dairy products, and olive oil. Its purpose is spiritual betterment, to avoid producing extra energy in the body, and instead to think of the spirit. Fasting is not necessary when ill. Religion should not harm one's health.

Demetrius retains the Eastern influence in his thinking. He envisions his soul as blending in with the spiritual cosmos and his actions as affecting the rest of creation. He is mystically inclined and believes that insights can be gained directly from God. He tells of sharing such an experience with a patient, Mrs. A., also Greek Orthodox.

Mrs. A. had experienced nine surgeries to build up deteriorating bones caused by rheumatoid arthritis. She faced another surgery. Demetrius saw Mrs. A. when he started working at 3:30 p.m. She was depressed, fearful, and crying. Later, at 6:30 p.m., he saw a changed person, fearless and calm, ready for surgery. She explained that she had seen Jesus in a vision, and that He had said, "Go ahead with the surgery. You'll have positive results. But call your priest and take Communion first." Demetrius called the priest, who gave her Communion. She went into surgery the next day with supreme confidence. She now walks.

In addition to Communion, other helpful symbols are prayer books, lighted candles, and holy water. Especially helpful to the Orthodox are **icons**, *pictures of Jesus, Mary, or a revered saint*. Saints can intercede between God and the person. One of the most loved is *Saint Nicholas*, a 3rd-century teacher and father figure who gave his wealth to the poor and became an archbishop. He is honoured on Saint Nicholas Day, December 6, and prayed to continuously for guidance and protection.

Every Sunday morning Demetrius participates in an hour-long liturgy. Sitting in an ornate sanctuary with figures and symbols on the windows, walls, and ceiling, facing the tabernacle containing the holy gifts and scripture, Demetrius finds renewal. He recites, "I believe in one God, the Father Almighty, Maker of Heaven and Earth and of all things visible and invisible; and in one Lord Jesus Christ, the only begotten Son of God."

**Protestantism** There are many Protestant denominations and sects. Jean Taylor is a member of the *Church of God*. She identifies the church by its headquarters because there are some 200 independent church groups in North America using the phrase "Church of God" in their title. Her group evolved late in the 19th century because members of various churches felt that organization and ritual were taking precedence over direction from God. They banded together in a drive toward Christian unity, toward recognition that any people who followed Christ's teachings were members of a universal Church of God and could worship freely together.

This example speaks of one of the chief characteristics of Protestantism: the insistence that God has not given any one person or group of persons sole authority to interpret His truth to others. Protestants use a freedom of spiritual searching and reinterpretation. Thus, new groups form as certain persons and their followers come to believe that they see God's teaching in a new and better light. Jean believes that reading the Bible for historical knowledge and guidance, having a minister to teach and counsel her, and relying on certain worship forms are all important aids. But discerning God's will for her life individually and following that will are her ultimate religious goals.

Jean explains that she "accepted Christ into her life" when she was eight years old. This identified her as personally following the church's teaching rather than just adhering to family religious tradition. A later experience, in which the *Holy Spirit gives the person more spiritual power and discernment*, is called **sanctification**.

Jean defines her corporate worship as free liturgical, with an emphasis on congregational singing, verbal prayer, and Scripture reading. A sermon by the **minister**, *the spiritual leader*, may take half the worship period. As with many Protestant groups, two sacraments or ordinances are observed: (1) baptism (in this case, **believer's**, or **mature**, **baptism** by *total immersion into water*); and (2) Communion. To Protestants, the bread and wine used in Communion are symbolic of Christ's body and blood rather than the actual elements. One additional ordinance practised in Jean's church and among some other groups is **foot washing**, *symbolic of Jesus' washing His disciples' feet*. These ordinances are practised with varied frequencies.

Because of the spectrum of beliefs and practices, defining Protestants, even within a single denomination or sect, is almost impossible (see Table 3-1). Some Protestant groups, retaining their initial emphasis on individual freedom, have allowed no written creed, but expect members to follow an unwritten code of behaviour. Jean does suggest some guidelines, however. She lists some of the main *Protestant bodies* in North America, beginning with the most formal liturgically and sacramental, the *Protestant Episcopal* and *Lutheran* churches. The in-betweens are the *Presbyterians, United Church of Christ, United Methodists*, and *Disciples of Christ (Christian Church)*. The liturgically most free and the least sacramental are the *Baptists* and *Pentecostals*. Bibby states that the established Roman Catholic and Protestant churches continue to monopolize the religion market. The Anglican Church and the United Church of Canada remain powerful religious corporations that are well established and have many followers.[23]

Among these groups, some of the opposing doctrines and practices are as follows: living in sin versus living above sin; predestination versus free will; infant versus believer's baptism; and loose organization versus tightly knit organization. Some uphold **fundamental precepts**, *holding to the Scriptures as infallible*, whereas others uphold **liberal precepts**, *using the Scriptures as a guide, with various interpretations for current living*. Recently, liberal and conservative Christians have become even more divided by subjects such as abortion, same-sex relationships, and what constitutes morality.

With this infinite variety, Jean believes that learning the individual beliefs of her Protestant client is essential. When and if a client wants Communion, whether or not an infant should be baptized, and what will be the most spiritually helpful attention for the patient—these factors are learned through careful listening. Generally, Jean believes that prayer,

a scriptural motto such as "I can do all things through Christ who gives me strength" (Philippians 4:13), or a line from a hymn can give strength to a Protestant. Some patients will also want to be anointed with oil as a symbolic aid to healing.

Jean has discovered that there are great differences within Protestantism, sometimes even within the same denomination, about the theology and rituals of death. Some Protestant theologies have come to grips with the realities and meaning of death, while others block authentic expression of grief by denying death and focusing on "If you are a Christian, you won't be sad."

Some Protestants view death as penalty and punishment for sins, while others see death as a transition when the soul leaves the body for eternal reward, and still others view death as an absolute end. All agree that death is a biological and spiritual event, a mystery not fully comprehended.

Rituals surrounding death vary widely. Some churches believe that the funeral service, with a closed casket, or memorial service with no casket present, is more of a testimony to the joy and victory of Christian life than is the open-casket service. Others believe that death is a reality to be faced, rather than denied. They believe that viewing the dead person promotes the grief process and represents confrontation with death in a Christian context.

Jean believes that, for most Protestants, the minister represents friendship, love, acceptance, forgiveness, and understanding. His or her presence seems to help the dying face death with more ease. She also believes that Protestants are becoming more active in ministering to the bereaved through regularly scheduled visits during the 12 to 18 months after the funeral, despite the fact that there are no formal rituals.

## Special Religious Groups of Interest

An understanding of, and an ability to participate in, practices or beliefs unique to certain groups and faiths should be part of every health provider's repertoire of previously prepared plans of nursing action.

**Seventh-Day Adventists** rely on Old Testament law more than do other Christian churches. As in Jewish tradition, the Sabbath is from sundown Friday to sundown Saturday. Like the Orthodox Jew, the Seventh-Day Adventist may refuse medical treatment and the use of secular items such as television during this period and prefer instead to read spiritual literature. Diet is also restricted. Pork, fish without scales and fins, tea, and coffee are prohibited. Some Seventh-Day Adventists are **lacto-ovo-vegetarians**: *they eat milk and eggs but no meat*. Tobacco, alcoholic beverages, and narcotics are also avoided. Because Adventists view the body as the "temple of God," health reform is high on their list of

## Table 3-1 Summary of Major Health Care Implications of Selected Religious Cultures and Subcultures

| Religion | Food Preference | Responsibility Related to Client Belief or Need |
|---|---|---|
| *Hinduism* | Vegetarian; no alcoholic beverages; other restrictions conform to sect doctrine; fasting important part of religious practice, with consequences for person on special diet or with diabetes or other metabolic diseases | Medical care is last resort; client considers help will come from own inner resources. Nurse should treat client with respect and convey sense of dignity. Reinforce need for medical care and explain care measures. Client may reject help and be stoic. Assess carefully for pain. Provide privacy. Assist to maintain religious practices. Cleanliness and dietary preferences are important. Certain prescribed rites are followed after death. The priest may tie a thread around the neck or wrist to signify blessing; the thread should not be removed. Immediately after death, the priest will pour water into the mouth of the corpse; the family will wash the body. They are particular about who touches their dead. Bodies are cremated. Loss of limb is considered sign of wrongdoing in previous life. |
| *Buddhism*<br>Zen, sect of Buddhist Shintoism, Japan's state religion | Vegetarian; no intoxicants; moderation in eating and drinking | Family help care for ill member and give emotional support. Religion discourages use of drugs; assess carefully for pain. Cleanliness important. Question about feelings regarding medical or surgical treatment on holy days. Prepare for death; help patient remain alert, resist confusion or distraction, and remain calm. Last rite chanting is often practised at bedside soon after death. Contact the deceased's Buddhist priest or have the family make contact. |
| *Islam* | No pork and pork-containing products; no intoxicants | Members are excused from religious practices when ill but may still want to pray to Allah and face Mecca. There is no spiritual advisor to call. Family visits are important. Cleanliness is important. After 130 days, fetus is treated as fully developed human. Members maintain a fatalistic view about illness; they are resigned to death, but encourage prolonging life. Patient must confess sins and beg forgiveness before death, and family should be present. The family washes and prepares the body, folds hands, and turns the body to face Mecca. Only relatives or friends may touch the body. Unless required by law, no autopsy and no body part should be removed. |
| *Black Muslim*<br>**(Nation of Islam)** | | There is no baptism. Procedure for washing and shrouding dead and performing funeral rites is carefully prescribed. Cleanliness is important. |
| *Judaism* | Orthodox Jews eat only kosher (ritually prepared) foods; milk consumed before meat, or meat eaten six hours before | There is no infant baptism. Baby boy is circumcised on eighth day if Orthodox. Preventative measures, avoiding illness, are important. Members are |

*(continued)*

Table 3-1 (continued)

| Religion | Food Preference | Responsibility Related to Client Belief or Need |
|---|---|---|
| | milk consumed; do not eat pig, horse, shrimp, lobster, crab, oyster, birds of prey. Others may restrict diet. Special utensils and dishes for Orthodox. Fasts on Yom Kippur and Tisha B'av; may fast other times but excluded if ill, pregnant, child, or elderly | concerned about future consequences of illness and medication. Some are preoccupied with health; will convey that pain is present and want relief. Nursing measures for pain are important. On Sabbath, Orthodox Jews may refuse freshly cooked foods, medicine, treatment, surgery, and use of radio or television. Orthodox male may not shave. Nurse should avoid loss of yarmulke, prayer books, or phylacteries. Nurse must arrange for kosher or preferred food; food may be served on paper plates. Check consequences of fasting on person's condition. Visits from family members are important. If patient is without family, notify synagogue so other people may visit. Family or friends should be with dying person. Artificial means should not be used to prolong life if patient is vegetative. Confession by dying person is like a rite of passage. Human remains are ritually washed following death by members of the Ritual Burial Society. Burial should take place as soon as possible. Cremation is not permitted. All Orthodox Jews and some Conservative Jews are opposed to autopsy. Organs or other tissues should be made available to the family for burial. Parts of the body are not donated to medical science or removed, even during autopsy. Donation or transplantation of organs requires rabbinical consultation. A fetus is to be buried, not discarded. |
| *Christianity* | | All will wish to see spiritual advisor when ill and to read Bible or other religious literature and follow usual practices. |
| Roman Catholic | Nothing special, except fasting or abstaining from meat on Ash Wednesday and Good Friday; some Catholics may fast every Friday and other holy days | Client finds comfort in having rosary, Bible, prayer book, crucifix, medals. Infant baptism is mandatory, and especially urgent if prognosis is poor. Baptism is demanded if aborted fetus may not be clinically dead. For baptismal purposes, death is a certainty only if there is obvious evidence of tissue necrosis. Tell priest if you baptize baby; it is done only once. Inquire about dietary preferences and fasting. Members may want information on natural family planning. The Rite for Anointing of the Sick is mandatory. If the prognosis is poor, the patient or his or her family may request it. In sudden death, priest is called to anoint and administer Viaticum, if possible, or special prayers are said. Amputated limb may be buried in consecrated ground; there is no blanket mandate but it may be required within a given diocese. Donation or transplantation |

*(continued)*

Table 3-1 (continued)

| Religion | Food Preference | Responsibility Related to Client Belief or Need |
|---|---|---|
| | | of organs is approved providing the recipient's potential benefit is proportionate to the donor's potential harm. |
| Orthodox | | |
|   Eastern Orthodox (Turkey, Egypt, Syria, Cyprus, Bulgaria, Romania, Albania, Poland, Czech Republic, Slovakia) | Fasting each Wednesday, each Friday, and 40 days before Christmas and Easter; avoid meat, dairy products, and olive oil | Prayer book and icons are important. Infant is baptized if death is imminent. Check consequences of fast days on health; fasting is not necessary when ill. Blessing for the sick (unction) is not last rite but a form of healing by prayer. Last rites are obligatory if death is impending; cremation is discouraged. |
|   Greek Orthodox | Fasting periods on Wednesday, Friday, and during Lent; avoid meat and dairy products | Prayer book and icons are important. Infant is baptized if death is imminent. Patient prepares by fasting for Holy Communion and Sacrament of Holy Unction. Fasting is not mandatory during illness. Members oppose euthanasia. Every reasonable effort should be made to preserve life until terminated by God. Cremation or autopsies that may cause dismemberment are discouraged. Last rites are administered for the dying. |
|   Russian Orthodox | Fasting on Wednesday, Friday, and during Lent; no meat or dairy products | Prayer book and icons are important. There is no baptism of infant. Check consequences of fasting on health. Cross necklace is important; it should be replaced immediately when patient returns from surgery. Do not shave male patients except in preparation for surgery. Patients do not believe in autopsies, embalming, or cremation. Traditionally, after death, arms are crossed, and fingers are set in a cross. Clothing at death must be of natural fibre so that the body will change to dust sooner. |
| Protestantism (Many denominations and sects) Baptist | Some groups condemn coffee and tea; most condemn alcoholic beverages; some groups may fast on Sundays or other special days, especially in Black Baptist churches | There is no infant baptism. Client may be fatalistic; may believe illness is punishment from God; and may be passive about care. Inquire about effect of fasting if client is on special diet, is a diabetic, or has disease dependent on dietary regulation. |
| Brethren (Grace) (Plymouth) | Most abstain from alcohol, tobacco, and illicit drugs | There is no infant baptism. Anointing with oil is done for physical healing and spiritual uplift. There are no last rites. |
| Church of Christ, Scientist (Christian Scientist) | Avoid coffee and alcoholic beverages | There is no infant baptism. If hospitalized or receiving medical treatment, guilt feelings may be intense. Be supportive. Allow practitioner or reader to visit freely as desired. Use nursing measures to alleviate pain. Patient may refuse blood transfusions as well as intravenous fluids and medication. There are no last rites or autopsy, unless sudden death. |
| Church of Christ | Avoid alcoholic beverages | There is no infant baptism. Anointing with oil and laying on of hands are done for healing. There are no last rites. |

(continued)

Table 3-1 (continued)

| Religion | Food Preference | Responsibility Related to Client Belief or Need |
|---|---|---|
| Church of God | Most avoid alcoholic beverages | There is no infant baptism. |
| Church of Jesus Christ of Latter Day Saints (Mormon) | Eat in moderation; limit meat; avoid coffee and tea; no alcoholic beverages; avoid use of tobacco | There is no infant baptism, but baptism of dead is essential; living person serves as proxy. Laying on of hands is done for healing. White undergarment with special marks at navel and right knee is to remain on; it is considered a safeguard against danger. |
| Episcopalian | May fast from meat on Friday | Infant baptism is mandatory, but not for aborted fetus or stillbirth. Patient fasts in preparation for Holy Communion, which may be daily; thus, check effects on disease. Rite for Anointing Sick (last rites) is not mandatory. |
| Society of Friends (Quakers) | Moderation in eating; most avoid alcoholic beverages and drugs | There is no infant baptism. Health teaching is important. Give explanations about medical technology used in care. Share information about condition as indicated. |
| Jehovah's Witnesses | Avoid food to which blood is added, e.g., certain sausages and luncheon meats | There is no infant baptism. Members are opposed to blood transfusion. (Hospital administrator or doctor may seek court order to be appointed guardian of child in times of emergency need for blood.) There are no last rites. |
| Lutheran | | Baptize only living infants shortly after birth, by pastor. Communion may be given before or after surgery or similar crisis. |
| Mennonite | Most avoid alcoholic beverages | There is no infant baptism. Shock therapy, psychotherapy, and hypnotism conflict with individual will and personality. |
| Methodist | | No baptism at birth. Communion may be given before surgery or similar crisis. |
| Nazarene | Avoid alcoholic beverages | There is no need to baptize infant. Stillborn is buried. Laying on of hands is done for healing. There are no last rites. |
| Pentecostal | Avoid alcoholic beverages | There is no infant baptism. Prayer, anointing with oil, laying on of hands, speaking in tongues, shouting, and singing are important for healing of patient. |
| Unitarian/Universalist | | Infant baptism is not necessary. Cremation is preferred to burial. Check before calling clergy to visit. |
| Seventh-Day Adventists | Vegetarian (no meat) or lacto-ovo-vegetarian (may eat milk and eggs but not meat); pork and fish without fins and scales prohibited; avoid coffee and tea; avoid alcoholic beverages | There is no infant baptism. Health measures, prevention, and health education are important. Some believe in divine healing and anointing with oil. Avoid administering narcotics and stimulants. Use nursing measures for pain; medication is last resort. Check on food preferences. Sabbath is Friday sundown until Saturday sundown for most groups. Client may refuse medical treatment and use of secular items, such as television, on Sabbath. |

priorities and they sponsor health institutes, cooking schools, and food-producing organizations. They are pioneers in making foods for vegetarians, including meat-like foods from vegetable sources. Much of their inspiration comes from Ellen G. White, a 19th-century prophet who gave advice on diet and food and who promoted Christ's return to earth.

The **Church of Jesus Christ of Latter-Day Saints (Mormon)** takes much of its inspiration from the **Book of Mormon**, *translated from golden tablets believed to have been found in what is now the U.S. by the prophet Joseph Smith*. The Mormons believe that this book and two others supplement the Bible. Every Mormon is an official missionary. There is no official congregational leader, but a **seventy** and a **high priest** *represent successive steps upward in commitment and authority*.

The church believes in a *whole-being approach* and provides education, recreation, and financial aid for its members. A health and conduct code called *Word of Wisdom* prohibits tobacco, alcohol, and hot drinks (interpreted as tea and coffee), and recommends eating, though sparingly and with thankfulness, herbs, fruit, meat, fowl, and grain—especially wheat.

The Mormon believes that disease comes from failure to obey the laws of health and from failure to keep the other commandments of God. However, righteous persons sometimes become ill simply because they have been exposed to microorganisms that cause disease. Mormons also believe that by faith the righteous sometimes escape plagues that are sweeping the land. They believe that often, having become sick, the obedient are restored to full physical well-being by the gift of faith. There is no restriction on the use of medications or vaccines and there is no restriction on the use of blood or blood components.[24]

The two groups discussed above (the Seventh-Day Adventists and the Church of Jesus Christ of Latter-Day Saints) generally accept and promote modern medical practices. The next two groups discussed, Jehovah's Witnesses and Church of Christ, Scientist, hold views that conflict somewhat with the medical field.

The first group, **Jehovah's Witnesses**, refuses to accept blood transfusions. Their refusal is based on the Levitical commandment, given by God to Moses, declaring that no one in the House of David should eat blood. If the person did so, he or she would be cut off from his or her people. In support, a New Testament reference (in Acts) prohibits the tasting of blood. Every Jehovah's Witness is a minister. The people who belong to Jehovah's Witnesses engage in door-to-door proselytizing, worship in Kingdom Halls, and promote the sale to the public of their magazines *Awake* and the *Watchtower*.[25] Today, they are most widely known for their refusal to accept blood transfusions—even when their own lives, or those of their children, are at stake.[26] They also refuse to donate blood.[27] Not surprisingly, some

have spoken out in criticism of the Watchtower Society Blood Policy.[28]

The second group, **Church of Christ, Scientist (Christian Scientists)**, turn wholly to spiritual means for healing. Occasionally, they allow an orthopedic surgeon to set a bone if no medication is used. Parents do not allow their children to undergo a physical examination for school; to have eye, ear, or blood pressure screening; or to receive immunizations. In addition to the Bible, Christian Scientists use as their guide Mary Baker Eddy's *Science and Health with Key to the Scriptures*, originally published in 1875. The title of this work indicates an approach to wholeness, and those who follow its precepts think of God as Divine Mind, of spirit as real and eternal, and of matter as unreal illusion.

Christian Scientists are not opposed to doctors in the health care delivery system. They exercise their own autonomy regarding treatment in any given situation. However, they usually choose to rely on spiritual healing because they have seen its effectiveness in the experience of their own family and fellow church members.[29]

One religious group, the Mennonites, has retained its lifestyle, geographic solidarity, and theological unity. Mennonites believe that each person is responsible before God to make decisions based on his or her comprehension of the Bible. The Mennonite faith encompasses a wide range of cultural circumstances, which are largely responsible for differences among individual Mennonites. For example, regarding health care practices, no generally held religious ritual is applied. The client, however, might ask for one that is personally meaningful to him or her.[30]

In Canada, the **Mennonites** settled mainly in southern Ontario and the western provinces, where they maintained their religious practices.[31] The Mennonites generally emphasize plain ways of dressing, living, and worshipping. They do not believe in going to war, swearing oaths, or holding offices that require the use of force. Many of them farm the land, while some are inclined toward service professions. They are well known for their missionary efforts. Another group, the **Amish**, split from the Mennonites. Amish people believe that the body is the temple of God and that people are the stewards of their bodies. Their belief is that medicine and health care should always be used with the understanding that it is God who heals.[32]

---

### CRITICAL THINKING

*What may be some barriers to health care for the Amish people?*

Choquette, in his book *Canada's Religions*, explains how globalization has generated much religious diversity in society. Further, Canada's largely Christian heritage has been transformed into both a multi-ethnic mosaic and a pluralistic society.[33] He claims that the alternative religions, with their two components of *new religious movements* and *new religions*, could be classified into two categories. The first category is composed of those religious movements that are rooted in traditional mainstream religions—Aboriginal spiritualities included—that continue to teach the fundamental doctrines of that religion. Such religions include Christian Scientists, Mormons, and Jehovah's Witnesses.

For many Aboriginal peoples, spirituality is the cornerstone to their way of living. It is not seen as solely a religion, but as a way of life intertwined in all aspects of daily living. It embraces the individual's values, ceremonies, songs, dances, and teachings.[34] In Aboriginal Canadian traditions, the medicine wheel is a powerful sacred symbol that expresses the four directions (east, west, north, and south) and the four elements (air, fire, water, and earth). The directions and elements are important to human existence and to the maintenance of proper balance.[35] In addition, the four quadrants of the wheel are physical, mental, emotional, and spirituality. The critical point is that each of these parts needs to be functioning, and in balance, in order to maintain health in mind, body, and spirit.[36] Healing is described as a process that results in the "coming together" of the body, mind, and spirit at a deep level of inner knowledge.[37] An ethnographic study was conducted to investigate the question *How do urban-based First Nations people use healing traditions to address their health issue?* The healing practices used were found to be extensive, both in number and in nature. They included smudging, talking circles, and drumming circles, as well as the use of sweat lodges. Elders within this study group were willing to share their knowledge at "circle" time and they used stories to make their points, which provided enriching realizations on how to act respectfully, responsibly, and honourably. For nurses, the main implication of these findings is that the concepts of balance, holism, and cultural healing can be incorporated into the health care procedures for Aboriginal people.[38]

Many Aboriginal people have been successful in incorporating Christian or other doctrines, teachings, and practices into their spirituality, and they have adopted an ecumenical approach to worship. Currently, various faiths and churches practise Aboriginal-based ceremonies as part of their services. These services also include Aboriginal teachings.[39]

Many Canadians have learned the practice of **yoga**. The term *yoga* is a form of activity designed to harness its practitioners to knowledge of the divine. Yoga refers to the various paths leading to spiritual liberation.

The **Baha'i faith** is a monotheistic religion led by an elected body called the Universal House of Justice. The faithful practise daily personal devotions, annual fasts, missionary activity, and regular communal gatherings, and they celebrate annual feast days.[40] Baha'i members believe that the main purpose of marriage is the procreation of children. They believe that to have children is the highest physical honour of one's existence. The Baha'i are encouraged to seek out competent medical care, follow the advice of those in whom they have confidence, and pray.[41]

Canada's **Pentecostals**, while remaining diversified, have become part of the mainstream of evangelical Protestantism. In fact, some of the key Pentecostal ideas have made inroads into several Christian churches, including the Roman Catholic Church. Pentecostalism has spread globally.[42]

The **Hare Krishna** is the eighth and the most famous incarnation of the god Vishnu and is the object of much devotion by the Hindu faithful.[43]

The second category of new religions is composed of religions that seem to be concerned with creating a new doctrine, a new revelation, or a new truth—frequently combined with elements drawn from a variety of traditions and cultures.[44] These new religions include some North American Aboriginal religions, Scientology, and New Age. Reason and Scripture have insignificant importance in new religions as sources of truth. Even though there is a rapid turnover in membership, these new religions exert a significant impact in the West, and particularly in Canada.

The **Native American Church** has spread with a desire to preserve Aboriginal people's ancestral lifestyle and customs. By consuming peyote (a stimulant from cacti), the devotees achieve an altered state of consciousness that they consider to be a religious experience.[45]

Meanwhile, the Church of Scientology originated from the writings of L. Ron Hubbard. He coined a new vocabulary that became part of **Scientology**. A few of his concepts are engram, reactive mind, and clear, auditing, and analytical mind. Scientology has been criticized in Canada and elsewhere.[46]

Although the New Age movement may be in decline, it has exerted a tremendous influence on contemporary culture. The followers of the **New Age** recognize a wide range of movements, customs, beliefs, and objects. Unlike most formal religions, it has no holy text, formal clergy, dogma, creed, or central organization.[47] It stands apart from Judaism and Christianity. In its monistic tradition, New Age is in the company of the occult sciences—spiritualism, Eastern religions, and psychology each have imparted an influence on its growth. Choquette explains that one of the New Age's foundational components is modern psychology, whose focus is on the inner self. This focus is the awareness of self, and the awareness of one's divinity that replaces conversion, while personal transformation replaces salvation. New Age dismisses religion as irrelevant and invites individuals to look inside themselves for wholeness and divinity. The best-known symbol of the New Age is the crystal. Crystals are embraced by

New Age individuals who consider them as instruments of transformation and healing, believing that they assist in healing by restoring the natural harmony between the physical and etheric (or spiritual) bodies.[48]

## CRITICAL THINKING

*How does the practice of health promotion affect someone who is a follower of the New Age?*

## Agnosticism and Atheism

To this point, the present chapter has concentrated on the worship of God, the divine, or other positive spirits, with an emphasis on traditional teaching. Some people live by ethical standards, considering themselves either **agnostic**, *incapable of knowing whether God exists*, or **atheistic**, *believing that a God does not exist*.

Wright[49] discusses ethical principles that must be practised with all people as follows:

1. **Beneficence:** *the duty to do no harm.* Give of self wholeheartedly in interactions with patients because this positive action is beneficial.

2. **Non-malfeasance** urges *constraint from doing harm to another*, but it also tends to render judgments that another's beliefs can be harmful. However, you can share your beliefs in a non-judgmental way as you provide care in the spiritual dimension.

3. **Autonomy:** *the right of patient self-determination.* Assess what patients desire regarding spiritual care, and avoid imposing your own ideas on the patient.

4. **Advocacy:** *actively assisting the patient in exercising autonomy.* Help the patient find meaning, hope, and clarification of personal beliefs and values.

## OTHER TRENDS IN SPIRITUAL DIMENSIONS

One trend that not only has been popular but also is an important treatment modality for addictions is the 12-step program (originally developed by Alcoholics Anonymous). Such programs help individuals overcome several types of addictions and help to build spiritual strength. This approach refers to "God" but may view God as a higher power, deity, spiritual force, or even the collective power of the group.[50]

## CRITICAL THINKING

*As a health professional, how can you approach an individual who is a substance abuser and inform him or her about either Alcoholics Anonymous or Narcotics Anonymous?*

## PROFILE OF CHANGING WORLD RELIGIONS IN CANADA

It is important to note that religious diversity has been increasing in Canada since the 1960s. Most of this shift has been attributed to the changing source of immigration in the country. The 2001 Census reports that Canada is still predominantly Roman Catholic and Protestant. (It should be noted here that the religion question is asked every ten years. Because it was asked in 2001, it was not asked in the 2006 Census.) The largest religious group in Canada is Roman Catholic. Religions of Asian origin have grown, and the number of Canadians who reported being affiliated with religions such as Islam, Hinduism, Sikhism, and Buddhism has increased substantially. Within the Orthodox denominations, the two largest being Greek Orthodox and Ukrainian Orthodox, slight declines have occurred. However, the numbers of two other Orthodox churches—the Serbian Orthodox and Russian Orthodox—have more than doubled. A slight increase of individuals of Jewish faith has occurred. There was also an increase in the number of people reporting "no religion" in Canada. This group accounted for 16 percent of the population in 2001, compared to 12 percent a decade earlier.[51] It is important to note that, on average, the people who reported that they had no religion were younger than the general population.

Many Canadian scholars, theologians, and writers have contributed to a comprehensive view of religions in contemporary Canada.[52] Each has contributed significantly toward understanding religious patterns and the belief systems that affect individual, as well as family, views and practices in everyday life.

Choquette claims that during the second half of the 20th century a number of diverse worldviews and theologies appeared in Canada. The descriptions of the world that accompany these views and theologies reflected not only radically different views of the East and West, but also a growing diversity within Catholic, Protestant, and Orthodox Christians. An increased visibility of Aboriginal religion also occurred during that time. Above all, the fundamental worldview put forth by the religions of the East constituted a radically new element in Canadian society.[53] In two of his earlier books,[54] Bibby claimed a steep descent in religious involvement and interest by Canadians. Now, in his more recent book *Restless Gods*, Bibby indicates that significant signs exist of renewed religious interest—both inside and outside churches. Bibby also explains that acceleration has occurred in the spiritual quest of Canadians, specifically since the 1980s.

One of the results from the Project Canada 2000 Survey indicated that generally Canadians have an interest in spirituality, and a solid majority indicate that they have

You are a registered nurse who has worked on a palliative care unit for five years. Joan, who recently graduated as a registered nurse, has been partnered with you by the nurse unit manager (NUM). As a result of a brief meeting with the NUM, you and Joan have agreed to work each shift together—first, for orientation purposes, and second, so you can assess Joan's work performance and provide feedback to both Joan and the NUM. You like Joan, and it appears that the two of you might become friends. However, one evening she informs you that her feelings were hurt a few months ago by certain members of her church. She shares with you how she has come to believe that institutionalized forms of worship do not promote spiritual growth, and that she doesn't really see spirituality as an identifiable entity. She states that she avoids making referrals to chaplains and clergy for her dying patients. She says that she firmly believes she is acting in the clients' best interests when she bypasses chaplains and clergy. She asks you not to share her beliefs and actions on spirituality with anyone on the unit because she thinks that most of the professionals might be "overly involved with religion." You have a deep conviction to your own faith and you consider yourself a spiritual person. Tomorrow is your first meeting with the NUM to review Joan's work performance.

1. What will you do with the information that Joan has shared with you regarding her views on religion and spirituality?
2. What will you say to the NUM regarding Joan's performance and convictions?
3. What do you consider to be the best way for you to approach Joan on the matter? What other realistic alternatives exist for you?

spiritual needs. More than half see themselves as spiritual.[55] Fay explains that social justice, interfaith ecumenism, Native people, and Canadian women are all meaningful dynamics in today's Roman Catholic Church.[56] He goes on to say that in order to enrich the Catholic community, women, the marginalized, and Native people, given an opportunity, will help to energize, universalize, and organize the church in the 21st century.

Clark and Schellenberg used data from the General Social Survey (GSS) and the 2002 Ethnic Diversity Survey to track religious views and practices of Canadians and to identify those groups most likely to be religious. They found that some Canadians who do not attend services still attach high significance to religion in their life. This indicates that, while attendance rates have declined, many Canadians continue to practise their religion in private. Consistent with other findings, this study found that young adults comprise the group with the weakest attachment to organized religion. However, even when other forms of religious behaviour such as praying and meditating are considered, almost half of Canadians aged 15 to 29 still have a low degree of religiosity.[57] In recent decades, a rising number of individuals are seeking spiritual development outside of established religious organizations. This phenomenon has led some analysts to conclude that people are becoming a post-denomination society.[58]

Recently, a number of religious organizations have turned to computer technology to disseminate their message. In fact, 5 percent of the national television audience tunes in to religious television. The current popularity of media ministries and the high levels of recent immigration will together result in diversification of the religious profile of Canadian society in the years to come.[59]

The growing presence of diverse religions constitutes a shift in political, social, and cultural life in Canada. Choquette claims that Canada's new immigrants have not only given the country a more religious outlook but also contributed to the development of a society much more open to change and difference.[60]

## HEALTH PROMOTION IN NURSING PRACTICE

You can use the foregoing concepts—basic beliefs, dietary laws, and ideas about illness and health, body, spirit, mysticism, pragmatism, pain, death, and family ties—as a *beginning*. Even more basic than understanding these concepts is respecting your client as a person with spiritual needs who has a right to have these needs met, whether or not he or she has formal religious beliefs. Critical thinking knowledge and skills will assist you to promote clients' spiritual well-being and health.[61] You can help clients as well as their families in their journey. *As a nurse, you are the transition, the key professional between the client and spiritual help.*

Several books are available for nurses that detail spiritual caregiving, including *Spiritual Care Nursing: Theory, Research and Practice*,[62] and *Spiritual Care in Nursing Practice*.[63] Both books explore the meaning of spirituality and the world of spiritual care. Each book can be used to assist the nurse in applying the concepts of spirituality to clients and their families. The *Journal of Christian Nursing* is another helpful resource. In particular, the Summer 1999 issue is devoted to the connection between faith and health.

### Assessment

Although you can learn much from selecting points in the case studies found in this chapter, you can also refer to Table 3-1 and to the questions posed in Tables 3-2 and 3-3.

## Table 3-2 Questions for Spiritual Assessment

1. What is your concept of God? What is your God like? (Or, what is your religion? Tell me about it.)

2. Do you believe that God, or someone, is concerned for you?

3. Who is the most important person to you? Is that person available?

4. Has being sick (what has been happening to you) made any difference in your feelings about God? In the practice of your faith? If it has, could you explain how it has changed?

5. Do you believe that your faith is helpful to you? If it is, how? If it is not, why not?

6. Are there any religious beliefs, practices, or rituals that are important to you now? If there are, could you tell me about them? May I help you carry them out by showing you where the chapel is? By telling the dietary department about your vegetarian preference? By allowing you specific times for prayer or meditation?

7. Is there anything that would make your situation easier? (Such as a visit from the minister, priest, rabbi, or chaplain? Someone who would read to you? Time for reading your religious book or praying? Someone to pray with you?)

8. Is prayer important to you? (If so, has being sick made a difference in your practice of praying?) What happens when you pray?

9. Do you have available religious books or articles such as the Bible, prayer books, phylacteries, or a crucifix that mean something to you?

10. What are your ideas about illness? About life after death?

11. Is there anything especially frightening or meaningful to you right now?

12. If these questions have not uncovered your source of spiritual support, can you tell me where you do find support?

However, each of these is only a basis from which to begin your quest to provide holistic care to clients and their families.

## CRITICAL THINKING

*What single concept from this chapter so far stands out for you as most meaningful as you think about providing spiritual care to your clients and their family members?*

Prior to beginning a spirituality assessment, the individual nurse should reflect upon and gather insight about her or his own spirituality.[64] To gather such insight, the nurse can read, be religiously involved, or engage in mediation activities. One such meditation activity is the use of the labyrinth, which is formal and ritualistic. Walkers in the labyrinth progress through three phases during the walk. The first phase, *releasing*, occurs during the walk to the centre at a normal walking speed. Walkers are encouraged to empty their minds and repeat a word or prayer, or recall a special dream to reflect upon. In the centre, walkers engage for a time in *receiving*, during which they remain still and quiet while inviting an opening to personal healing. The third phase, called *returning*, involves turning around and retracing one's steps in the opposite direction of the labyrinth. With each return step, walkers gradually come back to the day-to-day world, and in doing so they often experience a change of energy in mind, body, and spirit. The labyrinth walk is intended to bring about physiological, affective, and spiritual outcomes similar to those sought in a sitting meditation.[65]

*Spiritual beliefs and beliefs about purpose in life and life after death are important dimensions of high-level wellness.* Beliefs are related to feelings about self-worth, goals, interactions with others, philosophy of life, and interpretations of birth, life events, and death. The value and meaning of life are not judged by its length but by the purpose for which the person lives, the principles by which he or she lives, the reflection about a being greater than the self, and the love and joy obtained from relationships with others. All of these factors may directly affect health status.

Assessment of the spiritual needs of any client, not just the terminally ill or dying, should be part of the nursing history. **Spiritual need** is defined as *lack of any factor necessary to establish or maintain a dynamic, personal relationship with God, or a higher being, as defined by the individual.* Four areas of concern can be covered later in the interview as part of assessment after the client feels safe with the nurse in the therapeutic relationship. The following are the assessment areas:

- Person's concept of God or deity

- Person's source of strength and hope

- Significance of religious practices and rituals

- Perceived relationship between spiritual beliefs and current state of health

During this part of the assessment, be prepared for any answer. The agnostic or atheist may answer with as much depth and meaning from his or her perspective as someone with a specific religious background. The person who is part of a formal religion may not answer freely, reserving such conversation for the spiritual leader, or hesitating until the nurse is better known to the client.

When determining medical background, such as drug or food allergies, you could also ask about religious dietary

## Table 3-3 Religious and Spiritual Assessment Questionnaire

1. Are religious or spiritual issues important in your life?
   - ☐ Yes
   - ☐ Somewhat
   - ☐ No

2. Do you believe in God or a Supreme Being?
   - ☐ Yes
   - ☐ No

3. Do you believe you can experience spiritual guidance?
   - ☐ Yes
   - ☐ No

   If so, how often have you had such experiences?
   - ☐ Often
   - ☐ Occasionally
   - ☐ Rarely
   - ☐ Never

   Are you committed to it and actively involved?
   - ☐ Yes
   - ☐ Somewhat
   - ☐ No

4. How important was religion or spiritual belief to you as a child and adolescent?
   - ☐ Important
   - ☐ Somewhat Important
   - ☐ Unimportant

5. Are you aware of any religious or spiritual resources in your life that could be used to help you overcome your problems?
   - ☐ Yes
   - ☐ No

   If "yes," what are they?

   _____

   _____

   _____

   _____

   _____

   _____

6. Do you believe that religious or spiritual influences have hurt you or contributed to some of your problems?
   - ☐ Yes
   - ☐ No

   If "yes," briefly explain how.

   _____

   _____

   _____

   _____

   _____

   _____

*This questionnaire contributed by Sylvia Adams, MSN, RNC, and Pamela Talley, MSN, RN, CS, CSAC.*

laws, special rituals, or restrictions that might be an important part of the client's history. Recording and helping the client follow beliefs could speed recovery.

Perhaps *you could share with the chaplain the responsibility for asking questions related to spirituality as you give client care.* No specific set of questions will be right for every client, but the questions in Tables 3-2 and 3-3 may elicit helpful responses as you assess the client's spiritual realm.

Be sure to identify the person's strengths, not weaknesses. Allow the client to assume his or her own spiritual stance. Ensure that the assessment is relevant to the client's situation and demonstrate the ethic of care.[66]

Because your relationship with the person may be of short duration, be sure to document well the results of this interview. Later, when you or others care for the client, you should watch for religious needs that may be expressed through non-religious language. You must again let the client know what options are available for spiritual help. If you hide behind hectic activities and procedures, you may lose a valuable opportunity to aid in health restoration.

*You can now relate your understanding of social class and cultural differences obtained from Chapter 1 to comprehend more fully the religious and cultural differences related in this chapter.* Review both chapters and take time to reflect on how you can apply the various concepts and belief systems presented regarding the different groups in regions throughout Canada.

*Ideally, religion and spirituality provide strength, an inner calm, and faith with which to work through life's problems.* Healing, too, has varied meanings. Some will demand that God, or their Higher Power, provide a quick and miraculous recovery, whereas others will expect the process to occur through the work of the health team. Still others combine God's touch, the health providers' skill, and their own emotional and physical co-operation. Some even consider death as the final form of healing.

Sometimes you will be called upon to deal with your own values and negative reactions. Your personal background and nursing knowledge may provoke dismay at some religious practices. For instance, how will you react as you watch a postoperative Jehovah's Witness client die because she has refused a blood transfusion? Basically, she prefers to die. Should you dictate otherwise? You may need to think through and discuss such situations with a spiritual leader.

## CRITICAL THINKING

*What conflicts could arise in the health care delivery system because of different beliefs and values held by individuals?*

Clients may present issues. For example, a client may question his or her belief system, may be discouraged or despairing, may feel spiritually empty, or may be ambivalent, first asking for spiritual assistance, then rejecting it. On the other hand, the client may indicate strength—that is, be at peace within and calmly accept his or her medical diagnosis. Clients may desire prayer from a nurse to help them thank God for their life.

*As nurses become more attuned to these situations, perhaps meeting the client's spiritual needs will not be detached from other care.* At the same time, the spiritual dimensions must be thought of as something in addition to the psychosocial dimension. Specific measures must be taken for spiritual care—measures that are not necessarily included in psychosocial care. Olson and her researchers conducted a study to identify the extent to which the spiritual dimension was addressed in Canadian undergraduate nursing curricula. The results indicated that some educators view the spiritual dimension as part of the psychosocial dimension. These researchers concluded that it is time to engage in serious dialogue about the spiritual dimension in nursing education because there appears to be conceptual confusion in the area.[67]

It is interesting to note the concept of spirituality addressed in other health care disciplines. For example, a study was conducted to examine the manner and extent to which Canadian occupational therapy education addressed the concept of spirituality. Results indicated that although Canadian occupational therapy programs address spirituality in their curricula, the importance focused on the concept is low.[68] Grabovac and Ganesan surveyed 16 psychiatry residency programs in Canada to determine which types of psychiatry-related religion and spirituality training are being made available. Their findings indicated that most Canadian programs offer minimal instruction on issues pertaining to religion, spirituality, and psychiatry. These researchers propose a ten-session lecture series, with outlines, designed to introduce residents in psychiatry to religious and spiritual issues as they pertain to clinical practice.[69]

## NARRATIVE VIGNETTE

You are beginning your final year of studies as a student nurse in the Baccalaureate Nursing Degree Program. You have been asked to be a teaching assistant (TA) for the Introduction to Nursing Care course being taught at the first-year level of the program. While reviewing your TA responsibilities with you, the course leader asks you to share with her your opinion, as a senior student, on what you believe to be the more important aspects that first-year nursing students should realize about spirituality. Because the course leader knows that health care professionals conduct numerous teaching/learning experiences after graduation, she is interested in hearing what you believe, from a learner's point of view, to be effective approaches to teaching spirituality.

Reflect for a few minutes on what you believe to be important early in one's health care career regarding spirituality. Think about the teaching/learning methods used when you were taught spirituality.

1. What teaching/learning approaches would you prefer to have experienced regarding spirituality?

2. How will you respond to the course leader?

   a. What do you believe to be the more important aspects of spirituality for early-career health care professionals?

   b. What are the more effective approaches to use in teaching spirituality?

## Intervention

The Canadian Holistic Nurses Association (CHNA), a recognized interest group of the Canadian Nurses Association (CNA), emphasizes the development of holistic nursing practice.[70] The main goal of the CHNA is to further the development of holistic nursing practice to ensure that professional health maintenance and health promotion care are available to the people of Canada. The objectives of the CHNA include: to promote CNA Nursing Practice Standards of provinces and territories as applicable; to promote holistic nursing practice, education, research, and administration; and to adhere to the CNA Code of Ethics for Nurses.[71]

Spirituality is an integral part of *holistic health*.[72] There is a qualitative difference between giving spiritual care and supporting another person by sharing transcendent human qualities. Florence Nightingale described spiritual care as that which enables a person to be conscious of the presence of God, who is the creator and sustainer of the universe. In nursing, a few scholars, such as Wright, describe the ethical, professional, and legal responsibilities for spiritual care,[73] and Meyeroff, Van Hofwegen, Hoe Harwood, and Drury present the development of spiritual nursing interventions to restore meaning in the lives of clients and their families.[74] In addition, Lorraine Wright has added to the Canadian literature by writing a textbook called *Spirituality, Suffering, and Illness*. It is the first text for nurses and other health professionals that acknowledges the relatedness between spirituality and suffering and, at the same time, provides an analysis of the importance of these concepts within the context of illness.[75]

---

### CRITICAL THINKING

*What personal characteristics and qualities do you have that enable you to provide good spiritual care? (You might find some good ideas in Pesut.[76])*

---

Several other authors have written about how prayer and faith enable a better implementation of the nursing process, and help to provide holistic care—physical, emotional, sociocultural, and spiritual. Some say that when they pray, the tasks go more smoothly. Others say that when they pray with patients, they benefit as much as do the patients.[77] Others describe the barriers to giving spiritual care.[78] Wallace[79] writes about one family's effort to incorporate a holistic approach to care. When staff learned about the patient as he had been, staff became more responsive. The patient's recovery for three years was viewed as a miracle by all. Wright, in her clinical work with families, claims that her goal and obligation is to alleviate or heal emotional, physical, and spiritual suffering.[80]

## CASE SITUATION

### Spiritual Distress

Susan Santini is a 40-year-old, middle-class bank manager. She lives in a small town with her husband and four children. She also deals in real estate, works with civic and Roman Catholic church groups, and is developing an advertising company. She seems constantly busy. She discusses business over lunch and competes with friends when playing golf or bridge.

One evening, she started having severe chest pain. She was taken in an ambulance to a metropolitan hospital 120 kilometres away where a specialist successfully performed triple-bypass surgery.

For the first time in her life, Susan was stopped. She was away from family and friends and was confined. Good and bad memories flooded her mind. She began to evaluate her activities, her emphasis on material gain and competition, how her children were growing up so fast, how her religious activities were superficial, and how, without skilled surgery, she might have died.

At first, she tried being jovial with the staff to strike out these new and troubling thoughts. But she could not sleep well. She was dreaming about death in wild combinations with her past life. She began to mention these dreams, along with questions about how the surgery would affect her lifespan, diet, and activities. She mentioned a friend who seemed severely limited from a similar surgery. She also said she was worried about the problems her teenagers were beginning to face and about her own ability to guide them properly.

The staff members never forced Susan to express more than she wished but answered her questions and asked whether she would like to see the chaplain since her own priest was not available. Susan agreed. An appointed nurse then informed the chaplain of Susan's physical, emotional, and spiritual history to date. In the course of several sessions, the chaplain helped Susan work through a revised philosophy of life that put more emphasis on spiritual values, family life, and healthy use of leisure.

### Questions

1. If the chaplain had been unable to come to Susan, because, let's say, he had suffered a heart attack, what could the nurse have done to address Susan's spiritual needs?

2. What barriers might the nurse encounter when endeavouring to provide spiritual care to Susan and her family?

3. If you were Susan's nurse, to what sources of information could you turn to learn more about addressing spiritual needs?

## Role of Faith Communities in Intervention*

*Churches, or faith communities, contribute to health promotion. Churches have been a refuge for people of all faiths throughout the centuries, and they have been and still are a major centre for health promotion.*

*Faith communities have contributed to health promotion in two ways: by the generic nature of the faith community and by intentional, planned activities to address health issues in the faith community and in the larger community.*

Faith communities are excellent settings for health promotion.[81] In fact, they are considered to be competent in the spiritual area, a fact that is often overlooked in secular health promotion programs. In Canada, greater attention is being given to different ways that individuals and their families can take responsibility of their own well-being. Churches have begun to reclaim their heritage of providing for people's health-related needs—spiritual, physical, mental, social, emotional, and cultural.[82] These realizations cause one to wonder how the parish nurse relates to faith communities.

The concept of parish nursing began in Europe, arrived in the United States in the mid-1980s, and spread to Canada less than a decade later, as early as 1992.[83] A parish nurse, known sometimes as a faith community nurse, is a registered nurse who has specialized knowledge and is hired and acknowledged by a faith community to provide intentional health promotion ministry.[84] In fact, parish nursing is practised from a holistic framework that promotes the health of the whole person.[85] With specialized knowledge in health promotion, parish nurses capitalize on the strengths of individuals and their families. Through the expansion of the nurse role, more services can be brought to the faith community. In fact, faith community nursing can be expanded to include well-child care, adult care, and minor acute care.[86] To practise safely and effectively in health ministry, the Canadian Association for Parish Nursing Ministry has developed Parish Nursing Core Competencies for Basic Parish Nurse Educational Programs along with five standards of practice for parish nursing ministry: facilitation of spiritual care, health promotion, collaboration, advocacy, and professional accountability.[87]

### CRITICAL THINKING

*Compare the roles of a parish nurse in an urban community to those of a parish nurse in a rural community.*

**Guidelines for Intervention** Spiritual support can be given to the *ill and dying person* in various ways. Your warmth, empathy, and caring human relationship are essential. Your

*This section contributed by Frances Atkins, PhD, MS(N), RN, CS.

respect for the person's beliefs, your willingness to discuss spiritual matters and provide for rituals and sacraments of religion are important. Be open to religious and philosophic beliefs other than, or possibly opposed to, your own. You may be uncomfortable discussing spiritual matters; yet for the client, you must try to overcome personal reluctance to discuss spiritual concerns. Often, the intimacy of spiritual concerns is discussed by the client during the intimacy of physical care. Helping the person ask questions and seek solutions does not mean that you have to supply the answers. You may suggest bibliotherapy as a spiritual intervention.[88] Religious beliefs and activities have been linked with better immune functions, lower death rates from cancer, fewer incidences of heart disease, lower blood pressures and levels of cholesterol, better health behaviours, and improved compliance with medical treatment.[89]

With the *dying client*, the aspects of spiritual support considered most helpful are (1) calling the person directly by name; (2) talking directly to the person (realize that everything may be heard by the dying person); and (3) supporting the family by staying with them as they say goodbye. Let family members know they can touch their dying loved one, offer your condolences, and offer to help them in any appropriate way.

Spiritual care of the *psychiatric client* is often overlooked. Assessment must determine whether the person is describing a religious delusion, something most people would consider false, such as "I am Jesus Christ" or "I am Mohammed," or stating conflicts between religious beliefs and rituals and the current situation or feelings. Such statements may sound like, and be labelled as, delusions, but the *nursing diagnosis* of *spiritual distress* would be more appropriate. The spiritual components that you can address through listening and counselling include the person's sense of not being loved by others, of having no meaning or purpose in life, and of feeling unforgiven or not being able to forgive another. These issues take time to resolve, so referral to clergy may be indicated.

Be alert to subtle clues that indicate a desire to talk about spiritual matters, a need for expressions of love and hope, a desire for your silent presence, and an acceptance when the client labels himself or herself as unworthy.

*Communication is essential between health care providers and pastoral care representatives.* You can help to build that communication link. Good rapport can mean that the *whole* person is served rather than segmented parts of that person. Chaplains are especially helpful to clients and to nurses when they assist with expressions of anger, death, and grief. You and the chaplain need to know what to expect from each other. There is no substitute for talking about these expectations and coming to agreement on the strategies to be implemented, and altered if it becomes necessary to do so.

CRITICAL THINKING

*What are some reasons for nurse–chaplain consultation?*

*Nine combinations of client behaviour that call for conferring with, or referring to, a spiritual leader*, unless contraindicated by the care plan, are:

1. Withdrawn, sullen, silent, depressed
2. Restless, irritable, complaining
3. Restless, excitable, garrulous, wants to talk a lot
4. Shows, by word or other signs, undue curiosity or anxiety about self
5. Takes turn to worse, critical, terminal
6. Shows conversational interest or curiosity in religious questions and issues, reads scripture
7. Specifically inquires about chaplain, chapel worship, scripture
8. Has few or no visitors, has no cards or flowers
9. Has had, or faces, a particularly traumatic or threatening surgical procedure

With all of these aspects to consider, an *interdisciplinary team approach* that includes the client, family, health care providers, and chaplain or other spiritual leader is imperative. Assist with such measures as preparing the client for chapel service, or seeing that the Sabbath ritual is carried out. Work with the team to provide important factors, such as rituals, diet, quiet, group work, various articles, or family relationships.

Validate the appropriateness of proposed interventions with the client. For example, ask whether the person wishes you to pray with him or her about the concerns that have been voiced. The person can then accept or reject your offer.

*Consider the milieu.* If a client is confined to a room, you can prepare a worship centre or shrine by arranging flowers, prayer book, relics, or whatever other objects have spiritual meaning.

You should *keep one or more calendars of various religious holidays.* Eastern Orthodox Easter usually does not coincide with the Roman Catholic and Protestant Easter. Jewish and Muslim holidays do not fall on the same dates of the Western calendar in successive years. Remember, also, that holidays are family days and that ill people separated from the family at such times may be especially depressed.

*Maintain a list of available spiritual leaders.* Know when to call them, and know how to prepare for their arrival.

If a client cannot make the request, consult with the family. One woman said, "If my sister sees a priest, she will be sure she is dying." Once, a health care provider took the initiative to call an Eastern Orthodox priest who, unfortunately, represented the wrong nationality; the client's main source of comfort would have come from discussion and prayers in the native language.

Brief the spiritual leader on any points that might provide special insight and be sure that the client is ready to receive the spiritual leader. Prepare any special arrangements, such as having a clean, cloth-covered tray for Communion. Guard against interruption by health care providers from other departments who may be unaware of the visit. Finally, incorporate the results of the visit into the client's record.

CRITICAL THINKING

*What experience have you had with spiritual care leaders?*

Many clients will benefit from the sacraments, prayers, scripture reading, and counselling provided by the spiritual leader, but others will want to rely on their own direct communication with God. The Zen Buddhist, Hindu, Muslim, and Friend (Quaker) might be in the latter category. All may want reading material, however. Most will bring their sacred book with them, but if they express a desire for more literature, offer to get it. Some hospitals furnish daily and weekly meditations and a Bible.

Occasionally, it may be helpful to offer scripture references for various stated spiritual needs. For example, reference to *love* and *relatedness* can be found in Psalm 23. Reference to *forgiveness* can be found in Matthew 6:9–15, and reference to *meaning and purpose* is in Acts 1:8.

If you feel comfortable doing so, you can at times say a prayer, read a scripture, or provide a statement of faith helpful to the client. If you're not comfortable providing this kind of spiritual care, you can still meet the client's spiritual needs through respectful conversation, listening to the client talk about beliefs, referral to another staff member, or calling one of the client's friends who can bolster his or her faith. If spiritual leaders are not available, you could organize a group of health workers willing to counsel with, or make referrals for, clients of their own faiths.

*Shared prayer,* if it is accepted by the client, counteracts the loneliness of illness or dying by offering the person intimacy with a Supreme Being and another person without the need for confession. It can be a means of bringing both human and divine love. It holds transcendent qualities and conveys both present and future hope. Prayer can focus on the conditions or emotions that the client is unable to talk about, allowing the person to handle the matter or vent in another way. Prayer should promote closeness, through closed eyes and hands that touch. Prayer should not strip the person of defences. Nor should prayers be recited as a way to avoid the person or avoid questions raised by the person.

*Use of life review* can foster developmental, emotional, and spiritual maturity (not only in the elder and dying person). Encourage the person to reminisce about past life experiences. Memories can be pleasurable or painful, but recalling them with a skilled listener can help resolve those ridden with shame, guilt, anger, or other feelings. Past sources of strength can also be identified, and sometimes they are useful in the present situation. (Refer to Chapter 14.) Music can also be used to lift depression, convey calm, stimulate hope and joy, and promote physical and mental healing.

Counselling, along with mental and spiritual methods, can be combined to help the client overcome hurtful or traumatic memories, forgive self or others, work through unresolved grief, promote healing within self, and establish healthier relationships with others. You may refer to spiritual leaders or a counsellor to assist you with these aspects. Do not overlook needs not overtly expressed.

*Atheists* should not be neglected because they do not profess a belief in God. They have the same need for respect as everyone else and may need you to listen to fears and doubts. Moreover, just as health teaching is often omitted for health care providers who are clients, so is spiritual guidance often omitted for spiritual leaders who are clients. You must recognize that each person, regardless of religious stand or leadership capacity, may need spiritual help.

Various groups refuse medical or hospital treatment for illness, including members of Fundamentalist or Holiness groups, Jehovah's Witnesses, Amish, and Christian Scientists. Realize that if adults refuse treatment for themselves or their children, they are not deliberately choosing death. They are rejecting something objectionable, based on their beliefs. Nurses may teach nutritional therapy, or various stress-management or relaxation techniques. Sometimes parents accept the services of a home health nurse, even though they refuse hospital and formal medical treatment.

Although a hospital setting has been used as a point of reference throughout this chapter, you can improvise in your setting—nursing home, hospice, school, industry, clinic, home, or other health centre—to provide adequate spiritual assistance.

Table 3-1 summarizes interventions for many of the religions discussed in this chapter.

## Research in Spiritual Care

Research on spirituality and health continues to be carried out. However, knowing precisely how to assess and intervene, and realizing exactly what constitutes spiritual care all need further research. Yet, there are obstacles to carrying out a scientific study that is theologically sound (i.e., in keeping with the beliefs and needs of the person). There is no effective way to determine ahead of time whether an intervention, such as prayer, is going to be completely effective, regardless of who is saying the prayer. Similarly, it is difficult to know in which situation prayer might be helpful or even desired.

The article by O'Mathuna[90] discusses the importance of, and problems with, research on prayer and healing. Hudson[91] writes of the observed results of a hospital chaplain working with patients. The patient's sense of hope, renewed motivation to live, and unexpected recovery are all real and possible outcomes. An interesting study was conducted, first, to investigate how research on the concept of spirituality has been reported in the health literature in the last ten years and, second, to develop an ontological and theoretical understanding of spirituality. The researchers reported that their results identified essential elements of spirituality, the current use of operational definitions and instruments, conceptual frameworks used in spirituality research, and cultural aspects of spirituality.[92]

**Research with Nurses** Stranahan examined the attitudes, perceptions, and practices of nurse practitioners with regard to spiritual care. She found that 57 percent of the respondents stated that they rarely or never included spiritual care in their daily work, 45 percent stated that their ability to provide spiritual care was weak or limited, and 34 percent were uncomfortable providing spiritual care compared with 32 percent who reported feeling very comfortable. These nurses often used basic spiritual care interventions, such as standard documentation, reading religious material, praying, and reporting spiritual needs to colleagues. The nurses who scored high on the spirituality scale employed more complex interventions and provided spiritual care more frequently. The nurses in the study noted the lack of sufficient educational foundations in spiritual care at both the undergraduate and the graduate levels.[93]

Rankin and Delashmutt published an article that describes a nursing faculty's approach to support baccalaureate nursing students in their quest to explore and develop an understanding of the concepts of spirituality and nursing presence in light of their clinical practice. A clinical placement in a faith-community crisis centre for the homeless and poor served as part of their psychiatric/mental health clinical course. The students affirmed that this placement was an experience of self-discovery and maturation in understanding spirituality and nursing presence in nursing practice.[94]

## CRITICAL THINKING

*What findings from nursing research could you include when preparing to care for your clients and their families?*

**Evaluation** The nurse provides care to the client while evaluating the extent to which planned goals and interventions were achieved. The nurse compares the client's spiritual health with the perceptions and behaviours noted on assessment.[95] Spiritual care interventions can be evaluated best by using a combination of objective and subjective criteria, with spiritual well-being as the major criterion. The following questions, with positive answers, indicate a direction that is heading toward that criterion. Does this intervention: (1) bring peace or unity; (2) provide a source of help,

## EVIDENCE-BASED PRACTICE

# Health within Illness: Experiences of Chronically Ill/ Disabled People

The concept of health within illness is beginning to gain recognition in nursing. Although there has been little research to explore and describe this phenomenon, a recent study investigated the meaning of the experience of feeling healthy for people living with a chronic illness and/or disability. The results of that study provide the basis for this box.

An interpretive phenomenological study was undertaken with eight participants living with a variety of different chronic conditions. The results provide a rich mosaic of themes describing the participants' health experiences. These themes include (1) honouring the self; (2) seeking and connecting with others; (3) creating opportunities; (4) celebrating life; (5) transcending the self; and (6) acquiring a state of grace. These results are significant in that they provide for a reconceptualization of health and illness. Such a reconceptualization calls for a transformation in nursing practice from a problem focus and deficit perspective, to one that focuses on the client's capacity and the promotion of health and healing.

## Discussion

The results of this study are "phenomenologically informative" in that they provide guidance for understanding and promoting the health experience for people with chronic conditions. These research findings have been presented in workshops to people with chronic illnesses/disabilities, and the majority of these workshop participants say that they recognize many similarities between the study participants' experiences and their own. The author of the report, Dr. Elizabeth Lindsey, states, however, that some caution should be introduced here. This study, she asserts, is only one representation of health within illness. No claim should be made that all ill people with chronic conditions have similar experiences. Dr. Lindsey goes on to say that if the researcher asks about the illness experience, he or she will probably explore with the participants their experience of the illness. In contrast, if the researcher asks about the experiences of health within illness, the results are necessarily very different.

## Practice Implications

1. If nurses in clinical practice focus their questions and their care on problem identification and illness experience, they are likely to be aware of only some dimensions of the client's experience.

2. Nurse educators and practitioners need to become sensitized to the phenomenon of health within illness. Medicine and nursing have traditionally focused on problem identification, the alleviation of symptoms, and cure. Health professionals should abandon this problem orientation and adopt an approach that focuses on people's capacities.

3. Nurse educators must relinquish their emphasis on teaching students to investigate client problems and needs. Instead, they must consider other forms of client management that provide opportunities for the promotion of health and well-being. Such a shift is not merely a shift in orientation, but a fundamental transformation in philosophical perspective.

4. As nurses adopt a caring and health-promoting stance, they expand their own potential for promoting health and healing. This potential could be experienced on a personal and professional level. Not only will clients be provided the opportunity to expand their health potential, but the nurse will undoubtedly come to experience the power of this caring and health-promoting potential. Such a transformation will help facilitate the health and healing capacities for both nurses and clients.

Source: Lindsey, E., Health within Illness: Experiences of Chronically Ill/Disabled People, *Journal of Advanced Nursing, 24*(1996), 465–472. Used with the permission of Blackwell Science Ltd.

comfort, relief, or strength; (3) promote transcendent values such as meaning, purpose, love, relatedness, and forgiveness of self, God, and others; (4) decrease or alleviate symptoms, such as anxiety, withdrawal, helplessness, agitation, crying, hostility, guilt, shame, depression, and non-forgiveness; (5) bring integration to the personality; (6) help the person to cope and solve problems; and (7) promote hardiness, hope, and intrinsic spiritual values? Realizations and signs that at least some of these objectives have been achieved would provide satisfying evidence of spiritual well-being. These questions can be measured on a continuum of 1 to 10, rated by both nurse and patient. Objective measures alone are inadequate because the client must realize the positive value of the outcome.

Outcomes toward which we must strive are those that (1) enhance trust, (2) allow people to carry on spiritual practices not detrimental to health, (3) decrease feelings of anxiety and guilt, and (4) cause satisfaction with their spiritual condition. To ensure these responses, spiritual care should be considered part of quality assurance. Sister Rosemary Donley suggests that this incorporation—with the addition of some mystery and grace—will help foster support for poor, minority, and very rich people, who are sometimes blamed for their illnesses.[96]

## SUMMARY

1. Spirituality and the spiritual dimensions are inherent in all people, regardless of the presence of beliefs.

2. You will care for clients who adhere to beliefs different from your own.

3. The major world religions include Hinduism, Sikhism, Buddhism, Jainism, Shintoism, Confucianism, Taoism, Islam, Judaism, and Christianity.

4. Wide religious diversity exists in Canada today.

5. Some religious groups of interest include Seventh-Day Adventists; Church of Jesus Christ of Latter-Day Saints (Mormon); Jehovah's Witnesses; Church of Christ, Scientist (Christian Scientist); Mennonites; and Amish.

6. Alternative religions are divided into two components: religious movements and new religions.

7. You can practise principles of spiritual care based on concepts presented in this chapter in every health care setting.

8. Faith communities are ideal to promote health in individuals and their families.

9. You can now engage in lifelong learning about your own and others' beliefs to enable you to assess, plan, and provide holistic care to clients and their families.

## Interesting Websites

### Religions in Canada
www.forces.gc.ca/hr/religions/engraph/religions_toc_e.asp
From Baha'i and Buddhism through Christianity to Judaism, Sikhism, and Alternative Spirituality, this site provides information, book lists, and insights into Canada's religions.

### Statistics Canada's Overview of Religion
www12.statcan.ca/english/census01/Products/Analytic/companion/rel/canada.cfm

Head to this site for extensive information on religion from Statistics Canada, based on census data.

### Religion, Society & Culture in Newfoundland and Labrador
www.ucs.mun.ca/~hrollman/
This site, as presented by Dr. Hans Rollmann, Department of Religious Studies, Memorial University of Newfoundland, provides in-depth information on the religions of Newfoundland and Labrador.

## Key Terms

| | | | |
|---|---|---|---|
| advocacy (80) | atman (62) | beneficence (80) | Brahman (62) |
| agnostic (80) | Aum (62) | Bhagavad-Gita (62) | Buddhism (65) |
| ahimsa (65) | autonomy (80) | bhakti yoga (64) | burial (71) |
| Amish (78) | Baha'i faith (79) | Black Muslims (Nation of Islam) (68) | Christianity (70) |
| Analects (67) | baptism (71) | | Christmas (70) |
| Anointing of the Sick (71) | bar mitzvah (69) | Book of Mormon (78) | Chun-sui (67) |
| | bat mitzvah (69) | bracha (70) | Church of Christ, Scientist (Christian Scientists) (78) |
| atheistic (80) | believer's baptism (73) | Brahma (62) | |

Church of Jesus Christ of Latter-Day Saints (Mormon) (78)
Communion (72)
confirmation (71)
Confucian (65)
Confucianism (66)
Confucius (67)
Conservatives (69)
Divine Liturgy (72)
Easter (71)
Eucharist (71)
fasting (68)
Feast of Sacrifice (Eida-Fita) (68)
foot washing (73)
fundamental precepts (73)
funeral mass (71)
Good Friday (71)
Greek Eastern Orthodox faith (72)
Hadith (67)
Hare Krishna (79)
hatha yoga (65)
high priest (78)
Hindu (62)
Holy Orders (71)
icons (72)
inana yoga (64)

incarnations (62)
Islam (67)
Jainism (65)
Jehovah's Witnesses (78)
Jen (67)
Judaism (69)
karma yoga (64)
kosher (69)
lacto-ovo-vegetarians (73)
Lao-tzu (67)
Lent (70)
Li (67)
liberal precepts (73)
Lotus Sutra (65)
Mass (71)
matrimony (71)
mature baptism (73)
matzo (70)
Mennonites (78)
menorah (69)
mikvah (69)
minister (73)
mitzvah (70)
Nation of Islam (74)
Native American Church (79)
New Age (70)
Nirvana (65)

non-malfeasance (80)
Om (62)
Orthodox (69)
Passover (70)
Penance (71)
Pentecostals (79)
Pesach (70)
phylacteries (69)
Quran (67)
raja yoga (64)
Ramadan (68)
Ramakrishna (62)
Reform Jews (69)
religion (61)
Rosh Hashanah (70)
Sabbath (69)
Sacraments (71)
sanctification (73)
Scientology (79)
Seventh-Day Adventists (73)
seventy (78)
Shintoism (65, 66)
Shiva (62)
Siddur (69)
Sikhism (65)
sitting shiva (70)
Soka Gakkai (65)

spiritual dimension (61)
spiritual need (82)
spirituality (61)
Talmud (69)
Tao (66)
Taoism (66)
Tao-te-ching (67)
Te (67)
Tisha B'av (70)
Torah (69)
treyfe (69)
Unction of the Sick (72)
Upanishads (62)
Vedas (62)
Vishnu (62)
wake (71)
Wen (67)
yang (66)
yarmulke (69)
yin (66)
yin–yang symbol (66)
yoga (64, 79)
Yom Kippur (70)
Zen sect (66)
Zoroastrianism (67)

# Part II
## Basic Concepts Related to the Developing Person and Family Unit

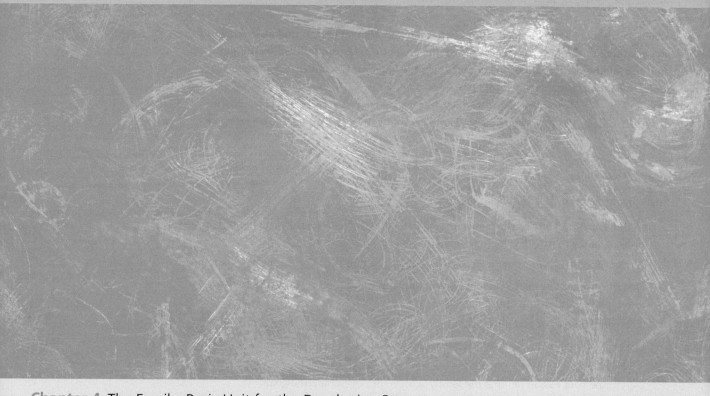

# Chapter 4

## The Family: Basic Unit for the Developing Person

*When we speak of "family" each of us reaches into our store of images and experiences to give meaning to the term. In every culture fundamental roles are fulfilled by the family. And the family instills values, the sense of what is important, what is worth preserving, protecting and, if necessary, fighting for.*

Marlene Brant Castellano (2002). Aboriginal Family Trends, Section 4. Reprinted from the Vanier Institute of the Family's website at www.vifamily.ca. Used with permission.

## Objectives

*Study of this chapter will enable you to:*

1 Define *family* and discuss the family as a system, and be able to identify the implications of family for the developing person.

2 Assess various theoretical approaches for studying the family.

3 Describe the trends, roles, and functions of the family and their relationship to the development and health of its members.

4 Compare and contrast family mechanisms, both adaptive and maladaptive.

5 List stages of family life cycle for the middle-class Canadian family and for other varied family forms.

6 Determine your role in helping the family achieve its developmental goals.

7 Relate the impact of feelings about the self and childhood experiences on later family interaction patterns.

8 List and describe the variables affecting relationships between parent and child, and general family interaction, including single parent, step-parent, and adoptive families.

9 Compare and contrast ways in which your family life has influenced your present attitudes about family.

10 Analyze the influence of 20th-century changes on family life and parenting practices in Canada.

11 Predict how a changing culture may affect the development and health of the family system.

12 Practise therapeutic communication methods to be used when working with a family or other clients.

13 Analyze characteristics and phases of a therapeutic relationship with a client such as the family.

14 Assess a family, constructing a genogram and ecomap using criteria provided in the chapter, to formulate a nursing diagnosis and plan of care.

15 Evaluate your role and various measures and resources to use in promoting physical and emotional health of a family in various situations.

It's an uncanny feeling—to suddenly know that I am answering my son's question with the same words— even the same tone—as my father used with me 30 years ago.

. . .

Even though I have a happy, successful marriage, two loving children, a nice home, and a profession in which I feel competent, I constantly fight a feeling of inferiority. A contributing factor must be that my parents never encouraged or complimented me. When I took a test, they emphasized the 2 wrong, not the 98 right.

. . .

I always admired my aunt. If my cousin, her son, had told her he wanted to build a bridge to the moon, she would have furnished the nails.

These three people are speaking of aspects of a social and biological phenomenon that is often taken for granted: the family. So strongly can this basic unit affect our development and health that we may live successfully or unsuccessfully because of its influence. Much that the person learns about loving, coping, and the various aspects of life is first learned in the family unit.

Some form of family exists in all human societies. Culture, not biology, determines family organization.[1] Between society and the individual person, the family exists as a primary system and social group, because most people share many of life's experiences with the family. Thus the family has a major role in shaping the person; it is a basic unit of growth, experience, adaptation, health, and illness.

The traditional family persists as a norm in the imagination. Today, however, norms hardly exist, considering the fragility of marriage, the high incidence of divorce (and remarriage), the many styles of family life, the diversity of roles held by members, and the increasing number of homeless families. Today's children are being shaped differently— sometimes negatively—by the family unit. For many youngsters, the pain of family life, a changing family scene, having no permanent home, and being separated from other family members is compounded by poverty and neglect.

This chapter is not an exhaustive study of families or family life. Rather, it is an overview of the various forms, stages, and functions of contemporary families and of how you can use this knowledge. Although various aspects of the family are discussed separately, keep in mind that family purposes, stages of development, developmental tasks, and patterns of interaction are all closely interrelated. They are all influenced by historical foundations, and are continually evolving into new forms. Thus the *family should be viewed as a system, affected by the culture, the environment, religious-spiritual dimensions, and other variables, which in turn affect the person and society.*

## DEFINITIONS

Families may have difficulty in maintaining the characteristics proposed in these definitions. Your support, teaching, and counselling may assist family members in promoting and maintaining health.

## Family

The **family** is *an institution, a social group, and an intergenerational group of individuals related to each other by blood, adoption, or marriage/cohabitation.*[2] The **family** also may be defined as *domestic partners, people who have chosen to share each other's life in an intimate and committed relationship of mutual caring.* This definition permits the extension of legal benefits usually accorded to traditionally married heterosexuals, such as health and life insurance and pension benefits, property rights, hospital and prison visitation rights, and bereavement leave, to homosexual or same-sex families or unmarried partners. Researchers and advocacy groups claim that a broad-brush definition of family should not be restricted to household membership but should include caring and enduring intimate relationships regardless of legal or blood ties.[3]

Many headlines declare the demise of the family. However, most of us live, or have lived, in a family unit. A family may exist in one of several forms: traditional, common-law, blended, lone-parent, or same-sex family.[4] We define our own family. The data from the 2001 Canadian Census clearly indicates that the family, while in transition, endures as society's oldest and most basic indestructible institution.[5]

Nurses who care for families should learn who it is that clients consider to be members of their family. These persons should be included in the planning of nursing care. The family may range from traditional notions (father, mother, child, grandparents, uncles, aunts, and cousins) to such "postmodern" family structures as stepfamilies, single-parent families, and same-sex families.[6] Understanding health as a contextual and social phenomenon and understanding that family is the primary social structure in society help direct health care workers to focus on the significance of family to ensure the health of individuals. The family's beliefs, values, and practices strongly influence the health-promoting behaviours of its members.[7] The health status of each member of the family influences the ways in which the family unit functions, and its ability to achieve goals.[8]

## CRITICAL THINKING

*Give your own definition of a family.*

Family may be defined, and viewed, differently by various cultures. Aboriginal families are adopting a variety of forms, for example. The extended family networks on reserves and in rural communities continue to contribute to a stable point of reference—especially for younger members, even though they may relocate while pursuing education and career opportunities. The nuclear family, a two-generation family consisting of parents and children, is steadily becoming the unit of family organization within the Aboriginal community.

Because Aboriginal community membership is becoming increasingly more heterogeneous in ethnic origin and cultural practices, a vigorous movement exists to conserve and revitalize traditional languages, teachings, and ceremonial practices. Spontaneous and self-directed ways to heal from the effects of trauma, past and present, constitute the most promising sign of what the future holds for Aboriginal families.[9] Healing circles have been adopted as preventative, supportive, and rehabilitative measures in dealing with family violence.[10] Due to the growing interdependence of individuals, families, and communities, efforts by the individual must be complemented by collective efforts to offset many of the structural disadvantages that Aboriginal families experience. The fact of these structural disadvantages is evident in statistics regarding income, education, and health. It is important to note that different challenges exist between subgroups of the Aboriginal population. A common theme prevails, however, in Aboriginal community efforts: institutions that collaborate with families to protect children, provide quality education, promote and restore health, and prevent disease must be responsive to the culture and identity of Aboriginal citizens.[11] According to Brant Castellano, a strong movement exists to re-establish Aboriginal control of public services, including health, education, and justice.[12]

The family is a group whose members rely on each other for daily services. With the family, the person can usually let down his or her guard and be more himself or herself than with non-family people. The family comprises a household (or cluster of households) that persists over years or decades and that is characterized by value, role, and power structures; communication patterns; affective socialization, family coping, and health care functions; and developmental stages and tasks.[13]

Sometimes families live together daily. Sometimes the adult partners are employed in different geographic areas, or one member is hospitalized or in prison. Family members maintain contact by telephone, correspondence, and visits. In the two-career family, the partners usually share the same residence on weekends, or at least on some consistent basis. These families carry out their functions and characteristics in their own unique way.

# Family Composition

The family takes several forms. Table 4-1 defines traditional as well as non-traditional family forms. Non-traditional forms may include *same-sex* or *homosexual families*. The family may be childless, have custody of and care for biological children from a previous heterosexual marriage, or have adopted children. Alternately, lesbian women may, through artificial insemination or contact with a selected man, bear a child, in which case the other woman in the relationship shares the parenting role, clearly acknowledging that she is not the mother. Alternately, a gay couple may contract with a woman to carry a baby to term for them. The homosexual person who has had a biological child now frequently seeks custody and/or visiting and caretaking rights and responsibilities after having established a same-sex relationship. Various authors describe the same-sex family.[14] Alderson's study appears be to the first phenomenological study of same-sex marriage. The results indicate that same-sex marriage is here to stay, and that increasing our understanding of this phenomenon is a critical new area of social science research.[15] Same-sex families are, in many respects, pioneering a "new" way of life, and they may need special social support from communities.[16] In addition, health systems, health institutions, and health care providers must play an active role in

---

**Table 4-1 Types of Family Composition**

1. **Nuclear family:** Mother, father, child(ren).
2. **Extended family:** Nuclear plus other relatives of one or both spouses. Relatives of the nuclear family may or may not live with the nuclear family. May include great-grandparents and great-great-grandparents.
3. **Single-parent family:** Mother or father, living with either biological or adopted children, possibly tied emotionally but not legally to a partner.
4. **Stepfamily:** One divorced or widowed adult with all or some of his or her children and a new spouse with all or some of his or her children, and often, also, the children born to this union so that parents, step-parents, children, and stepchildren (or stepsiblings) live together.
5. **Patrifocal/patriarchal family:** Man has main authority and decision-making power.
6. **Matrifocal/matriarchal family:** Woman has main authority and decision-making power.
7. **Same-sex/homosexual family:** Gay or lesbian partners live together.
8. **Single state:** Never married, separated, divorced, widowed.

combating prejudice and reducing barriers to care in partnership with gay, lesbian, bisexual, and Two-spirit people and communities.[17] (The term *Two-spirit* has been derived from interpretations of Native languages, and is used to describe people who display characteristics of both males and females.)

In 2005, Canada became the third country to legalize same-sex marriage after the Parliament approved landmark legislation despite strong opposition from the Conservative party and religious leaders.[18] The Conservative party's platform leading up to the January 2006 election stated that, if elected, a truly free vote on the definition of marriage would be held and, if the resolution passed, the government would introduce legislation to restore the traditional definition of marriage while respecting same-sex marriage.[19] In December 2006, this motion was defeated in Parliament.[20]

---

### CRITICAL THINKING

*What legal rights and spousal benefits, if any, are in place in your province or territory for lesbian and gay families?*

---

The family may be a *series of separate, but interrelated, families*. Some middle-aged parents are helping their adolescent and young adult offspring to be emancipated from the home, while simultaneously caring for increasingly dependent parents, and sometimes up to four pairs of grandparents plus older aunts and uncles! See Chapter 13 for further details.

The family group may be a **psychologically extended family** in which *people who are not biologically related consider themselves as siblings, "adopted" parent, child, aunt, uncle, or grandparent-in-spirit.* Conversely, related or unrelated family members may not live under the same roof.

Present-day mobility of people, the ease of communication over distance, the freedom to evolve and think independently, the freedom to develop in ways less restricted by strong or rigid ethnic or cultural mores, and the ease of transportation all help enable families in Canada to be geographically distant, yet emotionally close and often quite involved with each other.

Regarding divorce, the 2001 Canadian Census claims that the most appropriate way to measure the divorce rate is to compare the number of divorces to the number of marriages that occurred in the year that the couple married. Based on that premise, the Canadian rate is currently 31 to 36 percent.[21] The average "age" of a marriage at divorce is 13.7 years, with the highest rate of divorce resulting after five years of marriage.[22]

People are beginning to realize that divorce does not necessarily improve life. The allure of creativity, growth, and expanding oneself emotionally through divorce is not necessarily realistic. Family members frequently speak of trying harder, and of resolving to stay committed to each other in times of conflict.

## OVERVIEW OF FAMILY THEORETIC APPROACHES

Theoretic approaches to the study of families include developmental, structural-functional, interactional, role, family systems, and crisis theories (see Table 4-2). Refer to the endnote at the end of the text for more extensive explanation.[23]

## TRENDS, ROLES, AND FUNCTIONS OF THE FAMILY

Knowledge of the following sections will enhance a number of health care activities, including assessment, health promotion intervention, teaching, referral, and advocacy. Family structure, roles, and responsibilities have been influenced by communications technology, globalization of economy, globalization of marketing, bio-genetic engineering, and the resulting social changes, which are leading to a hurried culture.[24] The demands of time have entered into our contemporary descriptions of family life. Daly states that it is almost pure madness to think of families living without sophisticated scheduling tools.[25] The forces shaping this continuous growing pace are the following:

- *Changing family form.* The dual-earner family is the dominant family form, and it faces heavy demands in negotiating time for its members. Many such families, as well as other family forms, have too many responsibilities and not enough time.[26] Even as the Canadian population ages, the demand on families in their role as caregivers will rise.

- *Increasing effects of technology.* Technology has accelerated the family's lifestyle along many avenues. One such avenue is that of a general growing of impatience fuelled by the desire for immediate results brought on in part by such devices as cell phones, beepers, and even microwave ovens, to name a few.

- *Increasing workload.* Daly argues that the culture of overwork is flourishing in our society. Families are working more hours than ever before, and they are playing less.[27] This scarcity of available time to relax is felt not only by the adult members in the family, but by children as well.

Frederick claims that 15- to 17-year-old students report feeling anxious when their time is limited. Unfortunately, when they need more time, they tend to cut back on sleep.[28]

## Table 4-2 Summary of Major Family Theories and Approaches

| Family Theory | Definition of Family | View of Person | Approach/Focus |
|---|---|---|---|
| **Developmental theory:** compilation of several frameworks | *Series of interacting personalities, intricately organized into paired positions (father, husband, daughter, sister); norms for reciprocal relations prescribe role behaviour for each position; predictable natural history designated by stages.* | Person is a member of group; each new member adds to complexity of interaction. | **Study family** in terms of role behaviours for each family life-cycle stage, along with the changing ages of each person; study quality and type of interaction as age and member composition of family changes.<br>**Focus:** Analyze developmental needs and tasks of each family life-cycle stage; analyze family behaviours and changing developmental tasks and role expectations in terms of increasing complexity, analyze children, parents, and family units as a whole. Cultural influences at each stage of family life cycle are considered. |
| **Structural-functional theory:** focus on family as a system | *Social system open to outside influences and transactions; maintains boundaries by responding to demands of system or acting under family constraints, passively adapting to external forces rather than acting as an agent of change in itself.* | Person is seen as reactive in fulfilling roles and as having status in the social system. | **Study family** in relation to other social structures or social systems and in terms of roles.<br>**Focus:** Determine how family patterns are related to other institutions and overall society; study family functions (reproduction, socialization of children, provision of physical needs, economics). |
| **Interactional theory:** reflection of role theory and psychodynamic theory | *Defined in terms of individual members, a unity of interacting personalities with assigned position and roles, expectations, and norms of behaviour; seen as closed unit with little relationship to outside institutions, associations, or cultures.* | Person is seen as fulfilling roles and as an interacting being. Messages sent by members to each other have multi-level meanings. | **Study family** in terms of overt interactions, fulfillment of interacting roles and ways of communicating.<br>**Focus:** Analyze roles, interstatus relations, authority matters, and action taking communication processes, conflicts, problem solving and decision making. Teach most effective communication methods. |

## Table 4-2 (continued)

| Family Theory | Definition of Family | View of Person | Approach/Focus |
|---|---|---|---|
| **Role theory:** life is structured according to roles that are ascribed or assumed by the person in interaction with others; roles are learned through socialization | *Defined in terms of members' role interaction;* roles contribute in the following way to the family unit: Circumscribe behaviour Define social position, responses, and expectations Influence group associations Are purpose of interaction Provide norms for the family or group. | Person is seen in terms of roles, which are specialized or shared and depend on sex, age, social norms, status, and ability to complement. Roles change through development and negotiation, which depend on flexibility, stability, and congruence of expectations. Person experiences role reciprocity, being complemented, or strain.<br><br>**Role reciprocity:** *mutual exchange; sharing affects decision making and cohesion;* personal and family needs met; high mutual dependence in division of labour; potential for growth; commitment to family and reducing conflict.<br><br>**Role complementarity:** *family members differentiate and define roles in relation to each other;* opportunity for growth; sometimes not a sense of mutual-gratification; can confirm identity of one at expense of other; if rigid roles, transitions are difficult.<br><br>**Role strain:** *occurs when individuals have difficulty meeting others' or own expectations and the obligations of the role and is manifested as:*<br><br>1. **Role conflict:** *unclear, incomplete, contradictory elements in role; performing one role makes it impossible to perform another; conflicting norms.* | **Study family** in terms of role interactions, differentiation, allocation, role change, and role strain.<br>**Focus:** Analyze role reciprocity, complementarity, and strain. |

(continued)

Table 4-2 (continued)

| Family Theory | Definition of Family | View of Person | Approach/Focus |
|---|---|---|---|
| | | 2. **Role overload:** *must consider impact of distribution of power; the greater the control over negotiation of roles, the more the person can avoid role strain; person with less power assumes more unwanted burdens;* person with more power has less dependency needs and can make role demands. | |
| **Family systems theory** | *Integral unit in society, made up of parts or members, with individual and family characteristics that are interacting and interdependent. Maintain equilibrium by developing repetitive techniques of interaction.* | Person is member of system and subsystem. | **Study family** as a whole unit; sum of whole is greater than its parts or subsystems.<br>**Focus:** Analyze family's adaptive process, exchange between members and subsystems, and decision making, transactions, bargaining, cooperative, and coercive processes. Examine rules of family organization, patterns of interaction, traditions, whether boundaries are open and flexible or closed, and interaction with other systems. |
| **Crisis theory** | *Family made up of members who individually experience hazardous events.* | Problems or illness of one member is expressed in conflict or problems of that family. All family members are affected by inability of one to cope. | Brief therapy<br>**Study family** in terms of crisis impact on all, rather than just one.<br>**Focus:** Analyze present situation. Identify role and conflicts, general coping skills. Avoid blame; focus on perception and reality. Specific tasks are to be mastered. Alternate plans for coping are attempted until effective ways to reduce tension and disorganization are found. Ways to handle future crisis are explored. Therapist uses a variety of cognitive, educational, behavioural, and communication approaches to help family cope with crisis and become more functional. |

Sauvé, in his 2006 *Report on the Effects of the Changing Age Structure on Households and Families to 2026*, considers several significant projections as follows:

- The trend in families has seen rates of family formation fall for all age groups with the exception of those aged 65 and over.

- The growth in the total number of families is projected to slow significantly over the next two decades, with growth of only about 15 percent between 2005 and 2026.

- Families with a primary maintainer who is aged 65 or over will rise from 17 percent of all families recorded in 2005 to 30 percent in 2026. Furthermore, the actual number of maintainers 65 years or older will likely more than double over the next two decades.

- The current 84 percent of families that include both husbands and wives will continue to decline and represent 81 percent of the total by year 2026, compared to 87 percent in 1986.

- As more people live alone, families will make up a shrinking percentage of all households. This ratio is now at 70 percent and may decrease toward 62 percent by 2026.[29]

In Canada and other industrialized nations, balancing paid work and family activities is a pivotal issue that must be explored. Hall and Callery conducted a study using the grounded theory method to explain how dual-earner couples manage work and family life. The analysis of data produced a substantive theory whose outcomes, processes, and strategies offer a rich array of opportunities whereby health professionals can influence individual and family development and viability.[30]

## Roles of the Family

The family assigns **roles**, *prescribed behaviours in a situation*, in ways similar to that of society at large. In society, we have specialists who enforce laws, teach, practise medicine, and fight fires. In the family there are:

1. **Performance roles:** breadwinner, homemaker, handyman (or handywoman), the expert, political adviser, chauffeur, and gardener.

2. **Emotional roles:** leader, nurturer, protector, healer, arbitrator, scapegoat, jester, rebel, dependant, "sexpot," and "black sheep."

Family members may fill more than one role. The fewer people there are to fulfill these roles, as in the nuclear family, the greater the number of demands placed on any one person.

If a member leaves home, someone else must take up his or her role. Any member of the family can satisfactorily fulfill any role in either category unless he or she is uncomfortable in that role. Ideally, family members enjoy sharing roles, working together to get the tasks done without worrying about what is men's or women's work.

*The emotional response of a person to the role he or she fulfills should be considered.* Someone may perform the job competently and yet dread doing it. Changes in performance roles also necessitate emotional changes (e.g., the man who takes over household duties when his wife becomes incapacitated).

*The child learns the types of accepted emotional responses to family roles by observing and imitating adults.* The child experiments with various roles in play. The more pressure put on the child by the parents to respond in a particular way, the more likely that child is to learn only one role and be uncomfortable in others, as evidenced by the athletic champion who may be a social misfit. As a result of increasing

---

## NARRATIVE VIGNETTE

Your neighbours and friends Janet and Abe, along with their two school-age children, who are highly active in school and community activities, constitute a dual-earner family. Last evening, Janet called you and related that things are getting difficult for her at work. It seems that she is working longer hours this year, and is finding it increasingly difficult to juggle her time satisfactorily between work and family life. Janet wants to inform her supervisor that her (Janet's) mother has just been hospitalized and that she needs some time off work to care for her. However, Janet knows that her supervisor is also under heavy pressure due to recent layoffs in the business. Janet, realizing that you know her supervisor well, asked you to speak to the supervisor in support of Janet's upcoming request for time away from work. You listened to

Janet last evening, but told her, as a friend, that you were exhausted and would call her back this evening. You would like to help Janet, but you remember her habit of being late for appointments and her increasing anxiety about the daily activities of her family.

As a lone parent with two preschool children, you are also very busy balancing your nursing duties and family life.

As a health professional:

1. How will you respond to Janet?

2. In what ways can you help her to cope with the many issues she faces?

To help you to respond to these questions, see Hall and Callery (2003).[31]

pressure, the child often becomes less adaptive socially, even within the family.

*Major situational life events facing families unavoidably affect their role functioning.* These situations are usually stressful events such as natural disasters (e.g., tornados), unemployment, or changes in the health of family members, such as cancer.[32]

Exercising a capacity for a variety of roles, either in actuality or in fantasy, is healthy. The healthy family is one in which there is opportunity to shift roles intermittently with ease. Through these roles, family functions are fulfilled.

---

CRITICAL THINKING

*What are the various roles in your family?*

---

## Functions of the Family as a Social System

The *family meets the criteria of a system because it functions as a unit* to:

1. Fulfill its purposes, roles, and tasks.
2. Provide shelter, stability, security, and a setting for nurturance and growth.
3. Provide opportunity to experiment with the dynamics and role behaviours required in a system.
4. Provide a support system for individual members.
5. Adapt in order to meet individual needs and prepare its members to participate in the social system.

The *organization of a family system is hierarchal,* although it may not be directly observable. The usual family hierarchies are built on kinship, power, status, and privilege relationships that may be related to individual characteristics of age, sex, education, personality, health, strength, and vigour. We can infer a hierarchy by observing each person's behaviour and communication. For instance, who talks first? Last? Longest? Who talks to whom? When? Where? About what? If one family member consistently approaches the staff about the client's health care, he or she probably holds an upper position in the family and has the task of being the "expert." Your attempt to communicate with family members may meet with resistance if the communication inadvertently violates the family communication hierarchy.[33]

*Hierarchal relations in the family system determine the role behaviour of family members.* These hierarchal role relationships typically have great stability, and ordinarily family members can be counted on to behave congruently with their roles. When there are differences in behaviour from situation to situation, they are almost inevitably in response to the family's expectations for that particular situation or circumstance.[34] Families develop a system of balanced relationships. Roles and relationships are based on reciprocal interaction, with each member of the family contributing to the total unit in a unique and functional way.

Family functions cover many dimensions: physical, affectionate, emotional, social, and spiritual. Most families agree generally with the functions described below. Interestingly, Jones[35] found that there was no significant difference between deaf and hearing parents' perceptions of family function and that they agreed on seven of ten items ranked as most important.

**Physical functions** of the family are met by the parents' *providing food, clothing, and shelter; protection against danger; bodily repairs after fatigue or illness; and reproduction.* In some societies, these physical needs are the dominant concern. In Western societies, many families take them for granted.

**Affectional functions** are equally important. Although many traditional family functions, such as education, job training, and medical care, are being absorbed by other agencies, *meeting emotional needs and promoting adaptation and adjustment are still two of the family's major functions.* The family is the primary unit in which the child tests emotional reactions. Learning how to react and maintain emotional equilibrium within a loving and supportive family enables the child to repeat the pattern in later life situations. A healthy family has several dominant characteristics:

1. All persons are seen as unique, developing, and worthy of respect.
2. When a disturbing situation arises, members understand that many factors were involved—people were not simply trying to be difficult.
3. Members accept the notion that change is continuous.
4. Members share their thoughts and feelings with a minimum of blame, and generally they feel good about each other and themselves.

**Social functions** of the modern family include *providing social togetherness, fostering self-esteem and a personal identity tied to family identity, providing opportunities for observing and learning social and sexual roles, accepting responsibility for behaviour, and supporting individual creativity and initiative.* The family gives a name to the infant and hence indicates a social position or status in relation to the immediate and kinship-group families. *Parental socialization practices* arise from combinations of the following:

- Cultural and social environmental determinants, including poverty, and norms about what may be considered the "best" parenting practices.
- Parents' personalities as well as beliefs.
- Parental adaptation to children's behaviours, needs, and personalities.

In this interactional perspective, children contribute to the development of the socialization style of parents.[36] In fact, the child's genetic background may be at least as important in his or her development as the parenting style.[37]

The **spiritual function** to raise the child to be a moral person with a belief system of some kind is now discussed less frequently in texts. The authors believe, however, that much of society expects parents to continue to shoulder this responsibility. See Chapter 3 for further details on the matter.

The parent generation educates by literal instruction and by serving as models. Thus the child's **personality**, *a product of all influences that have and are impinging on him or her*, is greatly influenced by the parents.

---

CRITICAL THINKING

*What aspects of family culture would an Inuit family likely transmit to its children?*

---

## FAMILY ADAPTATION

The following information can be used in assessment and in health promotion. You can teach healthy adaptive patterns, assess for unhealthy or abusive patterns, and use the interventions introduced and discussed throughout the chapter.

**Adaptive responses in the family** represent the *means by which it maintains an internal equilibrium so that it can fulfill purposes and tasks, deal with internal and external stress and crises, and allow for the growth of individual members.* Some capacity for functioning may be sacrificed to control conflict and aid work as a unit. But the best functioning family keeps anxiety and conflict within tolerable limits and maintains a balance between effects of the past and new experiences. In the same ways that other social systems adjust, the family system must adjust as well.[38]

Ideally, the family achieves equilibrium by talking over problems and finding solutions together. Humour, problem-solving abilities, flexibility, the occasional acceptance of nonsense, shared work, and leisure all help to relieve tension. Strategies that extend outside the family include: (1) seeking information; (2) maintaining links with the extended family or with people or agencies in the community; (3) using self-help groups or informal or formal support networks; and (4) seeking spiritual support.[39]

## Designation of One Person as Family Healer

This mechanism involves using a "wise one" (most often in the extended family), "umpire," minister, storekeeper, bartender, or druggist to arrange a reconciliation between dissenting parties.

A variant of the healer role is that of the family "counsellor," who assists family members to cope with their stress.

The Aboriginal community is undergoing a cultural, traditional, and spiritual renewal. The inclusion of tradition and culture in Aboriginal healing practices has facilitated Aboriginal people to seek out healing. They view healing as a celebration of survival and triumph over one's human condition.[40] In the Aboriginal community, one of the roles of the elder is that of a healer. An elder's wisdom is seen as coming from deep within his or her being, and it reaches to the roots of the past to help link contemporary peoples with their ancestors and their traditions.[41] It is important to realize that to the Aboriginal people, family has a relatively broad meaning. Family encircles an extended network of grandparents, aunts, uncles, and cousins.[42] In essence, family and community represent the same network of resources.

---

CRITICAL THINKING

*How do Aboriginal traditional practices differ from your own family healing practices?*

---

## FAMILY MALADAPTATION

Dysfunctional or ineffective coping strategies used by families during stressful times include denial of problems; exploitation or manipulation of one or more family members; abuse of or violence toward children or adult members; use of authoritarianism or threats; changing to ineffective customs, traditions, or family myths; use of alcohol or drugs; and abandonment of the family by one member through separation, divorce, or suicide.[43]

*Signs of strained or destructive family relationships* include the following:[44]

- Lack of understanding, communication, and helpfulness between or among members, resulting in unclear roles and conflict
- Each family member alternately acting as if the other does not exist or harassing through arguments
- Lack of family decision making or lines of authority
- Parents' possessiveness of the children or the mate
- Children's derogatory remarks to parents or vice versa
- Extreme closeness between the husband and his mother or family or the wife and her mother or family
- Members not maintaining individuality, being too close or enmeshed or too distant with each other
- Parent being domineering about performance of household tasks
- Few outside friends for parents or children

- Scapegoating or blaming each other for difficulties
- High level of anxiety or insecurity present in the home
- Lack of creativity and stability
- Pattern of immature or regressive behaviour in parents or children
- Boundaries between generations not maintained; children carrying out parental roles because of a parent's inability to function, illness, or abandonment

Several recent texts provide in-depth information pertinent to the assessment of and intervention with families.[45]

## STAGES OF THE FAMILY LIFE CYCLE

Families are composed of individuals who have a shared history and future in terms of intergenerational connectedness. They go through a typical path known as the family life cycle.[46] Events in the typical life cycle are connected to the comings and goings of family members. Many of these events, such as the birth of a child or the death of a loved one, require formal reorganization of rules and roles within the family system.[47] That is, boundaries shift, psychological distances change between and among members, and roles in subsystems are constantly redefined.[48] Although families have roles and functions, the main emphasis is the set of irreplaceable relationships. Relationships that involve parents, siblings, and other family members go through noticeable transitions as the individuals travel along the life cycle.

Cultural and spiritual factors play a major role in the manner in which families go through the life cycle. Furthermore, each family member's worldview and attitudes toward life-cycle transition are influenced profoundly by the historical era in which they grew up and were socialized. Therefore, families must be examined both within their own context and in the larger cultural contexts, both of which can change over time.[49]

Over the last ten years, many tumultuous changes have occurred in the family life cycle. Some of those changes can be accounted for by lower birth rates, a longer life expectancy, the impact of terrorism, an increase in immigration, increases in divorce and remarriage, and differences in gender roles—especially the changing role of women.[50] Families are complex interactive systems that need to deal with smooth, as well as difficult, progressions. Frequently, in working with families, both change and stability must be addressed simultaneously.[51]

## Middle-Class North American Family Life Cycle

According to McGoldrick and Carter, the family life cycle of the North American middle-class family highlights the expansion, contraction, and realignment of relationships as entries, exits, and developments of family members occur. Table 4-3 illustrates the stages of this family life cycle, the emotional process of transition (key principles), and the second-order changes in family required to proceed developmentally. That is, the table indicates the tasks that often are accomplished during each stage. The family life cycle begins at the stage of "young adulthood." The primary task there is that young adults come to terms with their family of origin by remaining connected to the family yet separating without sharply cutting off or fleeing to a substitute emotional source. This phase is a cornerstone. It is a period during which the young adult can formulate personal life goals and become a "self" before joining with a partner to form a new family subsystem.[52] The other stages require transition and reconnection to a new way so the family can move developmentally.

Due to the variability of family forms and development, four types of family life cycles are discussed briefly, and outlined in table form. The last family life cycle to be considered—gay, lesbian, bisexual, and transgendered family life cycle—is discussed briefly. There is no unique framework for this family group because all of the stages of the traditional family life cycle can be applied to gays and lesbians, with some unique differences, outlined below.[53]

**Divorced Family Life Cycle** A relatively high level of divorce exists in our society today. A considerable amount of debilitating stress is experienced by members of families who experience the process of divorce.[54] Divorce is a painful transition. It can create extensive sadness, worry, and regret, all of which coexist with competent social and psychological functioning.[55] Table 4-4 illustrates some of the phases, emotional processes of transition, and developmental issues involved during divorce and post-divorce.

---

### CRITICAL THINKING

*What factors can contribute to a divorce? What are some of the negative outcomes of divorce for children?*

---

**Remarried Life Cycle** Today's stepfamilies are different from stepfamilies of the past.[56] Many fears beset the family during the transition to remarriage. Some of those fears consist of the struggles one experiences about investing in a new relationship; the fear of rearing children, possibly from both partners; and dealing with upset reactions from children, the extended family, or the ex-partner.[57] Table 4-5 summarizes the prerequisite attitudes and development issues for stepfamily formation.

**Professional and Low-Income Family Life Cycle Process: A Comparison** Several differences exist between two-career professional families and lower-income families that receive social assistance.[58] These two types of

Table 4-3 The Stages of the Family Life Cycle

| Family Life Cycle Stage | Emotional Process of Transition: Key Principles | Second-Order Changes in Family Status Required to Proceed Developmentally |
| --- | --- | --- |
| Leaving home: single young adults | Accepting emotional and financial responsibility for self | a. Differentiation of self in relation to family of origin<br>b. Development of intimate peer relationships<br>c. Establishment of self in respect to work and financial independence |
| The joining of families through marriage: the new couple | Commitment to new system | a. Formation of marital system<br>b. Realignment of relationships with extended families and friends to include spouse |
| Families with young children | Accepting new members into the system | a. Adjusting marital system to make space for children<br>b. Joining in child rearing, financial and household tasks<br>c. Realignment of relationships with extended family to include parenting and grandparenting roles |
| Families with adolescents | Increasing flexibility of family boundaries to permit children's independence and grandparents' frailties | a. Shifting of parent/child relationships to permit adolescent to move into and out of system<br>b. Refocus on midlife marital and career issues<br>c. Beginning shift toward caring for older generation |
| Launching children and moving on | Accepting a multitude of exits from and entries into the family system | a. Renegotiation of marital system as a dyad<br>b. Development of adult-to-adult relationships between grown children and their parents<br>c. Realignment of relationships to include in-laws and grandchildren<br>d. Dealing with disabilities and death of parents (grandparents) |
| Families in later life | Accepting the shifting generational roles | a. Maintaining own and/or couple functioning and interests in face of physiological decline: exploration of new familial and social role options<br>b. Support for more central role of middle generation<br>c. Making room in the system for the wisdom and experience of the elderly, supporting the older generation without overfunctioning for them<br>d. Dealing with loss of spouse, siblings, and other peers and preparation for death |

Source: Carter, B., and M. McGoldrick, Overview: The Expanded Family Life Cycle: Individual, Family, and Social Perspectives. In B. Carter and M. McGoldrick (eds.), *The Expanded Family Life Cycle: Individual, Family, and Social Perspectives*, 3rd ed (pp. 1–26). Toronto: Allyn and Bacon, 1999.

## Table 4-4 An Additional Stage of the Family Life Cycle for Divorcing Families

| Phase | | Emotional Process of Transition: Prerequisite Attitude | Developmental Issues |
|---|---|---|---|
| Divorce | The decision to divorce | Acceptance of inability to resolve marital tensions sufficiently to continue relationship. | Acceptance of one's own part in the failure of the marriage. |
| | Planning the breakup of the system | Supporting viable arrangements for all parts of the system. | a. Working cooperatively on problems of custody, visitation, and finances.<br>b. Dealing with extended family about the divorce. |
| | Separation | a. Willingness to continue cooperative co-parental relationship and joint financial support of children.<br>b. Work on resolution of attachment to spouse. | a. Mourning loss of intact family.<br>b. Restructuring marital and parent-child relationships and finances; adaptation to living apart.<br>c. Realignment of relationships with extended family; staying connected with spouse's extended family. |
| | The divorce | More work on emotional divorce: overcoming hurt, anger, guilt, etc. | a. Mourning loss of intact family; giving up fantasies of reunion.<br>b. Retrieval of hopes, dreams, expectations from the marriage.<br>c. Staying connected with extended families. |
| Post-divorce Family | Single parent (custodial household or primary residence) | Willingness to maintain financial responsibilities, continue parental contact with ex-spouse, and support contact of children with ex-spouse and his or her family. | a. Making flexible visitation arrangements with ex-spouse and family.<br>b. Rebuilding own financial resources.<br>c. Rebuilding own social network. |
| | Single parent (noncustodial) | Willingness to maintain financial responsibilities and parental contact with ex-spouse and to support custodial parent's relationship with children. | a. Finding ways to continue effective parenting.<br>b. Maintaining financial responsibilities to ex-spouse and children.<br>c. Rebuilding own social network. |

Source: Carter, B., and M. McGoldrick, The Divorce Cycle: A Major Variation in the American Family Life Cycle. In B. Carter and M. McGoldrick (eds.), *The Expanded Family Life Cycle: Individual, Family, and Social Perspectives*, 3rd ed (pp. 373–380). Toronto: Allyn and Bacon, 1999.

## Table 4-5 Remarried Family Formation: A Developmental Outline

| Steps | Prerequisite Attitude | Developmental Issues |
|---|---|---|
| 1. Entering the new relationship | Recovery from loss of first marriage (adequate emotional divorce). | Recommitment to marriage and to forming a family with readiness to deal with the complexity and ambiguity. |
| 2. Conceptualizing and planning new marriage and family | Accepting one's own fears and those of new spouse and children about remarriage and forming a stepfamily.<br>Accepting need for time and patience for adjustment to complexity and ambiguity of:<br>1. Multiple new roles.<br>2. Boundaries: space, time, membership, and authority.<br>3. Affective issues: guilt, loyalty conflicts, desire for mutuality, unresolvable past hurts. | a. Work on openness in the new relationships to avoid pseudomutuality.<br>b. Plan for maintenance of cooperative financial and co-parental relationships with ex-spouses.<br>c. Plan to help children deal with fears, loyalty conflicts, and membership in two systems.<br>d. Realignment of relationships with extended family to include new spouse and children.<br>e. Plan maintenance of connections for children with extended family of ex-spouses. |
| 3. Remarriage and reconstruction of family | Final resolution of attachment to previous spouse and ideal of "intact" family; acceptance of a different model of family with permeable boundaries. | a. Restructuring family boundaries to allow for inclusion of new spouse-stepparent.<br>b. Realignment of relationships and financial arrangements throughout subsystems to permit interweaving of several systems.<br>c. Making room for relationships of all children with biological (noncustodial) parents, grandparents, and other extended family.<br>d. Sharing memories and histories to enhance step-family integration. |

Source: Carter, B., and M. McGoldrick, The Divorce Cycle: A Major Variation in the American Family Life Cycle. In B. Carter and M. McGoldrick (eds.), *The Expanded Family Life Cycle: Individual, Family, and Social Perspectives,* 3rd ed (pp. 373–380). Toronto: Allyn and Bacon, 1999.

family pass the life cycle benchmarks at different ages. In a low-income situation, the family often begins with a mother and child, and a partner is added later. Meanwhile, the professional family begins with the couple, but they add children only after a substantial delay. Lower-income families are more predisposed to severe environmental pressure compared to professional families.[59] Table 4-6 illustrates a comparison of the family life cycle stages of professional and low-income families.

**Gay, Lesbian, Bisexual, and Transgendered Family Life Cycle** Society generally has either ignored gays, lesbians, bisexuals, and transgendered people in couple or family relationships, or delineated them as an invisible subculture.[60] Recently, the visibility of these individuals has grown, along with open discussions of same-sex marriage or union.[61] More attention is now being focused on the structure, developmental life cycles, strengths, and limitations of these relationships. Certainly, there are some differences from the traditional family life cycle. One such difference is that the adolescent who struggles with role identity within the family context often has a difficult time, but gays and lesbians, who also struggle with identity issues, are often without the support of their family or community. Another difference is that some gays and lesbians may opt for a split-self adaptation, which means straight to the world but gay to self. Although some may appear to adjust well, low to high anxiety related to fears of being found out may persist under the mask.[62] Health care services are needed to provide supportive environments and address the barriers and homophobia that persist in these settings.[63]

### CRITICAL THINKING

*What steps can you, as a nurse, take to promote the health of a gay or lesbian adolescent?*

## Table 4-6 Comparison of Family Life Cycle Stages

| Age | Professional Families | Low-Income Families |
|---|---|---|
| 12–17 | a. Prevent pregnancy<br>b. Graduate from high school<br>c. Parents continue support while permitting child to achieve greater independence | a. First pregnancy<br>b. Attempt to graduate from high school<br>c. Parent attempts strict control before pregnancy. After pregnancy, relaxation of controls and continued support of new mother and infant |
| 18–21 | a. Prevent pregnancy<br>b. Leave parental household for college<br>c. Adapt to parent–child separation | a. Second pregnancy<br>b. No further education<br>c. Young mother acquires adult status in parental household |
| 22–25 | a. Prevent pregnancy<br>b. Develop professional identity in graduate school<br>c. Maintain separation from parental household. Begin living in serious relationship | a. Third pregnancy<br>b. Marriage—leave parental household to establish stepfamily<br>c. Maintain connection with kinship network |
| 26–30 | a. Prevent pregnancy<br>b. Marriage—develop nuclear couple as separate from parents<br>c. Intense work involvement as career begins | a. Separate from husband<br>b. Mother becomes head of own household within kinship network |
| 31–35 | a. First pregnancy<br>b. Renew contact with parents as grandparents<br>c. Differentiate career and childrearing roles between husband and wife | a. First grandchild<br>b. Mother becomes grandmother and cares for daughter and infant |

Source: Fulmer, R.H., Lower-Income and Professional Families: A Comparison of Structure and Life Cycle Process. In B. Carter and M. McGoldrick (eds.), *The Changing Family Life Cycle: A Framework for Family Therapy*, 2nd ed (pp. 545–578). Toronto: Allyn and Bacon, 1989.

## FATHERHOOD

Becoming a father is a critical stage in adult life. The man experiences a variety of feelings on learning of the pregnancy, feelings that usually change during the pregnancy. For the father, the reality of the pregnancy increases with time. Concerns identified by fathers include caring for the infant, adequacy as a father, financial security, and the baby's effect on the marital dyad.[64]

Historically, men have been known as providers. Traditionally, men spend much time outside the home providing for the family in terms of economic security. Now, Dubeau argues, the pendulum has swung in the other direction. Men are becoming not only affectionate, but caring fathers.[65] Presently, fathers are emotionally involved in rearing, caring for, and communicating with their children. A paucity of literature and research exists on the experiences of men who take on the primary caregiving of children. More research and scholarly articles are needed to assist health professionals in obtaining necessary knowledge in this field.

One important area to examine, mainly due to the increased rate of immigration to Canada, is the role of immigrant fathers. Steinberg, Kruckman, and Steinberg conducted a transnational study of Japanese and Canadian families.[66] Their results suggest that the social meaning of fatherhood has been transformed, justifying the presence of the father in the household as a result of shifting extended family domestic structures, economic conditions, and the empowerment of women. The findings indicated other significant patterns. Canadian fathers, for example, participate in labour and delivery to a higher degree than do Japanese fathers.[67] Leininger, in writing about Japanese Americans and culture care, addresses important cultural information about the Japanese worldview, cultural values, and other pertinent issues.[68] As Canadian

## CASE SITUATION

Wan and his now 34-year-old Japanese-Canadian wife, Oniki, immigrated to Canada a few years ago. Initially, Wan was happy that Oniki was pregnant with their first child. Lately, however, he has been behaving in a somewhat stressed manner, presumably about the coming baby. He says he is hoping for a boy. At the clinic, he informs you shyly that he must be the provider, and that he fears he will not have much time to devote either to Oniki or to the baby. Both sets of future grandparents, who recently arrived to stay in Canada, are delighted that Oniki is pregnant.

1. According to the Steinberg, Kruckman, and Steinberg study on "Reinventing Fatherhood" in Japan and Canada, what is meant in this case by a "reciprocal cultural" barrier?

2. What other challenges might Wan be experiencing that should be considered in order to assist him in his adjustment to the role of fatherhood?

3. What can you say, and do, to assist Wan as he adapts to his role as a father?

See Steinberg, Kruckman, and Steinberg (2000),[69] and Leininger (2002).[70]

authors, we believe that the study of acculturation and value changes is a highly important issue for health professionals who strive to provide quality health care to the family.

## FAMILY INTERACTION

One of the most important activities in the family is the interactional relationship known as communication. As a social system, the family communicates continually with its internal and external environment. Healthy families and relationships are based on functional communication patterns and processes. The nurse needs to develop an awareness of the many different types of family communication patterns that can either enhance or impede family health and wellness.[71]

Interactions of the husband and wife, or of all adult members living under one roof, are basic to the mental, and sometimes physical, health of the adults, and to the eventual health of the children. Two factors strongly influence this interaction: (1) the sense of self-esteem, or self-love, of each family member, and (2) the different socialization processes for boys and girls.[72]

Many young adults are returning home to the family unit. These young people are known by some as the "boomerang" generation.[73] Table 4-7 lists suggestions for adult children and their parents that can make living together more harmonious.[74]

**Table 4-7 Guidelines for Parents When Young Adult Offspring Move Back Home**

1. Remember what it was like when a new baby came home. No matter how loved the child is, disruptions are bound to occur. Realize that another relative's homecoming will be the same.

2. Everyone involved should remember whose house it is.

3. Realize that no matter how long sons or daughters have been away, basic family procedures do not change significantly. Mom may still be critical. Dad may be a constant advice giver. Expect it.

4. Talk about resentments. Discuss problems if you think it will help.

5. Parents may say offspring are grown up, but that does not mean they believe it. Still, they cannot exert the same authority with a 30- or 40-year-old as they could with a youngster.

6. Offspring and elderly parents must be flexible. It is unfair to expect the middle-agers who are "hosts" to change their household and life routines too much.

7. Even if parents refuse money, adult offspring should insist on paying something, no matter how minimal. Otherwise, the offspring are reinforcing the idea that parents are taking care of them. Elderly parents can also contribute financially most of the time.

8. When grandchildren are involved, negotiate rules about who is in charge, and when. To decrease dependency, babysitters should be hired when possible. Then family members do not feel as obligated or constrained.

9. Determine the length of the adult offspring's stay. It need not be a precise date, but future plans about leaving the home should be explicitly stated.

10. Both adult offspring and older relatives should share responsibilities if possible. Do not upstage Mom or Dad, however. For example, if Mom loves cooking, do not make her feel useless by taking over in the kitchen.

11. Space permitting, privacy is important. The relative who has lived on his or her own is probably used to time and space alone.

12. Middle-agers should resist meddling in the affairs of either offspring or parents. They can advise, but grown offspring need to think for themselves, and older relatives expect to make their own decisions.

13. Realize that the living situation may be temporary. Living together may not be ideal for anyone, but some parents and offspring, or middle-agers and their parents, become closer during such periods.

## Importance of Self-Esteem

The most important life task for each person is to feel a sense of self-esteem; that is, to love the self and have a positive self-image. The self-image has evolved through interaction with the parents from the time of birth onward. In turn, the self-image affects how the person interacts in later life with others, including a spouse and offspring. You can help family members to realize the importance of respecting and loving one another. You can help them work through problems stemming from the low self-esteem of a family member.[75]

## Influence of Childhood Socialization

The second crucial influence on interaction among adults in the family is the difference in socialization processes for boys and girls. Important differences exist, even in our changing society. Within some cultural groups, the differences are obvious, especially among people in mainstream society who may deny that they socialize boys and girls differently. The girl may be loved simply because she exists and can attract attention, as shown by the admiration that pretty girls receive. The girl may be taught to be subtle because such behaviour is part of her attraction. The boy may be loved for what he can do, and for what he may become. He must prove himself. Boys, especially from school age on, are afforded less recognition than girls are for good looks. Instead, they receive much recognition for what they can do.[76]

In Canada, much of the child's socialization takes place in either public or private day centres. It is best to examine the parent–child relationship within the context of personalities involved and the sociocultural context in which the family is embedded.[77] You can help the couple to recognize the effect that the process of socialization has on their children. You can assist them as well, in planning health promotion strategies to help the children adapt to the community in healthy and meaningful ways.

---

**CRITICAL THINKING**

*What effects did your culture have on your socialization process during your formative years?*

---

## Variables Affecting Interaction in the Family

*Each critical period in the child's development reactivates a critical period in the parent.* Demands made on the parent vary with the age of the child. The infant needs almost total and constant nurturance. The baby's cry and behaviour evoke feelings of helplessness, dependency, and anger associated with the child's unacceptable dependency needs and feelings. Many mothers return to work while their infants are young and place the children in the care of supportive caregivers. Some experts believe that a mother and infant should have four to six months together before the mother either becomes employed or returns to her place of work.[78] The toddler struggles with individuality and autonomy, exploring and vacillating between dependency and independency. The parents may enjoy this explorative, independent behaviour of the child, even though the toddler leaves them feeling tired and frustrated. With your intervention, support, and teaching, the parent may be able to resolve personal conflicts and move to a more advanced level of integration as he or she works with, and comes to understand and accept, the developing child.[79]

Long before the child learns to speak, sensory, emotional, and intellectual exchanges are made between the child and other family members. Through such exchanges, and later with words, the child receives and tests instructions on how to consider the rights of others and how to respond to authority. The child also learns how to use language as a symbol, how to carry out certain routines necessary for health, how to compete, and what goals to seek. The games and toys purchased for the child, the books selected and read, and the television programs allowed can all provide key learning techniques.

Being an only child, or being part of multiple births, or being an adoptive child or stepchild—all affect individual experiences within family. One's birth position and sex both influence the strategies implemented by the child to secure parental favour and affect family dynamics and experiences.

*Parents tend to identify with their children, and they frequently treat their children according to how they were treated as children.* A parent can identify best with the child who matches his or her own sibling position. For example, a man from a family of boys may not know how to interact with a daughter; and he may not empathize well with her. In the process of identifying with the parent, the child picks up many of the parent's characteristics, especially if the child is the oldest or a lone child. Using family constellation theory, Sulloway[80] describes features of each child in a family, based on sex and ordinal position, and how that child feels about and interacts with people.

**Ordinal Position of the Child** Birth order is important to development. Table 4-8 lists characteristics of children in first, middle, and last ordinal positions, as well as characteristics of the only child. *Siblings, of both the same and opposite sex, have an important influence on each other as buddies, bullies, or heroes, and the early relationship often affects the adult relationship.* Whether the child has male or female siblings also affects personality development.[81]

Table 4-8 Influence of Ordinal Position on Child

Firstborn Children

1. Are most likely to be wanted
2. Enjoy advantages until second child comes along
3. Are subject to greater parental expectations for achievement in school, work at home, and adult success
4. Begin to speak earlier in life
5. Demonstrate higher intellectual achievement
6. Are more achievement-oriented and responsible
7. Are more goal-directed, plan better, and experience fewer frustrations
8. Identify more with parents than with peers
9. Are more dominant with siblings and peers
10. Have stronger superego or conscience, more self-discipline, and inner direction
11. Are more socially insecure
12. Engage in less risk-taking
13. Tend to have responsible leadership or high-level positions and be successful in adulthood

Middle Children

1. Are more difficult to characterize because of variety of positions in family
2. Receive less of the parents' time
3. Are praised less often
4. Are less stimulated toward achievement
5. Learn to compromise, handle conflict, and be adaptable because they are caught between jealousy of older sibling and envy of younger sibling
6. Develop sense of humour as adaptive mechanism
7. Learn double or triple roles and are prepared for more relationships in adulthood because of sibling coalitions
8. May succeed in role of mediator or negotiator in adulthood

Youngest Children

1. Benefit from parents' experience with childrearing
2. Tend to identify more with peer group than with parents
3. Are less tense, more affectionate, more good-natured, possibly to gain parental attention and sibling acceptance
4. Are popular with peers
5. Are more flexible in thinking
6. Have fewer expectations for household tasks or school achievement from parents
7. Are more dependent in relationships

Only Child

1. Resemble first-born children
2. Experience greater parental pressure for mature behaviour and achievement
3. Learn to fill many roles because fewer family members have more demands
4. May be forced to assume roles prematurely without adequate preparation
5. Are more mature, cultivated, serious, and goal-oriented than peers who have siblings
6. Are more assertive, responsible, and independent
7. May be adept at various roles but lack self-confidence
8. Are usually intellectually superior, curious, creative with rich fantasy life, and academically successful
9. May feel lonely but are able to entertain selves and find satisfaction in personal pursuits because of parental demands
10. Demonstrate superiority in use of language
11. Do not usually share feelings and experiences with someone close
12. Learn less about coping with jealousy, envy, and sibling rivalries and sharing adult attention than peers with siblings
13. Learn less about intimate interactions with opposite or same-sex peers
14. Develop into a well-adjusted, capable adult rather than the stereotype of spoiled, selfish child

As you counsel parents who plan for or have only one child, emphasize the need for peer activity and the danger of too much early responsibility and pressure.

**Family with a Large Number of Children** The dual-earner family with more than three or four children is less frequently seen now than it was in the past. The last-born child may be less wanted than the first- or middle-born, although parents feel more skilled and self-confident in rearing the younger children. Large families have advantages. Of necessity, the children learn thrift and conservation of resources and material goods. Children learn to share time, space, and possessions. In a loving home, they have not only their parents' love but also that of their siblings. They have a listening ear, respect, support, compassion, and help when they need it. If the parents do not have time to read to the three-year-old, an older sibling often does. In doing so, he or she gains additional experience in reading, gains increased self-esteem from being helpful, and learns responsibility and caring. Each child learns co-operation, compromise, tolerance, and how to handle peer pressure. For parents, the effort, work, expense, and self-denial of having a large family are usually offset by the rewards of watching children grow and develop, and by the resulting sense of contribution to the generations to come.

Although having many children within a family unit has its benefits, the reality is that family size has continued to decline in Canada. Most demographers project that low birth rate will be the norm in the near future for two reasons: first, children are costly to care for in urban environments; and second, combining work and family life is difficult when both partners are employed and must purchase child care. In fact, the Canadian labour force has changed dramatically as many more partnered women and mothers accept full-time positions. The impact of the double workload of women is now being felt in families. Disputes over housework or child care often occur within families. On the other hand, additional pressures often help to persuade the other partner to share housework and child care.[82]

Your teaching and support can influence how well parents cope with the daily responsibilities of a large family.

**Multiple Births** The increased use of assisted reproductive technology, as well as the increased frequency of multiple births, has had profound impacts on the family and Canadian society.[83] Twins, or other multiple births, have a considerable impact on family interactions. If ovulation has been inhibited with contraceptive pills, or if certain infertility drugs are used, multiple births are more likely to occur. Multiple fetuses in uteri often create problems for the parents regarding such things as the health of the mother and babies, financial strain, ethical decisions, and family relationships. The needs and tasks of multiple-birth parents will differ from those parents who have a single birth. Your health promotion strategies and support in assisting multiple-birth families can strongly influence how well the parents cope with their particular set of responsibilities.

Because multiple births are often premature, the first four or five months are very demanding on the parents in terms of the amount of energy and time they spend on child care. In such situations, the parents have little available energy and time, either for each other or for any other children. If there are more than two babies, the mother should have help for several months or longer from the husband, a relative, a friend, or a neighbour. Caring for multiples is more difficult and physically demanding than caring for one child, especially during infancy and childhood.[84] Financial worries and concerns about space and material needs often intrude on normal husband–wife relationships, as well as on relationships with other children in the family.

Although some source books tend to discourage the mother of twins from breastfeeding, and from using alternate breast- and bottle-feeding, the mother may actually be able to breastfeed both twins successfully by alternating breast-feeding with bottle-feedings. The babies will not necessarily be poor breast-feeders with this arrangement.

You can suggest shortcuts in, or realities about, types of care that will not be detrimental to twin babies, and that will give the parents more time to enjoy the children and each other. Each baby can be given a total bath every other day, instead of daily. Heating bottles before feeding is not necessary. Multiple offspring should be fun as well as work. Encourage the parents of twins (or other combinations of multiple offspring) to perceive the babies as individuals and to consider the long-term consequences of giving them similar-sounding names, dressing them alike, and expecting them to behave alike. Inform parents about different resources in Canada, such as Multiple Births Canada (MBC), whose vision is to improve the quality of life for multiple birth individuals and their families across Canada. MBC provides support, advocacy, research, and education.[85] Another support network is Mom2Many.com—Parents of Multiples across Canada, which provides parents with various resources and a lot of information.[86] One example of the type of information supplied is that on April 7, 2004, Canada became the first country to ban the selling, reselling, advertising, and importing of baby walkers.

Usually, multiple-birth children are closer emotionally than ordinary siblings. Because these children have lived with each other from before birth, experiences are different from those with various-aged siblings. With fraternal twins, authority preferences of parents tend to determine what age ranks the girl and the boy will be ascribed. In contrast, identical twins meet the world as a pair; it is difficult for them to imagine life without each other. It takes longer for twins to separate in adolescence and adulthood. In fact, they may never separate entirely, either emotionally or physically.

Siblings of a multiple birth tend to be more detached from other siblings, and even from parents, than are multiple-birth children or ordinary siblings. Multiple-birth children may each receive less parental affection and communication because parents have less time to devote to each child. Thus they are often slower to talk and many have slower intellectual growth unless parents work to prevent it.[87]

Compared to a single infant, the maternal and paternal attachment processes take longer and are more complex with two, three, or more babies.[88]

---

## CRITICAL THINKING

*What steps can you take to help a multiple-birth family from the Yukon obtain information on multiple births?*

---

**Sex of the Child** Temperamental stereotyping may influence the quality of the parent–infant relationship. A parent of a quiet girl may observe her behaviour as a sign of "girlness," and will respond to her behaviour with approval. Meanwhile, the parent of an active boy may tolerate his activity level, or even encourage it, because he or she sees it as evidence of masculinity. But sometimes girls and boys demonstrate opposite behaviours. If the girl is too active, or the boy is too quiet, what happens? The parent of an active girl may teach her to be less active; and the parent of a quiet boy may push him to be more active. Unfortunately, in such cases, parents may develop a disapproving attitude toward their child that may generalize to all aspects of their relationship with them. If this occurs, such a stereotype-based manner of responding to infants can lead to an undesirable quality of attachment.[89]

You can help parents understand ways in which their attitudes toward their own sexuality and their assessments of boys and girls can influence their relationships with their children. Emphasize the importance of encouraging the child's unique identity to develop naturally.

**Adopted Child** Adoption is the combination of a social and legal process whereby a parent–child relationship is created. The adopted child may experience some of the problems of the only child. In addition, the adopted child may need to work through feelings of rejection and abandonment stemming from the biological parents. Conversely, they will experience feelings of being wanted and loved by the adoptive parents. The child should be told that he or she is adopted as early as the idea can be comprehended. Usually by the preschool years, he or she can incorporate the idea of being a wanted child. Explanations will need to be repeated and expanded upon in the years ahead.

Adopted children bring to their adoptive family their own genes, birth experiences, biological family ties, and often an extensive life history. The adoptive family is not the same as a biological family. Both adoptive parents and adopted children tend to feel that they have less control over their situation than do the children and parents of non-adoptive families. Adoptive parents and adopted children are both likely to experience a sense of loss. It is not unusual for the adoptive child to seek his or her own biological parents in late adolescence or young adulthood, especially if the child was old enough to remember both parents when adopted. This strong desire can occur in the child even when the adoptive parents are truly considered to be the parents. This search may be perceived as a threat by the adoptive parents. On the other hand, the adoptive parent(s) and even one biological parent may feel sufficiently secure to assist the offspring in the search for a missing biological parent.

Some of the *major determinants* of the child's adjustment and development include the adoptive parents' personal qualifications, their marital harmony, their love of the child, their ability to communicate with the child about the adoptive process, their acceptance of the child, and the extent and quality of the child's friends. Factors that are not predictive of adjustment include socioeconomic status, occupational status, presence or absence of biological siblings, and the parents' age, health, religion, and experience with children.[90]

The definition of "suitable" adoptive parents has been liberalized. The adoptive parent may be a man, a homosexual couple, an infertile couple, or a relative. Additionally, couples today consider adoption even if they have their own children. Some believe that they have a responsibility and enough love to provide a home for an existing child rather than add to the world's population. Others are single or older persons who want to offer love and security to a child.

In Canada, each provincial government has a designated office that is responsible for adoptions, and each office has specific procedures for adoptions.[91] The process of adoption is carried out through either a public or a private agency. Public domestic adoption refers to any adoption arranged by a public, or government, agency. It is important to note that the focus of a public adoption is on meeting the needs of the child rather than on satisfying the needs of the adoptive couple.[92]

Usually, no costs are involved in adopting through a public agency. In the private system, there is a longer waiting period, especially for a healthy newborn. Biological mothers who are seeking to have a child put up for adoption find the private system easier to deal with and more responsive to their needs. However, social workers and psychologists now consider that giving up a child for adoption can be psychologically damaging for both the mother and the child.[93] Additional information is available from www.canadaadopts.com.

Recently, the number of foreign adoptions has increased, mainly because couples tend to be highly motivated to be parents and babies are quite readily available from abroad.[94] Many couples are concerned about the conditions of war, extreme poverty, or the exploitation of children. The guidebook *How to Adopt Internationally* was designed by Jean and Heino Erichsen to provide couples with the information they need. To see the features of the book, refer to www.internationaladoption.ezhoster.com.

You may have opportunities to educate adults about adopting an older child with special needs, or a foreign-born child, or to work with adoptive parents who have encountered needs and concerns.

The adoption of a child with special needs involves four phases: (1) commitment of adults and child; (2) honeymoon or placement period; (3) storm period; and (4) adaptation and adjustment. The phases do not begin or end abruptly. Each phase builds on the preceding phase and sometimes reversals occur. The phases, along with thoughts, emotions, and activities accompanying each phase, are summarized in Table 4-9. The adoptive process can terminate at any point. If termination is necessary, both sides—the family and child—need help to understand what happened and to understand that no one person is responsible. Future adoption procedures are enhanced if proper guidance is given with the first failure.[95]

*Stresses to adoptive families* include the following:[96]

- The parents may worry about the child's heredity.

- The parents choose to be parents; hence they are highly motivated to parent and invest considerable expense and time.

- The parents see themselves as a chosen group because someone thought they would be good parents; the chosen group idea leads to problems such as difficulty in setting limits, increased stress in the parenting role, and oversensitivity to problems observed in the child.

- Infertile couples may have feelings of hostility or inferiority that are projected onto the child. The child may be a constant reminder of the couple's inability to conceive.

- The adopted child or adolescent may project onto their adoptive parents normal feelings of anger. Parents may think that normal developmental problems are a fact of adoption.

- If one child is adopted and one is biological, favouritism, insufficient rewards to the adoptive child, or competition between the children may occur.

- Sanctions and regards for role performance differ from those for biological parents (e.g., the company may not have maternity leave for adoptive parents). Actually, there is little emotional support in society for adoptive parents.

- Role autonomy is lacking. Adoptive parents need someone (e.g., extended family, adoption agency) to agree with them that they will be good parents but they need someone else to bear a child for them. Such requirements inject dependence into a role considered independent, with the result that parental confidence is undermined.

- Community or school attitudes toward adoption may be negative. For example, one's "own" child may be spoken of as a biological child, hence "real." The child who encounters attitudes of differentiation between "real" and "adoptive" can begin to feel undermined in the sense of belonging. The emotional result can begin to drive a wedge between parents and child.

Parents often experience heightened stress when they adopt older children.[97] Most often, older children have special needs, or they tend to suffer from problems that relate to difficulties in their original or foster home placements. Older adopted children bring with them emotional, genetic, and contextual baggage that may make it difficult to form a strong and meaningful attachment to the adoptive parent.[98]

Adoption is a unique way of building families. Adoptive families are different from other families because of the circumstances that bring people to adoption and because of the way in which adoption affects their lives.[99] If the adoption was biracial or international, cultural differences must be acknowledged. The adopted child must be given opportunities to learn about his or her cultural background. A recent study conducted by Carriere explored the relationship among connectedness, health, and adoption among First Nations children. The results of the study suggest that connections to the birth family and community and to ancestral knowledge are very important for First Nations adoptees.[100]

Traditional social and legal forces have hindered the adoption of children by gay and lesbian individuals and couples. However, in Canada, adoption rights vary across provinces and territories.[101] Erich and his researchers conducted a study to examine adoptive families with gay and lesbian parents in terms of family functioning capabilities. The findings of the study suggest that these families usually have adequate assistance from their support networks.

Table 4-9 Adoptive Process of a Child with Special Needs

| Phases | Thoughts and Emotions | Activities |
| --- | --- | --- |
| **Commitment of Adults and Child** | *Adults* make general decision to adopt (stage 1), leading to decision to adopt specific child(ren) (stage 2). | *Adults* prepare for adoption through dialogue with helpful people and agencies and sometimes attend sessions on adoption given by adoption agency. |
| "Courting stage" | *Child* expresses desire for adoption (stage 1), leading to decision on specific family (stage 2). | *Child* is counselled for potential adjustment by adoption agency staff. Visits are arranged and made between potential family and child. All members involved (including existing children in family) get to know each other. |
| **Placement** | *Parents* are on an "emotional high"; excitement. | Household routines are altered to accommodate child. Limit setting is minimal. Parent(s) meet child's whims. |
| "Honeymoon period" (child comes to live with parents) | *Child* is excited but somewhat scared. "Can I trust these people?" "Will they send me away when I don't act my best?" | *Child* is put on best behaviour. Sometimes parents' show of affection for child is not accepted because of child's past negative parenting. |
| "Storm period" | *Parents* are tired of permanent houseguest, feel anger, disappointment and guilt, and displace these feelings on each other and the child. They may wish the child would leave.<br><br>*Child* can no longer keep up good behaviour but wants to be loved and accepted.<br><br>*Parents* may feel sense of failure. They may have expected too much of themselves and child and now may strike out at each other and other family members. Spouse may be jealous of time and energy mate gives to child.<br><br>*Child* may think, "They don't want me. What's going to happen to me?" and may live with anticipatory grief, fears of rejection, and insecurity, based on past hurts. Parents and child test each other. | *Parents* treat child or other family members with decreasing tolerance for behaviour not in family norm.<br>*Child* may have tantrums, run away, or try to reject parents before they reject him or her.<br>If the outcome is positive, the *parents* will use problem solving, limit setting with flexibility, sense of humour, ongoing empathy and caring, supportive others, and community resources. |
| **Adaptation and Adjustment Phase (Equilibrium Occurs)** | *All* believe they can live and work together; mutual trust is growing; family feels fused as a unit and able to handle frustrations and crisis. | Parents are consistent with child. *Parents* and *child* can attend to outside interests without threatening family status. |

*"Adults/parents" and "child" are used in this table; however, only one adult may be adopting (single parent), and more than one child may be adopted.*

Further, those gay and lesbian families who adopted siblings and older children with a history of abuse reported higher levels of good family functioning. Therefore, the results of this exploratory study, in combination with previous studies of gay and lesbian families, support the practice of adoption by gay and lesbian adults.[102]

Ambert suggests that the position of the adopted individual in our society is socially constructed, and is not an entirely positive one. She states that the "genetic linkage" has a positive orientation in our society. Genetic linkage is portrayed as being critical for a positive sense of self and personal completeness. Thus, adopted individuals are placed in an awkward position and may elicit negative responses to their circumstances. In fact, the more recent development of reunions of adopted children with their birth mothers well illustrates the theme of social construction of adoption. However, adoptive parents are usually equally attached to both their adopted and biological children. The results of studies vary regarding adjustments between adopted and non-adopted individuals. For example, adoptive mothers report considerably more child problems, whereas the reports of adoptive fathers and adopted children are more similar to those in biological families.[103]

Changes in the nature of adoptions have resulted in the realization that adoptive families have been seeking more professional assistance and that adoption professionals are now being called upon to consider the kinds of services the families need and how to deliver those services. The box entitled "Intervention Guidelines for Therapy with Adoptive Families" summarizes the therapy considerations.[104]

---

## CONTROVERSY DEBATE

# The Question of Adoption

You work as a nurse counsellor at a recently opened fertility clinic in a small town. The other health professional in the clinic is a social worker, who is scheduled to begin work in a few weeks. Today, a childhood friend, June, telephoned to arrange a counselling session with you. She informs you that she will bring her husband, Jay, to the session. You have agreed to see this couple because there is no other office in town to which you might refer them. During the brief telephone conversation, you learn that they have been transferred here from the city, but they must return to the city in a few days to pack their belongings and complete arrangements for the move. June relates that for a couple of years she has been taking physician-prescribed fertility drugs, but

has not been able to conceive. She advises you that Jay seems to strongly favour assisted human reproduction technology, while she really wants to adopt either a disabled child or a child from a foreign country. From the telephone conversation, you have become quite certain that Jay is not interested in adoption and that June wants to adopt a child.

Both June and Jay are scheduled to see you for counselling in your office tomorrow morning.

1. In what ways can you be therapeutically present to both June and Jay?
2. How can you help this couple to cope with, and adapt to, the stressors they seem to be experiencing?

---

## INTERVENTION GUIDELINES FOR THERAPY WITH ADOPTIVE FAMILIES

- Conventional treatment may not work well with adoptive families.
- Adoptive parents need validation as parents and validation of their decision to adopt.
- Adoptive parents must be included in therapeutic interventions to empower them further and to reinforce the adoptive commitment.
- In treating child-rooted problems, often the job will be to help parents modify their expectations.
- A child cannot successfully mourn the past and integrate it into present circumstances if preoccupied with emotional survival. Developing a sense of safety and security is of paramount importance.
- Child-rooted barriers can come from unfinished emotional business, attachment disorders, or poor preparation for adoption.

- Adult-rooted barriers may stem from unfinished business, marital problems, or individual pathologies.
- Environmental barriers include lack of support or active disapproval from the extended family or the broader community.
- Any assessment is useful only if the assessed family accepts it as valid.
- In deciding to terminate an adoption that is not working, one must be committed to preserving the family's integrity, yet be open to the removal of the child as a viable option.
- When an adoption is terminated, avoid judgment about reasons for its failure. Plans for adoption of another child should not be made until grief over the loss is resolved.

---

**Stepchild** When a family has a stepchild, or stepchildren, adults and children experience feelings of loss and disruption. These feelings can rise from several possible sources—psychological, social, and economical—through changed life patterns and roles with each restructuring cycle of the family: divorce, custody battles, remaining a single parent with the child(ren), choosing to live unmarried with a partner or remarriage, and possibly another divorce and remarriage. The resulting combinations of people may never be a truly compatible "blended family." Further, the adjustment may never be fully made. At best, it is likely to take several years for all involved. The child involved may express for years the desire for the biological parents to reunite, even after a divorce, and even if the union was abusive and dysfunctional.[105]

The stepchild grieves and mourns the loss of a biological parent, either from death or through divorce, and must also deal with the many problems associated with integration into a new family unit. The stepchild may have conflicting feelings of loyalty to the natural parent and to the step-parent, thinking that acceptance of the step-parent is rejection of the natural parent. The stepchild may also feel rejected by his or her remarried natural parent, seeing the step-parent as a rival for the parent's attention.

Health promotion strategies need to be developed and implemented so that health care professionals are able to work more effectively with parents, family members, lawyers, and judges surrounding the impact of divorce and conflict on children. Effective community resources and obtaining assurance of support from the father are critical to reduce the effects of poverty on divorced women who are awarded child custody.

## FAMILY LIFESTYLES AND PARENTING PRACTICES

There is no single type of contemporary Canadian family; but the lifestyles of many families correspond to the factors discussed in this section, including family structure, family cultural pattern, and the impact of the 21st century. These factors, in addition to those already discussed, influence family interaction. An understanding of them will assist you in family care.

## Parenting Culture

The biological and reproductive unit considered typical in North America is the mother–father–child group. However, today, single mothers, single fathers, dual-earner parents, step-parents, and gay and lesbian parents all share in the cultural mandate to support their children. In this context,

culture may be viewed as the way parents adapt to the changing conditions of their social and economic worlds that give rise to a changing parenting culture. Traditionally, parents were married to each other, had established a residence of their own, were viewed (along with their children) as an integral social unit, and lived in an intimate, monogamous relationship. Daly states that the most dramatic shift in the culture of parenting has been the dramatic rise in the number of women in the paid labour force. The once dominant patriarchal paradigm of the "sole provider role" has been shifted to the co-provider role whereby both parents contribute to the economic needs of the family.[106]

## Single-Parent Family

The *single-parent family* is becoming increasingly more common. In fact, Lynn states that one of the most notable changes in Canadian families over the past three decades is the increase in single-parent families.[107] Although death, or being born to a single parent, may cause the child to have only one parent, divorce of the natural parents is the more common reason. If the parents are divorced, the family may have experienced considerable disruption before the break-up. Sometimes, though, the single-parent family is a planned event. A woman lacking a suitable partner but wanting to be a mother may choose to have a child by artificial insemination, or a single man or woman may choose to adopt a child. Regardless of the reason for the situation, some of these families have undergone a considerable change in lifestyle. As a result they often encounter considerable stress, including financial strain and sometimes even poverty. Other families appear to survive. Many of the children whose parents live in separate households are not only spending time with, but also being cared for by each parent on a week-about basis—that is, one week with one parent and the next week with the other parent.[108]

Children living in a single-parent household often exhibit greater adaptability, responsibility, and maturity than do their peers. However, a child who lives with the parent of the opposite sex may have greater difficulty with adjustment to the divorce or death of the other parent, or to the remarriage of the parent, than a child living with the same-sex parent. Inappropriate social behaviour, difficulty with identity formation, depression, and poorer school performance may be manifested by the child. If there always was only one parent, the child may have evolved behaviour and roles appropriate to the available parent, regardless of the child's sex. This situation may result in later developmental problems.[109]

Often a series of open discussions concerning the changed lifestyle, along with support from relatives, friends, and other single-parent families, can together enhance the coping abilities of single parents. Family members may need professional help if they exhibit symptoms of more extreme dysfunction, grieving, or prolonged "acting-out" behaviours. The family may also need information about various community resources.[110]

Ford-Gilboe describes the strengths of single-parent families, and compares these strengths to those of two-parent families. This study presents families' explanations of the effect of self-identified strengths on health.[111] Her findings indicate that although structural differences exist between single-parent and two-parent families, the nature and pattern of strengths are more alike than different between these two groups. In essence, these findings challenge the stereotypical views of single-parent families that emphasize vulnerability and problematic issues and exclude their strengths.[112]

Stepfamilies The proportion of stepfamilies in Canada is lower than that in the United States due to lower rates of divorce and remarriage in Canada.[113] In the 2001 Canadian Census, stepfamilies were not counted in a formal manner. Participants were simply asked to list their stepsons and stepdaughters as "sons" or "daughters."[114]

Both the number and the variety of relationships are greater in stepfamilies than in nuclear, non-divorced families. Church states that in many instances there are no terms for some of the multiple relationships. For example, let's enter Heather's life for a moment. As a result of living with Harry, Heather has increased the number of her relationships. What does she call herself in relation to Harry's ex-wife, Sybil? In her study, Church found that many women who become stepmothers have no idea of the complications brought about by such a family.[115]

Although many stepfamilies are harmonious, they can pose problems for a variety of reasons. One reason is that couples who form stepfamilies after a divorce have many problems to solve (e.g., financial problems) even before the new family begins. Another reason is that most of the problems associated with stepfamilies have at their source the quality and quantity of changes a child must make in the new family. Adapting to new parents and to new siblings usually causes considerable confusion and turbulence for a child. Even if the child gets along well with the new siblings, he or she may feel in competition with near-strangers for the affection of his or her parent.[116]

Church states that increasing our acceptance of stepfamilies is important. On the positive side, the stepfamily can offer more choice of kin and a greater freedom in defining roles. Church also claims that we can use stepfamilies to assist us in examining some of our own unexamined beliefs of how a family should act.[117]

CRITICAL THINKING
*What effect do the media have on childrearing practices?*

Another type of family structure has been termed **apartners**, or as some investigators have termed it, **"living apart together" (LAT) couples**.[118] *Rather than getting married, a couple, who may have children by a previous marriage, may choose to maintain separate residences, take care of their own children, professional life, and everyday affairs but also choose to share special times with each other on a regularly scheduled basis.* Personal time and freedom, coupled with intimacy, are what the participants say they seek. Gay or lesbian couples may set up this type of arrangement, often because of social constraints rather than choice. It is necessary to point out that this type of arrangement is not just for young adults who may have children. For older individuals, an LAT arrangement may be an adequate arrangement whereby they can keep their own households, if they wish, and retain the relationship they desire.[119]

Single Person Family *The* **single state** *(never married, separated, divorced, or widowed)* is another form of family structure. Today, more Canadians are choosing singlehood than has been the case in the past. Society now accepts being single as an acceptable option rather than a deviant lifestyle. The following are some of the perceived advantages of being single:[120]

- *Privacy:* Being able to think and create in a peaceful atmosphere without interruption
- *Time:* Being able to travel, cultivate talents and interests, entertain and be entertained, and follow intellectual pursuits
- *Freedom:* Being able to choose and make decisions, form friendships, use time as desired, depend on self, have a healthy narcissism
- *Opportunity:* Being able to extend borders of friendship, develop skills and knowledge, enjoy geographic moves or job mobility and success (e.g., the single person is often preferred for certain jobs or positions)

Many single adults claim that personal freedom is one of the major advantages of being single.[121] Many Canadian singles hold values that are more individualistic than family oriented. Such individualistic values may intensify the longer the person remains unattached. Currently, there seems to be decreasing parental pressure to marry directed toward young sons and daughters, despite the fact that some parents admit disappointment when intimate relationships of their children do not result in marriage. Middle-aged divorced women who have a flourishing career may tend to look with skepticism at marriage, viewing it as a bad bargain once they have gained financial and sexual independence. One of the greatest challenges encountered by single people is the development of strong social networks to provide positive adjustments and satisfactions.[122]

## CRITICAL THINKING

*What do you see as the main components of a satisfying single life?*

**Stepgeneration Parents** The **stepgeneration family** develops when *the next generation (grandparents or great-grandparents) become the parenting people because the mother will not, does not, cannot, or should not care for her offspring.* Many children live in households (sometimes consisting of five generations) that are headed by one or both grandparents or great-grandparents. Circumstances that lead the grandparent generations to provide care for the grandchildren transcend race and economic level and reflect a number of factors that create instability in family life. The elder generation may be called upon to provide a home for grandchildren, as well as great-grandchildren, and their parent(s) if:

1. The parental generation is unemployed or in financial difficulty.
2. There has been separation, divorce, or death of one of the parents.
3. One or both parents are physically or mentally ill.
4. One or both parents are abusing, or addicted to, alcohol or drugs.
5. Physical, emotional, or sexual abuse of the child has occurred.
6. One or both parents are imprisoned or have abandoned the child.

How well the situation works depends, among other factors, on the degree of respect, love, and communication shown. Success depends upon how clearly rules are set and enforced in the home, who takes responsibility for child care and home maintenance tasks, and how effectively legal and financial problems are handled by the family unit. In a stable home, each generation can benefit from the other, and all can learn to appreciate each other. In a home with conflict, each person will carry scars. Conflicts will be inevitable as the children and grandparent generations each grow older and have different needs. Yet, it is possible that the grandparents can experience real peace of mind as they finally realize their successful contribution to the young ones. In Canada, several organizations provide assistance to grandparents who are caregivers (see the box entitled

## Canadian Organizations for Grandparent Caregivers

- CANGRANDS: www.cangrands.com/groups.htm
- Grandparents Support Groups in Canada: www.grandparentagain.com/community/support_canada.html

"Canadian Organizations for Grandparent Caregivers."[123] The real concern is that the grandparents may become ill or die before the child is reared. Most grandparents realize that the physical and emotional care and the moral and spiritual guidance they provide might prevent the grandchild from repeating the pattern into which the child was born.

## Family Size

Canadians have fewer children now than they did in earlier decades.[124] In the early 1900s, women gave birth to an average of 3.5 children, but by the 1990s the figure was 1.5 children.[125] The portrait of the family taken by the census at the outset of the 21st century indicates a continuation of the many changes that have been occurring in the family. The proportion of "traditional" families—dad, mom, and the kids—is continuing to decline, partially as a result of a much lower fertility rate. Regarding same-sex couples, there were more male same-sex couples than female same-sex couples, but more female same-sex couples had children living with them.[126]

## Family Cultural Pattern

*The ways of living and thinking that constitute the intimate aspects of family group life constitute the* **family cultural pattern**. The family transmits to the child the cultural pattern of its own ethnic background and class, together with the parents' attitudes toward other classes. It becomes the responsibility of health professionals to be aware of their own beliefs and attitudes about families and cultures in order to provide quality care. Dicicco-Bloom and Cohen claim that cultural competence is a significant aspect of health care delivery.[127]

## Influence of 20th-Century Changes

**Shift from an Agrarian to a Complex Technologic Society** A dramatic paradigm shift from primarily farm-based to primarily city-based families has produced noticeable changes in the North American family. A greater percentage of children now survive childhood than in 1900, and a higher percentage of mothers survive childbirth. Some women marry at a later age than in former generations because they first pursue a career or profession. Young adults believe they can manage both career and family. Typically, the husband-to-be encourages the young woman to be as committed to her profession as she is to him. Fewer children are born to most parents. Children are spaced closer together, and more first children are born to parents who are in their late thirties or early forties. An increasing number of women become single mothers by choice, whether they are teenagers or in their late thirties or early forties. Middle-aged couples now can look forward to more years together than their parents and grandparents could, after their children are grown and leave home. Because of an increased life expectancy, families now have more living relatives than former families did, especially elderly relatives, for whom the family may have responsibility.[128]

**Other Trends Related to Living in a Complex Industrial and Information Society** Primarily families live in urban or metropolitan areas. More families than ever are homeless or at risk for homelessness. More women work outside the home. The woman who formerly stayed home and was the "homemaker" is now quite different. If the woman stays home today and concentrates on "mothering," she may receive considerable criticism.[129] Her outside activities may include volunteer work so that she can control her hours and feel she has prime time at home while making significant contributions outside the family unit. Conversely, the father may be the house parent because he has an office in the home, or he is the unemployed member who thereby assumes child and home care responsibilities. Family members are now better educated. Greater individual freedom exists. Sexual mores are changing, with trial and serial partnerships and marriages. Value changes and different patterns of living are now apparently the norm.

Cheal claims that a shift has occurred toward a more diverse family, expanding a sense of individuality and personal autonomy. He claims that postmodernism has had a decisive influence on family life.[130] One such influence can be realized with the study of families regarding their appreciation of pluralism or diversity.[131] Because Canadians are so mobile and are increasingly living in smaller homes or apartments, or in townhouses or condominiums, many ties with kin, other than the immediate family, are loosened or at least geographically extended. Sometimes close friends become "the family." Many Canadians continue to strengthen kinship ties through email, telephone calls, and holiday and vacation visits. Religious influences affect family ties. For example, Jews and European Catholics, with their many family traditions, are generally more embedded in a network of relatives than are white Protestants. The

four- and five-generation family and great-grandparent–great-grandchild (as well as grandparent–grandchild) relationships are gaining the attention of researchers.

**Parenting Practices in Canada** Chan claims that good child care allows for the fact that each family and child is unique. That is, each child and family has their own social, physical, and developmental needs.[132] Research continues to show that children who experience consistent love, attention, and security will grow up to be adults who can survive change and stressors, with self-reliance, optimism, and their identities intact.[133]

Aboriginal cultures in Canada have allocated a significant role to the extended family regarding childrearing. Even if the child's grandparents, or other relatives, do not actively partake in caring for the child, they give advice on the child's welfare.[134] The recent move to Aboriginal self-government has been met with a growing self-respect, and many communities have taken over education and child welfare services.[135]

## Renewed Focus on the Family

Certainly, the health of a nation, and the world, depends on the health of the family. In fact, Health Canada supports Aboriginals in their recognition of children as the nation's most valuable resource.[136] It is important to consider the strengths of families in today's society. Schlesinger claims that despite the diversity in the patterns of family development and function, it is possible to define common aspiration, common needs, and common obligations of Canadian families. He says that, if we are to learn how to deal in a constructive manner with diversity and lend support to the families in Canada, it is necessary to understand the common elements that cut across different patterns of family formation and function.[137]

### CRITICAL THINKING

*In the light of so many languages and cultures in Canada, how can a health professional cope with language differences in giving support to families?*

## HEALTH PROMOTION IN NURSING PRACTICE

The family, as the basic unit for the developing person and health, cannot be taken for granted. The need for nurses to ensure that their focus of care includes family has never been greater.[138] Nurses have unique opportunities to work with families. They may be able to provide support directly to families or indirectly by assisting them to support their own members.[139]

You will frequently encounter the entire family as your client in the health care system, regardless of the setting. Increasingly, the *emphasis is on health promotion of the family*.[140] Rapid change, increasing demands on the person, technologic progress, and other trends seem to isolate people. The family may need your help in becoming aware of disruptive forces and maladaptive patterns, and in learning ways to promote an accepting home atmosphere. Assessing the strengths and needs of the family is fundamental to increasing the self-care abilities of the client/family.[141]

## Communication and Relationship Principles Basic to Client and Family Care

*Communication is the heart of the nursing process and health care* because it is one of the primary methods used to accomplish specific and general goals with most people.

It is used in assessing and understanding the client and family, and in intervention. The process of communication assists individuals to express thoughts and feelings, identify their strengths, clarify problems, receive information, consider alternate ways of coping or adapting, and remain realistic through feedback from the environment. Essentially, the client learns something about the self, then how to identify health needs, and shortly after that, if and how he or she wishes to meet these needs.[142] Family input, as you will undoubtedly come to realize, is very important in client care.

The nurse must have the ability to develop, maintain, and, when the time comes, close effectively the nurse–family working alliance. Crawford and Tarko state that "the term working alliance was first used by Greenson in 1976 (as cited in Egan, 2002)." The **therapeutic or helping relationship or alliance**, sometimes called the therapeutic nurse–client relationship, is a *purposeful interaction over time between an authority in health care and*

EVIDENCE-BASED PRACTICE

# Siblings' Experiences with Childhood Cancer: A Different Way of Being in the Family

A longitudinal qualitative research study guided by the philosophy of interpretive interactionism sought meaningful interpretations of the experiences encountered by siblings of children with cancer. The resulting challenges can be particularly stressful to the siblings due to the tremendous changes that occur in their lives. The 30 siblings who participated in the study took part in individual interviews, focus group interviews, and participant observation. For the siblings, cancer was experienced as a different way of being within the family. This "different way of being" was viewed by the siblings as undergoing a loss regarding the family way of life, which, in turn, revealed three related themes: *keeping my family together, being present, and enduring sadness*. In addition, siblings tended to experience a loss of self within the family.

### Practice Implications

The findings of the study support the following needs for siblings of children with cancer:

- Siblings need to be given frequent opportunities to talk about their feelings throughout the cancer trajectory.
- Siblings need to be assured that their own suffering is justified, that the childhood cancer experience is also their

experience, and that they are justified in wanting to spend more time with their parents.
- Siblings need to be provided with opportunities to express their own emotions. By doing so, they are provided with opportunities to gain reassurance and to reduce feelings of fear and guilt.
- It is important that siblings maintain a sense of presence around those significant in their lives.

### Implications for Nurses

Nurses should assess the emotional impact on the daily lives of siblings arising from the serious illness of a brother or sister. Ongoing talks with siblings allow the nurse to intervene in a timely and appropriate fashion.

Nurses can facilitate siblings to become involved in the health care of their brother or sister. Care can be provided in ways that meet the needs and wishes of both the siblings and the ill child.

Nurses need to focus on the changing nature of sibling and parent–child relationships throughout the complete cancer trajectory. In doing so, nurses are equipped to provide psychosocial support and targeted interventions, such as family therapy, that help to strengthen significant relationships.

Source: Woodgate, R.L., Siblings' Experiences with Childhood Cancer: A Different Way of Being in the Family, *Cancer Nursing, 29*(5) (2006), 406–414. Used with permission.

a person, family, or group with health care needs, with the focus on the needs of the client, while being empathic and using one's knowledge. The therapeutic relationship/alliance must be differentiated from mere social association. The relationship will be therapeutic when the nurse or helper uses a *caring, client-centred approach*. The capacity to be a helping person is strengthened by a genuine desire to be responsible and sensitive to another person. In addition, experience with a variety of people will increase your awareness of the reactions and feelings of others. The feedback you receive from others will teach you a great deal on both the emotional and the cognitive levels.

Table 4-10 and the box entitled "Application of Therapeutic Communication Skills to Client as Family" outline the facilitative interactive skills that enhance the nurse's ability to communicate effectively at different stages of the nurse–family alliance.[143] Table 4-11 lists some non-therapeutic communication techniques that are worth knowing about.[144]

**Table 4-10 Therapeutic Communication Processes and Skills Applied to Client as Family**

| Stage I | • Warmth |
| | • Respect |
| | • Empathy (basic) |
| Stage II | • Concreteness |
| | • Genuineness |
| | • Self-disclosure |
| | • Empathy (advanced) |
| Stage III | • Confrontation |
| | • Immediacy |
| | • Problem solving (interpersonal and situational) |
| | • Conflict resolution |

Source: Crawford, J.A., and M.A. Tarko, Family Communication. In P. Bomar (ed.), *Promoting Health in Families: Applying Family Research and Theory to Nursing Practice*, 3rd ed (pp. 162–186). Philadelphia: Saunders, 2004.

**Table 4-11 Non-therapeutic Communication Techniques**

| Technique | Detrimental Consequence | Example |
|---|---|---|
| Social responding | Engaging in superficial conversation that is not client centered | Client: "I'm glad I'm being discharged today." <br> Nurse: "Are you going to watch the football game tonight?" |
| Asking closed-ended questions | Questions that elicit a "yes" or "no" answer instead of allowing for wider exploration of the client's thoughts and feelings | Nurse: "Do you understand everything I've told you about electroconvulsive therapy?" |
| Changing the subject | Introducing an unrelated or peripherally related topic (usually to avoid sensitive issues or reduce the nurse's anxiety) | Client: "I don't think my husband finds me attractive since I had the mastectomy." <br> Nurse: "I didn't realize you had breast cancer. Does it run in your family?" |
| Belittling | Discounting the client's feelings or making comparisons that imply the client's problems are smaller than he or she perceives | Client: "My home was totally destroyed in the fire." <br> Nurse: "At least you are alive." |
| Making stereotyped comments | Offering platitudes or wise sayings that seem automatic or contrived | Client: "I can't get over the loss of my mother." <br> Nurse: "Time heals all wounds. Everything happens for a reason." |
| Offering false reassurance | Attempting to cheer up the client by suggesting there is no real problem | Client: "I'm afraid my boss will fire me if he finds out I have a substance abuse problem." <br> Nurse: "Don't worry. He wouldn't do that." |

*(continued)*

**Table 4-11** (continued)

| Technique | Detrimental Consequence | Example |
|---|---|---|
| Moralizing | Passing judgment by imposing one's own values on the client and implying that the client's thinking is wrong | Client: "I want a divorce."<br>Nurse: "Don't you think you owe it to your children to give the marriage another try?" |
| Interpreting | Making intrusive comments in an attempt to psychoanalyze clients | Client: "I don't want to take this medication."<br>Nurse: "I think you're in denial about your illness." |
| Advising | Making specific suggestions instead of offering information and asking clients what they think is most likely to work | Client: "I feel depressed."<br>Nurse: "You should do some volunteer work to take your mind off things." |
| Challenging | Denying the client's perception, forcing the client to prove what he or she is saying | Client: "Nobody cares about me."<br>Nurse: "What about your sister? I saw her visiting yesterday." |
| Defending | Arguing or justifying your position rather than attempting to hear the client's concerns | Client: "I can't get any help with this problem."<br>Nurse: "We are doing our best to help you but we are very busy." |

Source: Deering, C., and J. Fredrick, Therapeutic Relationships and Communication. In W. Mohr (ed.), *Johnson's Psychiatric–Mental Health Nursing*, 5th ed. (pp. 53–75). Philadelphia: Lippincott Williams & Wilkins, 2003.

# Application of Therapeutic Communication Skills to Client as Family

## STAGE I: INITIAL STAGE FOR DEVELOPMENT OF NURSE FAMILY ALLIANCE

Goals: Helping the family to tell their story; promoting self-exploration

### Warmth

Conveyed by the nurse through the use of attending behaviors such as the use of eye contact, tone of voice, maintaining an open and relaxed posture, use of touch if appropriate, facial expressions such as smiling, and active listening.

### Respect

Conveyed by the nurse through behaviors such as calling the family members by their preferred names, not interrupting others, being nonjudgmental, using the same language as the family member, offering undivided attention, use of regular eye contact if this is warranted culturally, and recognizing the care and support family members have offered each other in the family meeting, as well as during other times of stress and crisis.

### Basic Empathy

Conveyed by the nurse through accurate reflection of *surface feelings* or emotions associated with the *content* of the situation or context of the individual or family's story. Formula and natural responses are presented as exemplars.

> Formula response for basic empathy: *"You feel upset because your mother has taken ill."*
> Natural response for basic empathy: *"You're upset because your mother has taken ill."*

The nurse, through each stage of the nurse-family alliance, can use warmth, respect, and empathy. Further, the use of respect and empathy may assist the nurse in obtaining information and in dealing sensitively with families in the context of diversity (i.e., their unique qualities, needs, and behaviors). It is important for the nurse to understand diversity from the worldview of the family; to demonstrate self-awareness of his or her own cultural values, beliefs, attitudes, and biases related to diversity; and to alter communication interventions and strategies based on family culture (e.g., the appropriateness of self-disclosure varies among families and from one culture to another).

## STAGE II: TRANSITION STAGE FOR DEVELOPMENT OF NURSE-FAMILY ALLIANCE

Goals: Challenging the family's communication patterns and processes; promoting self-understanding and commitment to change

### Concreteness

Conveyed by the nurse by being specific and through the use of descriptive words and phrases, as opposed to use of abstract terms and generalizations.

The use of *open-ended questions* or probes and the use of clarifying, paraphrasing, and summary statements by the nurse facilitate concreteness and the exchange of information about the family.

Examples of open-ended questions or probes include questions such as the following: *"Tell me who . . ., what. . ., when. . ., where. . ., and how. . . . "* The use of open-ended questions by the nurse promotes the expression of feelings, thoughts, and ideas.

The use of *closed-ended questions* or probes by the nurse should be avoided because they tend to elicit a "yes" or "no" response, with little or no elaboration. The use of closed-ended questions by the nurse is less effective in facilitating the expression of feelings, thoughts, and ideas.

Examples of closed-ended questions or probes include questions such as the following: *"Are you . . ., Can you . . ., Do you . . ., Did you . . ., Will you . . ., Is it. . . . "* Closed-ended questions or probes should be avoided *except* during assessment for risk of suicide, homicide, abuse, incest, or family violence, that is, in situations in which the nurse needs a definitive answer in relation to issues of safety of family members, legal requirements, and ethical issues.

The use of *why questions* by the nurse should be avoided because they tend to imply blame, often elicit responses that attempt to justify the family's behavior (rationalization), and have the potential to weaken any gains made in the nurse-family alliance. For example, asking *"Why did the family miss our last meeting?"* is less effective than asking, *"What happened that the family was unable to attend our last meeting?"*

Statements that reflect *clarification* are referred to as paraphrasing and parroting information to the family as client.

> #### Parroting
> Family member: *"I cannot believe this has happened to our mother."*
> Nurse: *"You cannot believe this has happened to your mother."*

#### Paraphrasing
Family member: *"I cannot believe this has happened to our mother."*
Nurse: *"You're finding it hard to believe your mother has had a heart attack."*

*Summary statements* are intended to capture the content, themes, or essence of what was said by family members. Summarizing can be used at any time during a family assessment or meeting to clarify ideas or messages being conveyed and to enhance the nurse's understanding of the family's situation.

> Nurse: *"What I am hearing from everyone here is that the primary concerns are whether your mother is physically strong enough to cope with open heart surgery and whether she will have a full recovery."*

### Genuineness

Conveyed by the nurse through being sincere honest, and spontaneous and the use of "I" statements. For example, the nurse states, *"I'm concerned . . .," "I appreciate that each of you feels comfortable in sharing your concerns with me."*

### Self-disclosure

Conveyed by the nurse through use of personal information of a similar situation and related feelings currently being experienced by the family. Self-disclosure should be used only when it will benefit the family or family members and should be used with discretion so as not to shift the focus from the family's experience to that of the nurse. When self-disclosure is used, it is important for the nurse to be in the process of resolving the situation or for the situation to have been positively resolved. The use of self-disclosure is intended to validate family members' feelings and let them know they are not alone in their experience and that their situation has the potential to be resolved. It is common for family members to ask the nurse what strategies were used or how the situation was resolved. It is important for the nurse to ask family members what ideas they have for resolving their situation before disclosing what strategies were used to resolve the nurse's situation. In this way the nurse avoids the position of giving advice, and if the family chooses to employ strategies used by the nurse, family members are less likely to blame the nurse if the strategies do not work to resolve the family's unique situation because they were given an opportunity to present their own ideas first.

### Advanced empathy

Conveyed when the nurse accurately reflects the underlying feelings or emotions associated with the content, themes, or context of the individual's or family's story. Formula and natural responses are presented as exemplars.

> Formula response for advanced empathy: *"You feel scared/terrified because your mother's cancer has*

>

*spread, and you feel overwhelmed because she may die if she undergoes surgery."* Natural response for advanced empathy: *"I am sensing that you're scared/terrified about your mother's cancer spreading, and you are devastated that she may not be strong enough to survive the surgery."*

## STAGE III: ACTION STAGE FOR DEVELOPMENT OF FAMILY ALLIANCE

Goals: Focusing on family communication solutions; empowering families to manage communication issues through problem-solving strategies; and developing resources and opportunities

### Confrontation

Conveyed by the nurse through the use of empathy: a statement that describes the discrepancies in family member's communication related to feelings, behaviors, and/or actions and communicates the nurse's commitment to continue working with family members.

Discrepancies that the nurse can address through the use of confrontation include (1) discrepancies in family member's feelings and behavior (i.e., differences between what is currently being expressed verbally and what behavior is being observed); (2) what family members have stated previously and what they are saying currently; and (3) how family members behaved previously or what they did previously and how they are behaving currently or what they are doing now.

Prefacing each type of discrepancy statement with a basic empathic response and following the statement of discrepancy with a statement that reflects commitment to further involvement with family members reinforce the therapeutic nature of using such an advanced communication skill.

Basic Empathy: *"You are feeling worried about your mother's illness and her impending surgery."*

Discrepancy 1: *"You say you are not upset, but I notice that some of your feet are tapping, you have tears in your eyes, and some of you are tremulous."*

Commitment: *"I have some time to sit with you. Let's talk about what is bothering each of you right now."*

Discrepancy 2: *"When we met last week, I understood that each member of the family said he or she would take turns spending time with your mother at the hospital, and now I hear you saying that each of you hasn't been able to follow through with your commitment."*

Commitment: *"Let's talk about what is happening for each of you that is interfering with your ability to spend time with your mother."*

Discrepancy 3: *"Last week I noticed that each of you seemed really emotional about your mother, and today I notice that each of you seems more composed and relaxed, and you even have a sense of humor."*

Commitment: *"Let's talk about what has changed for each of you."*

### Immediacy

Conveyed by the nurse when calling attention to the relationship between the family and the nurse as to (1) what is happening "here and now" in the nurse-family alliance, that is, in the current interview or meeting and (2) what has been happening in the alliance with the family over time. Conveying how the nurse feels in the context of what is going on requires the nurse to express his or her own feelings or emotions in the context of any barriers to the maintenance and development of the nurse-family alliance.

Nurse:
(1) *"I am concerned that I may have upset some of you with the information I shared about the procedure for open heart surgery. My intent was to share information about what your mother is facing and in no way to make anyone feel more upset. What concerns do you have at this time with regard to your mother's situation?"*
(2) *"I am concerned about what has been happening in our last two meetings. I noticed that some of you are participating less, and I'm wondering if you may be questioning my ability to help you successfully work through your grief associated with your mother's illness. What do you think is happening? I'd appreciate knowing what you are thinking and feeling and how I can help."*

### Problem solving

Situational and interpersonal problem solving are two approaches that can be used to work toward resolving two different types of issues or problems.

*Situational problem solving* aims to explore with families: what events or stressors led to the problem situation; how family members responded to the problem situation; what previous experience the family has had in managing this type of problem situation; what coping strategies the family has used in the past and what has been effective and what has not been effective for the family; what coping strategies are currently effective for the family and what strategies are currently ineffective for the family; and what new or alternative coping strategies the family is aware of or interested in pursuing.

*Interpersonal problem solving* aims to resolve issues between two or more family members. Two considerations will guide the nurse in deciding whether to attempt to resolve the issue with each of the family members involved. (1) How important is it for the family member to solve the problem? (2) Is the problem solvable? If one or more of the family members are in agreement about attempting to resolve the problem or issue, the nurse has each family

>

member respond to each of the following requests for information in sequence: (1) *"Tell me how the problem looks to you right now."* (2) *"Describe for me how are you involved in the problem."* (3) *"Tell me how you feel about the problem."* (4) *"Tell me how you react to or behave in response to the problem."* and finally, (5) *"Tell me how you think that you contribute to the problem."*

Family members involved are encouraged to work through each step of the process individually and then to share their perceptions with each other. Exploration of options, alternatives, and contracting for change in ways of relating to each other may be outcomes of the process.

*Conflict Resolution*

The *win-win* problem-solving method of managing conflict is based on seven strategies. The nurse as facilitator and mediator invites the family to work through the series of seven strategies in an effort to promote effective family communication and to

reduce family conflict over the course of a few sessions. The strategies are as follows:

(1) Have each family member identify his or her issues and unmet needs.
(2) Establish a time for family members to share their identified issues and needs with the other family members involved.
(3) Have each family member describe his or her issues and needs to the other family members present.
(4) Have each family member listen to the points of views raised by the other family members involved.
(5) Have the family members generate and negotiate possible solutions.
(6) Have the family members implement the solutions.
(7) Follow up with the family by setting a time and date to revisit the effects of the solution (in 1-week or 1-month intervals).

Source: Crawford, J.A., and M.A. Tarko, Family Communication. In P. Bomar (ed.), *Promoting Health in Families: Applying Family Research and Theory to Nursing Practice*, 3rd ed (pp. 62–186). Philadelphia: Saunders, 2004.

The quality of any response depends on the degree of mutual trust in the relationship. Techniques can be very successful or they can be abused, depending on your attitude at the time, the other person's interpretation, and how they are used. Facilitative techniques are stepping stones to better understanding—an understanding that nurtures trust and the expression of feelings. We seek the realization of the feeling of caring, safety, and security in your company, and the feeling that you want to help the person help him- or herself. By using therapeutic principles, you will help the person and family identify you as someone to whom ideas and feelings can be safely and productively revealed. One of the common barriers to effective interactions by health professionals is making assumptions about client and family situations that may result in valuable data being omitted.[145]

## CRITICAL THINKING

*When you have experienced family problems professionally, what methods have you tried as you endeavour to assist the family to resolve them?*

You may find the following *guidelines helpful in evaluating your communication methods.* Do you:

■ Examine the purpose of your communications?

■ Consider the total physical and human setting?

■ Plan your communication, clarifying ideas and seeking consultation?

■ Analyze the methods used and their effectiveness?

■ Identify possible hidden meanings as well as the basic content of the message you conveyed?

■ Support communication with actions?

■ Follow up communication to determine whether your purpose was accomplished?

Your use of therapeutic communication and a client-centred approach will move you through the relationship with a family or individual. However, *certain constraints* may be experienced if you are not careful about your feelings and behaviours. Table 4-12 describes constraints or problems commonly encountered as you work closely with a family member or unit.[146]

## Family Assessment

*In doing a family assessment*, ask questions related to family structure and develop a **genogram**, *a diagram of family members and their characteristics and processes* (see Figure 4-1). Determine communication patterns and relationships, family health, access to health care, occupational demands and hazards, religious beliefs and practices, childrearing practices, participation in the community, and support systems. An **ecomap** may be drawn to *illustrate the contact that family members have with the larger systems*. Wright and Leahey state that "ecomaps shift the emphasis from the historical genogram to the current functioning of the family

**Table 4-12** Constraints in the Helping Relationship

- **Certain limits exist for you, the helper, and for the client. Relationship means involvement and commitment;** it takes time. The client's dependency may create demands for extra time or responsibility. You will have to consider feelings and needs, meet important demands, and set limits whenever necessary.

- **The client may not be willing to change sufficiently to resolve the problem.** The person may not be able to give up his or her discomforts because these may be a core part of his or her identity.

- **As the helper, you may experience the phenomenon of countertransference**—*an unconscious, inappropriate emotional response to the client as if he or she were an important figure in your life, or unconsciously based in past unresolved experiences with key people in your life.* The helpful measure in this situation would be to respond to the client realistically as he or she really is. Countertransference works in much the same ways as transference does for the client. You relate to the client based on your feelings toward someone from the past.

If you are *experiencing countertransference,* you may have *any of the following reactions.*

1. Overidentify with the client; you exert pressure on the person to act a certain way or to improve.

2. Attempt to make the person over in your own image.

3. Invite gifts or favours, dependence on the client's praise or affection.

4. Offer excessive reassurance or help that is not really necessary.

5. Feel a need to impress the client.

6. The wish to be the client's child, grandchild, or younger sibling may occur with older people, especially if they actually resemble your parents, grandparents, or siblings.

7. Realize that your thoughts wander from the client, or the client's words trigger unrelated thoughts.

8. Focus repetitively on one aspect or way of looking at the person's behaviour or statements. Be attentive to the client's verbal and nonverbal behaviour.

9. Defend interactions with the patient to others. Ignore behaviour; show lack of objectivity about the behaviour, or focus on one aspect of behaviour.

10. Be impatient with or have guilt about the client's lack of progress, insensitivity to, or lack of empathy for his/her needs, or feelings of being unable to help.

11. Experience conflicting feelings of intense affection, dislike, defensiveness, indifference, fear, or angry sympathy with the person.

12. Feel overconcern about the person between sessions, or have an overemotional reaction to the client's troubles, believing no one else can care for the person as well as you can.

13. Experience sexual or aggressive fantasies about the client.

14. Experience dreams about the client; be preoccupied with the client when awake.

Countertransference can be overcome through guidance from a supervisor and a willingness to examine your personal behaviour and comments.

- **You may feel anger toward the client.** Your anger may be a reaction to his or her overt behaviour and your fear of acting that way. Your anger may be a counterreaction to the client's anger that is related to something else but is directed toward you. You can stop the cycle by recognizing your own feelings, and the helplessness felt by the client, by talking with him or her to determine possible sources of anger, and by avoiding either a hostile or too sweet response. Do not joke about anger in yourself or the client, and do not reject or punish the client for anger. Make sure that you are not the cause of anger because of actions that demean, aggravate, or neglect him or her. If the person arouses anger in you, seek help from a skilled colleague to work through possible reasons for your anger, to talk about how you demonstrate anger in your behaviour, and to explore ways to handle such feelings.

- **You may think you are the only person who can care for the client** or that you can solve all of the problems. Such a feeling of omnipotence is unfounded.

- **You may have difficulty with dependence and independence within a relationship.** You may want to have others depend on you. Therefore, you do things for the client that he or she can do. Such smothering discourages independent behaviour. On the other hand, you may find it difficult to tolerate the person's dependency, clinging, helplessness, or need for total assistance. Seek help to work through your own feelings.

- **If you joke or tease in a harsh or belittling manner, if you use jestful sarcasm, if you laugh at the client's appearance or behaviour, if you play childish games to get him or her to co-operate or be pleasant, or if you use the client as a scapegoat,** you will be the cause of the client's anger, hate, despair, hopelessness, and finally complete withdrawal and regression.

**Figure 4-1** Genogram format

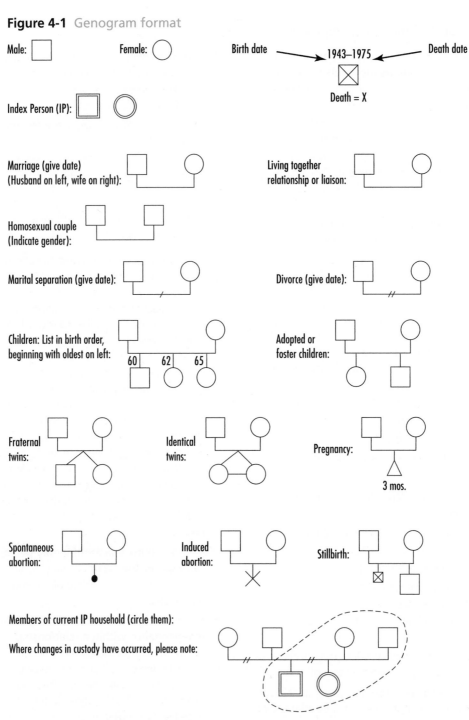

Symbols to describe basic family membership and structure (include on genogram significant others who lived with, or cared for, family members; place them on the right side of the genogram with a notation about who they are). Religion, education, or ethnic origin can be written in by oldest generation or other units. Health problems are noted by person.

and its environmental context."[147] An ecomap for a family is illustrated in Figure 4-2.

## CRITICAL THINKING

*After completing the ecomap for your family, what patterns did you notice?*

When you work with the family unit, the information in Figure 4-3 will help you assess the family's lifestyle and needs. Other criteria are listed in the box entitled "Criteria for Assessing Healthy Families."

The Calgary Family Assessment Model (CFAM), developed by Wright and Leahey, is a multidimensional model that incorporates developmental, structural, and functional

**Figure 4-2** Family ecomap

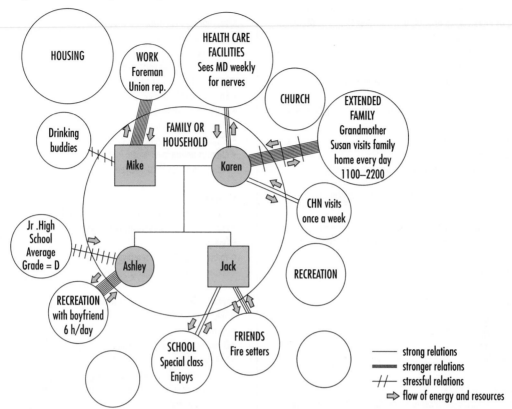

Source: Wright, L.M., M. Leahey, and A.G. Perry, Family Nursing. In P.A. Potter, A.G. Perry, J.C. Ross-Kerr, and M.J. Wood (eds.), *Canadian Fundamentals of Nursing* (pp. 295, 305). Toronto: Elsevier, 2006.

theory. It is based on systems–communication, cybernetics, change theory foundation, as well as postmodernism and the biology of cognition. Wright and Leahey claim that CFAM consists of three major categories: **structure, development**, and **function**. Further, each category comprises several sub-categories and the nurse decides which subcategories should be included in the assessment of the family (see Figure 4-4).

*In what ways are you able to obtain data regarding a family's emotional communication?*

In a hospital, health centre, or community setting, wherever the family unit is considered as part of the client, you may assess some important phenomena. These may be the issues, strengths, or healthy responses observable in the family. For example, you may assess the family's denial of the client's illness, or the open communication processes in the family system that benefit all lifestyle patterns of family members.

It is essential to note that every family has strengths and weaknesses. Family strengths are the cornerstone that assists the family to cope in times of transition and change. In the literature, common threads in healthy families seem to be open communication, an environment

that nurtures and sustains individual family members as well as the family unit, specific yet flexible definition of roles, and ability to express warmth, intimacy, and humour.[148] Wellness diagnoses that would reflect family strengths include:

- Progressive sharing by family members of thoughts, feelings, and perceptions

- Analyzing issues together; mutual problem-solving episodes that recognize individual and family needs

- Mutual love, trust, and respect for all family members[149]

CRITICAL THINKING

*In what ways can you develop insight into a family's strengths in order to develop a wellness diagnosis?*

## Formulation of Goals and a Plan of Care

The primary *goal* in working with families is to use yourself and your assessment in a way that allows the family to (1) bring issues into the open, (2) gain a new awareness, (3) learn new ways to facilitate balance in the family system, and (4) fulfill family functions in more healthful ways.

**Figure 4-3** Family assessment tool

**Meeting of Physical, Emotional, and Spiritual Needs of Members**
- Ability to provide food and shelter
  Space management as regards living, sleeping, recreation, privacy
  Crowding if over 1.5 persons per room
  Territoriality or control of each member over lifespace
  Access to laundry, grocery, recreation facilities
  Sanitation including disposal methods, source of water supply, control of rodents and insects
  Storage and refrigeration
  Available food supply
  Food preparation, including preserving and cooking methods, (stove, hotplate, oven)
  Use of food stamps and donated foods as well as eligibility for food stamps
  Education of each member as to food composition, balanced menus, special preparations or diets if required for a specific member
- Access to health care
  Regularity of health care
  Continuity of caregivers
  Closeness of facility and means of access such as car, bus, cab
  Access to helpful neighbours
  Access to phone
- Family health
  Longevity
  Major or chronic illnesses
  Familial or hereditary illnesses such as rheumatic fever, gout, allergy, tuberculosis, renal disease, diabetes mellitus, cancer, emotional illness, epilepsy, migraine, other nervous disorders, hypertension, blood diseases, obesity, frequent accidents, drug intake, pica
  Emotional or stress-related illnesses
  Pollutants that members are chronically exposed to such as air, water, soil, noise, or chemicals that are unsafe
- Neighbourhood pride and loyalty
- Job access, energy output, shift changes
- Sensitivity, warmth, understanding between family members
  Demonstration of emotion
  Enjoyment of sexual relations
    Male: Impotence, premature or retarded ejaculation, hypersexuality
    Female: Frigidity (inability to achieve orgasm), enjoyment of sexual relations, feelings of disgust, shame, self-devaluation; fear of injury, painful coitus
    Menstrual history, including onset, duration, flow, missed periods and life situation at the time, pain, euphoria, depression, other difficulties
- Sharing of religious beliefs, values, doubts
  Formal membership in church and organizations
  Ethical framework and honesty
  Adaptability, response to reality
  Satisfaction with life
  Self-esteem

**Childrearing Practices and Discipline**
- Mutual responsibility
  Joint parenting
  Mutual respect for decision making
  Means of discipline and consistency
- Respect for individuality
- Fostering of self-discipline
- Attitudes toward education, reading, scholarly pursuit
- Attitudes toward imaginative play
- Attitudes toward involvement in sports
- Promotion of gender stereotypes

**Communication**
- Expression of a wide range of emotion and feeling
- Expression of ideas, concepts, beliefs, values, interests
- Openness
- Verbal expression and sensitive listening
- Consensual decision making

**Support, Security, Encouragement**
- Balance in activity
- Humour
- Dependency and dominance patterns
- Life support groups of each member
- Social relationship of couple: go out together or separately; change since marriage mutually satisfying; effect of sociability patterns on children

**Growth-Producing Relationships and Experiences within and without the Family**
- Creative play activities
- Planned growth experiences
- Focus of life and activity of each member
- Friendships

**Responsible Community Relationships**
- Organizations, including involvement, membership, active participation
- Knowledge of and friendship with neighbours

**Growing with and through Children**
- Hope and plans for children
- Emulation of own parents and its influence on relationship with children
- Relationship patterns: authoritarian, patriarchal, matriarchal
- Necessity to relive (make up for) own childhood through children

**Unity, Loyalty, and Cooperation**
Positive interacting of members toward each other

**Self-Help and Acceptance of Outside Help in Family Crisis**

**Figure 4-4** Branching diagram of CFAM

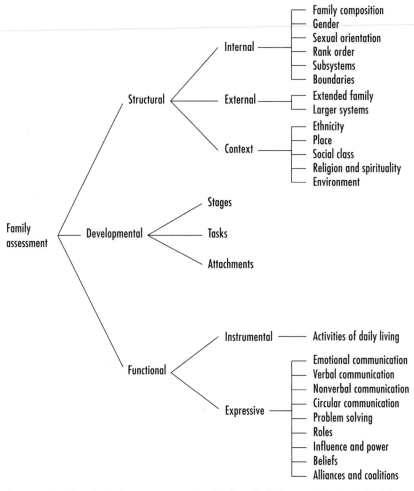

Source: Wright, L.M., and M. Leahey, *Nurses and Families: A Guide to Family Assessment and Intervention*, 3rd ed. Philadelphia: F.A. Davis, 2000, p. 68. Used with permission.

## Criteria for Assessing Healthy Families

- Ability to provide for the physical, emotional, social, and spiritual needs of the family
- Ability to be sensitive to the needs of family members
- Ability to listen and communicate effectively
- Ability to provide trust, support, security, affirmation, and encouragement
- Ability to initiate and maintain growth-producing relationships and experiences inside and outside the family
- Demonstration of mutual respect for family and others
- Commitment to teach and demonstrate moral code
- Concern for family unity, loyalty, and interfamily co-operation
- Capacity to use humour and to share leisure time with each other, to enjoy each other

- Commitment to strong sense of family where rituals and traditions abound
- Ability to perform roles flexibly and share responsibility
- Ability to maintain balance of interaction and privacy among the members
- Ability for self-help and helping other family members, when appropriate
- Ability to use crisis or seemingly injurious experience as a means of growth
- Ability to grow with and through children
- Capacity to maintain and create constructive and responsible community relationships in the neighbourhood, school, town, and local and provincial/state governments and to value service to others.

Sources: Friedman, M., V. Bowden, and E. Jones. *Family Nursing: Research, Theory and Family Practice*, 5th ed. Upper Saddle River, NJ: Prentice Hall, 2003.

*Short-term goals* could be stated as follows:

- Family system will convey support to the ill member through daily visits and empathic conversation.
- Family members will be able to describe special dietary needs and other self-care measures essential to client recovery.
- Family member (specific person) will continue to demonstrate correct techniques for rehabilitative care of client.

*Long-term goals* are appropriate if you will be working with a family over time. Such goals could include the following:

- Family system will identify key issues that contribute to hostile communication and withdrawal of members from participation in family life.
- Family members will practise daily (for an increasing amount of time) communication methods that promote cohesion.
- Parents will share their successes of achieving effective disciplinary measures for children.

You will write goals specific to the family systems with which you are working. Perhaps the examples given will stimulate your thinking.

## Intervention

*You can help families understand some processes and dynamics underlying interaction* so that they, in turn, learn to respect the uniqueness of the self and of each other. Certainly, members in the family need not always agree with each other. Instead, they can learn to listen to the other members about how they feel and why they feel as they do, accepting each person's impression as real for self. This attitude becomes the basis for mutual respect, honest communication, encouragement of individual fulfillment, and freedom to be. There is then no need to prove or defend the self.

Once the attitude "we are all important people in this family" is established, conflicts can be dealt with openly and constructively. Name calling and belittling are out of place. Families need to structure time together; otherwise individual schedules will allow them less and less time to meet. Parents need to send consistent messages to their children. To say "don't smoke" while lighting a cigarette is hardly effective.

*Times of communication are especially necessary* when children are feeling peer pressure; children, moreover, should be praised for what they do right rather than reprimanded for what they do wrong. Children need structure

but should be told the reason for the structure if they are old enough to comprehend it. As you help the family achieve positive feelings toward and with each other, you are helping them to fulfill their tasks, roles, and functions. Review the adaptive mechanisms of families described in this chapter.

**Models of Intervention** The Calgary Family Intervention Model (CFIM) highlights three types of family interventions that focus on *cognitive, affective, and behavioural levels* of family functioning and involve teaching and counselling. For example, family nursing interventions focusing on the cognitive level are intended to provide the family with fresh ideas about how family members communicate with each other. The choice of interventions used depends on how the family perceives the issue at hand. Interventions should be developed to address the family's perception and beliefs in relation to issues of how members interact with one another.[150]

The CFIM recommends nursing practices that promote family functioning, such as:

- Asking interventive questions
- Offering commendations
- Providing information
- Validating emotional responses
- Encouraging illness narratives
- Supporting family caregivers
- Encouraging respite

There are two types of interventive questions: *linear questions*, which provide the nurse with information about a client and family, and *circular questions*, which help determine changes that could be made in a client or family's life. Table 4-13 illustrates the four types of circular questions.[151]

### CRITICAL THINKING

*What interventions can you develop to change a family's affective domain of functioning?*

The person's health problems, especially emotional ones, may well be the result of the interaction patterns either in childhood or in the present family. Knowledge of the variables influencing family interaction—parents' self-esteem and upbringing, number of siblings, person's ordinal position in the family, cultural norms, family rituals—help you assist the person in talking through feelings related to past and present conflicts. You may assist families to cope with crises or various unexpected disorganizing events, such

**Table 4-13 Types of Circular Questions**

| Type of Question | Examples to Elicit Change in the Following Domains: | | |
| --- | --- | --- | --- |
| | **Cognitive Domain** | **Affective Domain** | **Behavioural Domain** |
| **Difference Question** | | | |
| Explores difference between people, relationships, time, ideas, or beliefs | What is the best advice given you about supporting your son with AIDS? What is the worst advice? | Who in the family is most worried about how AIDS is transmitted? | Which family member is best at getting your son to take his medication on time? |
| **Behavioural Effect Question** | | | |
| Explores connections between how one family member's behaviour affects other members | What do you know about the affect of life-threatening illness on children? | How does your son show that he is afraid of dying? | What could you do to show your son that you understand his fears? |
| **Hypothetical/Future-oriented Question** | | | |
| Explores family options and alternative actions or meanings in the future | What do you think will happen if these skin grafts continue to be painful for your son? | If your son's skin grafts are not successful, what do you think his mood will be? Angry? Resigned? | When will your son engage in treatment for his contractures? |
| **Triadic Question** | | | |
| Question posed to a third person about the relationship between two other people | If your father were not drinking daily, what would your mother think about his receiving treatment for alcoholism? | What does your father do that makes your mother less anxious about his condition? | If your father were willing to talk with your mother about solutions to his addiction, what could he say? |

Source: Wright, L.M., M. Leahey, and A.G. Perry, Family Nursing. In P.A. Potter, A.G. Perry, J.C. Ross-Kerr, and M.J. Wood (eds.), *Canadian Fundamentals of Nursing* (pp. 295, 308). Toronto: Elsevier, 2006.

as illness and natural disasters. Table 4-14 summarizes steps in crisis intervention or brief therapy.

*You may help families explore and resolve ethical dilemmas* related to their decisions about the use of newer technology for getting pregnant, or in dealing with an adoptive child. A technique that allows infertile couples to become pregnant is called in vitro fertilization. The consideration of this technology might, however, cause parents to face major ethical dilemmas when, for example, they endeavour to determine which of the fertilized embryos should be transplanted into the uterus and which should be frozen for future use. The careful and extensive exploration of feelings and implications is essential. Having children through human reproductive technology can force parents to face major and serious ethical dilemmas. In vitro fertilization can become an issue for families later when grown children wish to know who their biological parents are.

You may explore with the family the decision to use sperm donors who are paid for their service for artificial insemination. The donor should be screened carefully for a family history of inherited diseases and for current pathogens such as human immunodeficiency virus (HIV). Because some infections, such as HIV, are present long before they may be detected (as long as ten years), transmission of this disease via insemination may occur. The donor is also screened in terms of race, intelligence quotient, physical characteristics, and health. Recipients may choose the baby's sex. Some women become pregnant after the first insemination; others require several to many inseminations.

The *Developmental/Health Framework within the McGill Model of Nursing* provides basic knowledge consistent with Nightingale's vision of working with the "laws of nature" to promote health and healing. It provides substantive knowledge to guide nursing practice. For example, the working

| Table 4-14 | Family Crisis Intervention to Assist Families with Coping |
|---|---|

1. Encourage family to identify the stressor or hazardous life event.

2. Assess family's interpretation of event and its real impact.

3. Determine family's usual and current coping abilities and resources to handle the event.

4. Assess family's level of functioning as a whole, and the function of individual members.

5. Assist family members in communicating with each other.

6. Encourage all family members to be involved in finding a solution(s) or resources.

7. Be supportive but encourage the family to mobilize its own resources and extended family or community resources.

8. Empower families by indicating their strengths, reinforcing positive behaviour, helping them make sense of the event, and promoting a sense of being normal.

9. Explore possible ways to prevent and cope with future stressful experiences.

10. Teach coping strategies, ways to prevent or minimize future stressors, stress management, and lifestyle alterations.

11. Recognize members at risk for violence and intervene as necessary.

12. Either continue longer-term therapy as needed with the family unit or members or refer them to ongoing therapy if necessary.

definition of development is that it begins at conception and ends at the last stage of life, which is death. Development involves the appearance, over time, of physical structures, psychological traits, capacities, and competencies to adapt to life challenges. It involves balancing between change and stability. Gottlieb and Gottlieb state that the focus of nursing attention is both the individual and the family. That is, the individual within the context of the family, as well as the family as a unit, constitute the focus of care. In the McGill Model of Nursing, family is defined as any individual, or group of individuals, that the client identifies as family. Even though the nurse does not always care for the family as a unit, the nurse should always be *family-minded*. Many nurse interactions are considered through the family lens.[152]

The decision to hire a surrogate mother—a woman to become pregnant and bear a baby for the family—must be explored carefully because of implications for the surrogate mother and her feelings, consequent feelings of the childrearing family, and legal issues.

Other decisions may not be as difficult, but they are key to future family development and relationships. Examples include helping adoptive parents to relate with their child, or helping the homosexual family to explain "coming out" to the children from an earlier marriage. Such parents may require help in preparing to explain their child's origins when the child asks, or in assisting the child to understand that there are many different kinds of families. We do not yet know all of the consequences, developmentally and emotionally, for children who are raised without consistent parental guidance from the opposite sex, or who are raised by only one parent. Your assessment, exploration, and teaching with such families are important.

Admittedly, further research is desperately needed in all of these areas. To help families explore values and ethical principles, you must *first* explore and resolve these issues within yourself. You cannot give another *the* answer. You can, however, use good therapeutic communication skills to enable clients to find their own answers.

Through the *use of an empathic relationship and effective communication skills, thoughtful teaching, and insightful crisis therapy*, you can encourage family members to talk about their feelings with one another; and you can assist them in resolving their conflicts. Help them become aware of the need to work for family cohesiveness, just as they would work at a job or other important project. Refer them to a family counselling service if you determine that the problems are beyond your scope. Your work may help them to access and use other community resources, such as private family or psychiatric counselling or family and children's services.

One example of a family self-help resource is the formation of a group of four or five complete family units (including stepfamily, single-parent, cohabitation, or traditional units) who contract to meet together over an extended period for shared educational experiences that concern relationships within their families. This setting provides a positive approach and affirms family members because a commitment is made for all persons—no matter what their age—to have both power and input into the group.

Table 4-15 summarizes intervention measures for counselling or educating families to promote their health.

## Role of the Nurse in Well-Baby Care

You may care for well babies and mothers in a variety of settings—clinic, hospital, home, or doctor's office. Your actions will contribute significantly to their health.

Table 4-15 Summary of Intervention Measures

1. **Develop a therapeutic relationship.** Establish rapport and trust between yourself and the family by being open to the family structure or system and the cultural values and norms that are manifested. Use therapeutic communication principles. Use the family's language, but be a model for clear, effective communication. Remember the trust, influence, and impact that you have on the family unit. Be empathic, supportive, and impartial as you provide feedback to the family. By doing so you will enable the family members to identify and modify patterns that cause dysfunction and discomfort.

2. **Identify issues with the family.** Subjective issues are what the family members perceive as problem areas. Objective issues are what you see as limits or problems. Have each family member list or identify problems and areas for change. Refrain from challenging or questioning the accuracy of anyone's values or statements of problem areas. Do not side with any one particular member. Encourage family members to explore those areas that you see as dysfunctional.

3. **Encourage and assist members in their communication skills,** to listen to one another, to talk kindly, and to clarify their own perceptions and the feelings, thoughts, and behaviours of the others. If you confront gently and serve as a mirror for the family members, they will be able to gain increased understanding of themselves as a unit. As they learn to talk honestly to one another, members will have less need to deny the pain they feel, or to deny hurtful behaviours practised in family living.

4. **Establish a teaching plan for the family unit if it is appropriate,** either for the client as a member of the family or for the family as a whole. Help each one to find appropriate resources in the external environment and to identify their own personal strengths for managing a situation. Encourage the family to find ways to adapt the lifestyle or home situation so they can better manage an illness or crisis.

5. **Determine willingness of family members to participate in counselling and change.** Keep in mind that families, according to systems theory, strive to maintain their balance and are frightened and ambivalent about negotiating and enacting change. Have each member participate in defining the problem and in making the decision for change to enable family members to feel more in control of what is occurring and more willing to participate. Even so, some members may continue to be resistant to change during counselling, or they may choose not to participate at all. It is essential for you to remain objective, reassuring, and supportive. Considerable theoretical knowledge, communication skill, and supervised practice are necessary before you will be able to work with deep, long-term, or complex problems; resistant behaviour; power struggles; or coalitions.

6. **Negotiate a contract for the goals for treatment.** Identify with the family one or two goals that are crucial to work toward to begin to achieve some happiness and smoother function. Later, other goals may be added to the list. It is better to set small achievable goals that the family perceives as worthwhile than to inhibit family change through an extensive list of statements. Remember that the questionable behaviour of any one family member is a symptom of a problem in the family system.

7. **Negotiate a contract about specific behavioural changes that can be accomplished** and that will encourage family members to interact or behave in ways that break dysfunctional patterns or rigid structures. Assist members to disagree constructively and to contract with one another for change. Help the family to anticipate problem areas, work through alternatives, and explore the possible consequences of the alternatives.

8. **Be patient.** Do not expect great change. The family may change its behaviour, but only to the point that is comfortable and tolerable to all. Regression to previous patterns will occur. Your consistent kindness and encouragement may be the main factors in the family's ability to cope with stressors or crises, to adjust to the daily routines of the needs of an ill member, or to stay with therapy and modify troublesome behaviour.

**Prenatal Care** Prenatal care for the mother and her partner may include physical assessment, teaching healthful practices for mother and baby, listening to the mother vent frustrations or share fears, counselling her during periods of depression or uncertainty, and sharing her happy feelings about becoming a mother. You may conduct childbirth classes for mother and father so that they can better understand changes occurring in the mother and the nutrition and hygiene necessary during pregnancy. Help them to know what to expect during labour, delivery, and postpartum, and prepare the father for an active role during birth. A maternity nursing book will provide adequate detail to help you do prenatal assessment and care, as well as intrapartum and postpartum assessment and intervention.

If the mother-to-be is unwed, you may endeavour to work with the father-to-be, if both are willing. The father-to-be will likely need help in talking about his feelings, and he needs to know how to support the mother. He may also benefit from sex education.

To assist the unwed parents, it is helpful to gain a better understanding of the unwed father. The relationship between the unwed mother and the father-to-be is likely to be a meaningful one to both. If the parents-to-be are adolescents, they need to realize that a new life has been created as a result of their actions. They probably want to act responsibly and will be concerned about the child's well-being.[153]

The unwed father can be encouraged to stand by the unmarried mother. Although he may feel proud of fathering because he has proven his masculinity, the long-term consequences of having a child are such that alternate solutions regarding the future of the child should be thoroughly explored with and by both partners. Alternatives include marriage, placing the child for adoption, or assumption of the responsibility for rearing the child by either parent, or by the grandparents. The man probably needs help in understanding and accepting the fact that he will become a father, and in realizing the serious implications at hand for the mother, the child, and himself.

Adolescents may admit that their sexual experiences were unsatisfactory, leaving them depressed, guilty, and scared. The good relationship with the girlfriend may have begun to deteriorate when sexual relations were started. Pregnancy comes as a shock to both. They may have known about contraceptives, but may have used them sporadically, if at all. Some people believe that the spontaneity and sincerity of the sexual act are lessened by contraceptive preparations.[154]

*Sex education* must relate to the values of interpersonal relations and a profound concern for others if it is to be successful. The implications and responsibilities of sexual behaviour must be discussed with the teenagers. The difference between teenage love and a more mature relationship between people who are ready to meet the problems and responsibilities of adulthood should be discussed.[155]

Both parents of the unwed teen father should be involved in helping their son. Communication between the boy and his parents should be maintained, or re-established. In addition, parents should assert themselves by supportively helping the boy to take responsibility for his actions and assist him in the case of marriage.

Efforts to prevent unwed pregnancies must be directed toward improving and strengthening family life and developing a better respect for the father's role in the family. Fathers can help adolescent sons by talking with and listening to them, by being slow to judge, by taking them to the office or workplace so the youth can see how the father earns a living, and by being a role model in relating maturely to the spouse and other women. Fathers can be highly influential in creating an atmosphere in which his sons will want to talk about emerging sexual feelings and experiences.[156] If the adolescent son comes from a home where no father is present, the mother can work at listening to and discussing problems and feelings with the son. She may also be able to foster a bond between the son and another male member of the family.

*A pregnant 15-year-old informs you that she is frightened at the realization of being pregnant. What can you say and do to help her overcome her fears?*

**Childbirth Education Classes** If you conduct childbirth and parenting education classes, try to interview each couple in their home early in the pregnancy, by the fourth month if possible, to observe their relationship and determine their response to pregnancy. Their response may be different and more honest in their own home than in class. During the classes, include opportunities for both men and women to talk about their feelings, or the problems they feel are uniquely theirs. Provide anticipatory guidance about the couvade syndrome. *Couvade syndrome* refers to sympathetic pregnancy experienced by a man, usually the husband of a pregnant woman. Symptoms mimic those suffered by pregnant women, such as weight gain, fatigue, dizziness, nausea, vomiting, constipation, abdominal pain, cramping in the legs, unusual food cravings, and changed sexual appetite. Avoid pushing the father into participation, but provide support for him. Focus childbirth education on the known benefits to the baby and parents and not on overromanticized and dramatic statements about improved marital relationships. Educate both parents about family planning so that future pregnancies can be mutually planned. Refer either partner, or both, to psychological counselling when necessary, especially if antisocial behaviour is seen or if there has been fetal loss.

**Labour and Delivery** During labour and delivery, the nurse provides the necessary physical care. She might act as a coach for the mother, or support the father as he assists the mother. Flexibility in hospital routines for obstetric patients is usually possible and contributes to the parents' sense of control.

The physician and nurse, or nurse-midwife, can work as a team with the expectant couple. In some facilities, the nurse-midwife assumes primary responsibility for the family unit. Whenever a mother delivers, she has the right to capable, safe care by qualified caretakers. Home deliveries can be carefully planned and safe. Hospital deliveries can be more homelike. Maternity centres now provide families anticipating a normal childbearing experience with antepartum care that is educational in nature, labour and delivery in a homelike setting (but with adequate equipment), discharge to home whenever it is safe for mother and baby, and follow-up care by public health nurses in the home during the postpartum course. The labour and delivery rooms can be designed to accommodate the presence of the father or family during delivery and be less traumatic (less cold, with less intense lights) for the newborn. After the birth, the infant can remain with the mother, and the newborn's physical examination can be done in the mother's (and father's) presence. Childbirth should be a positive, maturing experience for the couple. Expectant parents have the right and responsibility to be involved in planning their care with the health team and to know what is happening. Cultural beliefs should be recognized, respected, and accommodated whenever possible. A positive childbearing experience contributes to a healthy family unit.

**Postpartum Period** Because of short hospital stays after delivery of the baby (6 to 48 hours), you may not be able to provide the traditional and essential physical or emotional postpartum care. Instead, the care will be delivered in the home by the family, with continuing support and assistance from a home health nurse or maternal–child advanced practice nurse who is a consultant.

The following guidelines must be taught to the family member(s) who will be caring for the new mother and baby or carried out by the nurse in the home. In the early postpartum period, assess mother and baby. Facilitate the mother's physical care; assist her as necessary, even if she looks well and able. The mother needs to be mothered to enhance attachment between her and the baby. Listen to the mother's (and father's) concerns; answer questions; support maternal and paternal behaviour. In a non-threatening way, teach the parents how to handle the baby. Help them begin to unlearn preconceived ideas about the baby and to perceive self and the baby positively. If the mother is breastfeeding, teaching and assistance are necessary. After the initial "taking in" period of having received special care and attention, the mother moves to the "taking hold" stage, in which she is able to care for the child.[157]

The interaction between the infant and primary caretaker is crucial. The mothering person helps the baby feel secure and loved, fosters a sense of trust, provides stimulation, reinforces certain behaviour, acts as a model for language development, and trains the baby in basic learning strategies. In turn, maternal behaviour is influenced by baby's cries, coos, smiles, activity, and gazes and by how well baby's behaviour meets the mother's expectations.

Your significant contributions to the family unit are to promote attachment between parents and baby and to encourage continuing contacts between the family and health professionals so that adequate health and illness care are received. As well, encourage parents to meet the baby's needs adequately. You can help the parents feel good about themselves and the baby.

You can be instrumental in continuing new trends in care to make the hospital or clinic environment more homelike, while providing safe, modern care.

**Continued Care in the Postpartum Period**
During the six or eight weeks after delivery, the mother needs assistance with child care and an opportunity to regain her former self, both physically and emotionally. The father also needs support as he becomes involved in child care responsibilities. In the nuclear or single-parent family, the parent may struggle alone. Continued visits by a home health nurse may be useful. Some communities have a crisis line for new parents. You may be able to suggest services or help the parent think of people who could be helpful.

As you assess the mother's functioning, consider her physical and emotional energy, support systems, and current level of parenting activity. If she apparently is not caring adequately for the child, assess for anemia, pain, bleeding, infections, lack of food or sleep, drug use, or other medical conditions that would interfere with her activity level and feelings of caring. Depression and postpartum blues are difficult to differentiate. In depression, the mother is immobilized and unable to do basic care for herself or the baby. With postpartum blues from hormonal shifts and the crisis of parenthood, she may cry but she cares for the baby's physical needs. Depression has a longer course and should be medically treated. The new mother usually has enough energy to do only top-priority tasks: eating, sleeping, baby care, and essentials for other family members.

The mother's support system is crucial for her energy maintenance, both physical and emotional. She needs direct support and assistance with daily tasks, plus moral support, a listener, and a confidant. Support comes from personal and professional sources: the partner, parents, friends, and other relatives, and the nurse, doctor, social worker, or pastor. Negative attitudes from others can drain emotional energy. Actual parenting skills can be manifested in various ways: touching; cuddling; a tender, soft voice tone; and loving gazes. Additional information about parents' feelings and the parenting process is provided in Chapter 7.

If the baby is progressing in normal fashion, focus on the mother's needs and concerns. Help her find non-professional support systems that can assist her when the professional is unavailable, or someone who can help with child care. In addition to concern over child care, we must help the mother grow developmentally. Helping her stay in good physical and emotional health ensures better parenting.

Certain *behaviour patterns in parents strongly suggest a disturbed parent–child relationship and future problems in parenting*, for example, if the parent:

■ Is unable to talk about feelings, fears, and sense of responsibility for the child

■ Makes little effort to secure information about the baby

■ Consistently misinterprets or exaggerates either positive or negative information about the baby

■ Receives no practical support or help from family or friends, and community resources are lacking

■ Is unable to accept and use help offered

You may be instrumental in suggesting *certain procedures that can be used to promote the parent–child relationship*:

■ Permit the mother to see and touch the baby as soon as possible, preferably in the delivery room.

■ Permit the mother's involvement in the baby's care as soon as possible.

■ Provide an atmosphere that encourages questions.

■ Encourage parents to talk with each other, family members, and friends, using others for support.

■ Recognize that parents' excessive questions, demands, and criticisms are a reaction to stress and not personal attacks on the professional worker or hospital.

■ Arrange for the father to visit the baby before discharge, calling him about the baby's progress at intervals when he is unable to visit.

■ Encourage the parents to handle the baby and do the baby's care before discharge; teach about baby care as necessary while the parents are engaged in care of their baby.

In addition, observe the interactions and relationship between the parents or between the mother and other members of the family. It will be difficult for the mother to remain caring if she is abused. A father who is abusive to the mother—verbally, physically, or emotionally—may become abusive to the child at some point. Chapters 6, 7, and 8 and other references can be helpful.[158]

## Care of Families with a Chronically Ill or Special-Needs Child

Families who have a child with chronic illness, or a special-needs child with developmental disabilities or chronic physical or emotional illness experience a number of stressors in addition to the physical, emotional, and social burdens and financial costs of continuing care. Parents may feel as if they want collaboration and control, but have no control over the care of and treatment consequences for their child, depending on the health care providers' approaches to the child and family. Some families passively depend on the professional providers for all directions. Parents experience a sense of loss, chronic sorrow, and ongoing grief and mourning related to the ideal or normal child they expected, as they adapt their expectations to fit the real child they have. Ongoing physical care and guidance problems are constant reminders of developmental lag, that the child will not achieve certain developmental tasks and will remain dependent on someone, perhaps for life. Continual, possibly lifelong adjustments will need to be made for the child and his or her care. Parents worry about the child's care and quality of life in the future when they are unable to continue care. All family members react to the time and energy demands of a special-needs child, realizing that their child's needs mean less time and energy for each other and for themselves. All family members will realize the effects that the inevitable financial drain will exert on their standard of living. Financial stress includes more than cost of care. It also includes the loss of employment or of educational opportunities when a parent must either stop or reduce these activities because of child care demands. McNeil examined the experience of fathers who have a child with juvenile rheumatoid arthritis. His findings indicated that based on the nature of fathers' experience and the extent of their involvement, more attention by health care practitioners to fathers' adaptation is undoubtedly warranted.[159]

Marital stress occurs as parents negotiate parental roles and responsibilities, time, energy, and finances, and reconcile career-versus-family demands. Career mobility, especially related to geographic moves, may occur because of dependence on a specific treatment agency or team or because of the employer's insurance plan. Divorce in families with special-needs children is not unusual.

*Families with special-needs children need a social support system to maintain an adequate level of family stability and care for the child.* Social support may include an extended family, close friends, religious affiliation, parents of other children with special needs, and access to empathetic professionals. Extra effort is often needed to encourage these parents to participate in self-help or other groups, because they often do not develop or maintain social contacts and consequently they tend to become more isolated. A family with adequate finances, who has lived in a community long enough to have developed contacts and friendships and have a house and a car, will likely have a good understanding of and collaboration with the health care system. If so, this family will fare better than a family without these characteristics.

*Health care professionals can develop family support groups to provide:*

- Education about the diagnosis, how to cope with it, and how to treat the condition
- A place where parents can discuss their feelings and concerns and receive acceptance and empathy as they grieve losses in the situation
- Information about available services and resources in the community
- Assistance with fulfilling role responsibilities and demands
- Assistance to parents to become advocates for their children in negotiating for services, education, and favourable legislation
- Social functions to reduce the sense of isolation the families may feel

Table 4-16 provides telephone numbers of organizations that can provide information for families with special-needs children.

## Parent Education

To combat the problems associated with the high adolescent birth rate, some junior and senior high schools are establishing creative programs in parenthood education. Some hospitals and health clinics are initiating specialized prenatal and postnatal services for the adolescent mother and her at-risk infant. You can initiate non-traditional programs in your own community.

Some health care agencies have established programs to help adolescent mothers become more effective parents. The adolescent mother who decides to keep her baby needs all the family and outside help she can get. She will probably fear that whatever personal ambitions she has will be thwarted by the baby. Unmarried and unprepared for employment, she finds it almost impossible to make her own way in the world. Anger, frustration, and ignorance may hamper her ability to attach to, and appropriately care for, the baby. Repeated pregnancies, child neglect and abuse, and welfare dependency often result.

Formation of a mothers' or parents' group, including women and men of various ethnic origins and income brackets, can provide parent education and support and foster talking about one's feelings. Be sure to educate parents about using community resources.

| Table 4-16 | Telephone Numbers and Websites for Special Needs Information |
|---|---|
| Canadian National Institute for the Blind | 1-800-563-2642 www.cnib.ca |
| Canadian Diabetes Association | 1-800-226-8464 www.diabetes.ca |
| Kidney Foundation of Canada | 1-800-361-7494 www.kidney.ca |
| Arthritis Society | 1-416-979-7228 www.arthritis.ca |
| Canadian Down Syndrome Society | 1-800-883-5608 www.cdss.ca |
| Canadian Hemophilia Society | 1-800-668-2686 www.hemophilia.ca |
| Canadian Mental Health Association | 1-613-745-7750 www.cmha.ca |
| Canadian Paraplegic Association | 1-613-723-1033 www.canparaplegic.org |
| Children's Wish Foundation of Canada | 1-800-267-9474 www.childrenswish.ca |
| Disabled Peoples' International | 1-709-747-7600 http://v1.dpi.org |
| Epilepsy Canada | 1-877-734-0873 www.epilepsy.ca |
| Heart and Stroke Foundation of Canada | 1-613-569-4361 www.heartandstroke.com |
| Multiple Sclerosis Society of Canada | 1-800-268-7582 www.mssociety.ca |
| Muscular Dystrophy Association of Canada | 1-866-MUSCLE-8 www.muscle.ca |
| Canadian Cystic Fibrosis Foundation | 1-800-378-2233 www.cysticfibrosis.ca |
| Canadian Society of the Investigation of Child Abuse | 1-403-289-8385 www.csicainfo.com |
| Fetal Alcohol Syndrome World Canada | 1-613-952-1220 www.phac-aspc.gc.ca/fasd-etcaf |
| Canadian Institute of Child Health | 1-613-230-8838 www.cich.ca |
| Spina Bifida and Hydrocephalus Association of Canada | 1-204-925-3650 www.sbhac.ca |

Your work with the mother may prevent maternal deprivation, insufficient interaction between mother and child, conditions under which deprivation or even abuse develops, and negative effects on the child's development.

## Family Care throughout the Life Cycle

You may be called on to assist families as they meet various developmental crises throughout the life cycle: school entry of the child, the adolescent period, children leaving home, divorce, retirement, or the death of a family member. Your goal is health promotion and primary disease prevention. Your intervention early in the family life cycle may help to establish a positive health trend in place of its negative counterpart. The care you extend to young parents lays the foundation for their children's health. You may even find yourself becoming an advocate for such families to promote legislation that affects families and child care.

Another way to improve the family as an institution is from within. Parents should teach their children not just to get ahead but to be altruistic—that is, to serve, to co-operate, and to be kind. We can teach our children to believe that family ties are the most rewarding values, that social, cultural, and community activities can be deeply satisfying, and that the gratification from income and jobs is not the main priority.[160]

Parents can make a profound difference by teaching spiritual values—helpfulness, co-operation, generosity, love—throughout childhood. Two-year-old children can be encouraged to help set the table, especially if they are then thanked and praised. Teenagers can be expected to work in hospitals and to tutor younger children. Such jobs should not be presented as distasteful. Children enjoy taking on adult jobs when they are presented as opportunities and their efforts are appreciated.

Just as vital is a family atmosphere in which parents treat each other and their children with respect, affection, and a smile. The best forum is still mealtime and the family meeting. When teenagers first give excuses for why they cannot make it to a family meal, parents should say very positively, "We like to have the whole family be together."

When parents are asked questions about sexual matters by two-, three-, and four-year-old children, they should advance from anatomy and physiology to emphasize the loving and caring aspects of sex and marriage. An even greater influence on children is their parents' behaviour toward, and commitment to, a partner and their admiration and respect for one another. Joking and disparaging remarks about marriage should be avoided. Parents can suggest that if young people want to claim the right to sexual freedom, they should be aware of the responsibilities. If a youthful marriage soon ends in divorce, parents can point out that no marriage succeeds by itself, that it must be continually cultivated, like a garden. It is wise to look for openings to discuss these topics when children are 9, 10, or 11 years of age. When they are 13 years old and beyond, they think their parents are hopelessly old-fashioned and consider peer opinions as the only truth.[161]

You have a role as educator and advocate as well as health care provider. You can assist parents as they guide children toward meeting developmental needs. You can assist adults to be mature parents who present a positive model for the future of the family and society.

**Canadian Military Families** The Canadian authors believe that tribute should be extended to Canadian military families for their enduring sacrifices for the national good. Unfortunately, paucity exists in Canadian scholarly writing and research about military families. We believe that enforced separations have a detrimental consequence on the family as a unit. Even civilians, such as journalists who travel to war zones and become exposed to political danger, frequently subject their families to similar separation dynamics. During all kinds of separation, and even in cases of unavoidable death, patterns of coping and adapting can play a central role in determining the final outcome of relationships within the family.

## SUMMARY

1. There are various types of family forms and systems.

2. You will care for clients who come from a family background quite different in structure and dynamic relationships from your own family system.

3. People who come from varied family forms—heterosexual or homosexual, for example—show both similarities and differences when compared to each other.

4. The view of a family life cycle for varied family forms depicts the complexity of life's transitions.

5. Family relationships are interacting dynamic processes, and the extent to which developmental tasks are met within the family is a major influence on development and health.

6. You will practise in all health care settings principles of health promotion within a family context, based on concepts considered in this chapter.

7. Engage in lifelong learning about your own and other family systems so you can assess, plan, and provide comprehensive care to the client and family.

## Interesting Websites

The Vanier Institute of the Family

**www.vifamily.ca**

Established in 1965 under the patronage of Governor General Georges P. Vanier and Madame Pauline Vanier, the Vanier Institute is a national charitable organization dedicated to promoting the well-being of Canadian families. It is governed by a volunteer board with regional representation from across Canada.

### Dads Canada

**www.dadscan.org**

The Dads Canada site is a gateway helping to identify individuals (researchers, professionals), organizations, and institutions interested in promoting fatherhood in Canada. This information is presented for all provinces and territories across the country.

### CANGRANDS

**www.cangrands.com/**

The CANGRANDS site welcomes all grandparents and family members who are raising grandchildren or extended family members. The organization's aim is to promote, support, and assist families in maintaining or re-establishing family ties—especially between grandchildren and grandparents and extended families.

### Multiple Births Canada

**www.multiplebirthscanada.org/**

This organization exists to improve the quality of life for multiple-birth individuals and their families. It offers an extensive network of local chapters, health care professionals, and organizations.

### Canada Adopts!

**www.canadaadopts.com/**

This site, aimed at adoptive parents, is backed by a support team of professionals specializing in adoption, infertility, social justice, law, education, new media, Web design, marketing, advertising, and journalism.

### Canadian Child Care Federation (CCCF)

**www.cccf-fcsge.ca**

The CCCF's mission is to improve the quality of child care services for Canadian families. This site includes news about child care in Canada and information about publications for parents and child care practitioners. For a partial list of provincial child care organizations, click on "Affiliates".

## Key Terms

**adaptive responses in the family** (103)

**affectional functions** (102)

**apartners** (118)

**countertransference** (127)

**development** (129)

**ecomap** (126)

**extended family** (96)

**family** (95)

**family cultural pattern** (119)

**function,** (129)

**genogram** (126)

**"living apart together" (LAT) couples** (118)

**matrifocal/matriarchal family** (96)

**nuclear family** (96)

**patrifocal/patriarchal family** (96)

**personality** (103)

**physical functions** (102)

**psychologically extended family** (97)

**roles** (101)

**same-sex family** (96)

**single state** (96, 118)

**single-parent family** (96)

**social functions** (102)

**spiritual function** (103)

**stepfamily** (96)

**stepgeneration family** (119)

**structure** (129)

**therapeutic or helping relationship or alliance** (121)

# Chapter 5

## Overview: Theories Related to Human Development

*No theory explains everything about the person.*
**Ruth Beckmann Murray**

## Objectives

*Study of this chapter will enable you to:*

1 Examine major theoretic perspectives for understanding the developing person.

2 Describe selected biological and evolutionary theories about aspects of the developing person.

3 Discuss ecologic theory and systems theory as they apply to the developing person.

4 Analyze the work of major psychological developmental theorists, according to their views about the developing person.

5 Compare and contrast major concepts of behavioural, psychoanalytic and neo-analytic, cognitive, existential, and humanistic theories.

6 Discuss the importance of eclecticism in the study of human development.

7 Differentiate major concepts between stress and crisis theories.

8 Apply concepts from at least three theories of development in promoting health of the client and family.

## PROGRESSION OF STUDY OF HUMAN DEVELOPMENT

Human development has been described for millennia. During the 18th century, the "nature versus nurture" argument began. The child was considered to be a little adult, the product of either heredity or environment. By the 19th century, child study was beginning to be more systematic. The science of **psychology**, *the study of human behaviour*, developed in the later 1800s, led people to understand themselves better by learning about child behaviour. Theories about human behaviour were being developed. The rise of Protestantism, with its emphasis on responsibility for self and others, led adults to feel more responsible for

how the child developed into an adult. With the Industrial Revolution, children became more important to their parents—if for unfortunate reasons. Gradually, child education occurred outside of the home. Until the 20th century, the study of child development and advice on child care were not based on the scientific method, but instead carried biases couched in folklore.

As the 20th century progressed, theories about human behaviour were developed. Study was expanded to include the child and the adult. Later, the adolescent became of interest, as did different stages of adulthood, including young and middle adulthood. Now, in the 21st century, when people are living longer, the elderly have become a particular focus. Several stages of older adulthood have now been described.

The lifespan is studied as persons are observed while they continue to develop or undergo change—physically, emotionally, cognitively, spiritually, and socially. Dying is seen as the last developmental phase, the final attempt to come to terms with self, others, and life in general. The study of the changes made by the individual and the family unit throughout the lifespan is the focus of this book. By learning more about ourselves and others, including how people respond to surrounding influences to meet basic needs, we hope to help people become better able to meet their individual potential and, in turn, create a better world.

Theories that are used to explain or account for the developing person and the person's behaviour use some combination of biological and evolutionary, ecological, systems, and psychological study. The psychological theories are divided according to their emphases: behaviourism, analytic, cognitive, and humanistic. Stress and crisis theories are addressed and a brief description of eclecticism is included along with an indication of its importance in the study of human development. *The whole person is best understood when several theories are combined to explain the person's total development.* Use the theories described in this chapter in assessment, goal-setting, and strategies for health promotion.

## CRITICAL THINKING

*Before reading this chapter, consider for a moment any theories of human development that come to your mind.*

Although this chapter focuses on an overview of theories of human development, it is important to note that the health promotion of the individual and the family throughout the lifespan is also pertinent. Therefore, it seems appropriate to outline and address briefly the main theoretical frameworks pertinent to health promotion.

Nutbeam and Harris state that four theories influenced the practice of health promotion: (1) the health belief model; (2) the theory of reasoned action; (3) the trans-theoretical (stages of change) model; and (4) the social cognitive theory.[1] The main thrust of these theories is that they explain health behaviour, and health behaviour change, by focusing on the individual. The health belief model is designed to explain health behaviour by better understanding beliefs about health. The usual progression is to move from the individual and the families to consideration of the relative costs and benefits of strategies to protect and improve health. The major assumption underlying the theory of reasoned action, developed by Ajzen and Fishbein, is that people are usually rational and will make predictable decisions, particularly in those circumstances that are well defined. The reasoned action model is based on the assumption that the intention to act is the most immediate determinant of behaviour, and that all other variables influencing behaviour will be mediated through behavioural intention. The trans-theoretical (stages of change) model, developed by Prochaska and DiClimente, is based on the premise that behaviour change is a process, not an event, and that individuals have different levels of motivation or readiness to change. Finally, the social cognitive theory has evolved from social learning theory and is one of the most widely applied theories for health promotion because it addresses both the underlying determinants of health as well as the methods to promote change. Many researchers have contributed to the social cognitive theory, but one of the most influential has been Albert Bandura. These four theories are becoming increasingly important to know in the implementation of health promotion because health professionals' demands are calling for theory-based decisions. We start with a brief consideration of biological and evolutionary theories.

## BIOLOGICAL AND EVOLUTIONARY THEORIES

The theories of nativism, ethology, behaviour genetics, and sociobiology all propose that, over time and through a series of genetic mutations and natural selection, the genetic and physiological processes that are basic to human behaviour gradually change.[2] Some specifics are considered first.

## Brain

Various areas of the brain control functions and influence development and behaviour. The brain controls behaviour—how we perceive, think, feel, behave, act, and interact. The two halves of the brain are mutually involved in all high levels of psychological functioning. Although each hemisphere functions independently in perception, learning, and memory (see Table 5-1), consciousness and the conscious self are single and unified, mediated by brain processes that span both hemispheres. A general consensus on the exact nature of consciousness remains elusive. Some recently proposed theories are built around the concept of working memory.[3]

Huge quantities and vast ranges of sensory information are transmitted to the cerebral cortex. The ways in which the brain sorts, classifies, organizes, and interprets sensory information, and the ways it handles input and output; considers expectations, past experiences, and other sources of information; and sends messages throughout the body are all well beyond the capability of any computer system. Research on the physiologic basis for behaviour has gained sophistication with advancing technology in studying the

## Table 5-1 Right Brain–Left Brain Information Processing Differences

| Mode | Left Brain (Controls Right Side of Body) | Right Brain (Controls Left Side of Body) |
|---|---|---|
| Thinking | Time bound<br>Rational, logical, sequential or linear, analytical, interpretive<br>Synthesis of sensory input<br>Spirituality | Space bound<br>Concrete, appears irrational<br>Artistic<br>Intuitive; holistic |
| Language | Hearing words<br>Writing words<br>Voice recognition<br>Reading<br>Speech comprehension<br>Verbal memory | Metaphoric<br>Singing songs<br>Face and form recognition<br>Draw figures<br>Body image |
| Mathematics | Algebraic functions, adding, subtracting, multiplying, dividing | Geometric, spatial, relational |
| Problem solving | Focus on specifics<br>Breaks problems into parts, linear, sequential<br>Details | Focus on generalities<br>Grasps problem in totality<br>Grasps relational dimensions<br>Patterns |
| Organizational | Action mode: primed to manipulate environment<br>Focal attention<br>Heightened boundary perception<br>Object-oriented<br>Dominance of formal over sensory | Receptive mode: primed to take in environment<br>Diffuse attention<br>Boundary fusion<br>Dominance of sensory over formal |
| Interactional | Controlled, consistent<br>Explicit, directed, objective, judgmental, evaluative | Emotive<br>Affect-laden<br>Tacit<br>Tolerant of ambiguity, subjective<br>Nonjudgmental, noncritical |
| Operational | Figures things out in stepwise order<br>One idea follows another<br>Comfortable with precise connotations, right/wrong<br>Computer-like functions<br>Memory for verbal and auditory stimuli | Makes leaps of intuition<br>Creativity<br>Pattern recognition and relationships form basis of ideas<br>Comfortable with alternatives and multiple explanations, nonlinguistic stimuli |

complexity of the brain and nervous system, endocrine and immune functions, and physiologic responses in a variety of situations. Findings obtained in these ways affect current beliefs about healthy growth and development throughout the lifespan. In the following discussion, factors related to genetic, biochemical, neurophysiologic, immunological and maturational factors are covered briefly. Also, Chapters 6 through 14 discuss physiologic factors that affect the person.

## Genetic Traits

Our understanding of the role of genetic factors has grown rather dramatically in recent years. Examples include the direct visual examination of chromosomes and the biochemical analyses of genetic material and enzymatic processes.[4] In fact, in the near future, genetic testing—along with the detection, treatment, and prevention of disorders—is expected to increase substantially in health care settings.[5] An urgent need exists for nurses and other health care professionals to be well informed about all of these issues and be involved in providing genetic services in particular to individuals and their families.[6]

The importance of a genetic foundation is paramount in the promotion of an understanding of this complex field. For example, the Mendelian Law of Inheritance states that a dominant gene for a trait or characteristic in at least one parent will cause, on average, 50 percent probability that any child of those parents will inherit it. If both parents have the dominant gene, each child has a 75 percent probability of inheriting the trait. When the trait is attributed to a recessive gene, the offspring does not inherit it unless the gene is received from both parents. If the gene is received from only one parent, the offspring is not affected, but will probably pass the gene to a child (the grandchild). If the spouses are **heterozygous** for a recessive gene (*both received the same gene type from only one of their parents*), each child has a 25 percent probability of being affected. If the spouses are **homozygous** for the recessive gene (*the same gene type was received from both of their parents*), all the children probably will inherit the trait or characteristic.[7]

The genetic system has several levels of complexity. For example, each neuron is genetically assigned to produce certain neurotransmitters. Genes produce many kinds of receptors for each neurotransmitter. A single cell may respond differently to the same receptor at different times, for unknown reasons. When a neuron "learns" or is altered by experiences, there is a radical change in its surface proteins as well as in the receptors. Thus, environment and experience can in fact alter genetic predisposition.[8]

To isolate environmental factors from genetic effects, researchers have used several methodological designs, such as the family resemblance method, the twin study method, and a combination of the two. The family resemblance method looks for similarities between a person with a disorder and his or her relatives.

The twin study method relies on differences between **monozygotic twins** (*from a single ovum and therefore identical*), and between **dizygotic twins** (*from two ova fertilized by two sperm and therefore not identical—that is, fraternal twins*). For example, one study indicates that the correlation for depressive symptoms is highest among identical twins. Twin studies indicate that there is a stable predisposition to temperament and that the environment of the child contributes little to adult depression.[9] Monozygotic twins, compared to dizygotic twins, have been found to resemble each other more in mood level and ability. Research is also being conducted on identical and fraternal twins reared apart.[10] For example, one recent Canadian study examined the correlation between genetic liabilities for alcohol and drug misuse with perceptions of the social environment of the family of origin. In Vancouver, a mail-out survey collected data from monozygotic and dizygotic twin pairs using newspaper advertisements and media stories. The researchers concluded that genotype–environment correlations (in particular, moral emphasis in the home) appear to be quite influential in the development of substance misuse.[11]

CRITICAL THINKING

*What other twin studies are you aware of? What were the results?*

Considerable interest has been expressed in the study of the respective contributions of environmental and genetic influences on an individual's body fat in order to control the "epidemic" of obesity. A York University study estimated the degree of familial resemblance in anthropometric indicators and fat distribution. Anthropometric indicators include body mass index, skin folds, and waist circumference. In this sample of 327 Caucasian participants from 102 nuclear families, the role of genes was found to explain at least part of the heritability.[12]

Simonen and her colleagues conducted a study on familial aggregation of physical activity levels, as part of the Quebec Family Study. They investigated 696 subjects from 200 Quebec families and found that physical activity is represented by a significant degree of familial resemblance. Physical inactivity has a slightly higher heritability level than does moderate to strenuous physical activity. These researchers concluded that familial practices that shared familial environmental factors, along with genetic factors, are important in accounting for the familial resemblance in physical activity levels.[13]

The Mendelian law explains the occurrence of various physical traits such as eye colour and height, and probably explains certain physiologic characteristics. However, the Mendelian law does not fully explain emotional or mental development, and it does not address social, moral, or spiritual development.

Specific genes cannot be linked with specific kinds of behaviour until the behaviour is precisely defined. This has not been done. In contrast, linking a gene with a specific disease, such as cystic fibrosis, has been done.[14]

Genes determine a foundation for reaction or predisposition. The exact behavioural expression depends on many prenatal, parental, and postnatal influencing factors. For example, a specific chromosomal aberration, such as the presence of an extra chromosome, is directly related to Down syndrome, with its resultant limited intellectual function. Unfortunately, the intellectual achievement may be lower than the inherited capacity if the person receives inadequate education. Conversely, the achievement may be somewhat greater than predicted by early testing when a loving family and appropriate education coexist to develop fully the inherited potential.[15]

Genes exert an effect on health and disease, as well as on human traits and behaviours. Only recently has science begun to unravel the complex pathways that underlie such attributes as cognition, handedness, diurnal rhythms, and certain behavioural characteristics. Often, it is claimed, research in behavioural genetics, such as on sexual orientation or intelligence, has been somewhat flawed in design. The ramifications are that some findings have been communicated in a way that oversimplifies and overstates the role of genetic factors. In many cases, serious problems have occurred for those who have been stigmatized by the suggestion that alleles, associated with so called "negative" physiological or behavioural traits, are more frequent in certain populations. Therefore, it is important to gather scientifically valid information about genetic and environmental factors to provide a good understanding of the contributions and interactions between genes and environment in these complex phenotypes.[16]

Thus, **polygenic** inheritance, the *combination or interaction of many genes acting together to produce a behavioural characteristic*, is believed to be a factor if certain characteristics or behavioural defects occur. Environmental effects contribute to the person's development of genetic potential from the moment of conception.[17]

Researchers in the emerging field of epigenetics have found that epigenetic factors play a critical role in development across the lifespan.[18] Epigenetics refers to the study of changes that influence the phenotype (observable characteristics of the individual) without causing alterations to the genotype (unique genetic blueprint of the individual). It involves changes in the properties of a cell that are inherited, but does not involve a change in the deoxyribonucleic acid (DNA) sequence.[19] Both genetic and epigenetic factors interact with the environmental variables to shape an individual's level of well-being across the lifespan.[20]

Hegele claims that in familial hypercholesterolemia (FH), early coronary heart disease (CHD) is a complex trait resulting from a large monogenic component of susceptibility due to elevated low-density lipoprotein (LDL). Not all subjects, however, with a LDLR gene mutation suffer from early coronary heart disease. In fact, the environment plays a large role in modulating expression of the genetic susceptibility to coronary heart disease.[21]

A brochure called *The Healthy Heart Kit* is sponsored by Health Canada, Population and Public Health Branch (PPHB), in partnership with the College of Family Physicians of Canada, Health and Social Services (Montreal), and the Heart and Stroke Foundation of Canada and Quebec. This widely supported brochure helps individuals understand cholesterol and its impact on heart disease.[22] It informs the individual of the nature of both "good" cholesterol, called HDL (high-density lipoprotein), and "bad" cholesterol, LDL (low-density lipoprotein). LDL tends to block arteries. Furthermore, the brochure outlines desirable cholesterol levels, measured in millimoles per litre, or mmol/L for short. The ideal level of LDL for people with heart disease is less than 2.5 mmol/L. In addition, the brochure informs individuals of ways to control their blood cholesterol regarding diet and exercise. It also emphasizes "no smoking" and following doctors' orders on prescription medication.[23] All provinces and territories have Heart and Stroke Foundation offices, and they all supply other useful and informative resources.

---

### CRITICAL THINKING

*What differences do you observe in the content of pamphlets among the provinces and territories?*

---

# Reproductive Screening

In a classroom debate, your colleagues are discussing reproductive screening tests. The situation at hand pertains to Jean, a pregnant young woman who has advised the nurse that both she and her partner are carriers of cystic fibrosis (CF). Based on the Mendelian Law of Inheritance, you understand that there are four possible combinations of genes from parents who are both carriers. Carriers will have both a dominant normal gene (N) for CF and a recessive gene (c) for CF. Each parent's gene pool for CF will be represented as (Nc). The CF gene combination possibilities for the offspring of these parents are as follows:

1. N/N (Normal), no CF in offspring
2. N/c (Carrier), no CF in offspring
3. N/c (Carrier), no CF in offspring
4. c/c (Disease), shows CF in offspring

You can predict that there is a 25 percent probability that the child will have CF.

1. What is your position on reproductive screening for this couple?

2. If pregnant women who are carriers of other autosomal recessive diseases wish to pay for reproductive screening, would you, as a health professional, support and possibly lobby for their cause?

A study determined the diagnostic performance characteristics of HNF1A genotyping for diabetes and impaired glucose tolerance (IGT) in Oji-Cree Aboriginal people in Canada.[24] The researchers had identified a private HNF1A mutation, G319S, which was associated strongly with type 2 diabetes in the Oji-Cree. The HNF1A S319 allele occurred in less than 40 percent of the Oji-Cree who had diabetes, and was linked with a younger age at onset of diabetes, adolescent-onset type 2 diabetes, and changes in plasma lipoproteins. All subjects in this study were genotyped for the HNF1A G319S mutation. The results indicated that the most specific genetic test developed to date for the prediction of a common multifactor disease using present-day standards of clinical epidemiology in molecular genetics is the HNF1A genotype. The result of a positive test had particular diagnostic value in the Oji-Cree. That is, a subject with HNF1A S319 was certain of having diabetes, or IGT, by age 50. On the other hand, a subject without HNF1A S319 had a decreased risk, compared with the age-specific prevalence, but was not totally risk-free. It is important to note that HNF1A S319 was not the only relevant factor for diabetes in the Oji-Cree. It was found that subjects without HNF1A S319 were still at some risk for diabetes or IGT.[25]

Young, Reading, Elias, and O'Neil reviewed the published literature on type 2 diabetes mellitus from the past two decades, and they focused on the First Nations people in Canada. (They excluded the Inuit and Métis, because diabetes is not a serious health problem for the Inuit, and few data exist for the Métis.) These investigators conclude that the current health and social effects of the disease are considerable and that genetic interactions are likely the cause.[26]

Virtually every disease has a genetic component based on a specific gene or gene mutation. Research with molecular techniques is helping us understand genetic contributions (the specific chromosomal regions) to such diseases as Alzheimer's disease, hypertension, diabetes, various cancers, heart and kidney diseases, and some mental illness or brain diseases. In the future, a genetic profile will be developed for each child at birth. However, genetic predisposition or causation is not immutable. Environmental factors can modify and affect the expression of a specific gene, or gene mutation. Even though an individual has a very strong genetic susceptibility to coronary heart disease (CHD), personal decisions and actions to modify the environment will create an effective impact on the unfavourable genetics in CHD.[27] Health professionals can play a significant role in promoting a healthy lifestyle through screening methods, and by teaching risk reduction measures to individuals and their families.

**Human Genome** A prime component of the Human Genome Project is the effort to construct a detailed map of human DNA and the genes that guide the development of a human being from a fertilized egg cell. Another interest of the project is the examination of the ethical, legal, and social implications of this recently discovered genetic knowledge. Also included within the mandate of the project is the development of policy options for public consideration regarding this genetic research strategy. The genome is the sum total of genes carried by all 46 chromosomes in the human being.[28] It is estimated that, during their lifespan, 60 percent of Canadians will experience an illness with some form of genetic component. Advances in human genomics will play an important role in predicting and preventing disease in the 21st century.[29] Genetic technologies hold the potential to assist a large majority of Canadians.[30] In fact, the combined effects of recent and anticipated genetics research hold the potential to redefine medicine within the lifetime of most Canadians. The recent plethora of knowledge of individual susceptibility to diseases raises questions about the types of related ethical issues. Included among

---

## CASE SITUATION

Ted Smith, a 40-year-old husband and father of three young children, is a sales manager with a well-known computer company. A few years ago, Ted was diagnosed with coronary heart disease (CHD). His father died of a heart attack a few months earlier. Over the last few weeks, Ted has mentioned several times to his wife, Sharon, that he has been experiencing "chest heaviness." He attributes this discomfort to work stress and assures Sharon that it will likely pass when business picks up. Sharon, however, is worried that Ted frequently eats packaged snacks and drinks a lot of canned drinks and coffee while "on the run" between appointments. Ted's usual twice-weekly stop at the gym for a workout has been neglected now for almost a year. With these observations in mind, Sharon has convinced Ted to stop at the Walk-In Clinic to check out the chest heaviness symptom.

You are a clinical nurse specialist at this clinic. When Ted arrives, you conduct the initial assessment. Sharon shares with you her concerns and observations about Ted. Ted then consults with the doctor, who recommends that he have his blood cholesterol checked. Ted makes arrangements with the lab to have his blood drawn. In a few days, the lab sends you his results of the three types of cholesterol and the triglycerides. You particularly notice that Ted's LDL reading is high—above 4.0 mmol/L. You know that Ted will return for the blood test results by the end of the week.

1. What is your understanding of blood cholesterol levels?

2. According to the *Healthy Heart Kit*, is Ted's LDL level borderline high or high? (See www.healthyheartkit.com.)

3. What health promotion strategies will you plan with Ted at this time?

these issues is the need to protect the privacy and safety of individuals and outlaw the use of genetic information in the place of employment. It is important to provide all health care professionals with the tools and knowledge they need to navigate this complex terrain. Those same health care professionals need to build in the community and in society generally a climate of understanding and acceptance of genetic innovation.[31]

## CRITICAL THINKING

*What is your understanding of Parkinson's disease and its management? See Guttman et al. (2003).*[32]

Genome Canada is a not-for-profit corporation whose aim is to develop and implement a national strategy to genomics and proteomics in Canada. With financial assistance from the federal government, Genome Canada has established five genome centres across the country. Together with these centres and other partners, Genome Canada invests and manages large-scale research projects in important areas such as agriculture, environment, fisheries, forestry, health, and new technology.[33]

As a matter of interest, in April 2004 the I.H. Asper Clinical Research Institute, at the St. Boniface General Hospital in Winnipeg, hosted Canada's first national, travelling, bilingual exhibition on DNA and genomics. It was called "The Geee!"[34]

## CRITICAL THINKING

*Will knowledge of the human genome lead to the development of a repair manual for the human body?*

As a partner with Genome Canada, the Ontario Genomics Institute (OGI) is dedicated to developing new preventative measures, diagnostics, and treatments that will affect the lives of people in Ontario and globally.[35] A project called "Strengthening the Role of Genomics and Global Health," led by Drs. Singer and Daar, is funded through the OGI. This project is examining the role of developing world biotechnology companies in meeting local health needs in genomic innovation. At the same time, the project seeks to ensure that advances in pharmacogenomics are appropriately used to address global health challenges. In addition, this project aims to ensure the mobilization of agricultural genomics knowledge through interventions to promote sustainable food security in developing countries.[36]

**Reproductive Screening** Reproductive screening can be conducted for carriers of autosomal recessive diseases, such as cystic fibrosis, in order to provide information to the partners. The information provided may be used regarding decisions about family planning. However, careful

counselling is necessary with carrier screening to make certain that individuals comprehend the limitations of testing and the implications of results.[37] Wilson and his associates assessed the role of cystic fibrosis (CF) testing within the Canadian health care system. They recommended that during pregnancy, CF testing should be indicated for individuals who may be at increased risk for CF because of family history or clinical manifestations. Prior to CF screening, each province/territory should review the ethnic diversity of its reproductive population to ensure that CF screening would be appropriate. The screening of all women for CF carrier status during pregnancy could not be recommended at this time.[38] Couples who are exploring reproductive technology, such as in vitro fertilization (IVF) and intracytoplasmic sperm injection (ICSI) when the man has obstructive azoospermia, should be offered genetic/clinical counselling for informed consent and genetic testing for alterations in genes associated with cystic fibrosis (CF) before attempting either IVF or ICSI.[39]

**Bioinformatics** As a result of biotechnology, another developing industry called **bioinformatics** *focuses on the storage and retrieval of biological information from a database in a biologically meaningful way. Practice applications* are apparent because of the rapidly advancing knowledge about genetics and health care.

**Role of the Nurse** The CNA position statement *The Role of the Nurse in Reproductive and Genetic Technologies* states that nurses will be called on to play a critical role in advocating the availability of helpful information. Nurses will be essential in encouraging public participation in developing policies about a number of highly significant issues. Some of the issues in which the nurses will play key roles include assisted human reproduction, genetic testing, genetic therapy, genetic enhancements, the human genome project, and privacy concerns—as well as human cloning.[40]

Even though the role of genetics in human health is complex, nurses are well situated to play an important role in genetics in their various practice settings.[41] In order to do so, nurses must take the responsibility to become knowledgeable about this rapidly changing field, and help clients make well-informed decisions about the risks and benefits of assisted human reproduction, and genetic testing.[42]

## CRITICAL THINKING

*What assessment tool would you use to gather information about those genetic factors considered important for health promotion?*

Bottorff et al. claim that the use of modern technologies is introducing a new kind of health care that focuses on the role of genetic factors in common adult-onset hereditary diseases, including cancer and heart disease. They synthesize the literature on genetic nursing roles to provide a foundation for Canadian nursing leaders as they take on the challenge of nursing in the genomic era. The findings of their literature review indicate a consensus that genetics and genomes are, in fact, important in nursing, and that genetics and genomes will soon become increasingly important in all areas of nursing practice.[43]

Recently, a Canadian planning forum was called to begin the identification of opportunities, priorities, and strategies to support the incorporation of genetics and genomics in the practice of nursing. Five recommendations were developed:

1. Identify and define genetic competencies to guide nursing practice and education
2. Heighten awareness about the relevance of genetics to nursing
3. Convey the integration of genetics into nursing education programs as a national priority
4. Heighten the capacity of nurse researchers to focus on topics related to genetics
5. Develop a national strategy to lobby for and support the development of genetic roles in Canada

The strategies attached to each recommendation are published in the Bottorff report. This initial work provides valuable direction for continuing the discussion on the future of genetics and genomics in nursing practice in Canada.[44]

## Biochemical Factors

Research on the relationship between biochemical factors and behaviour involves the areas of neurochemistry and hormones.

*Neurochemistry* is implicated in some behavioural development. The amount of biogenic amines, especially the **neurotransmitters**, *chemicals involved in the transfer or modulation of nerve impulses from one cell to another*, seems to be related to mood. Acetylcholine, norepinephrine, dopamine, serotonin, and gamma-aminobutyric acid (GABA) are important neurotransmitters in the brain. They are involved in such emotional states as arousal, fear, rage, pleasure, motivation, exhilaration, sleep, and wakefulness.[45] These emotional states, in turn, affect the reactions of others—especially parents of the child who displays the arousal condition. The child's moods may even affect the parents' subsequent childrearing plans.

*Hormonal factors* are based on changes in the endocrine system during stress, or on endocrine system disorders. Hormonal factors may contribute to certain physiologically based behaviours. Thyroid dysfunction, such as hypothyroidism, results from suboptimal levels of thyroid hormone.

The most common form is autoimmune thyroiditis, in which the immune system attacks the thyroid gland. Meanwhile, the second most prevalent endocrine disorder, after diabetes mellitus, is hyperthyroidism. Graves' disease, the most common type of hyperthyroidism, results from an excessive output of thyroid hormones caused by abnormal stimulation of the thyroid gland by circulating immunoglobulins. Clients with well-developed hyperthyroidism manifest a presenting symptom of nervousness. They are often emotionally hyperexcitable, irritable, and apprehensive.[46] As a matter of interest, between 1970 and 1996, Liu, Semenciw, Ugnat, and Mao examined time trends in thyroid cancer cases in Canada. They considered the following variables: age, time period, and birth cohort. Their findings indicated that increases in thyroid cancer incidence in Canada may be associated with more intensive diagnostic activities, and with changes in radiation exposure in childhood and adolescence. In addition, temporal changes in reproductive factors among young women may explain some of the gender differences observed.[47]

The hormone estrogen appears to play a highly relevant role in maintaining, and possibly improving, memory in encoding, storing, and retrieving data. It is known that the loss of estrogen after menopause is related to memory loss, and that this loss may be a factor in the increased risk of Alzheimer's disease.[48]

If the biochemical factors fluctuate too far from their set point values, the homeostatic balance of the body is threatened and various manifestations are exhibited by the client.

## Neurophysiologic Factors

*Neurophysiologic factors* mediate all physiologic processes and behaviour via the nervous system. However, neurophysiologic factors in behaviour and personality development are inconclusive. Some specific motor and speech functions and various sensations in different body parts can be traced to specific brain areas.

**Localization of brain function** means that *certain areas of the brain are more concerned with one kind of function than another*. It does not imply that a specific function is mediated by only one brain region. Specific brain function requires the integrated action of neurons located in many different brain regions.

The cerebrum, the largest and uppermost division of the brain, consists of the right and left cerebral hemispheres. The surface of the cerebrum, called the cerebral cortex, consists of grey matter 2 to 4 millimetres deep. Fissures divide each cerebral hemisphere into five lobes. Four of the lobes are named for the bones that lie over them: frontal lobe, temporal lobe, parietal lobe, and occipital lobe. The fifth lobe, the insula, lies hidden from view in the lateral fissure.[49]

Various areas of the cerebral cortex are necessary for normal functioning of the somatic, or general, senses as well as the special senses. The somatic senses include the sensations of touch, pressure, temperature, and body position. The special senses include vision, hearing, and other types of perception that require complex sensory organs such as the eye and ear. Mechanisms that control voluntary movements are complex and imperfectly understood. However, for normal movements to take place, many parts of the nervous system, including certain areas of the cerebral cortex, must function together systematically.

*The integrative functions of the cortex* consist of all events that take place in the cerebrum between the reception of sensory impulses and the sending out of motor impulses. Integrative functions include consciousness and mental activities of all kinds, such as the use of language, emotions, and memory.[50]

The limbic system is the seat of emotion and is involved in affective and cognitive function and motivation, feelings, and behavioural homeostasis.[51] However, to bring about the normal expression of emotions, part of the cerebral cortex, other than the limbic system, must function.[52]

Scientists have found severe depletion of key cells in the brains of people who died with depressive illness. A study of the brain tissue of seven people with depression, or manic depression, showed that 40 to 90 percent of glial cells in the anterior cingulate in the prefrontal cortex were gone! Glial cells support other cells and provide growth factors and nutrients to neurons. The brains of people who were not depressed did not show such depletion. Studies have shown that when reduced blood flow exists in this region of depressive or manic depressive patients, the condition does not go away with treatment.[53]

Children are born, apparently, with a predisposition to be outgoing or quiet. It is believed that there may be a chemical predisposition to seeking danger or high risk. Yet neurophysiology does not supply all of the answers. A supportive environment may cause further development of certain neurophysiologic rudiments, and even promote additional development of the desired neurophysiologic processes. Thus, environment helps to produce a well-adjusted child. A hostile home environment, especially in early life, usually produces the opposite result.

## Immunologic Factors

The *immune system* functions to protect the body against disease. It recognizes and distinguishes from the body's own tissue foreign substances such as bacteria, toxins, and cancer. Both immune suppression and stimulation are necessary at different times to maintain health. Sometimes, the system responds excessively and destroys normal tissues.

The operation of the immune system is closely interrelated with the workings of the central nervous system, endocrine system, perceptions, and behaviour.

A chronic inflammatory autoimmune collagen disease, resulting from disturbed immune regulation that causes the exaggerated production of autoantibodies, is called systemic lupus erythematosus (SLE).[54] In Manitoba, Peschken and Esdaile conducted the first study to examine the prevalence, disease course, and survival of patients with SLE. They studied a population of 120 000 North American Indians (NAI) and contrasted the results to those found in the non-Indian population. The researchers concluded that the prevalence of the disease was increased twofold in the NAI population. Further, NAI patients had higher SLE Disease Activity Index (SLEDAI) scores at the time of diagnosis. The NAI patients exhibited more frequent vasculitis and renal involvement. They also required more treatment later in the disease trajectory, accumulated more damage following diagnosis, and had increased fatality.[55]

A number of disorders can cause serious, often life-threatening, alterations within the body's immune system. One disorder that profoundly increases the anxiety level within the individual, family, and community is human immunodeficiency virus (HIV), and the subsequent development of acquired immunodeficiency syndrome (AIDS).[56] Canadians are at the forefront of the response to HIV/AIDS, and they continue to expand their involvement through collaborative initiatives at the local, regional, national, and international levels.[57]

---

### CRITICAL THINKING

*What initiatives are being taken in your province/territory to combat HIV/AIDS?*

---

The field of psychoneuroimmunology has shown the connections between stress in the environment and physical and emotional health. Certain mechanisms, not yet fully understood, produce greater physical health when emotional well-being abounds. The stress of rapid or unexpected change can negatively affect health.

## Maturational Factors

The maturational view emphasizes the emergence of developmental patterns of organic systems, physical structures, and motor capabilities that fall under the influence of genetic and maturational forces. Because of an inherent predisposition of the neurological, hormonal, and skeletal-muscular systems to develop spontaneously, *physiologic and motor development occurs in an inevitable and sequential pattern in children throughout the world.* The growth of the nervous

## How People with HIV/AIDS Manage and Assess Their Use of Complementary Therapies: A Quantitative Analysis

The results of this study provide a qualitative analysis of the practical concerns that people with HIV/AIDS have with regard to their use of complementary therapies. The authors cite studies that have identified therapies and activities most often used by people with HIV/AIDS: aerobic exercise, prayer, massage, needle acupuncture, meditation, support groups, visual imagery, breathing exercises, spiritual activities, and non-aerobic exercise. In-depth, semi-structured interviews were conducted with a diverse group of 46 people with HIV/AIDS. An inductive grounded approach was used to collect and analyze the data. There were five central concerns: (1) selecting which therapies to use; (2) judging which therapies work; (3) combining Western medicine with complementary therapies; (4) assessing the safety of complementary therapies; and (5) dealing with barriers to the use of complementary therapies. A better understanding of the practical dimensions of complementary therapy use highlights the treatment and care issues that people with HIV/AIDS face. This understanding also offers insights into the role that nurses might play in addressing some of the issues.

### Nursing Implications

1. Health care professionals can represent an important source of information, but typically respondents drew on other resources.

2. Many health care professionals with whom clients have contact do not seem to posses enough knowledge about, or interest in, complementary therapies to provide them with much advice.

3. Nurses can play an important role in assisting those people with HIV/AIDS who wish to take a complementary approach to health care.

   a. Nurses can inform themselves about the dominant complementary approaches, and they can encourage other health care providers to do so as well.

   b. Nurses can play a particularly supportive role with patients and physicians alike in encouraging a more open dialogue with regard to the broad range of health care approaches that people with HIV may be employing.

   c. Nurses can play an important role in linking patients to community supports that will help to involve them in actively making informed decisions about possible strategies for managing their health and in overcoming barriers to accessing the care they desire.

4. Health care professionals, and nurses in particular, can play a critical role as a resource and support person for people with HIV/AIDS, who are dealing with the practical challenges of integrating different types of health care options, both complementary therapies and Western medical treatments.

Source: Gillett, J., D. Pawluch, and R. Cain, How People with HIV/AIDS Manage and Assess Their Use of Complementary Therapies: A Qualitative Analysis, *Journal of the Association of Nurses in AIDS Care, 13*(2) (2000), 17–27.

---

system is critical in this maturation, unless the normal process is inhibited by severe environmental, physiologic, or emotional deprivation.[58]

Sex differences may be inherent for some characteristics. For example, women generally have a greater response to the intuitive and analytic side of the brain, whereas men have a greater response to the spatial side of the brain. Yet many characteristics are the result of sociocultural influences; women from certain cultures may demonstrate characteristics common to men in other cultures. Sex differences are described in Chapters 10 to 14.

## ECOLOGIC THEORIES

**Ecology** is the *science that is concerned with the community and the total setting in which life and behaviour occur.* A basic ecologic principle is that both the continuity and the survival of a person depend on a deliberate balance of factors influencing the interactions between the family, or person, and the environment.

*Family* is dependent on the resources and groups in the community to survive and continue its own development and to nurture adequately the development of offspring. Climate, terrain, and natural resources affect family lifestyles and the development and behaviour of individual family members. The neighbourhood may adversely affect development, especially if the person is reared in a family that lives in a deteriorating neighbourhood or in an area with poor schools, inadequate housing, and a high crime rate. Excessively crowded housing can create stresses within the family that contribute to sleep deprivation, bickering, incest, or other abuse. These stresses, in turn, affect developmental progress in all spheres of the person. Job loss, caused by a changing community and the resultant financial problems, may affect health care practices and nutrition and, in turn, physical growth and emotional security.[59]

*Urbanization*, rapid social changes, social stressors, discrimination, unemployment, poor housing, inadequate diet and health care, poverty, feelings of **anomie** (*not being part of society*), and negative self-image all contribute to stress and developmental difficulties in the vulnerable, immature person, or in a normal person who is without an adequate support system.[60]

*Sociologic variables*, including family socioeconomic level and position in the community, and the prestige related to birth, race, age, cultural ties, and power roles, affect development, behaviour, and adaptation of the person and family. Certain behaviours can be expected from a person because of their age, sex, race, religion, or occupation. The individual may experience role conflicts and developmental problems when discrepancies occur between norms and values and the demands of age, sex, occupation, or religion.[61]

*Cultures* vary in their definitions of normal and abnormal behaviour so that cross-cultural comparisons of developmental norms are difficult. Theorists in each culture describe their research findings about normal child or adult characteristics and behaviours based on the norms of their culture and on their cultural bias. For example, a research study was conducted to explore arthritis management strategies among Chinese immigrants in Calgary. They want to assess the factors that affected these arthritis management strategies. The findings illustrated that disease management strategies among Chinese immigrants are not only affected by the disease itself, but also by personal and cultural strategies. In fact, these factors suggest helpful guidelines to providing culturally sensitive care. These suggestions, in turn, can lead to greater satisfaction and well-being for Chinese immigrants with arthritis.[62]

## CRITICAL THINKING

*What question might you ask an Inuit client about his or her health beliefs and practices?*

*Geographic moves* create the need for many adjustments for the person as he or she attempts to meet norms of the new community. Developmental problems and dysfunctional behaviour may occur among those who migrate.[63] Persons who move, often as children, may never form "chumships" or close relationships later in adulthood. However, the mobile family or individual do learn coping skills that help them adjust to new, unfamiliar, or stressful situations.

DeWit explored the relationship between the number of geographic moves before the age of 16 and the timing of onset of drug use, and the subsequent progression to drug-related problems. The data were obtained from 3700 young adults aged 18 to 35 participating in the 1990–1991 Ontario Mental Health Supplement, a large random-probability survey of the residents in Ontario. The significant results indicated positive relationships between moving and the early initiation of illicit drugs, such as marijuana, hallucinogens, and crack/cocaine, and the illicit use of prescribed drugs. The relationship between moving and measures of alcohol use/problems (onset of first drink, onset of any alcohol-related problems) were either weak or nonsignificant. However, important sex differences were found. It was also established that progression occurred primarily among males. DeWit argues that further research is desperately needed: (1) to discover why drug use appears to be a more common response to relocation among boys, and (2) to test for possible mediating factors linking relocation with the onset of drug use, and to determine moderating influences.[64]

## CRITICAL THINKING

*After reading about the study conducted by DeWit,[65] what are your thoughts on why drug use appears to be a more common response to relocation among boys than among girls?*

One view of an individual's psychological problems is that they are the result of some personal circumstances, such as the deficient achievement of developmental tasks, immaturity, character defect, or maladjustment. An alternate approach is to view the individual problems as stemming from social causes. The broad economic, political, cultural, and social patterns of our society, and particular subcultures, can be viewed as determinants of individual developmental responses. In this case, the community is the place to begin making changes if individual dysfunction is to be decreased.[66]

Chapters 1 through 4 discuss cultural, environmental, religious, spiritual, and family variables, and Chapters 7 through 14 present the interrelationship of these variables on the person.

## SYSTEMS THEORY

First proposed by von Bertalanffy,[67] general systems theory presents a comprehensive, holistic, and interdisciplinary view. This theory proposes that the family, individual, various social groups, and cultures are all systems. Nothing is determined by a single cause, nor explained by a single factor. Nothing can be studied as a lone entity, be it the environment; various sociocultural components; political-legal, religious, educational, and other social institutions or organizations; the person, family, group, or community; or the health care delivery organization. All are believed to have interrelating parts, and all components interact with each other.[68] An interconnectedness, or interrelationship, exists at and between every system level. A complementarity exists among the parts of a system.

A **system** is an *assemblage, unit, or organism of interrelated, interdependent parts, persons, or objects that are united by some form or order into a recognizable unit. And these independent parts, persons and objects are in equilibrium.*[69]

The notion of **synergy** means that *the whole is greater than the sum of the parts or units.* Within a system, **subsystems** exist as *smaller units within the whole.* Examples include spouses and children in the family, or the mental health clinic as a subsystem within the larger health care centre. **Suprasystems** refer to *the large environment or community.* All systems need energy and activity to maintain self. Input of energy allows **differentiation**, *the tendency for the system to advance or mature to a higher level of complexity and organization.*[70]

The elements or components that are common to all systems are listed in Table 5-2. A given entity is not a system unless these characteristics are present.[71]

People satisfy their needs within social systems. The **social system** is a *group of people joined co-operatively to achieve common goals by using an organized set of practices to regulate behaviour.*[72] The person can occupy various positions and has defined roles in the social system. The person's development is shaped by the system. In turn, people create and change social systems. Active social systems include the family, church, and economic systems, as well as politico-legal and educational institutions and health care agencies.

All living organisms comprise an open social system. Change occurs constantly within, and between, the system and other systems. An **open system** is *characterized by the ability to exchange energy, matter, and information with the environment to evolve into higher levels of heterogeneity, organization, order, and development.*[73] Physically, there is a *hierarchy of components*, such as cells and organ systems. Emotionally, there are levels of needs and feelings. Cognitively, a person has memories, knowledge, and cognitive strategies. Socially, the person is in a relative rank in a hierarchy of prestige roles, such as boss, worker, adult, or child. Spiritually, the person may orient his or her life in terms of an inner awareness.[74] The *boundaries or environment*, such as one's skin, the limits set by others, social status, home, and community, influence the person's *needs* and *goal achievement.* To remain healthy, the person must be able to *communicate* and must have *feedback.* A constant *exchange of energy and information* must exist with the surrounding specified environment if the system is to be open, useful, and creative. If this *information or energy exchange does not occur*, the system becomes a **closed system** and ineffective. In this case, disorganization, disease, and sometimes death result.

Each person and family you care for is a system interacting with other systems in the community. Development and function are greatly affected by the interdependence and interrelationships of each component part and by all other surrounding systems. Best and his associates claim that although there is general agreement about the complex interplay among individual-, family-, organizational-, and community-level factors, as they affect health outcomes, a gap exists between health promotion research and practice. They suggest a few critical steps to close this gap: (1) investing in networks that promote, support, and sustain ongoing discussion and the sharing of experience; (2) finding common ground in an approach to community partnering; and (3) gaining consensus on the proposed integrating framework.[75]

Family systems theory has been derived from general systems theory. Relationships that exist between family members constitute a system, and a reaction in one family member is followed by a predictable reaction in others. *The smallest stable relationship system within a family or social system is the* **three-person system** *or* **triangle**. When a two-person relationship is unstable and anxiety increases, that relationship becomes uncomfortable. When the level of intensity reaches a certain level, the twosome involves a vulnerable third person. Often the issue is an emotional one. With the involvement of the third person, the level of anxiety decreases as it shifts from one to the other of the three relationships in the triangle. The triangle becomes more flexible and stable than that of the twosome. Further, the threesome has a higher tolerance of anxiety, and it is capable of handling more of life's stresses. The same emotional patterns are then repeated, so that family members develop fixed, often unchanging, roles in relation to each other.[76]

## CRITICAL THINKING

**What family situation can you think of whereby a twosome has triangulated someone new into the emotional issue at hand?**

## Bronfenbrenner Bioecological Systems Theory

Bronfenbrenner has formulated **bioecologic systems theory** to *describe how the person's development is influenced in terms of relationships between individuals and their environment or contexts*, as follows:[77]

1. **Microsystems.** *Face-to-face physical and social situations that directly affect the person*, such as family, schoolroom, workplace, church, peers, and health services.

2. **Mesosystems.** *Connections and relationships among the person's microsystems.*

3. **Exosystems.** *Settings or situations that indirectly influence the person*, such as the extended family, friends of the

## Table 5-2 Elements and Characteristics of a System

| Element | Definition/Example |
|---|---|
| Parts | *The system's components that are interdependent units.* None can operate without the others. Change in one part affects the entire unit.<br><br>The person as a whole system is composed of physical, emotional, mental, spiritual, cultural, and social aspects. Physically, he or she is composed of the body systems—neurological, cardiovascular, and so on. The health agency is one part of the health care system, and it, in turn, is composed of parts: physical plant, employees, clients, and departments that provide services. |
| Attributes | *Characteristics of the parts* such as temperament, roles, education, age, or health of the person or family members. |
| Information/communication | *Sending of messages and feedback, the exchange of energy*, which varies with the system but is essential to achieve goals. A system has input and output with the environment. |
| Feedback | *Monitoring of internal and external responses to behaviour* (output) that allows the system to readjust or change if needed. |
| Equilibrium | *Steady state or state of balance that is maintained through adaptive, dynamic, self-regulating processes*, and information input, transformation, output, and feedback. |
| Boundary | *A barrier or area of demarcation that limits or keeps a system distinct from its environment and within which information is exchanged.*<br><br>The skin of the person, home of the family, or walls of the health agency: each constitutes a boundary. The boundary is not always rigid. Relatives outside the home are part of the family. The boundary may be an imaginary line, such as the feeling that comes from belonging to a certain racial or ethnic group. |
| Organization | The *formal or informal arrangement of parts to form a whole entity so that the organism or institution has a working order that leads to an established hierarchy, rules, or customs.*<br><br>The person is organized into a physical structure, basic needs, cognitive stages, and the achievement of developmental tasks. Hierarchy in the family or health agency provides organization that is based on power (ability to control others) and responsibility. The specialization of medical practice is also a way of organizing care. Interdisciplinary teams are becoming important whereby the nurse, pharmacist, doctor, and physiotherapist can initiate health promotion strategies needed by the client and family.[78] Organization in an institution is also maintained by norms, roles, and customs that each member must follow. |
| Goals | *Purposes of, or reasons for, the system to exist.* Goals may be *long term or short term.* Goals include survival, development, and socialization of the individual member of the family or contributions to society. |
| Environment | The *social and physical world outside the system, boundaries, or the community in which the system exists.* The environment of the person or family may be a tribal enclave, farm, small town and surrounding area, or an urban neighbourhood and surrounding city. Environment of a health care system may be the city in which the agency is located, or it may extend to other regions for a major urban medical centre. |
| Evolutionary processes | *Changes within the person and the environment, proceeding from simple to complex*, occur at all times, in all systems. The person undergoes changes in physical, psychological, and social growth throughout the lifespan, within certain parameters. |

family, neighbours, spouse's workplace, mass media, legal services, the local government, and community agencies and organizations.

4. **Macrosystems.** *Sociocultural values, beliefs, and policies that provide a framework for organizing our lives and indirectly affect the person* through the exosystem, mesosystem, and microsystem.[79]

Bronfenbrenner's detailed analysis of the influences of the environment has suggested ways in which the development of children may be optimized. For example, at the level of the exosystem, health promotion strategies can be used by parents to improve their relationships with their children. This enhancement of the parent–child relationship can only occur if the community has parenting classes or groups where parents are able to express their concerns and learn from one another ways in which they can elicit more favourable reactions from their children.[80]

---

**CRITICAL THINKING**

*Explain how microsystems are dynamic contexts for the development of children.*

---

## PSYCHOLOGICAL THEORIES

A number of psychological theories have been formulated to explain human development, behaviour, and personality. A theorist who follows one perspective may disagree with another theorist from the same perspective. For example, some behaviourists would disagree with B.F. Skinner on some points. Further, no theorist or group of theorists has all of the answers about human behaviour, development, or learning. Realize that often theorists who sound very different in their theory may be stating basically similar concepts.

## BEHAVIOURAL THEORY
### Overview

**Behaviourists** *adhere to stimulus-response conditioning theories.* This scientific approach to the study of the person generalizes results from animal experiments to people. The **neo-behaviourists**—*contemporary behavioural theorists and the theorists in this school who have changed their ideas*—obtain data for laws of behaviour by observing the human's behavioural response to stimuli. The person is considered in terms of component parts. *The focus is on isolated, small units of behaviour, or parts of behavioural patterns, that are objectively observed and analyzed from the perspective of non-mental, physiologic associations.*

## View of the Human

Behavioural theorists view the living organism as a self-maintaining mechanism. Because the *focus is on physiologic processes and identifiable aspects of the person, subjective, unobservable, unique, and inner aspects of the human are not studied.* There are no concepts that explain self-concept; ideas; emotions such as love, joy, sadness, and anger; the meaning in a situation; memory; understanding; insight; empathy; the person initiating and being an active agency in his or her behalf; or variety in human behaviour. The person is explained by overt behaviour or physiologically, not in abstractions. There are no biases except for past conditioning. The learner or the client is considered deficient, which results in *activity or behaviour* called **learning**. Rest or cessation of behaviour follows reward.[81]

## View of Education and Therapy

The goals of education and treatment are to (1) control the person's behaviour; (2) help the person become more efficient and realistic, as defined by others in the environment; (3) move toward a goal set by external standards; and (4) create learning by forming bonds, connections, or associations. Responses that are appropriate are rewarded and therefore are stamped in to form habits.[82]

The teacher, health care provider, or therapist is at the centre of, and in control of, the educational process. The learner or client is passive. Programmed or computerized instruction is considered efficient education, with the teacher functioning as a reinforcer to help the learner achieve behavioural objectives.

Behavioural theorists propose that maladaptive behaviours are reinforced and learned. A treatment approach is to identify factors in the environment, or in prior learning, that must be modified to change the problem behaviour.

## Behavioural Theorists

**Early Theorists** Ivan Pavlov laid the foundations for the behavioural school. He was a Russian physiologist and pharmacologist of the mid-19th century who wrote about psychic processes during his study of salivation and flow of digestive juices in dogs. His experiments established **classical conditioning**: *An unconditioned, or new, stimulus is presented with a stimulus that is already known just before the response to the conditioned, familiar stimulus. The organism learns to respond to a new stimulus in the same way it responded to a familiar stimulus.* Associations are shifted from one stimulus to another, with the same response being made to the substituted stimulus.[83]

John B. Watson is considered the founder of **behaviourism**. His experiments showed that fears and phobias could result from classical conditioning in childhood and could, in turn, be unlearned in adulthood.[84]

Some *present-day relaxation methods used by health care providers are based on classical conditioning*. The client is trained to respond to a therapist's direction by relaxing a muscle group; music is then played while the therapist gives directions for relaxing. Later, the person is able to respond automatically by relaxing when music plays.[85] Classical conditioning is also used in the Lamaze preparation for childbirth, and in other kinds of childbirth education classes.

**Skinner: Operant Conditioning Theory** Skinner is well known for his operant conditioning theory, which used animal studies and built on the theories of Watson and Thorndike. According to Skinner, **behaviour** is an *overt response that is externally caused and is controlled primarily by its consequences*. The environmental stimuli determine how a person alters behaviour and responds to people or objects in the environment. Feelings or emotions are the accompaniments or result, not the cause, of behaviour. Innate or hereditary reflexes activate the internal glands and smooth muscles, but reflexive behaviour accounts for little of human behaviour.[86]

**Learning** is a *change in the form or probability of response as a result of conditioning*. **Operant conditioning** is the *learning process whereby a response (operant) is shaped and is made more probable or frequent by reinforcement*. **Transfer** is an *increased probability of response in the future*. A set of acts are called *operant responses* because they operate on the environment and generate consequences. The important stimulus is the one immediately following the response, not the one preceding it.

Operant conditioning occurs in most everyday activities, according to Skinner. People constantly cause others to modify their behaviour by reinforcing certain behaviour and ignoring other behaviour. During development, people learn to balance, walk, talk, play games, and handle instruments and tools because they are reinforced after performing a set of motions, thereby increasing the repetition of these motions. Social and ethical behaviours are learned as people are reinforced to continue them through their reinforcing of others for the same behaviours. Operant reinforcement improves the efficiency of behaviour, whether the behaviour is appropriate or inappropriate. Any attention, even if negative, reinforces the response to a stimulus.[87]

---

**CRITICAL THINKING**

*In what ways do you see operant conditioning used in your practice?*

---

**Positive reinforcement** occurs when the *presence of a stimulus* increases the probability that the response will reoccur. **Negative reinforcement** occurs when the *withdrawal of a stimulus strengthens the tendency to behave in a certain way*. A positive reinforcer can be food, water, a smile, or a pleasant, friendly interchange with another person. A negative reinforcer consists of removing noxious stimuli. Skinner's theory emphasizes positive reinforcement.[88] He rejected the use of negative reinforcement or aversive control, contending that this merely produces escape or avoidance behaviour. A **reinforcement schedule** is a *pattern of rewarding behaviour at fixed time intervals, with a fixed number of responses between reinforcements*. Reinforcement does not strengthen a specific response, but rather it tends to strengthen a general tendency to make the response, or a class of responses, in the future. Thus trial-and-error learning does not exist.[89]

**Punishment** *consists of presenting a negative stimulus or removing a positive one*. Experiments show that punishment does not reduce a tendency to respond. Apparently, reward strengthens behaviour because the response is stamped in. Punishment does not weaken behaviour, however, because the response cannot be stamped out. **Extinction**, *letting a behavioural response die by not reinforcing it*, is preferred instead of punishment for breaking habits. Extinction is a slower process than reinforcement in modifying behaviour.[90] Operant reinforcement covers most human behaviour. Imitative behaviour is an example. It arises over time because of discriminative reinforcement. A person waves to someone because of the reinforcement, not because of the stimulus of the other person's hand waving. Differentiation of responses improves motor skills. The person selects a motion because it was reinforced. In this process, reinforcement must be immediate.

**Behaviour modification** is the *deliberate application of learning theory and conditioning, thereby structuring different social environments to teach alternate behaviours and to help the person gain control over behaviour and environment*. **Shaping** (*the gradual modification of behaviour by breaking complex behaviour into small steps and reinforcing each small step that is a closer approximation to the final desired behaviour*) also achieves behavioural change.[91]

Recently, Garry Martin and Joseph Pear of the University of Manitoba wrote an authoritative and widely used text, *Behavior Modification: What It is and How to Do It*.[92] This text, with highly accessible format and hands-on experience, relates principles to applications in everyday situations. These experiences include clinical, home, school, and work settings. In this text, which is widely used in both Canada and the U.S., Martin and Pear explain that shaping is the development of a new behaviour by the successive reinforcement of closer approximations and the extinguishing of preceding approximations of the behaviour. They explain four factors that influence the effectiveness of shaping. In one interesting example, we meet Frank, who retired early at 55 and, as an admitted "couch potato," decided on the advice of his doctor to begin a regular exercise program. Frank, who had never been active in his life, decided he would jog one kilometre daily. After a couple of attempts, he became discouraged and returned to his couch-potato routine. He had expected too much, but a friendly neighbour suggested he use shaping. The factors influencing shaping, according to Martin and Pear, are as follows:

1. *Specify the final desired behaviour.* In Frank's case, the final desired behaviour was jogging one kilometre each day. Because this distance might have been too great for Frank to accomplish successfully, a shorter, more easily attainable distance would be better to select at the outset.

2. *Choose a starting behaviour.* Frank's neighbour encourages him to lace on his runners and walk around the outside of his house each day, as a start. On successful completion of this starting behaviour, the neighbour praises Frank for his good effort. He arranges to meet Frank the next day to do it again as a step toward the half-kilometre jog objective which, with the neighbour's guidance, Frank selected. It is important that, throughout the shaping steps, the activity and the successive approximations be enjoyable and attainable.

3. *Choose the shaping steps.* Frank's neighbour assists Frank in outlining the behaviours to approximate the final behaviour—jogging half a kilometre per day. Behaviours such as walking around the outside of the house, followed by walking around the block, and so forth, constitute successive approximations to the desired behaviour. So, when Frank walks around the house several times, the neighbour reinforces that approximation. Then, when Frank has progressed to walking around the block several times, the neighbour again reinforces that approximation. The shaping procedure continues while Frank progresses through the step of jogging, say, 10 strides followed by walking 20 steps. A next step might be that of jogging 100 strides followed by walking 100 steps, until he reaches the desired behaviour (also referred to as the terminal behaviour). The final desired behaviour is jogging half a kilometre each day.

In behaviour modification, the behaviour first must be reinforced each time it occurs. Once the desired response has been established and maintained by a continuous reinforcement schedule (i.e., each time the desired response is seen, it is reinforced), the next step is to switch to an **intermittent schedule of reinforcement**, *whereupon reinforcement is contingent on increasingly multiple emissions of*

## NARRATIVE VIGNETTE
# Shaping

You are trying to help a college friend, Judy, to lose 5 kg. Judy tells you that she eats a great number of chocolates each day, and that she is considering the low-carbohydrate diets she has read about in magazines. You recall, however, that in your psychology class the concept of behaviour modification seemed appealing to you, and that eating fruits instead of chocolates might be good for Judy. Together, you and Judy decide that through the process of shaping, she will seek to eat more fruits (and consequently lose 5 kg).

**Questions**

1. What is Judy's final desired behaviour?

2. What might be a starting behaviour for Judy?

3. List the shaping steps through which Judy might progress toward her desired behaviour.

*the desired behaviour.* After this, occasional reinforcement will keep the desired behaviour going. Behaviour that has been maintained by an intermittent schedule of reinforcement or partial reinforcement is highly resistant to extinction.[93]

Sometimes aversive methods (e.g., seclusion) are used to change behaviour. The purpose is not punishment but time out, as in allowing a tantrum to run its course, without accidental reinforcement and without triggering similar behaviour in other people. Operant techniques include the following:

- **Time out.** *Seclusion for examination of behaviours*
- **Assertion training.** *Using role playing, modelling, feedback, and social reinforcers to change communication patterns*
- **Token economies.** *Rewards or payments for behaviour improvement that are applied to an entire unit of patients*
- **Social skills training.** *Rehearsal of appropriate social behaviours*

Operant conditioning is used in many situations, including to:

- Replace undesirable behaviours of normal or developmentally disabled children
- Reduce abnormal or self-destructive behaviour
- Train parents, teachers, probation officers, and nurses to be more efficient in their roles
- Reduce specific maladaptive behaviours such as stuttering, tics, poor hygiene, and messy eating habits
- Control physical symptoms through biofeedback

Figure 5-1 illustrates how development is viewed by learning theorists. Table 5-3 lists key terms and definitions, with examples.

**Figure 5-1**

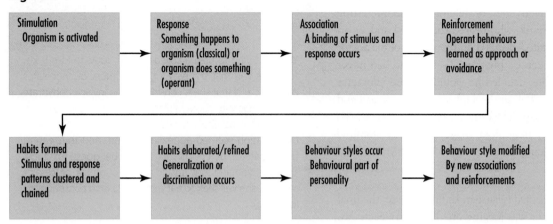

Development as viewed by learning theorists. Stimuli from inside or outside the organism are reinforced (positively or negatively) and on a particular schedule that determines their force and strength. Habits develop. The response processes of generalization and discrimination elaborate these habits and modify them. Effective habits are equated with effective development. This force rarely speaks about the whole organism but rather about situationally determined behaviours.

**Table 5-3** Selected Terminology Pertaining to Application of Behavioural Theory

| Term | Definition | Example |
|---|---|---|
| **Respondent conditioning** | *Pairing a neutral stimulus with a nonneutral stimulus until the person learns to respond to the neutral stimulus as to the nonneutral stimulus* | Baby learns to "love" a sibling (nonneutral stimulus) because the sibling shakes a rattle and offers other toys (neutral stimulus) while cooing, touching, and smiling at baby. |
| **Operant conditioning** | *Rewarding or punishing a response until the person learns to repeat or avoid that response in anticipation of positive or negative consequences* | Preschooler returns toys to the toy box at the end of the day because he remembers the consequences: doing so is followed by ten minutes of time with the parent; failure to do so results in sitting alone in his room for five minutes. |
| **Positive reinforcement** | *Rewarding desired behaviour to maintain that behaviour* | Parent buys a desired item for the child who earns an A in a course. |
| **Negative reinforcement** | *Removing an aversive stimulus in response to behaviour, which maintains that behaviour* | Parent allows the child to forgo household tasks if he complains when asked to do them, yet the child receives an allowance weekly. |
| **Extinction** | *Suppressing behaviour by removing reinforcers that are maintaining the behaviour* | Parent does not give the child who complains about doing household tasks the allowance at the end of the week and explains why. |
| **Punishment** | *Suppressing an undesirable behaviour by using an aversive stimulus in response to the person's behaviour* | Parent spanks the child for running into the street. |
| **Time-out** | *Suppressing maladaptive behaviour by removing the subject to a neutral environment, void of reinforcements when the behaviour is manifested* | Parent makes the four-year-old child sit facing a corner for five minutes after hitting a sibling. |

*(continued)*

**Table 5-3** (continued)

| Term | Definition | Example |
|---|---|---|
| Generalization | *Transferring a conditioned response from the conditional stimulus to another stimulus* | Child who is bitten by a dog fears all animals. |
| Systematic desensitization | *Pairing an anxiety-causing stimulus with an induced state of relaxation to extinguish fearful behaviour* | Parent remains with the child who has been bitten by a dog when the child is in the vicinity of animals, gradually helps the child to relax, and eventually to pet a very friendly dog. |
| Discrimination | *Responding only to a specific stimulus* | Toddler learns via punishing encounters with mother that playing in water in the bathtub is acceptable and playing in the water in the toilet is not. |
| Escape behaviour | *Initiating a response to escape an unpleasant or aversive stimulus* | Adolescent brings the parents a gift when returning late from a weekend with a friend. |
| Avoidance learning | *Arranging responses to avoid exposure to an aversive stimulus* | Adolescent verbally refuses the offer and walks away from the person offering a marijuana joint after a bad experience with it. |
| Chaining | *Developing complex behaviour by focusing on the individual components of the behaviour; this is done in a backward fashion* | Schoolchild learns to clean his room with the parent instructing and assisting with each step of the task and then verbally repeating in reverse order the steps after the task is finished. |
| Shaping | *Reinforcing successive approximations or small units of a desired response until that behaviour is gradually achieved* | Parent teaches the child to clean his room by praising him for doing every step of the process—vacuuming the rug, dusting each piece of furniture, and so on. |
| Fading | *Gradually removing the reinforcement given to the person* | Parent gives less and less verbal approval to the schoolchild for doing assigned household tasks. |
| Satiation | *Providing excessive amount of reinforcer, which causes loss of effectiveness* | Chocolate candy is reward for behaviour. Child is given extra candy and loses desire for candy and for behaviour change. |
| Token | *Object that serves as general reinforcer; may be exchanged for other reinforcers* | Client earns tokens for helpful behaviour on unit, exchanges 10 tokens for trip to Science Museum. |
| Contingency | *Relationship between behaviour to be changed and activities or consequences following behaviour* | Condition a desired response or suppress maladaptive response by drawing up contract indicating rewards and punishments contingent on or related to responses in the contract. |

# PSYCHOANALYTICAL AND NEO-ANALYTICAL THEORIES

Knowledge of genetics, developmental levels, and effects of internal stimuli, unconscious processes, social relationships, and environmental context are all used to understand, assess, and treat the person.

The **psychoanalytic theory**, or perspective, is divided into two groups: psychoanalytic and neo-analytic. The writings of Freud, Sullivan, and Erikson are discussed in this chapter. They are known as "*stage theorists*" because they emphasize that people develop in sequential stages. The **neo-analytic theorists** reinterpreted Freud's psychoanalytic theory in formulating their theories. Erikson, in his psychosocial theory, expanded understanding of normal developmental stages and tasks throughout the lifespan, emphasized sociocultural influences to a greater degree, and saw the person as capable of emotional growth throughout life.

## Overview

Psychoanalytic theorists include those who adhere to psychoanalytic and neo-analytic theories. These theorists generally believe *data for study about the person come from within the developing person, observation of interpersonal relationships, and knowledge of the impact on the person of social units, norms, and laws. Data from unconscious processes, early development, and the past are used to understand present behaviour and goal direction.* Psychoanalytic theorists share the assumption that adult personality and ongoing issues are formed primarily by experiences during early childhood.[94]

## View of the Human

Reality is external and interpersonal—what people agree on. The person is a social organism with a developmental past on which to build. Each person has a level of readiness that influences or contributes to their learning and behaviour. *The person has maturational and social needs that affect development, learning, and behaviour. He or she seeks social role satisfaction and reacts to social values and symbolic processes.* The person internalizes societal rules to gain approval, can understand cause-and-effect relationships and complex abstract issues, is capable of insight and emotions, and initiates action and makes choices. The goal of behaviour is seen as the reduction of symbolic, or internal, needs or tension.[95]

## View of Education and Therapy

The goal of developmental guidance and discipline is to help the person become an adaptive, effective social being who is aware of, and responsive to, social reality and patterns. The person is expected to learn and follow socially prescribed values, customs, and norms to fit into society. Development, learning, and behaviour are all influenced strongly by the person's developmental level, their personal history, their cognitive processes and intellect, and intrapsychic processes.

The health care provider, teacher, or therapist is the central figure—a social role model who directs the client. Emphasis is on bringing the person, even in the younger years, to understand self and his or her own behaviour. Increased insight promotes development and maturation. If the person is not ready to learn, or change behaviour, the parent, teacher, or another acts as an external motivator or facilitator of readiness to change. Rewards are given through approval, affiliation, and various verbal and nonverbal methods. Learning and self-observed behaviour changes can be self-reinforcing to the person.[96]

## Psychodynamic Perspective

The **psychodynamic perspective** is concerned with the *inner and unconscious processes of the person—drives, needs, motivations, feelings, and conflicts.*[97]

### Freud: Psychoanalytic Theory
Sigmund Freud, a Viennese neurologist, developed psychoanalytic theory, the first psychological theory to include a fully developed explanation of abnormal behaviour. He gave biological factors little emphasis but used the medical model of emphasizing pathology and symptoms.

Freud's *theory of personality* seems complicated because it *incorporates many interlocking factors.* The major components are psychic determination; psychic structures including the id, ego, and superego; primary and secondary process thinking; the conscious–unconscious continuum; libido or psychic energy; behaviour, anxiety, and defence mechanisms; transference; and psychosexual development. Some of Freud's theory is discussed here and referred to in the chapters on childhood. Table 5-4 summarizes these concepts.[98]

**Anxiety** is the *response of tension or dread to perceived or anticipated danger or stress. It is the primary motivation for*

| Table 5-4 Summary of Freud's Theory of Personality | |
|---|---|
| **Psychic determination** | **All behaviour determined by prior thoughts and mental processes** |
| **Psychic structures of the personality** | **Id**—*Unorganized reservoir of psychic energy;* furnishes energy for ego and superego<br>*Consists of instinctual forces, primitive biological drives, and impulses necessary for survival*<br>Operates on **pleasure principle** (*seeking of immediate gratification and avoidance of discomfort*)<br>Discharges **tension** (*increased energy*) through reflex physiologic activity and **primary process thinking** (*image formation, drive-oriented behaviour, free expression of feelings and impulses, inability to distinguish between reality and non-reality, dream-like* state) |

*(continued)*

Table 5-4 (continued)

| Psychic determination | All behaviour determined by prior thoughts and mental processes |
|---|---|
| | **Ego**—*Establishes relations with environment through conscious perception, feeling, action*<br>Controls impulses from id and the demands of the superego<br>Operates on **reality principle** (*external conditions considered and immediate gratification is delayed for future gains that can be realistically achieved*)<br>Controls access of ideas to conscious<br>Appraises environment and reality<br>Uses various mechanisms to help person feel emotionally safe<br>Guides person to acceptable behaviour<br>Directs motor and all cognitive functions<br>Assists with **secondary process thinking** (*delayed or substitute gratification; realistic thoughts; conscious processes; cognitive strategies*)<br>**Superego**—*Represents internalized moral code based on perceived social rules and norms; restrains expression of instinctual drives; prevents disruption of society*<br>Active and concrete in directing person's thoughts, feelings, actions<br>Made up of two systems:<br>**Ego ideal**—*Perfection to which person aspires; corresponds to what parents taught was good*<br>**Conscience**—*Responsible for guilt feelings; corresponds to those things parents taught were bad* |
| Conscious–unconscious continuum | **Conscious**—*All aspects of mental life currently in awareness or easily remembered*<br>**Preconscious**—*Aspects of mental life remembered with help; not currently in awareness*<br>**Unconscious**—*Thoughts, feelings, actions, experiences, dreams not remembered; difficult to bring to awareness; not recognized*<br>Existence inferred from effects on behaviour |
| Instincts (drives) | Basic force in personality and behaviour<br>*Inborn psychological representation or wish of inner somatic source of excitation*<br>Kinds of instincts: self-preservation, preservation of species, life, death; life and death instincts in conflict |
| Libido (sexuality) | *Sexual or psychic energy arising from hidden drives or impulses involved in conflict*<br>Desire for pleasure, sexual gratification<br>Not limited to biology or genital areas; includes capacity for loving another, parental love, and preservation of species |
| Anxiety | *Response to presence of unconscious conflict, tension, or dread; perceived or anticipated danger; and stress—primary motivation for behaviour*<br>Basic source is the unconscious, related to loss of self-image<br>Psychic energy accumulates if anxiety is not expressed; may overwhelm ego controls; panic may result<br>Kinds of anxiety: (1) neurotic—id–ego conflict; (2) realistic—in response to real dangers in world; (3) moral anxiety—id–superego conflict<br>Managed by direct action, coping strategies, or unconscious defence mechanisms |
| Transference | *Phenomenon of investing libido in another object; projection of feelings, thoughts, and wishes onto therapist, who represents significant person from the past (usually the parent); and based on unconscious and repressed material and therefore not realistic or appropriate to the situation* |
| Cathexis | *Energy responsible for behaviour* |

behaviour. If anxiety cannot be managed by direct action or coping strategies, the ego initiates unconscious defences by warding off awareness of the conflict to keep the material unconscious, to lessen discomfort, and to maintain the self-image. Because everyone experiences psychological danger, the use of defence mechanisms clearly is not a special characteristic of maladaptive behaviour. Such mechanisms are used by all people, either singly or in combination, at one time or another, and are considered adaptive.[99] Commonly used ego adaptive (defence) mechanisms are summarized in Table 5-5. They are described throughout the text in relation to the developmental era during which they arise.

## Table 5-5 Ego Adaptive or Defence Mechanisms

| | |
|---|---|
| **Compartmentalization** | *Separation of two incompatible aspects of the psyche from each other to maintain psychological comfort;* behavioural manifestations show the inconsistency. |
| | **Example:** The person who attends church regularly and is overtly religious conducts a business that includes handling stolen goods. |
| **Compensation** | *Overachievement in one area to offset deficiencies, real or imagined, or to overcome failure or frustration in another area.* |
| | **Example:** The student who makes poor grades devotes much time and energy to succeed in music or sports. |
| **Condensation** | *Reacting to a single idea with all of the emotions associated with a group of ideas;* expressing a complex group of ideas with a single word or phrase. |
| | **Example:** The person says the word *crazy* as a shorthand expression for many types of mental illness and for feelings of fear and shame. |
| **Conversion** | *Unconscious conflicts are disguised and expressed symbolically by physical symptoms involving portions of the body, especially the five senses and motor areas. Symptoms are frequently not related to innervations by sensory or motor nerves.* |
| | **Example:** The person is under great pressure on the job; awakens at 6 a.m. and is unable to walk but is unconcerned about the symptom. |
| **Denial** | *Failure to recognize an unacceptable impulse or an undesirable, but clearly obvious thought, fact, behaviour, conflict, or situation, including its consequences or implications.* |
| | **Example:** The alcoholic person believes that he or she has no problem with drinking even though family and work colleagues observe and reflect to the person the classic signs of alcoholism. |
| **Displacement** | *Release or redirection of feelings and impulses on a safe object or person as a substitute for that which aroused the feeling.* |
| | **Example:** The person punches a punching bag after an argument with the boss. |
| **Dissociation** | *Repression or splitting off from awareness of a portion of a personality, or of consciousness;* however, repressed material continues to affect behaviour (compartmentalization). |
| | **Example:** A client discusses a conflict-laden subject and goes into a trance. |
| **Emotional isolation** | *Repression of the emotional component of a situation, although the person is able to remember the thought, memory, or event,* dealing with problems as interesting events that can be rationally explained but have no feelings attached. |
| | **Example:** The person talks about the spouse's death and details of the accident that caused it with an apathetic expression and without crying or showing signs of grieving. |
| **Identification** | *Similar to, and the result of, introjections; unconscious modelling of another person so that basic values, attitudes, and behaviours are similar to those of a significant person or group; but overt behaviour is manifested in an individual manner.* (Imitation is not considered a defence mechanism per se, but imitation usually precedes identification. Imitation is consciously copying another's values, attitudes, movements, etc.). |
| | **Example:** The adolescent begins to manifest the assertive behaviour, and state ideas similar to those that she admires in one of her instructors. She is, however, unaware that her behaviour is similar to that of the instructor. |

*(continued)*

**Table 5-5** (continued)

| | |
|---|---|
| **Introjection** | *Symbolic assimilation of, or process of, taking attitudes, behaviour, wishes, ideals, or values of significant person into the ego and/or superego* (a part of identification).<br><br>**Example:** The client talks about how much she or he helps other people with their problems. |
| **Projection** | *Attributing one's unacceptable, or anxiety-provoking, feelings, thoughts, impulses, wishes, or characteristics to another person.*<br><br>**Example:** The person declares that the supervisor is lazy and prejudiced; work colleagues note that this person often needs help at work and frequently makes derogatory remarks about others. |
| **Rationalization** | *Justification of behaviour or offering a socially acceptable, intellectual, and apparently logical explanation for an act or decision actually caused by unconscious, or verbalized, impulses. Behaviour in response to unrecognized motives precedes reasons for it.*<br><br>**Example:** A student fails a course but maintains that the course was not important and that the grade can be made up in another course. |
| **Reaction formation** | *Unacceptable impulses repressed, denied, and reacted to by opposite overt behaviour.*<br><br>**Example:** A married woman who is unconsciously disturbed by feeling sexually attracted to one of her husband's friends treats her husband rudely and keeps him at a safe distance. |
| **Regression** | *Adopting behaviour characteristic of a previous developmental level; the ego returns to an immature, but more gratifying, state of development in thought, feeling, or behaviour.*<br><br>**Example:** The person takes a nap, curled in a fetal position, on arriving home after a stressful day at work. |
| **Repression** | *Automatic, involuntary exclusion from awareness of a painful or conflictual feeling, thought, impulse, experience, or memory.* The thought or memory of the event is not consciously perceived.<br><br>**Example:** The mother seems unaware of the date or events surrounding her child's death; and she shows no emotions when the death is discussed. |
| **Sublimation** | *Substitution of a socially acceptable behaviour for an unacceptable sexual or aggressive drive or impulse.*<br><br>**Example:** The adolescent is forbidden by her parents to have a date until she graduates from high school. She gives much time and energy to editorial work and writing for the school paper. The editor of the school paper and the faculty advisor are males. |
| **Suppression** | *Intentional exclusion of material from consciousness.*<br><br>**Example:** The husband carries the bills in his pocket for a week before remembering to mail in the payments. |
| **Symbolization** | *One object or act unconsciously represents a complex group of objects and acts,* some of which may be in conflict with, or unacceptable to, the ego; external objects or acts stand for any internal or repressed desire, idea, attitude, or feeling. The symbol may not overtly appear to be related to the repressed ideas or feelings.<br><br>**Example:** The husband sends his wife a bouquet of roses, which ordinarily represents love and beauty. But roses have thorns; his beautiful wife is hard to live with, but he consciously focuses on her beauty. |
| **Undoing** | *An act, communication, or thought that cancels the significance or partially negates a previous one; treating an experience as if it had never occurred.*<br><br>**Example:** The husband purchases a gift for his wife after a quarrel the previous evening. |

Freud proposed five stages of psychosexual development and contended that personality was formed by age five. The stages in psychosexual development, each resolved in turn, are summarized in Table 5-6 and referred to throughout the text.

Freud's ideas about psychosexual development are undoubtedly the most controversial aspects of his theory. His theory continues to influence thought and research, especially in Western cultures, in relation to the development and therapy of the ill person.[100] Freud made us more aware of the importance of unconscious thoughts, motivations, and feelings; the role of childhood in forming personality; the ambivalence of emotional responses, especially to parents; and ways in which later relationships are affected by earlier ones.[101]

## CRITICAL THINKING

*What are some criticisms of Freud's theory?*

### Table 5-6 Freud's Stages of Psychosexual Development: Libidinal Extension

| Stage (years) | Major Body Zone | Activities | Extension to Others |
|---|---|---|---|
| **Oral** $(0-1\frac{1}{2})$ | Mouth (major source of gratification and exploration) | Security—primary need<br>Pleasure from eating and sucking<br>Major conflict—weaning<br>Incorporation (suck, consume, chew, bite, receive) | Sense of *We*—no differentiation or extension<br>Sense of *I* and *Other*—minimum differentiation and total incorporation<br>Beginning of ego development at 4–5 months |
| **Anal** $(1\frac{1}{2}-3)$ | Bowel (anus) and bladder source of sensual satisfaction, self-control, and conflict (mouth continues in importance) | Expulsion and retention (differentiation, expelling, controlling, pushing away)<br>(Incorporation still is used)<br>Major conflict—toilet training | Sense of *I* and *Other*—separation from other and increasing sense of *I*<br>Beginning control over impulses |
| **Phallic** (4–6) | Genital region—penis, clitoris (mouth, bowel, and bladder sphincters continue in importance) | Masturbation<br>Fantasy<br>Play activities<br>Experimentation with peers<br>Questioning of adults about sexual topics<br>Major conflict—Oedipus complex, which resolves when child identifies with parent of same sex<br>(Mastery, incorporation, expulsion, and retention continue) | Sense of *I* and *Other*—fear of castration in boy<br>Sense of *I* and *Other*—strengthened with identification process with parents<br>Sense of *Other*—extends to other adults |
| **Latency** (6–puberty) | No special body focus | Diffuse activity and relationships<br>(Mastery, incorporation, expulsion, and retention continue) | Sense of *I* and *Other*—extends out of nuclear family and includes peers of same sex |
| **Genital** (puberty and thereafter) | Penis, vagina (mouth, anus, clitoris) | Develop skills needed to cope with the environment<br>Full sexual maturity and function<br>(Mastery, incorporation, expulsion, and retention continue)<br>Addition of new assets with each stage for gratification<br>Realistic sexual expression<br>Creativity and pleasure in love and work | Sense of *I* and *Other*—extends to other adults and peers of opposite sex |

## Major Neo-Analytic Theorists

Neo-Freudians or neo-analysts follow Freud's theory in general; but they disagree with, or have modified some of, the original propositions. They *maintain the medical model and share the view of intrapsychic determinism as the basis for external behaviour. Some take into account the social and cultural context in which the person lives.* Harry Stack Sullivan and Erik Erikson are considered briefly. Both Sullivan and Erikson are referred to throughout the text.

### Sullivan: Interpersonal Theory of Psychiatry

Harry Stack Sullivan[102] formulated the interpersonal theory of psychiatry. The theory focuses on relationships between and among people, in contrast to Freud's emphasis on the intrapsychic sexual phenomena and Erikson's focus on social aspects. Experiences in major life events are the result of either positive or negative interpersonal relationships. Personality development is largely the result of the mother–child relationship, childhood experiences, and interpersonal encounters. There are two basic needs: *satisfaction* (biological needs), and *security* (emotional and social needs).

Sullivan used the following biological principles to understand the person's development:[103]

- **Principle of communal existence.** *A living organism cannot survive if separated from the necessary environment for survival.* For example, the embryo must have the correct intrauterine environment to live. Similarly, the baby must have love and human contact to become socialized or human.

- **Principle of functional activity.** *Functional or physiologic activities and processes affect the person's interaction with the environment.*

- **Principle of organization.** *The person is systematically arranged physically, emotionally, and within society. This particular organization enables function.*

Sullivan implied that the *need to avoid anxiety* and the *need to gratify basic needs* are the two primary motivations for behaviour. One of his major concepts—the **concept of anxiety**—states that *anxiety has its origin in the prolonged dependency of infancy, the urgency of biological and emotional needs, and how the mothering person meets those needs. Anxiety is the result of uncomfortable interpersonal relationships, is the chief disruptive force in interpersonal relationships, is contagious through empathic feelings, and can be relieved by being in a secure interpersonal relationship.* Sullivan's other concepts are **satisfaction of needs**, which is *the fulfillment of requirements associated with an individual's psychochemical environment;* **interpersonal security,** *the feeling associated with relief from anxiety;* and self-system.[104]

The **self-system** is the *internal organization of experiences that exists to defend against anxiety and to secure necessary*

security. One aspect of the self-system is known as *good-me, bad-me,* and *not-me,* which refers to feelings about the self that begin to form in infancy.[105]

### Erikson: Psychosocial Theory of Personality Development

Erik Erikson[106] formulated the psychosocial theory. His theory explains step by step the unfolding of emotional development and social characteristics during encounters with the environment. Erikson's psychosexual theory enlarges on psychoanalytic theory in that it is not limited to any historical era, a specific culture, or personality types. It encompasses development through the lifespan and is universal to all people. It acknowledges that society, heredity, and childhood experiences all influence the person's development.[107]

The following are basic principles of Erikson's theory, based on cross-cultural studies:[108]

- Each phase has a specific developmental task to achieve or solve. These tasks describe the order and sequence of human development and the conditions necessary to accomplish them, but actual accomplishment is completed at an individual pace, tempo, and intensity.

- Each psychosexual stage of development is a developmental crisis because there is a radical change in the person's perspective, a shift in energy, and an increased emotional vulnerability. During this peak time, the potential in the personality comes in contact with the whole environment, and the person has some degree of success in solving the crucial developmental task of the specific era. How the person copes with the task and crisis depends on the person's previous developmental strengths and weaknesses.

- The potential inherent in each person evolves, if given adequate chance to survive and grow. Anything that distorts the environment essential for development interferes with the evolution of the person. Society attempts to safeguard and encourage the proper rate and sequence of the unfolding of human potential so that humanity is maintained.

- Each developmental task is redeveloped, reworked, and redefined in subsequent stages. Potential for further development always exists.

- Internal organization is central to development. Maturity increases as the tasks of each era are accomplished, at least in part, in proper order.

Erikson proposed eight stages of development and described the developmental task of crisis for each stage (see Figure 5-2). They are described in Chapters 7 through 14 in relation to each developmental era. This particular theory is widely accepted, and quite generally used in understanding the developing person and in

**Figure 5-2** Erikson's eight stages of the person

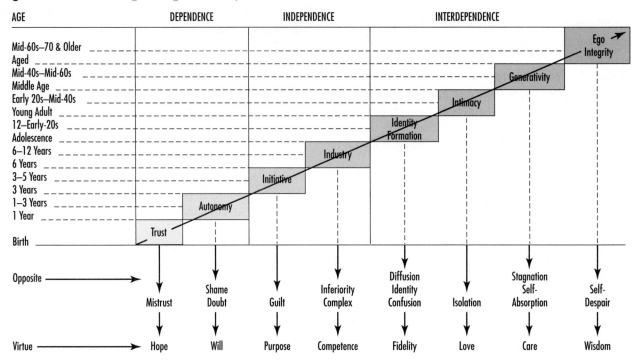

planning health promotion strategies and nursing care interventions.[109]

**CRITICAL THINKING**

*If an eight-year-old child is not able to resolve his or her developmental tasks at the expected stage, what may be the consequences for the child?*

# COGNITIVE THEORIES AND THEORISTS

**Cognitive theory** *deals with the person as an information processor and problem solver.* The cognitive perspective is concerned with internal processes, but it emphasizes the way that people attempt to acquire, interpret, and use information to solve life's problems and to remain normal or healthy. It emphasizes conscious processes, present thoughts, and problem-solving strategies. The cognitive perspective has grown out of relatively new directions in learning and psychodynamic theories. Relationships among emotions, motivations, and cognitive processes are being studied. Cognitive theorists can be divided into four groups:

1. Beck's cognitive theory
2. Behavioural-cognitive theorists
3. Social learning theorists
4. Cognitive development theorists

## Cognitive Theory: Beck

Aaron Beck originated cognitive theory and therapy. His premise was that psychological problems result from repetitive, automatic distorted or dysfunctional patterns of thinking that have evolved from faulty learning, making incorrect inferences on the basis of inadequate or incorrect information, and not distinguishing adequately between imagination and reality (see Table 5-7). Unrealistic thinking may be attributed to enduring negative attitudes (low self-esteem, hopelessness, and helplessness) about self, the world, and the future. The idiosyncratic, angry, or distorted thought patterns may become activated by life stresses, yet the responses are automatic, or based on past experiences, usually developed early in life and formed by relevant experience.[110]

Cognitive therapy is a short-term, structured therapy involving an active collaboration between the client and therapist toward achieving the therapy goals. It is usually conducted on an individual basis, but may also be used with groups. The *goals of therapy* are to:

1. Help the person identify erroneous beliefs in relation to stressful events or behaviours.
2. Help the person look at these thoughts, compare them with objective evidence, and correct distortions.
3. Give feedback to the person about the accuracy of the new thoughts.
4. Allow and encourage the person to rehearse new cognitions in therapy and at home.

## Table 5-7 Definitions of Cognitive Distortions

| Distortion | Definition |
|---|---|
| **All-or-nothing thinking or dichotomous thinking** | *Seeing events in black-and-white categories;* if performance falls short of perfect, the self is a total failure. |
| **Overgeneralization** | *Seeing a single negative event as a never-ending pattern of defeat.* |
| **Mental filter or selective inattention** | *Focusing on a single negative detail exclusively so that vision of all reality becomes darkened;* interpreting situation, or life, on basis of one incident. |
| **Disqualifying the positive** | *Rejecting positive experiences by insisting they "don't count" for some reason or other.* In this way, a negative belief that is contradicted by everyday experiences is maintained. |
| **Jumping to conclusions or arbitrary inference** | *Making a negative interpretation even though there are no definite facts that convincingly support the conclusion;* holding to beliefs without supporting evidence. |
| **Mind reading** | *Arbitrarily concluding that someone is reacting negatively to the self* and not checking this out. |
| **The fortune teller error** | *Anticipating that things will turn out badly,* and feeling convinced that prediction is an already established fact. |
| **Magnification (catastrophizing) or minimization** | *Exaggerating the importance of things* (such as a goof-up, or someone else's achievement), *or inappropriately shrinking things until they appear tiny* (own desirable qualities or the other person's imperfections). This is also called the "binocular trick." |
| **Emotional reasoning** | *Assuming that negative emotions necessarily reflect the way things really are:* "I feel it, therefore it must be true." |
| **Should statements** | *Trying to motivate self with "shoulds" and "should nots."* "Musts" and "oughts" are also offenders. The emotional consequence is guilt. Directing "should" statements toward others creates feelings of anger, frustration, and resentment. |
| **Labelling and mislabelling** | *An extreme form of overgeneralization.* Instead of describing the error, a negative label is attached to self: "I'm a loser." When someone else's behaviour rubs the wrong way, attaching a negative label to him: "He's a louse." Mislabelling involves describing an event with language that is highly coloured and emotionally loaded. |
| **Personalization** | *Seeing self as the cause of some negative external event for which there was no responsibility.* |

Cognitive therapy is short-term, highly structured, and goal-oriented therapy that consists of three major components: educational aspects, cognitive techniques, and behavioural interventions.[111] Cognitive therapy helps the patient to use problem-solving techniques to identify distorted thoughts, to correct dysfunctional thoughts, and to learn more realistic ways to formulate the experiences. The health care provider or therapist serves as a teacher or guide in the process, and is non-judgmental, objective, and empathetic. Questioning rigid beliefs and attitudes guides the person to refocus problems, alter errors in thinking, and rehearse new behaviour patterns.[112]

Donald Meichenbaum, at the University of Waterloo, developed a form of cognitive-behavioural therapy called *stress inoculation* to treat anxiety. Some degree of anxiety is normal. Excessive anxiety, however, can be crippling.

It can prevent the individual from finishing projects, and it can seriously interfere with work efficiency. Stress inoculation training was designed to reduce anxiety in both academic and non-academic settings. Three phases occur in stress inoculation:

- Education phase: the individual is taught about the nature of the anxiety

- Rehearsal phase: the individual is taught how to manage anxiety better

- Implementation phase: the person deals with anxiety-provoking stimuli in real-world situations

Stress inoculation has become a widely accepted technique for controlling anxiety.[113]

**Social-Cognitive Theory: Bandura**  Albert Bandura's social-cognitive theory states that learning occurs without reinforcement, conditioning, or trial-and-error behaviour because people can think and anticipate consequences of behaviour and act accordingly.[114] This theory emphasizes:

1. That cognitive processes, modelling, environmental influences, and the person's self-directed capacity all contribute to development, learning, and behaviour.

2. The importance of vicarious, symbolic, and self-regulatory processes in psychological functioning.

3. The capacity of the person to use symbols, represent events, analyze conscious experience, communicate with others at any distance in time and space, and plan, create, imagine, and engage in actions of foresight.

The person does not simply react to external forces: he or she selects, organizes, and transforms impinging stimuli and thus exercises some influence over personal behaviour. *Bandura's model of causation involves the interaction of three components: (1) the person, with cognitive, biological, and other internal events that affect perceptions and actions, (2) external environment, and (3) behaviour* (see Figure 5-3).[115]

Human nature is characterized as a vast potential that can be fashioned by knowledge and skill that results from direct and vicarious experience into a variety of forms of development and behaviour within biological limits. The level of psychological and physiologic development restricts what can be acquired at any given time.[116]

The person may be motivated by ideas or fantasies of future consequences or by personal goal-setting behaviour. If the person wants to accomplish a certain goal and there are distractions from the task, the person visualizes how he or she will feel when the goal is attained. After evaluating their behaviour, people usually respond to it and tend to persist until the behaviour or performance meets the goal.[117]

**Figure 5-3** Bandura's concept of reciprocal determinism.

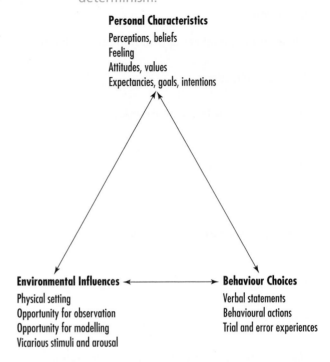

Bandura[118] proposes that learning occurs through **modelling**, *imitation of another's behaviour. Four interacting mental processes must be present:*

1. *Attention.* The learner must perceive the model.

2. *Memory.* The learner must encode the information obtained from observing the model in a form that can be used at a later time.

3. *Motor control.* The learner must be able to use this coded information to guide his or her own actions.

4. *Motivation.* The learner must have some reason or inducement to perform the modelled actions.

These processes must be involved in behaviour that depends on information gained from the environment. Learning is achieved primarily through interactions with other people. Social rewards, such as praise and acceptance, help motivate and reinforce such learning as do simple observations by other people. Bandura asserts that people learn, and thereby modify, their cognitive constructs throughout life as they interact with others. The person acts on the environment (and the environment on the person) in a continuous lifelong process.[119]

According to his theory, much of our daily behaviour is learned by modelling and by the perceptions that form in the process. Imitation is one of the most effective forms of learning. Bandura's research shows the power of media violence on people's behaviour. For some people, a model of aggressive behaviour will cause later acting-out behaviour.[120] This research is discussed further in Chapter 10.

## CRITICAL THINKING

*What behaviours have you learned through the modelling of others?*

Bandura identified self-efficacy as a particularly influential mediator in behaviour.[121] Self-efficacy is a judgment about one's ability to organize and execute action and to accomplish a certain level of performance in a situation. Self-efficacy is based on mastered experiences, vicarious experiences (or the observation of other people doing the behaviour), verbal persuasion from another to adjust behaviour, and physiologic states (or internal cues that are evidence of the capability or deficit). Bandura's theory is pertinent to implementing health promotion behaviour.[122]

## Cognitive Development: Piaget

Jean Piaget[123] formulated the theory of cognitive development. The bulk of his research was concerned with the child's thinking at particular periods of life, and with studying differences among well children of a specific age. He believed that development is neither **maturational**, an *unfolding of the innate growth process*, nor **learning**, an *accumulation of experiences*. Rather, development is an active process resulting from **equilibration**, an *internal force that is set in motion to organize thinking when the child's belief system develops sufficiently to contain self-contradictions*. **Intelligence** *is a basic life function that helps the individual to adapt to his environment*.[124]

Through interaction with the environment, the person constructs reality by assimilation, accommodation, and adaptation. **Assimilation** is *taking new content and experiences into the mind or cognitive structure*. **Accommodation** is the *revising, realigning, and readjusting of cognitive structure to take into account the new content*. **Adaptation** is the *change that results from the first two processes*. Piaget emphasizes the innate, inborn processes of the person as the essential force to start the process of equilibration or cognitive growth. Cognitive development proceeds from motor activity to interaction with the wider social world. Finally, cognitive development arrives at abstract ideas. Development is seen as solidly rooted in what already exists, and it displays continuity with the past. Adaptations do not develop in isolation; all form a coherent pattern so that the totality of biological life is adapted to its environment. The theory focuses on development of intellectual capacities with little reference to emotional or social development.[125]

The thinking process is explained by schematic mental structures of pictures formed in response to stimuli. A **schema** is a *cognitive structure, a complex concept encompassing both motor behaviour and internalized thought processes. A schema involves movement of the eyeballs, paying attention, and the mental picture that is formed as a result of the sensory process.* Thinking eventually involves using combinations of mental pictures, forming concepts, internalizing use of language or sub-vocal speech, drawing implications, and making judgments. When these internal actions become integrated into a coherent, logical system, they are considered logical operations.[126]

Piaget divided human development into four periods: sensorimotor, preoperational, concrete operations, and formal operations. Table 5-8 provides a summary of these

## Table 5-8 Summary of Piaget's Theory of Cognitive Development

| Period | Age | Characteristics |
|---|---|---|
| **Sensorimotor Period** | | |
| Stage 1: Use of reflexes | 0–1 month | Behaviour innate, reflexive, specific, predictable to specific stimuli<br>**Example:** sucking, grasping, eye movements, startle (Moro reflex) |
| Stage 2: First acquired adaptations and primary circula reactions | 1–4 months | Initiates, prolongs, and repeats behaviour not previously occurring<br>Acquires response to stimulus that creates another stimulus and response<br>Modifies innate reflexes to more purposeful behaviour; repeated if satisfying<br>Learns feel of own body as physiologic stabilization occurs<br>**Example:** Looks at object, reaches for it, and continues to repeat until vision, reaching, and mouthing are coordinated |
| Stage 3: Secondary circular reactions | 4–8 months | Learns from unintentional behaviour<br>Motor skills and vision further coordinated as infant learns to prolong or repeat interesting act<br>Interest in environment around self<br>Explores world from sitting position |

*(continued)*

**Table 5-8** (continued)

| Period | Age | Characteristics |
|---|---|---|
| | | Assimilates new objects into old behaviour pattern |
| | | Behaviour increasingly intentional |
| | | **Example:** Looks for object that disappears from sight; continues to drop object from different locations, which adult continues to pick up |
| Stage 4: Coordination of secondary schema acquisition of instrumental behaviour, active search for vanished objects | 8–12 months | Uses familiar behaviour patterns in new situation to accomplish goal |
| | | Differentiates objects, including mother from stranger (stranger anxiety) |
| | | Retains memory of object hidden from view |
| | | Combines actions to obtain desired, hidden object; explores object |
| | | Imitates others when behaviour finished |
| | | Develops individual habits |
| | | Cognitive development enhanced by increasing motor and language skills |
| Stage 5: Tertiary circular reactions and discovery of new means by active experimentation | 12–18 months | Invents new behaviour not previously performed |
| | | Uses fewer previous behaviours |
| | | Repeats action without random movements |
| | | Explores variations that occur when same act accomplished |
| | | Varies action deliberately as repeats behaviour |
| | | Uses trial-and-error behaviour to discover solution to problem |
| | | Differentiates self from object and object from action performed by self; increasing exploration of how objects function |
| | | Invents new means to solve problems and variation in behaviour essential to later symbolic behaviour and concept formation |
| Stage 6: Internal representation of action in external world | 18–24 months | Pictures events to self; follows through mentally to some degree |
| | | Imitates when model out of sight |
| | | Forms mental picture of external body, of body in same space with another object, and of space in limited way |
| | | Uses deliberate trial and error in solving problems |
| **Preoperational Period** | | |
| | 2–7 years | Internalizes schemata of more and more of the environment, rules, and relationships |
| | | Forms memories to greater extent |
| | | Uses fantasy or imitation of others in behaviour and play |
| | | Intermingles fantasy and reality |
| | | Uses words to represent objects and events more accurately; symbolic behaviour increases |
| | | **Egocentric** (*self-centred in thought*)—focuses on single aspect of object and neglects other attributes because of lack of experience and reference systems, which results in false logic |
| | | Follows rules in egocentric way; rules external to self |
| | | Is static and irreversible in thinking; cannot transform from one state to another (e.g., ice to water) |
| | | Develops story or idea while forgetting original idea so that final statements disconnected, disorganized; answer not connected to original idea in monologue |
| | | Tries logical thinking; at times sounds logical but lacks perspective so that false logic and inconsistent, unorganized thinking result |
| | | Is magical, global, primitive in reasoning |
| | | Begins to connect past to present events, not necessarily accurate |
| | | Links events by sequence rather than causality |
| | | Deals with information by recall; begins to categorize |

*(continued)*

Table 5-8 (continued)

| Period | Age | Characteristics |
|---|---|---|
| | | Is **anthropomorphic** (*attributes human characteristics to animals and objects*) |
| | | Unable to integrate events separated by time, past to present |
| | | Lacks reversibility in thinking |
| | | Unable to anticipate how situation looks from another viewpoint |
| Preconceptual stage | 2–4 years | Forms images or preconcepts on basis of thinking just described |
| | | Lacks ability to define properly or to denote hierarchy or relationships of objects |
| | | Constructs concepts in global way |
| | | Unable to use time, space, equivalence, and class inclusion in concept formation |
| Intuitive stage | 4–7 years | Forms concepts increasingly; some limitations |
| | | Defines one property at a time |
| | | Has difficulty starting definition but knows how to use object |
| | | Uses transductive logic (from general to specific) rather than deductive or inductive logic |
| | | Begins to classify in ascending or descending order; labels |
| | | Begins to do seriation; reverses processes and ordinality |
| | | Begins to note cause–effect relationships |
| **Concrete Operations** | | |
| **Period** | 7–11 years (or beyond) | Organizes and stabilizes thinking; more rational |
| | | Sees interrelationships increasingly |
| | | Does mental operations using tangible, visible references |
| | | Able to **decentre** (*sees other perspectives; associates or combines events; understands reversibility [e.g., add–subtract, ice–water transformation]*) |
| | | Recognizes number, length, volume, area, weight as the same even when perception of object changes |
| | | Develops conservation as experience is gained with physical properties of objects |
| | | Arranges objects in order of size and other characteristics |
| | | Fits new objects into series |
| | | Understands simpler relationships between classes of objects |
| | | Distinguishes between distances |
| | | Understands observable world, tangible situations, time, and tangible space |
| | | Retains essential idea when perceiving conflicting or unorganized data |
| | | Recognizes rules as essential; perceives mutually agreed on standards |
| | | Is less egocentric except in social relationships |
| **Formal Operations** | | |
| **Period** | 12 years and beyond | Manifests adult like thinking |
| | | Not limited by own perception or concrete references for ideas |
| | | Combines various ideas into concepts |
| | | Coordinates two or more reference systems |
| | | Develops morality of restraint and cooperation in behaviour |
| | | Uses rules to structure interaction in socially acceptable way |
| | | Uses probability concept |
| | | Works from definition or concept only to solve problem |
| | | Solves problem mentally and considers alternatives before acting |
| | | Considers number of variables at one time |
| | | Links variables to formulate hypotheses |
| | | Begins to reason deductively and inductively instead of solving problem by action |
| | | Relates concepts or constructs not readily evident in external world |
| | | Formulates advanced concepts of proportions, space, destiny, momentum |
| | | Increases intellectual ability to include art, science, humanities, religion, and philosophy |
| | | Is increasingly less egocentric |

periods. In each stage, the person demonstrates interpretation and use of the environment through certain behaviour patterns. These periods are discussed with development of the infant, toddler, preschooler, schoolchild, adolescent, and adult. You will find these stages pertinent to determining mental development of the person and corresponding educational approaches and activities.[127]

## Information Processing: Neo-Piagetian Theory

This neo-Piagetian *approach does not propose stages of cognitive development but, like Piaget, sees people as active thinkers about their world.* People learn by becoming efficient at processing information rather than through equilibration. These theorists *study mental processes underlying intelligent behaviour; perception, attention, memory, and problem solving; and how people acquire, transform, and use sensory information through active manipulation of symbols or mental images.* They look at the mind as a computer. Practice enables learning, since there is a limit to the number of schemes a person can keep in mind. *With practice, an idea or skill becomes automatic, which frees the person to learn additional information and do more complex problem solving.* These theorists believe that learning does not occur in demarcated stages but is more gradual and continuous. However, this theory neglects study of creativity, motivation, and social interaction as they relate to cognitive development.[128]

According to this theory, information is taken from the environment, through the senses, and held in memory: the first memory storage. If the person pays attention, the information is transferred to the short-term memory storage. The short-term memory can only hold about seven pieces of information at a time, so the information is either forgotten or processed to the long-term memory storage. To save information at this third level, organizing and hearing it is necessary. Retrieval may be difficult. As the child grows older, information is processed more efficiently and comprehensively. The child develops **metacognition**, *an awareness of how to think and learn, and an understanding of self as a learner.* Thus, a knowledge base is developed through the lifespan. However, knowledge is specialized, depending on the information and skills accumulated.[129]

## Moral Development Theories

**Kohlberg's Theory of Moral Development**  Lawrence Kohlberg formulated a theory of moral development that is related to cognitive and emotional development and to societal values and norms. It, too, is divided into stages.[130]

Moral reasoning focuses on ten universal values: punishment, property, roles and concerns related to affection, roles and concerns related to authority, law, life, liberty, distribution of justice, truth, and sexual behaviour. A conflict between two or more of these universal values necessitates a moral choice and its subsequent justification by the individual, requiring systematic problem solving and other cognitive capabilities.[131]

Kohlberg believed that both cognitive development and relevant social experience underlie the growth of moral reasoning.[132] Kohlberg theorized that a person's moral reasoning process and behaviour develop through stages over varying lengths of time. Each stage is derived from a prior stage and is the basis for the next stage. *Each moral stage is based on, or dependent on, the reason for behaviour. Each stage shows an organized system of thought by which the person is consistent in the level of moral judgment.*[133]

More advanced logical thinking is needed for each successive *moral stage.* One criterion of moral maturity, the ability to decide autonomously what is right and caring, is lacking in the *pre-conventional and conventional* levels because in each level the person is following the commands of authority figures. If the person's cognition is at the stage of concrete operations, according to Piaget, the person is limited to the *pre-conventional or conventional* levels of moral reasoning. Even the person in the stage of formal operations may not be beyond the *conventional* level of moral maturity. The transition to *post-conventional* morality represents only a minority of adults and even a smaller minority of adolescents. It is important to comprehend that what determines the stage or level of an individual's moral judgment is not any specific moral choice but the form of reasoning used to justify that choice.[134] Table 5-9 shows the three levels and six stages.[135]

---

## CRITICAL THINKING

*Who in the world, in your opinion, has progressed to the post-conventional stage? State your rationale.*

---

Development of moral judgment is stimulated whenever (1) the educational process intentionally creates cognitive conflict and disequilibrium so that the person can work through inadequate modes of thinking, (2) the person has opportunity for group discussion of values and can participate in group decision making about moral issues, and (3) the person has opportunity to assume responsibility for the consequences of behaviour. Kohlberg's theory has application to nursing, education, and family counselling.[136]

**Gilligan's Theory of Moral Development**  Gilligan's research on moral development has focused on women in contrast to Kohlberg's focus on men. Gilligan claimed that moral development proceeds through three levels and two transitions, with each level representing a more complex understanding of the relationship of self and others and each transition resulting in a crucial re-evaluation of the conflict between selfishness and responsibility. Women define the

Table 5-9 Progression of Moral Development

| Level | Stage |
|---|---|
| **Pre-conventional** | |
| The person is responsive to cultural rules of labels of good and bad, right or wrong. Externally established rules determine right or wrong actions. The person reasons in terms of punishment, reward, or exchange of favours. | I. *Punishment and Obedient Orientation* <br> Fear of punishment, not respect for authority, is the reason for decisions, behaviour, and conformity. Good and bad are defined in terms of physical consequences to the self from parental, adult, or authority figures. The person defers to superior power or prestige of the person who dictates rules ("I'll do something because you tell me and to avoid getting punished"). <br> Average age: toddler to 7 years |
| Egocentric focus | II. *Instrumental Relativist Orientation* <br> Conformity is based on egocentricity and narcissistic needs. The person's decisions and behaviour are usually based on what provides satisfaction out of concern for self: something is done to get something in return. Occasionally the person does something to please another for pragmatic reasons. There is no feeling of justice, loyalty, or gratitude. These concepts are expressed physically ("I'll do something if I get something for it or because it pleases you"). <br> Average age: preschooler through school age |
| **Conventional** | |
| The person is concerned with maintaining expectations and rules of the family, group, nation, or society. A sense of guilt has developed and affects behaviour. The person values conformity, loyalty, and active maintenance of social order and control. Conformity means good behaviour or what pleases or helps another and is approved. | III. *Interpersonal Concordance Orientation* <br> A. Decisions and behaviour are based on concerns about others' reactions; the person wants others' approval or a reward. The person has moved from egocentricity to consideration of others as a basis for behaviour. Behaviour is judged by the person's intentions ("I'll do something because it will please you or because it is expected"). <br> B. An empathic response, based on understanding of how another person feels, is a determinant for decisions and behaviour ("I'll do something because I know how it feels to be without; I can put myself in your shoes"). <br> Average age: school age through adulthood (Most North American women are in this stage.) |
| Societal focus | IV. *Law-and-Order Orientation* <br> The person wants established rules from authorities, and the reason for decisions and behaviour is that social and sexual rules and traditions demand the response. The person obeys the law just because it is the law or out of respect for authority and underlying morality of the law. The law takes precedence over personal wishes, good intentions, and conformity to group stereotypes ("I'll do something because it's the law and my duty"). <br> Average age: adolescence and adulthood (Most men are in this stage; 80% of adults do not move past this stage.) |
| **Post-conventional** | |
| The person lives autonomously and defines moral values and principles that are distinct from personal identification with group values. He or she lives according to principles that are universally agreed on and that the person considers appropriate for life. | V. *Social Contract Legalistic Orientation* <br> The social rules are not the sole basis for decisions and behaviour because the person believes a higher moral principle applies such as equality, justice, or due process. The person defines right actions in terms of general individual rights and standards that have been agreed on by the whole society but is aware of relativistic nature of values and opinions. The person believes laws can be changed as people's needs change. The person uses freedom of choice in living up to higher |

*(continued)*

Table 5-9 (continued)

| Level | Stage |
|---|---|
| | principles but believes the way to make changes is through the system. Outside the legal realm, free agreement and contract are the binding elements of obligation ("I'll do something because it is morally and legally right, even if it isn't popular with the group"). <br><br>Average age: middle age or older adult. No more than 20% of North Americans achieve this stage. |
| Universal focus | VI. *Universal Ethical Principle Orientation* <br> Decisions and behaviour are based on internalized rules, on conscience rather than social laws, and on self-chosen ethical and abstract principles that are universal, comprehensive, and consistent. The rules are not concrete moral rules but instead encompass the Golden Rule, justice, reciprocity, and equality of human rights, and respect for the dignity of human beings as individual persons. Human life is inviolable. The person believes there is a higher order than social order, has a clear concept of civil disobedience, and will use self as an example to right a wrong. The person accepts injustice, pain, death as an integral part of existence but works to minimize injustice and pain for others ("I'll do something because it is morally, ethically, and spiritually right, even if it is illegal and I get punished and even if no one else participates in the act"). <br><br>Average age: middle age or older adult. (Few people attain or maintain this stage. Examples of this stage are seen in times of crisis or extreme situations.) |

Source: Data used here are based on Kohlberg, L. (ed.). *Collected Papers on Moral Development and Moral Education.* Cambridge, MA: Moral Educational Research Foundation, 1973; Kohlberg, L., Moral Stages and Moralization: The Cognitive Developmental Approach. In T. Lickona (ed.), *Moral Development and Behavior* (pp. 31–53). New York: Holt, Rinehart, & Winston, 1976; Kohlberg, L. *Recent Research in Moral Development.* New York: Holt, Rinehart, & Winston, 1977; Kohlberg, L., The Cognitive-Developmental Approach to Moral Education. In P. Scharf (ed.), *Readings in Moral Education* (pp. 36–51). Minneapolis: Winston Press, 1978.

moral problem in the context of human relationships, exercising care, and avoiding hurt. In Gilligan's studies, women's moral judgment proceeded from initial concern with survival, to a focus on goodness, to a principled understanding of others' need for care. Table 5-10 summarizes the three levels and two transitions of moral development proposed by Gilligan.[137]

The care focus proposed by Gilligan is concerned with issues of abandonment, and the theory values ideals of attention and response to need. Some people may combine both Kohlberg's and Gilligan's perspectives and incorporate into moral development such values as honesty, courage, and community, which are implied in Kohlberg's postconventional level. More research in all age groups, men and women, and all races and ethnic groups is needed to understand fully moral development.[138]

Friedman[139] tested Gilligan's claim that men and women differ in moral judgments. College students read four traditional moral dilemmas and rated the importance of 12 considerations for deciding how the protagonist

should respond. There were no reliable sex differences on moral reasoning. Sex-typed personality measures also failed to predict individual differences in moral judgments.

## EXISTENTIAL AND HUMANISTIC THEORIES

### Overview

Existential and humanistic psychologies acknowledge the dynamic aspect of the person but emphasize to a greater degree the impact of environment.

**Existentialism** has its roots in philosophy, theology, literature, and psychology and *addresses the person's existence in a hostile or indifferent world and within the context of history.* It is phenomenological in nature; the context, uniqueness, and ever-changing aspects of events are considered. Existentialism regards human nature as unexplainable but emphasizes freedom of choice, responsibility, and satisfaction of ideals, the burden of freedom, discovery of inner

## Table 5-10 Gilligan's Theory of Moral Development

| Level | Characteristics |
|---|---|
| Orientation of Individual Survival | *Concentrates on what is practical and best for self*; selfish; dependent on others |
| Transition 1: From Selfishness to Responsibility | Realizes connection to others; thinks of responsible choice in terms of another as well as self |
| Goodness as Self-Sacrifice | *Sacrifices personal wishes and needs to fulfill others' wants* and to have others think well of her; feels responsible for others' actions; holds others responsible for her choices; dependent position; indirect efforts to control others often turn into manipulation through use of guilt; aware of connectedness with others. |
| Transition 2: From Goodness to Truth | *Makes decisions on personal intentions and consequences of actions rather than on how she thinks others will react*; takes into account needs of self and others; wants to be good to others but also honest by being responsible to self; increased social participation; assumes more responsibilities. |
| Morality of Non-violence | *Establishes moral equality between self and others; assumes responsibility for choice in moral dilemmas*; follows injunction to hurt no one, including self, in all situations; conflict between selfishness and selflessness; judgment based on view of consequences and intentions instead of appearance in the eyes of others. |

Sources: The data used here are based on C. Gilligan, In a Different Voice: Women's Conceptualization of Self and of Mortality, *Harvard Educational Review, 47*(4) (1977), 481–517; Gilligan, C. *In a Different Voice: Psychological Theory and Women's Development.* Cambridge, MA: Harvard University Press, 1982; Gilligan, C., and D. Attanucci, Two Moral Orientations: Gender Differences and Similarities, *Merrill-Palmer Quarterly, 34*(3) (1988), 332–333.

self, and consequences of action. Themes addressed include suffering, death, despair, meaninglessness, nothingness, vacuum, isolation, anxiety, hope, self-transcendence, and finding spiritual meaning. The transcendence of inevitable suffering, anxiety, and alienation is emphasized.[140]

**Humanism** *emphasizes self-actualization, satisfaction of needs, the individual as a rule unto himself or herself, the pleasure of freedom, and realization of innate goodness and creativity. Humanism shares the following assumptions with existentialism:* uniqueness of the person, potential of the person, and necessity of listening to or studying the person's perceptions, called the *phenomenological approach.*

Both existentialists and humanists seek to answer the following questions:

1. What are the possibilities of the person?

2. From these possibilities, what is an optimum state for the person?

3. Under what conditions is this state most likely to be reached?

These disciplines strive to maximize the individuality and developmental potential of the person.[141]

Because all behaviour is considered a function of the person's perceptions, *data for study of the person are subjective and come from self-reports,* including (1) feelings at the moment about self and the experience, (2) meaning of the experience, and (3) personal values, needs, attitudes, beliefs, behavioural norms, and expectations. Perception is synonymous with reality and meaning. All behaviour is pertinent to, and a product of, the phenomenal or perceptual field of the person at the moment of action. The **phenomenal field** is the *frame of reference and the universe as experienced by the person at the specific moment (the existential condition).*[142]

## View of the Human

The person is *viewed as a significant and unique whole individual in dynamic interaction with the environment, and continually in the process of becoming.* In addition, the person is seen as *holistic, with overall organizational complexity being more than the sum of the parts.* The person is constantly growing, changing, expanding perceptual processes, learning, developing potential, and gaining insights. Every experience affects the person, depending on the perceptions. The goals of the creative being are growth, feeling adequate, and reaching the potential. The person is active in pursuing these goals. Basic needs are the maintenance and enhancement of the self-concept and a sense of adequacy and self-actualization.[143]

Reality is internal; the *person's reality is the perception of the event*, rather than the actual event itself. No two people will view a situation in exactly the same way. *Various factors affect perception*:

1. The sensory apparatus and central nervous system of the person
2. Time for observation
3. Opportunities available to experience events
4. The external environment
5. Interpersonal relationships
6. Self-concept

What is most important to the person is conscious experience, what is happening to the self at a given time. The person is aware of social values and norms but lives out those values and norms in a way that has been uniquely and personally defined.[144]

Perceptions are crucial in influencing behaviour. Of all the perceptions that exist for the person, none is more important than those held about the self and the personal meaning and belief related to a situation. *Self-concept* is learned as a consequence of meaningful interactions with others and the world and has a high degree of stability at its core, changing only with time and opportunity to try new perceptions of self.

The *truly adequate person* sees self (and others) as having dignity, integrity, worth, and importance. Only with a positive view of self can the person risk trying the untried or accepting the undefined situation. The person can become self-actualized only through the experience of being treated as an adequate person by significant others.[145] This person is open to all experiences. The person develops trust in self, and dares to recognize feelings, live life fully, and express uniqueness. The person feels a sense of oneness with other people, depending on the nature of previous contacts.

## View of Education and Therapy

Education and therapy are:

1. Growth-oriented rather than controlling
2. Rooted in perceptual meaning rather than facts
3. Concerned with people rather than things
4. Focused on the immediate rather than the historical view of people
5. Hopeful rather than despairing

*The goals of education and therapy are the same goals as those of the person*: full functioning of the person, ongoing development, meeting the individual's potential, and movement toward self-actualization. Education and therapy are a process, not a condition or institution, and through the process the person achieves effective behaviour. The basic tenets of freedom and responsibility are essential focal points in this approach.[146]

*Characteristics of the learner or client* are as follows:

1. Is unique, has dignity and worth
2. Brings a cluster of understandings, skills, values, and attitudes that have personal meaning
3. Presents total self as sum of reactions to previous experiences and cultural and family background
4. Wants to learn that which has personal meaning; learns from experience
5. Wants to be fully involved; learning involves all dimensions of person
6. Believes finding the self is more important than facts[147]

The health care provider, teacher, or therapist is a unique, whole person with a self-concept that directly affects the philosophy and style of teaching or counselling. He or she does not consider self as central. Instead she or he is learner- or client-centred. Each sees the self as using the personality as an instrument, acting as a permissive facilitator, and providing a warm, accepting, supportive environment that is as free as possible from threat and obstacles. The teacher or therapist provides an enriched environment and a variety of ways for the person to perceive new experiences and to learn. The teacher, or therapist, realizes that all people need to be perceived and related to as empathic, co-operative, forward-looking, trustworthy, and responsible. These theorists reject the traditional, pessimistic, or mechanical view of people.[148]

Humanistic psychology emphasizes the natural tendency of all people, regardless of age or stage of life, to strive for self-actualization. Treatment approaches promote increased self-esteem and positive self-concept, problem solving to achieve goals, and helping the person achieve optimal functioning through a supportive therapeutic relationship characterized by warmth, non-possessive caring, and validation of the person's worth and dignity. Osachuk and Cairns claim that the therapist's characteristics contribute to successful outcomes.[149]

## Theory of Motivation and Hierarchy of Needs: Maslow

Maslow, in contrast to other developmental and personality theorists, studied normal people and mental health. One of his most important concepts is **self-actualization**, the *tendency to develop potentialities and become a better person*, and the need to help the person achieve the sense of self-direction implicit in self-actualization. Implicit in this concept is that people are not static, but are always in the process of becoming different and better.[150]

The needs that motivate self-actualization can be represented in a hierarchy of relative order and predominance. The basic needs, always a consideration in client care, are listed in Table 5-11.

Although Maslow ranked these basic human needs from lowest to highest, they do not necessarily occur in a fixed order. The physiological and safety needs (deficiency needs), however, are dominant and must be met before higher needs can be secured. Personal growth needs are those for love and belonging, self-esteem and recognition, and self-actualization. The highest needs of self-actualization, knowledge, and aesthetic expression may never be fully gratified as those at a lower level.[151] It is important for the therapist to understand the hierarchy of needs when working with clients.

| Table 5-11 Maslow's Theory of Hierarchy of Needs | |
|---|---|
| **Needs*** | **Characteristics** |
| **Physiologic** | Requirements for oxygen, water, food, temperature control, elimination, shelter, exercise, sleep, sensory stimulation, and sexual activity met |
| | Needs cease to exist as means of determining behaviour when satisfied, re-emerging only if blocked or frustrated |
| **Safety** | Able to secure shelter |
| | Sense of security, dependency, consistency, stability |
| | Maintenance of predictable environment, structure, order, fairness, limits |
| | Protection from immediate or future danger to physical well-being |
| | Freedom from fear, anxiety, chaos, and certain amount of routine |
| **Love and belonging** | Sense of affection, love, and acceptance from others |
| | Sense of companionship and affiliation with others |
| | Identification with significant others |
| | Recognition and approval from others |
| | Group interaction |
| | Not synonymous with sexual needs, but sexual needs may be motivated by this need |
| **Esteem from others** | Awareness of own individuality, uniqueness |
| | Feelings of self-respect and worth and respect from others |
| | Sense of confidence, independence, dignity |
| | Sense of competence, achievement, success, prestige, status |
| | Recognition from others for accomplishments |
| **Self-actualization** | Acceptance of self and others |
| | Empathetic with others |
| | Self-fulfillment |
| | Ongoing emotional and spiritual development |
| | Desire to attain standards of excellence and individual potential |
| | Use of talents, being productive and creative |
| | Experiencing fully, vividly, without self-consciousness |
| | Having peak experiences |
| **Aesthetic** | Desire for beauty, harmony, order, attractive surroundings |
| | Interest in art, music, literature, dance, creative forms |
| **Knowledge and understanding** | Desire to understand, systematize, organize, analyze, look for relations and meanings |
| | Curiosity; desire to know as much as possible |
| | Attraction to the unknown or mysterious |

*Needs are listed in ascending order. Physiologic needs are most basic, and self-actualization is highest level of needs.

Sources: Maslow, A. *The Farther Reaches of Human Nature*. New York: Viking Press, 1971; Maslow, A. *Towards a Psychology of Being*, 2nd ed. New York: D. Van Nostrand, 1968.

## Person-Centred Therapy: Carl Rogers

Carl Rogers is, along with Maslow, one of the leaders of humanistic-existentialist psychology. He developed a perspective on personality with a focus on self-concept. Self-actualization is a key concept in his theory. Rogers assumed that the person sees self as the centre of a continually changing world, and that he or she responds to the world as perceived. The person responds as a whole in the direction of self-actualization. The ability to achieve self-understanding, self-actualization, and perception of social acceptance by others is based on experience and interaction with other people. The person who, as a child, felt wanted and highly valued is likely to have a positive self-image, be thought well of by others, and have the capacity to achieve self-actualization. Optimal adjustment results in what Rogers calls the fully functioning person. The fully functioning person accepts self, avoids a personality facade, is genuine and honest, is increasingly self-directive and autonomous, is open to new experiences, avoids being driven by other people's expectations or the cultural norms, and has a low level of anxiety.[152]

Rogers's *technique of person-centred therapy* brings about behavioural change by conveying complete acceptance, respect, and empathy for the client. The therapist neither provides interpretations nor gives advice.[153] Providing this high degree of acceptance allows the person to meet basic needs that should have been met in childhood, to incorporate into the self-structure threatening feelings that were previously excluded, and to become aware of unconscious material that is controlling life. Rogers has given the therapist a more active role that includes sharing emotions and feelings in an interchange with the client.[154] *Chapter 4 discusses the use of Rogers's technique as it can be applied to the nurse–client relationship.*

## ECLECTICISM

The use of multiple perspectives is a current trend in the study of human development.[155] Instead of relying on one theoretical framework to enlarge their view of behaviour across the lifespan, developmentalists use ideas drawn from many theoretical concepts.

## STRESS AND CRISIS THEORIES

Stressors and crises are a part of development throughout the lifespan, and they do affect health. An understanding of stress and crisis theories is essential for health promotion assessment and interventions.

Two theories require consideration. One describes how a person responds to stressors, both routine and severe. The second relates to how people approach overwhelming events or crises. *The Theory of Stress and the General Adaptation Syndrome*, as formulated by Dr. Hans Selye, *described the physiologic adaptive response to stress*, the everyday wear and tear on the person.[156] Continued studies show, however, that the stress response has emotional, cognitive, and sometimes social effects as well. *Crisis theory was formulated to explain how people respond psychologically and behaviourally when they cannot cope adequately with stressors.* Responses to crises, or overwhelming events, also have physical effects. The two theories together explain a wide range of adaptive responses. Stress responses always occur to some extent in crisis. Not every stressor, however, constitutes a crisis.

## Theory of Stress Response and Adaptation

### Stress Response and Adaptation Syndrome

**Stress** is a *physical and emotional state that is always present in the person. Stress is influenced by various environmental, psychological, and social factors, but it is uniquely perceived by each individual person. Stress is intensified in response when environmental change or threat occurs either internally or externally and the person believes that he or she* must *respond.* The manifestations or results of stress are described as being overt and covert; purposeful; initially protective; and maintaining equilibrium, productivity, and satisfaction to the extent possible.[157]

---

### CRITICAL THINKING

*What stressors are you encountering today? What are you doing to cope with them?*

---

The person's survival depends on constant mediation between environmental demands and adaptive capacities. Various self-regulatory physical and emotional mechanisms are in constant operation, adjusting the body to a changing number and nature of internal and external stressors, agents, or factors, all of which cause intensification of the stress state. **Stressors** (*stress agents*) encompass a number of types of stimuli (see Table 5-12).[158] **Eustress** *is the stress that comes with successful adaptation. It is beneficial in that it promotes emotional development and self-actualization.* Eustress is *positive stress*, an optimum orientation to life's challenges coupled with the person's ability to regulate life and maintain optimum levels of stress for a growth-promoting lifestyle.[159] A moderate amount of stress, when regulatory mechanisms act within limits and few symptoms are observable, is constructive. **Daily hassles** are the *repeated and chronic strains of everyday life*. Daily hassles have a negative effect on both somatic health and psychological status.

## Table 5-12 Stimuli That Are Stressors

*Physical:* excessive or intense cold or heat, sound, light, motion, gravity, or electrical current

*Chemical:* alkalines, acids, drugs, toxic substances, hormones, gases, or food and water pollutants

*Microbiologic:* viruses, bacteria, moulds, parasites, or other infectious organisms

*Physiologic:* disease processes, surgery, immobilization, mechanical trauma, fever, organ hypo- or hyperfunction, or pain

*Psychological:* anticipated marriage or death, imagined events, intense emotional involvement, anxiety or other unpleasant feelings, distortions of body image, threats to self-concept, others' expectations of behaviour, rejection by or separation from loved ones, role changes, memory of negative past experiences, actual or perceived failures

*Developmental:* genetic endowment, prematurity, immaturity, maturational impairment, or the aging process

*Sociocultural:* sociocultural background and pressures, inharmonious interpersonal relationships, demands of our technologic society, social mobility, changing social mores, job pressures, economic worries, childrearing practices, redefinition of sex roles, or minority status

*Environmental:* unemployment, air and water pollution, overcrowding disasters, war, or crime

---

**Distress** is *negative, noxious, unpleasant, damaging stress* that results when adaptive capacity is decreased, or exhausted.

What is considered a stressor by one person may be considered pleasurable by another. The amount of stress in the immediate environment cannot be determined by examining only the stressor or the source of stress. *Certain principles, however, apply to most people:*[160]

- **The primary response to a stressor is behavioural.** When an event or situation is perceived as threatening, the person reacts in intensity and scope to meet the threat; physiologic impact is secondary.

- **The impact is cumulative.** Most stressors in the environment occur at levels below that which would cause immediate physical or emotional damage.

- **Circumstances alter the impact or harm done by a stressor.** The social and emotional context of an event and the attitude and previous experiences of the person are as important as the physical properties of the stimuli.

- **People are remarkably adaptable.** Each person has evolved a normal range of response or a unique pattern of defence. What may at first be considered uncomfortable or intolerable may eventually be perceived as normal routine. The immediate impact of a stressor is apparently different from long-term or indirect consequences, which are more difficult to detect.

- **Various psychological or social factors can ease or exaggerate the effects of a stressor.** If a stressor is predictable, it will not be as harmful as an unpredictable one. If the person feels in control of the situation or can relate positively or directly to the stressor, the effects are less negative. Studies show less stress response when people feel they are in control and actually have control over a stressful environment.

- **There are definite low points when stressors are poorly tolerated.** Time of day affects stress response. For example, in most people, hydrocortisone secretion normally peaks in the early morning and decreases throughout the day, until it is almost undetectable at night. Although diurnal rhythms vary from person to person, stressors may be better tolerated early in the day.

- **Conditioning is an important protection.** The person whose heart, lungs, and skeletal muscles are conditioned by exercise can withstand cardiovascular and respiratory effects of the alarm stage better than someone who leads a sedentary life.

- **Responses to stress throughout life are both local and general.** The **local adaptation syndrome**, typified by the inflammatory response, is the *method used to wall off and locally control effects of the physical stressors.* When the stressor cannot be handled locally, the *whole body responds to protect itself and ensure survival in the best way possible through the* **general adaptation syndrome.** The general body response augments body functions that protect the organism from injury, both psychological and physical, and suppresses those functions non-essential to life. The general adaptation syndrome is characterized by alarm and resistance stages and, when body resistance is not maintained, an end stage: exhaustion.[161]

**General Adaptation Syndrome** The **alarm stage** is an *instantaneous, short-term, life-preserving, and total sympathetic nervous system response* that occurs when the person consciously or unconsciously perceives a stressor and feels helpless, insecure, or biologically uncomfortable. This stage is typified by a "fight-or-flight" reaction. Perception of the stressor—the alarm reaction—stimulates the anterior pituitary to increase production of adrenocorticotropic hormone (ACTH). The adrenal cortex is stimulated by ACTH to increase production of glucocorticoids, primarily hydrocortisone or cortisol, and mineral corticoids, primarily aldosterone. Catecholamine release triggers an increase in sympathetic nervous system activity, which stimulates production of epinephrine and norepinephrine by the adrenal medulla, with their release at the adrenergic nerve endings. The alarm reaction also stimulates the posterior pituitary to release increased amounts of antidiuretic hormone.[162]

*Lazarus identified three psychological stages that occur during the alarm stage:* threat, warning, and impact. The psychological processes that occur when the stress stage is intensified begin with appraisal of the threat or potential degree of harm (warning). This process is cognitive and affective and involves perception, memory, thought, and a feeling response, such as anxiety, fear, anger, guilt, or shame, to the meaning of the impact of the threat.[163]

The **stage of resistance** is characterized by a number of different responses. *The adrenal cortex and medulla return to their normal rates of secreting hormones.* During the stage of resistance, the arousal changes that occurred during the alarm stage as a result of increased corticoid secretion disappear. Bodily responses eventually return to normal.[164]

If biological, psychological, or social stresses occur, either alone or in combination, over a long period without adequate relief, the stage of resistance is maintained. *With continued stressors, the person becomes distressed and manifests objective and subjective emotional, intellectual, and physiologic responses.* If adaptation occurs, the third stage is prevented or delayed.[165]

**Protective factors** *modify, ameliorate, or alter the person's response to stressors and to a potentially maladaptive outcome.* They are influenced by such factors as positive temperament; intelligence; the ability to relate well to others; participation in achievements; success in school or the job; family support, closeness, and safe family environment; and extended family, friends, and teachers.

The **stage of exhaustion** occurs when the *person is unable to continue efforts to adapt to internal and external environmental demands.* Physical or psychic disease, or death, results because the body can no longer compensate for, or correct, homeostatic imbalances. Manifestations of this stage are similar to those of the alarm stage except that all reactions now intensify at first, and then diminish in response. They show no inclination to return to an effective level of function. If stress continues to the stage of exhaustion, corticoid secretion and adaptation eventually decrease markedly.[166]

Hans Selye's contributions regarding the General Adaptation Syndrome have proved to be highly informative and helpful. Modern researchers are learning how some biological changes are adaptive in the short term, and can become hazardous in the long run.[167] When one is under stress, the brain's hypothalamus sends messages to the endocrine gland along *two major pathways.* One pathway activates the sympathetic division of the autonomic

nervous system, the *flight-or-fight* reaction, by producing the release of epinephrine and norepinephrine from the inner part of the adrenal glands. The second major pathway becomes active when the hypothalamus initiates activities along the *HPA axis* (hypothalamus–pituitary– adrenal cortex). The hypothalamus releases chemical messengers that communicate with the pituitary gland, which, in turn, sends messages to the cortex of the adrenal glands. The adrenal cortex secretes cortisol and other hormones that elevate blood sugar, which results in the protection of the body's tissues from inflammation in case of injury. See Figure 5-4 to view the brain and body under stress.[168]

Ideally, the best health promoting strategy is to identify all potential stressors that the person might encounter and then determine how to alter the stressors, or how to support the person's adaptive mechanisms and resources physically, emotionally, and socially. The relationship of stress to life

**Figure 5-4** The Brain and Body Under Stress

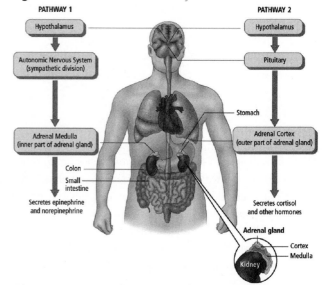

When a person is in danger or under stress, the hypothalamus sends messages to the endocrine glands along two major pathways. In one, the hypothalamus activates the sympathetic division of the autonomic nervous system, which stimulates the adrenal medulla to produce epinephrine and norepi nephrine. The result is the many bodily changes associated with "fight or flight." In the other pathway, messages travel along the HPA axis to the adrenal cortex, which produces cortisol and other hormones. The result is increased energy and protection from tissue inflammation in case of injury.

Source: Wade, C., Tavris, C., Saucier, D., Elias, L., *Psychology*, Second Canadian Edition, p. 545. Toronto: Pearson Prentice Hall, 2007. Reprinted with permission by Pearson Education Canada.

crises or changes must be considered whenever you are conducting health promotion measures or intervening with the ill person.[169]

Stress management involves the use of coping strategies in response to stressful situations. Coping strategies are adaptive when they protect the individual from harm, or if they strengthen the individual's ability to meet challenging situations. Meanwhile, coping strategies are considered maladaptive when the conflict being experienced is either intensified or remains unresolved.[170]

*Although responses to stressful situations vary, anxiety is a common response. Other responses include the adaptive mechanisms* described in Tables 5-5 and 5-13.

The **mind–body relationship**, the *effect of emotional responses to stress on body function and the emotional reactions to body conditions*, has been established through research and experience. Emotional factors are important in the precipitation, or exacerbation, of nearly every organic disease, and they are thought to increase susceptibility to infections. Stress and emotional distress, including depression, influence the function of the immune system via the central nervous system and endocrine mediation.

Winnipeg researchers MacPherson, Enns, and McWilliams investigated increased neuroticism and self-criticism in association with the presence versus absence of post-traumatic stress disorder (PTSD) in a nationally representative sample of adults who experienced a traumatic stressor. They concluded that self-criticism, and especially the broad personality domain of neuroticism, may represent robust psychological dimensions associated with the presence of PTSD. Further, these psychological dimensions are likely to be as important to assess as are more commonly assessed variables such as personal and familial psychiatric history.[171]

Another Winnipeg study by Iwasaki, Bartlett, and O'Neal revealed better understanding of the ways in which Aboriginal people with diabetes cope with stress. Focus groups were used to gather data. Based on the cross-thematic analysis of the data from a series of First Nations and Métis women and men with diabetes, three themes were identified. First, the strengths of Aboriginal people, either individual or collective, must be identified and used to facilitate healing from, or coping with, the experience of stress and trauma. Second, healing must be accomplished holistically by keeping a balance over mind, body, and spirit. Third, effective ways of coping with stress and healing caused by trauma can promote positive transformation for Aboriginal peoples and communities at both an individual and a community level.[172]

## CRITICAL THINKING

*What steps would you include in planning health promotion strategies for an Aboriginal client who has diabetes?*

Use of positive adaptive mechanisms, such as compensation, identification, and sublimation (described in Table 5-5), and positive coping strategies (described in Table 5-13), as well as visualization, imagery, and positive thinking, all promote a health response. Each of these strategies helps people to handle stressors.[173]

## Crisis Theory

**Definitions and Characteristics** **Crisis** is any *temporary situation that threatens the person's self-concept, necessitates reorganization of the psychological structure and behaviour, causes a sudden alteration in the person's expectation of self, and cannot be handled with the person's usual coping mechanisms.*[174]

*Crises always involve change and loss.* The changes or losses that occur usually result either in the person's inability to cope or, as a result of the crisis, in the person no longer being able to behave in the manner he or she once could. He or she must change certain behaviours to remain adaptive and functional. In the process, loss will be felt. The process of resolving the crisis followed by subsequent behavioural growth reveals that something is lost even while something else is gained.[175]

*During crisis, the person's ordinary behaviour is no longer successful—emotionally, intellectually, socially, or physically.*

| Table 5-13 | Positive Coping Strategies |
|---|---|
| **Affiliation** | Seek help and support from others. |
| **Altruism** | Dedicate self to meet the needs of others. |
| **Anticipation** | Prepare by thinking of future problems, realistic solutions, and consequences. |
| **Assertiveness** | Express one's feelings and thoughts directly. |
| **Humour** | Recognize the amusing aspects of a situation; maintain the ability to laugh. |
| **Self Observation** | Reflect on one's thoughts, feelings, motivations, and behaviour, and respond appropriately to self |

The person may refer to a crisis as a "tough time," or speak of the lack of coping ability by saying, "I'm at the end of my rope. I can't manage anymore." The usual coping skills, or adaptive mechanisms, do not work anymore. Old habits and daily patterns are disturbed. Thus, the person feels motivated to try new behaviour to cope with the new situation. Although behaviour during crisis is often inadequate or inappropriate to the present situation and may be different from normal, it should not be considered pathologic. For example, rage, bitterness, or prolonged crying by a usually jovial person may be anal forms of emotional release that pave the way for problem solving.[176]

Not all persons facing the same hazardous event will be in a state of crisis. *Some events or situations are viewed as a crisis by all persons*, of any age, in that some behavioural adjustment must be made by anyone facing that situation. *Crises vary in degree.* A situation may be perceived as major, moderate, or minimal in the degree of discomfort caused, and in the amount of behavioural change demanded. A person may view mild to moderate crises as stressful life situations, but the objective observer may see that the individual is being ineffective at coping.[177]

## CRITICAL THINKING

*What life events do you see as more stressful than others?*

Crisis differs from transition. **Transition** refers to a *passage, or movement, from one state or place to another that occurs over time, involving changes that can be managed.*[178]

**Types of Crises** Crises are divided into two broad categories: (1) developmental, maturational, or normative, and (2) situational, accidental, or catastrophic.[179] **Developmental crises** *occur during transition points, those periods that every person and family experience in the process of biopsychosocial maturation.* Examples are school entry, puberty, graduation, marriage, pregnancy, childbirth, menopause, retirement, and death. These are times in development when new relationships are formed and old relationships take on new aspects. New expectations are made of the person. Certain emotional tasks must be accomplished to move on to the next phase of development. The onset of the developmental or maturational crisis is gradual because it occurs as the person moves from one stage of development to another. The crisis resolves when the individual succeeds in new age-level behaviours; disruption does not last for the entire developmental phase.[180]

There are *three main reasons why someone may be unable to make role changes necessary to prevent a maturational crisis.*[181]

1. The person may be unable to picture self in a new role. Roles are learned, and adequate role models may not exist.

2. The person may be unable to make role changes because of a lack of intrapersonal resources (e.g., inadequate communication skills); the realization that, with life passing, certain goals will not be achieved; or the lack of past opportunities to learn how to cope with crises because of, say, overprotection.

3. Others in the social system may refuse to see the person in a different role. For example, when an adolescent tries to move from childhood to the adult role, the parent may persist in keeping him or her in the child role.

Several factors help the person adjust to a new life era: (1) desire for change and boredom with present experiences; (2) agenda for a life course—present versus future plans; (3) accomplishments in the present era; (4) past success in coping with turning points; (5) group support in meeting turning points; and (6) examples of how peers have coped with similar situations. The more clear-cut the cultural definitions, the less frightening is the future situation. This is true because the person has clear models of behaviour and can prepare in advance for change.

**Situational crisis** *is an external event or situation not necessarily a part of normal living, often sudden, unexpected, and unfortunate, that looms larger than the person's immediate resources or ability to cope and thereby demands a change in behaviour.* Life goals are threatened. Tension and anxiety are evoked if unresolved problems and crises from the past are reawakened. The amount of time taken for healthy, or even unhealthy, adaptation to occur usually ranges from one to six weeks, although resolution may take longer. A situational crisis may occur at the same time as a developmental crisis.

Situational crises include natural disasters, such as hurricane, tornado, earthquake, and flood; loss through separation, divorce, or death of a loved one; loss of one's job, money, or valued possessions; and a job change. Additions to the family, such as an unwanted pregnancy; return of a prisoner of war, a deserter, or someone taken as a hostage; adoption of a child; and remarriage resulting in a step-parent and stepsiblings, all can cause a change in lifestyle. Each is a potential crisis. Illness, hospitalization, or institutionalization; a power struggle on the job; a sudden change in role responsibilities; and a forced geographic relocation are other examples. Rape, suicide, homicide, and imprisonment can also be classified as this type of crisis.

Crisis always involves a sense of loss. Developmental and situational events that involve loss, in reality or symbolically, are listed in Table 5-14.[182]

| Table 5-14 | Loss Situations That Contribute to Crises |

1. Period of weaning in infancy; learning to wait
2. First haircut, even when it involves pride and anticipation
3. Period of increasing locomotion, exploration, and bowel and bladder control and resultant loss of dependency
4. Loss of baby teeth, baby possessions, toys, clothes, or pets
5. Change in the body, body image, self-concept, and self-attribute with ongoing growth and development
6. Change in body size and shape and in feelings accompanying pregnancy and childbirth; loss of body part or function, external or internal, through accident, illness, or aging
7. Departure of children from the home when they go to school or marry
8. Menopause and loss of childbearing functions
9. Loss of hearing, vision, memory, strength, and other changes and losses associated with old age
10. Changes and losses in relationships with others as the person moves from childhood to adulthood—loss of friends and lovers; separation from or death of family members; changes in residence, occupation, or place of business; promotions and graduations
11. Losses with symbolic meanings, such as the loss of a symptom that attracted others' attention; a loss or change that necessitates a change in body image; or "loss of face," honour, prestige, or status
12. Loss of home due to natural disaster or relocation projects; loss of possessions or money
13. Loss experienced with divorce or incapacitation of a loved one

**Phases of Crisis** All crises display a sudden and then a later restructuring of biopsychosocial integration before normal function can be restored. The phases involved are (1) shock, followed closely by general realization of the crisis; (2) defensive retreat; (3) acknowledgment; and, finally, (4) adaptation or disorganization.[183]

The paradigm set forth by Aguilera suggests that whether a person experiences a crisis in response to a stressful situation depends on the following three factors:

- *Perception of the event:* if the individual perceives the event realistically, he or she will likely draw upon adequate resources. On the other hand, if the event is distorted, the individual's attempts to problem solve will be largely ineffective.

- *Availability of situational supports:* the person's network of those who can be depended upon to help the individual cope.

- *Adequate coping mechanism:* the individual's ability to draw on coping strategies that have worked in the past. If coping mechanisms fail, tension and anxiety increase.[184]

Table 5-15 presents the feelings and behaviours that may be experienced by the person during the phases of crisis. These behaviours are normal when a crisis is encountered and you must be aware of that fact in your assessment. Grief and mourning processes are discussed further in Chapter 13.

Table 5-16 summarizes factors that influence how the person, family, or community will react to and cope with crisis and, thereby, the crisis outcome.[185]

The family unit undergoes essentially the same phases of crisis and manifests similar reactions as the designated client, although the intensity and timing may be different for each person. Furthermore, members of the family in crisis interact with each other, often compounding the crisis reaction and creating more intense or complex behavioural responses. Roles are disorganized; expectations of self, other family members, and outsiders change; and individual needs intensify. All families have problems, and all families have ways of managing them, successfully or otherwise.[186]

*Crisis events for the family include the developmental and situational crises previously discussed, which can be categorized as follows:*[187]

- **Dismemberment.** Medical emergencies; loss of family member through death, divorce, separation, marriage, or geographic move.

- **Accession.** Addition of family member through birth, adoption, marriage, or foster placement, or older relative moving into the home.

- **Demoralization.** Loss of morale in the family unit through delinquency, legal problems, economic problems, job loss, child or spouse abuse, certain illnesses such as AIDS, crimes, or events that cause alienation from the community or carry a social stigma.

- **A combination of the above.**

*Various factors influence how prone a group or community is to crisis:*[188]

1. Personal strengths, characteristics, and level of need satisfaction of its members
2. Social and economic stability of family units or groups versus social and economic inequities among ethnic, racial, or socioeconomic groups

Table 5-15  Individual Reactions in the Crisis Phases

| Phase and Duration | Feelings | Cognitive Manifestations | Physical Symptoms | Interpersonal/Social Behaviour |
|---|---|---|---|---|
| **Initial Impact; Shock** (duration of 1 to 24–48 hours) | Anxiety. Helplessness. Chaos. Overwhelmed. Hopeless. Incomplete. Detached. Despair. Depersonalized. Panic. Self-concept threatened. Self-esteem low. Anguish may be expressed by silent, audible, or uncontrollable crying<br><br>*Developmental Crisis*<br>Response more gradual. Feelings less intense. May feel anxiety, frustration, lack of confidence, discouragement, imperfection, unfamiliarity with self, loss of self-control as realizes new responsibilities. Cannot move emotionally into next stage or change life perception | Altered sensorium. Disorganized thinking. Unable to plan, reason logically, or understand situation. Impaired judgment. Preoccupation with image or hallucination of last object/person | Somatic distress. May suffer physical illness or injury and ignore symptoms. Shortness of breath. Choking. Sighing. Hyperventilation. Weakness. Fatigue. Tremors. Anorexia. Lump in throat or abdomen. Respiratory or other infection may develop | Disorganized behaviour. Habitual or automatic behaviours used unsuccessfully. Withdrawn. Docile. Hyperactive. May appear overtly as if happened or may be unable to carry out routine behaviour. Lacks initiative for daily tasks. May need assistance meeting basic needs. Very suggestible, even if contrary to values or well-being<br><br>*Developmental Crisis*<br>May try to do more than is biologically or emotionally realistic. Unable to achieve behaviour appropriate to role or to change inappropriate behaviour in relationships |
| **Denies Retreat** (duration of hours to weeks) | May feel tense and inadequate, but usually feels as if nothing is wrong because of use of repression and defence mechanisms. Apathetic or euphoric. Feelings displaced onto other objects | Tries habitual coping mechanisms unsuccessfully. States nothing is wrong. May try to redefine problem unrealistically. Fantasizes about what could be done, how well past problems handled. Avoids thinking about event. May be disoriented. Maintains rigid thinking. States same ideas over and over. May be unable to devise alternate courses of action or predict effects of behaviour | Denies symptoms including presence of physical illness | Tries habitual behaviours and defence mechanisms unsuccessfully. May seek support of others indirectly. Usually withdraws from others. Superficial response. May avoid reality with overactivity. Resistant to change suggested by others. Unwilling to initiate new behaviour. Ineffective, disorganized behaviour. May be unable to maintain daily |

*(continued)*

Table 5-15 (continued)

| Phase and Duration | Feelings | Cognitive Manifestations | Physical Symptoms | Interpersonal/Social Behaviour |
|---|---|---|---|---|
| | | Denies through rationalization cause for situation | | activities, work performance, or social roles. Denies through demands, complaints, or projections of inadequacy |
| | | *Developmental Crisis*<br>Denies that physical, emotional, or role changes are occurring or that different behaviour is expected; behaviour reflects earlier developmental stage; developmental tasks not worked out or met | | |
| **Acknowledgment of Reality** (duration varies) | Tension and anxiety rise. Loneliness. Irritable. Depressed. Agitated. Apathetic. Self-hate. Low self-esteem. Grief—mourning occurs. Gradually self-satisfaction increases. Self-concept becomes more positive. Gains self-confidence in ability to cope | Becomes aware of facts about change, loss, event. Asks questions about situation. Slowly redefines situation. Attempts problem solving. May be disorganized in thinking. Trial-and-error approach to problems. Gradually perceives alternatives. Makes appropriate plans. Gives up undesirable goals. Validates personal experiences and feelings. Coping skills improved | Symptoms may reappear or intensify. New symptoms may occur. May somatize feelings. Gradually regains physical health | Exhibits mourning behaviours. Gradually demonstrates appropriate behaviours and resumes roles. Uses suggestions. Tries new approaches. Greater maturity demonstrated |
| **Resolution Adaptation, Change** (duration of mourning and crisis work may be 6–12 months) | Painful feelings integrated into self-concept and sense of maturity. New sense of worth. Firm identity. Gradual increase in self-satisfaction about mastery of situation. Gradual lowering of anxiety. Does not feel bitter, guilty, or ashamed | Perceives crisis situation in positive way. Integrates crisis event into self. Problem solving successful. Discusses feelings about event. Organizes thinking and planning. Redefines priorities. Does not blame self or others. Remembers comfortably and realistically pleasures and disappointments of last relationship | Functions at optimum level | Discovers new resources. Uses support systems and resources appropriately. Resumes status and roles. Strengthens relations with others. Adaptive in relationships. Lifestyle may be changed. Initiates measures to prevent similar crisis if at all possible |

*Note: Temporary retreat emotionally, mentally, and socially is adaptive and protective from perceived stress and loss and overwhelming anxiety. Allows time to gradually realize what has happened; avoids debilitating effects of high anxiety or panic. Initially person fluctuates between the phases of Defensive Retreat and Acknowledgment of Reality.

Table 5-16 Factors Influencing the Outcome of Crisis

1. **Perception of the event.** If the event (or the implications or consequences of it) threatens the self-concept; conflicts with the value system, self-expectations, or wishes for the future; contributes to a sense of shame or guilt; or is demoralizing or damaging to self, family, or personal objects, the situation is defined as hazardous. The perception of the event is reality for the person or family, regardless of how others might define reality. How the event is perceived depends in large measure on past experience.

2. **Degree of perceived dependency on a lost object.** This is also crucial; the greater the dependency, the more difficult the resolution of loss.

3. **Physical and emotional status.** This includes level of health, amount of energy present, age, genetic endowment, and biological rhythms of the person or family, or the general well-being of the community. Working through crisis takes considerable energy.

4. **Coping techniques or mechanisms and level of personal maturity.** If adaptive capacities are already strained, or if the stress is overwhelming, the person will cling to old habits or existing defences, and behaviour will very likely be inappropriate to the task at hand. The person or family who has met developmental tasks all along and who perceives self as able to cope will adapt more easily in any crisis. The group or community that has mechanisms, policies, or procedures defined and in operation to cope with the unexpected event or disaster can better meet the crisis.

5. **Previous experiences with similar situations.** The person, family, or group needs to learn to cope with stress, change, and loss. If past crises were handled by distorting reality or by withdrawing, when similar crises arise, burdens of the prior failure will be added to the problem of coping with the new situation. Unresolved crises are cumulative in effect. The most recent crisis revives the denial, depression, anger, or maladaptation that was left unsettled from past crises. If the person, family, or group successfully deals with crises, self-confidence and self-esteem will thereby be increased, and future crises will be handled more effectively.

6. **Realistic aspects of the current situation.** These include personal, material, or economic losses, the extent to which group ties or community services are interrupted, and changes required in living pattern or family life necessitated by the loss.

7. **Cultural influences.** How the person is trained and socialized in the home to solve problems and meet crisis situations; the use of religious, cultural, or legal ceremonies or rituals to handle separation or loss and facilitate mourning; expectations of how the social group will support the person or family during crisis; and the method established by the community to provide help—all influence present behaviour.

8. **Availability and response of family and close friends, community groups, or other helping resources, including professional persons.** The less available the environmental or emotional support systems are to decrease stress or buttress the coping response, the more hazardous the event will be. The family system, by its influence on the development of the self-concept and maturity, can increase or decrease the person's vulnerability to crisis.

3. Adherence to versus rebellion against social norms by families and groups

4. Adequacy of community resources to meet social, economic, health, welfare, and recreational needs of individuals and families

5. Geographic, environmental, and climatic resources and characteristics that surround the group or community

The community can be affected by natural disasters, such as floods, tornadoes, hurricanes, earthquakes, volcanic eruptions, tsunami, and blizzards; by disasters resulting from advances in our civilization, such as chemical or radiation spills and electrical blackouts; and by disasters for which humans are responsible, such as sniping in a schoolyard or restaurant, fire, and war.[189] Reactions of a community to any of these disasters will be influenced by the factors listed in Table 5-17.[190]

A group in crisis demonstrates:

■ Acute unmanageable anxiety that interferes with daily function

■ Sudden alteration in perceptions of meaning, purpose, and goals—a turning point

■ Sudden disruption in cognitive, emotional, or physical alterations

Communities in crisis have characteristics in common with individuals and groups in crisis. The most immediate

## Table 5-17 Factors That Influence Community Response to Disasters

1. **Element of surprise versus preparedness.** If warnings are not given about an impending crisis—or if warnings are given without an action plan—panic, shock, denial, and defensive retreat are more likely to occur.

2. **Separation of family members.** Children are especially affected by separation. The family should be evacuated from a disaster area as a unit.

3. **Availability of outside help**, such as the sending of food, shelter, and workers.

4. **Leadership.** Someone must make decisions and give directions. Usually the police, Red Cross and Civil Defence workers, military, or professionals in a community are seen as authoritative persons. Coordination of the activities of all of these groups is essential to deliver effective services and avoid chaos.

5. **Communication.** Public information centres should be established to quickly avoid rumour, provide reassurance and direction, and ensure that all citizens get information about coping measures, evacuation, reconstruction, rehabilitation, and available financial aid. Otherwise, later, citizens will be bitter and suspicious when some learn that others benefited more than they did.

6. **Measures taken to help reorientation.** Communication networks lay the foundation for the re-identification of individuals into family and social groups, and for the registration of survivors.

7. **Presence of plans for individuals and social institutions to cope with disaster,** including evacuation of a population from a stricken area if necessary. Good emergency plans focus on the following concerns:
   a. Preservation of life and health through rescue, triage, inoculation, and treatment of the injured
   b. Conservation and distribution of resources, such as shelter, water, food, and blankets
   c. Conservation of public order by police surveillance to prevent looting and further accidents or injuries
   d. Maintenance of morale through the dispatching of health and welfare workers to the disaster scene
   e. Administration of health services

social consequence of a disaster is the disruption of normal social patterns and services; the community is socially paralyzed. Furthermore, one disaster such as a chemical spill may contribute to another disaster, such as an explosion or fire.

In a major disaster, many victims will be in shock. This is usually followed by the phase of defensive retreat, in response to warnings of disaster, orders of evacuation, destruction of homes, and disruption of water, electricity, heat, food supplies, communication, traffic, and transportation. Furthermore, there is potential inability of the health agencies to care for the injured and ill because of manpower and supply shortages or damage. In addition to individual reactions, an atmosphere of tension, fear, confusion, and suspicion exists; facts are distorted and rumours are rampant. Normal functioning is reduced because businesses, vital services, schools, and recreational areas may be closed. Yet, one may see all available community service providers, such as police officers, firefighters, construction workers, city planners, Red Cross volunteers, medical personnel, and corporation executives, co-operating to assist in rescue, cleanup, and the restoration of services and a sense of normality. Although some people are in shock or denial, a proportionate few will display altruism and heroic behaviour.

There will be a few who take advantage of the chaos to loot and steal, and a few businesses may profit.

### Bioterriorism and Emergency Preparedness

In Canada, all levels of government are involved in preparing for and responding to an emergency or disaster. At the federal level, if assistance is requested or if the emergency involves more than one province or territory, the Government of Canada will mobilize the resources.[191]

Response to external emergencies is often quicker than the response to internal stresses or crises. About 10 to 25 percent of the victims remain reality-oriented, calm, and able to develop and implement a plan of action. These people often are those with advanced training. However, they may experience their own crisis phases later.

## HEALTH PROMOTION IN NURSING PRACTICE

Table 5-18 summarizes how the theories discussed in this chapter can be applied in nursing and health care practice.

## Table 5-18 Health Promotion Implications of Selected Theories

| Theorist/Theory | Practice Implications |
| --- | --- |
| **General Systems Theory** | 1. Consider self as an individual system as well as part of other systems.<br>2. Consider client (individual, family, group, or community) as part of a system in implementing nursing process.<br>3. Consider client in totality and the relationships and interactions between parts: physiologic, psychological, spiritual, and sociocultural. Dysfunction in one part affects all parts.<br>4. Client, as a system, has definite range for absorption, processing, and retention of stimuli. Avoid overstimulation or deprivation of stimuli. Assess needs and intervene accordingly.<br>5. Help client determine resources and supportive systems that will maintain or return function and wellness. |
| **Skinner's Operant Conditioning Theory** | 1. In teaching or therapy, follow the guidelines previously described for a behaviour modification program.<br>2. The general procedure for behaviour modification is to:<br>  a. Plan what behaviour is to be established; plan what is to be taught and at what specific time. Objectives are specific. Follow the teaching or treatment plan explicitly.<br>  b. Determine available reinforcers. Feedback from physical sensations, excelling over others, or the teacher's affection—all may reinforce. The only way to determine whether a consequence is rewarding is to observe its effect on the behaviour associated with it.<br>  c. Identify the responses that can be made by the person.<br>  d. Plan how reinforcements can be efficiently scheduled so the behaviour is likely to be repeated. Reinforcements must immediately follow the desired behaviour. |
| **Freud's Psychoanalytic Theory** | 1. Insight into own behaviour can add to personal maturity and understanding of others.<br>2. Constructs of id, ego, superego, conscious–unconscious continuum, manifestations of anxiety and defence mechanisms, and psychosexual development are useful in assessment and therapy.<br>3. All behaviour is meaningful; outer behaviour may hide inner need or conflict.<br>4. Use knowledge of psychosexual development to teach parents about norms and meaning of child's behaviour.<br>5. Transference and resistance must be worked through in therapy. |
| **Sullivan's Interpersonal Theory** | 1. One Genus Postulate basic to nursing practice with clients from all settings and backgrounds.<br>2. Assess developmental stage and task; teach family about normal development and development of self-system.<br>3. Promote syntaxic, rather than parataxic, mode of experiencing through intervention.<br>4. Promote positive experiences for client so that "good-me," or positive self-concept, can develop. |
| **Erikson's Epigenetic Theory** | 1. Assessment of, and insight into, own stage of development.<br>2. Use knowledge of eight stages and psychosexual tasks in assessment, therapy, and teaching parents about child development.<br>3. Help clients and staff realize that emotional development is a lifelong process and that society influences health and behaviour. |
| **Beck's Cognitive Theory** | 1. Facilitate person's recognition of how thoughts influence emotions through questions, examples, examination of person's self-conversation. |

*(continued)*

Table 5-18 (continued)

| Theorist/Theory | Practice Implications |
| --- | --- |
| | 2. Facilitate person's recognition of irrational beliefs by having person tell what would happen if belief actually was true; enumerate reasons for problems created by the belief. |
| | 3. Facilitate person's recognition that rational beliefs influence emotional or physical distress by systematically exploring situations related to feelings of inadequacy, helplessness, aloneness, depression, or anger. Sort out facts in a supportive way. |
| | 4. Facilitate person's efforts to revise and contradict irrational beliefs through alternative self-messages, homework assignments, role-play, rehearsal, and invalidation of distorted belief. |
| | 5. Restructuring experience with person helps him or her recognize and revise unrealistic expectations and negative self-conversations, reduce sensitivity to other's response, and interact more flexibly and effectively. |
| | 6. Therapy lasts about six months and is divided into stages:<br>  a. Eliciting and answering automatic thoughts<br>  b. Discovering and testing underlying assumptions<br>  c. Cognitive restructuring |
| | 7. Basis for improvement is in change of basic philosophy of the person, not necessarily in removal of present symptoms. |
| | 8. Therapist is active in confronting person; person is expected to do homework assignments. |
| | 9. Therapist is to act as role model for person; as an authoritative, scientific helper who is highly trained and rational, and to show unconditional positive regard for the person. |
| **Bandura's Social Learning Theory** | 1. Your appearance and behaviour are a model for client. |
| | 2. Determine who significant adults were in the person's life and who role models were. |
| | 3. In teaching, demonstrate desired self-care behaviour. |
| | 4. Recovered person visiting an ill client can serve as model for rehabilitation and a normal life (e.g., person with mastectomy, colostomy, amputation, alcoholism). |
| | 5. Demonstrate nurturing approaches or discipline methods to child client so that parents can learn effective childrearing methods. |
| | 6. Nurse–client relationship is a behavioural model of trust and interpersonal relations for the client. |
| **Piaget's Theory of Cognitive Development** | 1. Teach parents about process of child's cognitive development and the implications for education, purchase of toys, and interactions. |
| | 2. Assess cognitive stage of client as basis for planning content and presentation in teaching sessions. |
| | 3. Assess cognitive development to determine language and abstraction level to use in therapy. |
| | 4. Use knowledge of cognitive development in play therapy. |
| **Kohlberg's Theory of Moral Development/Gilligan's Theory of Moral Development** | 1. Assess own level of moral development. |
| | 2. Assess client's level of moral development when working with children, adolescents, or adults. |
| | 3. Through your modelling, clarification, explanation, and validation, contribute to client's moral development. |
| **Existential Theory** | 1. Each person is in charge of own destiny; each person is primary agent of change and is responsible for own future. Destiny is not in hands of others. |

(continued)

**Table 5-18** (continued)

| Theorist/Theory | Practice Implications |
|---|---|
| | 2. In therapy, be concerned with basic conflicts that are outgrowths of confrontation with existence—death, freedom, helplessness, loss, isolation, aloneness, anxiety, and meaninglessness—and promote reflection about these life issues. |
| | 3. Nurse is facilitator who understands and accepts the person as being and becoming. Main themes of therapy are self-awareness, self-determination, search for meaning, and relatedness. |
| | 4. In therapy, assist person in learning how to confront self, how behaviour is viewed by others, how others feel about own behaviour, and how behaviour contributes to opinions about self. |
| | 5. In therapy, assist person to learn how to change; give support to reduce anxiety, low self-esteem, and loneliness. |
| | 6. Help person move to self-actualization and achieve maximum potential. |
| **Maslow's Theory of Motivation and Hierarchy of Needs** | 1. Assessment can be done around hierarchy of needs. Planning and intervention must consider need hierarchy and priorities in care. |
| | 2. Person is a unified whole, not divided into components of needs. |
| | 3. Higher-level needs can be met simultaneously with some lower-level needs. |
| | 4. Concepts of needs and motivation can be used in teaching and therapy. By meeting needs of client on one level, you can help client mature and feel motivated to meet growth needs. |
| **Carl Rogers's Theory on Self-Concept and Person-Centred Therapy** | 1. Assess own self-concept and self-actualization needs prior to counselling clients. |
| | 2. Assess client's self-concept; promote positive experiences and contribute to development of positive self-concept. |
| | 3. In therapy, assume as much as possible client's frame of reference to perceive world as she or he does. |
| | 4. Be accepting, warm, genuine, and empathic to help client discover self and mature. |
| **Stress and Adaptation Theory** | 1. Assess physical, emotional, and cognitive manifestations of stress response. |
| | 2. Assess level of anxiety. |
| | 3. Determine stage of adaptation. |
| | 4. Teach stress management methods. |
| | 5. Counsel as necessary. |
| | 6. Intervene as necessary to prevent exhaustion stage. |
| **Crisis Theory/Crisis Intervention (Brief Therapy)** | 1. Assess presence of emotional and physical symptoms. |
| | 2. Assess presence of emotional and physical symptoms. |
| | 3. Determine whether person is suicidal or homicidal. |
| | 4. Explore support system and usual coping patterns. |
| | 5. Clarify crisis event, its onset and impact. |
| | 6. Provide comfort measures for client. |
| | 7. Help client work through feelings about situation. |
| | 8. Develop plan with client to resolve crisis; develop alternative options to achieve goal. |
| | 9. Reinforce strengths and healthy adaptive patterns. |
| | 10. Involve client in decisions and working on specific tasks. |
| | 11. Help person establish necessary social relationships; assist person in seeking and accepting help. |
| | 12. Refer as necessary for additional services. |

# SUMMARY

1. Various theories describe aspects of the developing person. No theory describes all dimensions (physiologic, emotional, cognitive, cultural, social, moral, and spiritual) of development.

2. Biological theories include the study of genetics, biochemistry, neurophysiology, immunology, maturational factors, biological rhythms, and biological deficiencies.

3. Ecologic theories include study of sociologic variables, culture, geographic environments, and systems such as the family, school, community, and organization.

4. Behavioural theories study behaviour that is learned, or modified, through various kinds of conditioning, and shows a measurable outcome.

5. Psychoanalytic and neo-analytic theories include study of the intrapsychic processes, emotional life stage, and interpersonal development of the person; and the effect of these dimensions on behaviour of the person, family unit, or the broader society.

6. Cognitive theories include study of the stages of the person's cognitive development, the person as an information processor and problem solver, and effects of modelling or imitation on behaviour.

7. Moral theories study how the person learns to incorporate societal and philosophic norms into behaviour and the relationship of moral to cognitive and emotional behaviour.

8. Existential and humanistic theories study the needs, self-concept, and dynamic aspects of the person's existence and development within the self and in relation to the environment or society.

9. Stress and crisis theories study the person's responses to routine, severe, and overwhelming events. The local and general adaptation syndromes and phases of response to various types of crisis explain the reactions of the person to unexpected, situational, or developmental events.

10. The theories presented in this chapter form the basis for various approaches for therapy, nursing, and health care.

## Interesting Websites

### Huntington Society of Canada
www.hsc-ca.org
On this site you will find information about Huntington disease, the many ways the Huntington Society works to support the needs of people with the disease, and opportunities to support the organization's work.

### The Hospital for Sick Children
www.sickkids.on.ca
Affectionately called "Sick Kids," this is one of the largest paediatric academic health science centres in the world, with an international reputation for excellence in health care, research, and teaching.

### Genome Canada
www.genomecanada.ca
This is the primary funding and information resource relating to genetics and proteomics in Canada. To date, Genome Canada has invested more than $379 million across Canada. It has established five genome centres across the country and has a main objective to ensure that Canada becomes a world leader in genomics and proteomics research.

## Key Terms

accession (183)
accommodation (169)
adaptation (169)
alarm stage (179)
all-or-nothing thinking or dichotomous thinking (167)
anomie (152)
anxiety (161)
assertion training (157)
assimilation (169)
attributes (154)
behaviour (156)

behaviour modification (156)
behaviourism (156)
behaviourists (155)
bioecologic systems theory (153)
bioinformatics (148)
boundary (154)
cathexis (161)
classical conditioning (155)
closed system (153)
cognitive theory (166)

compartmentalization (162)
compensation (162)
concept of anxiety (165)
condensation (162)
conscience (161)
conscious (161)
conversion (162)
crisis (181)
daily hassles (178)
demoralization (183)
denial (162)

developmental crises (182)
differentiation (153)
dismemberment (183)
displacement (162)
disqualifying the positive (167)
dissociation (162)
distress (179)
dizygotic twins (145)
ecology (151)
ego (161)
ego ideal (161)

emotional isolation (162)

emotional reasoning (167)

environment (154)

equilibration (169)

equilibrium (154)

eustress (178)

evolutionary processes (154)

existentialism (174)

exosystems (153)

extinction (156)

feedback (154)

fortune teller error (167)

general adaptation syndrome (179)

goals (154)

heterozygous (145)

homozygous (145)

humanism (175)

id (160)

identification (162)

information/ communication (154)

instincts (drives) (161)

intelligence (169)

intermittent schedule of reinforcement (157)

interpersonal security (165)

introjection (163)

jumping to conclusions or arbitrary inference (167)

labelling and mislabelling (167)

learning (155, 156, 169)

libido (sexuality) (161)

local adaptation syndrome (179)

localization of brain function (149)

macrosystems (155)

magnification (catastrophizing) or minimization (167)

maturational (169)

mental filter or selective inattention (167)

mesosystems (153)

metacognition (172)

microsystems (153)

mind reading (167)

mind–body relationship (181)

modelling (168)

monozygotic twins (145)

negative reinforcement (156)

neo-analytic theorists (159)

neo-behaviourists (155)

neurotransmitters (149)

open system (153)

operant conditioning (156)

organization (154)

overgeneralization (167)

parts (154)

personalization (167)

phenomenal field (175)

pleasure principle (160)

polygenic (146)

positive reinforcement (156)

preconscious (161)

primary process thinking (160)

principle of communal existence (165)

principle of functional activity (165)

principle of organization (165)

projection (163)

protective factors (180)

psychoanalytic theory (159)

psychodynamic perspective (160)

psychology (142)

punishment (156)

rationalization (163)

reaction formation (163)

reality principle (161)

regression (163)

reinforcement schedule (156)

repression (163)

satisfaction of needs (165)

schema (169)

secondary process thinking (161)

self-actualization (176)

self-system (165)

shaping (156)

should statements (167)

situational crisis (182)

social skills training (157)

social system (153)

stage of exhaustion (180)

stage of resistance (180)

stress (178)

stressors (178)

sublimation (163)

subsystems (153)

superego (161)

suppression (163)

suprasystems (153)

symbolization (163)

synergy (153)

system (153)

tension (160)

three-person system or triangle (153)

time out (157)

token economies (157)

transfer (156)

transference (161)

transition (182)

unconscious (161)

undoing (163)

# Chapter 6

## The Developing Person: Principles of Growth and Development

*Nothing has a stronger influence on their children than the unlived lives of their parents.*

Carl Jung

## Objectives

*Study of this chapter will enable you to:*

1 Define growth, development, and related terms.

2 Explore general insights into and principles of human behaviour.

3 Examine various influences that have an effect on the developing person: prenatal variables involving father, mother, and fetus; variables related to childbirth; early childhood variables, including child abuse; sociocultural experiences; and environmental factors.

4 Relate information in this chapter to yourself as a developing person.

5 Apply knowledge from this chapter when assessing the person through the lifespan cycle.

6 Teach the person and family about factors that influence the development of self or offspring, when appropriate.

Developmental theory, the study of the person throughout the lifespan, centres on certain principles of the person's growth and development. Although growth and development are usually thought of as a forward movement, a kind of adding on such as an increase in height and weight or the self-actualizing personality, the model can also apply to reversal, decay, deterioration, or death. Three kinds of reversals occur: (1) loss of some part, such as occurs with catabolism (changing of living tissue into wastes or destructive metabolism); (2) purposefully changing behaviour when it is no longer useful; and (3) death.[1]

Growth and development are generally characterized by the following:[2]

- Direction, goal, or end state
- Identifiable stage or era
- Forward progression, so that once a stage is worked through, the person does not return to the same position
- Increasing specialization
- Causal forces that are either genetic or environmental
- Potentialities and capabilities for various behaviours and achievements

## DIMENSIONS OF TIME

Theories about time dimensions, including assumptions about behaviour, and principles of growth and development are used in assessment and in health promotion interventions. This theory is applicable to all age eras.

Lifetime, or chronologic age, is frequently used as an index of maturation and development, but it is only a rough indicator of the person's position on any one of the numerous physical or psychological dimensions. Furthermore, society itself is a reference point for understanding behaviour. What is appropriate for a 14-year-old individual in one society is not appropriate in a different society.

**Social time**, or *social expectations of behaviour for each age era*, is not necessarily synchronous with biological time. Neither chronologic age nor maturational stage are in themselves a determinant of aging status. They can only signify the biological potentiality on which a system of age norms and age grading can operate to shape the life cycle.[3]

Historical time shapes the social system, and the social system creates a changing set of age norms and a changing age-grade system that shapes the person's life cycle. **Historical time** refers to a *series of economic, political, and social events that directly shape the life course of the person*, such as industrialization and urbanization, which create the social cultural context and changing definitions of the phases of the life cycle.[4] A *group of people born at a certain calendar time* (cohort) has, as a group, a particular background and demographic composition so that most of the people of that specific age or generation will have similar experiences, level of education, fertility and childrearing patterns, sexual mores, work and labour force participation patterns, value systems, leisure patterns, religious behaviour, consumer behaviour, and general ideas about life.[5]

*Social time* is prescribed by each society in that all societies rationalize the passage of lifetime, divide life into socially relevant units, and transform calendar or biological time into social time. Thus, age grading occurs; the life cycle consists of a succession of formally age-graded, descriptive norms. Duties, rights, and rewards are differentially distributed to age groups. In societies in which division of labour is simple and social change is slow, a single age-grade system becomes formalized. When this happens, family, work, religious, and political roles are all allocated by society. A modern, complex, rapidly changing society, which has several overlapping systems of age status, has some tasks and roles that are tied to chronologic age and some that are more fluid or less clearly defined. In every society there is a time to be a child and dependent, a time to be educated to whatever level is needed, a time to go to work, to form a partnership, to have a family, to retire, and finally a time to die. The members of the society have a general consensus about these age expectations and norms, although perceptions may vary somewhat by age, sex, or social class. Patterns of timing can play an important role with respect to self-concept and self-esteem, depending on the person's level of awareness about his or her fit to social age norms and the rigidity in the culture. The young are more likely to deny that age is a valid criterion by which to judge behaviour. Middle-aged and older adults, who see

greater constraints in the age-norm system than do the young, have learned that to be too far ahead or behind in one's developmental stage involves negative consequences. Many of the major marks in the life cycle are ordered and sequential. They are social rather than biological, and their time is socially regulated.[6]

*This book is organized along chronologic lines, with the life cycle divided into different periods, rather than organized around a topical approach.* The person's life is divided into the following chronologic stages: the prenatal period (from the moment of conception to birth); infancy (birth to 1 year); toddlerhood (1 to 3 years); preschool (3 to 6 years); school years (6 to 12 years); adolescence (12 to 20 or 25 years); young adulthood (20 or 25 to 45 years); middle age (45 to 65 or 70 years); and late maturity (65 or 70 years and older). *The divisions are somewhat arbitrary because it is difficult to assign definite ages; individual lives are not marked off so precisely.*

The study of development is not merely a search for facts about people at certain ages. Development study involves finding *patterns*, or *general principles*, that apply to most people most of the time.

People are often at one level in one area of development and at another level in another area. For example, an 11-year-old girl may have begun to menstruate—an activity that marks her physical transition from childhood to puberty—before she has outgrown many childish feelings and thoughts. A 48-year-old man who took several years to find his career direction, who married in his thirties, and who became a father in his forties may, in many important psychological ways, be in the young adulthood period. On the other hand, his 49-year-old neighbour, who settled early on a professional direction and into family life, may already be a grandfather and may act and feel more like a middle-aged man. The individual differences among people are so great that they enter and leave these age periods at different times of life. People are aware of their own timing and are quick to describe themselves as "early," "late," or "on time" regarding developmental tasks.

Ideal **norms**, *standards* or *expectancies*, for different behaviours vary among different groups of people. The entire life cycle is speeded up for the poor and working classes, who tend to finish their education earlier than middle- or upper-class people. The poor and working take their first jobs sooner, marry younger, have children earlier, reach the peak of their careers earlier, and become grandparents earlier. These differences are related to financial needs that make it imperative for poor and working-class people to get paying jobs earlier in life. People from more affluent backgrounds can pursue their educations for a longer time. They can use young adulthood to explore options, and then delay becoming financially independent and beginning a family.

# PRINCIPLES OF GROWTH AND DEVELOPMENT

## Definitions

Certain words are basic to understanding the person, and they are used repeatedly. They are defined below for the purpose of this book.

**Growth** refers to *increase in body size or changes in structure, function, and complexity of body cell content and metabolic and biochemical processes up to some point of optimum maturity.*[7] Growth changes occur through incremental or replacement growth. **Incremental growth** refers to *maintaining an excess in growth over normal daily losses from catabolism, seen in urine, feces, perspiration, and oxidation in the lungs.* Incremental growth is observed as increases in weight or height as the child matures. **Replacement growth** refers to *normal refills of essential body components* necessary for survival.[8] For example, once a red blood cell (erythrocyte) has entered the cardiovascular system, it circulates for an average of 120 days before disintegrating, when another red blood cell takes its place. Growth occurs through **hypertrophy**, an *increase in the size of cellular structures*, and **hyperplasia**, an *increase in the number of cells.*[9] Growth during the fetal and infancy periods is achieved primarily through hyperplasia, which is gradually replaced by hypertrophic growth. Each body organ has its own optimum period of growth. Body tissues are most sensitive to permanent damage during periods of the most rapid hyperplastic growth.

**Development** refers to the *patterned, orderly, lifelong changes in structure, thought, feelings, and behaviour that evolve as a result of maturation of physical and mental capacity, experiences, and learning and results in a new level of maturity and integration.*[10] Development should permit the person to adapt to the environment by either controlling it or controlling responses to it. Developmental processes involve interplay among the physiologic characteristics that define the person; the environmental forces, including culture, that act on him or her; and the psychological mechanisms that mediate between them. Psychological processes include the person's perception of self, others, and the environment, and the behaviours he or she acquires in coping with needs and the environment. Development combines growth, maturation, and learning and involves organizing behaviour throughout the life cycle.

**Maturation** refers to *the emergence of genetic potential for changes in form, structure, complexity, integration, organization, and function, both physically and mentally.*[11]

**Biological age** is *the level of physical growth and development and how the body functions over time.* **Psychological age** is *the person's perception of aging processes.* **Social age** refers to *society's expectations of the person at a specific age or stage.*[12] **Chronologic age** is the *time since birth* and is not always exactly in step with the other ages.

**Learning** is *the process of gaining specific knowledge, or skill.* It involves *acquiring habits and attitudes as a result of experience, training, and behavioural changes.* Maturation and learning are interrelated. No learning occurs unless the person is mature enough to be able to understand and change his or her behaviour.[13]

## General Principles of Development

The following statements apply to the overall development of the person.

**Childhood is the foundation period of life.** Attitudes, habits, patterns of behaviour and thinking, personality traits, and health status established during the early years (the first five years determine to a large extent how successfully the person will continue to develop and adjust to life as he or she gets older). Early patterns of behaviour persist throughout life, within the range of normalcy.[14]

**Development follows a definable, predictable, and sequential pattern and occurs continually through adulthood.** Each person progresses through similar stages, but the age for achievement varies because achievement depends on inherent maturational capacity interacting with the physical and social environment. The different areas of growth and development—physical, mental, emotional, social, and spiritual—are interrelated, proceed together, and affect each other; yet these areas mature at their own pace. The stages of development overlap, and the transition from one stage to another is gradual.[15]

**Growth and development are continuous, but they occur in spurts rather than in a straight upward direction.** At times, the person will appear to be at a standstill, or even to have regressed developmentally.

**Growth is usually accompanied by behaviour change.** As the child matures, he or she retains earlier ways of behaving, but there will be a developmental revision of habits. For example, the high-activity infant becomes a high-activity toddler or adult, but the object of the activity changes from diffuse interests, to concentrated play, to work. The young child's temperament is a precursor of later behaviour, although the person is adaptable and changes occur throughout life. Behaviour changes occur sometimes because of the reactions and expectations of others, which tend to change as the person matures physically.

**Human behaviour has purpose, or is goal directed.** Therefore, the behaviour is commonly preceded by imagining the desired result. The person visualizes the future and tries to bring it about. Behaviour is directed toward meeting needs and goals.

**When one need or goal is met, the person has energy to pursue another need, interest, or goal.** Behaviour changes direction, but does not come to an end.

**Critical periods** in human development *occur when specific organs and other aspects of a person's physical and psychosocial growth undergo marked rapid change and the capacity to adapt to stressors is underdeveloped. During these critical periods, when tremendous demands are placed on the person, the individual has an increased susceptibility to adverse environmental factors* that may cause various types and degrees of negative effects. For example, implantation is a critical period, and at certain times during pregnancy certain substances are more likely to damage fetal structures.[16] The form of the brain is established by the twelfth week of gestation. Critical periods of brain growth occur during early formation (organogenesis) from the third to ninth weeks of gestation, during brain growth spurt from 12 to 20 weeks of gestation, and during the time of rapid neuronal additions from 30 to 40 weeks of gestation and during the first 18 to 24 months after birth. Exposure of the nervous system to a teratogen during these time frames may affect specific brain regions that are growing most rapidly at that time. During adolescence, the rapid physical growth may negatively affect social relationships or feelings about self. Middle or old age may be another critical period.[17]

If appropriate stimuli and resources are not available at the critical time, or when the person is ready to receive and use particular stimuli for the development of a specific psychomotor skill, the skill may be more difficult to learn later in the developmental sequence. Learning of any psychomotor skill, however, is influenced by sociocultural factors. The extent to which any skill is influenced by genetics, environmental opportunity, cultural and family values and patterns, and emotional status is not yet fully known.

**Mastering transitions during a life cycle stage is the basis for mastering the second-order changes required to proceed physically and emotionally.** Certain periods occur when the task can be best accomplished. The task should be mastered at that time. If the time is delayed, the person will have difficulty in accomplishing the task. Each phase of development is usually accompanied by characteristic traits,

along with a period of equilibrium when the person adjusts rather easily to environmental demands. Usually, as well, there will be a period of disequilibrium, when he or she experiences difficulty in adjustment. Developmental hazards occur in every era. Some are environmental and interfere with adjustment; others come from within the person.[18]

**Progressive differentiation of the self from the environment results from increasing self-knowledge and autonomy.** The young child first separates as an object apart from mother. Gradually, he or she becomes less dependent emotionally on the parents. As the child matures into adulthood, an increase in cognitive development enables increased control over their own behaviour. The person can think and act on his or her own and becomes increasingly more autonomous.

**The developing person simultaneously acquires competencies in four major areas:** physical, cognitive, emotional, and social. **Physical competency** includes *various motor and neurological capacities* to attain mobility and manipulation and the ability to care for self physically. **Cognitive competency** includes *learning how to perceive, think, solve problems, and communicate thoughts and feelings* that, in turn, affect emotional and social skills. **Emotional competency** includes *developing an awareness and acceptance of self as a separate person, responding to other people and factors in the environment because others have been responsive to him or her.* The person is now able to work at coping with inner and outer stresses, and at becoming increasingly more responsible for their personal behaviour. **Social competency** includes *learning how to affiliate securely, first with the family, and then with various people in various situations.* These four competencies constantly influence one another. The health of one domain or the extent of competency affects the other domains or competencies. The person develops toward using personal assets optimally. Inner resources, competencies, and abilities are called upon by the body to keep energy expenditures at a minimum while focusing on the attainment of a goal.[19]

**Readiness and motivation are essential for learning to occur.** Hunger, fatigue, illness, pain, and the lack of emotional feedback or opportunity to explore all inhibit one's readiness and lower motivation.[20]

**Many factors contribute to the formation of permanent characteristics and traits,** including the child's genetic inheritance, undetermined prenatal environmental factors, family and society when he or she is an infant and young child, nutrition, physical and emotional environment, and the degree of intellectual stimulation that is accessible in the environment.

*Progressive differentiation of the self from other people and the environment,* the **Principle of Development toward Self-Knowledge and Autonomy,** is made apparent with the individual's increasing self-awareness and emergent self-concept. The young child achieves increasing ability to perceive himself or herself as an initiator of action on the environment. An increasing ability develops to regulate his or her own behaviour, to think and act in an individual and unique way, and to become more autonomous. The ability to be autonomous and interdependent is reworked continually throughout life.[21]

CRITICAL THINKING

*What situations might increase the likelihood of a negative developmental outcome for the individual?*

## Principles of Growth

Several principles of growth are emphasized in the following pages. The primary determinant of normal growth is the development of the central nervous system, which, in turn, governs or influences other body systems.

The **Principle of Readiness** states that the *child's ability to perform a physical task depends on the maturation of neurological structures in the brain, and on the maturation of the muscular and skeletal systems*.[22] Until a state of physiologic readiness is reached, the child cannot perform a function, such as toilet training, even with parental training or planned practice.

The **Principle of Differentiation** means that *development proceeds from simple to the complex, from homogeneous to heterogeneous, and from general to specific*.[23] For example, movement from *simple to complex* is seen in mitotic changes in fetal cell structures as they undergo cell division immediately after ovum fertilization by a sperm. Androgens or steroids administered prenatally can "masculinize" a genetic female brain.[24] *Differentiation from simple to complex* motor skill is seen after birth as the baby first waves his or her arms and later learns to control finger movements. The general body configurations of males and females at birth are much more similar than during late adolescence, thus indicating *movement from homogeneity to heterogeneity*. The mass of cells in the embryo is at first homogeneous, but the limbs of the five-week-old embryo show considerable differentiation as the elbow and wrist regions become identifiable and finger ridge indentations outline the progressive protrusion of future fingers from the former paddle-shaped arm bud.[25] *General to specific* development is observed in motor responses, which are diffuse and undifferentiated at birth and become more specific and controlled later. Baby first moves the whole body in response to a stimulus. Later, he or she reacts with a specific body part.[26]

The **Cephalocaudal**, **Proximodistal**, and **Bilateral Principles** all indicate that *major physical and motor changes invariably proceed in three bipolar directions*. **Cephalocaudal** (*head to tail*) means that the *upper end of the organism develops with greater rapidity than and before the lower end of the organism*. Increases in neuromuscular size and maturation of function begin in the head and proceed to hands and feet.

Auditory, visual, and other sensory mechanisms in the head develop sooner than the motor systems of the upper body. At the same time, the arm buds, first appearing paddle shaped, continue to change in shape and size more rapidly than do the lower limbs. After birth, the infant will be able to hold the head erect before being able to sit or walk. **Proximodistal** (*near-to-far*) means that *growth progresses from the central axis of the body toward the periphery or extremities*. **Bilateral** (*side to side*) means that *the capacity for growth and development of structures is symmetric*.[27] Growth that occurs on one side of the body occurs simultaneously on the other.

The **Principle of Asynchronous Growth** focuses on *developmental shifts at successive periods in development*. A comparison of pictures of persons of different ages indicates that the young child is *not* a "small adult." The proportional size of the head to the chest and of the torso to the limbs of younger and older persons is vastly different. Length of limbs in comparison to torso length is smaller in the infant than in the schoolchild. The same comparison is greater in the aged than in the adolescent because of the biological changes of aging.

The **Principle of Discontinuity of Growth Rate** refers to the *different rate of growth changes at different periods during the lifespan*. The *whole* body does not grow simultaneously as a total unit. Instead, various structures and organs of the body grow and develop at different rates, reaching their maximum at different times throughout the life cycle. For instance, in its rudimentary form the heart and circulatory system begin to function during the third week of embryonic life, continue to mature slowly compared with the rest of the body, and after the age of 25 years remain fairly constant in size. Before birth, the head is the fastest growing body part. The brain grows and develops according to a different pattern. This vital organ grows very rapidly during fetal life and infancy, reaching 80 percent of its maximum size at the age of two years. Full growth is seen at approximately six years of age.[28] Body growth is rapid in infancy and adolescence and relatively slow during school years.

All body systems normally continue to work in unity throughout the lifespan. Some physiologic characteristics, such as oxygen concentration in the blood, remain fairly stable throughout life. Others, such as body temperature, undergo minor changes, depending on age, hormonal balance, or time of day. Some characteristics, such as pulse rate and fluid intake, that are affected by changes in body surface, organ size, or maturity change markedly during the life cycle. Age-related changes occur at varying chronologic periods. Structural deterioration usually precedes functional decline. Some organs and systems deteriorate more rapidly than others. In late life, the capacity for adaptation changes and finally decreases. Before death, decline or deterioration usually affects most structural, and many functional, centres in the aged person.[29]

The study of growth and development processes must focus on the complete continuum of the life cycle—from conception through death—to acquire a comprehensive understanding of the complexity of these processes, and to know how these principles are activated throughout the lifespan.

## LIFESPAN DEVELOPMENTAL PSYCHOLOGY

Lifespan developmental psychology encompasses the study of the individual from conception to old age. As you probably know, development is not completed at adulthood but extends across the lifespan. Lindenberger and Baltes claim that, across the lifespan, adaptive processes such as acquisition, maintenance, transformation, and attrition all take place in the psychological structures and functions of the individual.[30] As a result, the ontogenesis of mind and behaviours in the individual's development involves the following constructs:

- *Lifelong:* Development spans the years from conception to old age. Each stage has its own unique experiences, and none is more important than the others.

- *Dynamic:* Development involves much change throughout the years as well as a series of challenges. Development is always being constituted by gains and losses. Many individuals maximize their gains to minimize their losses.

- *Multidimensional:* Development consists of connections and interplays among the physical, cognitive, social, psychological, and spiritual dimensions, each of which varies in its rate of development.

- *Multifunctional:* Many abilities of the individual throughout the lifespan can be either improved upon or redirected. For example, cognitive performance may be portrayed as the combined outcome of biological and cultural systems of influence.

- *Non-linear:* The progression of development in many instances is either circular or reversible in nature, depending on cultural contexts and age-related changes. For example, parental roles may change from that of childrearing to contending with an empty nest syndrome.

These constructs can serve as a framework for the study of lifespan development. A central theme in lifespan developmental psychology concerns malleability. For example, the effects of cohort, historical period, and environmental differences on age changes and differences in cognitive performance are indications of malleability.[31]

Research that is informed by lifespan psychology is intended to generate knowledge about three components of individual development: (1) interindividual similarities (regularities) in development; (2) interindividual differences in development; and (3) intraindividual plasticity (malleability) in development. The joint attention directed toward each of these components, and the specification of their age-related interplays, creates not only the conceptual, but also the methodological foundations of developmental psychology.[32]

This brief introduction to lifespan developmental psychology will help you to examine more closely individuals and their families throughout the lifespan as you find them in diverse cultures. The understanding you attain will undoubtedly help you to recognize the importance of health promotion and disease prevention so that you might help to enhance the quality of life in the young as well as the old.

---

### CRITICAL THINKING

*Give a few examples of how development is influenced by both biology and culture throughout the lifespan.*

---

## DEVELOPING PERSON: PRENATAL STAGES AND INFLUENCES

Use the following information in prenatal assessment, teaching, other health promotion measures, and advocacy for public policy related to health.

### The Beginning

The cell, the basis for human life, is a complex unit. Refer to an anatomy or physiology text for a review of cell structure and function. This chapter presents a brief overview of the prenatal period as the beginning of life. For an in-depth study of the biological differences of the male and female; the reproductive process, including fertilization and development of the unborn child in utero; inheritance patterns; and the process of labour and delivery, refer to an anatomy and physiology developmental text and to a maternity nursing text.[33]

All body cells have 22 pairs of rod-shaped particles, non-sex **chromosomes** (*autosomes*), and a pair of sex chromosomes. The biological female has two X chromosomes; the biological male has one X and one Y chromosome. Each of the chromosomes contains approximately *20 000 segments strung out like lengthwise beads* called **genes**. The genes, apparently located according to function, are made up of deoxyribonucleic acid (DNA), which processes the information that determines the makeup and specific function of every cell in the body. The genes play a major role in determining hereditary characteristics.[34]

The female reproductive cycle is more regular and easier to observe and measure than the male reproductive cycle.[35] In contrast to the normal ovulatory cycle, spermatogenesis normally occurs in cycles that continuously follow one another.

Approximately 14 days after the beginning of the menstrual period, fertilization may occur in the outer third of the fallopian tube. The sperm cell from a male penetrates and unites with an **ovum** (*egg*) from a female to form a *single-cell* **zygote**. The sperm and ovum, known as **gametes** (*sex cells in half cells*), are produced in the reproductive system through **meiosis**, a *specialized process of cell* division and chromosome reduction.[36]

A newborn girl has approximately 400 000 immature ova in her ovaries; each is in a **follicle**, or *small sac*. **Ovulation**, *the expelling of an ovum from a mature follicle in one of the ovaries*, occurs approximately once every 28 days in a sexually mature female.[37]

Spermatozoa, much smaller and more active than the ovum, are produced in the testes of the mature male at the rate of several hundred million a day and are ejaculated in his semen at *sexual climax* (**orgasm**). For fertilization to occur, at least 20 million sperm cells must enter a woman's body at one time. They enter the vagina and try to swim through the **cervix** (*opening to the uterus*) and into the fallopian tube. Only a tiny fraction of those millions of sperm cells makes it that far. More than one may penetrate the ovum, but only one can fertilize it to create a new human. The sex of the baby is determined by the pair of sex chromosomes; the sperm may carry either an X or a Y chromosome, resulting in either a girl (XX zygote) or a boy (XY zygote).

Spermatozoa maintain their ability to fertilize an egg for a span of 24 to 90 hours; ova can be fertilized for approximately 24 hours. Thus, there are approximately 24 to 90 hours during each menstrual cycle when conception can take place. If fertilization does not occur, the spermatozoa and ovum die. Sperm cells are devoured by white blood cells in the woman's body; the ovum passes through the uterus and vagina in the menstrual product.[38]

If fertilization does occur, the zygote travels to the uterus for implantation or imbedding in the uterine wall. Progesterone secretion has prepared the uterus for the possible reception of the fertilized ovum. The continued secretion of ovarian estrogen and progesterone develops the uterus for the nine-month nurturance of the developing embryo and fetus in pregnancy. Continued secretion of estrogen during this period increases the growth of the uterine muscles and eventually enlarges the vagina for the delivery of a child. Continued secretion of progesterone during pregnancy serves to keep the uterus from prematurely contracting and expelling the developing embryo before the proper time. In addition, progesterone prepares the breast cells in late pregnancy for future milk production.[39]

**Multiple Births** Multiple births may occur. For example, with twins, two ova are released within a short time of each other; if both are fertilized, **fraternal** (*dizygotic or two-egg*) **twins** will be born. Created by different eggs and different sperm cells, the twins are no more alike in their genetic makeup than other siblings. They may be of the same or different sex. If the ovum divides in two after it has been fertilized, **identical** (*monozygotic or one-egg*) **twins** will be born. At birth, these twins share the same placenta. They are of the same sex and have exactly the same genetic heritage; any differences they will later exhibit are the result of the influences of environment, either before or after birth. Other multiple births—triplets, quadruplets, and so forth—result from either one or a combination of these two processes.[40]

Multiple births have become more frequent in recent years as a result of the administration of certain fertility drugs that spur ovulation and often cause the release of more than one egg. Twins have a limited intrauterine space and are more likely to be premature and of low birth weight. They therefore have a lower rate of survival at birth.[41] Mariano and Hickey claim that Canadian women are two-and-a-half times more likely to have triplets, quadruplets, or even quintuplets today than they would have been 20 years ago.[42] Thirty to 50 percent of the world's twin pregnancies, and at least 75 percent of triplet pregnancies, occur in industrialized countries among women using fertility treatments.[43] Reasons for multiple births include increasing maternal age and the use of fertility drugs and other reproductive technologies.[44]

In Canada, National Multiple Births Awareness Day is both a celebration and an opportunity for the multiple-birth community to speak to Canadians about issues and challenges unique to their families. It commemorates annually, on May 28, the birth date of the Dionne quintuplets. Each year, members of Multiple Births Across Canada are encouraged to unite and draw attention to that year's chosen theme.[45]

In Canada, Bill C-6 (An Act Respecting Assisted Human Reproduction and Related Research) became law in March 2004. This law prohibits human cloning and other unacceptable activities, while protecting the health and safety of Canadians who use assisted human reproduction (AHR). Furthermore, this law provides controls for AHR-related research and will lead to the establishment of the Assisted Human Reproduction Agency of Canada (AHRAC), which will be responsible for licensing, inspecting, and enforcing activities controlled under the Act.[46]

On January 12, 2006, AHRAC was established in Vancouver, British Columbia. It is a federal regulatory organization responsible for administering a regulatory framework and regime to oversee controlled AHR activities and to enforce prohibition under the Act. The legislation and the establishment of AHRAC put Canada into a leadership

Sue, age 35, comes to the clinic for an appointment with a nurse clinician. She informs the nurse that she and her partner, after a second cycle of in vitro fertilization and embryo transfer, just received news from the gynecologist that she is expecting a multiple birth—possibly triplets. Sue and her partner have two young adopted children at home, and she is quite anxious about how she will manage to care for the multiples as well as the rest of the family. She is wondering if she should expect annoying bouts of "morning sickness," and whether they will be more intense with a multiple pregnancy. Sue also states that she learned from a neighbour that the risk of preterm delivery is higher with a multiple pregnancy.

1. What would be the nurse's response regarding Sue's concern about "morning sickness"?
2. What risk factors are specific to multiple pregnancies? How could the nurse counsel Sue?
3. What health promotion strategies could the nurse consider for Sue in caring for herself and her family, both now and after delivery?

capacity internationally as a regulator of this sector. During 2007, AHRAC focused on many activities, such as management and governance structures and staffing required to become an operation.[47]

## Stages of Prenatal Development

Life in utero is usually divided into three stages of development: germinal, embryonic, and fetal. The **germinal stage** lasts *approximately ten days to two weeks after fertilization*. It is characterized by rapid cell division and a subsequent increasing complexity of the organism and its implantation in the wall of the uterus. The **embryonic stage**, *from two to eight weeks*, is a time of rapid growth and differentiation of major body systems and organs. The **fetal stage**, *from eight weeks until birth*, is characterized by rapid growth and changes in body form caused by different rates of growth of different parts of the body.[48]

The fetus is a very small, but rapidly developing, human being who is influenced by the maternal and external environment and to whom the mother responds, especially when fetal movement begins. Table 6-1 summarizes some major

**Table 6-1 Summary of the Sequence of Prenatal Development**

| Time Period after Fertilization | Developmental Event |
| --- | --- |
| **Germinal Stage** | |
| 30 hours | First division or cleavage occurs. |
| 40 hours | Four-cell stage occurs. |
| 60 hours | **Morula,** *a solid mass of 12 to 16 cells;* total size of mass not changed because cells decrease in size with each cleavage to allow morula to pass through lumen of fallopian tube. Ectopic pregnancy within fallopian tube occurs if morula is wedged in lumen. |
| 3 days | Zygote has divided into 32 cells; travels through fallopian tube to uterus. |
| 4 days | Zygote contains 70 cells. Morula reaches uterus; forms a **blastocyst,** *a fluid-filled sphere.* |
| 4.5–6 days | Blastocyst floats in utero. **Embryonic disk,** *thickened cell mass from which baby develops,* clusters on one edge of blastocyst. Mass of cells differentiates into two layers: (1) **ectoderm,** *outer layer of cells* that become the epidermis, nails, hair, tooth enamel, sensory organs, brain and spinal cord, cranial nerves, peripheral nervous system, upper pharynx, nasal passages, urethra, and mammary glands; (2) **endoderm,** *lower layer of cells* that develops into gastrointestinal system, liver, pancreas, salivary glands, respiratory system, urinary bladder, pharynx, thyroid, tonsils, lining of urethra, and ear. |
| 6–7 days | **Nidation,** *implantation of zygote* into upper portion of uterine wall, occurs. |
| 7–14 days | Remainder of blastocyst develops into the following: (1) **Placenta,** *a multipurpose organ connected to the embryo by the umbilical cord* that delivers |

*(continued)*

**Table 6-1** (continued)

| Time Period after Fertilization | Developmental Event |
|---|---|
| | oxygen and nourishment from the mother's body, absorbs the embryo's body wastes, combats internal infection, confers immunity to the unborn child, and produces the hormones that (a) support pregnancy, (b) prepare breasts for lactating, and (c) stimulate uterine contractions for delivery of the baby. Placenta circulation is evidenced by 11 to 12 days. (2) **Umbilical cord**, *a structure that contains two umbilical arteries and an umbilical vein and connects embryo to placenta*. It is approximately 55 cm long and 3.8 cm in diameter. Rapid cell differentiation occurs. (3) **Amniotic sac**, *a fluid-filled membrane that encases the developing baby*, protecting it and giving it room to move. |
| 2–8 weeks | Period during which embryo firmly establishes uterus as home and undergoes rapid cellular differentiation, growth, and development of body systems. This is a *critical period when embryo is most vulnerable to deleterious prenatal influences*. All development birth defects occur during *first trimester (3 months)* of pregnancy. If embryo is unable to survive, a **miscarriage** or **spontaneous abortion**, *expulsion of conceptus from the uterus*, occurs. |
| **Embryonic Stage** | |
| 15 days | Cranial end of elongated disk has begun to thicken. |
| 16 days | **Mesoderm**, the *middle layer*, appears and develops into dermis, tooth dentin, connective tissue, cartilage, bones, muscles, spleen, blood, gonads, uterus, and excretory and circulatory systems. Yolk sac, which arises from ectoderm, assists transfer of nutrients from mother to embryo. |
| 19–20 days | Neural fold and neural grove develop. Thyroid begins to develop. |
| 21 days | Neural tube forms, becomes spinal cord and brain. |
| 22 days | Heart, the first organ to function, initiates action. Eyes, ears, nose, cheeks, and upper jaw begin to form. Cleft palate may occur if development is defective. |
| 26–27 days | Cephalic portion (brain) of nervous system formed. Leg and arm buds appear. Stubby tail of spinal cord appears. |
| 28 days | Crown to rump length, 4–5 mm. Cardiovascular system functioning. Heart beats 65 times per minute; blood flows through tiny arteries and veins. Lens vesicles, optic cups, and nasal pits forming. By end of first month, new life has grown more quickly than it will at any other time in life. Swelling in head where eyes, ears, mouth, and nose will be. Crown to rump length, 7–14 mm. |
| 30 days | Rudimentary body parts formed. Limb buds appear. |
| 31 days | Eye and nasal pit developing. Primitive mouth present. |
| 32 days | Paddle-shaped hands. Lens vesicles and optic cups formed. |
| 34 days | Head is much larger relative to trunk. Digital rays present in hands. Feet are paddle shaped. Crown to rump length, 11–14 mm. |
| 35–38 days | Olfactory pit, eye, maxillary process, oral cavity, and mandibular process developing. Brain has divided into three parts. Limbs growing. Beginning of all major external and internal structures. Crown to rump length, 15–16 mm. |
| 40 days | Elbows and knees apparent. Fingers and toes distinct but webbed. Yolk sac continues to (1) provide embryologic blood cells during third through sixth weeks until liver, spleen, and bone marrow assume function; (2) provide |

*(continued)*

Table 6-1 (continued)

| Time Period after Fertilization | Developmental Event |
| --- | --- |
| | lining cells for respiratory and digestive tracts; (3) provide cells that migrate to gonads to become primordial germ cells. |
| 42 days | Crown to rump length, 21–23 mm. |
| 50 days | All internal and external structures present. External genitalia present but sex not discernible; yolk sac disappears, incorporated into embryo; limbs, hands, feet formed. Nerve cells in brain connected. |
| 55–56 days | Eye, nostril, globular process, maxilla, and mandible almost completely formed. Ear beginning to develop. |
| 8 weeks | Stubby end of spinal cord disappears. Distinct human characteristics. Head accounts for half of total embryo length. Brain impulses coordinate function of organ systems. Facial parts formed, with tongue and teeth buds. Stomach produces digestive juices. Liver produces blood cells. Kidney removes uric acid from blood. Some movement by limbs. Weight, 1 g. Length, 2.5–3.75 cm. |
| **Fetal Stage** | |
| 9–40 weeks | Remainder of intrauterine period spent in growth and refinement of body tissues and organs. |
| 9–12 weeks | Eyelids fused. Nail beds formed. Teeth and bones begin to appear. Ribs and vertebrae are cartilage. Kidneys function. Urinates occasionally. Some respiratory-like movements exhibited. Begins to swallow amniotic fluid. Grasp, sucking, and withdrawal reflexes present. Sucks fingers and toes in utero. Makes specialized responses to touch. Moves easily but movement not felt by mother. Reproductive organs have primitive egg or sperm cells. Sex distinguishable. Head one-third of body length. Weight, 30 g. Length, 7.5–9 cm at 12 weeks. |
| 13–16 weeks | Much spontaneous movement. Sex determination possible. **Quickening**, *fetal kicking or movement*, may be felt by mother. Moro reflex present. Rapid skeletal development. Meconium present. Uterine development in female fetus. **Lanugo**, *downy hair*, appears on body. Head one-fourth of total length. Weight, 120–150 g. Length, 20–25 cm. Foetus frowns, moves lips, turns head; hands grasp, feet kick. First hair appears. Ova formed in female. |
| 17–20 weeks | New cells exchanged for old, especially in skin. Quickening occurs by 17 weeks. Vernix caseosa appears. Eyebrows, eyelashes, and head hair appear. Sweat and sebaceous glands begin to function. Skeleton begins to harden. Grasp reflex present and strong. Permanent teeth buds appear. Fetal heart sounds can be heard with stethoscope. Weight, 360–450 g. Length, 30.5 cm. |
| 21–24 weeks | Extrauterine life, life outside uterus, is possible but difficult because of immature respiratory system. Fetus looks like miniature baby. Mother may note jarring but rhythmic movements of infant, indicative of hiccups. Body becomes straight at times. Fingernails present. Skin has wrinkled, red appearance. Alternate periods of sleep and activity. May respond to external sounds. Weight, 720 g. Length, 35.5 cm. |
| 25–28 weeks | Jumps in utero in synchrony with loud noise. Eyes open and close with waking and sleeping cycles. Able to hear. Respiratory-like movements. Respiratory and central nervous systems sufficiently developed; some babies survive with excellent and intensive care. Assumes head-down position in uterus. Weight, 1200 g. |

*(continued)*

Table 6-1 (continued)

| Time Period after Fertilization | Developmental Event |
|---|---|
| 29–32 weeks | Begins to store fat and minerals. Testes descend into scrotal sac in male. Reflexes fully developed. Thumb-sucking present. Mother may note irregular, jerky, crying |
| 33–36 weeks | Adipose tissue continues to be deposited over entire body. Body begins to round out. May become more or less active because of space constriction. Increased iron storage by liver. Increased lung development. Lanugo begins to disappear from body. Head lengthens. Brain cells number same as at birth. Weight, 2800 g. Length, 46–60 cm. |
| 37–40 weeks | Organ systems operating more efficiently. Heart rate increases. More wastes expelled. Lanugo and vernix caseosa disappear. Skin smooth and plump. High absorption of maternal hormones. Cerebral cortex well-defined; brain wave patterns developed. Skull and other bones becoming more firm and mineralized. Continued storage of fat and minerals. Glands produce hormones that trigger labour. Ready for birth. Weight, 3200–3400 g. Length, 51–53 cm. Baby stops growing approximately 1 week before birth. |

milestones in the sequential development of the **conceptus**, *the new life that has been conceived.* However, *being precise about the exact timing is difficult.*[49]

## Prenatal Influences on Development

**Heredity** Genetic information is transmitted from parents of offspring through a complex series of processes. The *basic unit of heredity* is the **gene**. Each cell in the human body contains about 100 000 genes, which are made up of DNA. DNA carries the biochemical instructions that tell the cells how to make the proteins that enable them to carry out specific body functions. Each gene is located in a definite position in the rod-shaped **chromosome**. Twenty-three pairs of chromosomes in the human germ cells divide into two gametes by meiosis, giving to each of these mature germ cells (female ovum and male spermatozoon) one-half of the genetic material necessary for producing a new individual.

Table 6-2 summarizes physiologic changes in the woman during pregnancy.[50]

At conception, the single-celled zygote has all of the biological information necessary to develop into a baby through the process of **mitosis**, a process whereby the cells

**Table 6-2 Summary of Major Physiological Changes in Woman during Pregnancy**

| Physiological Characteristics | Change Related to Pregnancy |
|---|---|
| **Weight** | First trimester: increases by 0.9 to 1.8 kg. <br> Second and third trimester: increases by 0.36 to 0.45 kg per week. |
| **Skin** | Warmed by increased blood flow. <br> **Linea nigra**: *dark vertical line from sternum to symphysis pubis.* <br> Stretch marks on abdomen with increasing **chloasma**: *dark brown patches on face or over bridge of nose.* |
| **Musculoskeletal System** | Centre of gravity changes, tilting pelvis forward, causing lower back pain. <br> Fatigue and aches caused by increasing weight in abdomen and breasts. |
| **Cardiovascular System** | First trimester: blood volume increases gradually. <br> 6–8 weeks: may hear systolic ejection murmur on auscultation. Heart displaced upwards and to the left by rising diaphragm. <br> Orthostatic hypotension during pregnancy because blood pools in lower limbs; varicose veins and hemorrhoids are common. |

*(continued)*

Table 6-2 (continued)

| Physiological Characteristics | Change Related to Pregnancy |
|---|---|
| | 14–20 weeks: pulse gradually increases by 10 to 15 beats per minute; cardiac output increases 30 percent to 50 percent. |
| | Last half of pregnancy: drop in colloid osmotic pressure shifts fluid into extra vascular space, causing edema in lower limbs. |
| | 32–34 weeks: blood volume increases to 40 percent to 50 percent above baseline; 40 weeks: blood volume gradually declines. |
| **Respiratory System** | Diaphragm rises and waistline expands even before enlarging uterus exerts much upward pressure. |
| | 24th week: thoracic rather than abdominal breathing; mild dyspnoea; nasal mucosa swells as a result of higher estrogen level; nasal stuffiness, epistaxis (nosebleeds) common. |
| | Costal ligaments relax because of rising estrogen levels; chest can expand and deeper breathing for increasing oxygen requirements. |
| | Respiratory rate increases slightly. |
| | Respiratory volume increases 26 percent, decreasing alveolar carbon dioxide concentration, compensated respiratory alkalosis. |
| | Alkalosis facilitates diffusion of nutrients to and wastes from the fetus through placenta. |
| **Renal System** | Kidneys excrete additional bicarbonate to compensate for drop in alveolar carbon dioxide concentration. |
| | Second trimester: increase in renal plasma flow (35 percent) and glomerular filtration rate (50 percent); both drop in late pregnancy. |
| | Urinary stasis caused by enlarging uterus and increasing blood volume. |
| **Gastrointestinal System** | First trimester nausea and vomiting resulting from increased human chorionic gonadotropin and estrogen. |
| | Gastric reflux as uterus enlarges and progesterone relaxes smooth muscle. |
| | Reduced bowel sounds; intestinal transit time increases, causing better nutrient absorption and constipation. |
| **Hematological System** | Second trimester: physiologic anemia with hemoglobin level and hematocrit slightly lower, proportionate to increased plasma volume. |
| | White blood cell count increases during pregnancy. |
| | Platelets remain normal. |
| **Reproductive System** | Uterus enlarges 20 times normal size to hold fetus, placenta, and amniotic fluid. |
| | 12th week: uterus expands out of pelvis into abdominal cavity. |
| | 16th week and after: supine position causes uterus to compress vena cava and iliac veins, decreasing blood flow to uterus and lower extremities (left lateral position recommended for sleeping). |
| | Vagina: pH more acid in mucus, which acts as barrier against infection to uterus. |
| | Breasts begin to feel full and tingly at second month; gradually enlarge as number and size of milk ducts and lobules increase; breast may leak colostrum. |

divide in half over and over. Each cell, except the **gamete** (*sex chromosomes* X *or* Y), is identical to the original zygote in normal development.[51]

**Congenital anomalies**, *physical handicap or intellectual impairment* that occur before birth for a variety of reasons, are discussed in the following pages. However, sometimes disorders or defects are **genetic**, *the result of dominant or recessive transmission of abnormalities in the genes or*

*chromosomes.* An example of a sex-lined disorder is **fragile X syndrome**, which *involves an abnormal fragile section of DNA at a specific location on the X chromosome.* This is a sex-linked inherited disorder. The female is usually a carrier, and the male is more likely to demonstrate the effects. It is estimated that 5 to 7 percent of all intellectual impairments are caused by this syndrome.[52] Recessive genes may cause inherited autosomal disorders, such as sickle-cell disease, phenylketonuria (PKU) disease, and Tay-Sachs disease.[53] An example of a disorder caused by dominant genes is Huntington's disease. This disease, which causes the brain to deteriorate and affects both psychological and motor functions, is not diagnosed until adulthood.[54]

An example of a common congenital anomaly, known as a chromosomal abnormality, is **Down syndrome (trisomy 21)** *in which the child has three of the chromosome 21 instead of the normal two.* Various factors contribute to the chromosomal break, discussed in later sections. The level of intellectual impairment varies.[55]

---

### CRITICAL THINKING

*In what ways can you help a family with a Down syndrome infant to cope?*

---

An inherited predisposition to a disorder may interact with an environmental factor before or after birth and lead to the expression of the disorder. Some abnormalities or diseases that are inherited appear months or years later.[56] The sense of danger, anxiety, and uncertainty that lives on in the family affects the biological system of the child. Thus, the gene for a predisposition has to be "turned on" by an outside force before it can do its job, but the offspring's behaviour reflects the stresses that its mother lived through. High levels of stress activate a variety of genes, including those involved in shyness, panic disorder, and schizophrenia, which are some of the diseases that can occur in offspring.

Hereditary factors do not by themselves fully determine what the person will become. There is a **reaction range**, *a range of potential expression of a trait* (e.g., weight), *that depends on environmental conditions.* Then, there are certain traits, such as eye colour, that are so strongly programmed by genes that they are **canalized**. That is, *there is little variance in their expression.*[57]

Genetic endowment with respect to any trait may be compared to a rubber band. The rubber band may remain unstretched because of environmental influences and therefore remain dormant. Or the rubber band may be stretched fully, causing the person to excel beyond what seems to be his or her potential. The person in later maturity, for example, has had many years of changing environmental influences. What he or she has become is no doubt an expression of innate genetic potential, environmental supports, and the wisdom to take advantage of both.[58] Thus, judgments cannot be made at birth. Whatever the genetic background, the child deserves the opportunities to master the trait, turn it into an advantage, or learn how to cope with it.

**Parental Age** The age of the mother and father and the number of previous pregnancies all tend to affect the health of the fetus:

- The most recent ten-year period for which data are available in Canada (1992–2002) indicates a persistent and steady decline in teen pregnancy rates for both younger (15- to 17-year-old) and older (18- to 19-year-old) teens. The trend continues. In 2003, the number of teenage women who gave birth also declined, from 16.8 live births in 1997 to 12.1 in 2003. Although not scientifically conclusive, the increased use of the birth control pill by females has corresponded with the drop in teen pregnancy rates.[59] Pregnancy during the teen years, especially before age 17, is associated with infants who are premature, are of low birth weight, have neurological defects, have higher mortality rates during the first year, and have more developmental problems during preschool and school years. Pregnant teens are more likely to have inadequate income, poor diet, and inadequate prenatal care.[60]

- A baby born to a woman who has had three or more pregnancies before age 20 is less likely to be healthy.[61]

- In recent years, the proportion of women who delay childbearing to later in life has increased markedly in Canada.[62] This delay may be associated with adverse outcomes for the infant, as well as for the mother. As a woman's age increases, her risk of having a baby with Down syndrome also increases.[63] Antepartum complications associated with delayed childbearing include increased risks of spontaneous abortion, gestational diabetes, hypertension, pre-eclampsia, placenta previa, and prenatal hospital admission. Further labour and delivery complications that arise with advanced maternal age include malpresentation, fetal distress, prolonged labour, operative deliveries, and postpartum hemorrhage.[64]

- The more pregnancies a woman has had, the greater the risk to the infant. Maternal physiology cannot support many pregnancies in rapid succession, and as age increases, the ability to cope with the stresses of pregnancy decreases.[65]

- When fathers are age 40 or older, they are at risk because sperm cells have divided so many times that there are more opportunities for errors. Anomalies linked to autosomal dominant mutations include Down syndrome, dwarfism, bone malformations, and Marfan's syndrome.[66]

---

### CRITICAL THINKING

*What do you believe the rate of live births to teen mothers is in Nunavut?*

---

## Prenatal Endocrine and Metabolic Functions

Fetal growth and development depend on maternal endocrine and metabolic adjustments during pregnancy. The placenta helps to provide necessary estrogens, progesterone, and gonadotropin to sustain pregnancy and trigger other endocrine adjustments that primarily involve the pituitary, adrenal cortex, and thyroid. Fetal endocrine function is regulated independently from the mother, but endocrine or hormonal drugs, such as birth control pills, progestin, diethylstilbestrol (DES), androgens, and synthetic estrogens, which are given to the mother, may produce undesirable effects in the fetus.[67]

*The fetal period is the first critical period for sexual differentiation.* Although the fetus has a chromosomal combination denoting male or female, it must be exposed to corresponding hormones during pregnancy. If the male fetus is insensitive to androgen (a hormone that promotes male sex characteristics), and is exposed to large amounts of estrogen (a feminizing hormone), the child may possess many female characteristics.[68] Testicular inductor substance causes the production of fetal androgens that suppress anatomic precursors of the oviducts and ovaries and, in turn, cause the male genital tract to develop during the seventh to twelfth weeks. The male embryo's testosterone offsets the maternal hormone influences. Unless androgens are present, the external genitalia of the fetus will appear female regardless of the chromosomal pattern. Estrogens are released in the genetically female embryo and are necessary for the fetus to develop female genitalia. Likewise, inspection of the external genitalia of a newborn female may show abnormal fusion of the labia and enlargement of the clitoris caused by an androgen agent taken by the mother early in her pregnancy.[69]

*The second critical period for sexual differentiation occurs just before, or just after birth, when sex typing of the brain occurs.* Testosterone may influence the hypothalamus so that a noncyclic pattern for the release of pituitary hormones, the gonadotropin, will occur in males; and a cyclic pattern of gonadotropin release will occur in females.[70]

Fetal and placental growth, nourishment, waste excretion, and total function all depend on the adequacy of the mother's metabolism.[71]

Maternal diabetes continues to play a significant role in neonatal morbidity and mortality. This role exists despite a better understanding of maternal and fetal metabolism, better control of maternal diabetes, and improved obstetrical and neonatal care. Infants of diabetic mothers (IDMs) and infants of gestational diabetic mothers (IGDMs) are at some risk for complications. The excessive fetal growth of the IDM is caused by exposure to high levels of maternal glucose, which readily crosses the placenta. In early pregnancy, fluctuations in blood glucose levels and episodes of ketoacidosis are believed to cause congenital anomalies.

The most frequently occurring anomalies involve the cardiac, musculoskeletal, and central nervous systems. Hyperinsulinemia accounts for many of the problems of the fetus or infant. In addition to fluctuating glucose levels, maternal vascular involvement or superimposed maternal infection adversely affects the fetus.[72] Prenatal management is directed toward controlling maternal glucose levels, which if successful minimizes the complications of IDMs.

Current evidence indicates certain nutritional and health concerns among today's Aboriginal women of childbearing age. The prevalence of diabetes among Aboriginal people is twice to five times the national average.[73] It becomes important to assess early in pregnancy whether the woman's eating patterns follow the revised Canada's Food Guide.[74]

**Maternal Nutrition** Nutrition is a most important variable for maintaining fetal health and preventing prenatal and intrapartum complications. In fact, the physiological changes of pregnancy call for extra nutrients and energy to meet the demands of the expanding blood supply and factors. These other factors include the growth of maternal tissues, a developing fetus, and the loss of maternal tissues at birth, as well as preparation for lactation.[75] Even before pregnancy, women should follow the revised food guidelines outlined in *Canada's Food Guide to Healthy Eating* (available at Health Canada's website). These new guidelines organize foods into four major food groups: (1) vegetables and fruits; (2) grain products; (3) milk and alternatives; and (4) meat and alternatives. These guidelines give direction regarding the amount and selections of foods that individuals need each day. The revised Food Guide recommendations are flexible enough to be adapted for age, gender, activity level, and pregnancy.[76]

As a matter of interest, the revised Food Guide has many strengths, including simplicity, flexibility, visual appeal, widespread awareness, and consistency with current science. Released early in 2007, it concentrates on nutrient standards and the prevention of chronic disease as key scientific inputs into the revision. It promotes a pattern of eating based on meeting nutrient needs, promoting health, and minimizing the risk of nutrition-related disease.[77] A *Cultural Adaptation of Canada's Food Guide to Healthy Eating* exists for use by culturally diverse individuals and families. This guide features culturally specific foods and full-colour illustrations (see the Interesting Websites section at the end of this chapter). For example, a *Northwest Territories Food Guide* and a *Nunavut Food Guide* are both available along with the general publications. All may be accessed on the Internet through the Health Canada portal website.

The Dietary Reference Intakes (DRIs) is a comprehensive set of nutrient reference values for healthy populations that can be used to assess and plan diets. They are based on the amount of vitamins, minerals, and other substances (such as fibre) that an individual needs—not only to prevent deficiencies, but also to lower the risk of chronic disease. The DRIs were established by Canadian and American scientists through a review process overseen by the National Academy of Sciences, an independent, non-governmental body.[78] Health Canada uses the DRIs in policies and programs that benefit the health and safety of all Canadians. (Check the Health Canada website for Using the Dietary Reference Intakes.)

## CRITICAL THINKING

*Who uses the Dietary Reference Intakes (DRIs)?*

Regarding gestational weight gain and pregnancy outcomes, current recommendations suggest that weight gain ranges be based on pre-pregnancy Body Mass Index (BMI). The BMI is an index of weight to height ($kg/m^2$). It is the most useful indicator to date of health risks associated with overweight and underweight individuals:[79]

■ *Pre-pregnancy BMI under 20:* Low pre-pregnancy weight is a critical determinant of intrauterine growth retardation and premature birth. Pregnant women with a low pre-pregnancy BMI should be referred to a registered dietician/nutritionist for dietary assessment and counselling. Weight gain by the woman should be monitored at each visit.[80]

■ *Pre-pregnancy BMI between 20 and 27:* Healthy-weight women are at lowest risk for giving birth to either a low-birth-weight baby or a high-birth-weight baby. Women with pre-pregnancy weight in this range should gain between 11.5 and 16.0 kg overall, or approximately 0.4 kg per week during the second and third trimesters.[81]

■ *Pre-pregnancy BMI above 27:* Women with a high BMI are more likely to develop gestational diabetes mellitus and to give birth to high-birth-weight infants, defined as over 4000 g. Although mean birth weights have been increasing, the differences between the proportions of

babies over 4000 g in the First Nations population and the general population remains significant.[82] Pregnant women with a BMI over 27 should be referred to a registered dietician/nutritionist for dietary assessment and counselling. Encourage women to gain between 7.0 and 11.5 kg overall—approximately 0.3 kg per week. A suggestion can be made for them to optimize the quality of eating patterns rather than to "diet" to restrict weight gain.[83]

Refer to Table 6-3 for guidelines for gestational weight gain ranges.

## CRITICAL THINKING

*What may be some contributing factors for the occurrence of high BMI rates among First Nation mothers?*

Pregnancy itself exerts a very powerful and lasting influence on the health and well-being of the mother, her infant, future children, and her family.[84]

During the first two months of pregnancy, the developing embryo consists mostly of water. Later, more solids in the form of fat, nitrogen, and certain minerals are observed. Because of the small amount of yolk in the human ovum, growth depends on nutrients obtained from the mother.[85] Although nutritional requirements for the embryo/fetus are quantitatively small during the first trimester, nutritional deprivations can negatively affect placental structure and the ultimate birth weight. Evidence suggests that a daily supplement containing folic acid (a form of folate) is important during the periconceptual period. Folic acid reduces the risk of neural tube defects.[86] It is important to note that taking a supplement containing folic acid does not preclude the need to eat a healthy diet in accordance with the revised *Canada's Food Guide to Healthy Eating*. In 1998, Health Canada made mandatory the addition of folic acid to flour and bread.[87]

## CRITICAL THINKING

*What are alternate food sources of folic acid?*

## Table 6-3 Guidelines for Gestational Weight Gain Ranges

| BMI Category | Recommended Total Weight Gain (kg) | Approximate Weekly Weight Gain (kg) |
| --- | --- | --- |
| BMI < 20 | 12.5–18.0 | 0.5 per week during 2nd and 3rd trimesters |
| BMI 20 > 27 | 11.5–16.0 | 0.4 per week during 2nd and 3rd trimesters |
| BMI > 27 | 7.0–11.5 | 0.3 per week |

Source: Adapted from Health Canada. *Nutrition for a Healthy Pregnancy—National Guidelines for the Childbearing Years,* p. 207. Ottawa: Author, 2002. Adapted and reproduced with the permission of the Minister of Public Works and Government Services Canada.

# High-Gestational-Weight Client

Jean is four months pregnant with her first child. Her pre-pregnancy BMI was high (over 27). Since her last visit to the prenatal clinic she has gained weight—more than the recommended 0.3 kg per week. She informs you that she "hates milk" and has been drinking milkshakes as a source of calcium.

**Questions**

1. What nutritional counselling does Jean need?
2. What better sources of calcium can you suggest for her?
3. What risks of high gestational weight gain, and a possible high-birth-weight baby, might you share with Jean?

*Caloric* and *protein* intake are of particular importance. Calories are needed for cell multiplication, and protein is believed to be primarily related to enlargement of these cells. Therefore, failure of the cells to receive sufficient protein and calories during critical periods of growth can lead to a slowing down and ultimate cessation of the ability of these cells to enlarge, divide, and develop specialized functions. The lack of protein also affects later intellectual performance. Finally, sufficient calories from fats and carbohydrates are needed so that protein is not used for energy.[88]

*Caloric requirements* for pregnant woman suggest that women should increase daily energy intake by approximately 100 kcal (400 kj) in the first trimester and by 300 kcal (1300 kj) in the second and third trimesters. Of course, energy requirements depend on basal metabolic rate and activity patterns, which vary markedly from one individual to another. Normally, women in the first trimester gain between 1.0 and 3.5 kg. Women who lose weight during the first trimester should be carefully assessed. Women with a large weight gain, particularly those with a pre-pregnancy BMI over 27, should be assessed. Their weight gain should be approximately 0.3 kg per week. For women with a BMI under 20, larger weight gains in the first trimester may be desirable. It is important to emphasize that most women can achieve normal weight gain by following the revised *Canada's Food Guide to Healthy Eating* (now called *Eating Well With Canada's Food Guide*), and by emphasizing nutrient-dense and lower-fat food choices. After the first trimester, weight gain is usually steady and increased, indicating a gain of both lean and fat tissues.[89] Patterns of either weight gain or weight loss must be evaluated thoroughly throughout the pregnancy.

Notably, low maternal weight at conception followed by little weight gain during pregnancy are associated with delivering a child who has low birth weight (less than 2500 g). Low birth weight is associated with neonatal morbidity, mortality, and developmental problems. Excessive gestational weight gain may be associated with high birth weight (defined as more than 4000 g). The possible consequences of gestational weight gain and high birth weight may include prolonged labour and birth, induced hypertension, gestational diabetes, birth asphyxia, birth trauma, caesarean birth, and increased risk of perinatal mortality.[90]

*Protein requirements* increase to support fetal growth and development, the formation of the placenta and amniotic fluid, the growth of maternal tissues, and the expanded blood volume. High-protein diets have not demonstrated improvement in birth weight and are not recommended prenatally.[91]

*Mineral and vitamin supplementation*, the preferred way to meet nutrient requirements during pregnancy, is to follow a healthy eating pattern according *Eating Well With Canada's Food Guide*.[92] When the diet does not provide sufficient calcium and vitamin D, and sun exposure is limited, effort must be directed toward increasing the dietary intake of these nutrients. Vitamin D is needed for calcium absorption.[93] Calcium and vitamin D supplements may be necessary for some women. The best sources of calcium are dairy products: milk, cheese, and yogurt. Regarding considerations for supplemental formulations of other minerals such as iron, the amount should be discussed with either the physician or the dietician. The publication *Nutrition for a Healthy Pregnancy—National Guidelines for the Childbearing Years* should be consulted. It is important to note that when a nutrient supplementation is chosen, not only must the supplements' formulation be considered, but the inhibitory factors and potential toxicities must be examined as well. For example, women who are taking supplements in a multi-vitamin/multimineral form should be cautioned against potential toxicity for vitamin A (retinol).[94]

*Folic acid supplementation* is used to prevent fetal malformations, especially neural tube defects, and maternal anemia. Health Canada indicates that abundant folic acid needs to be available in early gestation while the neural tube is closing—from 21 to 28 days after conception.[95] Folic acid (folate) is also necessary to build new cells and genetic material and to prevent stunted growth.[96] A study by House and colleagues, conducted in Newfoundland and Labrador, provided evidence to support the effectiveness of folate fortification programs, as well as prenatal education programs. The province was selected because it had one of the highest rates of neural tube defects in North America (1976–1991: 3.2 per 1000 births).[97] The findings of the study revealed that the status of both folate and cobalamin had significantly improved in the post-fortification era. These results were concurrent with a significant reduction in the number of neural tube defects from 4.67 (1992–1996) to 1.01 (1998–2002) per 1000 births. A folic acid supplement taken throughout pregnancy will help to meet the additional needs for fetal development.[98] During pregnancy, special attention should be given to folate, calcium, vitamin D, iron, and essential fatty acids intakes because of the risk of inadequate intakes in some groups of women.[99] The effects of inadequate nutrition are most severe for the pregnant adolescent, who herself has growth requirements. Nutritional deficiencies of the mother during her own fetal and childhood periods contribute to structural and physiologic difficulties in supporting a fetus. Improvement of the pregnant woman's diet, when she has previously been poorly nourished, does not appreciably benefit the fetus. *The fetus apparently draws most of its raw materials for development from maternal body structure and lifetime reserves*.[100] You have a significant role in teaching proper nutrition to children and adolescents.

The fetus with intrauterine growth restrictions (IUGRs) has a much greater illness and death rate compared to its normal counterpart. The long-term cost of some survivors illuminates the importance of prevention and prediction of pregnancies with fetal growth problems. Better education and nutrition to promote healthy pregnancies and the use of diagnostic ultrasonography as a technique are important in antepartum surveillance.

It is important for pregnant women to include a sufficient amount of the essential fatty acids linoleic and alpha-linolenic acid (one of the omega-3 fatty acids) in their daily diets. Omega-3 fatty acids are important to ensure neural and visual function development in the fetus.[101]

## CRITICAL THINKING

*What is a source of omega-3 fatty acid?*

**Anemia** The effects of maternal anemia on the fetus are less clear than those on the mother. Anemia denotes a decrease in the oxygen-carrying capability of the blood, which is directly related to a reduction in hemoglobin concentration and the number of red blood cells. The normal mean hemoglobin is 140g/L (SD 20g/L) for women. Clients whose hemoglobin counts fall two standard deviations (SD) below the mean should be considered anemic.[102]

*Iron deficiency anemia (IDA)* accounts for 75 percent of anemia diagnosed during pregnancy. The extra iron requirements of pregnancy are needed for the fetus and placenta

and to expand the maternal hemoglobin mass.[103] Willows and her colleagues assessed the prevalence of anemia and the associated risk factors among nine-month-old Cree infants in northern Quebec. They found that iron-deficiency anemia is highly prevalent among James Bay Cree infants.[104] Another study was conducted with Inuit infants in Nunavik, the northern part of Quebec. These results indicated that iron-deficiency anemia was a problem in Inuit infants as young as six months of age. The researchers concluded that breastfed infants were better protected against iron-deficiency anemia than were infants fed cow's milk or low-iron formula.[105]

*Sickle cell anemia* in the mother, associated with sickle cell disease, which is seen predominantly among blacks, may show a number of negative effects on the developing fetus. Changes in the mother's pathophysiologic state may lead to IUGR, premature labour, a reduction of 250 to 500 g in average birth weight, and even stillbirth, related to the "sickling" or clumping of misshaped erythrocytes within the placental vascular system.[106]

**Pica** One nutritional tradition is pica, a craving to eat non-food substances such as clay, unprocessed flour, cornstarch, laundry starch, coal, soap, toothpaste, mothballs, petrol, tar, paraffin, wood, plaster, soil, chalk, charcoal, cinders, baking powder, baking soda, powdered bricks, and refrigerator frost scrapes. Pica is common in children and women of all cultures who are hungry, poor, malnourished, and desire something to chew.[107] Women who practise pica are often ashamed of the compulsion and hesitate either to admit to the practice or to share their concern about it.[108]

## CRITICAL THINKING

*What are some health promoting strategies for women with pica?*

## Environmental Hazards to the Fetus: Teratogenic Effects

**Teratogen** A teratogen is an environmental substance, or agent, that interrupts normal development and causes malformation.

Teratogenesis is a development of abnormal structures. It is time-specific. The stimulus is non-specific and timing is more important than the nature of the insult or negative stimulus. The first trimester is the most critical. Development is characterized by a precise order. The timing, intensity, and duration of insult, injury, teratogen, or abnormal stimulus or event are important for the consequence. Teratogenic agents affect genes in several ways: (1) genes cease protein production so that development ceases; (2) genes fail to complete the development they have begun; or (3) excess growth of part of the organism occurs.[109]

Prominent environmental factors that have the potential to damage the fetus include radiation; chemical wastes; contaminated water; heavy metals, such as lead; certain food additives; various pollutants; chemical interactions; nicotine from smoking tobacco; pica; medicinal and non-medicinal drugs; alcohol; maternal and paternal infections; and maternal stress. The timing of fetal contact with a specific teratogen is a crucial factor (see Figure 6-1). Susceptibility to teratogens in general decreases as organ formation advances.[110]

Once implantation has occurred (seven or eight days after fertilization), the embryo undergoes very rapid and important transformations for the next four weeks. The sequence of embryonic events shows that each organ (brain, heart, eye, limbs, and genitalia) undergoes a critical stage of differentiation at precise times. For example, during the third week, teratogens can harm basic structures of the heart and central nervous system. During the individual critical periods, the embryo is highly vulnerable to teratogens, producing specific gross malformations. Each teratogen acts on a selected aspect of cellular metabolism.[111]

There is no evidence that congenital anomalies will always be produced when a teratogen is present because the embryo has the inherent capacity to replace damaged cells with newly formed cells. However, the higher the dose (intensity), the more harmful influences that are present, and the longer the exposure, the greater the chance that the baby will be harmed. The harm will be more severe than if dose and duration are less. Finally, the biogenetic vulnerability of the mother and infant influence the effects of a teratogen.[112]

A complicated interplay exists among the father, mother, offspring, and teratogen. In addition to the critical period of developmental stage and genetic susceptibility, the degree to which a teratogen causes abnormalities depends on its dosage, absorption, distribution, and metabolism; the physical state of the mother; and excretion by the separate body systems of mother and fetus. A teratogen that enters a mother's system also enters the system of her developing child, meaning that the so-called *placental barrier is practically non-existent*.[113]

**External Environmental Factors** Prenatally, environmental teratogens may interfere with the development of the embryo or fetus directly, or they may cause hormonal, circulatory, or nutritional changes in the mother that in turn damage the organism. Examples include the following:[114]

- Excess heat, such as soaks in hot tubs or sauna baths in early pregnancy, which may cause fetal neural tube defects
- High levels of noise
- Crowding and the consequent stressors
- Radiation from multiple sources at work or from diagnostic tests—most procedures cause low-level fetal x-ray exposure if performed accurately, but the pregnant woman should inform diagnosticians
- Ultraviolet light from excessive sun or a sunlamp
- Air, water, and soil pollutants, including lead, mercury, and pesticides or chemicals
- Trace minerals or chemicals linked to the work setting

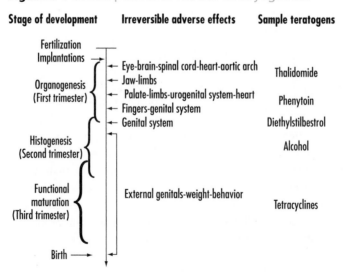

**Figure 6-1** Critical periods in human embryogenesis

| Stage of development | Irreversible adverse effects | Sample teratogens |
|---|---|---|
| Fertilization Implantations | | |
| Organogenesis (First trimester) | Eye-brain-spinal cord-heart-aortic arch | Thalidomide |
| | Jaw-limbs | |
| | Palate-limbs-urogenital system-heart | Phenytoin |
| | Fingers-genital system | |
| | Genital system | Diethylstilbestrol |
| Histogenesis (Second trimester) | | Alcohol |
| Functional maturation (Third trimester) | External genitals-weight-behavior | Tetracyclines |
| Birth | | |

Source: Reprinted from Wong D.L., M.J Hockenberry, S.E. Perry, D.L. Lowdermilk, and D. Wilson, *Maternal Child Nursing Care*, 3rd ed. (p. 843). Philadelphia: Mosby Elsevier, 2006. Used by permission.

- Chemicals and drugs in food
- Chemotherapeutic (anti-neoplastic) medications

Depending on dosage, radiation can be responsible for cell destruction that is linked to embryonic death, gross malformations, growth retardation, and an increased risk of malignancy in later life.[115]

Occupational hazards include the transfer of drugs and chemicals from the male to the female during intercourse—an action that later can negatively affect fertilization or implantation. If the woman is already pregnant, the same hazards can have teratogenic effects on the developing person. For example, decreased sperm count and infertility are related to paternal exposure to dibromochloropropane (DBCP). Paternal exposure to toxic agents is most likely to result in male infertility or spontaneous abortions. Anaesthetic gases, vinyl chloride exposure, chloroprene, or other hydrocarbons have all been connected to spontaneous abortions. Lead present in the environment directly increases sperm abnormalities, induces male infertility, and facilitates spontaneous abortion through either affected sperm or indirect contamination. Persistent environmental contaminants, such as dioxin and polychlorobiphenyls (PCBs), alter the activities of several different hormones.[116]

---

## CRITICAL THINKING

*In what ways can paternal exposure to toxins cause birth defects?*

---

There is no conclusive evidence that physical activity via employment promotes preterm birth and low birth weight, although causes could include prolonged standing, long working hours, high speed, bending, and lifting heavy objects. Health care providers should be sensitive to the presence of occupational fatigue associated with workload during pregnancy.[117]

Environmental hazards such as radiation, chemicals, and other pollutants in our industrialized world can endanger the fetus. For example, radiation from x-rays can seriously affect the developing fetus. The most critical time is during the first several weeks after conception, when women do not know they are pregnant.[118] Markowitz states that exposure to lead affects the child's mental development. However, because lead can enter any cell, toxicity may occur in any tissue or organ.[119] It is vital that preconception care begin with an assessment of the workplace, home, and leisure activity environments for exposure to toxins or hazardous conditions.[120] Researchers have found that industrial wastes such as polychlorinated biphenyls (PCBs) are harmful to prenatal development. Ayotte and his research team conducted a study to investigate factors influencing plasma PCB levels in Inuit infants during their

first year of life. One of their findings indicated that exposure to these lipophilic compounds, through breastfeeding, has a major and long-lasting influence on the offspring's body burden.[121] That is, the infants were affected by the PCBs in breast milk.

Mercury, like lead, has major implications for the health of the mother and offspring. Mercury-contaminated water results from medical wastes, industrial byproducts, incinerator emissions, and dumpsite leakage. Inorganic mercury converts to the more harmful organic form, methyl mercury, which is absorbed by fish and then consumed by humans. When ingested during pregnancy, nervous system impairment, compromised immune function, and a congenital syndrome similar to cerebral palsy may occur.[122]

**Smoking Tobacco** The primary mission of the Federal Tobacco Control Strategy (FTCS) is for all Canadians to reduce tobacco-related disease and death. The FTCS has five 10-year (2001–2011) objectives. One of these is to reduce the number of people who smoke from 25 percent to 20 percent of the population. This strategy is directed at Canadians of all ages, with a particular emphasis on high-risk groups such as youth (whose smoking prevalence is 25 percent), young adults (32 percent), Inuit (72 percent), and First Nations (62 percent).[123]

Smoking is associated with numerous detrimental effects:

- Higher percentage of spontaneous abortions, stillbirths, and preterm or premature births (decreased gestational age)[124]
- Lower birth weight (less than 2.5 kg, or 5.5 pounds) as the number of cigarettes smoked daily increases[125]
- Increased possibility of sudden infant death syndrome (SIDS)[126]
- Deficits in learning skills (reading, mathematics) in the child[127]
- Increased respiratory disease, pneumonia, bronchitis, and allergy in infancy and childhood[128]

Ideally, women should stop smoking prior to conception. Maximum reduction of risk is believed to occur if the woman quits smoking by 16 weeks gestation. However, quitting smoking at any stage of gestation is advisable.[129]

Johnson and her colleagues conducted a study with women who quit smoking during pregnancy and gave birth at one of five hospitals. These participating women were interviewed six months after delivery and were assessed using biochemical methods to determine their smoking status. The objective of the study was to test a program developed to prevent smoking relapse in the postpartum period by comparing the rates of continuous smoking abstinence, daily smoking, and smoking cessation self-efficacy in treatment and control groups. The researchers concluded that smoking cessation interventions centring on the pre-natal period have failed to achieve long-term abstinence. These same researchers continue to claim that interventions can be strengthened if they are extended into the postpartum period.[130]

A CNA position statement on tobacco—*The Role of Health Professionals in Smoking Cessation*—was developed co-operatively across many health care professional disciplines. Because health professionals are in a unique position to assist smokers, this position statement focuses on smoking cessation as part of a comprehensive strategy.

The relapse rate is very high due to two powerful variables: the addictive nature of tobacco, and social pressures on the smoker. However, most smokers attempt to quit several times before they finally succeed.[131] Therefore, do not reduce your effort to encourage smokers to quit.

A concern is growing surrounding the potential adverse reproductive health effects and pregnancy outcomes that result from exposure to second-hand tobacco smoke. Although exposure to second-hand tobacco smoke is preventable, the harmful effects are particularly prevalent among women who are pregnant.[132] For pregnant women who smoke, health education programs or self-help groups are advisable.

## CRITICAL THINKING

*What steps can a nurse take to develop a smoking cessation program in the community?*

## Drug Hazards to the Fetus: Teratogenic Effects

New drugs are almost never tested in pregnant women to determine the effects on the fetus. As a result, most drugs are not labelled for use in pregnancy. Many agents may cause toxic, rather than teratogenic, effects.[133] All of a woman's medications should be reviewed by her physician with regard to the optimal dosage.[134] The Motherisk site (www.motherisk.org) is an up-to-date source for evidence-based information about the safety or risk of drugs during pregnancy.[135]

## CRITICAL THINKING

*What health promotion strategies would you use for a pregnant client who is using an antidepressant called lorazepam?*

**Substance Abuse and Addiction** During pregnancy, drug abuse and addiction continue to manifest themselves as major psychosocial and physical problems for both mother and child. Substances commonly abused during pregnancy, taken individually or in combination, are known to have multiple effects on the developing person, on the outcome of pregnancy, and on neonatal neurobehaviour.[136] Infants exposed to addictive drugs in utero throughout pregnancy are at great risk for congenital malformations, obstetric complications, and perinatal mortality.[137]

Drugs of any kind may affect both the mother and the fetus because they: (1) impinge upon the mother's overall health and nutrition; (2) often interfere with motivation to obtain prenatal care; and (3) interfere with blood flow to the placenta by means of vasoconstriction and increasing uterine contractibility. Such substances include over-the-counter drugs (Aspirin, cold remedies, antihistamine, anti-nauseants, codeine, large doses of vitamins), prescription medication, herbal and plant products, caffeine, marijuana, narcotics (methadone, heroin, cocaine), and solvents.[138]

**Marijuana** Fried and Smith state that despite marijuana being the most widely used illegal drug among women of reproductive age, a scarcity of data exists on the neuro-behavioural consequences in the offspring, particularly the long-term effects. Further well-controlled investigations are needed in this area.[139] However, a significant association has been reported between marijuana use and the decrease of fetal growth and infant birth weight.[140] The Ottawa Prenatal Prospective Study (OPPS) was designed to explore the effects on offspring of soft drug use during pregnancy. Marijuana use was recorded in terms of the number of joints smoked per week. Cigarette use was also recorded by deriving a nicotine score. The findings indicated that fetal exposure to marijuana and cigarettes may have a significant impact on the initiation of marijuana use and cigarette smoking during adolescence.[141]

**Cocaine** Cocaine has been recognized for many years for its stimulant effects. However, crack, a free-base form of cocaine, became available in the late 1980s.[142] Cocaine crosses the placenta easily and rapidly and is found in breast milk.[143] Cocaine-dependent neonates do not experience the process of withdrawal seen in narcotic-exposed infants, but they do show a neurotoxic effect of the drug (see Figure 6-2).[144]

Over the last ten years, numerous controlled studies have identified developmental and behavioural differences associated with prenatal cocaine exposure.[145] Infants exposed to cocaine in utero score below their non-exposed counterparts in many areas of neurodevelopment. These effects seem to persist well beyond the newborn period.[146] Miller-Loncar and her researchers examined the pattern of motor development across 18 months of life in infants with in utero exposure to cocaine to determine how prenatal drug effects and levels of exposure relate to motor development. Their findings indicated that infant exposure to cocaine affected their motor development, but no effects of the level of cocaine use on change in motor skills were demonstrated.[147]

**Figure 6-2** Neonatal effects of maternal cocaine use

**PHYSICAL**
Preterm birth
Decreased length
Decreased head circumference
Intrauterine growth restriction
Ileal atresia
Hypospadias
Hydronephrosis
Seizures
Fever
Congenital heart disease
Skull defects
Hypertension
Cerebral infarction
Vomiting
Diarrhea
Sudden infant death syndrome
Tachypnea

**BEHAVIORAL**
Irritability
Tremors
Poor feeding
Abnormal sleep patterns
Increased startles
Disorganized behavior
Poor visual processing
Difficult to console

Source: Fraser Asken, D., Acquired Problems of the Newborn. In D.L. Lowdermilk and S.E. Perry, *Maternity and Women's Health Care*, 8th ed., pp. 1051–1074 Philadelphia: Mosby, 2004. Used with permission.

Koren states that exposure to cocaine, determined by hair analysis, is associated with extensive perinatal risk. In fact, if cocaine exposure were not detected through hair tests, most of the cocaine-exposed infants not only would have perinatal complications, but also would go home to be looked after by drug-dependent mothers, further increasing their health risk.[148]

**Ecstasy** During the past decade, a sharp increase has occurred in Ecstasy (MDMA = methylenedioxy–methamphetamine) use by pregnant women who are young, single, and experience mental distress. These pregnant women tend to exhibit a clustering of risk factors that often compromise pregnancy and the fetus.

Ho and her associates found that compounding the issue of Ecstasy is smoking, heavy alcohol intake, and multiple drug use. These threats combined with a higher than expected rate of unplanned pregnancies increase the risk of fetal exposure to potentially harmful substances.[149]

CRITICAL THINKING

*Who is at liberty to use the Motherisk Laboratory for Drug Exposure at the Hospital for Sick Children?*

**Narcotics** *Addiction to narcotics, such as heroin, morphine, or codeine, can create another problem: fetal addiction.* Withdrawing the drug from the addicted woman before delivery causes the fetus to experience withdrawal distress as a result of visceral vasoconstriction and reduced circulation to the uterus. Intrauterine death may occur. However, when addiction continues through pregnancy, the infant is born with drug addiction. The addicted newborn is twice as likely as the non-addicted baby to die soon after birth. If the newborn does not die, it will experience withdrawal in two to four days. This is the *acute* period. The baby may require up to 40 days of treatment during the *withdrawal* period. The limited ability of the newborn to metabolize and eliminate these fat-soluble drugs may be responsible for the postponement of withdrawal symptoms. However, the withdrawal does not end the problems. Babies born addicted to opiates may suffer the effects of addiction until at least age six.[150]

The Brazelton Neonatal Behavioural Assessment Scale can be used to evaluate the normality of responses to environmental stimuli.[151] Finnegan's Neonatal Narcotic Abstinence Syndrome (NSA) is useful for assessing neonatal withdrawal.[152] The specific pattern of symptoms depends on (1) the type, amount, and combination of drugs used by the mother, (2) the length of time between drug exposure and delivery, and (3) the fetal ability to metabolize the drug.

The effect of addictive drugs on the child extends beyond the neonatal and infancy periods. In early childhood, babies who were addicted at birth may weigh less and be shorter than the norm, and overall may be less well adjusted. These children score lower on perceptual and learning ability tests, are more anxious, and do not perform well in school.[153]

Clinical assessment for substance abuse should include the evaluation of physical appearance, since demeanour and hygiene may give clues. A thorough history and physical examination, along with a substance abuse interview, may reveal multiple drug use or exposure to more than one teratogen. Urine samples of mothers are effective to screen for the ingestion of illicit drugs.

*The effects of drug use on the fetus, neonate, and child depend on the type of drug ingested, the dose, duration of drug use before and during pregnancy, and the state of maternal nutrition.* There are fewer infant symptoms when the pregnant woman stops drug use in the first trimester of pregnancy than if drug use continues. Thus, it is imperative to prevent drug use, to support the mother's efforts to stop drug use, and to encourage adequate prenatal care and nutrition.[154]

Prenatal care must include increased surveillance for drug-related complications in coordinated, comprehensive, family-oriented drug treatment programs. Rehabilitation and support efforts should continue after delivery and address issues that lead to and maintain patterns of abuse.

**Alcohol**  Heavy drinking by pregnant women can cause devastating effects in their offspring.[155] According to the National Population Health Survey, women in their thirties were more likely than women in their twenties to report alcohol consumption during pregnancy.[156]

For women who are (or may become) pregnant, the smart choice is to abstain totally from alcohol. In a study of 11 698 Danish women, alcohol consumption of more than 120 g per week was associated with a five times greater reduction in average birth weight in babies of smokers versus babies of non-smokers.[157]

Prior to the identification of fetal alcohol spectrum disorder (FASD), the conditions fetal alcohol syndrome (FAS) and fetal alcohol effects (FAE) were used solely to describe birth defects caused by the maternal ingestion of alcohol.[158] It has been recorded that the rate of FAS/FAE in some First Nations and Inuit communities is much higher than the national average due to their history of colonization and the devaluation of their culture.

*FAS manifests itself through the following characteristics:*[159]

■ Low birth weight
■ Small head
■ Flat facial profile or deformity
■ Ear and eye abnormalities
■ Poor motor coordination
■ Disturbed sleep patterns
■ Extra digits
■ Heart defects

FAE refers to the cognitive and behavioural problems of children exposed to alcohol while in utero but who lack the typical diagnostic characteristics of full-blown FAS.[160] Investigations of children with FAE have demonstrated that they will have better cognitive abilities than those with FAS; however, their behavioural functions, such as poor social skills, have been termed secondary disabilities.[161]

Continued use of alcohol by the mother who breastfeeds undoubtedly impedes the motor development of the infant. Alcohol-induced damage to the developing brain carries devastating effects with a long developmental time frame. Alcohol affects more cell populations, occurs at lower levels of exposure, produces greater numbers of permanent effects, and is modulated by more factors than were initially suspected in earlier studies.[162] Community education, treatment for the alcohol-abusing mother, parenting education, and early identification and intervention with the alcohol-affected child are all essential.[163]

One of the recommendations to reduce the number of infants with FAS is to conduct further research into: (1) discovering why some women drink alcohol so heavily during pregnancy; (2) assessing drinking patterns more extensively; and (3) assisting women to avoid the consumption of alcohol during pregnancy.[164]

A recent Health Canada document entitled *Fetal Alcohol Spectrum Disorder: A Framework for Action* was produced in collaboration with a number of organizations and individuals nationwide.[165] **Fetal alcohol spectrum disorder (FASD)** is an umbrella term used increasingly to describe the spectrum of disabilities (and diagnoses) associated with prenatal exposure to alcohol. The diagnoses grouped under the FASD umbrella include fetal alcohol syndrome (FAS), partial FAS (pFAS), alcohol-related neurodevelopmental disorder, and alcohol-related birth defects. The Health Canada document not only encourages people to understand FASD, but also includes the basic building blocks required for concerted action within communities, provinces, and territories, as well as within the federal government.[166] The document reflects ideas and advice for the prevention of FASD and the treatment of those with the disability (see Figure 6-3). Its five broad goals for action are as follows:

1. Increase public and professional awareness and understanding of FASD as well as of the impact of alcohol use during pregnancy.

2. Develop and increase the capacity to identify and meet the needs of children, youth, adults, and families affected by FASD.

3. Create effective national screening, diagnostic, and data-reporting tools and approaches.

4. Expand the knowledge base and facilitate information exchange between people and professionals in all types of settings.

5. Increase commitment and support for action on FASD.

The Addictions Foundation of Manitoba, through the efforts of Zenon Lisakowski, Pat Hayward, and members of the Adult Education Service Team, has developed a *Participant Manual for Alcohol-Related Birth Defects*. The diagnostic criteria found in the manual have been developed through the work of Dr. Ann Streissguth and her colleagues from the University of Washington and the University of Victoria. For more information regarding FASD, visit the Addictions Foundation of Manitoba's website at www.afm.mb.ca or call 1-866-877-0050.

**Figure 6-3**

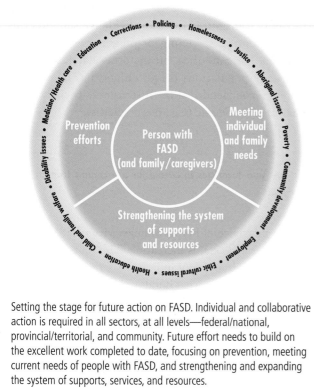

Setting the stage for future action on FASD. Individual and collaborative action is required in all sectors, at all levels—federal/national, provincial/territorial, and community. Future effort needs to build on the excellent work completed to date, focusing on prevention, meeting current needs of people with FASD, and strengthening and expanding the system of supports, services, and resources.

## CRITICAL THINKING

*What types of questions (linear, convergent, divergent, and circular) can a health professional ask the family for the purpose of circumventing denial regarding prenatal alcohol exposure?*

## Maternal Infections: Hazardous Influence on the Fetus

The pregnant woman is more susceptible to infections. The placenta cannot screen out all infectious organisms. Infectious diseases in the vaginal region can travel up to the amniotic sac and penetrate its walls and infect the amniotic fluid. Viral, bacterial, and parasitic diseases that have a mild effect on the mother may have a profound effect on the development of the fetus, depending on gestational age.[167]

**Rubella** (*German measles*) *can manifest as a maternal infection that may occur with harmful effects during the first trimester*. At the preconception visit, women at risk for rubella should be identified and, if not actively trying to become pregnant, should be immunized.[168] Rubella may go unnoticed by the mother, but it can cause severe effects and even death.[169] Screening by serology at the first prenatal visit is indicated. In fact, screening of serologic-negative women should be performed after exposure, or if the women have a possible rubella infection. Women who have negative serology should be immunized postpartum.[170]

New cases of congenital rubella are fewer now, compared to years past. However, surviving victims of the epidemic

continue to deal with its effects.[171] The fetus suffers an abnormal decrease in the absolute number of cells in most organs because of the viral interference with cell multiplication. The virus also causes adverse changes in the small blood vessels of the developing fetus and causes profuse damage to the placental vascular system as well, thus interfering with fetal blood flow and oxygenation.[172]

**Rubeola** ("*red measles*") is associated with abnormalities. If a pregnant woman has been exposed to measles, and her immunity status is in doubt, she should be tested for measles antibodies. Immune globulin (0.25ml/kg for a healthy adult; 0.5 ml/kg if immuno-compromised) is recommended within six days of the last exposure to measles. A number of conditions accompany this recommendation: (1) if the client is immuno-compromised; (2) if measles immune status is unknown or questionable; and (3) if measles IgG serology is either negative or cannot be obtained before six days from the last exposure. Immune globulin is not recommended if the woman was born before 1957, if she has had documented natural measles, or if she has had two doses of vaccine at a minimum of one month apart.[173]

**HIV** and **AIDS**, in both men and women, is a worldwide concern because of transmission between sexual partners, as well as in non-partnered sexual relationships. The number of HIV-infected women of childbearing age is rising worldwide. Because of the long incubation period (at least five years), the pregnant woman may be unaware that she has the virus. Transmission appears more likely when the mother has full-blown AIDS than when she is HIV-positive but not yet experiencing AIDS symptoms. Infection may depend on the strain of virus to which the fetus is exposed.

Three concepts support the idea of offering HIV testing to every pregnant woman during pregnancy: (1) the increasing rates of HIV infection in women; (2) the devastating effect on the baby of vertical transmission from the mother; and (3) the proven efficacy of AZT in reducing vertical transmission.[174] Therefore, it is recommended that HIV testing be offered to all pregnant women. Women should be provided with basic information about HIV testing. Normally this includes, first, learning of the risks and benefits of discovering a positive result and, second, stressing the success of treatment in reducing vertical transmission.[175]

Katz states that the care for the pregnant woman who has HIV is highly complex.[176] It is important for health professionals to become aware of certain issues in caring for the woman. One such issue, due to the major focus on treatment, has been the reduction of the risk of perinatal transmission. Therefore, the decision to initiate drug therapy is important. Nurses must be aware of the dosage levels and adverse effects, and they must help the woman deal with adherence issues.[177]

## CRITICAL THINKING

*What are some of the social aspects of HIV infection among pregnant women?*

Screening for **syphilis** by serology, at either the preconception or early pregnancy visit, is indicated according to provincial and territorial regulations. For women at risk, a repeat test in the third trimester is indicated.[178] It is essential that maternal syphilis be identified, before or early in pregnancy, to prevent devastating consequences for the neonate. Poor prenatal care and the lack of maternal treatment for syphilis contribute to these consequences.[179] Although necrosis of the umbilical cord (vein) is a clear indication that the newborn is infected, other symptoms may not appear until the fourteenth week of life. Alternatively, the child may appear healthy at birth, with symptoms appearing in two to six weeks. Occasionally, symptoms may not appear for up to two years.[180] Treatment of the mother also ensures treatment of the ill fetus because penicillin, or erythromycin, readily crosses the placenta.

**Chlamydia trachomatis** and **gonorrhea** are two genital infections that are easily transmitted and can produce pelvic inflammatory disease (PID). Tubal adhesions resulting from PID are an important factor in the occurrence of ectopic pregnancies.[181] Both diseases affect the fetus and neonate. For chlamydia, health care professionals should offer screening to women who are believed to be at increased risk, such as women younger than 20,

those with multiple sexual partners (or who have partners with multiple sexual partners), and women with a history of sexually transmitted diseases. Evidence supports the policy of routine screening of pregnant women with chlamydia. For gonorrhea, on the other hand, screening of high-risk populations (as for chlamydia) by cervical culture is recommended at the first visit—especially if the woman is symptomatic (e.g., has cervicitis).[182]

## CRITICAL THINKING

*What are your priorities in caring for a pregnant woman with chlamydia?*

The incidence of **herpes simplex virus (HSV)**, *infection of the genital area*, is increasing. The routine prenatal screening by culture is not indicated for those with a positive history. However, what is indicated is a single culture to confirm diagnosis when lesions are present.[183] Caesarean section is indicated in women with clinically apparent HSV infection at time of delivery to protect the newborn against infection. The primary source is maternal in nature in that genital herpes infections are sexually transmitted. Therefore, most affected women are in the childbearing age group. The majority of genital infections are asymptomatic and difficult to recognize on clinical examination. This makes the identification of a mother whose fetus is in jeopardy very difficult.

Congenital and neonatal HSV infections often prove lethal. Drug therapeutic measures taken thus far to cure the mother and newborn have been largely ineffective. Research in prevention and treatment of the infectious disease continues.[184]

No pregnancy screening is indicated for **cytomegalovirus (CMV)**. The potential public health effect of preconception screening remains to be determined because of the frequency of recurrent infections.

**Toxoplasmosis** is an infection contracted by eating infected meat or eggs that are either raw or undercooked, or through contact with the feces of an infected cat. Due to the high prevalence and seriousness of maternal infection and prenatal transmission, there exists a definite potential health benefit to routine preconception tests. For example, should the mother become infected during pregnancy, there is a good possibility that the parasite will cross the placental barrier. The presence of antibodies provides reassurance about immunity. The absence of antibodies underscores the need for education and vigilance.[185] Health promoting strategies on how to avoid contact with the parasite should be emphasized by the nurse. For example, pregnant women should use good handwashing techniques and avoid cat litter boxes.

**Fetal Infection** Intrauterine fetal infection caused by group B Streptococcus species probably occurs with greater frequency than is clinically diagnosed. In Canada, regarding group B Streptococcus (GBS), the Society of Obstetricians and Gynaecologists of Canada (SOGC) states that an urgent need exists for research in this area. They recommend that processes for the identification and management of women whose newborns might be at increased risk of GBS disease be initiated by one of the following methods: (1) universal screening of all pregnant women at 35 to 37 weeks gestation with a single combined vaginal-anorectal swab and the offer of intrapartum chemoprophylaxis to all GBS-colonized women;[186] or (2) no universal screening, but intrapartum chemoprophylaxis for all women with identified risk factors. This strategy should also be used in cases where universal screening is the policy, but either the screening was not done or the test results are not available.[187]

---

## CRITICAL THINKING

*What research question can a health professional develop regarding the effect upon a neonate of group B Streptococcus?*

---

**Immunologic Factors** The fetus is immunologically foreign to the mother's immune system, yet it is sustained. Selected antibodies of measles, chickenpox, hepatitis, poliomyelitis, whooping cough, and diphtheria are transferred to the fetus. The resulting immunity lasts for several months after birth. Antibodies to dust, pollen, and common allergens do not transfer across the placenta.[188] *Incompatibility between maternal and infant blood factors* is the most commonly encountered interference with fetal development resulting in various degrees of circulatory difficulty for the baby. When the blood of a fetus contains a protein substance, the Rh factor (Rh-positive blood), but the mother's blood does not (Rh-negative blood), antibodies in the mother's blood may attack the fetus and possibly cause spontaneous abortion, stillbirth, jaundice anemia, heart defects, mental retardation, or death. Usually, the first Rh-positive baby is not affected adversely; however, with each succeeding pregnancy the risk becomes greater. A vaccine can be given to the Rh-negative mother within three days of childbirth or abortion which will prevent her body from making Rh antibodies. Babies affected by the Rh syndrome can be treated with repeated blood transfusions.[189]

**Maternal Emotions** Most mothers find deep gratification in the maternal role, despite its challenges. The maternal role is critical to ensure the infant's safety, survival, and well-being. Several key infant and health variables may affect maternal role functioning.[190]

The physical–psychological interdependence between mother and fetus continues to be studied. The effects of the mother's elation, fear, and anxiety on the behaviour and other developmental aspects of the baby remain poorly understood. Anxiety and fear resulting from physical abuse, worries about the current living situation or finances, or violence in the neighbourhood or community produce a variety of physiologic changes in the mother. *Maternal stress, therefore, may be considered a teratogen resulting in physical and psychological alterations of the developing person before and following birth.*

Women employed outside the home continue to be exposed to many environmental stressors that affect their mothering role. One important decision-making experience elicits great conflict and anxiety in many women: whether the mother should return to work after the child is born. The decision is most difficult for women who are not forced to return to work for financial reasons. These women see their work as central to their identity. Women who believe that mothering is more important than their work, and whose identity does not depend on their work, have little trouble leaving their employment. Mothers who must return to work for financial reasons experience less conflict because they see their return to work as a responsibility rather than a choice.[191]

*Domestic violence is a severe and common stressor for the pregnant woman.* Physical abuse during pregnancy has been associated with unemployment, substance abuse and addiction, poverty, and family dysfunction, either in the past, the present, or both. Thus, it is difficult to determine the relative contribution of each of these risks.[192] The results of a Canadian study found that 95 percent of women who were abused during the first trimester of their pregnancies were also abused in the three-month period after delivery. The study also indicated that the abuse increased after the baby was born.[193] Battering a pregnant woman may represent an extreme response of jealousy toward the unborn baby and anger at being displaced from the centre of the woman's attention. Men may, in fact, fear or envy women's reproductive power. Such men deal with fear and envy by asserting physical power over women, often forcing themselves sexually on women to the extent of manifesting sexual addiction or rape.[194]

Maternal anxiety reactions are sometimes related to the physiologic responses of pregnancy, such as nausea and vomiting, backaches, and headaches, which in turn affect the fetus. The woman who begins pregnancy with relatively few psychic reserves is especially vulnerable to the stresses and conflicting moods that accompany pregnancy.[195]

---

## CRITICAL THINKING

*What questions would you ask an abused pregnant woman?*

---

**Direct** (occur at conception)

- Damage to spermatozoa caused by chemicals such as fumigants, solvents, vinyl chloride, methyl mercury, hypothermia, radiation, pesticides, diethylstilbestrol (DES), alcohol, or lack of vitamin C.
- Alterations in seminal fluid.
- Factor or agent affects chromosomes or cytogenic apparatus in sperm cells or their precursors.
- Drugs and chemicals cross into testes and male accessory reproductive organs for secretion in semen.

**Indirect** (occur before conception)

- Genetic constitution contributed by father to fetus may make fetus more susceptible to environmental factors to which it is later exposed. (Responses to teratogens may depend in part on genotype of exposed individual.)
- Transmission of chemicals to the pregnant woman through the man's skin, hair, or contaminated clothing.

**Examples of Paternal Contributions to Causes of Fetal Defects**

- Down syndrome (trisomy 21): paternal non-disjunction and extra chromosome; 20 to 30 percent of cases occur when father is 55 years or older at time of conception.

- Sex chromosome disorders in child.
- Adverse outcomes such as spontaneous abortion and perinatal death (stillbirth) due to methadone and morphine dependency and chemicals such as fumigants, solvents, and vinyl chloride.
- Infertility in the couple due to drugs or other chemicals.
- Hemophilia: coagulation disorder in child; deficiency of factor VIII.
- Marfan syndrome: connective tissue disorder with elongated extremities, hands.
- Progeria: premature aging, growth deficiency.
- Decreased neonatal survival due to methadone and morphine dependency.
- Birth defects if father is epileptic (especially if taking phenytoin) or if father is exposed to lead, waste, anaesthetic gases, Agent Orange, or dioxin.
- Tumours of nervous system if father is miner, printer, pulp or paper mill worker, electrical worker, or auto mechanic.

**Birth Defects Transmitted by the Father** Genes of both mother and father, and the prenatal maternal environment, may cause birth defects. Genetic mutations or abnormalities in sperm are being found in an increasingly growing percentage of the population. It is interesting to note that more male than female cells undergo genetic mutation. Mutations may be caused by exposure to irradiation, infection, drugs, and chemicals. These mutations occur more frequently in men as they age, and they may be responsible for various inborn disorders and congenital anomalies (see the box entitled "Causes of Paternal Contributions to Birth Defects in the Child"). For males, this "cut-off" is at about 45 years of age. Risks for chromosomal abnormalities may double when the male is 55 years or older.[196] The male may affect the unborn child in other ways as well.

## VARIABLES RELATED TO CHILDBIRTH THAT AFFECT THE BABY

Use the following information in assessment of, and intervention with, mother and baby.

## Medications

Analgesics and general anaesthetics given during childbirth cross the placental barrier, affecting the newborn for days after delivery. Respiration after birth is negatively affected and artificial resuscitation may be needed for severe respiratory depression. Motor skills tend to be less developed and more crying irritability is seen after birth as a result of analgesic and general anaesthetics.

Consequently, **analgesics**, or *drugs to reduce pain*, and sedatives, or mild tranquilizers to reduce anxiety, tend to be given in early labour. Epidural block, one form of local anaesthesia, is being used with increasing frequency rather than general anaesthesia. However, all drugs and local anaesthetics tend, indirectly, to affect the fetus by reducing blood flow to the uterus, thus affecting the fetal heart rate. The APGAR score may be low (see Chapter 7). Drugs given during labour remain in the infant's bloodstream for up to a few days.[197]

Childbirth without drugs was first introduced in 1914 by Grantly Dick Read, who was followed by a more familiar name, Dr. Fernand Lamaze. The natural childbirth method has become popular with both mothers and fathers because they can both participate actively in the birth of their child. During natural childbirth classes, the mother and father (or partner) learn about the physiology of pregnancy and childbirth, exercises that strengthen the mother's abdominal and perineal muscles, and techniques of breathing and relaxation during labour and delivery. The father or partner acts as encourager and coach throughout the prenatal classes, as well as during labour and delivery. In doing so, the birth experience is shared by the couple. An equal benefit of the Lamaze approach is the child who comes into the world without any ill effects from medication.

## Method and Place of Delivery

Birth can be difficult, even dangerous. Forceps may be needed to withdraw the baby, for either of maternal or fetal reasons. The use of forceps is safe if the cervix is completely dilated and the head is within 5 cm of the mouth of the vagina. Abdominal surgery, or caesarean section, is carried out when the baby cannot be born vaginally for a number of reasons. This major surgery should not be done unless absolutely necessary. No evidence exists to indicate that the site at which the baby is born has any effect on long-term development.[198] Adequate prenatal care and safety for mother and baby are the important factors.

---

**CRITICAL THINKING**

*What are some special features of home delivery available to the mother and newborn that may not be available in a family birthing centre?*

---

## Inadequate Oxygenation

**Anoxia,** *decreased oxygen supply,* and increased carbon dioxide levels may result during delivery. Some degree of risk occurs almost routinely from compression of the umbilical cord, reduced blood flow to the uterus, or placental separation. Fortunately, newborn babies are better able to withstand periods of low oxygenation than are adults. Other causes of asphyxia, however, such as drug-induced respiratory depression or apnea, kinks in the umbilical cord, wrapping of the cord around the neck, very long labour, and malpresentation of the fetus during birth, have more serious effects. Longitudinal studies of anoxic newborns revealed lower than normal performance scores on tests of sensorimotor and cognitive-intellectual skills and personality measures compared to children with minimal anoxia at birth. Anoxia is the principal cause of perinatal death, and it is a common cause of mental retardation and cerebral palsy.[199]

## Premature or Preterm Birth and Low Birth Weight

Prematurity may have long-term consequences for the child. **Preterm** birth is defined as *birth before 38 weeks of gestation.*

**Prematurity** is defined as *the birth at a gestational age of 37 weeks or earlier, combined with birth weight of less than 2500 g.* Risk of death is greater for premature or low-birth-weight babies. The causes of such death have been discussed earlier in this chapter.

Later developmental and behavioural problems, such as physical and mental retardation and hyperactivity, may also be correlated with prematurity.[200] Treatment of the premature neonate in sterile, precisely controlled incubators causes an absence of environmental and sensory stimuli. These conditions also contribute to later retardation. Research shows that hourly gentle rubbing promotes positive effects immediately and later for infants in isolettes. Babies who receive such stimulation tend to be more active and gain weight faster, and later they perform better on tests of motor development, while appearing healthier and more active than premature children who suffer tactile and sensory deprivation.

**Low-birth-weight** *infants weighing less than 2500 g* may not be premature; some are simply small for gestational age. The baby may have completed the thirty-eighth week in utero.[201] The **very-low-birth-weight (VLBW)** *baby weighs less than 1500 grams.* The **extremely-low-birth-weight (ELBW)** *baby weighs less than 1000 grams.* Both the VLBW and ELBW babies will be of low gestational age, or premature.[202] The **small-for-date** baby may be born after nine months' gestation but be too small because of a slowdown in prenatal growth.[203]

See Chapter 7 for further details.

The following *maternal factors contribute to a higher risk of low-birth-weight babies:*[204]

- Underweight before pregnancy
- Less than 21 pounds gained during pregnancy
- Inadequate prenatal care
- Age of 16 years or younger or 35 years or older
- Low socioeconomic level
- Poor nutrition during pregnancy
- Smoking cigarettes during pregnancy
- Use of addictive drugs or alcohol during pregnancy
- History of abortion
- Complications during pregnancy, poor health status, exposure to infections
- High stress levels, including physical or emotional abuse

The risk of low birth weight is often associated with financial problems, or living in high-crime areas, irrespective of the variables of race, poor health habits, and complications during pregnancy.[205]

Heaman states that at the Canadian Consensus Conference on Preterm Birth Prevention, held in 1998, consensus was reached on the facts regarding preterm birth prevention. Beyond that, suggestions were made for research, community, and clinical action. The recommendations for action emphasized the adoption of a population health approach to prevent preterm birth.[206]

*What is the main thrust of a population health approach?*

Premature children differ from full-term infants in a number of ways, including sleep patterns, which are poorly organized with poorly differentiated sleep states. Shorter and less regular periods of each sleep state are exhibited and may persist beyond infancy. Because more growth hormone is released during sleep, disturbed sleep patterns in the premature infant may generally affect physical growth and size.[207]

# EARLY CHILDHOOD VARIABLES THAT AFFECT THE PERSON

Use the following information in assessment of, and health promotion interventions with, the child and adults in the childbearing years.

## Nutrition

Nutrition exerts a powerful influence on growth and development, especially if nutritional deficiency diseases occur. Inadequate nutrition may slow normal growth, and apparently causes a permanent effect in low intellectual ability. Children who suffer starvation do not catch up with growth norms for their group. Later in life, however, adequate nutrition and socioemotional support do help to offset the differences. *In your nutritional counselling, emphasize that there must be enough calories to support adequate growth, so that the protein that is consumed by the body is not used primarily for energy, instead of for growth and repair.*[208]

## EVIDENCE-BASED PRACTICE

# Risk Factors for Spontaneous Preterm Birth (SPB)

In Manitoba, the incidence of preterm birth has been increasing and the rate is higher among Aboriginal than non-Aboriginal women. The purpose of this study was to identify risk factors for spontaneous preterm birth in Manitoba women, and to compare risk factors among Aboriginal and non-Aboriginal women. In this case-control study, cases delivered a live singleton infant at less than 37 weeks gestation (n = 226; 36 percent Aboriginal), while controls delivered between 37 and 42 weeks gestation (n = 458; 38 percent Aboriginal). An interview was conducted with each subject on the postpartum unit, and information was collected from the health record. Using stratified analyses to control for race/ethnicity, several risk factors for preterm birth had a uniform effect measure across strata, while others demonstrated heterogeneity. After adjusting for other maternal characteristics in a multivariate logistic regression model, significant risk factors emerged.

Significant risk factors for all women included:

1. previous preterm birth
2. two or more previous spontaneous abortions
3. vaginal bleeding after 12 weeks gestation
4. gestational hypertension
5. antenatal hospitalization, and
6. prelabour rupture of membranes

Potentially modifiable risk factors included:

1. low weight gain during pregnancy for all women
2. inadequate prenatal care for all women
3. high levels of perceived stress for Aboriginal women

### Practice Implications

1. Strategies to increase women's access to, and utilization of, prenatal care should be implemented. There should be more use of outreach into the community by a multidisciplinary team for the provision of prenatal care to Aboriginal women.

2. Prenatal care providers should consider women with low pregnancy weight gain at increased risk for preterm delivery.

3. Women need to be counselled about appropriate rates of weight gain in pregnancy based on national guidelines.

4. The need exists to develop culturally appropriate stress reduction strategies.

Source: Heaman, M.I. Risk Factors for Spontaneous Preterm Birth among Aboriginal and Non-Aboriginal Women in Manitoba. Ph.D. dissertation, University of Manitoba, 2001. Used with permission.

Increases in child overweight and obesity have become a major public health problem in industrialized nations, including Canada.[209] In Canada, rates of overweight and obesity among children have more than doubled in past decades. About 30 percent of children are either overweight or obese.[210] Children with excess cell mass from excessive caloric intake develop adult adipose cells early in life. Adipose stores continue to increase because of the increased number of adipose cells.[211]

Breast milk is considered the food of choice for the newborn and infant for at least six months. Yet, breastfeeding is not completely safe. Many substances and drugs ingested by the mother are excreted in human milk. The newborn is susceptible to foreign substances because the body's principal detoxifying mechanisms are not functional, the enzyme system is immature, and kidney function is incompletely developed.[212]

## Stress

Stress comes in various forms to young children as it does to individuals of any age. There may be illness and hospitalization; day-to-day frustrations; neglect, abuse, or abandonment by parents; emotional and sensory deprivation; natural disasters; and wars. Children need attention, love, and support in nurturing psychosocial and cognitive skills. Through a life of abundant affection children can develop, learn, cope, and be healthy.

## Effects of Practice on Neuromuscular Development

The effects of exercise or practice on developing early motor skills remain contradictory in reports. Certain motor behaviours tend to appear at such time when the body has the neuromuscular maturity for that behaviour to occur. Practice of the behaviour before its natural appearance does little to speed up long-term development, even though it may appear that the child can perform an activity earlier. Unpractised children catch up, often demonstrating the same activity only a few days later.[213]

## Endocrine Function

The mediation of hormones is crucial to the child and person throughout life. A **hormone** is a *chemical substance produced by an endocrine gland and carried by the bloodstream to another part of the body (the target organ), where it serves to control some function of the target organ.* The major functions of hormones include integrative action, regulation, and morphogenesis. **Integration,** *permitting the body to act*

*as a whole unit in response to stimuli, results from hormones travelling throughout the body and reaching all cells of the body.* For example, the response of the body to epinephrine during fright is generalized. Estrogen, which is more specific in its action, affects overall body function. **Regulation,** *maintaining a constant internal environment called homeostasis,* results from the action of all hormones. The regulation of salt and water balance, metabolism, and growth are examples. In **morphogenesis,** the *rate and type of growth of the organism,* some hormones play an important part.

*Growth hormone (GH),* or *somatotropic hormone (STH),* secreted by the anterior pituitary gland and regulated by a substance called *growth hormone–releasing factor (GHF)* produced in the hypothalamus, affects morphogenesis by promoting the development and enlargement of all body tissues that are capable of growing. Growth hormone has three basic effects on the metabolic processes of the body: (1) protein synthesis is increased; (2) carbohydrate conservation is increased; and (3) the use of fat stores for energy is increased.

Growth hormone is secreted in spurts instead of at a relatively constant rate. The lowest concentrations of plasma GH are found in the morning after arising. The highest concentrations occur between 60 and 90 minutes after falling asleep at night. The peak of GH is clearly related to sleep. Consequently, the folk belief that sleep is necessary for growth and healing has been supported.[214]

## Environmental Pollution

Children are especially affected by environmental pollution. The incidence of childhood asthma and cancer has increased sharply. Increases in both diseases are attributed in part to environmental hazards. A pilot study was conducted to determine the prevalence of impaired lung function in school-aged First Nations children. The results indicated that many children in the study had already established airflow obstruction, and were already at risk for asthma or chronic obstructive pulmonary disease (COPD). Somewhat surprisingly, exposure to mould appeared to be protective. The researchers claim that further research is needed to evaluate the lung health concerns of this population.[215]

---

### CRITICAL THINKING

*In what ways might mould be a protective factor, as found in the pilot study conducted with school-aged First Nations children? (See Williams, 1999.)*[216]

---

Asthma is caused in part by air pollution, and air pollution can prolong asthma attacks. The main causative factors, however, are allergens that are inhaled. Note that today's children spend considerable time in tightly sealed buildings, where they have high exposure to mould, dust mites, and animal dander. A child who has asthma has an underlying immune system dysfunction, making him or her overreactive to substances in the environment. The child's early experience can change the relative proportion of T-cells and the development of the immune system. Contaminant exposure before birth has been linked to altered T-cells: the higher the mother's level of PCBs and dioxin, the greater the change in the T-cells. The result can be immune suppression, allergy, or autoimmunity.[217]

## SOCIOCULTURAL FACTORS THAT INFLUENCE THE DEVELOPING PERSON

Use the following information with the information in Chapter 1 for assessment and health promotion.

## Cultural and Demographic Variables

Culture, social class, race, and the ethnicity of the parents; foods eaten by the pregnant woman; prenatal care and childbirth practices; childrearing methods; expected patterns of behaviour; language development and thought processes during childhood and adulthood; and health practices—all affect the person from the moment of conception. Refer to Chapter 1 for an in-depth discussion of cultural effects.

The health care provided to the child by the parents is related to one's sociocultural status. In urban areas, parents of children who are adequately immunized are likely to have the following characteristics: (1) they perceive childhood diseases as serious; (2) they know about the effectiveness of vaccination; (3) they are older; (4) they are better educated; (5) they have a smaller family size (number of children); and (6) they read newspapers, watch television promotions of immunizations, use the Internet, and respond to community educational efforts. Inadequately immunized children in urban areas are usually found in families in which the parents are young, poor, and minimally educated. These parents do not perceive childhood diseases as serious. They do not know about the effectiveness of vaccines, nor do they pay much attention to health education in the mass media.[218] A child's genetic potential depends on an extensive list of relevant variables.

Child–caregiver interaction; lifestyle factors such as adequate rest, smoking, and drug and alcohol use; use of

health promotion measures; poor food habits that result in either malnutrition or obesity; along with toxic factors in the environment and infections are, all together, major determinants of how closely the genetic potential can be reached. All of these factors affect the child's growth and development, learning ability, functional capacity, and health. Eventually, these factors affect the health and longevity of adults.

## Socialization Processes

**Socialization** is *the process by which the child is transformed into a member of a particular society and learns the values, standards, habits, skills, and roles appropriate to that person's sex, social class, and ethnic group or subculture to become a responsible, productive member of society.*

All humans experience socialization, the shaping of the person into a socially acceptable form, especially during the early years of life. Because of this fact, heritage and culture are perpetuated. The newborn is a biological organism with physical needs and inherited characteristics that will be socialized or shaped along a number of dimensions: emotional, social, cognitive, intellectual, perceptual, behavioural, and expressive. During the period of socialization, various skills, knowledge, attitudes, values, motives, habits, beliefs, needs, interests, and ideals are learned, demonstrated, and reinforced. Various people are key agents in the socialization process: parents, siblings, relatives, peers, teachers, and other adults. Certain forces will impinge on the person and these forces will interact with all that the individual is and learns. These forces include culture, social class, religion, race or ethnicity, the community, the educational system, mass media, and various organizations. Certain factors may limit or enhance the socialization process: age, sex, rate and stage of development, general constitution, and innate intelligence. The final integration of all of the various individual and socializing forces will form the adult character, personality traits, role preferences, goals, and behavioural mode.

The success of the socialization process is measured by the person's ability to perform in the roles that he or she attempts, and in how he or she responds to rapid social change, and a succession of life tasks. The person learns to think and behave in ways consonant with the roles to be played. That person's performance in a succession of roles leads to predictable personality configurations.[219]

## Community Support System

*Community relationships* influence the parents most profoundly, but they also influence the child. If the parents are unable to meet the child's needs adequately, other people or organizations in the community may make the difference between bare survival and eventual physical and emotional normalcy and well-being.

Cultures vary in the degree to which the new mother is extended help. Prenatal classes can bring together women and families who are often otherwise isolated.

## Family Factors

Several aspects of the family combine their effects to influence the child's development and well-being before birth and afterwards. The most significant influenced aspects within the family include the family structure, developmental level and roles of family members, their health and financial status, their perception of the baby, and community resources for the family. Social and environmental factors that produce low birth weight, for instance, are likely to continue to operate on the infant, and then on the child as well. The child learns to behave in his or her own way and, as an adult, will have specific values and expectations depending upon whether he or she is reared in a single-parent, nuclear, dual-earner, or extended family, or in a family whose socioeconomic status varies. The number of siblings, their sexes, and birth order influence how the child is cared for and perceives himself or herself. The family's presence or absence of work, leisure, travel, material comforts, habits of daily living, and the facade put on for society will all influence and affect the child's self-concept, learning, physical well-being, and eventual lifestyle. Refer to Chapter 4 for more information.

A study was conducted by Ford-Gilboe to determine which variables would predict *choice of health promotion options in single-parent and two-parent families*. The convenience sample in a mid-size city in southern Ontario consisted of 138 families (68 single-parent families, 70 two-parent families) with at least one preadolescent child. The majority of subjects were Caucasian, identifying with the Canadian culture, but they were from a variety of ethnic backgrounds. Mothers and children closest to age 12 completed questionnaires. The mother's education was the only demographic variable significantly related to choice of health options. Family pride, family cohesion, mother's non-traditional sex role orientation, general self-reliance, network support, and community support were significantly related to choice of health options. Single-parent families and two-parent family types were similar on all demographic variables. Two-parent families, however, were found to have more community support, higher income, and more resources.[220]

### Vulnerable and Resilient Children
Both vulnerable and resilient children can develop within the same family system. Siblings brought up under chaotic situations, with alcoholic or drug-using parents, or in impoverished circumstances do not all develop the same personality traits. One becomes physically or emotionally ill, while the sibling thrives. No single set of qualities or circumstances characterizes such resilient children, but they seem to be different from their vulnerable siblings, right from birth. Children who are exposed to more than one adverse factor, or long-term crisis, or who do not have a consistent caring adult, are less able to offset the negative effects of stress and maintain resiliency.[221]

**Resilient children** appear to be *endowed with innate characteristics that insulate them from the pain of their families, allow them to reach out to some adult who provides crucial emotional support, and are able to bounce back from adverse circumstances.* Characteristics of these children include the ability to:[222]

- Use some particular talent or personality trait to draw some adult to them as a substitute parent; experience some type of compensating events
- Recover quickly from stressors; be adaptable, resourceful, and creative
- Be more alert to their surroundings from birth
- Establish trust with the mother, or with the mothering person
- Have warm and secure relationships with the mother or mother surrogate, regardless of other circumstances
- Be more independent, easygoing, friendly, enthusiastic for activities, and able to tolerate frustration by age two
- Be more cheerful, flexible, and persistent in the face of failure, and be able to seek help from adults by age three-and-a-half
- Be sensitive to others
- Feel that they can exert some control over life
- Demonstrate good school performances and good problem-solving skills

**Vulnerable children** *are closest, emotionally, to the distressed parent and are most likely to show signs of distress.* These children are more likely to be self-derogatory, anxious, depressed, and physically ill. However, hardships can leave even the resilient children with psychological scars, although they tend not to become emotionally disabled. Even apparently well-adjusted, successful, resilient children may pay a subtle psychological cost. In adolescence, they are more likely to cling to a moralistic outlook. In intimate relationships they are apt to be disagreeable and judgmental. They tend to be constricted and overcontrolled. If the disturbed parent is of the opposite sex, the resilient person is often emotionally distant in intimate relationships, breaking off relationships as they become more intimate. Some seek partners with problems, possibly with the idea of rescuing or curing them.[223]

**Child Maltreatment** The 2003 Canadian Incidence Study (CIS) examined the incidence of reported child maltreatment and characteristics of the children and families investigated by Canadian child welfare services. The rate of substantiated maltreatment in Canada, excluding Quebec, has increased 125 percent from 9.64 cases per thousand in 1998 to 21.7 cases in 2003.[224] Child abuse is a negative influence on the developing person. It is currently an epidemic, and children are suffering more serious and brutal injuries. Parents who abuse their children may be from any race, creed, ethnic origin, or economic level.[225] You, as a nurse, are crucial in preventing child abuse through your assistance to parents. **Child maltreatment** is *physical abuse, neglect, sexual abuse, and emotional maltreatment of children.*[226] Abused children range in age from neonate through adolescence.

You may be the first professional health worker to encounter such a child in the community. Be alert for signs of child abuse as you assess the injured or ill child. Non-accidental physical injury includes multiple bruises or fractures from severe beatings, poisonings or overmedication, burns from immersion in hot water or from lighted cigarettes, excessive use of laxatives or enemas, and human bites. The trauma to the child is often great enough to cause permanent blindness, scars on the skin, neurological damage, subdural hematoma, and permanent brain damage or death. **Sexual abuse**, *exploitation of the child for the adult's sexual gratification,* includes rape, incest, exhibitionism to the child, and fondling of the child's genitals. **Emotional maltreatment** includes *excessively aggressive or unreasonable parental behaviour toward the child,* placing unreasonable demands on the child to perform above his or her capacities, verbally attacking or constantly belittling or teasing the child, or withdrawing love, support, or guidance. **Neglect** includes *failure to provide the child with the basic necessities of life* (food, shelter, clothing, hygiene, or medical care), *adequate mothering, or emotional, moral, or social care.*[227] The parent's lack of concern is usually obvious. Abandonment may occur. In all forms of abuse, the child frequently acts fearful of the parent, or of adults in general. The child is usually too fearful to tell how he or she was injured.

*There are a number of characteristics of the potentially or actually abusive parent.* Typically, the abuser:

- Is young
- Is emotionally unstable, unable to cope with the stress of life or even usual personal problems
- Was insufficiently mothered, rejected, or abused as a child
- Is lonely, has few social contacts, and is isolated from people
- Is unable to ask for help, lacks friends or family who can help with child care
- Does not understand the development or care needs of children
- Is living through a very stressful time such as unemployment, spousal abuse, or poverty
- Has personal emotional needs previously unmet, and has difficulty in trusting others
- Is angered easily, has negative self-image and low self-esteem
- Has no one from whom to receive emotional support, including the partner
- Expects the child to be perfect and to cause no inconvenience
- May perceive the child as different, too active, or too passive, even if the child is normal or only mildly different

Sometimes the child has mild neurological dysfunction and is irritable, tense, and difficult to impossible to hold or cuddle. The child may have been the result of an unwanted pregnancy, or be premature, or have a birth defect. Usually only one child in a family becomes the scapegoat for parental anger, tension, rejection, and hate. The child who does not react in some way that makes the parent feel good about his or her parenting behaviour will be the abused one.[228]

Additional information about child and adolescent abuse is found in Chapters 7 through 11.

**Prolonged Separation** Early separation, for more than three months, from a mothering person leads to serious consequences because from approximately 3 to 15 months of age, the presence of a consistently loving caretaker is essential. As a result of separation, both physical and intellectual growth are impaired and the baby will not learn to form and maintain trust or a significant relationship. He or she will either withdraw or precociously try to adapt by seeking attention from as many people as possible.

**Maternal Deprivation and Failure to Thrive**
**Maternal deprivation** and **failure to thrive** are the terms used to describe *infants who have insufficient contact with a mothering person, and who do not grow as expected in the absence of an organic defect.* Deprivation during the second six months occurs when a previously warm relationship with the mother is interrupted. This half-year of deprivation is more detrimental to the child than is the lack of a consistent relationship during the first six months. Another cause for failure to thrive is **perceptual deprivation**, *lack of tactile, vestibular, visual, or auditory stimuli,* resulting from either organic factors or the lack of mothering.[229] Touch and cuddling are essential for the infant. The sensations experienced through the skin are the primary means by which baby comes to know self and the environment.

Although damage to the child from maternal deprivation may be severe, not every deprived child becomes delinquent or a problem adult. Some infants who have lacked their mother's love appear to suffer little permanent damage. The age of the child when deprived or abused, the length of separation or duration of abuse, the quality of the parent–child relationship before separation or in later childhood, the type of care received from other adults during separation from the parents, and the stress produced by the separation or abuse all affect the long-range outcome for the child.

**Spiritual Factors**   Religious, philosophic, and moral insights and practices of the parents (and of the overall society) influence the manner in which the child is perceived, cared for, and taught. These early underpinnings—or their lack—will continue to affect the person's self-concept, behaviour, and health as an adult, even if he or she purposefully tries to disregard these early teachings. Refer to Chapter 3 for more information on this matter.

## Macroenvironmental Factors That Influence the Developing Person

Frequently it can be observed that the overall environment of the region in which the person lives affects the person's development and health. The everyday emotional climate that the person learns to tolerate, the availability of water and food, demands for physical and motor competency, social relationships, and opportunities for leisure—all can affect one's development and health. Added to these effects are the hazards from environmental pollution that affect all societies, whether it is excrement from freely roaming cattle or particles from industrial smokestacks. No part of the world remains uncontaminated by pesticides. All parts of our world have disease related to problems of waste control.

## HEALTH PROMOTION IN NURSING PRACTICE

*Your support, assistance, and teaching expertise with the pregnant woman and her significant support system will contribute to more nurturing ways of parenting. Throughout this chapter, ways and methods have been considered to overcome, or at least deter, harmful agents that act against normal development. Refer to texts on maternal–child nursing for additional information about nursing care of the woman during pregnancy, labour, delivery, and after delivery. Information is also provided in this text in Chapters 2 and 7 through 11 that can be shared with the pregnant woman and parents for health promotion.*

The following health promotion strategies are useful:

- Consider the principles of growth and development as you assess people in different developmental eras.

- Carefully assess pregnant women to determine whether they are at risk because of any of the negative influencing factors.

- Consider the sociocultural and religious backgrounds and the lifestyle of the person you are caring for so that you do not overlook or misinterpret factors that are significant to the pregnant woman and her family.

- Help those who are at risk to obtain the care necessary to prevent fetal damage and maternal illness.

- Teach potential parents about the many factors discussed in this and following chapters that can influence the welfare of their offspring.

- Be aware of community services such as genetic screening and counselling, family planning, nutritional programs, prenatal classes, counselling for prevention of child abuse, and medical services.

- Join with other citizens in attempts to reverse the hazards of environment and child abuse.

Your role with the child-abusing parent and the maltreated child is a significant one. To help parents and child, you must first cope with your own feelings as you provide necessary physical care to the child, or assist parents in getting proper care for the baby. Often, parents who feel unable to cope with the stresses of childrearing will repeatedly bring the child to the emergency room with a variety of minor complaints, vague illnesses, or injuries.

Finally, co-operate with legal, medical, and social agencies to help the parent(s) and to prevent further child abuse—and the possible death or permanent impairment of the child. Child maltreatment is against the law in every province and territory. Any citizen or health worker can report anonymously to authorities a case of child maltreatment without fear of recrimination from the abuser. An investigation by designated authorities of the danger to the child is carried out shortly after reporting. The child may be placed by court order in a foster home or institution if the child's life is threatened. The goal of legal intervention is to help the parents and the child—not to punish.

### CRITICAL THINKING

*What other health promotion strategies would you develop to use with a culturally diverse population?*

The use of health promotion strategies for the pregnant woman and her partner is critical for the nurse during this sensitive period. The main goal of the nurse and health team is to assist the family to adapt continually to the various changes that occur during pregnancy, and to achieve a healthy birth outcome.

# SUMMARY

1. Childhood is the foundation period of life, and development follows a definable, predictable, sequential pattern.

2. The person is unique, yet similar to other people in patterns of development, characterized by holism (physical, emotional, cognitive, social, and spiritual/moral dimensions).

3. Development, developmental tasks, maturation, and learning are key terms to understanding the developing person throughout the lifespan.

4. Several principles of growth are required to explain the pattern of development.

5. Prenatal influences on development include heredity, various physiologic processes, and the age, health,

and nutritional status of both the mother and the father.

6. Environmental hazards, drugs, alcohol, infections, and other conditions are teratogens that may adversely affect the developing organism, especially during the critical period of the first trimester.

7. Certain variables, such as medication and substance abuse in the mother, may negatively affect the fetus during labour and delivery.

8. Early childhood variables that affect the developing person include nurturance from the parents, nutrition, stressors, physiologic functions in the infant, and various sociocultural and family characteristics.

## Interesting Websites

### Folic Acid

**www.hc-sc.gc.ca; click on A-Z Index, and find folic acid**
Folic acid, or folate, is one of the B vitamins important for healthy growth of an unborn baby. It is essential to the normal development of the baby's spine, brain, and skull, especially during the first four weeks of pregnancy. This site provides information and several related links.

### Canada Prenatal Nutrition Program

**www.phac-aspc.gc.ca/dca-dea/programs-mes/cpnp-bunsa_e.html**
If you're young and pregnant in Ottawa, feel overwhelmed and lonely and aren't always able to eat nutritiously, then one place to go is Buns in the Oven. This program offers food ideas, peer support, and prenatal and parenting education. It is sponsored by a coalition of four Ottawa agencies. Through a community development approach, the CPNP aims to reduce the incidence of unhealthy birth weights, improve the health of both infant and mother, and encourage breastfeeding.

### Eating Well with Canada's Food Guide
### (formerly Canada's Food Guide to Healthy Living)

**www.hc-sc.gc.ca/fn-an/food-guide-aliment/index_e.html**
Canada's Food Guide was revised in the spring of 2007. The Nutrition Resource Centre presents the *Cultural Adaptations of Canada's Food Guide to Healthy Eating*. The adaptations are available for use by the Chinese, Portuguese, Punjabi, Spanish, Tamil, Urdu, and Vietnamese communities. These guides feature culturally specific foods and full-colour illustrations. Each adaptation has been produced in three languages: the language of the cultural group (e.g., Chinese), English, and French.

### Fetal Alcohol Syndrome/Fetal Alcohol Effects

**www.hc-sc.gc.ca; click on A-Z Index, and find fetal alcohol syndrome (FAS/FAE)**
Fetal alcohol syndrome (FAS) is the medical term used to describe certain birth defects that result from drinking alcohol during pregnancy. Fetal alcohol effects (FAE) is a similar condition that has some, but not all, of the characteristics of FAS. It is estimated that every day in Canada, at least one

child is born with FAS, which can lead to a variety of lifelong disabilities. Both FAS and FAE are preventable. The smart choice for women who are, or may become, pregnant is to abstain totally from alcohol. Explore this site and learn much more.

### First Nations & Inuit Health

**www.hc-sc.gc.ca/fnihb**
The Primary Health Care and Public Health (PHCPH) Directorate is responsible for primary health care delivered in partnership with First Nations and Inuit health authorities. All PHCPH activities have as their goals the support of knowledge and the building of capacity, among First Nations and Inuit, to facilitate First Nations and Inuit control of health programs and resources. This site provides current news, links, and general information.

### Canadian Centre on Substance Abuse

**www.ccsa.ca**
The Canadian Centre on Substance Abuse (CCSA) is an arm's-length national agency that promotes informed debate on substance abuse issues; encourages public participation in reducing the harm associated with drug abuse; disseminates information on the nature, extent, and consequences of substance abuse; and supports and assists organizations involved in substance abuse treatment, prevention, and educational programming.

### Motherisk

**www.motherisk.org**
This site is a source of evidence-based information about the safety or risk of drugs, chemicals, and disease during pregnancy and lactation.

### Fetal Alcohol Spectrum Disorder

**www.cnfasdpartnership.ca**
The Canada Northwest Fetal Alcohol Spectrum Disorder Partnership is an alliance for the development and promotion of an interprovincial/territorial approach on the prevention, intervention, care, and support of people affected by fetal alcohol spectrum disorders. This new site offers "single-window" access to related sites around the country.

# Key Terms

AIDS (215)

amniotic sac (201)

analgesics (218)

anoxia (219)

bilateral (197)

biological age (195)

blastocyst (200)

canalized (205)

cephalocaudal (197)

Cephalocaudal, Proximo-distal, and Bilateral Principles (197)

cervix (199)

child maltreatment (224)

chlamydia trachomatis (206)

chloasma (203)

chromosomes (198, 203)

chronologic age (195)

cognitive competency (196)

conceptus (203)

congenital anomalies (204)

critical periods (196)

cytomegalovirus (CMV) (216)

development (195)

Down syndrome (trisomy 21) (205)

ectoderm (200)

embryonic disk (200)

embryonic stage (200)

emotional competency (196)

emotional maltreatment (224)

endoderm (200)

extremely low birth weight (ELBW) (219)

failure to thrive (224)

fetal alcohol spectrum disorder (FASD) (214)

fetal stage (200)

follicle (199)

fragile X syndrome (204)

fraternal twins (199)

gametes (199, 204)

genes (198, 203)

genetic (204)

germinal stage (200)

gonorrhea (216)

growth (195)

herpes simplex virus (HSV) (216)

historical time (194)

HIV (215)

hormone (221)

hyperplasia (195)

hypertrophy (195)

identical twins (199)

incremental growth (195)

integration (221)

lanugo (201)

learning (195)

linea nigra (203)

low birth weight (219)

maternal deprivation (224)

maturation (195)

meiosis (199)

mesoderm (201)

miscarriage (201)

mitosis (203)

morphogenesis (221)

morula (200)

neglect (224)

nidation (200)

norms (194)

orgasm (199)

ovulation (199)

ovum (199)

perceptual deprivation (224)

physical competency (196)

placenta (200)

prematurity (219)

preterm (219)

Principle of Asynchronous Growth (197)

Principle of Development toward Self-Knowledge and Autonomy (196)

Principle of Differentiation (197)

Principle of Discontinuity of Growth Rate (197)

Principle of Readiness (197)

proximodistal (197)

psychological age (195)

quickening (202)

reaction range (205)

regulation (221)

replacement growth (195)

resilient children (223)

rubella (215)

rubeola (215)

sexual abuse (224)

small for date (219)

social age (195)

social competency (196)

social time (194)

socialization (222)

spontaneous abortion (201)

syphilis (216)

toxoplasmosis (216)

umbilical cord (201)

very low birth weight (219)

vulnerable children (223)

zygote (199)

# Part III

## The Developing Person and Family: Infancy through Adolescence

# Chapter 7

## Assessment and Health Promotion for the Infant

**THE GREAT SPIRIT GAVE US CHILDREN. . . .** *That is why we must love them.*

*Elder, Awasis Training Institute of Northern Manitoba (1994)*

## Objectives

*Study of this chapter will enable you to:*

1 Examine second-order changes in family status required to proceed developmentally in family life cycle stages: *the new couple* and *families with young children*.

2 Define terms and give examples of basic developmental principles pertinent to the neonate and the infant.

3 Comprehend the issue of birth as a crisis for the family. Identify factors that influence parental attachment for the neonate and infant. Ascertain details of your role in assisting the family to adapt to the challenges and joys of the birth crisis.

4 Identify and describe the adaptive physiological changes that occur at birth for the mother and for the child.

5 Assess the neonate's physical characteristics and the manner in which psychosocial needs begin to be fulfilled.

6 Determine the normal or expected characteristics of a neonate and infant regarding physiology, motor activity, cognitive abilities, emotional responses, and social characteristics including adaptive mechanisms.

7 Determine the normal range of sleep, movement, and play patterns of an infant.

8 Interpret an immunization schedule, and discuss with a parent safety and health promotion measures.

9 Discuss in a health care team setting your role in assisting parents: to foster the development of trust with each other, and to develop positive self-concepts regarding the new baby.

10 Compare thriving parent–infant behaviours to faltering parent–infant behaviours.

11 Discuss your role in promoting parental attachment.

12 Begin to implement health promoting strategies with parents and baby after delivery and during the first year of life.

This chapter discusses the normal growth and development of the baby during the first year of life, baby's effect on the family, and the family's influence on baby. Measures to promote the infant's well-being that are useful in health promotion and nursing practice and that can be taught to parents are described throughout the chapter.

In this chapter, the terms **neonate** and **newborn** refer to the *first four weeks of life*. **Infant** refers to the *first 12 months* (or, in some texts, 15 months). Practices vary from culture to culture. In most Asian cultures, the child is considered one year old at birth. Traditional Chinese custom adds one year to an infant's age on January 1, regardless of the birthday.[1] **Mother** or **parent(s)** is the term used to denote *the person(s) responsible for the child's care and long-term well-being*.

You can refer to an embryology and obstetric nursing textbook for detailed information on fetal development, prenatal changes, and the process of labour and delivery. This chapter builds on information presented in Chapters 4 and 6, and focuses on the family life cycle stage. The authors remind the readers that some characteristics and developmental processes of the infant and family described here may vary among cultures.

## FAMILY DEVELOPMENT AND RELATIONSHIPS

## Family Life Cycle

Table 4-3 illustrates the stages of the family life cycle, the emotional processes of transition (key principles), and the second-order changes in the family required to proceed developmentally. Review the family life cycle stages: the new couple and families with young children.

The coming of the child is a **crisis**, a *turning point in the couple's or at least the mother's life in which old patterns of living must be changed for new ways of living and new values*.[2] The crisis will be less severe if the baby is wanted than if the couple had planned not to have children. Many couples look forward to starting a family, and they make plans to accommodate a pregnancy. But having a baby is always a crisis—a change. The woman may first feel the crisis as she recognizes body changes and experiences new emotional responses. For example, Sally, age 28, who has just become pregnant, may wonder about losing her slim figure, question how long she can work, and worry about balancing work and childrearing. She may be concerned about making spatial changes in the home, or worried about moving to a new home to accommodate the baby. She might be anxious, too, about balancing the budget to meet additional expenses.

The crisis is greater when the baby is not planned, or not wanted. Such may be the case with Jane, who was devastated when she learned she was pregnant. Although she did not deliberately seek an abortion, she began to skip meals and to exercise vigorously in an effort to maintain a slim figure. Jane did not have anyone to talk to about her feelings and felt very much alone. She was frightened and eventually became ill at work. Jane's co-workers helped her to find medical attention.

At times, even though the pregnancy may have been planned, the man becomes fearful of fatherhood because of the consequent responsibility and loss of freedom due to the birth of the baby. When John learned that his wife, Nancy, was pregnant, he withdrew emotionally, was apathetic about the baby, and spent more time with his male friends and work associates. Nancy, in turn, spent much time alone and felt increasingly rejected, abandoned, depressed, and angry. These behaviours may cause John and Nancy to separate unless they find help, admit to their problem, work through their feelings, and recommit their love for one another.

Whether perceived as positive or negative, change always involves a sense of loss of the familiar, loss of the way it used to be. The vacuum created by the loss is a painful one and one for which new parents are usually ill-prepared. The couple's life will never again be "normal" as they once knew it, but together the family now needs to find a "new normal."

If pregnancy and parenting create a crisis for a couple who may want a baby, these events are even more stressful for the adolescent or for the single woman—either unmarried or, if married, left by her husband to face pregnancy, birth, and childrearing alone. This adolescent, or woman, needs the support of, and help from, at least one other person during this period. A parent, relative, or friend can be a resource. Often, the support and help of a number of people are needed. You may be the primary source of support. Your empathetic listening, acceptance, practical hints for better self-care and baby care, and general availability can make a real difference in the outcome of the pregnancy and in ability of the mother and the father to parent effectively and to handle future crises as they arise.

In Canada, a publication called *Family-Centred Maternity and Newborn Care: National Guidelines* has been developed through a collaborative process involving health care providers and consumers. It is a multidimensional, dynamic, and complex process that responds to the physical, emotional, and psychosocial needs of women and families. These guidelines not only view pregnancy and birth as normal, healthy events (a celebration), but also consider pregnancy and birth to be unique for each woman. One of the guiding principles stresses that health care providers form a trusting relationship between women and their families based on respect in order for the woman to give birth safely and with dignity.[3] Referral to other resources and self-help groups (such as Parents Without Partners), as well as to a counsellor, may be of great help to the mother. Another Canadian prenatal resource is Motherisk, which has a useful website (www.motherisk.org).[4]

CRITICAL THINKING

*Assume that you are working in a remote community in northern Canada. What steps could you take to access resources for a pregnant woman and her family?*

## Growth and Development of Parents

Parenting is an inexact science. An increasing number of people are not prepared either intellectually or emotionally for family life, possibly because of the difficult family life they experienced in childhood. Every parent hopes that their child will grow up to be an independent and happy adult. However, creating and maintaining a family unit is difficult in today's society. Therein lies the challenge for every parent. Many occupations demand travel, frequent changes of residence, and working on Sundays and holidays, the traditional family days. The rapid pace of life and available opportunities often interfere with family functions. For example, Gloria and Don, who both work, seem always to be on the go with their three young school-age children. At times, they take turns driving the children to dancing or piano lessons or to important sports activities. They find that their dinner schedule varies from day to day.

For Aboriginal people, the term **family** denotes the *biological unit of both parents and children residing together in a household*.[5] However, Aboriginal children receive nurturing not only from their family of origin, but also from the elders, extended family, and the community. Because children are valued and hold a special place in the Aboriginal community, the task of fostering child development in a healthy way becomes very important.[6] Even though Aboriginal communities are evolving and are in the process of demographic change in Canada, the centrality of the family remains important.[7] In fact, health care providers need to promote and reinforce Aboriginal parenting skills and traditional teachings.[8] Brenda and Fred, who reside in a northern community, maintain their traditional beliefs and cultural practices. Brenda, who is pregnant with their first child, views her pregnancy as a natural event. She is somewhat anxious and shy about attending a prenatal clinic, but soon realizes that the health professionals are approachable and display culturally sensitive and caring practices that are meaningful to her. Following are some general guidelines for health professionals who might interact with Aboriginal families:

1. Demonstrate friendliness during the visit with the family and show a genuine interest in topics that come up for discussion.

2. Demonstrate a nonjudgmental attitude.

3. Respect the child and family as they are.

4. Listen, listen, and listen again, as Aboriginal people have a strong oral tradition and stress the value of observing.

5. Learn to recognize the rights of the family and extended family who might be caring for the child.

6. Give everyone an opportunity to speak regarding the well-being of the child and, mainly, learn to recognize that "the child must be understood as a whole being in the total context of his or her family, culture, community and physical environment."[9]

Pregnancy is preparation for the birth event, whereas parenting is a process that continues for many years. Becoming a parent involves grieving the loss of one's own childhood and former lifestyle. The person must be in touch with, and be able to express and work through, feelings of loss before he or she can adapt and move on to a higher level of maturation. Being aware of the tremendous influence of parents on their children's development, parents may feel challenged to become the best persons they are capable of being. New parents may need to develop a confidence that they do not feel, an integrity that has been easy to let slide, and values that can tolerate being scrutinized. To grow and develop as a parent, the person needs to make peace with his or her past so that unresolved conflicts are not inflicted on the child.

After a baby joins the family, a number of problems must be worked through. The mother must deal with the fact of separation from a powerful symbiotic relationship with the baby. The reality of child care and managing a household may be disillusioning after exposure to the ideals inculcated by the mass media and advertising. Even though many parents exhibit strengths, problems always exist. It is important for you, as a health professional, to validate the couple's strengths to promote their health and well-being.

One of the potential problem areas that you can explore with parents is that of re-establishing a mutually satisfying sexual relationship. This task is not a simple process. It has intricate psychological overtones for both the man and the woman. You may also need to address the couple's desire for family planning. (See Table 11-6 for information on contraceptive measures.) Sexual relationships usually decrease during pregnancy, childbirth, and the postpartum period. However, couples can resume sexual intercourse once the episiotomy has healed and the lochia flow has stopped. This usually occurs by the end of the third week. Prior to the six-week checkup, it is important that the woman and her partner be informed about what to expect regarding sexual activity. For example, the couple should be informed that since the vaginal vault is dry (hormone poor), some form of lubrication may be necessary during intercourse.[10] By six weeks after birth, the woman's pelvis is back to normal, lochia has ceased, and involution is complete. Whether she is ready physically for an active sex life depends on the person and the situation. The mother may be so absorbed in, and fatigued by, the challenges and responsibilities of motherhood that the father becomes pushed into the background. He may feel in competition, somehow, with the baby, resenting both the baby and his wife.

Either parent may take initiative in renewing the role of lover, in being sexually attractive to the other. The woman may choose to do this by getting a new hairdo, or stylish clothes for her now slimmer figure. Inwardly, she can strengthen flabby perineal muscles through prescribed exercises. Patience on the part of the man is necessary because if an episiotomy was done before delivery, healing continues for some time and the memory of pain in the area may cause the woman involuntarily to tense the perineal muscles and wish to forgo intercourse. Happy couples who have a sound philosophy and communication system soon work out such problems, including the fact that the needs of the baby will sometimes interrupt intimacy. For couples whose earlier sex life was unsatisfactory and who do not work together as a team, such problems may be hard to surmount. Your support, suggestions, and assistance in helping the couple seek and accept help from family and friends will foster their ability to manage.

Given the whole realm of stresses and life changes associated with a baby's birth, it is understandable that, at least initially, parenting is at best a bittersweet experience. Parents may have strongly ambivalent thoughts and feelings toward this child, whom they have created together and who now, unknowingly, makes such heavy demands on them.

The following stress indicators may be used in your assessment to predict the likelihood of postpartum difficulties:[11]

- Woman is having her first baby (primipara).
- No relatives are available to help with baby care.
- Complications occurred during pregnancy.
- Woman's mother has passed away.
- Woman is ill apart from pregnancy.
- Woman was ill on bed rest during pregnancy.

- Woman has distant relationship, or conflict, with own mother.
- Male partner is often away from home, or not involved with pregnancy or childrearing.
- Woman has no previous experience with babies.

Postpartum difficulties are more likely to occur if the parent is an adolescent or has suffered child abuse, especially sexual abuse or incest. Strass claims that the assessment and treatment of postpartum depression is seriously overlooked. She says that all geographical health regions in Canada should offer appropriate assessment and health promoting strategies to such families.[12]

Parenting is a risky process. It involves facing the unknown with faith because no one can predict the outcome when the intricacies of human relationships are involved. Parents grow and develop by taking themselves, and their child, one day at a time. Parents grow in special ways by realizing the joy that can be part of those crazy, hectic early weeks and months. The feelings of joy and involvement increase as the parent–child attachment becomes more cemented.

Because establishing this attachment is crucial to the long-term nurturing of, and interest in, the child, the process is explored here in depth to assist you in assessment and intervention.

---

**CRITICAL THINKING**

*Differentiate between the type of health care information on pregnancy and delivery that you would provide a couple living in an urban area and that you would provide to a couple living in Nunavut.*

---

## Infant–Parent Attachment

John Bowlby's attachment theory can exert a tremendous effect on the way we perceive parent–child relationships and on the way young infants are cared for. Bowlby observes that children appear to function better when they have a sense that someone who cares about them is near. Moreover, children seek confirmation that someone is there to help them out when they are anxious or distressed.[13]

**Attachment** is *an emotional tie between two persons.* Thus, it is a *human phenomenon characterized by certain behaviours*. It is described as *a close, reciprocal relationship between two people that involves contact with, and proximity to, another that endures over time*. It is only when these behaviours are directed to one or a few persons, rather than to many persons, that the behaviours indicate attachment. Health care professionals often use the term *attachment* to describe behaviours between caregivers and their infants. On the other hand, scholarly writers and investigators often use the term *attachment* interchangeably with the term *bonding*. The term **bonding** first appeared in behavioural research, and it referred to the *sensitive period for the establishment of a tie between animal mothers and their offspring*. The term now *refers to the initial maternal feeling and attachment behaviour immediately following delivery*.[14] When considering infant behaviour, *temperament* is a concept frequently linked with attachment. **Temperament** is described as *a behavioural style* and is defined as *a characteristic way of thinking, behaving, or reacting in a given situation*. While it is believed that, from birth, children are predisposed to respond to the environment in different ways, these different ways of responding influence the ways that others actually respond to them and to their needs. Temperament is believed to have a major impact on behaviour and development because it influences the dynamic interactions, including attachment behaviours, between children and other people in their environment.[15]

Table 7-1 outlines some behaviours of the infant, mother, and father in the typical order of progression in establishing this initial relationship.[16]

In view of the beliefs of the general public concerning bonding, health care workers—especially childbirth educators—must present scientific information in an objective manner to decrease the possibility that parents will experience guilt, or disappointment, concerning their role in the intrapartum or postpartum period. It is important that childbirth educators inform parents that early contact with the infant during the immediate postpartum period can be fulfilling, but that is neither a necessary nor a sufficient experience.[17]

Realize also that there are cultural differences in expressions of attachment. In some cultures, the parents of either the new mother or the new father may take care of both the newborn and the mother for a designated time.

The state of the infant is a strong predictor of the relative frequency with which fathers display interactive, affectionate, and comforting behaviour toward the infant. One study found that fathers are most likely to stimulate by touch those infants who are awake but not crying. Fathers are as likely to talk in a stimulating manner to infants who are either crying or not crying and, similarly, to infants who are sleeping or awake. Perhaps fathers perceive talking as less soothing to crying infants than touch, and talking as less disturbing than touch to sleeping infants. Recently, a study found that fathers are less consistent than mothers at responding to infant cues. Sometimes fathers respond and at other times they do not.[18]

Bonding and attachment behaviours, especially for the male, are sometimes different in other racial and

## Table 7-1 Infant–Parent Attachment Behaviours

| Infant | Mother | Father |
|---|---|---|
| Reflexively looks into mother's face, *establishes eye-to-eye contact* or *"face tie"*; moulds body to mother's body when held | *Reaches* for baby; *holds high against breast-chest-shoulder area*; handles baby smoothly | Has great *interest in baby's face and notes eyes* |
| *Vocalizes, cries,* and *stretches out arms* in response to mother's voice; responds to mother's voice with *"dance"* or *rhythmic movements* | Talks softly in *high-pitched voice* and with intense interest to baby; puts baby face-to-face with her (*en face position*); eye contact gives baby sense of identity to mother | *Desires to touch, pick up, and hold baby;* cradles baby securely; shows fingertip touching and smiling to male baby; has more eye contact with infant delivered by forceps or caesarean section |
| *Roots, licks,* then *sucks* mother's nipple if in contact with mother's breast, cries, smiles | *Touches* baby's extremities; examines, strokes, massages, and kisses baby shortly after delivery; puts baby to breast if permitted; oxytocin and prolactin released | *Looks for distinct features;* thinks newborn resembles self; perceives baby as beautiful in spite of newborn characteristics |
| *Reflexively embraces, clambers, clings,* using hands, feet, head, and mouth to maintain body contact | *Calls baby by name;* notes desirable traits; *expresses pleasure* toward baby; *attentive* to reflex actions of grunts and sneezes | *Feels elated,* bigger, proud after birth; has strong *desire to protect and care for child* |
| *Odour* of mother distinguished by breastfeeding baby by fifth day | *Recognizes odour* of own child by third or fourth day | |

Note: Similar behaviours are seen with a premature baby but the timing will vary.

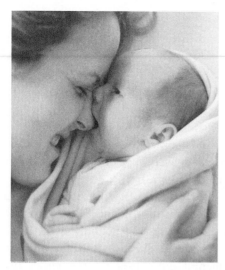
Mother–infant attachment develops mutually over the first year of life.

cultural groups. Some cultures emphasize the mother as caretaker of the infant. The bond or attachment between father and child is less overt and may be emphasized and demonstrated later in childhood. For Aboriginal people, "the family is the recognized cornerstone of First Nations cultures, and a distinctive feature of that cornerstone is the central position of the child." In that culture, a close relationship with the child is important, and the display of affection and kindness to the child is paramount. For example, the time period during the construction of cradleboards provides opportunities for bonding to occur between the mother and the child. The activities of designing and decorating the cradleboard give special attention to the child, and they help to keep his or her spirit happy. Although cradleboards are not as common in current generations of Aboriginal peoples, the significance of the time and effort taken during cradleboard construction exemplifies the continuing importance of teaching nurturing behaviour and recognizing the importance of child development.[19]

The development of attachment between parent and baby continues through infancy. What is essential is the opportunity for parent and infant to develop a mutual, interlocking pattern of attachment behaviours, called synchrony.[20] Developmentalists have indicated that six- to eight-month-old infants whose interactions are highly synchronous with their parents tend to have a larger vocabulary at age two and higher intelligence scores at age three than their counterparts whose interactions are less synchronous.[21]

## Mother–Infant Interaction: Achieving Synchrony

Twenty-nine first-time mothers were randomly assigned to either an intervention or a control group. Extra education, received by the intervention group about two weeks prior to their expected due date, consisted of a 45-minute videotape based on the Keys to Care Giving program about infant behaviour. The videotape contained information on infant states, communication cues, and ways to increase social and cognitive growth-fostering behaviours. The control group attended routine teaching sessions only, consisting of information on cord care, infant bath, and risk factors with early discharge. The purpose of the research was to study differences in mother–infant interaction within the first 24 hours following birth. The Nursing Child Assessment Teaching Scale was the questionnaire used to test the mother's sensitivity to, and understanding of, the infant's behaviour. In addition, the mother was videotaped when teaching her child to look at a rattle. The scores between groups were compared to determine the effect of education on the interaction that occurred between the dyads.

The results showed that:

1. In the treatment group there was a high correlation between the infant's clarity of cues and responsiveness to the care given.

2. There was a moderate correlation between the infant's responsiveness to the caregiver and caregiver total scores in both treatment and control group.

3. Based on t-test analysis, the education provided during the prenatal period did affect the quality of interaction that occurred between mother and infant.

### Practice Implications

Prenatal classes need to include information about how the baby communicates, cues to respond to, and ways to respond to different infant states. Doing so, coupled with the reinforcement of such behaviour postnatally in community health clinics and well baby clinics, would facilitate mother–infant synchrony.

Source: Leitch, D., *Mother–Infant Interaction: Achieving Synchrony, Nursing Research*, 48(1) (1999), 55–57. Used with the permission of Lippincott, Williams & Wilkins.

*Observe for maternal–child attachment.* Research indicates that educating the mother prenatally via videotape about infant behaviours, developmental norms, and communication cues facilitates a more positive mother–infant interaction in the postpartum period. The infant develops effective reciprocal interactions with the caregiver when the caregiver is responsive to the infant.[22]

An article by Byrd[23] gives suggestions on how to approach maternal–child home visits, and how to ask questions during the home visit about the quality of caregiving.

## Factors Influencing Maternal Attachment

Variables that are difficult, or impossible, to change include the woman's level of emotional maturity, how she was reared, what her culture encourages her to do, relationships with her family and partner, experience with previous pregnancies, and planning for and experiencing events during the course of this pregnancy.[24] Episodes of depression experienced by the mother may be another event related to attachment quality. When mothers are depressed, the infant's own facial expressions and behaviours frequently suggest that they feel depressed as well.[25]

*Deterrents to adequate mothering* include the mother's own immaturity or lack of mothering, stress situations, fear of rejection from significant people, loss of a loved one, financial worries, lack of a supportive partner, and even the sex and appearance of the child. Assess for these deterrents. Your nurturing of the mother and your assistance to her in seeking additional help may offset the negative impact of these factors.

*Discharge planning* begins when the expectant mother is admitted. During the hospital stay, although much time is spent teaching about newborn care, the mother must be taught to recognize physical manifestations that may cause her problems, such as vaginal bleeding or infection.[26] When the mother returns home, the community health nurse is one support system. Relatives or friends will likely be there too, as needed, to help. The nurse's assessment regarding the mother's physical and emotional status and her need for information about child care are critical, and it is also essential to determine as quickly as possible the status of the newborn.

*Parenting skills* can be demonstrated in various ways. Although eye contact, touch, and cuddling are important, love can be shown by a tender, soft voice and loving gazes. *Observe for other indications of warm parenting feelings:*

- Calls the baby by name
- Expresses enjoyment of the baby and indicates that the baby is attractive or has other positive characteristics
- Looks at the baby and into baby's eyes
- Talks to the baby in a loving voice
- Takes safety precautions for the baby
- Responds to the baby's cues for attention or physical care

## Factors Influencing Paternal Attachment

*Fatherly feelings do not necessarily accompany fatherhood.* Bonding and attachment feelings in the father appear to be related to various factors: general level of education, participation in prenatal classes, sex of infant, role concept, attendance at delivery, type of delivery, early contact, and feeding method for the baby.

Increasingly, the father is being recognized as an important person to the infant and young child. Specifically, the father is regarded not only as a breadwinner, but also as a nurturer.[27] The lack of a father figure can cause developmental difficulties for the child. Just as the mother is not necessarily endowed with nurturing feelings, the father is not necessarily lacking nurturing feelings. Some fathers seem to respond better to this role than the mothers do.[28] Lorne, for example, is assuming the basic childrearing responsibilities while his wife, Gwen, pursues the major family career. Both parents are content in carrying out their individual family responsibilities. Today, such undertakings by couples are generally accepted.

### NARRATIVE VIGNETTE
## Attachment in a Remote Area

You are a nurse in a northern community. A month ago, after completing a generous maternity leave, you managed to regain your full-time appointment at the local hospital and, as before, you are frequently called in for overtime work. You and your spouse, an RCMP officer at the local detachment, have a ten-month-old infant, Sarah, your first child. For the times when you and your spouse are working simultaneously, you have hired a local grandmother, Clara, to look after Sarah in her home. All seems well for your family, except when disruptions occur—which can happen at any time. For example, you are called to the hospital frequently on weekend evenings when the emergency ward is very busy. Weekends are especially demanding for the police force and overnight flights into the interior are routine for all RCMP members. Clara has not been too enthusiastic recently about having Sarah overnight two or three times per week. As well, it seems that Sarah is becoming less regular at sleeping through the night and is fussing more.

1. What issues will you take into consideration?
2. What plans will you make to facilitate your own, and your spouse's, attachment with Sarah?

Jones studied 30 adolescent fathers in Manitoba to explore variables that may influence teen fathers' participation in parenting. The findings indicated that unrealistic expectations and the inability to combine the developmental tasks of adolescence with the responsibilities of fatherhood increased their vulnerability to parenting failure.[29]

## CRITICAL THINKING

*On repeated occasions, you experience that an older mother readily hands her baby to you as you begin a home visit. What possible reasons might the mother have for doing this?*

# Health Promotion Strategies to Promote Attachment

Certain health promoting strategies directed to the parents will help them to develop attachment with the infant:

■ Call the child, mother, and father by their names during your care.

■ Inquire about the mother's well-being; too often, all of the focus is on the baby. She is in a receptive state and must be emotionally and physically cared for.

■ The father also needs nurturance before he can show caring and be helpful to the mother and baby.

■ Make favourable comments about the infant's progress.

■ Compliment the mother on her intentions or ability to comfort, feed, or identify her baby's needs. Speak of the pleasure baby shows in response to the parent's ministrations.

■ Reassure parents that positive changes in baby are a result of their care, and avoid judgmental attitudes or guilt statements.

■ Encourage both parents to cuddle, look at, and talk to the baby; if necessary, demonstrate how to stroke, caress, and rock baby.

■ Encourage parents to be prompt and consistent in answering the infant's cry.

■ Assist parents in gaining confidence in responding effectively to baby's cry through recognizing the meaning of the cry, meeting the child's needs, and using soothing measures such as rocking, redundant sounds, and swaddling.

■ Explain the infant's interactive abilities and help the parents develop awareness of their own initial effective responses to the newborn's behaviour.

■ Explain the basis of early infant learning as the discovery of associations, connections, and relationships between self and repeated occurrences. Explore how to provide variety; a gradually increasing level of stimulus complexity, sights, sounds, smells, movements, positions, temperatures, and pressure all provide learning opportunities and opportunities for emotional, perceptual, social, and physical development.

■ Call attention to baby and those behaviours that indicate developmental responsiveness, such as reflex movements, visual following, smiling, raising chin off bed, rolling over, and sitting alone. Pupil dilation in the presence of the parent begins at approximately four weeks of age. During the first few weeks of life, baby prefers the human face to other visual images.

■ Differentiate between contact stimulation and representative behaviours present in fetal life. Pressure and touch sensation is present a few months before birth. Thus, the newborn responds well to touch and gentle pressure. Rooting and hand–mouth activity occur in fetal life and are major adaptive activities after birth.

■ Emphasize the importance of visual and auditory skills for developing social behaviours during the first two months of life.

■ Encourage mutual eye contact between parent and baby. All the infant's efforts to vocalize should be reinforced. Eye contact between the parent and baby increases during the first three months of life and is soon accompanied by other social responses: smiling and vocalization.

■ Encourage regular periods of affectionate play when the infant is alert and responsive. Mother and father may pick up and hold the baby close, encourage visual following and smiling, and talk to the infant, repeating sounds. Rhythm and repetition are enjoyed. Often baby is most alert after a daytime feeding.

■ Promote awareness of baby's competencies in other family members so that they, too, can respond to and reinforce the infant.

Incorporate the parents' cultural beliefs, values, and attitudes into your nursing care and modern health care practices whenever possible.[30] Maintaining important cultural traditions is one way to individualize care. Listen attentively for information and signs that give you clues to the parents' feelings about themselves, where they are in their own developmental growth, whom they rely on for strength, their ideas about child discipline, and their expectations of the new child. As you see weaknesses, or gaps, in essential understanding, you can instruct. If your approach is right, the parents will recognize you as a helpful friend. Mothers are receptive to your information and to your reinforcement of mothering skills.

Help parents to realize that soon the complete focus on mother–father–new baby will be gone. Other roles will be re-established: husband, wife, employer or employee, student, daughter, son, friend. The new parents should be encouraged to allow for all aspects of their personalities to function again. Baby will fit in.

## Infant's Influence on Parents

Some babies have a high activity level and warm up readily to the parent. Others are quiet and withdrawn, with low activity levels, and various other mixtures of activity level and temperament are found.[31]

It is easy to love a lovable baby, but parents must work harder with babies who are not highly responsive. Assess the reactions between baby and parents because the style of child care that will develop has its basis here. A highly active mother who expects an intense reaction may have a hard time mothering a low-activity, quiet baby because she may misinterpret the baby's behaviour, feel rejected, and in turn tend to reject the child. If this happens, the baby will be denied the stimulation necessary for development. If the mother is withdrawn, quiet, and inexpressive and has a high-activity baby, she may punish the baby for normal energetic or assertive behaviour and ignore the baby's normal bids for affection and stimulation. The child needs to feel that his or her behaviour will produce an effect or he or she will stop contacting the parents.

Help parents to understand the *mutual response* between the baby and themselves. Help them, too, to learn to read the baby's signals and to give consistent signals to the baby. All parents feel incompetent and in despair at times when they are unable to understand the child's cues and meet needs. If self-confidence is consistently lacking, the parent's despair may turn to anger, rejection, and even abuse.

## Expansion of Intrafamily Relationships

Grandparents-to-be and other relatives frequently become more involved with the parents-to-be (bringing gifts and advice) than is necessarily desired. Yet their gifts and supportive presence can be a real help if the grandparents respect the independence of the couple, if the couple has resolved any earlier adolescent rebellion and dependency conflicts, and if the grandparents' advice does not conflict with the couple's philosophy or the doctor's advice. The couple and grandparents should collaborate rather than compete. Grandparents should be reminded not to take over the situation, and the couple's autonomy should be encouraged in that they can listen to the various pieces of advice, evaluate

the statements, and then, as a unit, make their own decision. In addition, parents should refrain from expecting the grandparents to be built-in babysitters and to rescue them from every problem. Grandparents usually enjoy brief, rather than prolonged, contact with baby care. For the single parent, the grandparents or other relatives can be a major source of emotional and financial help, and they can also provide help with child care.[32] You may assist the parent(s) in working with grandparents, resolving feelings of either being controlled or not adequately helped, understanding grandparents' feelings, accepting help, and avoiding excessive demands. Nurses who are sensitive to the needs and responsibilities of grandparents and grandchildren can help to reduce stress and increase the wellness of these families.[33]

In some cultures, the maternal grandmother has a major role in taking care of the pregnant and postpartum daughter, and in caring for the infant. The grandmother may give to the daughter advice about nutrition, self-care, or baby care. However, the advice may be contrary to present-day scientific and medical knowledge and practices. Establish rapport with both the grandmother and the mother, or the mother-to-be. Respect the role of the grandmother. Often, the advice she gives is culturally based—the practices she advocates will have maintained the family for centuries.

### CRITICAL THINKING

*What would you say to a grandfather who insists that his only daughter remain in the maternity unit with her healthy baby for a week?*

## Child Maltreatment

A common area of concern for the nurse who cares for infants and their families is **child maltreatment** (*physical abuse, neglect, sexual abuse, and emotional maltreatment*). Brief descriptions of these four categories of child maltreatment are provided below:

- **Physical abuse** is *the application of force to any part of the child's body. This may involve shaking, choking, biting, burning or poisoning a child, or any other dangerous use of force.*[34]

- **Sexual abuse** is the *use of a child for sexual gratification, such as touching and fondling the genitals, including exposure to pornographic material.*[35]

- **Neglect** *occurs when the caregiver does not give appropriate attention to the child's needs, such as physical neglect, abandonment, and educational and medical neglect.*[36]

- **Emotional maltreatment** *involves threatening, intimidating, terrorizing, and socially isolating a child.*

The Canadian Incidence Study of Reported Child Abuse and Neglect (CIS) was the first Canada-wide study to examine incidence of child maltreatment based on 7672 investigations from 51 sites in all provinces and territories.[37] The results of substantiated cases indicate the following: inappropriate punishment (69 percent) and shaken baby syndrome (1 percent) were related to physical abuse; touching and fondling of the genitals (68 percent) were related to sexual abuse; exposure to family violence (58 percent) was related to emotional maltreatment; and failure to supervise leading to physical harm (48 percent) was related to neglect. The primary category of abuse was physical in nature. In Canada, an estimated 21.52 cases of child abuse and neglect per 1000 children occurred. Of these, 9.71 cases per 1000 were confirmed or verified. Data collection for the second cycle of the study commenced in the fall of 2003.[38]

The 2003 Canadian Incidence Study of Reported Child Abuse and Neglect (CIS-2003) was the second Canada-wide study to examine the incidence of reported child maltreatment and the characteristics of the children and families investigated by child welfare services. The rate of substantiated maltreatment in Canada, excluding Quebec, has increased 125 percent from 9.64 substantiated cases per thousand children in 1998 to 21.71 cases in 2003. There are several reasons for the increase, one being the development of a more precise system to identify victimized siblings. Currently, there is greater awareness of both emotional maltreatment and exposure to domestic violence.[39]

The three primary categories of substantiated maltreatment were neglect (30 percent), exposure to domestic violence (28 percent), and physical abuse (24 percent). Emotional maltreatment accounted for another 15 percent of the cases, while sexual abuse cases represented only 3 percent of all substantiated investigations.[40]

In Canada, all individuals in jurisdictions with reporting statutes are obliged to report suspected child abuse to the appropriate child protection authorities. For health professionals, the reporting statute overrides statutory rules regarding confidentiality.[41]

Child maltreatment is not a simple phenomenon. It is a complex sequence of events that lead to children being hurt. Theorists have proposed numerous models to explain child maltreatment, but no single theoretical framework has yet been recognized as the definitive explanation of child abuse and neglect. Instead, models include a complex interaction of personal, social, and environmental factors.

Whenever the developing person and family, and influences on development and behaviour, are considered, the microsystem, exosystem, and macrosystem are all found to be contributors. Each of these rather important components is discussed in relation to child abuse, maltreatment, and neglect.

The **microsystem** *consists of the family*. Maltreating parents are angry and anxious, have poor impulse control and low self-esteem. They are under great stress, and are lonely and depressed. In general, they cannot cope with the demands of childrearing. They do not understand normal child development. They become enraged because the child does not meet their expectations for behaviour: to not cry, or to stay clean. Many of the parents, especially the mothers, are young and hold a lone-parent status. They tend to become highly stressed, for example, by child behaviours that most parents take in stride. Some of these parents are emotionally ill, have antisocial personalities, or have experienced a history of child abuse. Sometimes the pregnancy has been unplanned, or a negative attitude has developed toward the pregnancy. These people are less effective at resolving problems with their children, or with the spouse, or even with other family members. Often these parents are cut off from any support system; they are lonely and isolated. In such cases, the child may need more care than normal because of some disability or a demanding nature. When children are abused, some become more aggressive, which causes even more abuse from the parent. In contrast, neglectful parents tend to be apathetic, incompetent in relationships, irresponsible, and emotionally withdrawn.[42] Children who are sexually abused generally reside in a family without a natural parent, usually a stepfather. These children tend to relate poorly with their parents.[43]

The **exosystem**—*the outside world*—can be a contributor. Poverty, unemployment, job dissatisfaction, social isolation, and lack of assistance from others all contribute to stress, rage, and withdrawal. The low-income neighbourhood, with little sense of community, criminal activity, lack of facilities or resources, inadequate safety overall, and poor political leadership profoundly affects families and their ability to cope and care for themselves. A neighbourhood may be poor, but if there are strong social support networks and a sense of community, there is less child abuse.[44] Increasingly, the social support system may also be an obstacle. For example, individuals within a social support system may protect the abuser instead of the abused.[45]

The **macrosystem**—*cultural values and patterns of punishment*—is key. In Canada, high rates of violence exist in various forms and child abuse rates are especially high. In one-third of physical abuse cases, the victims are under one year of age. In countries where violent crime is less frequent, such as Japan, China, and Tahiti, child abuse is rare.[46]

The Hollow Water First Nation Holistic Healing Circle (CHCH) is a mature healing process that is widely acclaimed in Canada. The goal is that the community takes responsibility of their own offender and the offending actions. CHCH has facilitated a strong relationship between the community and the justice system.[47] For a summary of the theoretical models of abuse and neglect of children, see Baker.[48]

Professionals must be aware of the parent who has difficulty with attachment where maltreatment can result. Further information about maltreatment is presented in Chapters 6, 8, 9, and 10.

MacMillan describes the Preventive Interventions for Child Maltreatment:

1. Perinatal and early childhood programs aimed primarily at prevention of child physical abuse or neglect:
   a. Home visitation by nurses during perinatal period through infancy for the first-time mothers of low socioeconomic status, single parents, or teenage parents
   b. Comprehensive health care program and parent education or support program
   c. Combination of services including case management, education, and psychotherapy
   d. Intensive pediatric contact with home visits
   e. Extended parent–child contact
   f. Free access to health care centre

   *Note:* Of the strategies listed, only home visitation to first-time disadvantaged mothers has been shown effective in preventing physical abuse and neglect.

2. Educational programs aimed primarily at prevention of sexual abuse:
   a. Sexual abuse and abduction prevention programs for children

   *Note:* Improved knowledge of sexual abuse, and enhanced awareness of safety skills; no studies have determined the effectiveness of programs in reducing the incidence of sexual abuse or abduction.[49]

Other preventative approaches include the Kids Help Phone (1-800-668-6868), which is a national toll-free confidential hotline for children and adolescents who are in need of help and support.[50] The Population Health Perspective (PHP), which takes into account the determinants of health, can be used as a good framework in studying child maltreatment. Child maltreatment is a serious population health problem because its consequences early and later in life are widespread and detrimental to health. The most significant contribution of PHP is its holistic approach—taking into consideration both societal and personal factors.[51]

**Shaken baby syndrome (SBS)** *is a form of child abuse that is caused by vigorous shaking of the child, with or without impact. It produces rapid acceleration and deceleration forces in the head. Frequently, consequent damage results, with little or no evidence of external cranial trauma.* Because of the nature of the situation, there are no accurate statistics regarding the incidence of SBS in Canada. There is consensus, however, that head trauma is the leading cause of death of abused children, and that shaking is involved in many of these cases. Most perpetrators are male. Infants who have been shaken display symptoms ranging from irritability or lethargy and vomiting, to seizures or unconsciousness with interrupted breathing or death. Many survivors of SBS suffer brain damage, resulting in lifelong impairments. Victims of SBS are usually less than one year of age, with the majority being under six months.[52]

## CONTROVERSY DEBATE

You have recently graduated with your baccalaureate degree in nursing, and you are pleased to have obtained a position ten months ago in the pediatric respiratory unit of a large children's hospital in a major city in Saskatchewan.

During the past week, you have been caring for Ricki, an infant in the hospital with asthma. When Ricki's mother comes in each day with Ricki's five-year-old brother, Shawn, you notice that she is very caring and attentive to Ricki, while Shawn spends most of his time talking quietly to himself and exploring the room near Ricki's bed by touching and manipulating things. Strangely, Shawn does not seem to be very interested in Ricki.

Two days ago, you happened to see his mother grab Shawn rather roughly by the arm. Mother shook Shawn two or three times quickly, telling him harshly to leave the tissue box alone. Shawn struggled, cried out in apparent pain, and sobbed for a few minutes while sitting on the floor. Soon, he pulled a small ball from his pocket and held it as he slowly cruised about the room looking at, but not approaching, any of the other children. Mother had immediately turned her attention back to Ricki.

Today, a few minutes ago, when Shawn and his mother came to visit, you noticed a fresh bruise on Shawn's cheek. When you cheerfully asked about it, Shawn cowered and his mother quickly mentioned a fall from his tricycle and moved on. You are concerned that Shawn might be a victim of physical abuse. The unit chart shows that Shawn's mother is professionally employed and lives with her husband.

1. What are your options now, as a health care professional, while the mother and Shawn are still in Ricki's room and you must attend to other children on the ward?

2. Your nurse unit manager is not available to you for at least two hours. What is your plan of action?

Prevention efforts should be built on a population health basis. Strategies should be provided to the general public regarding the adverse effects of shaking a baby along with guidance for coping with such a baby.[53] Health professionals also need to be provided with guidelines to ensure appropriate and consistent care to SBS victims. These guidelines must ensure that health promoting strategies are provided for families regarding the care of an infant. Susan, a nurse unit manager on a paediatric unit, always makes certain that the staff handbook on the unit is up to date on shaken baby syndrome.

Teach parents, both mother and father (or step-parent if involved), to better understand normal infant behaviour and how to manage their frustrations to avoid abusive behaviour. If the parent feels angry, he or she should avoid touching the baby. They should step back and leave the room to calm down. Consider causes for crying: the child may be hungry, soiled, teething, tired, ill, injured, or frightened. The need behind the crying usually needs to be addressed.

## PHYSIOLOGIC CONCEPTS

The following information will assist you in assessment and intervention with the neonate and in parental education.

## Neonate: Physical Characteristics

The neonatal period of infancy includes the critical transition from parasitic fetal existence to physiologic independence. The normal newborn is described in the following pages.[54] The transition begins at birth with the first cry. Air is sucked in to inflate the lungs. Complex chemical changes are initiated in the cardiopulmonary system so that the baby's heart and lungs can assume the burden of oxygenating the body. The *foramen ovale* closes during the first 24 hours, and the *ductus arteriosus* closes after several days. For the first time, the baby experiences light, gravity, cold, and firm touch.

The newborn is relatively resistant to the stress of anoxia and can survive longer in an oxygen-free atmosphere than an adult can. The reason for this fact is unknown, as are the long-term effects of mild oxygen deprivation.

General Appearance The newborn does not match the baby ads and may be a shock to new parents. The misshapen head, flat nose, puffy eyelids and often undistinguished eye colour, discoloured skin, large tongue and undersized lower jaw, short neck and small sloping shoulders, short limbs and large rounded abdomen with protruding umbilical stump that remains for three weeks, and bowed skinny legs may result in disappointment if the parents are unprepared for the sight of a newborn. The head, which accounts for one-fourth of the total body size, appears overly large in relation to the body.

The **anterior fontanel**, a *diamond-shaped area at the top of the front of the head*, and the **posterior fontanel**, a *triangular-shaped area at the centre back of the head*, are often called soft spots. These unossified areas of the skull bones, along with the suture lines of the bones, allow the bones to overlap during delivery, and they also allow for the expansion of the brain as they gradually fill in with bone cells. The posterior fontanel closes by 2 or 3 months; the anterior fontanel closes between 8 and 18 months. These **soft spots** may add to the parents' fear that the newborn is too fragile to handle.

Reassure the parents that the newborn, although in need of tender, gentle care, is also resilient and adaptable. The head and fontanels can be touched gently without harm, although strong pressure or direct injury should be avoided. Reassure them that the baby will soon take on the features of the family members, and will look more as they had expected.

Apgar Scoring System The physical status of the newborn is determined with the Apgar tool one minute after birth, and again five minutes later. The newborn's respirations, heart rate, muscle tone, reflex activities, and colour are observed. A maximum score of 2 is given to each sign, so that the Apgar score could range from 0 to 10, as indicated in Table 7-2. A score of less than 7 means that the newborn is having difficulty adapting, needs even closer observation than usual, and may need life-saving intervention.[55]

Gestational Age Assessment In addition to using the Apgar score, assessment includes estimating gestational age to use parameters other than weight to assess the infant's level of maturity. By considering both *birth weight* and *gestational age*, you can categorize infants into one of several groupings. Problems can then be anticipated and, if present, be identified and treated early. Assessment can be carried out as early as the first day of life, and should be done no later than the fifth day of life because external criteria such as hip abduction, square window, dorsiflexion of foot, and size of breast nodules change after five to six days of life. If the neonate is examined on the first day of life, he or she should be examined again before the fifth day to detect neurological changes. The score can be affected by asphyxia or maternal anaesthesia.

To assess gestational age, several scales can be used. From Wong and Hockenberry's *Nursing Care of Infants and Children*, the *Classification of Newborns by Intrauterine Growth and Gestational Age* scale uses weight, length,

## Table 7-2 Assessment of the Newborn: Apgar Scoring System

| Sign | 0 | 1 | 2 |
|---|---|---|---|
| Heart rate | Absent | Less than 100 beats/min | More than 100 beats/min |
| Respirations | Absent | Slow, irregular | Cry; regular rate |
| Muscle tone | Flaccid | Some flexion of extremities | Active movements |
| Reflex irritability | None | Grimace | Cry |
| Colour | Body cyanotic or pale | Body pink; extremities cyanotic | Body completely pink |

Source: Wong, D., and M.J. Hockenberry, *Wong's Nursing Care of Infants and Children*, 7th ed. St. Louis: Mosby, 2003.

and head circumference to determine normal values for gestational age.[56] The "new" Ballard *Gestational Age Assessment*, which is a revision of the original scale, determines neuromuscular and physical maturity in relation to gestational age. This tool includes scores that reflect signs of extremely premature infants (see Figure 7-1).[57] To ensure accuracy, it is recommended that the initial examination be completed within the first 48 hours of life.

**Skin** The skin is thin, delicate, and usually mottled. It varies from pink to reddish, and becomes very ruddy when the baby cries. **Acrocyanosis**, *bluish colour of the hands and feet*, is the result of the sluggish peripheral circulation that normally occurs for only a few days after birth. **Lanugo**, *downy hair of fetal life*, most evident on shoulders, back extremities, forehead, and temples, is lost after a few months and is replaced by other hair growth. The *cheesy skin covering*, **vernix caseosa**, is left on for protective reasons. It rubs off in a few days. **Milia**, *tiny white spots that are small collections of sebaceous secretions*, are sprinkled on the nose and forehead and should not be squeezed or picked. They will disappear. **Hemangioma**, *pink spots* on the upper eyelids, between eyebrows, on the nose, upper lip, or on the back may or may not be permanent. **Mongolian spots** are *slate-coloured areas* on the buttocks, lower back, thighs, ankles, or arms of children of colour, especially black (90 percent), Asian (80 percent), and Aboriginal (80 percent). In contrast, only about 9 percent of Caucasian children have Mongolian spots. The dark areas usually disappear by the end of the first year.

If a birthmark is present, parents should be assured it is not their fault. **Jaundice**, *yellowish discolouration of skin*, should be noted. If it occurs during the first 24 hours of life, it is usually caused by blood incompatibility between mother and baby and requires medical investigation, and possibly treatment. **Physiologic jaundice** normally appears on the third day of life *because the excess number of red blood cells present in fetal life that are no longer needed are undergoing hemolysis, which, in turn, causes high levels of*

*bilirubin (a bile pigment) in the bloodstream*. The jaundice usually disappears in approximately one week, when the baby's liver has developed the ability to metabolize the bilirubin. If bilirubin levels are excessively high, the neonate is placed under full-spectrum lights (phototherapy) to promote bilirubin breakdown.[58] Parents should be reassured about these and other conditions of the skin that normally occur. Foot or hand prints are taken for permanent identification. **Desquamation**, *peeling of skin*, occurs in two to four weeks.

**Umbilical Cord** The *bluish-white, gelatinous structure that transports maternal blood from placenta to fetus* is the **umbilical cord**. It is cut 3.8 to 7.5 cm (1.5 to 3 inches) from the baby's abdominal wall. Because of its high water content, the stump of the cord dries and shrinks rapidly, losing its flexibility by 24 hours after birth. By the second day, it is a very hard yellow or black (blood) tab on the skin. Slight oozing where the cord joins the abdominal wall is common and offers an excellent medium for bacterial growth.

A Canadian study compared alcohol cleaning and natural drying of newborn umbilical cords and concluded that evidence does not support continued use of alcohol for newborn cord care, but that natural drying is preferred.[59] These results are supported by a U.S. study that demonstrated natural drying to be a safe and effective means of umbilical cord care in preterm infants.[60] Dry care consists of spot cleaning the soiled skin with soap and water in the periumbilical area, wiping it with a dry cotton swab or cloth, and allowing the area to air dry.[61] The cord and surrounding area should be observed for potential omphalitis. Parents should be informed of the normal process of cord separation, as well as the dry care procedure of cord care.[62]

**Circumcision** You may inform parents that in Canada, the Canadian Paediatric Society does not recommend circumcision as a routine procedure for newborns because the benefits and harms of circumcision are so evenly

**Figure 7-1** Ballard scale for newborn maturity rating

## NEUROMUSCULAR MATURITY

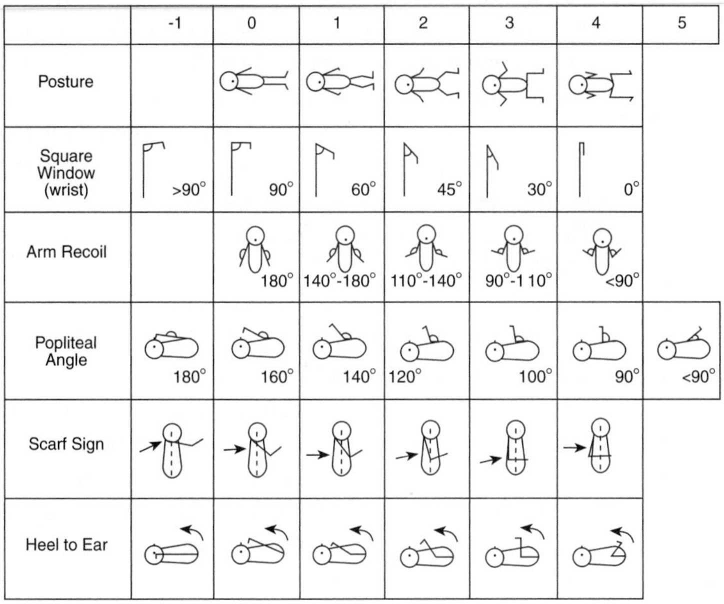

| | -1 | 0 | 1 | 2 | 3 | 4 | 5 |
|---|---|---|---|---|---|---|---|
| Posture | | | | | | | |
| Square Window (wrist) | >90° | 90° | 60° | 45° | 30° | 0° | |
| Arm Recoil | | 180° | 140°-180° | 110°-140° | 90°-110° | <90° | |
| Popliteal Angle | 180° | 160° | 140° | 120° | 100° | 90° | <90° |
| Scarf Sign | | | | | | | |
| Heel to Ear | | | | | | | |

### MATURITY RATING

| score | weeks |
|---|---|
| -10 | 20 |
| -5 | 22 |
| 0 | 24 |
| 5 | 26 |
| 10 | 28 |
| 15 | 30 |
| 20 | 32 |
| 25 | 34 |
| 30 | 36 |
| 35 | 38 |
| 40 | 40 |
| 45 | 42 |
| 50 | 44 |

## PHYSICAL MATURITY

| | | | | | | | |
|---|---|---|---|---|---|---|---|
| Skin | sticky; friable; transparent | gelatinous; red; translucent | smooth; pink; visible veins | superficial peeling &/or rash; few veins | cracking; pale areas; rare veins | parchment; deep cracking; no vessels | leathery; cracked; wrinkled |
| Lanugo | none | sparse | abundant | thinning | bald areas | mostly bald | |
| Plantar Surface | heel-toe 40-50 mm: -1 <40 mm: -2 | >50 mm; no crease | faint red marks | anterior transverse crease only | creases ant. 2/3 | creases over entire sole | |
| Breast | imperceptible | barely perceptible | flat areola; no bud | stippled areola; 1-2 mm bud | raised areola; 3-4 mm bud | full areola; 5-10 mm bud | |
| Eye/Ear | lids fused loosely: -1 tightly: -2 | lids open; pinna flat; stays folded | sl. curved pinna; soft; slow recoil | well-curved pinna; soft but ready recoil | formed & firm; instant recoil | thick cartilage; ear stiff | |
| Genitals male | scrotum flat; smooth | scrotum empty; faint rugae | testes in upper canal; rare rugae | testes descending; few rugae | testes down; good rugae | testes pendulous; deep rugae | |
| Genitals female | clitoris prominent; labia flat | prominent clitoris; small labia minora | prominent clitoris; enlarging minora | majora & minora equally prominent | majora large; minora small | majora cover clitoris & minora | |

### SCORING SECTION

| | 1st Exam=X | 2nd Exam=O |
|---|---|---|
| Estimating Gest Age by Maturity Rating | _____Weeks | _____Weeks |
| Time of Exam | Date _____ <br> Hour _____ am pm | Date _____ <br> Hour _____ am pm |
| Age at Exam | _____Hours | _____Hours |
| Signature of Examiner | _____ <br> _____ <br> M.D./R.N. | _____ <br> _____ <br> M.D./R.N. |

Source: Ballard, J., et al., New Ballard Score Expanded to Include Extremely Premature Infants, *Journal of Pediatrics, 119(3)* (1991), 417.

balanced.[63] Parents are advised to seek advice on the current state of medical knowledge regarding the benefits and harms of circumcision. Often, the parents' decision will reflect their personal, religious, or cultural beliefs.

**Weight, Length, and Head Circumference** In newborns, these measurements provide an accepted index to the normality of development. In Canada, most babies weigh between 2500 and 4499 g at birth.[64] Healthy birth weight indicates a probable healthy development in utero, and subsequently in the first year of life.[65] Newborn infants of African, Aboriginal, and Asian population groups are smaller, on the average, at birth. Atypical growth patterns can be indicators of pathological processes.[66]

Maternal age, parity, lifestyle, and the woman's previous state of nutrition and prenatal care also influence birth weight. In all instances, female babies are somewhat smaller than males. Shortly after birth, the newborn loses weight, up to 10 percent of birth weight, because of water loss. Parents should be told that this loss is normal before a steady weight gain begins in one or two weeks. Tissue turgor shows a sense of fullness because of hydrated subcutaneous tissue.[67] In Canada, the rate of low birth weight is defined as the number of live births under 2500 grams per 100 live births.[68] Infants less than 1500 grams are considered to be of very low birth weight.[69] According to the Manitoba Population-Based Study (2001) compiled in the Manitoba provincial health database, low-birth-weight infants may be at greater risk for developmental problems, and they are a relatively high cost to health services due to neonatal care costs.[70] Low-birth-weight outcomes in Canada focus on very young and older mothers. The *First Nations and Inuit Regional Health Survey* claims that the rate of low birth weight among Aboriginal people in 1996–1997 did not differ significantly from the national norms in 1994–1995. However, the rate of high birth weight associated with neonatal mortality was significantly higher.[71] One explanation proposed that Aboriginal people have a genetic predisposition to heavier babies. More research is needed to understand this pattern of heavy birth weight and to explore the role of nutrition. The prevention of low birth weight is a public health challenge because no clearly defined medical at-risk group exists. However, multiple risk factors such as smoking, drinking, drug use, physical and emotional abuse, and other stresses contribute to low birth weight.[72] Health promotion strategies in the community hold great promise for all families. Resources must be made available in all communities, stressing the importance of support for the mother and family.

Length is measured by placing the child supine on a hard surface, extending the knees, placing the soles upright, and measuring from the soles of the feet to the vertex (tip) of the head. In Canada, the average length at birth is between 50 and 52 cm.[73] The bones are soft, consisting chiefly of cartilage. The back is straight and curves with sitting. The muscles feel hard and are slightly resistant to pressure.[74]

The measurement of head circumference is important in assessing the rate of head growth to determine if any abnormalities, such as too rapid or too slow growth, are present. The measurement is taken over the brow, just above the eyes, and across the posterior occipital protuberance. This standard measure of head size averages approximately 31 to 37 cm at birth, but variations of 1 to 3 cm are common. In Canada, the average head circumference is 33 to 35 cm.[75] Chest circumference is almost 2 cm less than the head circumference.[76] Parents should be prepared for moulding of the skull during vaginal delivery. **Caput succedaneum**, *irregular edema of the scalp*, disappears at approximately the third day. Another irregularity is **cephalohematoma**, a *collection of blood beneath the fibrous covering of the skull bones*, usually the parietal bones.[77]

The baby's characteristic *position* during this period is one of flexion, closely imitating the fetal position. Fists are tightly closed and arms and legs are drawn up against the body. The baby is aware of disturbances in equilibrium and will change position, reacting with the Moro reflex.

It is recommended that the physical assessment of the newborn be conducted with the parents present.[78] Their presence provides the health professionals with the opportunity to reassure the parents of their newborn's normality, and to answer any questions that the parents might have. At the same time, health promoting strategies for the parents and newborn can be discussed. One strategy is to ensure that the mother and family know how to obtain emergency help and parent information.

## CRITICAL THINKING

*What is the role of a health professional, such as the nurse, in genetic diagnostic testing and counselling?*

**Neonate—Other Characteristics** Several other characteristics are normal and resolve themselves shortly after birth. They include swollen breasts that contain liquid in both boys and girls; swollen genitalia with undescended testicles in boys; and vaginal secretions in girls, caused by maternal hormones. Genital size varies for both boys and girls. Urine is present in the bladder, and the baby voids at birth. Obstruction of the nasolacrimal duct is also common, and the excessive tearing and pus accumulation usually clear up when the duct opens spontaneously in a few months.

**Vital Signs** In the newborn, vital signs are not stable.

**Respiratory Efforts** Respiratory efforts at birth are critical and immediate adaptations must occur to counter the decreasing oxygen level and increasing carbon dioxide level in the blood. Causes of respiratory initiations include cutting of the umbilical cord, which causes hypoxia, resulting in carbon dioxide accumulation; physical stimulation of the birth process; the sudden change in baby's environment at birth; the exposure to firm touch; and the cool air. If the mother was medicated during labour, or if the baby is premature, the respiratory centre of the brain is less operative, and the baby will have more difficulty with breathing. The average respiratory rate is 40 breaths/min but will vary between 30 and 60 breaths/min. The respiratory rate may be higher than 60 breaths/min if the newborn is very active or crying.[79] Respirations are irregular, quiet, and shallow and may be followed by an intermittent five- to ten-second pause in breathing.

**Body Temperature** Normal body temperature ranges from 36.5°C to 37.2°C because:

- The heat-regulating mechanism in the hypothalamus is not fully developed.
- Shivering to produce heat does not occur.
- There is less subcutaneous fat.
- Heat is lost to the environment by evaporation, conduction, convection, and radiation.[80]

At birth, amniotic fluid increases temperature loss by evaporation from the skin. Therefore, diligent efforts to dry the skin are necessary. Baby should be placed initially next to mother's abdominal skin or breast, and then wrapped well in blankets before being placed in a warm crib. Several mechanisms occur to help the newborn conserve heat:

- Vasoconstriction, by which constricted blood vessels maintain heat in the inner body
- Flexion of the body to reduce total amount of exposed skin (the premature baby does not assume flexion of the extremities onto the body)
- Increased metabolic rate, which causes increased heat production
- Metabolism of adipose tissue that has been stored during the eighth month of gestation

Body temperature of the baby normally drops approximately 1°C immediately after birth. In a warm environment, the body's temperature begins to rise slowly after eight hours. It is critical to maintain the birth area at 23°C to 25°C, with a draft-free environment.[81] Therefore, the prevention of heat loss, especially during the first 15 minutes, is crucial to adaptation to extrauterine life. Babies who have lost excessive amounts of heat cannot produce surfactant. **Surfactant** is *a thin lipoprotein film produced by the alveoli that reduces surface tension of the alveoli, allows them to expand, and allows some air to remain in alveoli at end of expiration.* The result is that it takes less effort to re-expand the lungs.[82]

The temperature should be taken at the axillary site for five minutes. Although the axilla is the method of choice,[83] a tympanic thermometer probe may be inserted into the auditory canal.

**Heart Rate** Heart rate ranges from 80 to 100 beats (sleeping) of the immature cardiac regulatory mechanism in the medulla. The heart rate may increase to 180 beats per minute when the newborn cries, but will drop to 90 beats per minute during sleep. The pulse rate gradually decreases during the first and subsequent years.

**Blood Pressure** Systolic blood pressure may range from 60 to 80 mm Hg and the diastolic may range 40 to 50 mm Hg. At ten days, the systolic ranges from 95 to 100 mm Hg and the diastolic slightly increases.[84]

**Meconium** Meconium, *the first fecal material*, is sticky, odourless, and tarry, and is passed from 8 to 24 hours after birth. Transitional stools, which last for a week, are loose, contain mucus, are greenish-yellow and pasty, and have a sour odour. There will be two to four stools daily. If the neonate takes cow's milk, the stools will become yellow and harder and average one to two daily. Once feeding begins the stools change in colour.[85]

**Reflex Activity** Reflex activity is innate, or built in through the process of evolution, and it develops while the baby is in utero. **Reflex** is an *involuntary, unlearned response elicited by certain stimuli*, and it indicates neurological status or function. Individual differences in the newborn's responses to stimulation are apparent at birth. Some respond vigorously to the slightest stimulation. Others respond slowly, and some fall somewhere between the extremes. Several types of reflexes exist in the neonate and young infant: consummatory, avoidant, exploratory, social, and attentional. **Consummatory reflexes**, *such as rooting and sucking, promote survival through feeding.* **Avoidant reflexes** are *elicited by potentially harmful stimuli* and include the Moro, withdrawing, knee jerk, sneezing, blinking, and coughing reflexes. **Exploratory reflexes** *occur when infants are wide awake and are held upright so that their arms move without restraint.* A visual object at eye level elicits both reaching and grasping reflexes. **Social reflexes**, such as smiling, *promote affectionate interactions between parents and infants* and thus have a rather high survival value. Crying, in response to painful stimuli, loud noise, food deprivation, or loss of support; quieting in response to touch, low soft tones, or food; and smiling in response to changes in brightness, comforting stimuli, or escape from uncomfortable stimuli are all examples of innate reflexes that can be modified by experience and that persist throughout life. **Attentional reflexes**, including orienting and attending, *determine the nature of the baby's response to stimuli* and have continuing importance through development.[86] The nervous system of the newborn is both anatomically and physiologically immature. Reflexes should be observed for their presence and symmetry. These reflexes are described in Table 7-3.[87]

## Table 7-3 Assessment of Infant Reflexes

| Reflex | Description | Appearance/Disappearance |
|---|---|---|
| Rooting | Touching baby's cheek causes head to turn toward the side touched. | Present in utero at 24 weeks; disappears 3–4 months; may persist in sleep 9–12 months |
| Sucking | Touching lips or placing something in baby's mouth causes baby to draw liquid into mouth by creating vacuum with lips, cheeks, and tongue. | Present in utero at 28 weeks; persists through early childhood, especially during sleep |
| Bite | Touching gums, teeth, or tongue causes baby to open and close mouth. | Disappears at 3–5 months when biting is voluntary, but seen throughout adult years in comatose person |
| Babkin | Pressure applied to palm causes baby to open mouth, close eyes. | Present at birth; disappears in 2 or 4 months |
| Pupillary response | Flashing light across baby's eyes or face causes constriction of pupils. | Present at 32 weeks of gestation; persists throughout life |
| Blink | Baby closes both eyes. | Remains throughout life |
| Moro or startle | Making a loud noise or changing baby's position causes baby to extend both arms outward with fingers spread, then bring them together in a tense, quivery embrace. | Present at 28 weeks of gestation; disappears at 4–7 months |
| Withdrawing | Baby removes hand or foot from painful stimuli. | Present at birth; persists throughout life |
| Colliding | Baby moves arms up and face to side when object is in collision course with face. | Present at birth or shortly after; persists in modified form throughout life |
| Palmar grasp | Placing object or finger in baby's palm causes his or her fingers to close tightly around object. | Present at 32 weeks of gestation; disappears at 3–4 months, replaced by voluntary grasp at 4–5 months |
| Plantar grasp | Placing object or finger beneath toes causes curling of toes around object. | Present at 32 weeks of gestation; disappears at 9–12 months |
| Tonic neck or fencing (TNR) | Postural reflex is seen when infant lies on back with head turned to one side; arm and leg on the side toward which he or she is looking are extended while opposite limbs are flexed. | Present at birth; disappears at approximately 4 months |
| Stepping, walking, dancing | Holding baby upright with feet touching flat surface causes legs to prance up and down as if baby were walking or dancing. | Present at birth; disappears at approximately 2–4 months; with daily practice of reflex, infant may walk alone at 10 months |
| Reaching | Hand closes as it reaches toward and grasps at object at eye level. | Present shortly after birth if baby is upright; comes under voluntary control in several months |
| Orienting | Head and eyes turn toward stimulus of noise, accompanied by cessation of other activity, heartbeat change, and vascular constriction. | Present at birth; comes under voluntary control later; persists throughout life |
| Attending | Eyes fix on a stimulus that changes brightness, movement, or shape. | Present shortly after birth; comes under voluntary control later; persists throughout life |

*(continued)*

Table 7-3 (continued)

| Reflex | Description | Appearance/Disappearance |
|---|---|---|
| Swimming | Placing baby horizontally, supporting baby under abdomen, causes baby to make crawling motions with his or her arms and legs while lifting head from surface as if he or she were swimming. | Present after 3 or 4 days; disappears at approximately 4 months; may persist with practice |
| Trunk incurvation | Stroking one side of spinal column while baby is on his or her abdomen causes crawling motions with legs, lifting head from surface, and incurvature of trunk on the side stroked. | Present in utero; then seen at approximately third or fourth day; persists 2–3 months |
| Babinski | Stroking bottom of foot causes big toe to rise while other toes fan out and curl downward. | Present at birth; disappears at approximately 9 or 10 months; presence of reflex later may indicate disease |
| Landau | Suspending infant in horizontal, prone position and flexing head against trunk cause legs to flex against trunk. | Appears at approximately 3 months; disappears at approximately 12–24 months |
| Parachute | Sudden thrusting of infant downward from horizontal position causes hands and fingers to extend forward and spread as if to protect self from a fall. | Appears at approximately 7–9 months; persists indefinitely |
| Biceps | Tap on tendon of biceps causes biceps to contract quickly. | Brisk in first few days, then slightly diminished; permanent |
| Knee jerk | Tap on tendon below patella or on patella causes leg to extend quickly. | More pronounced first 2 days; permanent |

Sources: Sherwen, L., M. Scoloveno, and C. Weingarten, *Maternity Nursing: Care of the Childbearing Family* (3rd Ed.). Norwalk, CT: Appleton & Lange, 1999; and Wong, D., *Wong's Nursing Care of Infants and Children* (7th ed.). St. Louis: Mosby, 2003.

**Perceptual Abilities** The newborn has a greater number of highly developed sensory abilities than was once supposed. Apparently a moderately enriched environment, one without stimulus bombardment or deprivation, is best suited for sensory motor development. The infant's use of the senses, innate abilities, and motor activity lay the groundwork for intellectual development.[88] Moderate, gentle kinesthetic stimulation daily results in a baby who is quieter, gains weight faster, and shows improved socioemotional function.

The first impressions of life, security, warmth, love, and pleasure—or lack of them—come to the infant through touch. Knowledge of the people around him or her, initially of mother, is gradually built from the manner in which the baby is handled. He or she soon learns to sense mother's self-confidence and pleasure as well as her anxiety, lack of confidence, anger, or rejection. These early touch experiences, and the infant's feelings through them, apparently lay the foundation for feelings about people throughout life.[89]

**Sensitivity to Pain, Pressure, and Temperature** Sensitivity to pain, pressure, and temperature extremes is present at birth. Pain is shown by a distinct cry. The baby is especially sensitive to touch around the mouth and on the palms and soles. Females are more responsive than males to touch and pain than males. Visceral sensations of discomfort, such as hunger, overdistension of the stomach, passage of gas and stool, and extremes of temperature apparently account for much of the newborn's crying. At first the cry is simply a primitive discharge mechanism that calls for help. He or she wails with equal force regardless of stimulus. In a few weeks, baby acquires subtle modifications in the sound of the cry that, in turn, provide clues to the attentive parent about the nature of the discomfort so that response can be adjusted to the baby's need.[90]

**Vision** Vision is the least well-developed sense at birth. The eyes of the newborn are smaller than those of the adult. The retinal structures are incomplete; the optic nerve is underdeveloped. The visual abilities of the baby change from birth to four months of age.[91]

The infant maintains contact with the environment through visual fixation, scanning, and tracking, and he or she pays more attention to stimuli from the face than to other stimuli. The newborn looks at mother's face while feeding and while sitting upright follows the path of an object. He will cry or pull backwards, though, if it comes too close to his face.

The newborn has the following visual abilities:

1. Able to fixate on moving objects in a range of 45 degrees when held 20 to 25 centimetres away

2. Can look at face of mother while feeding or sitting upright

3. Prefers human face to mobile toy

4. Pulls back if object comes too close to face

5. Has pupillary and corneal reflex

6. Prefers black and white to bright colours; prefers strong contrasts

7. Can focus attention on patterned object, such as geometric, symmetrical, and complex shapes; large circles, dots, and squares

8. Prefers to scan edges and contours of complex shapes; has peripheral vision to 180 degrees[92]

By the age of one month, baby can distinguish between the face of mother and a stranger.

Teach parents that baby needs eye contact and the opportunity to see the human face and a variety of changing scenes and colours. Providing a mirror or chrome plate

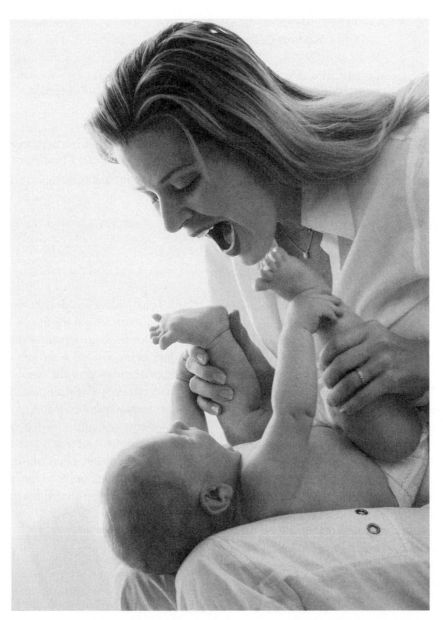

Infant has the ability to fix on the mother's face beginning one day after birth and finds geometric objects interesting.

that reflects light and objects and rotating the bed help the baby to use both eyes and avoid one-sided vision. Hang cardboard black-and-white mobiles, especially those that make sound, and have them within reach of baby's kicking feet. Later, the infant enjoys other colours and designs that are within grasp. By age two months, baby can see the ceiling and the decorations on it. As baby grows older, the crib should be low enough for baby to see things beyond it.

**Hearing** Hearing is developed in utero when the fetus is exposed to internal sounds of the mother's body, such as the heartbeat and abdominal rumbles (heard at five months), and external sounds, such as voices, music, and a cymbal clap (heard at seven months). The neonate cannot hear whispers but can respond to voice pitch changes. A low pitch quiets and a high pitch increases alertness.[93] Baby responds to sound direction—left or right—but responds best to mother's voice, to sounds directly in front of his or her face, and to sounds experienced during gestation. Baby often sleeps better with background songs or a tape recording of mother's heartbeat.[94] By three days of age, the newborn discriminates between the voice of mother and another female's voice. Differentiation of sounds, and the perception of their source, take time to develop, but startle reactions are present. The baby withdraws from loud noise. In Canada, hearing loss is estimated to occur in 1.5 to 6.0 cases per 1000 live births.[95] It is advocated that babies who are at increased risk for hearing loss should have screening completed in their place of birth. However, other appropriate arrangements should be made within three months of birth.[96] Some factors associated with increased hearing loss are birth weight less than 1500 g, congenital infections such as rubella, herpes, syphilis, and a family history of childhood sensory hearing loss.[97] It is important that health care professionals assist the parents to locate appropriate resources.

---

### CRITICAL THINKING

*What steps would you take to assist parents of a child with hearing loss to learn about resources available to them in their province or territory?*

---

**Taste and Smell** Taste is not highly developed at birth, but acid, bitter, salt, and sweet substances evoke a response.

## Checklist to Detect Presence of Hearing in Infancy

From Birth to 2 Weeks, Does Baby:

- Jump or blink when there is a sudden loud sound
- Stop crying when you start to talk
- Seem aware of your voice
- Stir in sleep when there is continuous noise close by
- Jump or blink when there is a sudden soft click such as a light switch or a camera click when the noise is otherwise quiet
- Stop sucking momentarily when there is a noise or when you start to talk
- Look up from sucking or try to open eyes when there is a sudden noise

From 2 to 10 Weeks, Does Baby:

- Stop crying when you talk to him or her
- Stop movements when you enter the room
- Seem aware of your voice
- Sleep regardless of noises
- Waken when the crib or bassinet is touched
- Respond to comforting only when held against mother or familiar caretaker

- Cry at sudden loud noises
- Blink or jerk at sudden loud noises

From 10 Weeks to 6 Months, Does Baby:

- Always coo with pleasure when you start to talk
- Turn eyes to the speaker
- Know when father comes home and wriggle in welcome (if awake)
- Startle when you bend over the crib after awakening
- Seem to enjoy a soft musical toy (e.g., a crib musical toy)
- Cry when exposed to sudden, loud, unexpected noise
- Stop movements when a new sound is introduced
- Try to turn in the direction of a new sound or a person who starts to talk
- Make many different babbling sounds when alone
- Try to "talk back" when you talk
- Start wriggling in anticipation of a bottle when you start preparing it (if the baby is awake and the preparation is out of sight, as the refrigerator door opens and so on)
- Know own name (smiles, turns, or otherwise gives an indication)

Note: The Hearing Foundation of Canada supports a broad range of services for deaf and hard of hearing children and adults across Canada.

Taste buds for sweet are more abundant in early life than in late life. Breathing rhythm is altered in response to fragrance, showing some ability to smell. The sense of smell is well developed in the newborn. Infants can discriminate the smell of mother's body from the smells of other bodies or objects, and they can sense the odours that adults sense.[98]

Neonates differ in their appearance, size, function, and response. Girls are more developmentally advanced than boys and blacks more so than Caucasians. The most accurate assessment is made by comparing the neonate against norms for the same sex and race.[99]

### Special Considerations in Physical Assessment of the Neonate
When a newborn is examined, the primary concerns are neurological status, congenital deformities, and metabolic disturbances. Any history of hereditary diseases and pregnancy and delivery information is essential. Reflex status indicates neurological development and some congenital deformities. The following are particular aspects to check when conducting a physical assessment of the neonate.

Ear position is important because there is a strong association between low-set ears and renal malformation or a chromosomal aberration such as Down syndrome. The top of the ear should be aligned with the inner and outer canthi of the eyes. The eustachian tube is shorter and wider than in the adult. To examine the neonate with an otoscope, the head should be stabilized and the pinna of the ear pulled back and up.

Discharges from the eye may result from chemical irritation. A mongoloid slant in a Caucasian infant may suggest a chromosome abnormality.

Check to determine whether pupils are unequal, constricted, dilated, or fixed. This may suggest intracranial pressure.

The nose should be patent (open or exposed). Flaring of the nares usually represents respiratory distress. A thick bloody discharge from the nose suggests congenital syphilis.

The mouth should be inspected for cleft lip and cleft palate. Although spitting up is common in the newborn, projectile vomiting is not. The newborn should have very little saliva, and tonsillar tissue should not be present at birth.

Check for bulging of the chest and unequal movement. Check the abdomen for bleeding and oozing around the umbilical cord. The umbilical cord should have two arteries and one vein. Auscultation of bowel sounds should precede palpation for masses, an extremely important procedure in the newborn.

The genitalia are examined for deformities. Only the external genitalia are examined in children. In uncircumcised males up to three months of age, the foreskin should not be retracted, thereby avoiding tearing of the membrane.

The testes should be palpated in the scrotum, although sometimes they are still undescended. A **hydrocele**, a *collection of watery fluid in the scrotum, or along the spermatic cord,* and **hernia**, a *protrusion of part of the intestine through the abdominal muscles,* are common findings in males.

A bloody, or mucus, vaginal discharge may be present in girls. Fused labia are a serious anomaly, but simple adhesion may be due to inflammation.

Taking temperatures rectally can rule out **imperforate anus** (*lacking normal anal opening*).

The spine should be palpated for **spina bifida**, a *congenital neural tube defect characterized by anomaly in posterior vertebral arch*. Observation for symmetric bilateral muscle movements of the hips and knees is essential. The hips should be examined for dislocation by rotating the thighs with the knees flexed.

Extremities should be checked for the right number of fingers and toes and bilateral movements, and position of hands and feet should be checked.

Signs of prematurity include low birth weight and small size, thick lanugo, excess vernix, slow or absent reflexes, undescended testicles in the male, and nipples not visible.[100]

## Infant—Physical Characteristics

### General Appearance
The growing infant changes in appearance as he or she changes size and proportion.[101]

The face grows rapidly; trunk and limbs lengthen; back and limb muscles develop; and coordination improves. By one month, the baby can lift the head slightly when prone and hold the head up briefly when the back is supported. By two months, the head is held erect but it bobs when he or she is sitting unsupported.

Skull enlargement occurs almost as rapidly as total body growth during the first year and is determined mainly by the rate of brain expansion. From birth to six months, the head size increases approximately 2 cm per month in the first three months, then 1 cm per month from four to six months. The head size growth rate drops to 0.5 cm increase per month during the second six months. The average size is 43 cm at 6 months and 46 cm at 12 months. At 3 months, expect about 39.5 cm, at 20 weeks about 41 cm, and at 30 weeks about 43 cm. By the end of the first year, the head will be two-thirds of adult size.[102]

### Physical Growth and Emotional, Social, and Neuromuscular Learning
Physical growth and these areas of learning are concurrent, interrelated, and rapid in the first year. The first year of life is one of the two periods of rapid physical growth after birth. (The other period is prepuberty and postpuberty.) Infants gain about 680 g per month until five months, when the birth weight has at least

doubled. By one year, the infant's birth weight has tripled, to an average weight of 9.75 kg. Baby grows approximately 30.5 cm (12 inches) in the first year.[103] The skeletal system should be assessed for any orthopedic problems.

Physical and motor abilities are heavily influenced by genetic, biological, and cultural factors; nutrition; maturation of the central nervous system; skeletal formation; overall physical health status; environmental conditions; stimulation; and consistent loving care.

Do you have any photographs of yourself as an infant? If you do, examine the photographs carefully. Note, if you can, the physical growth characteristics that you have attained in each of them.

Table 7-4 divides further developmental sequence into three-month periods for specific assessment.[104] *It is only a guide*, not an absolute standard. Great individual differences occur among infants, depending on their physical growth and emotional, social, and neuromuscular responses. Girls usually develop more rapidly than boys, although the activity level is generally higher for boys. Even with these cautions, the table can be a useful tool if you observe overall behaviour patterns rather than isolated characteristics.

## Table 7-4 Assessment of Physical Characteristics of the Infant

| 1–3 Months | 3–6 Months | 6–9 Months | 9–12 Months |
|---|---|---|---|
| Many characteristics of newborn, but more stable physiologically | Most neonatal reflexes gone Temperature stabilizes at 37.5°C (99.4°F) | | Temperature averages 37.7°C (99.7°F) |
| Heartbeat steadies at about 120–130 beats/min | | Pulse about 115/min | Pulse about 100–110/min |
| Blood pressure about 80/40; gradually increases | | Blood pressure about 90/60 | Blood pressure 96/66 |
| Respirations more regular at 30–40/min; gradually decrease | | Respirations about 32/min | Respirations 20–30/min |
| Appearance of salivation and tears | | | |
| Weight gain of 141.75–198.45 g (5–7 oz.) per week | Weight gain of 85–141 g (3–5 oz.) per week | | Weight gain of 85–141.75 g (3–5 oz.) per week |
| Weight at 3625–5900 g (8–13 lb.) | Weight at 7–7.3 kg (15–16 lb.) by 6 months | Birth weight doubled by 6 months | Birth weight tripled; average 10 kg (22 lb.) |
| Head circumference increases up to 40 cm (16 in.) | Head size increases 2.5 cm (1 in.) | Head size 43.2 cm (17.8 in.) | Head size increases slightly more, to 45–46 cm (18.3 in.) |
| Chest circumference 40 cm (16 in.) | Chest size increases more than 2.5 cm (up to 43–44 cm or 17.3 in.) | Chest circumference increases by 1.25 cm (to 44–45 cm or 17.8 in.) | Chest circumference increases to 45–46 cm (18.3 in.) |
| Body length: Growth of 2.5 cm (1 in.) monthly | Growth of 1.25 cm (½ in.) monthly | Growth of 1.25 cm (½ in.) monthly | Growth of about 1.25 cm monthly; height 72.5–75 cm (29–30 in.), increased by 50% since birth |
| Tonic neck and Moro reflexes rapidly diminishing | Most neonatal reflexes gone Palmar reflex diminishing | | |
| Arms and legs found in bilaterally symmetrical position | | | |

*(continued)*

**Table 7-4** (continued)

| 1–3 Months | 3–6 Months | 6–9 Months | 9–12 Months |
|---|---|---|---|
| Limbs used simultaneously, but not separately | Movements more symmetric | | |
| Hands and fingers played with | | | |
| Clenched fists giving way to open hands that bat at objects | | | |
| Reaches for objects | Reaches for objects with accurate aim and flexed fingers | Palmar grasp developed<br>Picks up objects with both hands; bangs toys | Throws objects |
| Plays with hands | Objects transferred from one hand to another by 6 months<br>Bangs with objects held in one hand<br>Scoops objects with hands<br>Begins to use fingers separately | Holds bottle with hands; holds own cookie<br><br>Preference for use of one hand<br><br>Probes with index finger<br>Thumb opposition to finger (prehension) by 7 months | Puts toys in and out of container<br><br><br><br>Points with finger<br>Brings hands and thumb and index finger together at will to pick up small objects<br>Releases objects at will |
| Can follow moving objects with eyes when supine; begins to use both eyes together at about 2 months | Binocular depth perception by about 5 months<br>Looks for objects when they are dropped<br>Improving eye–hand coordination<br>Eruption of one or two lower incisors | Explores, feels, pulls, inspects, tastes, and tests objects<br><br><br>Hand–mouth coordination<br>Feeds self cracker and other finger foods<br>Begins weaning process | Makes mark on paper<br><br><br>Eats with fingers; holds cup, spoon<br><br>Has 6 teeth, central and lateral incisors; eruption of first molars at about 12 months |
| Attends to voices | Binaural hearing present | | |
| Raises chin while lying on stomach at 1 month | Turns head to sound | Turns to sounds behind self | |
| Raises chest while lying on stomach at 2 months; raises head and chest 45° to 50° off bed, supporting weight on arms | | | |
| Holds head in alignment when prone at 2 months; holds head erect in prone position at 3 months | | | |

*(continued)*

**Table 7-4** (continued)

| 1–3 Months | 3–6 Months | 6–9 Months | 9–12 Months |
|---|---|---|---|
| Supports self on forearms when on stomach at 3 months | Rolls over completely by 6 months | | Rolls over easily from back to stomach |
| Sits if supported | Sits with support at 4 months<br>Holds head steady while sitting<br>Pulls self to sitting position<br>Begins to sit alone for short periods | Sits erect unsupported by 7 months | Sits alone steadily |
| | Plays with feet<br>Kicks vigorously<br>Begins to hitch (scoot) backward while sitting | Creeps or crawls by 8 or 9 months | Pivots when seated<br>Puts feet in mouth<br>Hitches with backward locomotion while sitting |
| | Bears portion of own weight when held in standing position | Pulls self to stand by holding onto support | Sits from standing position without help |
| | Pushes feet against hard surface to move by 3 or 4 months | Cruises (walking sideways while holding onto object with both hands) by 10 months | Stands alone for a minute |
| | | | Walks when led by 11 months |
| | | Begins to walk with help | Walks with help by 12–14 months |
| | | | Lumber and dorsal curves developed while learning to walk |
| | | | Turning of feet and bowing of legs normal |
| | | | Beginning to show regular bladder and bowel patterns; has one or two stools per day; interval of dry diaper does not exceed 1 to 2 hours |
| | | | Not ready for toilet training |
| Smiles reflexively at comforting person | Smiles at person deliberately during interaction | Experiences separation anxiety about 7–9 months | Attachment to caregiver |
| | Displays joy, frustration, rage | Engages in social play; elicits response from others | Sociable increasingly with others |
| Coos, chuckles, laughs | Babbles; plays with sounds | | Begins to co-operate in dressing; puts arm through sleeve; takes off socks |
| | | | Improves previously acquired skills throughout this period |

**Neurological System** The neurological system is immature, but it continues the fetal pattern of developing into a functional capacity at a rapid rate. Consistent stimulation of the nervous system is necessary to maintain growth and development; otherwise function is lost and cannot be regained.[105]

**Vision** *By two months of age*, the infant can:[106]

1. Focus both eyes on object steadily
2. Look longer at colours of medium intensity (yellow, green, pink) than at bright (red, orange, blue) or dim (grey, beige) colours
3. Distinguish red from green
4. Accommodate better; lenses have become more flexible
5. Use broader peripheral vision, which has doubled since birth
6. Follow path of an object

*By four months of age*, the infant can:[107]

1. Distinguish between red, green, blue, and yellow, and prefers red and blue
2. Use binocular vision (both eyes focus), which allows perception of depth and distance and ability to distinguish stripes and edges
3. Accommodate on an adult level

*Under four months of age*, baby does not look for an object hidden after seeing it, and when the same object reappears, it is as if the object were a new object. The infant has no knowledge that objects have a continuous existence: the object ceases to exist when it is not seen.[108] The baby coordinates both eyes and attends to, and prefers, novel stimuli. *At four months*, he or she can focus for any distance and perceive shape constancy when the object is rotated at different angles. Infants look longer at patterned stimuli of less complexity than at stimuli that have more complex designs, or no lines or contours, and she or he can detect a change of pattern.[109] The infant prefers faces but is attracted by checkerboard designs, geometric shapes, and large pictures (circles, dots, and squares at least 7.5 cm high and with angles rather than contours). By the first birthday, the infant's acuity is essentially the same as that of an adult with normal vision.[110]

**Vital Signs** During infancy, vital signs (temperature, pulse, respirations, and blood pressure) stabilize, as shown in Table 7-4.

**Intersensory Integration** At birth, perceptual skills are more acute than was previously believed. In infancy, information from two sense modalities is interrelated. Four-month-old infants respond to relationships between visual and auditory stimuli that carry information about an object. Six-month-old infants look longer at television when both picture and sound are on than when only the picture is on. They look longer at patterns on television than they look at other types of stimuli. The debate centres on whether such skill is inborn or learned.[111]

**Touch** The haptic system is the body system pertaining to the perception of tactile stimulation. There are different types of neural receptors for heat, warmth, cold, dull pain, sharp pain, deep pressure, vibration, and light touch. At birth, all humans possess central nervous system ability to register and associate sensory impressions received through receptor organs in the skin and from kinesthetic stimuli that originate with neuromuscular stimulation from their contact with other humans. Sensory pathways that subserve kinesthetic and tactile activities are the first to complete myelinization in infancy, followed by auditory and visual pathways.[112]

The sensations experienced by the infant as a result of being touched from birth onward provides the basis for higher-order operations in the neurological, perceptual, muscular, skeletal, and cognitive systems. Each tactile act carries a physiologic impact with psychological and sociocultural meaning. Much information is gained by discriminating one physical stimulus from another. It has been determined that, in infants, the form or quality of touch they receive changes the perception of the tactile experience. Tactile stimulation is essential for both beginning body image development and other learning. Encourage parents to stroke, massage, and cuddle baby; to talk and sing to baby; and to provide toys that have primary colours, different textures, and movement.[113]

**Endocrine System** The endocrine system begins to develop primarily in infancy and childhood. The lack of homeostatic control, because of various functional deficiencies, renders the infant especially vulnerable to imbalances in fluid and electrolytes, glucose concentration, and amino acid metabolism. Thus, the child is very susceptible to stress, including fluid and electrolyte imbalance, and metabolism of fats, proteins, and carbohydrates, during the first 18 months because the pituitary gland and adrenal cortex do not function well together and the adrenal gland is immature.[114] The pituitary gland continues to secrete growth hormone and thyroid-stimulating hormone (begun in fetal life), which influence growth and metabolism.[115]

**Respiratory System** The structures of the upper respiratory tract remain small and relatively delicate and they provide inadequate protection against infectious agents. Many of the body parts located in the head are very close to one another. Situated in close proximity are the middle ear, wide horizontal eustachian tube, throat, short and narrow trachea, and bronchi. The main result is a rapid spread of infection from one structure to the other. Mucous membranes are less able to produce mucus, causing less air humidification and warming, which also increases susceptibility to infection. The rounded thorax, the limited alveolar surface for gas exchange, and the amount of anatomic dead air space in the lungs, or portion of the tracheobronchial tree, where inspired air does not participate in gas exchange, means that more air must be moved in and out per minute than later in childhood. This causes an increased respiratory rate.[116]

**Gastrointestinal System** The gastrointestinal system matures somewhat after two to three months, when the baby can voluntarily chew, hold, or spit out food. Saliva secretion increases and composition becomes more adult-like. The Canadian Medical Association recommends that from the age of four to six months, the baby will be ready to sample solid food.[117] For example, iron-fortified cereal should be added as a first supplement at age four to six months (one grain type at a time).[118] During infancy, the stomach enlarges to accommodate a greater volume of food. By the end of the first year, the infant is able to tolerate three meals a day and an evening bottle, and may have one or two bowel movements daily. However, with any gastric irritation, the infant is vulnerable to diarrhea, vomiting, and dehydration.[119] Tooth eruption begins at approximately six months and stimulates saliva flow and chewing. Peristaltic waves mature by slowing down and reversing less after approximately eight months. At that time, stools are more formed and baby spits up or vomits less. By two months, baby usually has two **stools** (*bowel movements*) daily. Breastfed babies usually have soft, semi-liquid stools that are light yellow in colour. Breastfed babies may vary more than bottle-fed babies in the bowel movement pattern. The breastfed baby may have three or four watery stools a day or may go several days without a bowel movement. The stools of the formula-fed baby are more brown and formed.

**Colic**, a term that indicates *daily periods of distress*, usually occurs between two to three weeks and two to three months and seems to have no remedy. Apparently, colic disappears as digestive enzymes become more complex, and normal bacterial flora accumulates as the baby ingests a larger variety of food. It is important that health professionals assist the mother and family to cope with colic. It is also important that mothers do not resort to medications, but instead try to soothe the baby by cuddling, keeping the baby in motion, or rubbing the stomach in a rhythmic motion. It may be especially helpful for the mother to have an occasional evening out, and leave her partner or a competent caregiver in charge of the baby.[120]

**CRITICAL THINKING**

*What other health promoting activities can you suggest for a mother who is having a difficult time coping with her baby who is experiencing colic?*

Throughout infancy, the liver is the most immature of all the gastrointestinal organs. The ability to conjugate bilirubin and secrete bile is achieved after the first couple of weeks of life. However, the capacities for gluconeogenesis, formation of plasma protein and ketones, storage of vitamins, and deaminization of amino acids is somewhat immature for the first year of life.[121]

**Muscular Tissue** At birth, muscular tissue is almost completely formed. Growth results from the increasing size of the already existing fibres under the influence of growth hormone, thyroxin, and insulin. As muscle size increases in childhood, strength increases as well. In fact, changes in muscle composition lead to increases in strength that enable one-year-olds to walk, run, jump, and climb, all with notable exuberance.[122] Muscle fibres need continual stimulation to develop to full function and strength.

**Skin** Thermoregulation in infancy becomes more efficient. The skin acquires the ability to contract and muscles increase the ability to shiver in response to cold. The peripheral capillaries respond to changes in ambient temperature to regulate heat loss. The capillaries constrict in response to cold, thereby conserving core body temperature, and they dilate in response to heat, decreasing internal body temperature. Shivering causes the muscles and muscle fibres to contract, generating metabolic heat that is then distributed throughout the body.[123]

**Urinary System** The immaturity of the renal structures predisposes the infant to dehydration. Complete maturity of the kidney occurs during the latter half of the second year. Urine is voided frequently and has a low specific gravity.[124]

**Immune System** Components of the immune system undergo numerous changes during the first year.[125] The ability to produce antibodies is limited. Much of the antibody protection is acquired from the mother during fetal life. The development of immunologic function depends on the infant's gradual exposure to foreign bodies and infectious agents.

**Red Blood Cell and Haemoglobin Levels** The anemias are the most common hematologic disorders of infancy and childhood. Actually, they are not a disease but a manifestation of an underlying pathologic process. Iron deficiency anemia becomes apparent around six months of age if the physiologic system does not function adequately to sustain red blood cell and hemoglobin levels. Total blood hemoglobin primarily depends on the number of circulating red blood cells, and also on the amount of hemoglobin in each cell.[126]

Increasingly, studies show that the health of the adult is influenced considerably by the person's health status in early life. Obesity, discussed in Chapters 10, 11, and 12, is an example.

## Nutritional Needs

The feeding time is a crucial time for baby and mother: a time to strengthen attachment, for baby to feel love and security, for mother and baby to learn about self and each other, and for baby to learn about the environment. Meeting the nutritional needs of infants is well recognized as critical for the infant's healthy growth and development. For the best possible start in life, the Public Health Agency of Canada (PHAC) supports and promotes breastfeeding as the best way to provide optimal nutritional, immunological, and emotional nurturing of infants. The PHAC makes certain

that health professionals, such as nurses, have the information they need to assist parents and significant caregivers in meeting the growing nutritional needs of children from birth to two years of age.[127] See Table 7-5 for a stage-by-stage guide to infant feeding.

**Breastfeeding** Health Canada promotes breastfeeding as the optimal method of feeding infants because it provides optimal nutritional, immunological, and emotional benefits for the growth and development of infants.[128] The guideline promoted by Health Canada is that exclusive breastfeeding is recommended for the first six months of life for healthy term infants. Furthermore, infants should be introduced at six months to nutrient-rich solid foods with particular attention to iron. The mother should continue to breastfeed for up to two years and beyond. Health Canada encourages all health professionals at the national, provincial, and community levels to promote and implement this recommendation.[129]

Several research studies have been conducted to examine the initiation and discontinuation of breastfeeding. For example, Sheehan and her researchers found that discontinuation before four weeks post-discharge was associated with maternal

### Table 7-5 A Stage-by-Stage Guide to Infant Feeding

| Stage/Age | What to Do | Drinks | Meals and Feedings | | | | |
|---|---|---|---|---|---|---|---|
| | | | EARLY AM | BREAK-FAST | LUNCH | DINNER | BED-TIME |
| Weeks 1 and 2 Age 6 months (ages are guidelines only) | Give small tastes of baby cereal or fruit or vegetable puree at lunchtime, halfway through the breast- or bottle-feeding. Give the same food for three days to accustom your baby to it. | If you are bottle-feeding, offer your baby occasional drinks of cooled boiled water. | ☐ | ☐ | ☐■☐ | ☐ | ☐ |
| Weeks 3 and 4 Age 6½ months | Introduce solid food at breakfast, halfway through the feeding; baby cereal or other single-grain cereal is ideal. Increase the amount of solid food at lunchtime to 3-4 teaspoonfuls. | Offer cooled boiled water or diluted fruit juice in a bottle. Don't worry if your baby doesn't want any | ☐ | ☐■☐ | ☐■☐ | ☐ | ☐ |
| Weeks 5 and 6 Age 7 months | Introduce solid food at dinner, halfway through the feeding. A week later, offer two courses at lunch; follow a vegetable puree with a fruit one, giving 2-3 teaspoonfuls of each. | Introduce a trainer cup, but don't expect your baby to be able to drink from it yet—it's just a toy. | · | ☐■☐ | ☐■■☐ | ☐■☐ | ☐ |

*(continued)*

Table 7-5 (continued)

| Stage/Age | What to Do | Drinks | Meals and Feedings | | | | |
|---|---|---|---|---|---|---|---|
| | | | EARLY AM | BREAK-FAST | LUNCH | DINNER | BED-TIME |
| Weeks 7 and 8<br>Age<br>7½ months | Offer solid food as the first part of lunch then give breast or bottle to top up. She can have two courses at dinner now, a vegetable and a piece of banana, for example. At breakfast and dinner, continue giving the feeding first. She may eat 5-6 teaspoonfuls of solid food at each meal now. | You can start to give your baby drinks in her cup, but hold it for her as she drinks from it. | · | □■□ | ■■□ | □■■□ | □ |
| Weeks 9 and 10<br>Age<br>8 months | After lunch solids, offer a drink of formula or breast milk from a cup. After a few days with no lunchtime breast or bottle, offer solid food as the first part of dinner. | Offer formula or breast milk in a cup at each meal and water or diluted juice at other times. | · | □■□ | ■■ | ■■□ | □ |
| Weeks 11 and 12<br>Age<br>8½ months | Offer your baby a drink of breast or formula milk in a cup instead of a full feeding after her dinner. You may find she often refuses her breast or bottle feeding after her breakfast solids now. | As before | · | □■ | ■■ | ■■ | □ |
| Week 13 onwards<br>Age<br>9 months | Offer a drink in a cup instead of the feeding before breakfast; now your baby is having solids at three meals a day. Breast or formula milk should be the main milk drink until one year. She can have cow's milk from 12 months. | As before. Your baby may possibly be able to manage her own trainer cup now. | · | ■ | ■■ | ■■ | □ |

Key    □ feeding    ■ solid food

Source: Canadian Medical Association, *Complete Book of Mother and Baby Care: Parents Practical Handbook from Conception to 3 Years*, 3rd ed. Toronto, Tourmaline Eds. Inc., 2001, p. 113. Copyright Dorling Kindersley Limited.

preferences toward breastfeeding, formula feeding, or supplementation in hospital; infant readmission; and the use of walk-in clinics for infant care. The results suggest that continuing education about the benefits of breastfeeding should encourage women to value it for longer periods.[130] In another study, Clifford and her researchers found that a number of factors affected the successful continuation of full breastfeeding. One such factor was employment status. That is, a women's return to outside employment was linked to the cessation of breastfeeding. These researchers recommend that workplaces be made mother- and baby-friendly.[131] Dennis claims that other predictors that can affect full breastfeeding initiation or discontinuation include maternal age, marital status, educational level, and socioeconomic status.[132] It is important that health professionals carefully assess high-risk women so that any factors, conditions, and variables that

**Figure 7-2**

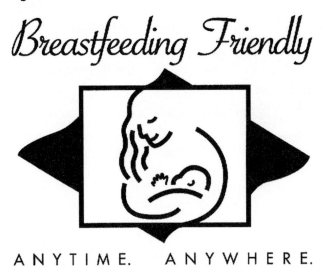

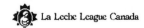

The Breastfeeding Friendly logo, developed with La Leche League Canada, is posted in areas to indicate that breastfeeding is welcome and encouraged on the premises.

Source: Health Canada/La Leche League Canada, Copright © Reproduced with the permission of the Minister of Public Works and Services, 2007

might be detrimental to breastfeeding can be made amenable to intervention.[133]

The Registered Nurses Association of Ontario (RNAO) developed the Nursing Best Practice Guidelines to be used as a resource tool. The RNAO believes that the document will provide timely guidance to nurses to improve breastfeeding outcomes for mothers and infants. The document includes the concepts of promotion, protection, and support of breastfeeding.[134]

*Breastfeeding is not recommended* in Canada for babies whose mothers are HIV-positive, or who have AIDS or active tuberculosis. Breastfeeding is not advised if the mother is receiving long-term chemotherapy or is using street drugs (heroin, cocaine, marijuana, or methadone). In Canada, infants who have galactosemia should not be breastfed. Alcohol and nicotine *pass into the milk and to the infant.* Currently, a limited number of drugs are contraindicated with breastfeeding. One key resource is the Motherisk Program at the Hospital for Sick Children in Toronto (www.motherisk.org). The mother should be informed of these hazards to her baby if she breastfeeds. Hopefully, she will then avoid harmful substances.[135] The occasional use of coffee has been approved by the American Academy of Pediatrics.[136] Women who choose to breastfeed should be provided with the appropriate resource contacts, in the event that any such issues or concerns should arise. One of the main health promoting

strategies for the mother is encouraging healthy lifestyle choices. Strategies include following a healthy eating pattern in accordance with *Eating Well with Canada's Food Guide.* A particularly interesting guide entitled *Eating Well with Canada's Food Guide: First Nations, Inuit and Métis* is available from Health Canada's website (http://hc-sc.gc.ca/fn-an/pubs/fnim-pnim/index_e.html).[137]

*Human milk is considered ideal* because it is sterile, digestible, available, and economical; it also contains the necessary nutrients, except for vitamins C and D and iron. Further, even in undernourished women, the composition of breast milk is adequate, although vitamin content depends heavily on the mother's diet. Breast milk is sufficient for all that baby needs during the first four months of life. It contains higher levels of lactose, vitamin E, and cholesterol, and less protein than cow's milk. The additional cholesterol may induce the production of hormones required for cholesterol breakdown in adulthood. Breast milk has a more efficient nutritional balance of iron, zinc, vitamin E, and unsaturated fatty acids.[138]

Because of the host-resistant factors in human milk, breast milk offers many advantages to the infant. Breastfed babies are ill less often because breast milk contains the mother's antibodies. Breastfed babies are less prone to diarrhea and constipation.[139] Breastfed babies are also less prone to allergies. Human milk is the ideal food for preterm babies. Human milk contains minerals (zinc and copper), vitamins (folic acid and vitamins B2, B6, C, D, E, and K), and the electrolytes (calcium, magnesium, phosphorus, and sodium) necessary to support growth and metabolism in the preterm infant.[140] Breastfeeding also promotes maternal–infant attachment, and it may even provide some protection against sudden infant death syndrome (SIDS).[141]

Health professionals can influence the mother in a positive manner regarding her attitude toward breastfeeding. The need for health professionals to promote and support breastfeeding as the healthiest choice for both infant and mother is well recognized.[142] Teach the mother the benefits to the baby of breastfeeding, how to express milk to be used by other caregivers, and suggestions given by community resources such as La Leche League Canada. Breastfeeding information should reflect Canada's multicultural population and be part of health promotion practices.

Several investigators describe: (1) the specific procedure for pumping the breasts; (2) how the mother can maintain a milk supply; (3) ways to enhance the experience for the mother, baby, and intensive care nursery staff; and (4) continuation of breastfeeding after discharge.[143]

*Preparation for breastfeeding begins during pregnancy.* An adequate diet during pregnancy is the initial step toward successful lactation and breastfeeding. The woman may consult La Leche League literature for help. The Canada Prenatal Nutrition Program (CPNP) provides long-term funding to community groups to develop or enhance programs for vulnerable pregnant women. Through a community development approach, the CPNP aims to reduce the incidence of unhealthy birth weights, improve the health of both the mother and the infant, and encourage breastfeeding. As a comprehensive program, the services provided include food supplementation, nutritional counselling, emotional support, education, referral, and counselling on health and lifestyle issues.[144]

*The baby should be put to breast immediately after delivery* and fed within eight hours of birth to reduce hypoglycemia and hyperbilirubinemia. In fact, it would be beneficial to breastfeed during the first half-hour after birth because the baby is most alert at that time.[145] The first nourishment the baby receives after delivery from breastfeeding is **colostrum**, a *thin yellow secretion* that lasts for two to four days after delivery. Colostrum has higher levels of antibodies than the later milk. Colostrum is rich in carbohydrates, which the newborn needs, and it serves as a laxative in cleaning out the gastrointestinal tract. Colostrum, fed immediately after birth, prevents against infection because it triggers antibody production. Depending on how soon and how often the mother nurses, true milk comes in the first few days.[146]

If a mother nurses after delivery, the pituitary gland secretes prolactin. The high levels of estrogen from the placenta that inhibited milk secretion during pregnancy are gone. As the baby sucks, the nipple is in the back of the mouth, and the jaws and tongue compress the milk sinuses. These tactile sensations trigger the release of the hormone oxytocin from the pituitary gland, which in turn causes the "let-down" response. The sinuses refill immediately, and milk flows with very little effort to the baby. This is the crucial time to learn breastfeeding. Oxytocin also causes a powerful contraction of the uterus, lessening the danger of hemorrhage.[147]

Every effort should be directed toward making breastfeeding a comfortable, uninterrupted time. Effective techniques to help mother get into a comfortable position, hold the baby, and put the baby to nipple are described in the following services: La Leche League literature from a lactation consultant, maternal child nursing and other child care books, and some booklets prepared by formula companies. Some babies take time to orient to the breast; others will latch and suckle well. Mother needs an encouraging partner or family member, knowledgeable and supportive nursing and medical personnel, or other successful nursing mothers to be with her for feeding when the baby is hungry and her breasts are full. The mother whose milk does not let-down may need oxytocin, a period of relaxation, or perhaps a soothing liquid before feeding. She should, in any case, be encouraged to increase her fluid intake and meet the increased recommended dietary allowances for lactating women.[148]

The baby may nurse every hour or two at first or on demand, perhaps 15 to 30 minutes each time. Following that, the baby will graduate to three- to four-hour intervals by four months, obtaining more milk in shorter feeding sessions. If anxieties, excessive stimuli, and fatigue are dealt with appropriately, the mother's milk supply will increase, or decrease, to meet the demand. Alternating breasts with each feeding and emptying the breasts will prevent caking. The infant should grasp the areola completely to avoid excess pressure on the nipples. Generally, breastfeeding babies get enough to eat. The child whose growth and weight are within the norm is being breastfed adequately. The large or active infant may need supplemental feeding in addition to breast milk, even when mother's supply is not compromised. Usually, however, extra formula or baby food is not necessary before the fourth to fifth month. Food, in addition to breast milk (or formula), should be introduced at six months.[149] Recent research suggests that the introduction of food before the age of four months may increase the risk of child obesity, cardiovascular disease, food allergies, and insulin-dependent diabetes in children who may be susceptible.[150]

**Infant Formulas** It is important for all health care facilities to be "breastfeeding-friendly." Health care facilities should not be centres for marketing infant formulas because they then come into conflict with the baby-friendly initiative.[151]

In Canada, the composition, processing, packaging, and labelling of all infant formulas are regulated under the Canadian Food and Drug Regulations (Department of National Health and Welfare).[152] Commercial infant formula that is fortified with iron is now the standard recommendation for all infants who are fed formula from birth.[153] The nutrient content of iron-fortified infant formula is designed to meet the nutritional needs of healthy term infants until 9 to 12 months of age.[154] If an infant is not exclusively, or is partially, breastfed, then commercial formulas are the most acceptable alternative to breast milk. For information regarding infant formulas, see the Health Canada website (www.hc-sc.gc.ca/).

Homemade formula containing canned evaporated milk, whether cow's or goat's milk, is not recommended as an alternative to breast milk or commercial infant formula because it is nutritionally incomplete.[155]

Various brands and styles of bottles and nipples are available. Most babies feed well with any nipple or bottle. It is critical that bottles and nipples be washed in warm soapy water using a bottle and nipple brush to facilitate thorough cleaning.[156]

**Cow's Milk** The Canadian Paediatric Society states that babies under 9 to 12 months of age should not be given cow's milk.[157] The quality and quantity of nutrients in cow's milk differs greatly from those of human milk. Furthermore, cow's milk does not contain many of the various growth and immunological factors found in human milk. Whole cow's milk is the main milk drink from 10 to 12 months. Low fat (2 percent milk fat) or skim milk should not be fed to infants because the lack of fat can be difficult for the kidneys to handle.

Before parents make the switch from breast milk, or formula, to cow's milk, they should check with their baby's doctor. If a mother in Canada is unable to provide her own breast milk for her baby, she should contact a breastfeeding support clinic (contact the local hospital or health clinic for referral). If the mother feels unable to breastfeed, one option, particularly for an ill or high-risk infant, is to receive pasteurized human milk from Canada's human milk bank in Vancouver. The mother is required to pay a processing fee and the cost of transportation for the milk. For information about milk banking call 604-875-2282 for donor information or 604-875-2424, extension 7634, for recipient information.[158]

**Water** Normally, healthy term breastfeeding babies should receive only breast milk, without other foods and fluids, unless a medical situation exists. Supplementation interferes with milk production.[159] In fact, supplemental foods intended to minimize dehydration are not routinely required. Failure of the baby to void (at least three times daily during the first two days, and six times per day subsequently) may indicate dehydration. Dehydration may be confirmed by the identification of weight loss and examination of the anterior fontanel, skin turgor, and skin perfusion.[160] Infants become dehydrated more quickly than adults because they have a smaller total fluid volume in the body compared with body size.[161] Health teaching should be implemented to the parents regarding the *signs of dehydration*.

Fluoridated drinking water does not harm the fetus, and it is beneficial to the mother's teeth during pregnancy, when hormonal changes may lead to possible dental problems. Breast milk is relatively low in fluoride, but this fluoride still benefits the infant's teeth. In Canada, some individuals may assume that bottled water is safer than municipal tap water, but no evidence exists to support this. Prepackaged water (bottled water) is considered to be food and is regulated under the Food and Drug Regulation.[162]

**Nutrient Requirements** Infants are encouraged to obtain nutrition in a pattern that encourages friendly and supportive social interaction with parents and caregivers. The average daily requirement is 115 kcal/kg during the first year of life, although there is some variation from one child to another. The average caloric content of breast milk and formulas is 20 kcal/oz or 67 kcal/100m. Adequacy of intake is best determined by observing weight gain. Expected gain is as follows:

- 30 g/day in the first three months
- 15 to 20 g/day in the second three months

Six well-soaked diapers and yellowish stool daily are also indicators of adequate nutritional intake.

**Feeding Comfort** Mothers frequently need instruction about times and methods of **burping** (*bubbling, or gently patting baby's back*) the baby to reduce gaseous content of the stomach during feeding, because the cardiac sphincter is not well developed. Young babies must be bubbled after every ounce and at the end of a feeding. Later, they can be bubbled halfway through and again at the end. The infant should be moved from a semi-reclining to an upright position while the feeder gently pats the back. Because a new infant's gastrointestinal tract is unstable, milk may be eructated with gas bubbles. Adequate bubbling should occur before the infant is placed into the crib to prevent milk regurgitation and aspiration. The infant should be positioned on his or her back or on the side.

**Solid Foods** There is no rigid sequence in adding solid foods to the infant's diet. Whatever solid food is offered first, or at what time, is largely a matter of individual preference of the mother or of the pediatrician. Iron-fortified infant cereal is generally introduced first because of its high iron content. New foods should be added one at a time. Fruit juice can be offered from a cup, for its rich source of vitamin C, as a substitute for milk for one feeding a day. Giving baby large quantities of certain juices—for example, apple, pear, prune, cherry, peach, and grape—is to be avoided because these juices may cause abdominal pain, bloating, or diarrhea.[163] Ideally, the infant's needs and developmental achievements, such as eye–hand–mouth coordination and fine pincer grasp, should be considered when introducing solids. The mother or nurse introducing the baby to solid foods should make it a pleasant experience. The foods offered should be smooth and well-diluted with milk or formula. The infant should not be hurried, coaxed, or allowed to linger more than 30 minutes. *Honey should not be added to feedings* during the first year because of the possibility of infant botulism.

Teach parents that when the baby is first fed pureed foods with a spoon, he or she expects and wants to suck. The protrusion of the tongue, which is needed in sucking, makes it appear as if baby is pushing food out of the mouth. Parents misinterpret this as a dislike for the food, but it really is the result of immature muscle coordination and possibly surprise at the taste and feel of the new items in the diet.

Teach parents to avoid overfeeding—either milk or foods. Theories hold that babies who are fed more calories than they use daily develop additional fat cells to store unused energy sources.[164]

In addition to discussing the food quantities, quality, and nutrients needed by the baby, teach parents that food and mealtime are learning opportunities. The baby gains motor control and coordination in self-feeding and he or she learns to recognize colour, shape, and texture. The use of mouth muscles stimulates the ability to make some of the movements necessary for speech development. He or she continues to develop trust with the consistent, loving atmosphere of mealtime. Food should not be used as reward or punishment (by withholding food). The child should learn moderation in feeding quantity, and between-feeding snacks should be avoided or, if used, should be healthful, small in quantity, and given because the child is hungry despite eating well at mealtime.[165]

**Weaning** The *gradual elimination of breastfeeding, or bottle-feeding, in favour of cup and table feeding* (**weaning**) is usually completed by the end of the first year. The ideal time to wean is when mother and baby are both ready. Baby shows signs of making this transition: muscle coordination increases, teeth erupt, and he or she resists being held close while feeding. The two methods should overlap and allow baby to take some initiative and allow mother to guide the new method. Mother's consistency in meeting the new feeding schedule is important to the development of a sense of trust.

The most difficult feeding to give up is usually the bedtime feeding because baby is tired and is more likely to want the "old method." After the maxillary central incisory teeth erupt, a night bottle should contain no carbohydrates, to reduce decay in the deciduous teeth. During periods of stress the baby will often regress. Baby is also learning to wait longer for food and may object vigorously to this new condition of receiving food only three or four times daily.

The need to suck varies with different children. Some children, even after weaning, will suck a thumb or use a pacifier (if provided). The baby should not be shamed for either of these habits because they are not likely to cause problems with the teeth or mouth during the first two years.

---

### CRITICAL THINKING

*How would you explain the process of weaning to a first time mother with a limited understanding of English?*

---

**Cultural Influences on Infant Nutrition** In Canada, university-educated Caucasian women are more likely to breastfeed than are other groups.[166] Members of subcultures vary in the extent to which they engage in breastfeeding. Cultural values influence: (1) women's perceptions about breastfeeding in terms of nutritional importance; (2) the father's beliefs and preferences; (3) acceptance of breast exposure; (4) sexuality issues; and (5) considerations related to convenience. For immigrant groups, bottle-feeding may be viewed as more modern and prestigious. In Canada, breastfeeding rates are positively related to maternal education.[167] Breastfeeding trends vary across Canada. For example, the First Nations and Inuit Regional Health Survey (FNIRHS) reports that the mothers in its survey were less likely to initiate breastfeeding than were the mothers in the National Longitudinal Survey on Children and Youth (NLSCY).[168] This suggests that we need to encourage Aboriginal women to increase the initiation rate of breastfeeding.

## Sleep Patterns

One of the most frequent concerns of a new mother is when, where, and how much baby sleeps. Awake or alert periods are altered by different types of feeding schedules. Sleep patterns are unique to each infant, but some generalizations can be made.

The infant exhibits at least six states, or levels, of arousal:[169]

- Regular or quiet sleep: Eyes are closed, breathing is regular, and the only movements are sudden, generalized startle motions. Baby makes little sound. This is the low point of arousal; infant cannot be awakened with mild stimuli.

- Irregular, active rapid eye movement (REM) sleep: Baby's eyes are closed, breathing is irregular, muscles twitch slightly from time to time, and there are facial responses of smiles or pouts in response to sounds or lights. Baby may groan, make faces, or cry briefly.

- Quiet wakefulness: Eyes are open, the body is more active, breathing is irregular, and varying spontaneous responses to external stimuli occur.

- Active wakefulness: Eyes are open; there is visual following of interesting sights and sounds, body movements, and vocalizations that elicit attention.

- Crying.

- Indeterminate state: Transition from one state of alertness to another.

Sleep patterns vary among children. By 3 to 4 months of age, most infants have developed a nocturnal pattern of

## Impressions of Breastfeeding Information and Support among First-Time Mothers within a Multi-Ethnic Community

A telephone survey was conducted to a sample of 108 immigrant and Canadian-born mothers (average age 29.4 years) in an ethnically diverse local community service centre in Quebec. All participants were primiparous, breastfeeding mothers at three weeks postpartum. The purpose of the study was to examine the mothers' perceptions of breastfeeding information and support they had received from health professionals within a multi-ethnic community.

Overall, mothers' evaluations of professional breastfeeding support were found to be positive, despite their reports of what breastfeeding experts would consider less than optimal standards of hospital and community-care practice concerning breastfeeding.

Additional findings from the survey revealed the following:

1. Immigrant and Canadian-born mothers differ in their perceptions of breastfeeding support:
   a. Immigrant mothers were more likely to experience practices detrimental to breastfeeding success (e.g., in-hospital formula supplementation).
   b. Immigrant mothers' evaluations of in-hospital breastfeeding support were more positive than those of Canadian-born mothers.
   c. Immigrant mothers were more likely than Canadian-born mothers to receive breastfeeding support from community health services.

   d. Immigrant mothers were less positive than Canadian-born mothers about the follow-up care that was provided.

2. Overall, the breastfeeding information that was provided tended to focus more on the successful initiation of breastfeeding rather than on strategies to incorporate breastfeeding into the lifestyle of the mother.

3. Despite evidence in the literature claiming that "perceived inadequate milk supply" is the most common reason for early termination of breastfeeding, mothers were provided with minimal information on ensuring adequate milk production.

4. As good sources of information, both books and nurses (hospital and community-based), were identified by both types of mother as valuable; nurses in particular were identified as significant by the immigrant mothers.

5. Canadian-born mothers were more likely to use fee-for-service lactation consultants.

### Practice Implication

Nurses must continue to provide support to mothers along with complete information on breastfeeding.

Source: Loiselle, C., S. Semenic, B. Cote, M. Lapointe, and R. Gendron. Impressions of Breastfeeding Information and Support among First-Time Mothers within a Multiethnic Community, *Canadian Journal of Nursing Research, 33(3)* (2001), 31–46. Used with permission.

sleep that lasts 9 to 11 hours. The total daily sleep time is approximately 15 hours. The number of naps per day varies, but infants may take one or two naps by the end of the first year.[170]

Help parents understand that when a baby goes through the stage of separation anxiety at about eight months of age, bedtime becomes more difficult because he or she does not want to leave mother or other people. Because the baby needs sleep, the parent should be firm about getting the child ready for bed. Prolonging bedtime adds to fatigue.

The infant should at least have a consistent place for sleeping (be it box, drawer, or crib), and a clean area for supplies. A baby can sleep comfortably in an infant crib or bassinet during the first few weeks, but as soon as active arms and legs begin to hit the sides, he or she should be moved to a full-sized crib. Note that cribs manufactured only after September 1986 are considered safe. Cribs made before this date do not meet current standards, and they put children at risk.[171] No pillows should be used. The crib should have a crib border placed at the bottom of the slats to prevent catching the head between the bars. It should be fitted with a firm, waterproof, easy-to-clean mattress and with warm light covers loosely tucked in. The sides of the crib should fit closely to the mattress so that the infant will not get caught and crushed if he or she should roll to the edge. Thin plastic sheeting can cause suffocation and should never be used on or around the baby's crib. Teach these safety measures to the parents.

Caressing or singing softly while holding baby in a sleeping position in bed is calming. If the mother is available when the baby first awakes, he or she anticipates this pleasure, and sleep is associated with mother's return. If the baby awakes and cries during the night, the parent should wait briefly. Many times the crying will subside with the baby's growing ability to control personal anxiety feelings. Persistent crying indicates unmet needs and should be attended.

**Co-sleep,** *when baby sleeps in the bed with the parent(s),* is never recommended. However, this practice is considered normal in some cultures. Co-sleep can help the baby regulate respiration, heart rate, and body temperature in cold climates, and it is convenient for breastfeeding. Because of the baby's movements, it may be difficult for the parents to sleep, and baby between the parents decreases their intimacy. Further, it can be difficult to get the child to break this habit. The Canadian Child Care Federation claims that bed sharing is a common practice for many families. Further, no evidence exists that a baby who shares the bed with a parent or sibling has a reduced risk of sudden infant death syndrome (SIDS). The risk of SIDS increases if the individual who shares the bed is a smoker, or has taken alcohol or other drugs that may alter responsiveness.[172]

Rates of SIDS are lower because parents are following recommendations for positioning the infant during sleep. However, in Canada, three children per week die from SIDS.[173] Health Canada recommends placing the child on the back, and on a firm (not soft and fluffy) mattress. SIDS probably has other causes; the occurrence is higher in infants whose mothers smoke tobacco or use cocaine. Other health promoting strategies include keeping the baby warm, not hot, and promoting breastfeeding strategies.

## Play Activity

The infant engages in self-play: with the hands or feet, by rolling, by getting into various positions, and with the sounds he or she produces. Baby needs playful activity from both mother and father to stimulate development in all spheres. Share the following information with parents. You may need to teach the parents how to touch, cuddle, talk to, and play with the baby.

Certain toys are usually enjoyed at certain ages because of changing needs and developing skills. The box entitled "Guide to Play Activities" lists age, characteristics that influence play interest and activities, and suggested activities, toys, and equipment.[174]

The baby can remain satisfied playing with himself or herself for increasing amounts of time, but prefers to have people around. Baby enjoys being held briefly in various positions, being rocked, swinging for short periods, and being taken for walks.

Because much of baby's play involves putting objects into the mouth, a clean environment with lead-free paint is important. A small object that baby swallows, such as a coin, is passed through the digestive tract. However, small batteries used in cameras, calculators, and other electronic equipment may be hazardous if swallowed because they can rupture and release poisonous chemicals. Surgical removal may be necessary. Children gradually build immunity to the germs encountered daily on various objects. However,

health may be threatened by that which goes unnoticed. Sitting and playing in dirt or sand that has been contaminated by dioxin, other pesticides or herbicides, or radiation is dangerous to the developing physiologic systems. Children's or parents' reading material, which can become play objects, may also be hazardous.

Toys need not be expensive, but they should be colourful (and without leaded paint), safe, sturdy, and easily handled and cleaned. They should be large enough to prevent aspiration or ingestion. They should be without rough or sharp edges or points, detachable parts, or loops to get around the neck, and some should make sounds and have moving parts. In Canada, the Canadian Toy Testing Council is responsible for conducting research to ensure the appropriateness and value of toys.[175]

Baby needs an unrestricted play area, such as the floor, that is clean and safe, although use of a playpen may be necessary for short periods. Excess restriction, or lack of stimulation, inhibits curiosity, learning about self and the environment, and the development of trust. Therefore, baby should not wear clothing that is restraining, and he or she should not be kept constantly in a playpen or crib.

Stationary play stations—an exersaucer play gym that turns, rocks, and bounces—should be used no more than 20 minutes a day. If overused, the baby is likely to have poor posture and weak back and stomach muscles. A delay in beginning to walk could also occur. Children learn through activity. They need supervised "tummy time" and "scoot time" and a clean, safe floor to develop back, neck, abdominal, and buttock muscles. Baby needs play objects and a loving parent who provides stimulating surroundings.

Parents should know the dangers of overstimulation and rough handling. Fatigue, inattention, and injury may result. The playful, vigorous activities that well-intentioned parents engage in, such as tossing the baby forcefully into the air or jerking the baby in a whiplash manner, may cause bone injuries or subdural hematomas and cerebrovascular lesions that later could cause mental retardation. Premature infants and male babies are twice as vulnerable as full-term girls because of the relative immaturity of their brains.

For Aboriginal people, toys and playthings are important tools through which the child can become better acquainted with the world around him or her. Any parent buying a toy should look for those that will enhance positive social-emotional development, help to build pride in identity, provide fun and enrich the child's growth, and help to encourage creative and dramatic play. Hammersmith and Sawatsky state that ways to socialize the child toward his or her identity may include the use of cultural events, puppets, music, dance, and body movement.[176]

| Age | Characteristics Development | Suggested Activities and Equipment |
| --- | --- | --- |
| 4 weeks | Tonic neck reflex position<br>Rolls partway to side<br>Disregards ring in midplane<br>Eyes follow ring in midplane<br>Hand clutches on contact<br>Drops rattle immediately<br>Attends bell<br>Activity diminishes<br>Marked head lag when pulled to sitting position<br>Head sags forward; back evenly rounded<br>Head rotation; in prone position<br>Startles easily to sudden sounds or movements | Much tender loving care<br>Mobiles and other hanging objects that can be followed by eyes but that cannot be grasped—bright in colour musical mobiles |
| 16 weeks | Head position in midplane<br>Plays with hands at midplane<br>Regards ring immediately, arms activate<br>Holds rattle in fist<br>Head fairly steady in sitting position<br>On verge of rolling<br>Rattles, bells, musical toys<br>Laughs aloud; coos; carries on "conversation"<br>Large wooden or non-splintering plastic toys, beads, spools<br>Spontaneous social smile<br>Knows mother; stares at strangers<br>Smiles at strangers who are friendly | Enjoys cuddling and motion<br>Cradle gym for brief periods (20 to 30 minutes)<br>Rattles<br>Soft, stuffed, small toys to touch and squeeze<br>Soothing music (humming, singing, CDs)<br>Crinkling paper, clap, or snap of fingers |
| 28 weeks | Transfers small toys (blocks, bells, etc.) from one hand to the other<br>Soothing music<br>Mouths objects<br>Lifts head in supine position<br>Peek-a-boo<br>Reaches with one hand<br>Sits momentarily by self leaning on hands<br>Feet to mouth<br><br>Regards image in mirror<br>Polysyllabic vowel sounds<br>Bounces actively<br>Prompt grasp<br>Pivots in prone position<br>Plays contentedly alone | Small toys<br>Cradle gym (30 to 40 minutes)<br>Pat-a-cake<br>Noise makers (bells, squeak toys)<br>Use of mirror to see self and others<br>Moderately active bouncing on lap<br>Outdoor excursions—walks<br>Splashing in water, water toys<br>Reading to child, letting child touch and pat books<br>Small (2.5 cm) square blocks |
| 40 weeks | Knocks blocks together in hands<br>Approaches objects with index finger<br>Pretends pellet, inferior pincer grasp<br>Grasps bell by handle and waves it<br>Sits with good control<br>Goes from sitting to prone position<br>Creeps<br>Pulls to standing position<br>Waves bye-bye | Soft, small toys<br>Peek-a-boo<br>Assorted objects of varying colour having interesting texture<br>Pat-a-cake<br>Rides in buggy or stroller<br>Parallel play<br>Nesting, stock, or climbing boxes and blocks<br>Kitchen utensils |

>

| Age | Characteristics Development | Suggested Activities and Equipment |
|---|---|---|
| | Increasing imitation | Bath toys |
| | Adjusts to simple commands | Cups and boxes to pour (water, sand) and fill |
| | Is fascinated with words and other sounds | |
| 12 months | Walks with help | Open and close simple boxes |
| | Throws and rolls ball | Empty and fill toys |
| | Offers objects, but frequently does not release them | Push-pull toys |
| | | Small, brightly coloured blocks |
| | Strongly strung large beads | Rag and oil cloth books |
| | Vocabulary of 3 to 10 words | |
| | Vigorous imitative scribble | |
| | Balls, bells, floating bath toys | |
| | Cuddle toys | |
| | Nursery rhymes | |
| | Music and singing to child | |

## Health Promotion and Health Prevention

In addition to measures already discussed, including the safety measures in the previous section on play activity, the following measures also promote health.

At birth, the neonate should have an antibiotic ointment instilled in the eyes to prevent gonococcal or chlamydia ophthalmia neonatorum. The possibility of blindness in the infant, along with the low cost and effectiveness of the treatment, makes this procedure mandatory.[177]

Injecting 0.05 to 1 mg of vitamin K is effective in preventing hemorrhagic disease, which is caused in 1 of 2000 to 1 of 3000 live births by a transient deficiency of factor VIII production. Sickle cell screening can be obtained from in-cord blood.[178]

**Immunizations** Immunizations, *promoting disease resistance through injection of attenuated, weakened organisms or products produced by organisms,* are essential to every infant as a preventive measure. The Conference of Deputy Ministers of Health in Canada endorsed the National Immunization Strategy, and the Government of Canada committed $45 million over five years to implement it. The federal government provided $300 million directly to the provinces and territories to support the introduction of new and recommended childhood and adolescent vaccines:

- Conjugate pneumococcal vaccine
- Conjugate meningococcal vaccine
- Varicella (chicken pox vaccine)
- Acellular pertussis vaccine (a new whooping cough vaccine for adolescents)[179]

A harmonized national immunization schedule would have great merit because it would reduce the risk of missed doses, increase cost savings through larger purchases, and provide more uniform teaching of vaccine schedules for physicians, nurses, and families. It is important that health professionals encourage parents to check with their local health departments concerning provincial and territorial variations.[180] For updates and supplements to the Canadian Immunization Guide, or for more information about the National Advisory Committee on Immunization (NACI), visit the website at www.naci.gc.ca.[181]

Before birth, baby is protected from certain organisms by the placental barrier, and by mother's physical defence mechanisms. Birth propels baby into an environment filled with many microorganisms. Baby has protection against common pathogens for a time, but as he or she is gradually exposed to the outside world and the people in it, further protection is needed through routine immunizations. Immunizations have been considered the most effective health promotion intervention, and they have had a positive impact on health in Canada. See Chapter 10 regarding parental concerns about immunization and ways of approaching these concerns. The NACI initiated a process to develop guidelines for childhood immunization practices. The original guidelines were officially endorsed by many professional bodies, and were modified slightly in the seventh edition of the Canadian Immunization Guide.[182] Table 7-6 outlines the routine immunization schedule for infants and older children.

Table 7-6 Routine Immunization Schedule for Infants and Children

| Age at vaccination | DTaP-IPV | Hib | MMR | Var | HB | Pneu-C-7 | Men-C | Tdap | Inf |
|---|---|---|---|---|---|---|---|---|---|
| Birth | | | | | Infancy 3 doses | | | | |
| 2 months | ○ | ✦ | | | | ⊠ | ◎ | | |
| 4 months | ○ | ✦ | | | | ⊠ | (◎) | | |
| 6 months | ○ | ✦ | | | | ⊠ | ◎ or | | 6-23 months |
| 12 months | | | ■ | ● | | ⊠ 12-15 months | ◎ if not yet given | | |
| | | | | | or | | | | 1-2 doses |
| 18 months | ○ | ✦ | ■ | | | | | | |
| 4-6 years | ○ | | or ■ | | | | | | |
| 14-16 years | | | | | Pre-teen/teen 2-3 doses | | ◎ if not yet given | ▲ | |

Notes

( )  Symbols with brackets around them imply that these doses may not be required, depending upon the age of the child or adult. Refer to the relevant chapter for that vaccine for further details.

○  **Diphtheria, tetanus, acellular pertussis and inactivated polio virus vaccine (DTaP-IPV):** DTaP-IPV(±Hib) vaccine is the preferred vaccine for all doses in the vaccination series, including completion of the series in children who have received one or more doses of DPT (whole cell) vaccine (e.g., recent immigrants). In Tables 1 and 2, the 4-6 year dose can be omitted if the fourth dose was given after the fourth birthday.

✦  *Haemophilus influenzae* **type b conjugate vaccine (Hib):** the Hib schedule shown is for the *Haemophilus* b capsular polysaccharide – polyribosylribitol phosphate (PRP) conjugated to tetanus toxoid (PRP-T). For catch up, the number of doses depends on the age at which the schedule is begun (see *Haemophilus Vaccine* chapter). Not usually required past age 5 years

■  **Measles, mumps and rubella vaccine (MMR):** a second dose of MMR is recommended for children at least 1 month after the first dose for the purpose of better measles protection. For convenience, options include giving it with the next scheduled vaccination at 18 months of age or at school entry (4-6 years) (depending on the provincial/territorial policy) or at any intervening age that is practical. In the catch-up schedule (Table 2), the first dose should not be given until the child is ≥ 12 months old. MMR should be given to all susceptible adolescents and adults.

●  **Varicella vaccine (Var):** children aged 12 months to 12 years should receive one dose of varicella vaccine. Susceptible individuals ≥ 13 years of age should receive two doses at least 28 days apart.

★  **Hepatitis B vaccine (HB):** hepatitis B vaccine can be routinely given to infants or pre-adolescents, depending on the provincial/territorial policy. For infants born to chronic carrier mothers, the first dose should be given at birth (with hepatitis B immunoglobulin), otherwise the first dose can be given at 2 months of age to fit more conveniently with other routine infant immunization visits. The second dose should be administered at least 1 month after the first dose, and the third at least 2 months after the second dose, but these may fit more conveniently into the 4 and 6 month immunization visits. A two-dose schedule for adolescents is an option (see *Hepatitis B Vaccine* chapter).

⊠  **Pneumococcal conjugate vaccine – 7-valent (Pneu-C-7):** recommended for all children under 2 years of age. The recommended schedule depends on the age of the child when vaccination is begun (see *Pneumococcal Vaccine* chapter).

◎  **Meningococcal C conjugate vaccine (Men-C):** recommended for children under 5 years of age, adolescents and young adults. The recommended schedule depends on the age of the individual (see *Meningococcal Vaccine* chapter) and the conjugate vaccine used. At least one dose in the pimary infant series should be given after 5 months of age. If the provincial/territorial policy is to give Men-C to persons ≥ 12 months of age, one dose is sufficient.

▲  **Diphtheria, tetanus, acellular pertussis vaccine – adult/adolescent formulation (Tdap):** a combined adsorbed "adult type" preparation for use in people ≥ 7 years of age, contains less diphtheria toxoid and pertussis antigens than preparations given to younger children and is less likely to cause reactions in older people.

Source: Public Health Agency of Canada, *Canadian Immunization Guide,* 7th ed., 2006. Copyright © Reproduced with the permission of the Minister of Public Works and Government Services Canada, 2007.

*Teach parents about the importance of immunizations.* Parents should keep a continuing record of the child's immunizations. Your teaching, encouragement, community efforts, and follow-up are vital.

A mailed reminder about the date for immunization of the infant increases the chances that baby will receive the scheduled immunization, especially in families that have a record of failing to keep clinic appointments. A telephone reminder will usually help in ensuring that mothers return for well-baby immunizations.

As a result of efforts around the globe, worldwide immunization of children is now increasing, according to the World Health Organization. Currently, 80 percent of the world's children are immunized against six diseases: diphtheria, measles, pertussis, poliomyelitis, tetanus, and tuberculosis. About 25 percent of child deaths in the developed world could be prevented by immunization. In Manitoba, registered First Nations children, both "on-reserve" and "off-reserve," have far lower complete immunization rates than all other Manitoba children at ages one (62 percent versus 89 percent) and two (45 percent versus 77 percent).[183]

## CRITICAL THINKING

*Regarding immunization, what would you tell a mother who has an infant born prematurely?*

**Safety Promotion and Injury Control** Safety promotion and injury control are based on the understanding of infant behaviour. Health Canada has concluded that baby walkers pose significant and unnecessary risks to infants. In fact, Health Canada's Consumer Product Safety Bureau is seeking the views of Canadians on a proposal that, under the *Hazardous Products Act*, would legally ban the sale, advertisement, and importation of baby walkers into Canada.[184]

Canada has had a dramatic decline in infant mortality rates in the past 35 years. In 1996, the infant mortality rate in Canada was 5.6 per 1000 live births compared with a rate of 27.3 per 1000 live births in 1960; it has decreased steadily since the early 1960s, tapering off somewhat in the mid-1980s. Differences in infant mortality are noted in terms of socioeconomic and educational variables. Substantial differences in infant mortality between the various ethnic and racial groups have been documented.[185]

Infants should be transported in an approved automobile infant seat. Furthermore, as the baby is helpless in water, he or she should never be left alone, or with an irresponsible person, while in water. The home and car have many, often unnoticed hazards; thus, the baby should never be left alone in either; and should never be allowed to roam freely in the car while it is in motion. Parents should use an approved car infant seat.

Falls can be avoided if the parents, or nurse, take responsibility for doing the following:

- Keep crib rails up and securely fastened.
- Maintain a firm grasp on the baby while carrying or caring for him or her, and support the head during the first few months.
- Use a sturdy highchair and government-approved car infant seat.
- Strap child securely in grocery cart, if used.
- Lock windows if infant can climb onto windowsills.
- Have a gate at the top of the stairs, or in front of windows or doors, that are above the first storey.
- Keep room free of loose rugs or trailing cables or cords so that child does not fall over them as he or she becomes mobile.
- Keep furniture, lamps, and heavy or breakable objects secure so child does not pull them on self after becoming mobile.
- Clean up spills immediately from floor.

Suffocation at home and in the health care setting can be avoided:

- Remove all small objects from floor or accessible surroundings that could be inhaled or ingested (safety pins, small beads, coins, toys, paper clips, nuts, raisins, popcorn, chips, parts of broken toys, balloons, etc.).
- Keep plastic bags, window blind cords, and all other cords out of reach.

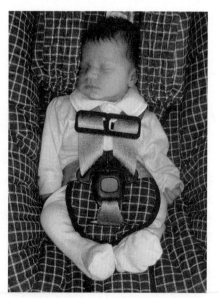

Infants should be transported in an approved automobile infant seat or harness.

- Avoid the use of pillows in the crib, as well as excessively tight clothing or bedcovers.
- Choose stair gate with opening too small for head; avoid accordion or expandable gates.

Burns can also be avoided:

- Place the crib away from radiators or fireplaces.
- Use warm-air vaporizers with caution.
- Disconnect unused appliances; cover electric outlets.
- Avoid having tablecloths that hang over the table edge.
- Place crib, play materials, and highchair away from heater and fans.
- Turn pot handles inward on the stove.
- Avoid excessive sun exposures; use sunscreen.
- Avoid smoking around the baby.
- Use sturdy screens in front of fireplace; keep child away from stoves.

*Encourage parents to take a first-aid course* (one directed toward cardiopulmonary resuscitation, preventing airway obstruction, and other home and family concerns) that enables them to recognize hazards and take appropriate measures to avoid injury to loved ones. Teaching parents about the child's normal developmental pattern will enable them to foresee potential accidents and take precautions. Because some infants are quite mobile by 10 or 12 months, the safety precautions discussed in Chapter 8 may also apply.

Parents must consider another threat to the safety of the child and to the integrity of their family unit: stealing, kidnapping, or abduction of their infant. Burgess and colleagues describe characteristics of the abductor and legal ramifications of the crime.[186]

## Common Health Problems: Health Promotion and Prevention

Various conditions are common in the infant. Table 7-7 summarizes the problems, their signs or symptoms, and methods to prevent or treat them. Refer also to Chapters 2 and 6 for illnesses that can result from various teratogens or infectious diseases in the mother (see Figures 6-1 and 6-2).

Because of their contact with a variety of microorganisms, infants who are in daycare centres have about twice as many respiratory infections as those who are reared entirely at home. Nationally, in 2002–2003, about 54 percent of Canadian children aged six months to five years were in some type of non-parental care.[187] Counsel parents about the careful selection of daycare services in relation to hygiene measures that are followed, the number of children

being served, and policies related to whether sick children are kept home for the day. However, when children raised entirely at home go to school, their illness rates are higher because of exposure to new germs.

Advise parents against the harmful effects of smoking. Discuss both active and passive effects of smoking. A study was conducted by Blizzard and her researchers to determine the effects of parental smoking on infant risk of respiratory tract infection in the first 12 months of life. The researchers concluded that parents who smoke should not smoke with their infants present in the same room.[188]

## PSYCHOSOCIAL CONCEPTS

The following information will facilitate assessment and intervention with the infant and parents.

The *intellectual, emotional, social, and moral components can be combined into what is often referred to as* **psychosocial development**. The separation of these facets of growth is artificial because they are so closely interrelated. Similarly, psychosocial, physical, and motor developments greatly influence each other. Babies are born cognitively flexible, rather than with preset instinctual behaviour. A level of physiologic maturation of the nervous system must be present before environmental stimulation and learning opportunities can be effective in promoting emotional and cognitive development. In turn, without love and environmental stimuli—tactile, kinesthetic, verbal, and others—some nervous system structures do not develop fully. Babies adapt and react to the environment with which they are confronted.

## Cognitive Development

**Intelligence** is the *ability to learn and understand from experience, to acquire and retain knowledge, to respond to a new situation, and to solve problems.* It is a system of living and acting developed in a sequential pattern through relating to the environment. Each stage of operation serves as a foundation for the next.[189] **Cognitive behaviour** includes *thinking, perceiving, remembering, forming concepts, making judgments, generalizing, and abstracting.* Cognitive development is learning, and it depends on innate capacity, maturation, nutrition, gross and fine motor stimulation, touch, appropriate stimulation of all senses through various activities, language, and social interaction.[190]

**Sequence in Intellectual Development** The sequence described by Piaget corresponds rather roughly in time span to those described for emotional development. The infant is in the *sensorimotor period of cognitive development.*[191] The infant arrives in the world with great

Table 7-7 Common Health Problems in Infancy

| Problem | Definition | Symptoms/Signs | Prevention/Treatment |
|---|---|---|---|
| Atopic dermatitis | Chronic inflammatory disease of skin, characterized by itching | Family history of allergic disease, especially asthma. Onset usually after 2 months. Rough, red, papular scaling areas, mainly on scalp, behind ears, on forearms and legs | Use warm water for baths. Apply lotions. Use soft cotton clothing. Keep fingernails short. |
| Diaper dermatitis | Inflammation of skin covered by diaper | Itching, irritability. Redness on buttocks, genitalia; papules, vesicles, and pustules | Keep area clean and dry. Allow air to circulate. Apply bland ointment or Burrow's solution. |
| Seborrheic dermatitis ("cradle cap") | Oily, scaly condition occurring in areas with large numbers of sebaceous glands | Scaly eruptions spreading to eyebrows, eyelids, nasolabial folds | Shampoo and massage scalp. More severe cases may require a selenium sulphide (e.g., Selsun) shampoo. |
| Oral candidiasis ("thrush") | Fungal infection found in mouth of infants | White, irregular plaques found in mouth | Administer oral medication (e.g., nystatin [Mycostatin]). |
| Constipation | Difficulty in passing stool; excessive firmness of stool; decreased frequency of defecation | Straining on defecation, lack of stool passage. Sometimes anal or perianal abscess | Give warm sitz bath. Apply petroleum jelly to anus. Give additional water to drink. |
| Iron deficiency anemia | Anemia associated with inadequate supply of iron for synthesis of hemoglobin | Hematocrit value less than 30. Pallor, lethargy. Anorexia. Poor weight gain. Splenomegaly | Discontinue whole cow's milk and substitute commercial formula. Increase intake of foods high in iron content. Give ferrous sulphate. |
| Colic | Periods of unexplained irritability, usually in first 3 months; apparently associated with abdominal pain | Intense crying, legs drawn up to abdomen, hands clenched, passes flatus | Reassure parents. Consider formula change. If breastfeeding, review mother's intake. Review feeding and feeding technique. Apply warmth to abdomen. Put to sleep in prone position. Hold with rhythmic movement. Feed warm water during attack. Try Mylicon drops. |

Sources: Sherwen, L., M. Scoloveno, and C. Weingarten, *Maternity Nursing: Care of the Childbearing Family, 3rd ed.* Norwalk, CT: Appleton & Lange, 1999; Wong, D., and M.J. Hockenberry, *Wong's Nursing Care of Infants and Children, 7th ed.* St. Louis, MO: Mosby, 2003.

potential for intellectual development, but at birth intellectual capacities are completely undifferentiated.

**Stage 1: The Reflex Stage** This stage covers the neonatal period when behaviour is entirely reflexive. Yet all stimuli are being assimilated into beginning mental images through reflexive behaviour and from human contact.

**Stage 2: Primary Circular Reactions** Primary circular reactions are response patterns, where a stimulus creates a response and gratifying behaviour is repeated. At one to four months life is still a series of random events, but hand–mouth and ear–eye coordination is developing. The infant's eyes follow moving objects; eyes and ears follow sounds and novel stimuli. Responses to different objects vary. Baby does not look for objects removed from sight. He or she spends much time looking at objects in the environment and begins to separate self from them. The beginning of intented behaviour is seen. He or she reproduces behaviour previously done. For example, the eight-week-old infant can purposefully apply pressure to a pillow to make a mobile rotate, smile at familiar faces, and anticipate a routine such as diapering.

### Stage 3: Secondary Circular Reactions

Stage 3 covers four to eight months. Baby learns to initiate and recognize new experiences and to repeat pleasurable ones. Intentional behaviour can be observed. Increasing mobility and hand control help him or her to become more oriented to the environment. Reaching, grasping, listening, and laughing all become better coordinated. Memory traces are apparently being established: baby anticipates familiar events, or a moving object's position. The child repeats or prolongs interesting events. Activities that accidentally brought a new experience are repeated. Behaviour becomes increasingly more intentional. Habits developed in previous stages are incorporated with new actions. Baby will imitate another's behaviour, if it is familiar and not too complex.

### Stage 4: Coordination of Secondary Schemata

In this stage, from 8 to 12 months, baby's behaviour is showing clear acts of intelligence and experimentation. Baby uses certain activities to attain basic goals. He or she realizes for the first time that someone other than self can cause activity, and that activity of self is separate from the movement of objects. He or she searches for, and retrieves, a toy that has disappeared from view. The shapes and sizes of familiar objects are recognized, regardless of the perspective from which they are viewed. Because of the baby's ability to differentiate objects and

people from self, and because of the increased sense of separateness, he or she begins to experience separation anxiety (eighth month) when the mothering figure leaves. Baby is more mobile; sitting, creeping, standing, or walking gives a new perception of the environment. Baby understands words that are said. Thus the coordination of schema involves using one idea, or mental image, to attain a goal, and a second idea or image to deal with the end result. Baby systematically imitates another while observing that person's behaviour.[192]

Reaffirm with parents that they can greatly influence the child's later intellectual abilities through the stimulation they provide for baby, including the loving attention they give, and the freedom they allow for baby to explore and use his or her body in the environment. Use the box entitled "Examples of Educational Toys for the Infant" as a guide for teaching parents.

Piaget's views have been challenged by some researchers, who suggest that very young babies have more understanding of object permanence than Piaget has indicated.[193]

---

### CRITICAL THINKING

*How do you differentiate between a good learning toy and a poor learning toy?*

---

## Communication, Speech, and Language Development

Communication between people involves facial expressions, body movements, nonverbal behaviour, vocalizations, speech, and the use of language. When a newborn is ready to communicate, the parents and caretakers need to know how to read the baby's messages. The first communications are through eye contact, crying, and body movements.[194]

---

### Examples of Educational Toys for the Infant

**1 to 3 Months**—Mobiles, unbreakable mirrors, and large colourful rings attached over crib; rattles of various sizes and geometric shapes; stuffed animals with black and white patterns; music boxes or tapes of music—need to change the tune and words from time to time.

**4 to 6 Months**—Plastic or paper streamers attached over crib, so child sees but cannot chew or choke on them; squeaky toys; colourful stuffed animals that are not too large; small beach ball or soft plastic ball; chunky bracelets; books made of cloth or vinyl; small barriers that encourage playing peek-a-boo.

**7 to 9 Months**—Larger stuffed animals, without buttons or small parts that can be detached and cause choking; nesting cylinders of various size, unbreakable cartons; pop-up toys; cloth blocks; large dolls and puppets; bath toys; mirror available so child can see self during adult play of "so big" and pat-a-cake.

**10 to 12 Months**—Push-pull toys; household objects like empty egg cartons or large spoons; stacked rings on a spindle; balls—soft, of various sizes and colours.

**Note:** Toys or items like a music box, CD, or audiotape that were enjoyed in the prior months continue to be enjoyed throughout infancy, especially if they are not continuously available.

**Speech** is the *ability to utter sound*. **Language** refers to *the mother tongue of a group of people, or the combination of sounds combined into a meaningful whole to communicate thoughts and feelings*. Speech development begins with the cry at birth, and the cry remains the basic form of communication for the infant. The newborn cries an average of one to four hours a day. *Baby's cry is undifferentiated for the first month.* Initially, the adult listener cannot distinguish between cries of hunger, pain, fear, and general unhappiness. Parents learn to distinguish the meanings of different cries and grunts the baby makes in the first two or three months.[195] Baby responds, with similar sounds at first, to both soothing and distressing stimuli. Then, other pre-speech sounds to come from the baby are as follows:

- **Cooing**, the soft murmur or hum of contentment, beginning at two to three months
- **Babbling**, incoherent sounds made by playing with sounds, beginning at two to three months. The number of sounds produced by babbling gradually increases, reaches a peak at eight months, and gives way for true speech and language development.
- Squealing and grunting
- **Lalling**, the movement of the tongue with crying and vocalization, such as "m-m-m"
- Sucking sounds
- Gestures

Smiles, frowns, and other facial expressions often accompany the baby's vocalizations, as do gestures of reaching or withdrawing to convey feelings.[196]

There is a biological basis for speech. The brain has the amazing ability to process and interpret verbal expressions over an infinite range. However, parent–child interaction is essential for the child to learn language and conversation. Further, a critical period arrives during which young children need environmental stimuli, or they will not learn to speak even when their deprived sensory environment is exchanged for stimulation rich environment.[197]

At first, vocalizations are reflexive. No difference exists between the vocalizations of hearing babies and deaf babies before six months of age. Later, vocalizations are self-reinforcing. That is, the baby finds pleasure in making and hearing his or her own sounds, and the responses from others provide further reinforcement. Reinforcement is necessary, when desired sounds are made and when certain sounds are omitted, for the infant to progress to language development. The child must hear others speak to reinforce further the use of the sounds and language of the culture. Effective mothers speak to their children frequently, even while they are doing their housework.[198]

## CASE SITUATION

### Infant Development

Michael, eight months old, is sitting on the lap of his babysitter, Aunt Jennifer, who is reading a story to him. As she reads to Michael, Aunt Jennifer smiles and chuckles. Michael responds by mimicking her mouth movements. She says, "Ooooohh" with a widened O-shaped mouth, and Michael imitates the O-shape of her mouth while she speaks. Michael makes a long, loud "Ooooohh" sound. Aunt Jennifer responds with smiles and exclamations of enthusiasm, recognizing his achievement. Michael smiles and continues to repeat "Ooooohh."

Michael then attempts to imitate Aunt Jennifer's actions in reading the book. He reaches toward the book and makes babbling sounds as he swats at it. Michael's coordination of vision, hearing, and tactile senses as he repeatedly imitates his aunt's facial expressions, reaches for the book, and engages in pre-speech babbling demonstrates a common behaviour of children in this age group. These behaviours demonstrate Piaget's Stage 3, secondary circular reactions of the sensorimotor stage of cognitive development.

### Questions

1. Suppose that you have been asked to observe this episode with Michael and Aunt Jennifer. Using your knowledge of Piaget's Stage 3, secondary circular reactions, what information about Michael's intellectual development would you be able to relate to his mother?

2. In what ways would you reinforce Aunt Jennifer's behaviour regarding Michael's intellectual development, especially regarding secondary circular reactions? Can you think of any suggestions, or insights, you might provide to Aunt Jennifer on Michael's behalf?

3. What new sensorimotor behaviours would you expect Michael to exhibit in the next two or three weeks? In the next two or three months?

4. What challenges or criticisms of Piaget's sensorimotor stages theory have you found?

At every age, the child comprehends the meaning of what others say more readily than he or she can put thoughts and feelings into words. In speech comprehension, the child first associates certain words with visual, tactile, and other sensations aroused by objects in the environment. Between 9 and 12 months, baby learns to recognize his or her name and the names of several familiar objects, responds to "no," echoes and imitates sounds, repeats syllables, and may occasionally obey the parent.[199]

Baby tries to articulate words from sounds heard. Words are invented, such as *didi* to mean a toy or food.

Language is **autistic;** *he or she associates meanings with sounds made by the self, but the sounds are not meaningful to others,* often even to the parents. By trial and error, by imitation, and as a result of reinforcement from others, the baby makes the first recognizable words, such as *mama, dada, no,* and *bye-bye,* between 10 and 18 months. (If the correct sound is directed to the appropriate parent, the sound is reinforced and the baby continues speech.) Words such as *mama* and *nana* are universal to babies in every culture because they result from the sounds the infant normally makes in babbling. By age one, the baby has a vocabulary of approximately six words. Nouns typically are learned first. He or she learns to associate meaning with an object, such as its name, size, shape, use, and sound; then a word becomes a symbol or label for the object. Learning to speak involves pronouncing words, building a vocabulary, distinguishing between sounds such as "pet" and "pat" or "hear" and "near" and then making a sentence. The baby's first sentence usually consists of one word and a gesture.

Teach parents that many factors influence speech and language development: innate intelligence, ability to hear, modification of the anatomic structures of the mouth and throat, sense of curiosity, parental verbal stimulation and interest, and encouragement to imitate others.

## Emotional Development

Eight psychological stages in the human life cycle are described by Erikson.[200] He elaborates on the core problems, or crisis, with which each person struggles at each of these levels of development. In addition to these problems, the child has other tasks to accomplish that relate to the psychosocial crisis, such as learning to walk. Emotional or personality development is a continuous process.

**Developmental Crisis** According to Erikson, the psychosexual crisis for infancy is trust versus mistrust.[201] **Basic trust** involves *confidence, optimism, acceptance of and reliance on self and others, faith that the world can satisfy needs, and a sense of hope or a belief in the attainability of wishes in spite of problems and without the overestimation of results.* A sense of trust forms the basis for a sense of hope and for later identity formation, social responsiveness to others, and the ability to care about and love others. The person accepts self, develops reachable goals, assumes life will be manageable, and expects people and situations to be positive. A sense of trust may be demonstrated in the newborn and infant through the ease of feeding, the depth of sleep, the relaxation of the bowels, and the overall appearance of contentment. **Mistrust** is *a sense of not feeling satisfied emotionally or physically, an inability to believe in, or rely on, others or self.* Security and trust are fostered by

the prompt, loving, and consistent response to the infant's distress and needs, and by the positive response to happy, contented behaviour. Parents should understand the meaning they convey through such care as changing diapers. Even if the techniques are not the best, baby will sense the positive attitude if it exists. If the parents repeatedly fail to meet primary needs, fear, anger, insecurity, and eventual mistrust will result. If the most important people fail him or her, there is little foundation on which to build faith in others or self and little desire to be socialized into the culture. The world cannot be trusted. If the baby is abused, neglected, or deprived, he or she may suffer irreversible effects, as discussed in Chapter 6.

The infant who is in a nurturing, loving environment and who has developed trust is a happy baby most of the time. He or she is sociable and responsive to others. Attachment to the parent has been formed so that separation, or stranger, anxiety is experienced at approximately 7 to 9 months of age and may extend to 10 to 12 months. After a time, the infant will again respond to strangers. Sociable babies have sociable mothers, and sociable, friendly babies score higher on cognitive tests than less sociable or mistrusting infants.[202]

The working mother may want to discuss her situation with you. The emotional development of the infant is not compromised by the working mother if she has time and energy to maintain consistent, loving, and stimulating responses when she is with baby. It is the quality of care rather than the quantity of time that is the essence of parenting and promoting emotional development. When work is not stressful and is a source of personal satisfaction for the mother, she is a more contented mother and gives the baby better care. The father's nurturance is also important, and often he is highly involved in caring for the child if the mother works, which contributes to quality care.[203]

Because so many mothers work outside the home today, an important subject to discuss is child care arrangements, or babysitting services. Even if the parent does not work, some time away from the baby is rejuvenating and enhances the quality of parenting. Each parent has different ideas about how often, if at all, to leave the baby with a sitter. Discuss characteristics to consider in a sitter. Point out that parents will probably be most satisfied with a sitter whose childrearing philosophy and guidance techniques coincide closely with theirs and who has had some child care training or experience.

If possible, parents should keep the baby with the same person consistently, especially around seven or eight months, when baby recognizes mother and familiar people and is experiencing separation anxiety. The sitter or nanny should have exact instructions about where the parents can be reached; special aspects of care; telephone numbers of doctor, police, and fire department; name and telephone number of another family member; and telephone number of a poison control centre. As more mothers return to the workforce shortly after childbirth, there has been an increasing trend toward infant daycare centres. Factors to consider in choosing daycare services are discussed in Chapter 9. As a point of interest, remote communities may not have the standard 911 system for emergencies. Therefore, ensure that visitors are aware of the local communication system if they are left in charge of a baby.

---

## CRITICAL THINKING

*What factors do you think are needed within a family unit for building trust in an infant?*

---

**Self-Concept** When the baby is creating an internal model of attachment and expressing his or her own individual temperament, he or she is also developing an internal model of self. Freud suggested that the infant needs to develop a sense of separateness from his or her mother before she or he can develop a sense of self. An infant can differentiate between images of itself, other infants, and dolls between five and eight months of age.[204]

The child's first task is to realize that he is separate from others and that this separate self endures over space and time. This aspect is called the *subjective self*. The second major task is for the toddler to come to understand that he or she is an object in the world. This self-awareness marks the second aspect of identity known as *categorical self* or *objective self*. As self-awareness develops, the infant begins to refer to himself or herself by name; near the second year, the infant begin to label himself or herself as a boy or girl. The development of the *emotional self* begins when the baby learns to identify changes in emotions in others' faces.[205]

The infant's initial experiences with his or her body, determined largely by maternal care and attitudes, are the basis for a developing self-concept and how he or she later likes and handles the body and reacts to others.

**Adaptive Mechanisms** **Adaptive mechanisms** are *learned behavioural responses that aid adjustment and emotional development.* At first, the baby cries spontaneously. Soon baby learns that crying brings attention. Consequently, he or she cries when uncomfortable, hungry, or bored. Other tools besides crying used in adaptation are experimentation, exploration, and manipulation. Baby uses the body in various ways to gain stimulation. He or she grabs and plays with whatever is within reach, whether it is

father's nose or a toy. By the end of infancy, emotions of anger, fear, delight, and affection are expressed through vocalization, facial expression, and gestures. The quality of the home environment and the passage of time significantly affect the outcome.[206]

Research indicates that the education of the mother about infant behaviours, emotional states, and communication cues facilitates mother–infant interaction, which has a positive effect on attachment, nurturing, and the child's development and adaptation.[207]

While peers are important at a later age, the nurturing that occurs during infancy and the first years of life is critical.[208]

## Gender Effects

Gender, or sex assignment, occurs at birth. The parents' first question is usually "Is it a boy or a girl?" The answer to this question often stimulates a set of adjectives to describe the newborn: soft, fine-featured, little, passive, weak girl; robust, big, strong, active boy, regardless of size or weight. The name given to baby also reflects the parents' attitudes toward the baby's sex and may reflect their ideas about the child's eventual role in life. Mothers maintain more physical and visual contact with infant daughters than they do with sons.[209]

When babies are six months old, mothers imitate the verbal sounds of their daughters more than their sons, and mothers continue to touch, talk to, and handle their daughters more than their sons. Throughout infancy and childhood, female children talk to and touch their mothers more. Boys are encouraged to be more independent, exploratory, and vigorous in gross motor activity.[210]

By 9 to 12 months, baby responds to his or her name, an important link to sex and role. Research indicates that girl babies are more dependent and less exploratory by one year than boys are because of different parental expectations. Parents appear to reinforce sex-coded behaviour in infancy so that sex role behaviour is learned on the basis of parental cues.[211]

Infants receive stimulation of their erogenous zones during maternal care. Initially, the mouth and lower face are the main erogenous zones, providing pleasure, warmth, and satisfaction through sucking. Both sexes explore their genitalia during infancy. Erection in the male and lubrication in the female occur.

Explore gender identity with parents. Help them to be aware of the importance for gender identity of their tone of voice, touch, behaviour, and feelings toward the boy or girl. Use health promotion strategies to assist them in developing ways to relate optimally with the child in order to promote trust and well-being.

## HEALTH PROMOTION IN NURSING PRACTICE

Your role with the infant and family has been discussed in each section throughout this chapter. You can be instrumental in establishing or working with community agencies that assist parents and infants. You may be called on to work with families who have adopted a child, or with the single parent, or with the stepfamily that then has their own child (see also Chapter 4). You may work with a family whose child is not healthy, or is born prematurely (see also Chapter 4), or you may work with a family who experiences the sudden death of an infant.

## Establishment and Use of Community Resources for Continuity of Care

Some sources of help that may be found in your community are summarized in the box entitled "Community Resources for Parents."

Although nurses work with many ill infants and their families in hospitals, they have many opportunities to care for well infants and their families in the community. It is necessary for the nurse to observe and listen to any issues of concern that the family may have regarding their child. Of equal importance is that the nurse observes, and listens to, the strengths and healthy responses of the family and the child.

## Care of the Premature Baby and the Baby with Congenital Anomalies

The principal threats to infant health are low birth weight—with its major antecedent, preterm delivery—and birth defects. The infant mortality rate in Canada has declined dramatically in the last 35 years.[212] Babies born of adolescent mothers, particularly young adolescent mothers, are at higher risk of low birth weight and infant mortality than are babies born of older mothers. Poverty is strongly and consistently associated with low birth weight, but the precise social and environmental conditions that produce preterm delivery are not yet understood.[213]

Several individual factors, such as cigarette smoking, the use of drugs, and diet, influence fetal growth. The cessation of smoking during pregnancy is the single largest modifiable factor affecting low birth weight and infant mortality. Other behaviours, such as diet and the abuse of alcohol and other drugs, while important in reducing the rates of low birth weight and preterm birth, do not have nearly the impact that cigarette smoking has. Thus, a woman can adopt healthful lifestyle changes that will significantly increase her chances of having a healthy, normal-weight child. Refer to Chapter 6 for more information on the negative effects of cigarette smoking, alcohol and drug use and abuse, and inadequate diet on prenatal and infant development.

While low-birth-weight infants are at a higher risk of death or long-term illness and disability than are infants born at normal weight, most low-birth-weight infants have normal outcomes. The sequelae associated with prematurity include higher rates of subnormal growth, illnesses, and neurodevelopment problems. Beyond that, problems with cognition, attention, and neuromotor problems may occur, and they might still be apparent in adolescence.[214]

Cultures vary in how they care for the premature. Premature babies in some countries are placed with their mothers two to three hours after birth, and are sent home soon after birth because of the economic status of the parents, problems with cross-infections, and deep respect for natural processes. In some countries, the premature child has little to no chance of survival.

In 2000, Health Canada brought together participants from every province and territory to discuss **congenital anomalies** (*defects in physical structure or function*).[215] Of the 350 000 children born in Canada each year,

---

### Community Resources for Parents

**Classes on Parenting, Prenatal or Postnatal Care, Lamaze or Psychoprophylaxis Method of Childbirth**

- Canadian Parents Online (www.canadianparents.com)
- Hospitals
- Community health nursing services

**Breastfeeding Information**

- La Leche League

**Parent Support**

- Canadian Association of Midwives
- Perinatal bereavement services
- Support groups for children who are challenged
- SIDS Canada Bereavement Support
- Health Canada Shaken Baby Syndrome
- Parents of Multiple Birth

**Crisis Attendance or Counselling**

- Crisis hotlines
- Clergy or other counsellors

2 to 3 percent will be born with a serious congenital anomaly.[216] Infant mortality due to congenital anomalies has decreased significantly in Canada. In spite of the frequency of occurrences of congenital anomalies, the underlying causes for most remain obscure.

The prevalence of maternal substance abuse has escalated over the last quarter-century. Infants exposed to drugs may exhibit many physical and psychological effects, including those discussed in Chapter 6, related to the effects of medications, the effects of addictive drugs, the narcotic abstinence (withdrawal) syndrome in the neonate, effects of alcohol use and abuse, and FASD (a set of birth defects associated with the maternal consumption of alcohol during pregnancy).

A generation of babies has already been affected, and these babies will present major problems to our society because of their developmental disabilities, uncontrollable behaviour and rage, learning deficits, and lack of values and remorse. There are not enough treatment centres and foster homes. Mothers or grandmothers are likely to bear the brunt of this crisis. For many parents and their families, the birth of a baby will not bring joy, but instead will bring fear, grief, and depression—for a long time. Supportive nursing care is a key factor for these families.

Parents of the baby with congenital anomalies always need the same extent of consideration as parents of the premature infant. They should be encouraged to see their infant as soon as possible to head off fantasies that are often worse than the anomaly. The manner in which the nurse presents the infant to the parents may well set the tone for the early parent–child relationship.

Show them the normal parts and emphasize the baby's positive features. Above all, show your acceptance of the infant: hold, cuddle, and look at the infant as you talk to him or her. Give information about the anomaly and the possible prognosis. This is a difficult time for parents, and they will need ample time to express their grief, guilt, and worries. Your patience and support will be most helpful. Various references provide more in-depth information to share with parents pertinent to the specific disability.[217] Refer to Chapter 4 for additional information on nursing practice with the family.

Numerous ethical issues arise in the context of care of the infant born with a congenital anomaly and the preterm or low-birth-weight infant. This is especially true if the infant has a severe congenital anomaly, is born extremely early, or weighs very little. The values of the individuals involved (health care professionals and parents) in caring for infants influence their clinical decision-making outcomes. In this group of infants, these values include preserving life, decreasing morbidity, and relieving pain and suffering.[218]

Parents and members of the health care and judicial systems continue to debate hotly the anticipated length and quality of many infant lives. Some infants who are saved will continue as a financial and care burden on their parents for the rest of the parents' lives.

The advanced technology required to maintain life has posed a major ethical dilemma for parents and professionals: Should life be continued with machines? When and how should the critically ill infant or child be allowed to die? Schloman and Fister describe the perspectives of parents in their study.[219]

It is becoming more imperative that nurses understand both the questions and the legal and ethical responses related to withholding life-sustaining treatment from infants. Nurses must be prepared to participate in this type of decision making, based on adequate knowledge of the issue.

## Care of the Family Experiencing Adoption and Infant Death

### Mothers Who Give Their Newborns for Adoption
These mothers are confronted with a crisis that involves bereavement. Ambivalence prevails during the prenatal period: love for baby, guilt about abandonment, and concern for the baby's future. Therapeutic intervention begins prenatally by exploring, with the mother, the anticipatory grief, anger, depression, decisions about seeing the baby, and choice of postdelivery care. To promote bonding would be cruel, but the mother should have the opportunity—the reality—of holding and inspecting. Not to recognize the infant is to deny the pregnancy. Seeing the infant gives concrete focus to the mother's grief. A maternity nurse-specialist should consult the relinquishing mother on a scheduled basis to promote the woman's personal growth, self-respect, and dignity. Refer to Chapter 4 for more information on the adoptive process and the family.

### Parents Whose Infant Dies
If the newborn dies, there are no magic words. Certain actions are helpful: (1) give parents mementos, such as a footprint sheet, identification band, or photograph; (2) be patient and compassionate; and (3) help the family to say goodbye. Parents must work through the affection-symbiotic bond developed in anticipation of the baby as perfect. Full expression of the grief, guilt, and anger is necessary.

Parents should, if they desire, be permitted to view, touch, and hold their deceased infant. In accordance with the beliefs of the parents, traditional fitting bereavement service should be arranged to enable grieving and help to make the death real. The spirituality of the parents influences their emotional, mental, and physical responses to bereavement.[220] Meeting with the parents after the death of an infant or attending the funeral can assist them through the mourning. Contact, or meet with, the parents within the next two to three weeks, and again in three to six months. During these visits you can effectively listen, encourage the expression of feelings, and assist the parents in working through their feelings and reactions.[221]

## CRITICAL THINKING

*If the parents were to approach you wondering whether they should take their dying child home from the hospital, how would you counsel them?*

## SUMMARY

1. Childbirth is a crisis for the parents. Life is changed with the birth of a baby.

2. The development of infant–parent attachment is essential for the child's total development.

3. Infant and parent behaviours are reciprocal.

4. Maltreatment of the infant by parents or others must be reported. Intervention is essential.

5. The neonatal period, the first 30 days of life, and infancy, the first year of life, constitute an era that is a critical period for the child.

6. Physiological adaptations are necessary to survive after birth.

7. The first year is a period of rapid physical growth and essential cognitive development.

8. Adequate nutrition, play, safety, health promotion, and illness prevention and treatment are essential for the infant's growth and development.

9. Culture influences all areas of the child's growth and development.

10. The first year is emotionally critical in order to thrive, to learn to trust, and to achieve developmental tasks. The infant must be consistently loved and cared for as a whole person.

11. The box entitled "Considerations for the Infant and Family in Health Care" summarizes what you should consider in assessment and health promotion with the infant.

## Weblinks

### Canadian Child Care Federation (CCCF)
www.cccf-fcsge.ca
The CCCF is recognized as the largest pan-Canadian child care organization based on its reach, relationships, resources, and reputation. Over the years, the CCCF has adopted various strategies in order to function within the changing dynamics of the child care sector. Today, the CCCF is restructuring once again to build a financially more sustainable organization and to fill the funding gap due to vanishing resources and growing competition.

### Canadian Incidence Study of Reported Child Abuse and Neglect
www.phac-aspc.gc.ca/cm-vee/cis-eng.php
The Canadian Incidence Study of Reported Child Abuse and Neglect (CIS) is the first nationwide study to examine the incidence of reported child maltreatment and the characteristics of children and families investigated by Canadian child welfare services. The CIS addresses the four principal forms of maltreatment: physical abuse, sexual abuse, neglect, and emotional maltreatment.

### First Nations and Inuit Health (FNIH)
www.hc-sc.gc.ca/fnih-spni/index_e.html
Detailed information is available at this site about FNIH: its organization, mandate and priorities, and the branch organization.

### Family-Centred Maternity and Newborn Care: National Guidelines
www.phac-aspc.gc.ca/dca-dea/prenatal/fcmc1_e.html
These national guidelines were established in 2000 by Health Canada, the Canadian Institute of Child Health, and 70 Canadian professionals and consumers. They are designed to help achieve the objective that we all share: a healthy and satisfying pregnancy, birth, and postpartum experience for all mothers, babies, and families.

### Joint Statement on Shaken Baby Syndrome
www.phac-aspc.gc.ca/dca-dea/publications/jointstatement_web_e.html
This site provides the Joint Statement on Shaken Baby Syndrome. The 11-page document contains the statement of purpose, what can be done, recommendations, and an extensive bibliography.

# Considerations for the Infant and Family in Health Care

- Cultural background and experiences of the family of the infant
- Reactions of the mother and the father to the crisis resulting from the baby's birth
- Attachment behaviours and the binding-in process of the mother, attachment of father and other family members
- Parental behaviours that indicate difficulty in establishing attachment or potential/actual abuse of the infant
- Physical characteristics and patterns, such as eating, sleeping, elimination, and activity in the neonate/infant, that indicate health and are within the age norms for growth
- Cognitive characteristics and behavioural patterns in the neonate/infant that indicate age-appropriate norms for intellectual development
- Communication characteristics and behavioural patterns in the neonate/infant that indicate intact neurological and sensory status, speech awareness, and the ability to respond with age-appropriate sounds (prespeech)
- Overall appearance and behavioural and play patterns in the neonate/infant that indicate the development of trust, rather than mistrust, and continuing age-appropriate emotional development
- Behavioural patterns and characteristics that indicate the infant has achieved developmental tasks
- Parental behaviours that indicate adequate knowledge about how to care physically and emotionally for the neonate/infant
- Parental behaviours that indicate they are promoting positive self-concept and sexuality development in the infant
- Evidence that the parents provide a safe and healthful environment and the necessary resources for the neonate/infant
- Parental behaviours that indicate they are achieving their developmental tasks for this era

## Key Terms

acrocyanosis (242)
adaptive mechanisms (273)
anterior fontanel (241)
attachment (233)
attentional reflexes (245)
autistic (272)
babbling (271)
basic trust (272)
bonding (234)
burping (260)
caput succedaneum (244)
cephalohematoma (244)
child maltreatment (238)
cognitive behaviour (268)
colic (255)
colostrum (259)
congenital anomalies (274)

consummatory reflexes (245)
cooing (271)
co-sleep (262)
crisis (231)
desquamation (242)
emotional maltreatment (238)
exosystem (239)
exploratory reflexes (245)
family (232)
hemangioma (242)
hernia (250)
hydrocele (250)
immunizations (265)
imperforate anus (250)
infant (231)
intelligence (268)

jaundice (242)
lalling (271)
language (271)
lanugo (242)
macrosystem (239)
meconium (245)
microsystem (239)
milia (242)
mistrust (272)
Mongolian spots (242)
mother (231)
neglect (238)
neonate (231)
newborn (231)
parent(s) (231)
physical abuse (238)
physiologic jaundice (242)

posterior fontanel (241)
psychosocial development (268)
reflex (245)
sexual abuse (238)
shaken baby syndrome (SBS) (240)
social reflexes (245)
soft spots (241)
speech (271)
spina bifida (250)
stools (255)
surfactant (245)
temperament (234)
umbilical cord (242)
vernix caseosa (242)
weaning (261)

# Chapter 8

## Assessment and Health Promotion for the Toddler

*Train up a child in the way he should go, and when he is old, he will not depart from it.*

Proverbs 22:6

## Objectives

*Study of this chapter will enable you to:*

1 Examine second-order changes in family status required to proceed developmentally in family life cycle stage: families with young children.

2 Explore the reciprocal effects of family and toddler within a family system.

3 Describe the significance of attachment behaviour and parenting practices.

4 Assess a toddler's physical and motor characteristics and related needs, including nutrition, rest, exercise, play, safety, and health protection measures.

5 Assess a toddler's cognitive, language, emotional, and sexuality development.

6 Evaluate specific methods of guidance and discipline for the toddler, and consider the significance of the family's philosophy about guidance and discipline.

7 Discuss with parents their role in contributing to the toddler's cognitive, language, emotional, self-concept, and moral development.

8 Describe the commonly used adaptive mechanisms that promote autonomy of the toddler, and analyze your role in assisting parents to promote the development of the child's autonomy.

9 Work effectively with a family and toddler in the health care and nursing situation, in either a hospital or a community setting.

In this chapter, the development of the toddler and family relationships are discussed. Nursing and health care responsibilities for the promotion of health for the child and family in many settings are discussed throughout the chapter.

Within the first year of life, children make remarkable adaptations to their environment. They sit, walk, remember, recognize others, and begin to socialize, communicate more purposefully with speech, and show more specific emotional responses.

The **toddler stage** *begins when the child takes the first steps alone at 12 to 15 months, and it continues until approximately three years of age.* The family is very important during this short span of the child's life when he or she acquires language skills, increases cognitive achievement, improves physical coordination, and achieves greater control over bladder and bowel sphincters. These factors lead to new and different perceptions of self and the environment, new incentives, and new ways of behaving.

# FAMILY DEVELOPMENT AND RELATIONSHIPS

## Family Life Cycle

Refer to Table 4-3, which illustrates the stages of the family life cycle, the emotional processes of transition (key principles), and the second-order changes in the family required to proceed developmentally. Stage 3, families with young children, is the relevant stage for the family with a toddler.

Behaviourally, the toddler changes considerably between 12 months and 3 years, and these changes, in turn, affect family relationships. Because of new skills, the child begins to develop a sense of independence, establishes physical boundaries between self and mother, and gains the sense of a separate, self-controlled being who can do things on his or her own. From the age of two years, the child moves toward independence—from the protracted dependency of childhood toward adulthood independence, self-reliance, and object relations. The child promotes self-education by engaging the parents and others to help when necessary. Without the myriad attempts to do things for himself or herself, the child would attain only a small degree of autonomy in skills. The periods of practice that foster the development of reliable performance and skills are often periods of independent action. However, frequent states of dependence on others and the feeling of gratification arising from dependency needs are essential for optimum ego development. Dependency does not mean passivity, because the child is quite active in obtaining help by crying, screaming, taking an adult by the hand and pulling him or her to another area, or by asking how to do something. The toddler should neither be kept too dependent, nor forced too quickly into independence.

The family of a toddler can be quiet and serene one minute and in total upheaval the next, resulting from the imbalance between the child's motor skills, lack of experience, and mental capacities. One quick look away from the toddler can result in a broken object, a spilled glass of milk, or an overturned dish. Teach parents that this behaviour is a normal and necessary part of maturation. Expecting, planning for, and trying to handle each situation patiently will help to reduce parent frustration.

Having a new baby arrive in the toddler's world is a crisis. Prepare the child for the arrival by explaining why mother's shape is becoming larger and changing. Prepare the toddler to sleep in a different bed if the crib is needed for the baby. Emphasis on the positive features of becoming a "big girl" or "big boy" is helpful. When baby arrives, the toddler will need more attention, especially while baby is receiving care and attention.

The toddler is frequently jealous of younger siblings because of now having to vie for the centre of attention that was once his or her own. Older siblings are sometimes resented because they are permitted to do things he or she is not permitted to do. Power struggles, focusing on feeding and toilet training, tend to occur between parent and child. Family problems may arise when the toddler's activities are limited because of parental anxieties concerning anticipated physical harm, or because of the parents' low tolerance of the child's energetic behaviour.

Inform parents that their social teaching will likely centre primarily on issues of cleanliness and on establishing reasonable controls over anger, impulsiveness, and unsafe exploration.

# INFLUENCE OF THE FAMILY

The chief moulder of personality is the family unit, and home is the centre of the toddler's world. Family life nurtures in the child a strong bond of affection, a social and biological identity, intellectual development, attitudes, goals, ways of coping, and ways of responding to daily life situations. The family life process is paramount for imparting tools such as language and an ethical system in which the child learns to respect the needs and rights of others. A loving, attentive, healthy, responsible family is essential for maximum physical, mental, emotional, social, and spiritual development in childhood. The importance of the father's role with both the child and the mother is being affirmed.[1] In fact, in recent years fathers have become more involved with their children, and fathers are no longer considered merely providers. The greater number of women in the job market, the higher divorce rate, and the more egalitarian division of roles and responsibilities are all factors that account for why men now play a more active role as fathers.[2]

Parents with high self-esteem provide the necessary conditions for the toddler to achieve trust, self-esteem, and autonomy (self-control) through allowing age-appropriate behaviour. Parents with low self-esteem tend to provoke feelings in the child of shame, guilt, defensiveness, decreased self-worth, and "being bad." These undesirable feelings in the child have been attributed to overestimating the child's ability to conform, inappropriately or forcefully punishing or restraining the child, denying him or her necessities, and withdrawing love.[3]

## Attachment Behaviours

Infant attachment behaviour has been observed since the early 1950s. Infant attachment refers to the deep emotional connection that an infant forms with her or his significant caregiver, usually the mother. The theory is based on the notion that a baby's main caregiver in the first year of life becomes the infant's primary attachment figure, a protector and a secure base from which he or she can explore the world. A new Health Canada resource, *First Connections . . . make all the difference*, has been developed to raise public awareness about the utmost importance of secure attachment, setting the stage as it does for healthy physical, emotional, and social development. *First Connections . . . make all the difference* can be downloaded at www.phac-aspc.gc.ca/mh-sm/mhp-psm/pub/fc-pc/index-eng.php.[4]

Attachment behaviour is very evident during the toddler years. Children need to be touched, cuddled, hugged, and rocked. All young mammals need physical contact for normal brain tissue development and for the brain to develop receptors that inhibit secretion of adrenal hormones (glucocorticoids)—the stress hormones. Thus, both the immune and neurological systems are affected positively by touch and by emotional attachment.[5]

The toddler shows attachment behaviour by maintaining proximity to the parent. Even when out walking, the child frequently returns part or all of the way to the parent for reassurance of the parent's presence, to receive a smile, to establish visual, and sometimes tactile, contact, and to speak before again moving away.[6]

Although attachment is directed toward several close people such as father, siblings, babysitter, and grandparents, it is usually greatest toward one person: mother. Attachment patterns do not differ significantly between children who stay home all day versus those who go to daycare centres, because attachment is related to the intensity of emotional and social experience between child and adult, rather than to physical care and more casual contacts. Attachment is as great, or greater, if the mother shows warm affection less frequently than if she is present all day but not affectionate. Schneider, Atkinson, and Tardif, a group of Canadian researchers, found that early

attachment for children seems to affect later social functioning. The researchers state that the child–mother attachment literature lends itself to rich speculation, but presently there is insufficient literature regarding implications of child–father attachment on children's later peer relations.[7] Further, Pederson and Moran, researchers from the University of Western Ontario, claim that for the study of attachment behaviours, the home setting is more natural to measure such behaviours than using the "Strange Situation," which measures mother–infant interactions in a laboratory setting. They developed a new, more natural setting, claiming that the richer fabric of a home environment may reveal differences in the relationships that are not observed in the Strange Situation. By using both methods to compare expressions of attachment relationships between the infant and the mother, the researchers determined that in a secure type of relationship, mothers were more sensitive to the needs of their infants, and infants displayed less fussy behaviour and enjoyed physical contact with the mother.[8]

**Separation anxiety**, the *response to separation from mother*, intensifies at approximately 18 and 24 months. Anxiety can be as intense for the toddler as it is for the infant, if the child has had a continuous warm attachment to a mother figure, because he or she thinks an object ceases to exist when it is out of sight. The child who is more accustomed to strangers will suffer less from a brief separation. When separated, the child experiences feelings of anger, fear, grief, and revenge. An apathetic, resigned reaction at this age is a sign of abnormal development. The child who is separated from the parent for a period, as with hospitalization, goes through three phases of *grief and mourning*—protest, despair, and denial, which may merge somewhat—as a result of separation anxiety.[9]

During **protest**, *lasting a few hours or days and seen during short or long separations, the need for mother is conscious, persistent, and grief laden. The child cries continually, tries to find her, is terrified, fears he or she has been deserted, feels helpless and angry that mother left him or her, and clings on her return.* If he or she is also ill, additional uncomfortable body sensations assault the toddler.[10] The child desperately needs mother at this time.

**Despair** *is a quiet stage, characterized by hopelessness, moaning, sadness, and reduced activity. The child does not cry continuously, but is in deep mourning. He or she does not understand why mother has deserted him or her. The child makes no demands on the environment, nor responds to overtures from others, including at times the mother. Yet the child clings to her if permitted.* Mother may feel guilty and want to leave to relieve her distress, because she might feel her visits are disturbing to the child, especially when the child does not respond to her.[11]

Parents need help in understanding that both the child's and their reactions are normal and that the child desperately needs parental presence.[12] If mothers can be present, you can promote family-centred care through your explanations to the mother and child, by not being rigid about visiting hours, by attending to the comfort and needs of mother (or father), and by letting the parent help care for the child. Protests, in the form of toddlers' screams and crying, will thus be less intense. Be accepting if a parent cannot stay with the child. Parents may live great distances from the hospital, or have occupational or family responsibilities that actually prevent them from visiting the child as often as they desire. The parent may also be ill or injured. Be as nurturing to the toddler as possible while the parent is away. Tell the toddler how much Mommy and Daddy love him or her and want to be present but cannot. If possible, have the parent leave an article with the child that is a familiar representation of the parent.

**Denial**, *which occurs after prolonged separation, defends against anxiety by repressing the image of, and feelings for, mother. Such behaviour might be misinterpreted as recovery.* The child now begins to take more interest in the environment, and eats, plays, and accepts other adults. Anger and disappointment at mother sometimes run so deep that the child acts as if he or she does not need mother and shows revenge by rejecting her, sometimes even rejecting gifts she brings. To prevent further estrangement, mother should understand that the child's need for her is actually more intense than ever.[13]

Continue the above interventions that promote family-centred care. Give the mother, or father, and child time together undisturbed by nursing or medical care procedures. Provide toys that help the child to act out the fears, anxiety, anger, and mistrust experienced during the hospitalization and separation. Encourage the parent to talk about and work through feelings related to the child's illness and absence from the family.

With prolonged hospitalization, the child may fail to discover a person to whom he or she can attach for any length of time. If the child finds a mother figure and then loses her, the pain of the original separation is re-experienced. If this happens repeatedly, the child will eventually avoid involvement with anyone, and invest love in self. Later, this child might value material possessions more highly than any exchange of affection with people.

Teach parents that the immediate after-effects of separation might include changes in the child's behaviour: regression, clinging, and seeking out extra attention and reassurance. If extra affection is extended to the child, trust is usually restored. If the separation has been prolonged, the child's behaviour can be rather extensively changed and somewhat disturbed for months after his or her return to the

## Physical Signs of Abuse of a Child

- An injury for which there is no explanation, or for which an implausible explanation is offered.
- Injury is not consistent with the type of accident described (e.g., child would not suffer both feet burned by stepping into a tub of hot water; he or she would step in with one foot at a time. A child who tips a pot of hot coffee on his or her hand has a splash-effect burn, not a mitten appearance.)
- Inconsistencies appear in the parents' stories about the reason for the child's injuries.
- Parents quickly blame a babysitter or neighbour for an accidental injury.
- Child does not have total appearance of an accident: dirty clothes, face smudged, hair tousled.
- Large number of healed, or partially healed, injuries is observed.
- Large bone fracture, multiple fractures, or tearing of periosteum caused by having limb forcibly twisted are evident.
- Child flinches when your fingers move over an area not obviously injured, but tender due to abusive handling.
- Human bite marks are evident.
- Fingernail indentations, or scratches, are noted.
- Old or new cigarette burns are evident.
- Loop marks from belt beating are present.
- Soft tissue swelling and hematomas are noted.
- Clustered or multiple bruises are observed on trunk or buttocks, in body hollows, on back of neck, or resembling hand prints or pinch marks.
- Bald spots are observed.
- Retinal hemorrhage appears, possibly from being shaken or cuffed about the head.
- History of unusual number of accidents exists.

Sources: Papalia, D., S. Olds, and R. Feldman, *Human Development*, 9th ed. Boston: McGraw-Hill, 2004; Seifert, K., R. Hoffnung, and M. Hoffnung, *Lifespan Development*. Boston: Houghton Mifflin, 1997; Wong, D., S. Perry, M. Hockenberry, D. Lowdermilk, and D. Wilson, *Maternal Child Nursing Care*, 3rd ed. St. Louis, MO: C. V. Mosby, 2006.

parents. The parent needs support in accepting the child's expressions of hostility and in meeting his or her demands. Counteraggression, or withdrawal from the child, will cause ever further loss in trust and regression.[14] Parenting can be hard work.

*Child maltreatment* may either begin or continue at this age. Even when parents seem concerned and loving,

## Interaction Signs of Parental Abuse of a Child

- Child flinches or glances about nervously when you touch him or her.
- Child seems afraid of parents or caregivers and is reluctant to return home.
- Parent issues threat to crying child such as "Just wait till I get you home!"
- Parent remains indifferent to child's distress.
- Parent blames child for his or her own injuries (e.g., "He's always getting hurt" or "He's always causing trouble").
- Parental behaviour suggests role reversal; parent solicits help or protection from child by acting helpless (when child cannot meet parent's needs, abuse results).
- Parent repeatedly brings healthy child to emergency room and insists child is ill (parent feeling overwhelmed by parental responsibilities and may become abusive).
- Child has had numerous admissions to an emergency room, often at hospitals some distance from the child's home.

Sources: Papalia, D., S. Olds, and R. Feldman, *Human Development*, 9th ed. Boston: McGraw-Hill, 2004; Seifert, K., R. Hoffnung, and M. Hoffnung, *Lifespan Development*. Boston: Houghton Mifflin, 1997; Wong, D., S. Perry, M. Hockenberry, D. Lowdermilk, and D. Wilson, *Maternal Child Nursing Care*, 3rd ed. St. Louis, MO: C. V. Mosby, 2006.

a child is not immune from abuse. Children today are exposed to a variety of potential abusers: babysitters, daycare workers, the parent's live-in lover or occasional friend, step-parents, extended family members, and neighbours. The results of one study, conducted by Onyskiw, indicated that children exposed to domestic violence had lower health status and more conditions or health problems. Theses factors, in turn, limited the child's participation in normal age-related activities compared to children in non-violent families. In addition, child witnesses of violence regularly used prescription medication more frequently than children who were not exposed to violence at home.[15]

In most cases, one must be very patient and observant to detect child maltreatment because the child does not have the language skills to tell you what has happened. The child's nonverbal behaviour, play, and artwork may provide clues. Observation of the latter takes time and patience as well as the parent's presence.[16] The boxes entitled "Physical

Signs of Abuse of a Child," and "Interaction Signs of Parental Abuse of a Child" present assessment data to aid you in recognizing signs of abuse.

### CRITICAL THINKING

*Kari, a toddler, has multiple bruises on her body. There is evidence that she has been beaten by her mother. What health promoting strategies can you employ with this family?*

## PHYSIOLOGIC CONCEPTS
## Physical Characteristics

Information in this section will assist you in assessment of the toddler, and in teaching the parents about normal development and health promotion measures.

**General Appearance**  The appearance of the toddler has matured from infancy. By 12 to 15 months of age, he or she has lost the roly-poly look of infancy with abdomen protruding, torso tilting forward, legs at stiff angles, and flat feet spaced apart. Limbs are growing faster than the torso, giving a different proportion to the body. By 12 to 15 months, the chest circumference is larger than the head circumference. The child increasingly looks like a family member as face contours fill out with the set of deciduous teeth. By age two, he or she has 16 teeth. Gradually, the chubby appearance typical of the infant is lost. Muscle tone becomes firmer as the fat-storing mechanisms change. Less weight is gained as fat. More weight is gained from muscle and bone.[17]

**Rate of Growth**  During toddlerhood, *growth is slower than in infancy but it is balanced, and development follows the cephalocaudal, proximodistal, and general-to-specific principles discussed in Chapter 6*. Although the rate of growth slows, bone growth continues rapidly with the development during the second year of approximately 25 new ossification centres.[18]

Between the first and second years, the average height increase is 10 to 12 cm. Average height increase during the third year is 6 to 8 cm. Weight gain averages 2.25 to 2.75 kg between the first and second years. *Birth weight is quadrupled by age two.* The two-year-old child stands 81 to 84 cm and weighs 11 to 13 kg; at 30 months, average height is 91.5 cm and weight is approximately 13.6 kg. *By age two, the girl has grown to 50 percent of final adult height. By age two-and-a half, the boy has grown to 50 percent of adult height.*[19]

The Indian and Inuit Health Committee of the Canadian Paediatric Society believes that no single growth chart for all Native children should be produced due to regional variation. They make the following recommendations:

- The growth charts prepared from the U.S. National Ambulatory Health and Nutrition Survey are suitable for use in Native communities.
- Throughout childhood, measurements of height and weight, and of head circumference for the first three years, should be taken at all well-child contacts and plotted.
- The Medical Services Branch should catalogue areas where head circumference tends to be larger than in Caucasian children.
- Health care workers must first comprehend how to use growth charts. Second, as part of their orientation they must be made aware of local variations in weight or head circumference.[20]

---

## CRITICAL THINKING

*What other factors, besides the child's environment and family history, should be taken into account in assessing growth abnormalities?*

---

**Neuromuscular Maturation** Neuromuscular maturation and the repetition of movements help the child further develop motor skills. **Myelinization**, *covering of the neurons with the fatty sheath called myelin,* is almost complete by two years. This enables the child to support most movements and their increasing physical activity, and to begin toilet training. Additional growth occurs as a greater number of connections form among neurons and the complexity of these connections increases. Lateralization, or specialization of the two hemispheres of the brain, has been occurring and evidence of signs of dominance of one hemisphere over the other can be seen. The left hemisphere matures more rapidly in girls than in boys; the right hemisphere develops more rapidly in boys. These differences may account for more adept language ability in girls and letter spatial ability in boys. Handedness is demonstrated, and spatial perception is improving.[21] (Spatial ability will be complete at approximately age ten.) The limbic system is mature; sleep, wakefulness, and emotional responses become better regulated. The toddler responds to a wider range of stimuli, responds voluntarily to sounds, and has greater control over behaviour. The brain reaches 80 percent of adult size by age two. The growth of the glial cells accounts for most of the change.[22]

**Motor Coordination** Increasing gross motor coordination is demonstrated by leg movement patterns and by hand–arm movements. Table 8-1 summarizes the increasing motor coordination skills manifested during the toddler years.[23]

**Vision** Visual acuity of 20/40 is considered acceptable during the toddler years. Visual perceptions are frequently similar to an adult's, even though the child is too young to have acquired the richness of symbolic associations. The child's eye–hand coordination also improves. At 15 months, he or she reaches for attractive objects without superfluous movements. Between 12 and 18 months, the toddler looks at pictures with interest and identifies forms.[24]

**Endocrine System** Endocrine function is not fully known. Production of glucagons and insulin is labile and limited, causing variations in blood sugar. Adrenocortical secretions are limited, but they are greater than they were in infancy. Growth hormone, thyroxin, and insulin remain important secretions for regulating growth.[25]

**Respiratory System** Respirations continue to be abdominal and average 20 to 30 per minute. The internal structures of the ear and throat continue to be short and straight, and the lymphoid tissue of the tonsils and adenoids continue to be large. Consequently, otitis media, tonsillitis, and upper respiratory tract infections are common.[26]

**Cardiovascular System** The pulse decreases, averaging 105 beats per minute. Blood pressure increases, averaging 80 to 100 systolic and 64 diastolic. The size of the vascular bed increases, thus reducing resistance to flow. The capillary bed has increased ability to respond to hot and cold environmental temperatures, thus aiding thermoregulation. The body temperature averages 37.2°C.[27]

**Gastrointestinal System** Foods move through the gastrointestinal tract less rapidly, and digestive glands approach adult maturity. Acidity of gastric secretion increases gradually. Liver and pancreatic secretions are functionally mature. The stomach capacity increases to allow for the schedule of three meals a day.[28]

**Skin** The skin becomes more protective against outer invasion from microorganisms, and it becomes tougher, with more resilient epithelium and less water content. Less fluid is lost through the skin as a result.[29]

**Urinary System** By age three, the bladder has descended into the pelvis, assuming adult position. Renal function is mature; except under stress, water is conserved, and urine is concentrated on an adult level.[30]

**Immune System** Specific antibodies have been established to most commonly encountered organisms, although the toddler is prone to gastrointestinal and respiratory infections when he or she encounters new microorganisms. Lymphatic tissues of adenoids, tonsils, and peripheral lymph

## Table 8-1 Motor Coordination during the Toddler Years

| Age (months) | Characteristics |
|---|---|
| 12–15 | Walks alone; legs appear bowed<br>Climbs steps with help; slides down stairs backwards<br>Stacks two blocks; scribbles spontaneously<br>Grasps but rotates spoon; holds cup with both hands<br>Takes off shoes and socks |
| 15–18 | Runs but still falls at times<br>Walks backwards and sideways (17 months)<br>Climbs to get to objects<br>Falls from riding toys or in bathtub<br>Hammers on pegboard<br>Grasps with both hands<br>Picks up small items from floor; investigates electric outlets; grabs cords and tablecloths (15 months)<br>Clumsily throws ball<br>Unzips large zipper<br>Takes off easily removed garments<br>Stacks three to four blocks (18 months) |
| 18–24 | Frequently falls from outdoor play equipment<br>Walks stairs with help (20 months)<br>Walks up and down stair steps alone, holding rail, both feet on step before ascending to next step<br>Can reach farther than expected, including for hazardous objects<br>Fingers food<br>Brushes paint; finger-paints<br>Takes apart toys; puts together large puzzle pieces |
| 24–30 | Runs quickly; falls less<br>Walks downstairs holding rail; does not alternate feet<br>Jumps off floor with both feet (28 months)<br>Throws ball overhand<br>Puts on simple garments<br>Stacks six blocks<br>Turns door handles<br>Plays with utensils and dishes at mealtimes; pours and stacks<br>Turns book pages<br>Uses spoon with little spilling; feeds self<br>Brushes teeth with help |
| 30–36 | Walks with balance; runs well<br>Balances on one foot; walks on tiptoes (30 months)<br>Jumps from chair (32 months)<br>Pedals tricycle (32 months)<br>Jumps 25 to 30 cm off floor (36 months)<br>Climbs and descends stairs, alternating feet (36 months)<br>Rides tricycle<br>Sits in booster seat rather than highchair<br>Stacks 8 to 10 blocks; builds with blocks<br>Pours from pitcher<br>Dresses self completely except tying shoes; does not know back from front<br>Turns on faucet<br>Assembles puzzles<br>Draws; paints |

Sources: Bee, H., D. Boyd, and P. Johnson. *Lifespan Development*, 2nd Canadian ed. Toronto: Pearson Canada, 2006; Papalia, D., S. Olds, and R. Feldman, *Human Development*, 9th ed. Boston: McGraw-Hill, 2004; Seifert, K., R. Hoffnung, and M. Hoffnung, *Lifespan Development*. Boston: Houghton Mifflin, 1997; Wong, D., S. Perry, M. Hockenberry, D. Lowdermilk, and D. Wilson, *Maternal Child Nursing Care*, 3rd ed. St. Louis, MO: C. V. Mosby, 2006.

nodes undergo enlargement, partly because of infections and partly from growth. By age three years, the adenoid tissue reaches maximum size and then declines, whereas tonsils reach peak size around seven years.[31]

**Overall Development** Development does not proceed equally, or simultaneously, in body parts and maturational skills. Sometimes a child concentrates so intently on one aspect of development (e.g., motor skills) that other abilities (e.g., toilet training) falter or regress. Illness or malnutrition may slow growth, but a catch-up growth period occurs later so that the person reaches the developmental norms. The brain is more vulnerable to permanent injury because destroyed cells are not replaced, although certain brain cells may take over some functions of missing cells. Most children show seasonal spurts in growth. Cultural differences in growth and development can be observed. Teach parents about the physical characteristics of the toddler to help them adjust to his or her changing competencies.

# Physical Assessment of the Young Child

The last approach to the physical examination depends on the age of the individual. Adequate time should be spent in becoming acquainted with the child and the accompanying parent. A friendly manner, quiet voice, and relaxed approach help make the examination more fruitful. Hands should always be warmed before giving an examination, but especially so in the case of the child.

No assessment is complete without knowing the antenatal, natal, and neonatal history. When the child is old enough, let him or her tell what conditions surround the visit, even if the message is only "stomach hurt."

---

**CRITICAL THINKING**

*Which details should a pediatric history include, as compared to an adult history?*

---

Usually, you will be learning about the young child from the mother, and at the same time you will be learning about the mother's attitude. If other siblings are present, observe the interaction among the family members.

What are the mother's facial expressions? In what tone of voice does she talk? Does she look away, or comfort the child, if the child seems disturbed with a procedure?

What are the other siblings' reactions toward the toddler, the mother, and the health care worker? What are the siblings' reactions in general?

Although the child may not talk much, general appearance can reveal a considerable amount of information. Does

the child look ill or well? What is the activity level? How do you describe his or her coordination? Gait, if walking? What are the child's reactions to parents, siblings, and the examiner? What is the nature of the child's cry? What do you learn from the child's facial expressions?

Before six months of age, the infant usually tolerates the examining table. Between six months and three to five years, most of the examination can be done from the lap of the mother or caretaker. After age four, much depends on the relationship you have established with the child.

The sequence of the examination with the young child should be from least discomfort to most discomfort. Undressing can be a gradual procedure, as children are often shy about this process. Some examiners prefer to go from toe to head, or at least to start with auscultation, which is painless and sometimes fascinating to the child. Measurement of length and height should be part of every health maintenance visit (along with the measurement of head circumference in the first two years of life). It is necessary to record these parameters on gender-appropriate growth curves, so measurements may be compared to the appropriate norm. These measurements should form part of the child's health record.[32]

It is best to leave the ears, nose, and mouth to the end because examination of these areas often initiates a negative response. Generally, the temperature should be taken rectally during the first years of life. Blood pressure should be taken with the cuff that will snugly fit the arm. The first reading is recommended at age three. The inflatable bladder should completely encircle the arm but not overlap. Artificially high indications of blood pressure result if the cuff is too narrow or too short.[33] Because this procedure causes some discomfort, and it is important to get readings in a low-anxiety state, sensitive timing is needed to obtain the desired results. It sometimes helps to make a game out of the procedure by allowing the toddler to help pump up the bulb or read the numbers on the gauge.

The skin can be examined for turgor by feeling the calf of the leg, which should be firm. **Spider nevi**, *pinhead-sized red dots from which blood vessels radiate*, are commonly found, as are **Mongolian spots**, *large, flat black or blue-and-black spots*. One or two *patches of light brown, non-elevated stains*, called **café au lait spots**, are within normal findings, but more than two may be indicative of fibromas or neurofibromas. **Bruises** (*ecchymoses*) are not abnormal in healthy active children, but their location is important. Bruises not on the extremities or not on areas easily hit when falling may indicate child abuse. Excessive bruising may indicate blood dyscrasias.[34]

Lymph nodes are palpable in almost all healthy young children. Small, mobile, non-tender nodes often point to previous infection.[35]

When examining the head region, consider the following:

- The auricles of the ears should be pulled back and down in young children, and back and up in older children.

- A complete hearing test with an audiometer should be completed before a child enters school. Before that, the whisper technique, or the use of a tuning fork, is adequate.

- A Snellen E-chart can be used for testing visual acuity before the child knows the alphabet. Visual acuity at three years is 20/40, and at four to five years is 20/30.

- Other aspects of the visual examination depend on the child's age, and on the suspected problem (e.g., after surgery for congenital cataracts).

- Teeth should be examined for their sequence of eruption, number, character, and position.[36]

When examining the thorax and lungs, remember that the breath sounds of young children are usually more intense and more bronchial, and expiration is more pronounced than it is in adults. The heart should be examined with the child erect, recumbent, and turned to the left. Sinus arrhythmia and extrasystoles can be benign, and are not uncommon.[37]

When standing, a child's abdomen may be protuberant; when lying down, it should disappear. The skilled examiner should be able to palpate both the liver and the spleen.[38]

When examining the male genitalia, the testicles should be examined while the male is warm and in a sitting position, holding his knees with heels on the seat of the chair or examining table. Without warmth and abdominal pressure, the testes may not be in the scrotum.[39]

Examination of the female genitalia is basically visual unless a specific problem in the area has developed.

When examining the extremities, the examiner may note bowlegs, which are common until 18 months. Knock-knees are common until approximately age 12. The toddler may appear flat-footed when first walking. All these characteristics are usually short term.[40]

The neurological examination is conducted throughout and is not much different from the sequence in the adult examination. However, the appropriate maturation level must be kept in mind.

## Nutritional Needs

Toddlerhood is an exciting time for changes. Attitudes are forming. Bodies are growing and maturing. Skills are being mastered. Youngsters get to know their world by using their senses, such as smelling and tasting.[41] Most two- and three-year-olds take pleasure in experimenting with new food. Two- and three-year-olds are striving for greater autonomy. They practise controlling their environment by deciding whether or not to eat something. For example, one day they may really like a particular food, and the next day they may reject it. It is important to understand that these whims are normal. Many toddlers insist on having their milk in a certain cup, or their food arranged or cut up in certain shapes. Most prefer meals and snacks on a regular schedule because they seek a sense of security. Serve small nutritious meals and snacks every day to meet their daily recommended Canada Food Guide servings. In addition, do not restrict nutritious foods because of their fat content. Offer a variety of foods from the four food groups.[42] When hungry, young children will focus on eating. When satisfied, their attention will turn elsewhere. *Eating Well with Canada's Food Guide* has been adapted for children by taking into account the smaller portions of food they eat. Consequently, the guide has become a useful tool for everyone in the family over two years of age.[43] See Figure 8-1 for a sample menu for a three-year-old girl.

The Food Guide gives a lower and higher number of servings for each food group. The range of these servings allows the Food Guide to be sufficiently flexible to use with family members with different energy and nutrient needs.[44] The following are general guidelines for children two to three years of age:

- Four servings per day of vegetables and fruits and three servings per day of grain products.

- Two servings per day of milk products. Toddlers and preschoolers should drink 500 mL (2 cups) of milk every day because it is their main dietary source of vitamin D. This amount can be counted as two

NARRATIVE VIGNETTE
## Toddler Checkup

You are working in a nursing station in rural Nova Scotia. A mother has brought in her three-year-old son for his yearly checkup. He has been sitting quietly on the floor playing, but looks up wide-eyed and appears somewhat anxious as you approach.

1. How will you begin your assessment?

2. What information will you seek from the mother?

3. Which of the child's behaviours might be noteworthy? For what reason(s)?

4. What significant health issues will you ensure that the mother comprehends?

**Figure 8-1** Sample one-day menu for Olivia, a three-year-old girl

| | Recommended Daily Food Guide Servings | | | |
|---|---|---|---|---|
| | **Vegetables and Fruit** | **Grain Products** | **Milk and Alternatives** | **Meat and Alternatives** |
| Girl 2 - 3 years | 4 | 3 | 2 | 1 |

| Foods | Number of Food Guide Servings | | | | |
|---|---|---|---|---|---|
| | **Vegetables and Fruit** | **Grain Products** | **Milk and Alternatives** | **Meat and Alternatives** | **Added Oils and Fats** |
| Breakfast<br>• ½ bowl of whole grain cereal (15 g)<br>• 125 mL (½ cup) of 2 % milk | | 1/2 | 1/2 | | |
| Snack<br>• 60 mL (¼ cup) carrots sticks and broccoli florets with salad dressing<br>• water | 1/2 | | | | ✔ |
| Lunch<br>• ½ salmon sandwich on whole wheat bread (made with 30 g or 1 oz of canned salmon and mayonnaise)<br>• 60 mL (¼ cup) red pepper strips and cucumber slices<br>• 125 mL (½ cup) milk<br>• 1 peach | 1/2<br><br>1 | 1 | 1/2 | 1/2 | ✔ |
| Snack<br>• oat rings cereal (15 g)<br>• 125 mL (½ cup) milk | | 1/2 | 1/2 | | |
| Dinner<br>• 125 mL (½ cup) spaghetti with tomato and meat sauce (about 40 g or 1 ½ oz of meat)<br>• 125 mL (½ cup) milk<br>• 125 mL (½ cup) applesauce | 1/2<br><br>1 | 1 | 1/2 | 1/2 | ✔ |
| Snack<br>• ½ banana | 1/2 | | | | |
| **Total Food Guide Servings for the day** | **4** | **3** | **2** | **1** | |

Source: Health Canada. E*ating Well with Canada's Food Guide: A Resource for Educators and Communicators*, Appendix A: Sample One-Day-Menus (p. 44). Ottawa: Health Canada, 2007.

**Figure 8-2** What amount of food should people eat?

| | Children | | | Teens | | Adults | | | |
|---|---|---|---|---|---|---|---|---|---|
| **RECOMMENDED NUMBER OF FOOD GUIDE SERVINGS PER DAY** | **2–3** | **4–8** | **9–13** | **14–18 Years** | | **19–50 Years** | | **51 + Years** | |
| | Girls and Boys | | | Females | Males | Females | Males | Females | Males |
| **Vegetables and Fruit** | 4 | 5 | 6 | 7 | 8 | 7–8 | 8–10 | 7 | 7 |
| **Grain Products** | 3 | 4 | 6 | 6 | 7 | 6–7 | 8 | 6 | 7 |
| **Milk and Alternatives** | 2 | 2 | 3–4 | 3–4 | 3–4 | 2 | 2 | 3 | 3 |
| **Meat and Alternatives** | 1 | 1 | 1–2 | 2 | 3 | 2 | 3 | 2 | 3 |
| The eating pattern also includes a small amount (30 to 45 mL or about 2 to 3 tablespoons) of unsaturated fat each day. | | | | | | | | | |

Source: Health Canada. *Eating Well with Canada's Food Guide: A Resource for Educators and Communicators*, Section 2: A Healthy Eating Pattern for Canadians (p. 5). Ottawa: Health Canada, 2007.

servings. In addition, parents may choose to include a child-size serving of other milk products such as cheese and yogurt.

■ Parents can choose one child-size serving of meat and alternatives each day. See Figure 8-2 and look at the 2–3 years column under Children.

See Figure 8-3 for tips that can help young children to follow Canada's Food Guide.

Malnutrition may lead to slower growth, tooth decay, lowered resistance to disease, and even death. Signs of malnutrition include abdominal swelling, lethargy, lack of attention to stimuli, lack of energy, diminished muscle strength and coordination, changes in skin colour, and hair loss. Apparently females are buffered better against the effects of malnutrition or illness than males are. Malnutrition delays growth, but children have great recuperative powers if malnutrition does not continue too long. When nutrition improves, growth usually takes place rapidly until norms for weight, height, and skeletal development are reached. For example, children who suffered early malnutrition but were provided good nutrition later performed as well on intellectual tests as did their peers.[45]

A hospitalized toddler frequently regresses. Refusing to feed self is one manifestation. The child needs a lot of emotional support. Children need to feel some kind of control over their destiny, and that they are not totally helpless and powerless. One way of ensuring some measure of control is by permitting the child to choose foods and by encouraging the child to feed himself or herself.[46]

## Play, Exercise, and Rest

**Play and Exercise** Children use play to experience their world and bring meaning to it. Play models the social framework that builds relationships for life, and it kindles imagination. It is through play that children learn best.[47]

Play is the business of the toddler. During play he or she exercises, learns to manage the body, improves muscular coordination and manual dexterity, increases awareness and organizes the surrounding world by scrutinizing objects, and develops beginning spatial and sensory perception. The child learns language, learns how to pay attention, and releases emotional tensions as he or she channels unacceptable urges, such as aggression, into acceptable activities. At the same time, the child translates feelings, drives, and fantasies into action and learns about self as a person. Through play, the toddler becomes socialized and begins to learn right from wrong. The child learns to have fun and to master things. See Figure 8-4.

The child has little interest in other children, except as a curious explorer. **Play**, at this age, is solitary and **parallel**; *he or she plays next to, but not with, other children.* There is little overt exchange, but there is satisfaction in being close to other children. The toddler is not interested in sharing toys, and is distressed by demands to share because he or she has a poorly defined sense of ownership. The toddler will play co-operatively with guidance, however.

Play time and positive relationships with the parents, siblings, and other family members help the toddler learn how to interact and be sociable and, over time, how to make friends. By the end of two years, most children imitate adults

**Figure 8-3** Tips for consumers: Help young children to follow Canada's Food Guide

## TIPS FOR CONSUMERS...

Help young children to follow Canada's Food Guide.

- ✔ Prepare meals that include foods from each of the four groups. For children, one Food Guide Serving from a food group such as Meat and Alternatives can be divided up into smaller amounts of food served throughout the day.

- ✔ Make sure to offer children a total of two cups of milk or fortified soy beverage every day. This will help meet their requirement for vitamin D.

- ✔ Offer a variety of nutritious foods, including some choices that contain fat such as milk and peanut butter.

- ✔ Make time for healthy eating so that children don't feel rushed. Set regular times for meals and snaks. This helps to establish a healthy routine.

- ✔ Sit down and eat with children. Provide a pleasant setting. Leave the television off during meal times.

- ✔ Let children help with simple food-related tasks. Ask them to set the table or help to wash the vegetables.

- ✔ Keep in mind that while parents and caregivers are responsible for what children eat, children are responsible for how much they eat. Offer suitable portions with options for seconds.

- ✔ Be patient. If an unfamiliar food is rejected the first time, it can be offered again later. The more often children are exposed to new foods, the more likely they are to accept them.

- ✔ Be a positive role model for children. They will be more likely to enjoy a variety of foods and to try new foods if you do.

- ✔ Organize fun and easy physical activities such as bicycling, walking, dancing, games of ball or tag in the summer and sledding or building a snowman in the winter. Young children rely on parents and caregivers to provide opportunities for physical activity.

Source: Health Canada. *Eating Well with Canada's Food Guide: A Resource for Educators and Communicators.* Ottawa: Health Canada, 2007. © Adapted and reproduced with the permission of the Minister of Public Works and Government Services Canada, 2008.

in dramatic play by doing such things as setting the table and cooking. When selecting play materials for the toddler, remember his or her likes and dislikes. Choose a variety of activities because the attention span is short. (The safety and durability aspects of toys, as discussed in Chapter 7, must be considered.)

Father is likely to continue the same kind of play pattern with the toddler as with the infant. Fathers tend to jostle the young child more and to devote more time to play, than do mothers.[48] Fathers are more likely than mothers to use their own body as a portable, interactive monkey bar or rocking horse. From infancy on, father helps the child to individuate by being willing to let the child move out of sight and will let a child crawl or move twice as far as mother allows before retrieving the child. When a child confronts a novel situation, a new toy, a stranger, or a dog, mothers move closer to support the child and offer reassurance with their presence. Meanwhile, fathers tend to stay back and let the child explore by him- or herself. The child needs to be exposed to both the comfort and the challenges.[49]

**Figure 8-4** The link between play and learning

> **The Link Between *Play* and *Learning***
>
> - Play nurtures children's creativity and problem solving capabilities.
> - Play is health promoting. It builds children's strength and coordination and is beneficial for children's emotional health.
> - Play stimulates the healthy development of children's brains.
> - Play allows children to acquire competence and skills that help them feel good about themselves.
> - Play provides the context in which caring adults teach children how to behave, how to treat others, and the social conventions of the community.
> - Play provides the opportunity to learn essential social skills: to take turns, to share, and to cooperate.
> - Play helps children develop friendships with their peers: good interpersonal skills are essential to children's lifelong success.
> - Play environments produce natural opportunities for children to learn self-respect and how to treat others with respect.
> - Play promotes a child's development and their development enhances their play, creating an upward spiral.

Source: Canadian Child Care Federation. Supporting Children to Learn through Play, Resource Sheet #77. Ottawa: CCCF, 2005. Used with the permission of Canadian Child Care Federation.

However, when the father is the primary caregiver, he interacts with the young child in much the same way as the mother does, by smiling frequently and imitating the child's facial expressions and vocalizations. The father continues to be quite physical with the child during interaction. As fathers assume greater responsibility for young child care due to changing social and cultural conditions and expectations, mothers and fathers are likely to interact more similarly with their young children.[50]

Table 8-2 presents suggested play activities and equipment for the child 18 months or 2 years of age.

*Teach parents the importance of play and safety.* A relationship exists between the quality of attachment between mother and baby and the quality of play and problem-solving behaviour at two years of age. Toddlers who are securely attached at 18 months are more enthusiastic, persistent, co-operative, and able to share than if secure attachment has not developed. There is also more frequent and sophisticated interaction with peers at three years when secure attachment has formed in infancy.[51] Discuss play patterns and toys with the parents.

Help parents to realize the importance of offering playthings that can transform into any number of toys, depending on the child's mood and imagination at the time. The adult can be available, but initially should start a play activity with the child. Soon, however, the child should be encouraged to play independently, developing mastery, autonomy, and self-esteem in the process.

## CRITICAL THINKING

*What role does gender play in the parental choices of play activities for toddlers?*

---

**Table 8-2** Suggested Play Activities and Equipment for Toddlers

| Age (months) | Toy, Equipment, or Activity |
| --- | --- |
| 18 | Push-pull toys (cars, trucks, farm tools) |
| | Boxes and toys for climbing |
| | Empty and fill toys (plastic food containers, kitchen utensils, small boxes, and open-close toys) |
| | Big picture books—thick-paged, colourful, sturdy (child will turn two or three pages at a time, tear at thin pages, can identify one picture at a time) |
| | Stuffed animals with no detachable parts |
| | Baby dolls, large enough to hug, carry, cuddle, dress, and feed |
| | Big pieces of plain paper or newspaper layers and crayons for scribbling |
| | Small blocks—builds a tower of two or three at a time |
| | Shape-sorting blocks or cubes |
| | Small chair; small furniture to play "house" |

*(continued)*

Table 8-2 (continued)

| Age (months) | Toy, Equipment, or Activity |
|---|---|
| | Toy farm animals or equipment |
| | Rubber or soft ball; throws overhand |
| | Phonograph record, preferably sturdy plastic that child can manipulate by self; musical and sound toys; musical instruments simple to use |
| | Rocking horse; rocking chair |
| 24 | All of the above are enjoyed; child now turns book or magazine pages singly—still tears; builds tower of seven blocks and aligns cubes |
| | Makes circular strokes with crayon, enjoys fingerpaints |
| | Puppets |
| | Pedal toys; dumping toys (dump trucks) |
| | Sandbox toys |
| | Play dough and clay; mud |
| | Jungle gym for climbing; sand box; small water pool for waterplay |
| | Pounding toys—hammer and pegs, drums, small boards |
| | Picture puzzles—two to four pieces (wooden or thick cardboard) |
| | Large, coloured wooden beads to string |
| | Simple trains, cars, boats, planes to push–pull or sit on and pedal |
| | Kicks ball |
| | Likes to run |

**Rest** Rest is as essential as exercise and play. Although a child may be tired after a day full of exploration and exerting boundless energy, bedtime is often a difficult experience. Bedtime means loneliness and separation from fun, family, and, most importantly, the mother figure. The toddler needs an average of 12 to 14 hours of sleep nightly plus a daytime nap no longer than 3 hours.[52] The sleep schedule may be as follows:

| 15 months | Morning nap is shorter; needs afternoon nap. |
|---|---|
| 17 to 24 months | Will have trouble falling asleep. |
| 18 months | Brings stuffed toy or pillow. |
| 19 months | Sleeps fairly well, tries to climb out of bed. |
| 20 months | May awaken with nightmares. |
| 21 months | May rest quietly and, at times, sleep for shorter periods during afternoon nap. |
| 24 months | Total sleep time reduced, tries to delay bedtime; continues to need afternoon nap or rest. |
| 2 to 3 years | Can be changed from crib to bed. Needs rails on side to prevent falling out. |

*Teach the following guidelines to parents for establishing a bedtime routine for the toddler:*

■ Set a definite bedtime routine and adhere to it. If the child is overly tired, he or she becomes agitated and difficult to put to sleep.

■ Establish a bedtime ritual, including bath, a story, soft music (some young children prefer classical), quiet talking and holding, and a tucking-in routine. Reduce noise and stimuli in the house. Avoid television, movies, or videos that show loud or aggressive scenes. Begin approximately 30 minutes before bedtime. The tucking-in should be caring and brief.

■ If the child cries, which most children do, briefly return in a few minutes to provide reassurance. Do not pick up the child, or stay longer than 30 seconds. If the crying continues, return in five minutes and repeat the procedure. Thus, the parent can determine whether there is any real problem, and ensure that the child feels secure.

■ If extended crying continues, lengthen the time to ten minutes before returning to the child. Eventually, fatigue will occur, the cry will turn to whimpers, and the child will fall asleep.

■ The child should remain in his or her bed, rather than sleep for all or part of the night with the parents. Bedtime routine becomes a precedent for other separations. However, if the parents make an occasional

### Toddler Development

The setting is an urban daycare centre. The grassy play area outdoors has a sandbox, a variety of climbing and swing play equipment, and wheeled toys. It looks inviting. Indoors, we find wide hallways and a cubicle for each child's clothing and personal items. There is a large room where the children can play. All of these facilities indicate that this is a busy centre. The large room has several distinct play areas: a house corner, a large block corner, a music area with piano and other children's instruments, a reading corner with books, and an art area with large sheets of paper and crayons, pencils, chalk, and finger-paints. Tables in the middle of the room are piled with toys. Large windows face the playground; potted plants and an aquarium add life to the bustling room.

Luis, 18 months of age, is a typical toddler: 11 kg (24 pounds) and 70 cm (28 inches) tall. Occasionally, he falls as he walks around the room, but he rises to his feet without help. He pulls a toy truck, then sits on a tractor and pushes himself with his feet. In a few minutes a pink ball on a shelf catches his attention, and he runs to it, grasping it with hands and forearms. He repeatedly sets the ball on the shelf to play with a nearby toy, but returns again for the ball.

While Luis is holding the ball, another toddler approaches him to get it. Luis yanks away, displaying the typical toddler's egocentricism and inability to share. The other child hits Luis, who cries to get the teacher's attention and support. The teacher talks to each child. She encourages them to hug each other and be friendly. She then plays with the two children briefly as they share the ball. In a few minutes, each child has been distracted to engage in another activity in the room.

Before lunch, the teacher calls the group together for story time, which is limited to ten minutes because of the short attention spans of toddlers. During this time the toddlers repeat a nursery rhyme that was part of the story and then sing the rhyme, demonstrating rote memory. Luis and the other toddlers enjoy music and rhyming play.

1. After assessing this situation, how would you describe the teacher's behaviour toward the toddlers?
2. How would you describe Luis's behaviour?
3. What type of attachment does Luis display? State your rationale.
4. Give another example of an appropriate activity exercise for the toddlers.

exception, such as during a family crisis of major loss, trauma, or transition, or if the child is ill, neither the marriage relationship nor the child's development will be hindered. It is important that the exception not become the routine.

As the child grows older, limit the number of times the child can get up, for any reason, after going to bed.

Sleep problems during hospitalization may show up through restlessness, insomnia, and nightmares. Increasingly, hospitals are permitting parents to spend the night in the child's room to lessen fears and separation anxiety. Cuddling is still important to a toddler, especially if hospitalized. If a parent cannot remain with a frightened child, you can hold and rock him or her while he or she holds a favourite object.

### CRITICAL THINKING

*What other strategies might you pursue with a frightened child who is unable to sleep?*

## Health Promotion and Health Prevention Routine Immunizations

Immunizations remain a vital part of health care. The toddler needs to continue the immunization process that was begun in infancy. See Table 7-6 for a routine immunization schedule for infants and children, or consult the *Canadian Immunization Guide* (2006) for more information regarding immunization schedules.

**Safety Promotion and Injury Control** Accidents, at the toddler stage, are common health threats. The main causes of accidents include motor vehicles, burns, suffocation, drowning, poisoning, and falls. Accidents are a major cause of death.[53]

Because children delight in exploring the world around them, they are vulnerable to injuries when they are in a vehicle or to being hit by a moving vehicle.[54]

Safety, both outdoors and indoors, is a must for the toddler. It is necessary to childproof the home. *Teach parents that they can prevent injury from furniture by:*

- Selecting furniture with rounded corners and a sturdy base
- Packing away breakable objects
- Putting safety catches on doors to prevent the child from opening furniture doors, or from pulling furniture on self
- Disconnecting unused appliances, coiling and tying up cords, and securing cords that are in use

*They can prevent falls by:*

- Avoiding hazardous waxing
- Discarding throw rugs
- Keeping traffic lanes clear

- Placing gates at tops of stairways and screens on the windows
- Placing toys and favourite objects on a low shelf
- Using appropriate child safety seats in the car and grocery cart

Burns are prevented by blocking access to electric outlets (safety plugs for wall sockets can be purchased), heating equipment, matches, lighters, hot water or hot food, stoves, fireplaces, and appliances that heat. Handles of pans should be turned to the back of the stove. Electric cords attached to appliances that heat should not drape over the top edge of a work surface or counter. Fireworks should never be used when a young child is nearby. Placing tools and knives high on the wall, or in a locked cabinet, can prevent lacerations or more serious injury. Any surface that is sharp may cut the child and should be covered, or kept out of the sight of the child. It is important to note that areas outside the home—the yard, the street, the grocery cart—have higher hazard because today there is considerable contact with them.

Due to the numerous accidental fires occurring in homes, it is important to make certain that the home is well equipped with working smoke alarms and carbon monoxide detectors. Further, it is highly recommended that families develop, and practise, a fire escape plan together.

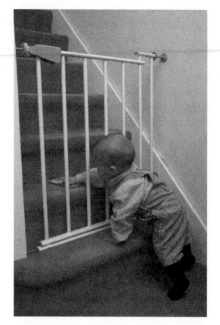

Toddlers should be prevented from climbing stairs, for example, by a portable gate.

## CRITICAL THINKING

*How would you go about teaching a family home fire safety in a rural area?*

Parents may call you to help when their child has been injured or is ill. *Know emergency care.* Many cities have poison-control centres to treat and give information to parents and professionals. Suggest that parents call Safe Kids Canada (1-888-SAFE-TIPS) or the Infant and Toddler Safety Association (519-570-0181). The local Canadian Red Cross is also a source of first-aid information, as is the St. John Ambulance. To find the contact information for the St. John Ambulance branch nearest you, visit www.sja.ca.

Explore thoroughly safety promotion with the parents, because the following normal developmental characteristics make the toddler prone to accidents. He or she:

- Moves quickly and is impulsive
- Is inquisitive and assertive
- Enjoys learning by touch, taste, and sight
- Enjoys playing with small objects
- Likes to attract attention
- Has a short attention span and unreliable memory

- Lacks judgment
- Has incomplete self-awareness
- Imitates the actions of others

Educate parents to teach the toddler to swim. Always stay with and constantly watch the child when he or she is near water. Boisterous play and sharp objects should not be allowed near a swimming pool, jungle gym, or sandbox. Provide safety equipment and supervision. Regarding product safety, urge adults to keep cleaners and other poisons away from toddlers. It is important to keep all cleaners in their original containers and to show children the hazard symbols.[55] See the box entitled "Parent Teaching to Prevent Poisoning."

## Common Health Problems: Promotion and Prevention

The child must be carefully assessed for infections and other disease conditions because he or she lacks the cognitive, verbal, and self-awareness capacities to describe discomforts. Table 8-3 summarizes common conditions.[56]

Consult pediatric nursing texts for additional information on childhood illnesses and their assessment, care, and prevention.[57]

## PSYCHOSOCIAL CONCEPTS

The following information will assist you to understand the toddler's behaviour, plan and give developmentally based care, promote health, and teach parents about the child.

Table 8-3 Common Health Problems of Toddlers

| Problem | Definition | Signs/Symptoms | Prevention/Treatment |
|---|---|---|---|
| **Myopia** | Nearsightedness | Squinting, not seeing far away | Prescribed glasses, use cards to check vision; 30 ft (9 m) represents maximum distance at which child should identify object; if identified at 15 ft (4.5 m), vision is 15/30 |
| **Astigmatism** | Unequal curvature in the refractive surfaces of the eyes | Cannot clearly focus | Prescribed glasses, use Allen cards to check vision; 30 ft (9 m) represents the maximum distance at which child should identify object; if identified at 15 ft (4.5 m), vision is 15/30 |
| **Strabismus** | Eyes are not straight or properly aligned | One or both eyes may turn in, turn out, turn up or down; may be consistent or come and go | Prescribed treatment to bring the deviating eye back into binocular vision before age 6 by wearing a patch over the better aligned eye |
| **Hearing impairment** | Hearing less than normal for age group | Inability to speak by age 2; failure to respond to out-of-sight noise; tilting the head while listening | Observe child carefully for appropriate hearing; check with practitioner to see if ear or upper respiratory problem is to blame; teach lip reading and sign language if appropriate |
| **Otitis media** | Infection of middle ear with accumulation of seropurulent fluid in middle ear cavity | Earache; fever; upper respiratory infection; decreased hearing; bulging tympanic membrane; disappearance of landmarks | Medication (antibiotic), sometimes decongestant; follow-up examination |
| **Dental caries** | Tooth decay often related to excess concentrated sweets or bottle mouth syndrome | Obvious dark places or breakdown of teeth; pain | Supplemental fluoride; avoidance of sweets; directions to parents for cleaning teeth on (hydrogen peroxide gauze before 18 months then a soft toothbrush) Prepare for first dental visit with explanation, role play, and positive image If problem with discoloured teeth, infection, chipping, see dentist immediately |

*(continued)*

Table 8-3 (continued)

| Problem | Definition | Signs/Symptoms | Prevention/Treatment |
|---|---|---|---|
| **Malabsorption syndrome** | Lactose intolerance | Chronic vomiting; diarrhea; abdominal discomfort; flatulence, irritability; poor sleep pattern | Try other products besides milk (e.g., soybean formula) |
| **Impetigo** | Lesions caused by micro-organism (usually *Streptococcus Species*), often a complication of insect bites, abrasions, or dermatitis | Upper layers of skin have honey-coloured, fluid-filled vesicles that eventually crust, surrounded by a red base | Identification of lesions significant because acute glomerulonephritis can follow if not properly treated; trim fingernails to avoid scratching; wash and scrub lesions gently three times daily; wash towels used on infected areas separately; oral or topical antibiotics |
| **Pharyngitis** | Inflammation of pharynx or tonsils, or both, caused by virus or group *A Streptococcus Species* and rarely *Mycoplasma pneumonia* and *Corynebacterium diphtheria* | Red throat, exudates, enlarged lymph nodes; fever; other upper respiratory infectious symptoms | Get specific diagnosis with throat culture; treat with antibiotic if bacterial cause to avoid further disease complications; antipyretic medicine if fever present. Do not give salicylates to children because of possible Reye's syndrome, a rare but sometimes fatal disease. Warm saline gargle if able; increased fluid intake |
| **Acute nonspecific gastroenteritis** (*simple diarrhea*) | Inflammation of the gastrointestinal tract during which stools are more liquid and frequent than usual | May cause dehydration with signs of sunken eyes, dry mucous membranes, decreased skin turgor, and weight loss | Discontinue milk; give small amounts of clear liquids such as flat soda (at room temperature) alternating with an electrolyte solution; add simple foods slowly |
| **Varicella** (*chickenpox*) | Acute, highly contagious disease caused by varicella zoster virus | Rash consisting of lesions that appear in crops and that go from flat macules to fluid-filled vesicles that crust in 6–8 hours; spread is from trunk to periphery and sometimes into the mouth; itching; fever; headache; general malaise; loss of appetite | Give vaccine when available; keep fingernails short; use lotions or prescription drug if itching intense; antipyretic drug if fever; isolate until lesions are all crusted |

*(continued)*

Table 8-3 (continued)

| Problem | Definition | Signs/Symptoms | Prevention/Treatment |
|---|---|---|---|
| **Rubella** (*3-day measles*) | Viral disease characterized by rash and lymph node enlargement | Rash on face or neck, spreading to trunk and extremities; rash usually gone in 3 days | Prevention: immunization—a very serious disease during pregnancy, associated with high degree of congenital malformation; mild disease treated symptomatically for the toddler, but to be avoided by all |
| **Pinworms** (*Enterobius vermicularis*) | Most common parasite infestation in North America; cycle begins with oral infection of pinworm eggs which pass through intestinal tract in 15–28 days, hatch into larva and then into adult worms | Possibly asymptomatic; itching around anus; 2.5 cm (1-inch) white thread-like worms visible on perineum, especially when child at rest | Medication (treat all family members); personal hygiene; washing all laundry and bedclothes in hot water; clean favourite stuffed animals, chairs, and rugs, which may harbour eggs |
| **Miliaria rubra** (*"heat rash"* or *"prickly heat"*) | Erythematous papular rash distributed in area of sweat glands | Fine red, raised rash; itching, pustules in neck and axillary region | Keep environment cool and dry; use air conditioner/fan; tepid baths; light clothing; use Caldesene powder; use sparingly 1% hydrocortisone cream |
| **Viral croup** (*laryngotracheo-bronchitis*; usually caused by Parainfluenza virus in late fall or early winter) | Inflammation of the respiratory mucosa of all airways; edema of the larynx and subglottic area | Gradual onset of upper respiratory infection; inspiratory stridor; low-grade fever; barking cough; wheezing; hoarseness; high-pitched sound on inspiration | Keep child well hydrated; use cool mist vaporizer; force liquids; take child in bathroom and turn on hot water; take child outside; if airway obstruction present, seek help immediately |

## Cognitive Development

The intellectual capacity of the toddler is limited. The child has all of the body equipment that allows for an assimilation of the environment, but his or her intellectual maturity is just beginning.

Learning occurs through several general modes:[58]

■ Natural unfolding of the innate physiologic capacity

■ Imitation of others

■ Reinforcement from others as the child engages in acceptable behaviour

■ Insight, gaining understanding in increasing depth as he or she plays, experiments, or explores

■ Identification, taking into self values and attitudes like those with whom he or she is closely associated through use of the other modes

The toddler's attention span lengthens. He or she likes songs, nursery rhymes, and stories, even though he or she does not fully understand simple explanations of them. He or she can name pictures on repeated exposure, plays alone sometimes but prefers being near people, and is aware of self and others in a new way.

Part of the toddler's learning is through imitation of the parents, helping them with simple tasks such as bringing an object, trying new activities on his or her own, the ritualistic repetition of an activity, experimenting with language,

- Teach the child that medication and vitamins are not candy; keep them locked away. Discard old medicine.

- Keep medicines, polishes, insecticides, drain cleaners, bleaches, household chemicals, garage products, and other potentially toxic substances in a locked cabinet out of the child's reach. Do not store them in containers previously used for food.

- Store non-food substances in original containers with labels attached, not in food or beverage containers.

- If you are interrupted while pouring or using a product that is potentially harmful, take it with you. The toddler is curious and impulsive, and moves quickly.

- Keep telephone numbers of the physician, poison control centre, local hospital, and police and fire departments by the telephone.

- Teach the child not to eat berries, flowers, or plants; some are poisonous.

and expressing self emotionally. According to Piaget, the toddler completes the fifth and sixth stages of the sensorimotor period and begins the preoperational period at approximately age two.[59]

In the **fifth stage of the sensorimotor period** (12 to 18 months), the child consolidates previous activities involving body actions into *experiments* to discover newly realized properties of objects and events and to achieve new goals, instead of applying previously habitual behaviour. He or she no longer keeps repeating the same behaviour to achieve a goal,

## CONTROVERSY DEBATE

# Safety with Cleansers

You are conducting a home visit with a young lone parent, Susan, who has a three-year-old toddler and an infant. Susan proudly shows you that she has placed each of her cleaning agents in its own container, which is identical to all the others. She states that it took her a lot of time to label each container with felt marker and to cut out the hazard labels from the original containers and attach them to the new containers.

1. How should you respond to Susan?

2. What health promoting strategies will you teach Susan?

but performs familiar acts with fewer random manoeuvres. The child differentiates self from objects in the environment. Understanding of *object permanence*, *space perception*, and *time perception* can be observed in new ways. The child is now aware that objects continue to exist even though they cannot be seen. He or she accounts for sequential displacements and searches for objects where they were *last* seen. The toddler manipulates objects in new and various ways to learn what they will do. For the first time, objects outside the self are understood as causes of action. Activities are now linked to internal representations or symbolic meaning of events or objects (memories, ideas, and feelings about past events).[60]

The **sixth stage of the sensorimotor period** (18 to 24 months) seems primarily to be a transitional phase to the preoperative period. Now the child does less trial-and-error thinking, and uses the memory of a past experience, and imitation, to appear as if he or she arrived at an answer. He or she is now able to imitate another who is out of sight. The toddler begins to solve problems, to foresee manoeuvres that will succeed or fail, and to remember an object that is absent and search for it until it is found.[61]

In the **preoperational period** (two to seven years), thought is predominantly symbolic. Memory continues to form, and the child internalizes mental pictures of people, the environment, and ideas about rules and relationships. The child begins to arrive at answers mentally, instead of through physical activity, exploration, and manipulation. Symbolic representation is seen in:

1. Use of language to describe (symbolize) objects, events, and feelings.

2. Beginning of symbolic play (crossing two sticks to represent an airplane).

3. Delayed imitation (repeating a parent's behaviour hours later).[62]

The toddler can understand simple abstractions, but thinking is basically concrete (related to tangible events) and literal. He or she is **egocentric** (*unable to take the viewpoint of another*). The ability to differentiate between subject and object, the real object and the word symbol, is not yet developed. He or she knows only one word for any object and cannot understand how the one word *chair* can refer to many different styles of chairs. If the flower is called *flower* and *plant*, the child will not understand that more than one word can refer to the same object. The concept of time is *now*, and the concept of distance is whatever can be seen. The child imitates the thinking and behaviour observed in another, but lacks the past experience and broader knowledge that is essential for logical thought. This level of learning will continue through the preschool era.[63]

Over the past decade, a considerable body of literature has been generated toward understanding cognitive development in infancy. Piaget's views on infancy have dominated the field for many years. Recent research suggests, however, that infants have the ability to conceptualize earlier than previously believed.[64] In fact, Aguiar and Baillargeon conducted a study to examine whether 8.5-month-old infants take into account the width and compressibility of an object when determining whether it can be inserted into a container. Their results indicated that by 8.5 months of age, infants are already capable of sophisticated reasoning about containment events.[65]

Pushing children to read and write at an early age has not been shown to produce long-lasting positive effects. Pushing may cause the child to lose initiative, curiosity, the desire to use ingenuity, and the ability to cope with ordinary life stresses. The child knows inside what he or she can do. If the parents to whom the child looks for support and guidance are manipulating him or her to meet their needs, the child may come to mistrust parents and self. Before parents put the child in a preschool that emphasizes formal academics, they should consider what the child might not be learning from missed playtime. Play that is parallel to and co-operative with peers helps the child to develop language, motor, cognitive, nonverbal, and social skills; positive self-esteem; a sense of worth as an individual; and unique problem-solving skills in the face of stress.[66]

Teach parents about this aspect of development. See the box entitled "Examples of Educational Toys and Play for the Toddler." This period can be trying and should be tempered by supportive guidance and discipline: parents' saying what is meant, providing environmental stimulation, showing interest in the child's activities and talking and working with the child, reinforcing intellectual attempts, and showing a willingness to teach with simple explanations. Much of the child's intellectual development as a toddler depends on the achievements of infancy. It matters how parents used the baby's potential, and the *quality of parent–child interaction rather than the amount of time, per se, that is spent with the child*.[67] The interactive system between the mother and the child is important. It depends on the mother's development of an emotional synchronization with her child. That is, the mother's ability to be in tune with the infant's states and to respond accordingly is significant. This process enables the mother and infant to engage in meaningful teaching/learning interaction. Lipari[68] provides a particularly insightful explanation of emotional synchrony.

## CRITICAL THINKING

*On a biological level, what might be the effects of emotional synchronization?*

# Language Development

Learning to communicate in an understandable manner begins during toddlerhood. Through speech, the toddler will gradually learn to control unacceptable behaviour, exchange physical activity for words, and share the views of reality held by society. The child is capable of considerable learning, including more than one language, and words of simple songs and prayers. Long before they can speak, children are initiated into their culture and speech by the language and words of their parents and significant caregivers.[69]

The ability to speak words and sentences is not governed by the same higher centre that controls understanding. The child understands words before they are used with meaning, and some children develop adequate comprehension but cannot speak.[70]

Various theories explain language acquisition. Although behavioural or learning theory explains some language learning through receiving reinforcement for the imitation of language sounds, the number of specific stimulus-response connections that would be necessary to speak even one language could not be acquired in a lifetime. Nor do behaviourists explain the sequence of language development, regardless of culture; however, learning principles can be used to modify acquired language deficits.[71]

Interactionist theory is used by most theorists to explain language development. Language develops through interaction between heredity, maturation, encounters with people and environmental stimuli, and life experiences. Humans are biologically prepared for language learning, but experience with the spoken word and with loving people who facilitate language acquisition are equally essential. Further, the child has an active role rather than a passive one in learning language. Adults usually modify their speech when talking to a child, and as a result the child is more attentive to the simplified speech. Mothers and fathers use different conversational techniques to talk with the child, which in turn teaches the child language in a broader way.[72] At York University in Toronto, researchers related mothers' scaffolding efforts to their toddlers' vocabulary at 15 months. It was concluded that greater efforts at scaffolding were associated with toddlers having larger vocabularies.[73] Scaffolding refers to the structuring of a child's learning experience.[74]

*Speech* and *language* are two of the major adaptive behaviours developed during the second year. Speech enables the child to become more independent and to make needs known more effectively. Speech is the mediation for thought processes. The greater the comprehension and vocabulary a child has, the further a child can go in cognitive processes. As the child and parents respond verbally

**13 to 15 months**
Toy telephone
Toy horse for rocking, rocking chair
Carriage, or other toys, for pushing and pulling
Household objects, such as pots or pans and unbreakable cups, or food cartons of various sizes for nesting and stacking
Pot lids for banging together
Wooden blocks of various sizes and shapes for stacking
Large plastic clothespins
Large balls and stuffed animals
Toys that encourage acrobatic movement

**16 to 18 months**
Sandbox, and toys that can be pushed through sand
Simple musical instruments, such as a tambourine and drum
Large coloured beads
Jack-in-the-box
Equipment for blowing bubbles, with adult help

**19 to 21 months**
Rocking horse
Kiddie cars
Toys to take apart and fit together
Small rubber balls
Digging toys
Large crayons, large sheets of paper
Easy puzzles, with large and few pieces, colourful pictures of animals, foods, and other objects in the environment made of sturdy material or wood

Dirt for making mud pies
Big cardboard boxes to play hide and seek (self and others)

**22 to 24 months**
Kiddie lawn mower
Kitchen sets for make-believe play, including toy utensils
Modelling clay
Construction blocks or sets
Action toys (e.g., toy trains, dump trucks, cars, and fire engines)
Old magazines that can be used to point out pictures and can be torn up
Baskets, boxes, and tubes of various sizes have multiple uses in action and fantasy play
Containers (e.g., pots, pans) with lids

**2 to 3 years**
Dolls, male and female, various ethnicities, with accessories such as clothing, strollers, baby bottle, feeding utensils
Beginner tricycle
Kiddie swimming pool
Mini-trampoline
Age-appropriate roller skates
Swing set, mini-basketball hoop
Dress-up clothes (parents' and older siblings' clothing no longer used) for male and female
Crayons, markers, fingerpaints, large sheets of paper
Colouring books, not too detailed in design
Easel or chalkboard and chalk
Kiddie woodworking bench

Note: Toys played with at an earlier age continue to be enjoyed, especially if they can be used in different ways or with different actions. Puppets and age-appropriate musical devices and cloth or vinyl books should be available throughout toddlerhood.

---

and nonverbally to each other, the child learns attitudes and values, and behaviours and ideas. The child first responds to patterns of sounds rather than to specific word sounds. If others speak indistinctly to the child, he or she will also speak indistinctly. The normal child will begin to speak by 14 months, although some children may make little effort to speak until after two years of age. By age three, children may still mispronounce more than half of their sounds.

The toddler speaks in the present tense initially, using **syncretic speech**, in which *one word stands for a certain object, and has a limited range of sounds*. Single words represent entire sentences; for example, "go" means "I want to go." By 18 to 20 months, he or she uses **telegraphic speech**, *two- to four-word expressions that contain a noun and verb and maintain word order*, such as "go play" and "go night-night." Variety of intonation also increases. A two-year-old will introduce additional words and say "I go play" or "I go night-night."

Conversation with parents involves contraction and expansion. The *child shortens into fewer words what the parent says but states the main message* (**contraction**); the *parent elaborates on, uses a full sentence, and interprets what the child says* (**expansion**). Expansion helps the child's language development. The toddler frequently says "no," perhaps in imitation of the parents and their discipline techniques, but may often do what is asked even while saying "no." Stuttering is common because ideas come faster than the ability to use vocabulary.

Recognizable language develops sequentially. See Table 8-4 for a summary of language and speech development.[75]

The toddler's speech is **autistic** because *vocalizations have specific meaning only to the child*. He or she plays with sounds and incorrectly produces the majority of consonant sounds.

Apparently the child learns to speak in a highly methodical way, breaking down language into its simplest

## Table 8-4 Assessment of Language and Speech Development

| Characteristics | 1 Year | 1½ Years | 2 Years | 2½ Years |
|---|---|---|---|---|
| Language understanding and basic communication | Understands "no-no" inhibition; knows "bye-bye" and pat-a-cake; says "mama," "dada," or some similar term for caretakers | Understands very simple verbal instructions accompanied by gesture and intonation; identifies 3 body parts; points to 5 simple pictures; points for wants | Identifies 5 body parts; finds 10 pictures; obeys simple commands | Points to 15 pictures; obeys 2 or 3 simple commands |
| Appearance of individual sounds | 10 vowels, 9 consonants in babbling and echoing | *p, b, m, h, w* in babbling | | *t, d, n, k, g, ng* in words |
| Auditory memory imitation and repetition | Lalls; imitates sound; echoes or repeats syllables or some words (may not have meaning) | | Meanings increasingly becoming associated with words | Repeats 2 digits; remembers 1 or 2 objects |
| Numerical size of vocabulary | 1 or 2 words | Adds 10–20 words a week | 50–300 words if consistently spoken to | 400–500 words |
| Word type | Nouns | Nouns, action verbs, some adjectives | Nouns, verbs, adjectives, adverbs | Pronouns, "I" |
| Sentence length | Single word | Single words expanding to 3 or 4 words, noun and verb | 2–5 words; elemental sentence | Basic sentence |
| Description of vocalization and communication | Babbling, lalling, echolalia (repeating sounds) | Leading, pointing, jargon, some words, intonations, gestures | Words, phrases, simple sentences | Developmental language problems first seen |
| Purpose of vocalization and communication | Pleasure | Attention getting | Meaningful social control; wish requesting | Interaction; express needs; convey yearnings |
| Speech content and style | | | Possessive "mine"; pronouns last grammar form learned; grammar depends on what is heard | |
| Percent intelligibility | | 20–25% for person unfamiliar with child | 60–75%; poor articulation of some words | Vowel production— 90% |

Sources: Santrock, J.W., A. MacKenzie-Rivers, K. Ho Leung, and T. Malcomson, *Life-span Development*, 2nd Canadian ed. Toronto: McGraw-Hill Ryerson, 2005; Papalia, D., S. Olds, and R. Feldman, *Human Development*, 9th ed. Boston: McGraw-Hill, 2004; Seifert, K., R. Hoffnung, and M. Hoffnung, *Lifespan Development*. Boston: Houghton Mifflin, 1997; Wong, D., S. Perry, M. Hockenberry, D. Lowdermilk, and D. Wilson, *Maternal Child Nursing Care*, 3rd ed. St. Louis, MO: C.V. Mosby, 2006.

parts and developing rules to put the parts together. Children proceed from babbling to one- and two-word sentences. They begin to use word order, plurals, and negative sentences, and phonetics and sounds become important. To communicate effectively, the child must learn not only the language and its rules, but also the use of social speech, which takes into account the knowledge and perspective of another person.[76] This complicated process begins in toddlerhood and continues to develop through childhood as the child gains interpersonal and social experiences.

CRITICAL THINKING

*What are a few strategies adults can use to help the child use more words?*

Teach parents that speech is facilitated when they teach social language strategies to the child as they introduce him or her to new life experiences. Through conversation with the family, both at mealtimes and in other activities, vocabulary is enlarged, and the child learns family expressions that aid in his or her socialization. Mealtime provides a miniature society in which the toddler can feel secure in attempting to imitate speech. He or she gets positive reinforcement for speech efforts, especially for words that are selected, repeated frequently, and reinforced by eager parents.

In addition, being talked with, using adult words rather than baby talk frequently throughout the day, being read to, and having an opportunity to explore the environment all help to increase the child's comprehension of words and rules of grammar. These activities help the child to organize and increase the size of vocabulary and the use of correct word inflections.[77]

Researchers from Carleton University in Ottawa claim that shared book reading provides a rich source of linguistic stimulation for young children.[78] The findings from their two experiments suggest that storybook experiences during the preschool years (ages three to six) may be the single most important influence on the development of language skills for children.[79]

*Language development requires a sense of security, as well as verbal and nonverbal stimulation.* For a child to speak well, he or she must have a loving, consistent relationship with a parent or caretaker. Unless the toddler feels that this person will respond to his or her words, the toddler will not be highly motivated to speak. The toddler may not speak when separated from mother, such as during hospitalization or the first day at daycare. When being prepared for hospital procedures, the toddler needs simple and succinct explanations, with gestures pointing to the areas of the body being cared for, and verbal and physical displays of affection.

If a child is delayed in speech, carefully assess the child and family. Causes for the delay of speech may include deafness or the inability to listen, mental retardation, emotional disturbance, maternal deprivation or separation from the parents, lack of quality verbal communication within the family and to the child, inconsistent or tangential responses to the child's speech, the presence of multiple siblings, or parents anticipating the needs of the child before he or she has a chance to communicate them.[80]

Verbal interaction, an environment with a variety of objects and stimuli, and freedom to explore are crucial to help the young child use his or her senses and emerging motor skills, and thereby are necessary to be able to learn most effectively during the sensorimotor and preoperational stages.

In Canada, most Aboriginal people are adamant that language be promoted, protected, preserved, and practised, especially at an early age.[81] Kirkness firmly states that language is the principal means by which culture is transmitted from one generation to the next. Language is culture and culture is language.[82]

CRITICAL THINKING

*In health care settings, how can you help to preserve Aboriginal languages?*

# Emotional Development

The toddler is a self-loving, uninhibited, dominating, energetic little person absorbed in self-importance, always seeking attention, approval, and personal goals. Sometimes the toddler is cuddly and loving. At other times, he or she bites or pinches and looks most unhappy, feeling no sense of guilt or shame. There is little self-control over exploratory or sadistic impulses. The toddler realizes only later that he or she cannot have everything desired, and that some behaviours annoy others. He or she experiments with abandon in the quest for independence, yet becomes easily frightened and runs to the parent for protection, security, reassurance, and approval.

Because the toddler relies so heavily on the parents and wants their approval, he or she gradually learns to curb negativism but to retain drive, to co-operate increasingly, and to develop socially accepted behaviour. The need for attention and approval is one of the main motivating forces in ego development and socialization in the toddler.

Parents should bestow sufficient attention to the child but not encourage the child to show off for an audience, verbally or physically, and they should not overstimulate too frequently with laughter or games. Finally, adults must realize that the child fears separation, strangers, darkness, sudden or loud noises, large objects and machines, and hurtful events such as traumatic procedures.

**Developmental Crisis** According to Erikson, the psychosexual crisis for the toddler is autonomy versus shame and doubt.[83] **Autonomy** *is demonstrated in the ability to gain self-control* over motor abilities and sphincters; to make and carry out decisions; to feel able to cope adequately with

## EVIDENCE-BASED PRACTICE

# Children in Crashes: Mechanisms of Injury and Restraint Systems

Motor vehicle crashes (MVCs) are the leading cause of injury, disability, and death in Canadian children. The objective of this study was to explore the levels of protection offered to children involved in motor vehicle collisions. This joint study by Children's Hospital of Eastern Ontario (CHEO) in Ottawa and Transport Canada was conducted in two phases. The retrospective phase from 1990 to 1997 involved the analysis of a series of 45 children who had been involved in MVCs. The analysis was based on the injury type—spinal versus seatbelt type. The second phase was a prospective study of 22 children injured in 15 MVCs. Interventions included a biomechanical assessment of the vehicle and its influence on the injuries sustained. The main outcome measurements were the nature and extent of injuries sustained, the vehicle dynamics, and associated occupant kinematics.

### Results

The odds ratio of sustaining a spinal injury while wearing a two-point belt versus a three-point belt was 24, indicating a much higher incidence with a lap belt than a shoulder strap.

### Conclusions

Proper seatbelt restraint reduces the morbidity in children involved in MVCs. Children under the age of 12 years should not be front seat passengers until the sensitivity of airbags is improved. Three-point pediatric seatbelts should be available for family automobiles to reduce childhood trauma in MVCs.

### Practice Implications

1. Because all chance fractures in this study were associated with a poorly fitting lap belt, the ideal position for the belt is on the anterior inferior iliac spines.

2. Proper belt fit with a lap belt is sometimes impossible to achieve. This occurs when seat depth is greater than femur length, forcing the child into a slouched position. A booster seat allows better fit of the belt across the bony pelvis, using either two-point or three-point devices, preventing a slouched position.

3. The addition of a crotch strap would prevent submarining and would maintain the belt on the pelvis in the younger child.

4. Airbags used as supplemental restraints have worked to prevent injury; they have also been implicated in its cause. For example, children have suffered injuries both directly from airbag inflation and indirectly by contact with the gear shift after being pushed into it. Therefore, children under 12 years should not be seated in the front passenger seat until airbags are rendered more sensitive to smaller occupants.

Source: Lapner, P.C., M. McKay, A. Howard, B. Gardner, A. German, and M. Letts, Children in Crashes: Mechanisms of Injury and Restraint Systems, *Canadian Journal of Surgery, 44*(6) (2001), 445–449. Used with permission. © 2001 Canadian Medical Association.

problems, or get the necessary help; to wait with patience; to give generously or to hold on, as indicated; to distinguish between possessions or wishes of self and of others; and to have a feeling of goodwill and pride. Autonomy is characterized by the oft-heard statement, "Me do it." Mastery accomplished in infancy sets the basis for autonomy.

*The toddler demonstrates his or her developing autonomy while maintaining a sense of security and control through the following behaviours:*

1. Using negativism

2. Displaying temper

3. Dawdling

4. Using rituals

5. Exploring even when parents object

6. Developing language skills; saying "no" although he or she may do as asked

7. Increasing control over his or her body or functions

The performing of ritualistic behaviour is normal and peaks at about 2.5 years, especially at bedtime and during illness. Although autonomy is developing, emotions are still contagious. The toddler reflects others' behaviours and feelings. For example, if someone laughs or cries, the toddler will imitate for no apparent reason.

Teach parents that reasonable limits help the toddler to gain positive experiences and responses from others and to build a sense of self and autonomy. Accepting the toddler's behaviours and allowing some self-expression and choice fosters autonomy.

### CRITICAL THINKING

*What type of ritualistic behaviours can the parents initiate when the toddler is ill?*

Shame and doubt are felt if autonomy and a positive self-concept are not achieved.[84] **Shame** is *the feeling of being* *fooled, embarrassed, exposed, small, impotent, dirty, wanting to hide, and rage against self.* **Doubt** *is fear, uncertainty, mistrust, lack of self-confidence, and the feeling that nothing they do is any good, and that one is controlled by others rather than being in control of self.*[85]

There is a limit to how exposed, dirty, mean, and vulnerable one can feel. If the child is pushed past the limit, disciplined or toilet trained too harshly, or abused, he or she can no longer discriminate about self, what he or she should be and can do. If everything is planned and done *for* and *to* the child, he or she cannot develop autonomy. The toddler's self-concept and behaviour will try to measure up to the expectations of such demanding parents and others, but there is no close attachment to an adult.

Discourage parents from creating an emotional climate of excessive expectations, criticism, blame, punishment, and over-restriction for the toddler, because within the child's consciousness, a sense of shame and doubt may develop that will be extremely harmful to further development. The child should not be given too much autonomy, or he or she will feel all-powerful. When a toddler fails to accomplish what he or she has been falsely led to believe could be achieved, the self-doubt and shame that result can be devastating. Aggressive behaviour results if the child is severely punished, or if parents are aggressive. With the proper balance of guidance, support, and discipline, the toddler gains a sense of possessing a number of personal abilities and thus has the potential to deal with the next set of social adjustments.

**Toilet Training** Toilet training is a major developmental accomplishment and relates directly to the crisis of autonomy versus shame and doubt, or to what Freudian theorists call the **anal stage**. Independence and autonomy (self-control), not cleanliness, are the critical issues in teaching the child to use the toilet. For the process to work, the parents must do little more than arrange for the child to use the toilet easily. The parent supports, rather than acts as a trainer, and is interested in the child, not just the act. The toddler is interested in the products he or she excretes. Toilet learning readiness should not be dictated by a child's chronological age. The child-oriented approach advocates that a child must be physiologically and psychologically ready to begin the process.[86] By the time the child reaches 18 months of age, reflex sphincter control has matured and the myelinization of extrapyramidal tracts has occurred; both processes are necessary for bowel and bladder control.[87]

In some cultures, the mother begins toilet training before the child is one year old, and the child is expected to achieve dryness by 18 months. In other cultures, the child is not expected to be toilet trained until about five years of age.[88] The Canadian Paediatric Society recommends a child-oriented approach, where the timing and method of toilet training are individualized as much as possible.[89]

Parents and all caregivers should be prepared to begin toilet training by ensuring that time is set aside for the process and that the arrangements are suitable for the entire family. The process should not be initiated at a stressful time in the child's life (e.g., after a traumatic event or after the birth of a new sibling). Parents should be prepared emotionally for the unavoidable accidents that will occur before the process is completed.

A few signs of the child's toilet readiness include:

- Able to walk to the potty chair
- Able to remain dry for several hours in a row
- Able to follow one or two simple instructions
- Able to use expressive language skills to communicate the need to use the potty
- Desire for independence and control of bladder and bowel function[90]

Parents can facilitate a child's toilet training by:

- Deciding on what vocabulary to use
- Encouraging the child to inform the parent when he or she needs to void
- Praising the child and avoiding negative reinforcement and punishment
- Ensuring a consistent approach to toilet training from all caregivers[91]

If toilet training does not work, it is usually because the child is not ready. Further, if the child refuses to use the potty, a break from potty training should be taken for about one to three months. For a child with special needs, a consultation with a physician is warranted.[92]

---

### CRITICAL THINKING

*What other strategies can you teach parents to use if toilet training with their toddler does not work?*

---

## Body Image and Self-Concept Development

**Body Image** Body image development gradually evolves as a component of self-concept. The toddler has a dim self-awareness, but with a developing sense of autonomy, he or she becomes more accurately aware of the body as a physical entity and one with emotional capabilities. The toddler is increasingly aware of pleasurable sensations in the genital area and on the skin and mouth and is learning control of the body through locomotion, toilet training, speech, and socialization.

**Self-Concept** **Self-concept** is also made up of *feelings about self, adaptive and defensive mechanisms, reactions from others, and one's perceptions of these reactions, attitudes, values, and many of life's experiences.*

The sense of self as a separate being continues to develop; the individuation process is complete between 24 and 36 months. When the child is able to sustain a mental image of the loved person who is out of sight, separation anxiety is resolved.[93]

As the child incorporates approval and disapproval, praise and punishment, gestures that are kind and those that are forbidding, he or she forms an opinion about self as a person. Experiences of discomfort are felt first with mother, and then these feelings are generalized to other people. As a result, much behaviour becomes organized to avoid, or minimize, discomfort around others. Thus, he or she gradually evolves adaptive and defensive behaviours and learns what to do to get along with others.

Self-awareness is demonstrated as the child says "mine" and "me" more often, beginning at about 18 to 24 months. Possessiveness with toys and the inability to share that as typical of the two-year-old may be a reflection of greater awareness of self, not just selfishness. The action may actually be an attempt to be sociable with another child.[94]

The child's significant caretaker should have a positive self-concept and feel good about being a mother (or father). If others in the family or society generally debase the mothering one, injury results to the child's self-esteem. Be mindful of body image and self-concept formation as you care for toddlers, because the two together determine the child's reaction. Only through repetitious positive input can you change a negative self-concept to one that is positive. By stimulating a positive self-image, you are promoting emotional health. Teach parents to provide an environment in which the child can successfully exercise skills such as running, walking, and playing and feel acceptance of his or her body and behaviour. Help them realize that as the child's autonomy develops so too will a more appropriate mental picture of his or her body and their emotions.

## Adaptive Mechanisms

Before the child is two years old, he or she is learning the basic response patterns appropriate for the family and culture. The child develops a degree of trust and confidence, or lack of it, in the parents. The child learns how to express annoyance and impatience, love and joy, and how to communicate his or her needs.

The toddler begins to adapt to the culture because of **primary identification**. He or she *imitates the parents* and responds to their encouragement and discouragement. With successful adaptation, the child moves toward independence. Other major adaptive mechanisms of this era include repression, suppression, denial, reaction formation, projection, and sublimation.[95]

**Repression** *unconsciously removes from awareness the thoughts, impulses, fantasies, and memories of behaviours that are unacceptable to the self.* The *not-me* discussed earlier is an example and may result from child abuse. **Suppression** *differs from repression in that it is a conscious act.* For example, the child forgets that he or she has been told not to handle certain articles. **Denial** is *not admitting, even when warned, that certain factors exist,* for example, that the stove is hot and will cause a burn. **Reaction formation** is *replacing the original idea and behaviour with the opposite behaviour characteristics.* For example, the child flushes the toilet and describes feces as dirty instead of playing in them, thus becoming appropriately tidy. **Projection** occurs when *he or she attributes personal feelings or behaviours to someone else.* For example, if the babysitter disciplines the toddler, he or she projects dislike for the babysitter by saying, "You don't like me." **Sublimation** is *channelling impulses into socially acceptable behaviour, rather than expressing the original impulse.* For example, he or she plays with mud, fingerpaints, or shaving cream, which is socially acceptable, instead of playing with feces.

Teach parents that the child's adaptive behaviour is strengthened when he or she is taught to do something for self and permitted to make a decision *if that decision is truly his or hers to make.* If the decision is one that must be carried out regardless of the toddler's wish, it can best be accomplished by giving direction rather than by asking the child if he or she wants to do the task.

## Sexuality Development

Traditionally, parents have handled sons and daughters differently during infancy, and the results become evident in toddlerhood.

Because parents encourage independent behaviour in boys, and more dependency in girls, by 13 months the boy ventures farther from mother, stays away longer, and looks at or talks to his mother less than does the girl. The girl at this age is encouraged to spend more time touching and staying near mother than is the boy. However, the separation process later seems less severe for girls. Perhaps boys should be touched and cuddled longer.[96]

Boys play more vigorously with toys than do girls, and they play more with non-toys such as doorknobs and light switches. Yet, basically, there seems to be no sexual preference for toys, although parents may enforce a preference.

A boy responds with more overt aggression to a barrier placed between him and his mother at 13 months of age than a girl does. Boys show more exploratory and aggressive behaviours than girls, and this type of behaviour is encouraged by the father. The female remains attentive to a wide variety of stimuli and especially to complex visual and auditory stimuli. The female demonstrates earlier language development and seems more aware of contextual relationships, perhaps because of the more constant stimulation from the mother.[97]

**Primary identification**, *imitation and observation of the same-sexed parent*, contributes to sex identity. By 15 months, child is interested in his or her own and others' body parts. Both boys and girls achieve sexual pleasure through self-stimulation, although girls masturbate less than boys (possibly because of anatomic differences).

By 21 months, the child can refer to self by name, an important factor in the development of identity. By two years of age, the child can categorize people into boy and girl and has some awareness of anatomic differences, especially if he or she has had opportunities to view them.[98]

By the end of toddlerhood, the child is more aware of his or her body, the body's excretions, and his or her actions, and he or she can be more independent in the first steps of self-care. Ability to communicate verbally expands to the point that he or she can ask questions and talk about sexual topics with parents and peers.

Help parents to understand the developing sexuality of their child and to be comfortable with their own sex identification and sexuality so that they can cuddle the child and answer questions. Help them understand that a wide variety of play experiences will prepare the child for adult behaviour and competence. They may talk through their concerns about a son's becoming a "sissy" if he plays with dolls or wears mother's high heels in dramatic play. Help parents to realize that a daughter's playing with trucks does not mean she will become a truck driver.

---

### CRITICAL THINKING

*What types of play experiences may help the child to be comfortable with his or her own sexuality later in life?*

---

## Guidance and Discipline

**Discipline** is *guidance that helps the child learn to understand and care for himself or herself and to get along with others*. It is not just punishing, correcting, or controlling behaviour, as is commonly assumed.

Everything in the toddler's world is new and exciting and meant to be explored, touched, eaten, or sat on, including porcelain figurines from Spain or boiling water.

In moving away from complete dependency, the toddler demonstrates energy and drive and requires sufficient restrictions to ensure physical and psychological protection and at the same time enough freedom to permit exploration and autonomy. Because mother must now set limits, a new dimension is added to the relationship established between mother and toddler. Before, mother met his or her basic needs immediately. With the toddler's increasing ability, freedom, and demands, the parent sometimes makes him or her wait, or even denies a wish, if it will cause harm. The transition should be made in a loving, consistent, yet flexible manner so that the child maintains trust and moves forward in the quest for independence. Excessive limitations, overwhelming and constantly steady pressure, or hostile bullying behaviour might serve to create an overly rebellious, negativistic, or passive child. Complete lack of limitations can cause accidents, poor health, and insecurity.[99] Through the parent's guidance and helpful reactions to the child's behaviours, the child is being socialized, learning what is right and wrong. Because the child cannot adequately reason, he or she must depend on, and trust, the parents as a guide for all activities. He or she can obey simple commands. Later, the child will be capable of internalizing rules and mores and will become self-disciplined as a result of having been patiently disciplined. Setting limits is not easy. Parents should not thwart the toddler's curiosity and enthusiasm, but they must protect him or her from harm. Parents who oppose the toddler's desire of the moment are likely to meet with anything from a simple "no" to a temper tantrum.

Teach parents the importance of constructive guidance and discipline. Temper tantrums result because the toddler hates being thwarted and made to feel helpless. Once the feelings are discharged, the child regains composure, usually quickly and without revenge. If temper tantrums, a form of negativism, occur, the best advice is to ignore the outburst; it will soon disappear. The parent's calm voice, expressing understanding of feelings, and the introduction of an activity to restore self-esteem are important in teaching self-control.

Because parents are sometimes confused about handling the toddler's behaviour, you can assist them by teaching some *simple rules for guiding the toddler*:[100]

- Provide an environment in which the child feels comfortable.

- Decide what is important, and what is not worth a battle of will. For example, the child may not be wearing matched clothing, but resists parental attempts to change. Avoid negativism and an angry scene by deciding that today it is all right for the child to wear an unmatched outfit.

- Changing one's mind, pursuing an alternate activity, or letting the child have his or her way is not giving in, losing face, being a poor parent, or letting the child be manipulative. When limits are consistent, changing a direction of behaviour can be a positive learning experience for the child. The child is becoming aware of being a separate person, able to assert self and influence others.

- Remove or avoid temptations such as breakable objects within reach, or candy that should not be eaten, to avoid having to say "no" repeatedly.

- Try not to ask open-ended questions for the child to decide about an activity when the decision is not really one the child can make.

- Consider limits as more than restrictions; think of them as a distraction *from* one prohibited activity *to* another in which the child can freely participate. A distraction with alternatives, or a substitute, is effective with the toddler because the attention span is short.

- Reinforce appropriate behaviour through approval and attention. The child will continue behaviour that gains attention, even if the attention is punitive, because negative attention to the child is better than no attention to the child.

- Set limits consistently so that the child can rely on the parent's judgment rather than testing the adult's endurance in each situation.

- State limits clearly, concisely, simply, positively, and in a calm voice. For example, if the child cannot play with a treasured object, he or she should not be allowed to handle it. Say "Look with your hands behind your back," or "Look with your eyes, not your hands," rather than "Don't touch."

- Set limits only when necessary. Some rules promote a sense of security, but too many rules confuse the child.

- Provide a safe area where the child is free to do whatever he or she wants to do.

- Do not overprotect the child; he or she should learn that some things have a price such as a bruise or a scratch.

- Do not terminate the child's activity too quickly; tell him or her that the activity is ending.

Each situation will determine the extent of firmness or leniency needed. The toddler needs gradations of independence.

## Moral-Spiritual Development

The period from birth through the toddler era might be termed the *pre-religious stage*. This label does not deny religious influences, but simply points out that the toddler is absorbing basic intellectual and emotional patterns regardless of the religious conviction of the caretakers. The toddler may repeat some phrases from prayers while imitating a certain voice tone or body posture that accompanies those prayers. The child only knows that when he or she imitates or conforms to certain rituals, affection and approval come that add to the child's sense of identification and security. Teach parents that the toddler can benefit from a nursery-school type of church program where emphasis is on positive self-images and appropriate play and rest rather than on a lesson to learn. The toddler also needs to have others to imitate who follow the rules of society, and he or she needs a lot of rewards and reinforcement for good or desirable behaviour. The development of moral integrity is increased if toddlers believe they are valued.[101]

The constantly sensitive situation of the toddler, gaining autonomy and independence—at times overreaching and needing mother's help, at times needing the freedom from mother's protection—is one you can help parents understand. The child's future personality and health will depend partially on how these many opportunities are handled during toddlerhood. *Your role in teaching and support is critical.*

### CRITICAL THINKING

*What may be some consequences for the child who is unable to perform a few developmental tasks?*

## HEALTH PROMOTION IN NURSING PRACTICE

Your role with the toddler and family has been discussed in each section throughout this chapter. It is important that you observe and listen to the child and family regarding issues, strengths, and healthy responses. Interventions include your role ability to model caring behaviour; parent and family education, support, and counselling; and direct care to meet the toddler's physical, emotional, cognitive, and social needs.

# SUMMARY

1. The toddler grows at a slower pace physically than the infant, but physical growth is steady and there is considerable gain in neuromuscular skills.

2. Emotionally, socially, and behaviourally, the toddler makes great strides in development during these two years.

3. The child gains control over basic physiologic processes, such as toileting, and gains competency in behaviour patterns.

4. Developmental, or autonomy tasks, are achieved in his or her own unique way as parents and family members provide consistent love and guidance, and adequate resources to foster physical, cognitive, emotional, social, and moral development.

5. The box entitled "Considerations for the Toddler and Family in Health Care" summarizes what you should consider in assessment and health promotion with the toddler.

6. The unique toddler characteristics of curiosity, impulsivity, the advancement of motor skills beyond verbal and cognitive development, and the assertion of will must be considered by parents and health care professionals in relation to safety and health promotion measures.

## Considerations for the Toddler and Family in Health Care

- Family cultural background and support systems for the family of the toddler
- Attachment behaviours of the parents; separation reactions of the toddler
- Parental behaviours that indicate difficulty with attachment, or potential/actual abuse of the toddler
- Physical characteristics or patterns, such as eating, toilet training, sleep/rest, and play, that indicate health and are within age norms for growth
- Cognitive characteristics and behavioural or play patterns in the toddler that indicate age-appropriate norms for intellectual development
- Communication patterns and language development that indicate age-appropriate norms for the toddler
- Overall appearance and behavioural or play patterns in the toddler that indicate development of autonomy rather than shame and doubt, positive self-concept, sense of sexuality, and continuing age-appropriate emotional development
- Behavioural patterns that indicate the toddler is beginning moral-spiritual development
- Behavioural patterns and characteristics that indicate the toddler has achieved developmental tasks
- Parental behaviours that indicate knowledge about how to provide physical and emotional care for the toddler
- Parental behaviours and communication approaches that indicate the effective guidance of the toddler
- Evidence that the parents provide a safe and healthful environment and the necessary resources for the toddler
- Parental behaviours that indicate they are achieving their developmental tasks for this era

## Interesting Websites

### First Nations Child and Family Caring Society of Canada
www.fncfcs.com
The purpose of the Caring Society is to promote the well-being of all First Nations children, youth, families, and communities, with a particular focus on the prevention of and response to child maltreatment.

### First Nations Research Site Online Journal
www.fncfcs.com/pubs/onlineJournal.html
The First Peoples Child & Family Review is an online journal published jointly by the First Nations Research Site, Centre of Excellence for Child Welfare, and the First Nations Child and Family Caring Society of Canada. This e-journal focuses primarily on First Nations and Aboriginal child welfare practices, policies, and research. It privileges the "voice and perspectives" of First Nations and Aboriginal child welfare scholars, researchers, practitioners, trainers, students, volunteers, and community developers.

### Canadian Paediatric Society
www.cps.ca
This site has information on programs and issues related to children's health, including immunization, healthy eating, childhood infections, choosing car seats, and injury prevention.

Canadian Coalition for Immunization Awareness and Promotion
**www.immunize.cpha.ca**
This site has information on types of immunization, schedules, and Canadian statistics on rates of immunization, as well as discussions of facts and myths related to the subject.

Children's Safety Association of Canada
**www.safekid.org**
Visit this site for information on a wide variety of safety topics.

## Key Terms

anal stage (303)

autistic (299)

autonomy (301)

bruises (285)

café au lait spots (285)

contraction (299)

denial (280, 304)

despair (280)

discipline (305)

doubt (303)

egocentric (297)

expansion (299)

fifth stage of the sensorimotor period (297)

Mongolian spots (285)

myelinization (283)

parallel play (288)

preoperational period (297)

primary identification (304, 305)

projection (304)

protest (280)

reaction formation (304)

repression (304)

self-concept (304)

separation anxiety (280)

shame (302)

sixth stage of the sensori motor period (297)

spider nevi (285)

sublimation (304)

suppression (304)

syncretic speech (299)

telegraphic speech (299)

toddler stage (278)

# Chapter 9

## Assessment and Health Promotion for the Preschooler

*If the child is safe, the people are safe.*

Marian Wright Edelman

## Objectives

*Study of this chapter will enable you to:*

1 Examine the second-order changes in family status required to proceed developmentally in family life cycle stage: families with young children.

2 Compare and contrast the family relationships in the preschool and previous developmental eras.

3 Differentiate among the types of influence exerted upon the preschooler by parents, siblings, and non-family members.

4 Evaluate the values and services available to parents and the child from daycare centres and nursery schools.

5 Discuss the types of adaptations required by the preschooler in daycare and nursery school settings.

6 Assess physical, motor, mental, language, play, and emotional characteristics of three-, four-, and five-year-olds.

7 Describe (1) the health needs of the preschooler, including nutrition, exercise, rest, safety, and immunization; and (2) measures to be taken to meet these needs.

8 Examine with parents their role in contributing to the preschooler's cognitive, language, self-concept, sexuality, moral-spiritual, and emotional development, and physical health.

9 Analyze measures to diminish the traumatic effects of hospitalization for this age group.

10 Explore with parents effective ways to enhance the development of the preschooler by means of communication, guidance, and discipline.

11 Describe (1) the developmental crisis of initiative versus guilt; (2) the adaptive mechanisms commonly used to promote a sense of initiative; and (3) the implications of this crisis for the child's later maturity.

12 Demonstrate the process of working effectively with a preschooler in a nursing situation.

In this chapter, the development of the preschool child and the family relationships are continued. Nursing and health care responsibilities for health promotion for the child and family are discussed throughout the chapter. The information regarding the child's normal development and needs is intended to serve as a basis for assessment. Your role is to use the information provided in this textbook as information for assessment and health promotion in health education counselling of families, and care of the preschooler in communities and various other health settings.

The **preschool years**, *ages three through five*, along with infancy and the toddler years, form a crucial part of the person's life. The preschool child is emerging as a social being. He or she participates more fully as a family member, but begins at this stage slowly to grow out of the family, spending more time with **peers**, children of the same age. Physical growth is slowing, but the body is well proportioned and control and coordination are increasing. Emotional and intellectual growth are progressively apparent in the ability to form mental images. The expression of self is shown through a range of emotions. The child identifies with the play group, follows rules, controls primitive (*id*) impulses, and begins to be self-critical with reference to a standard set by others (*superego formation*).

You can explore with parents the ways they can begin to separate themselves from their growing child, and how they might revise their decisions about how much free expression and initiative to permit the child while setting certain limits. Gradually promoting more independence during the preschool years allows both the child and the parents to be more comfortable about the separation that occurs when the child goes to school.

# FAMILY DEVELOPMENT AND RELATIONSHIPS

## Family Life Cycle

Refer to Table 4-3, which illustrates the stages of the family life cycle, the emotional processes of transition (key principles), and the second-order changes in the family required to proceed developmentally. Stage 3, families with young children, is the relevant stage for the family with a preschooler.

Assist parents to be cognizant of these changes. Encourage them to share their thoughts, feelings, and practical aspects related to fulfilling these changes.

The family unit, regardless of the specific form, is important to the preschooler, and in turn the preschooler affects relationships within the family through his or her personality and behaviour. The close relationship of the baby to the mother and father gradually expands to include other significant adults living in the home—siblings and other relatives—and they, too, will have a considerable effect on the child's personality.

There are several *dominant parenting styles:*[1]

- **Authoritarian**: *Demanding, impose many rules, expect instant obedience, and do not give reasons for rules.* No consideration given to the child's view. Rely on physical punishment to gain compliance.

- **Authoritative**: *Exert control, demanding but responsive to and accepting of child.* Give reasons for rules. Expect mature behaviour. Encourage independence and child meeting own potential. Maintain balance between control, socialization, and individualization.

- **Permissive**: *Accepting of and responsive to child. Rarely make demands or exert control. Indulgent.* Encourage child to express feelings and impulses.

- **Neglectful**: *Low in demand and control, but also low in acceptance and responsiveness. Uninvolved* in child's upbringing. May even reject child. So involved in own needs and problems that they have no energy to set and enforce rules.

## CRITICAL THINKING

*What effects do you think that the parenting styles of your own parents had on your development?*

Parenting behaviours vary with the culture. It is interesting that the child's temperament affects the parent's behaviour.[2] A cross-cultural study was conducted on child-rearing attitudes and behavioural inhibition in Chinese and Canadian toddlers. The Chinese toddlers were significantly more inhibited than were their Canadian counterparts. In the Canadian sample, inhibition was associated positively with mothers' punishment orientation, and negatively with mothers' acceptance and encouragement of achievement. In the Chinese sample, however, the directions of the relations were opposite. Child inhibition was associated positively with mothers' warm and accepting attitudes and negatively with rejection and punishment orientation. In summary, the researchers claim that the results indicate the existence of different adaptation meanings of behavioural inhibition across cultures.[3]

Research has indicated that maternal interaction patterns differ on the basis of the child's medical history. Mothers developed a pattern of higher involvement with the child if he or she was preterm or at high risk, medically, at birth than if he or she was normal and healthy at birth. Mothers of very ill preterm babies demonstrated high-quality and appropriate involvement that did not contribute to the child's developmental delay. Generally speaking, all of the children who were most competent in cognition, linguistics, and problem solving had mothers with higher interaction scores who were more responsive and who used appropriate control styles. The qualities of maternal interaction patterns appear to diminish adverse effects of medical morbidity or maternal education deficits.[4] Canadian researchers Magill-Evans and Harrison concluded that early parent–child interactions contributed to the child's development in both healthy preterm and full-term infants.[5]

The interactions of mothers and fathers with their child are similar in many aspects. For example, Harrison, Magill-Evans, and Benzies concluded that mothers and fathers of infants aged 2 to 12 months were equally sensitive to their infant's cues. However, fathers were less contingent in interaction with their infants.[6] In another study, Broom used three subscales of the Nursing Child Assessment Scale (NCATS) with first-time parents. The results did not show any differences among white, well-educated, middle-class mothers and fathers when their child was three months old.[7] Meanwhile, Harrison, Magill-Evans, and Sadoway observed fathers of 49 Canadian children (ages 13 to 24 months) interacting with their child at home using the NCATS. They concluded that when compared with the NCATS reference data for 164 mothers of similar ethnicity and marital status with similar–aged children, mothers were more responsive than fathers in the interactions.[8] It appears that to reach confident generalizations, further research is warranted regarding fathers' interaction with their children. The possibility of comparing maternal and paternal traits seems to have led to a somewhat negative image of fathers. Dubeau states that (1) future research must focus on fathers' strengths and motivations, and (2) we must interpret these traits in a different cultural and historical context than we do for mothers.[9]

## CRITICAL THINKING

*What is one research question you might pose regarding fathers and their interactions with their young children?*

The effects of parenting styles on preschoolers can be divided into several categories of behaviour, as depicted in the box entitled "Effect of Parenting Style on Child's Behaviour."[10]

## Relationships with Parents

Attachment continues to develop during the preschool years. The attachment that began with parents in infancy was extended to others in toddlerhood. Parallel, and then co-operative, play with other children is a continuation of the attachment learned in infancy. By age three, the child realizes that others may not think like him or her, but the child wants to interact. Thus, the child learns to share or play, even when there are differences of opinion. The four- or five-year-old has a best friend, likes to participate in many social activities, and plays with peers because of their earlier growth experiences with attachment, and as a result of their parental guidance with socialization. In the process, a child learns to like and accept self, and then the same occurs with others. Moss and her associates examined a sample of 121 French-Canadian school-aged children. The contributions of attachment, maternal reported stress, and mother–child interaction to the prediction of teacher-reported behaviour problems were examined. The researchers' results support the importance of attachment in explaining school-aged adaptation, and they promote the validity of attachment coding for children of this age.[11]

## Effect of Parenting Style on Child's Behaviour

| Parent's Behaviour | Child's Behaviour |
|---|---|
| Controlling, detached, rather than loving and warm | Discontented, withdrawn, moody, unhappy, easily annoyed, aimless, lacks self-reliance, lacks confidence in own decision-making abilities |
| More controlling, demanding, loving overtly than most parents | Friendly, self-controlled, self-reliant, cheerful, socially responsible, co-operative with adults and peers |
| Highly permissive, warm and friendly | Low levels of self-reliance and self-control, rebellious, low levels of independence and achievement orientation |
| Relatively demanding, loving | Self-reliant, more independent, better adjusted |
| Warm, loving, expect a great deal of child at early age, demanding of child, show interest in child's activities | Highly creative, high need for achievement, independent, highly competent, works toward set goals |

It seems reasonable to conclude that a non-responsive, neglectful, or abusive environment produces angry, depressed, or hopeless children by two, three, or four years of age.

## CRITICAL THINKING

*What events in a preschooler's life might be associated with insecure attachments?*

*Parental nurturing* cannot be overemphasized. If the child has been neglected in infancy, or has had traumatic experiences, brain scans show that the brain region responsible for emotional attachments may never have fully developed.[12] *Without early close relationships, there may be biological, as well as learned, reasons for the child to be unable later to form full and effective relationships and to demonstrate caring social behaviour.* In fact, recent neurological studies have found that severe maltreatment of the child is related to molecular and neurological damage in the emotional and memory areas of the brain that are still developing.[13]

## Relationships in One-Parent or Step-parent Families

In the *one-parent or step-parent family* (or in the abusive home), achieving identification may be quite difficult. In the *one-parent home*, the little girl raised by a male may not fit in with other girls at school, or may not feel comfortable at relating to women later in life. The boy raised by a woman may relate better to women than to men.

The 2001 Census collected information for the first time on the number of same-sex couples across Canada.[14] Today, gay and lesbian parents are becoming more visible in society, and they are being seen at child care centres, soccer fields, and school concerts. Research has made it clear that fears about the negative outcomes for children who are raised in gay and lesbian families have been refuted.[15] However, despite these findings, gay and lesbian couples and their children continue to be confronted by public and private homophobia.

## CRITICAL THINKING

*How can homophobia be considered in the health care system? What health promoting strategies might be implemented to address homophobia?*

Let us shift our consideration from children of gay and lesbian families to children of divorced parents. Children of divorced parents manifest higher levels of depression and lower levels of self-esteem compared to samples of children with intact parents. Preschoolers have a limited ability to understand separation and divorce. Very young children can sense the feelings of an upset parent and can become upset themselves. In fact, at any age, children are highly vulnerable to the anxious and troubled feelings of their parents. Separation from a parent is difficult regardless of the circumstance. Interestingly, it has been found that children who hold irrational beliefs and feelings about divorce are most likely to develop behavioural and psychological problems.[16] Recently, the study of the impact of divorce on young children has expanded to consider the longer-term consequences of divorce through longitudinal studies of young adult children. A recent investigation has looked at studies of intergenerational ties between young adult children and their divorced parents.[17] In one example, Connidis, from the University of Western Ontario, conducted a qualitative study involving 86 adults from 10 three-generation families to illustrate the extensive reach of divorce across time and generations. She concluded that multiple voices from three generations demonstrate: (1) the complexity of family relationships over time, and (2) the reverberation of life course transitions of individuals throughout family networks.[18]

## Gender Identity

Cognitive development theory emphasizes that, in regard to gender identity, self-perceptions come before behaviour. During the preschool years, children first acquire a cognitive appreciation of the permanence of their sex. They develop gender constancy and the understanding that sex is biologically based and remains the same event even though clothing, hairstyles, and play activities change. Following the attainment of gender constancy, children use these concepts to guide their behaviour.[19] The sex of the child is a strong determinant in personality development because each sex has different tasks and roles in every culture. However, you cannot predict the child's personality traits by knowing only the sex. Achieving a firm identity as a man or a woman is basic to emotional stability and ego development, and cultural expectations and influences are important. These are expressed by the family socialization.[20]

Explain parental reactions to and expectations of the child. Help parents clarify their feelings and behaviour and convey their respect to the child, regardless of sex. The feelings and needs of the parents strongly influence their reactions to the child so that sex assignment within the family can override biological factors.

## Teaching Sexuality

Preschoolers develop curiosity about their own and others' bodies and sexual functions. Their questions should be answered simply and factually. Parents and others should avoid teasing the preschooler about this interest; nor should adults imply that the child's sexual information is unacceptable.[21] The *Canadian Guidelines for Sexual Health Education* can be used by parents to gain an appreciation of sexual health. Sexual health education is an integral component of health promotion that allows all individuals, regardless of age, to be healthy.[22]

Although sex education must be tailored to the individual child's needs and interests and to the cultural, religious, and family values, *the following suggestions are applicable to all children and can be shared with parents:*

■ Recognize that education about the self as a sexual person is best given by example in family life through parents' showing respect and love for the self, mate, and the child.

■ Understand that the child who learns to trust others and is able to give and receive love has begun preparation for satisfactory adulthood, marriage, and parenthood.

■ Observe the child at play. Listen carefully to statements of ideas, feelings, and questions and ask questions to understand better his or her needs.

■ Respond to the child's questions by giving information honestly, in a relaxed, accepting manner and on the child's level of understanding. Avoid isolated facts, myths, or animal analogies. The question, "Where does baby come from?" could be answered, "Mommy carried you inside her body in a special place," rather than saying "The stork brought baby," "Baby was picked up at the hospital after a special order," or "God makes babies." Religious beliefs can be worked into the explanation while acknowledging human realities.

■ Teach the child anatomic names, rather than other words, for body parts and processes. Parents may hesitate to do this because they do not want the child to blurt out *penis* or *vagina* in public. Parents can teach the child that certain topics such as sexual and financial matters are discussed in the home, just as certain activities such as urinating are done in private.

■ Grabbing the genitals and some masturbation are normal. Children explore their bodies, especially body parts not easily seen and that give pleasurable sensations when touched. Masturbation is acceptable to many families if it occurs in the home. The child should be taught that this is not normal behaviour in public.

■ Playing doctor, or examining each other's body parts, is normal for preschool children. Parents should not overreact and should calmly affirm that they want the children to keep their clothes on while they play. Diversion from "playing doctor" is useful. If children seem to be using each other in a sexual way, they should be instructed that this is not acceptable.

■ Realize that sex education continues throughout the early years. The child's changing self motivates the same or different questions again and again. Remain open to his or her ongoing questions. Explanation about reproduction may begin with a simple statement, for example: "A man and a woman are required to be baby's father and mother. Baby is made from the sperm in the daddy's body and an egg in the mother's body." A simple explanation of sperm and egg would be needed. Later, the child can be given more detail.

### CRITICAL THINKING

*How can you respond to the question, "How does the baby get started?"*

## Relationships with Siblings

An attachment for the child that began with the parents extends to siblings in late infancy and continues to deepen during the toddler and preschool years. Often, parents are emotionally warmer to subsequent children after the first-born. Possibly they feel more experienced and relaxed after the first birth. In the following discussion, you should realize that the relationships described could occur at other developmental eras in childhood, but in the preschool years siblings begin to make a very definite impact.[23]

The preschool child often has **siblings**, *brothers or sisters*, either younger or older, so that family interaction is complex with many **dyads**, *groups of two people*. Siblings become increasingly important in directing the child's early development, partly because of their proximity but also because the parents change in their role with each additional child. Downey and Condron analyzed a sample of kindergartners. They endeavoured to replicate the often-noted negative relationship between the number of siblings and cognitive outcomes. They then demonstrated that this pattern does not extend to social skills. These researchers concluded that the findings were consistent with the view that children negotiate peer relationships better when they grow up with at least one sibling.[24] Gass and her researchers examined the protective effect of positive sibling relationships on child adjustment for children experiencing stressful life events. They concluded that positive sibling relationships are an important source of support for children who experience stressful life events, regardless of mother–child relationship quality.[25]

**Preschooler and New Baby** The arrival of a new baby changes life. The preschooler is no longer the centre of attention but is expected by the parents to delight in the baby. Preschoolers often become demanding and clingy for a time and engage in naughtiness.[26] It is important for parents to prepare the young child (toddler or preschooler) for a new arrival. Although a space of three to four years is ideal, such ideal spacing does not always occur.

*When pregnancy is apparent, there are some recommended ways for parents to prepare the older child:*

- Share the anticipation through discussions and planning. Let the child feel fetal movements. Show the child a picture of when he or she was a newborn. Talk about what he or she needed as a baby and the necessary responsibilities. Read books that explain reproduction and birth on his or her level.

- Include the child as much as possible in activities such as shopping for furniture for the baby or decorating baby's room. The preschool child likes to feel important, and being a helper enhances this feeling.

- Accept that the child may act out, regress, or express dependency or separation anxiety during the pregnancy as well as after the new baby arrives.

- Have the child attend sibling preparation classes, if available. Encourage relatives and friends to bring a small surprise gift for the older child when they visit and bring a gift for the baby. Have them spend time with the older child also, rather than concentrate only on the new baby.

- Prepare the child to be with mother during birth, if family considers this appropriate and if permitted by the birthing centre. Have the child visit mother and baby at the hospital, if rules permit, or suggest that the older child can talk to mother by phone.

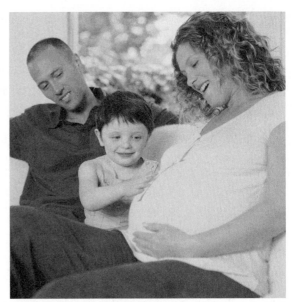

As birth approaches, parents can help prepare the preschooler for the arrival of the new sibling.

Accepting the family's affection toward the baby is difficult for the firstborn, and jealousy is likely to occur if more attention is focused on the baby than on him or her. The following behaviours may result:

1. The preschooler may regress, overtly displaying a need to be babied. He or she may ask for the bottle, soil self, have enuresis, lie in the baby's crib, or demand extra attention.

2. The child may harm the baby, directly or indirectly, through play or handling baby roughly.

3. He or she may appear to love the baby excessively, more than is normal.

4. The child may show hostility toward the mother in different ways: direct physical or verbal attacks, ignoring or rejecting her, or displacing anger onto the daycare, nursery, or Sunday school teacher.

Teach parents that these outward behaviours and the underlying feelings should be accepted, for they are better handled with overt loving behaviour than repressed through punishment. *Jealousy can be handled by the parents in a variety of ways:*

1. Tell the child about the pregnancy, but not too far in advance, because a young child has a poor concept of time.

2. Involve him or her in preparing for the new baby. Although the preschooler may have to give up a crib, getting him or her a new big bed can seem like a promotion rather than a loss.

3. Convey that the child is loved as much as before. Provide a time for him or her only, and give as much attention as possible.

4. Emphasize pleasure in having the child share in loving the new arrival and give increasing responsibility and status without overburdening him or her.

5. Encourage the child to talk about the new situation, or to express hostility in play.

6. Reading stories about the feelings of children with new siblings can help the child to express personal feelings.

Here are a few additional pieces of advice you can give about ways to handle jealous behaviour:

1. Do not leave the preschooler alone with the baby.

2. Give the child a pet or doll to care for as mother cares for the baby.

3. Encourage the child to identify with the parents in helping to protect the baby because he or she is more grown up.

4. Avoid overemphasizing affection for the baby.

**Older Sibling and Preschooler** An older sibling in the family who is given much attention for accomplishments may cause feelings of envy and frustration in the preschooler as the preschooler tries to engage in activity beyond his or her ability in endeavours to gain attention also. If the younger child can identify with the older sibling and take pride in the accomplishments of the older child while simultaneously receiving recognition for his or her own self and abilities, the child will feel positive about self. If the younger child feels defeated and is not given realistic recognition, he or she may stop emulating the older sibling and regress instead. In turn, the older sibling can be helpful to the younger child if the older child does not feel deprived or is not reprimanded because of the preschooler.

Naturally, disagreements occur among all siblings. However, the extent to which siblings can work out these disagreements depends on the quality of the sibling relationship. Ram and Ross, at the University of Waterloo, conducted a study where siblings could rate their relationship quality. They were asked to negotiate the division of six attractive toys. When siblings rated their relationships as negative, negotiations were destructive and resulted in a failure to reach an agreement. On the other hand, when sibling's relationships were positive, negotiations were usually constructive and led to fair approaches.[27]

Explore the matter of sibling relationships with parents. Provide suggestions for preventing conflicts. Positive feelings often exist between siblings. Quarrels are quickly forgotten if parents do not get overly involved. Because siblings have had a similar upbringing, they tend to have considerable empathy for each other. They have similar values, similar superego development, and related perceptions about situations. Sibling values may be as important as the parents' values in the development of the child. Recognition and other feelings

of the sibling are sometimes of such importance to the child that he or she may conceal ability rather than appear to move into an area in which the sibling has gained recognition. Alternatively, he or she may intentionally engage in an activity to keep the sibling from being unhappy. Children tend to learn to develop roles, such as "the boss" or "the angry monster," or they regulate space among themselves to avoid conflicts. Problems can arise if conflictual behaviour is given undue attention, or if the children are somehow manipulated against each other by adults.[28] A warm sibling relationship and play promotes a definition of self, helps the child learn to take others' perspectives, and enhances the child's ability to form relationships later because he or she has learned to co-operate, compete, negotiate, and be sociable.

### CRITICAL THINKING

*What interpersonal skills can the preschooler gain from the presence of older brothers and sisters?*

## Relationship with Grandparents

According to Rosenthal and Gladstone, grandparenting is a complex social process that carries different types of meanings for grandparents.[29] This process is reflected both in the feelings that grandparents have toward their grandchildren and in the ways they interact with their grandchildren. Sometimes the relationship with the grandparent is deeper than with either parent, especially if the parents: (1) are somewhat abusive or neglectful; (2) are busily employed professionals; (3) travel a great deal as part of a job, or (4) have separated or divorced.

Grandparents participate in different types of activities with their grandchildren, and they are valuable resources to children in both instrumental and symbolic ways.[30] They serve as babysitters and pass down traditions whereby the child learns about "olden days," family history, the meaning of old pictures and objects, and the child's own roots. Grandparents are ideal mentors, if they take the time and trouble: the child can learn to fix, to build, and to create. Grandparents can often provide spiritual sustenance to children of indifferent parents, and they can answer questions about God. Their ability to provide emotional or financial help may be especially useful if the parents are experiencing marital problems, separation or divorce, disability or health issues, or other stressful situations. Interesting books and courses are available to help grandparents develop a sense of competency in their role.[31] An example is that grandparents may need to be taught the importance of boundary issues regarding "parenting" limits.

Nurses practise in many settings, such as pediatric units in hospitals or community health clinics, where they may encounter grandparents who are raising grandchildren. It is

# Grandmother as Parent

Jody is a preschooler who started care with you yesterday on the pediatric unit. You met Jody's grandmother, Mrs. Jones, who informed you that because of her daughter's recent separation from her husband, she will be taking full parenting responsibilities for the next few months. During your interaction with Mrs. Jones, you learned that she has recently had a mastectomy. She also informed you that Jody loves to be picked up and cuddled often. It is clear to you that Mrs. Jones enjoys a deep and emotional closeness with Jody.

You wonder whether Mrs. Jones has received discharge teaching regarding lifting activities.

1. Design the plan of action you will take with Mrs. Jones regarding her recent surgery.
2. Because of Mrs. Jones's emotional closeness with Jody, how will you address the matter of "taking full parental responsibilities"?

important to be aware of the issues that the grandparents face and to conduct appropriate assessments of the needs of the grandparents, the children, and the home.[32]

A growing number of grandparents are losing contact with their grandchildren as a result of parental divorce, conflict between parents, the death of an adult child, or the adoption of a grandchild after remarriage. After divorce, the grandparent may wish to be the child's legal custodian but may not be permitted by his or her own child or the courts. Increasingly, in cases of divorce, grandparents are seeking legal means to ensure visitation rights and sometimes to gain custody.[33] Further, recent trends in fertility among today's young adults result in slightly lower percentages of individuals experiencing grandparenthood in the future. It does seem apparent, however, that most people will still have grandchildren.[34]

## CRITICAL THINKING

*How do grandchildren benefit their grandparents?*

## Influence of Other Adults and Non–Family Members

Help parents to realize that other people may be significant to the child, depending on frequency and duration of contact, the warmth of the relationship, and how well the parents meet the child's needs.[35]

*Other significant adults* may include relatives, especially grandparents, aunts, uncles, and cousins who are peers; the teacher at the daycare centre or nursery school; the babysitter; or neighbours. Relatives and friends also contribute to the development of a child's identity, if contact is frequent. *Guests* in the child's home introduce the child to new facets of family life and to their parents' behaviour. Visits to the home of others help the child to become socialized through

the comparison of households, the ability to separate from home, and interactions with people in new places. *Domestic pets* can be particularly useful in meeting certain needs: loving and being loved, companionship, learning a sense of responsibility, and learning about sex in a natural way. See www.bcchildrens.ca for more information regarding pets. This website provides guidelines for parents that range from choosing a pet to teaching children how to be with pets.[36]

Child Care If the family uses daycare, nursery school, or other early schooling for the child, the adults in the agency may exert a strong influence on the child. The child learns a variety of skills that are often not available in home life. These skills can, in turn, form a foundation for extracurricular activities in the school years, or even for a later vocation. The advantage of the year-round program is that the child retains and adds to learning; children who are not in a structured program during summer lose some of what was learned unless they have parents who continue to engage them in new experiences and with new resources.

In 2002–2003, about 45 percent of Canadian children aged six months to five years were in some type of non-parental child care. This rate represented an increase from the 42 percent of children in non-parental child care eight years earlier.[37] According to the Canadian Child Care Federation (CCCF), the child care environment must not only protect a child's health and safety, but also promote optimal child development. The CCCF is a bilingual, non-profit, member-based organization established in 1987. It is committed to improving the quality of child care services for families in Canada, and based on its reach, relationships, resources, and reputation it is recognized as the largest pan-Canadian child care organization. Over the years, the CCCF has adopted various strategies in order to function within the changing dynamics of the child care sector. It does so by strengthening the infrastructure of the child care community at both the national and the grassroots levels. In addition, it provides a national focus for commentary, information, and dialogue on current issues relating to child care.[38]

*Interaction* is CCCF's bilingual flagship magazine. It is available online and has engaging articles on emergent issues in early childhood development. The magazine contains narratives from child care and early learning practices across the country, as well as news on the latest research, resources, and government policy in the field.[39]

National Child Day is held on November 20, when people across the country take time to celebrate Canada's precious resource: our children. Past National Child Day themes have been:

- 2006: "I have the right to be heard"
- 2005: "I have a right to play"

National Child Day was proclaimed by the Government of Canada on March 19, 1993, to commemorate two historic events for children: the adoption of the *United Nations Declaration on the Rights of the Child* in 1959 and the UN adoption of the *Convention on the Rights of the Child* in 1989.[40]

## CRITICAL THINKING

*What ideas do you have, as a nurse, for celebrating National Child Day?*

There are three main types of child care available in Canada:

- Care provided in one's own home, called *own-home care*
- Care provided in the caregiver's home, called *other-home care*
- Care provided in a centre, or *centre care*[41]

It is important to note that no single type of child care is considered to be right for all infants or toddlers. All three types of child care may be good if they provide the warmth, supervision, individual attention, and activity that each child needs.

In Canada, child care may be licensed or unlicensed. The provincial or territorial government must license all centres, as well as some other-home facilities. Each province and territory sets its own licensing standards. These standards vary from province to province, but usually the standards specify the number and ages of children. Included in the standards are health, safety, and nutritional requirements, group size, and staff–child ratios. The requirements also include a program of child-focused activities. A licence is not a guarantee of quality care. It is only an indicator that at least the minimum standards that can be enforced by law are being met. A licence means that the program can be inspected at any time. However, in

some parts of Canada, inspection may be minimal or infrequent.[42] For specific information about licensing regulations, call your provincial/territory licensing authority.

The CCCF and its affiliate organizations recognize their responsibility to promote ethical practices and attitudes on the part of the child care practitioners.[43] The CCCF Code of Ethics is intended to guide child care practitioners to protect the children and families with whom they work. The eight ethical principles are as follows:

1. Promote the health and well-being of all children.
2. Enable children to engage to their full potential in carefully planned environments and facilitate the child's progress in a holistic way.
3. Demonstrate a caring attitude to all children.
4. Work in a collaborative way with parents in meeting their responsibilities to the children.
5. Work in partnerships with colleagues and other service providers.
6. Work in ways that enhance human dignity in trusting, caring, and co-operative relationships that respect the worth and uniqueness of the individual.
7. Pursue the knowledge and skills that are needed to be professionally competent.
8. Demonstrate integrity in all professional relationships.

Ethical practice must reflect these eight principles. In situations where ethical dilemmas occur, the practitioner must carefully think through the likely consequences of giving priority to any particular principles.[44]

## CRITICAL THINKING

*What are some ethical dilemmas with which a child care practitioner might be confronted?*

Parents may ask you about different child care agencies: the differences between them, their significance for the child, and the criteria for selection. Share the following information to the best of your ability. You may also assist in agencies with primary prevention and health consulting to teachers, children, and parents.

Generally speaking, **daycare** is *a licensed, structured program that provides care daily for some portion of the day, for 13 or more children away from home, five days a week year-round, for compensation.* The age of the children can range from infancy to 13 years, but most children will be of preschool age. Daycare is child-oriented both in program, and in the physical structure of the facilities.

**Family daycare** is *the arrangement by a caregiver to provide care for a small group of mixed-age children in his or her home while the parent works.* In some jurisdictions, if there are more than four children, the family daycare must meet licensing requirements, and many caregivers choose to avoid undergoing the regulations, procedures, and remodelling that would be involved in licensing.[45]

**Home daycare** is *the provision of child care in the child's home by someone (father or mother, other relative, non-relative) during the parent's working hours. The number of children tends to be small (one to four).* Thus, there is little opportunity, in such a case, for diverse peer interaction, and there will be limited adult contact as well. *There is usually no structured program.*

**Nursery school** is usually a *half-day program that emphasizes an educational, socialization experience for the children to supplement home experiences.*

**Early school experiences** may include a *Montessori program*, a *compensatory program*, or *kindergarten*, which has now become the first step before school entry for most children. **Montessori programs** evolved from the Italian educator Maria Montessori, who developed preschool education in Europe. They *emphasize: (1) self-discipline of the child; (2) intellectual developmental through training the senses; (3) freedom for the child within a structure and schedule; and (4) meaningful individual cognitive experiences that are provided in a quiet, pleasant, educational environment.*[46]

**Compensatory programs** *focus on making up for deprived conditions in the child's life.* They might include: (1) giving physical care (good nutrition, dental care, immunizations); (2) fostering curiosity, exploring creativity, and learning about the self and environment; (3) promoting emotional health through nurturing, positive self-concept, self-confidence, and self-discipline; and (4) teaching social skills and behaviours, and how to interact with peers, teachers, and parents.[47]

In the **child-centred kindergarten**, *education involves the whole child and includes concern for the child's physical, cognitive, and social development.* It could be a *half- or whole-day educational program* for the five-year-old child, and it may be either an extension of a nursery school or a part of the public elementary school system. The instruction is organized around the child's needs, interests, and learning styles. Play is critical in the child's total development. Therefore, strategies such as experimenting, exploring, discovering, and trying out are emphasized.[48]

More organizations are recognizing the need to address the child care needs of employees to reduce parental anxiety and missed workdays, and to enhance productivity. You can be an advocate for such programs.

Criteria for the selection of a daycare centre, or nursery school, may be discussed with parents as they seek assistance with child care and education. Some of the same criteria are useful in selecting family daycare, Montessori, or compensatory programs (see Table 9-1).

---

### Table 9-1 Criteria for Selection of Daycare Facility

1. Operated by reputable person, agency, or industry. Either profit or non-profit programs can offer quality care.

2. Licensed or certified by local and provincial regulatory bodies. Note that licensure ensures only that minimum standards are met.

3. Located convenient to home or workplace, open at the hours needed by the parent(s).

4. Committed to a philosophy of, and beliefs about, childrearing and discipline that are similar to those of the parents.

5. Staffed with certified daycare providers and other workers in appropriate staff–child ratio. Provider and staff have low turnover rates in employment.

6. Provision of an environment in which children and staff are happy and interacting. Children are having fun and learning.

7. Provision for grouping children according to age and developmental level so that children are safe and can learn from each other.

8. Provision of adequate space that is safe with well-controlled temperature; attractive; clean (but not sterile in appearance) and appropriate for age of child; psychomotor and sensory stimulation (height of windows, level floor); colourful but simple decor.

9. Provision of safe space and a variety of equipment, materials, and supplies for different types of play, such as:
   • Creative: art, music, reading, water play
   • Quiet: games, puzzles
   • Active: pedal toys, blocks
   • Outdoor: jungle gym, balls
   • Dramatic: Playhouse, farm, fire station

10. Provision of place for child to keep personal belongings.

*(continued)*

Table 9-1 (continued)

11. Provision for snacks and mealtime. Kitchen facilities meet health department standards. Tables and chairs are available for children and staff to sit and eat together.

12. Provision for child to be alone for short period, if desired, and for midday rest (floor mats provided).

13. Provision of age-appropriate toilet facilities and sinks.

14. Provision of separate room supplied to give emergency health services to an impaired or ill child until parents, or their designate, or emergency medical services can arrive.

15. Provision for occasional extra event, or short trip, such as a visit by a firefighter or trip to the local fire station.

16. Operated at a cost comparable to other similar facilities or programs or on a sliding scale basis.

17. Willingness by staff for anyone to visit unannounced.

18. Daily interaction of staff with parents including talk with parents about child's behaviour, progress, or health, as desired.

19. Discussion, well in advance, among providers, administrator(s), and parents about the contract for services, policies and procedures and their rationale, and explanation of planned changes.

20. Satisfaction among parents, child, providers, administrator(s), and staff with decision to have child attend the program.

The criteria in Table 9-1 are applicable, as well, to home daycare, although they would be applied to one adult in a home setting. The following questions should be asked:

■ Is there backup help available to the adult if it is needed (e.g., in case the daycare provider becomes ill, or if his or her child or another child was injured or became ill)?

■ Does the adult take the children for trips in a vehicle? If so, are there child safety seats or seatbelts appropriate to the child's age?

■ Is care provided on weekends, holidays, or in the evening?

The nursery school, operated by a reputable person or organization, provides the aforementioned, except for a full noon meal. Usually, only a mid-session snack is served. In any centre, the parent should observe the program to learn about the philosophy of the staff regarding childrearing, care, and discipline; administrative policies; the use of professional consultants for educational, social, or medical concerns; and the educational qualifications of the staff. They should note the warmth, emotional characteristics, and competence of the staff as they and children work and play together. The cost of the program, when the services are available, and the parents' obligations to the agency are other aspects worthy of consideration.

In either program, the child, under the guidance of qualified staff, will have many valuable experiences and will develop many skills, such as the following:

■ Following rules

■ Socializing with others; being co-operative in peer play

■ Investigating the environment

■ Doing imaginative experimentation with a variety of toys

■ Developing creative abilities

■ Carrying out basic problem solving

■ Becoming more independent, secure, and self-confident in a variety of situations

■ Handling emotions, broadening self-expression

■ Learning basic hygiene patterns

■ Learning about the surrounding community

Whether or not parents feel well-informed, they are the ones who ultimately decide which child care arrangements they will trust and support.[49]

In a paper entitled "Developing Cross-Cultural Partnerships: Implication for Child Care Quality Research and Practice,"[50] Pence and McCallum claim that working across cultural and institutional differences is a significant challenge. They provide an example of the partnership experience with Meadow Lake Tribal Council in Saskatchewan and the School of Child and Youth Care at the University of Victoria. They conclude that caring was an especially important element in the dynamic process inherent in the partnership.[51]

There are no accurate predictors of later academic success for preschool children. Some studies show that when infants and young children from poor families are given a planned educational experience aimed at preventing retardation and promoting parental interaction, environmental stimulation, and experiential opportunity, the experimental group showed superior cognitive abilities at age 5.5, compared with children in a control group raised in the usual way. Other studies showed that three-year-old children who were given special educational opportunities showed better intellectual performance at the end of grade two than did children in a control group.[52] Other authors say that pushing the child too early to develop reading and mathematics skills will create unnecessary problems: fatigue, stress-related illnesses, disciplinary problems, and parental burnout.[53]

If parents use a daycare centre, family daycare, nursery school, or early school program, help them understand that they remain the most important people to the child and that their love and involvement with the child are crucial for later learning and adjustment to life. The parents must have confidence in the agency so that they can convey a feeling of pleasurable expectation to the child. Help the working mother to realize that her working does not necessarily deprive the child. Many career women tend to do better parenting than full-time homemakers. They do not see the child as an end in itself; they allow the child to develop autonomy and initiative in creative ways because they have a sense of self-fulfillment in their own lives.

You can help the parents and child to prepare for the anxiety of separation if the child becomes enrolled in a nursery school or daycare centre. Help the parents realize, too, that the child's emotional and social adjustment and overall learning accomplishments depend on many factors. Because each child interprets entrance into the agency on the basis of his or her own past experience, each differs in adjustment. Being with a number of other children can be an upsetting experience. The child can often benefit from some form of preparation to avoid feeling abandoned or rejected.

---

## CRITICAL THINKING

*As a parent, what other criteria would you include in choosing a child care centre?*

---

# PHYSIOLOGIC CONCEPTS

The following information will be useful in the assessment of the child and in teaching the parents.

## Physical Characteristics

**Growth** Growth during the preschool years is relatively slow, but changes occur that transform the chubby toddler into a sturdy child who appears taller and thinner. Limb growth is greater in proportion to trunk growth. Although development does not proceed at a uniform rate in all areas or for all children, development follows a logical, precise pattern or sequence.[54] The preschool child grows approximately 6.75 to 7.5 cm and gains less than 2.2 kg per year. The child appears tall and thin because he or she grows proportionately more in height than in weight. The average height of the three-year-old is 94 cm; of the four-year-old, 104 cm; and of the five-year-old, 110 to 130 cm. At three,

the child weighs approximately 14.6 kg; at four years, 16.7 kg; and at five years, approximately 18.7 kg.[55]

**Vital Signs** The *body temperature* is 36.7° to 37.2°C. The *pulse rate* is normally 80 to 110 and the *respiratory rate* approximately 30 per minute. Normal *blood pressure* is approximately 90/60 mm Hg.

**Other Characteristics** *Eye–hand coordination* improves. By age 4.5, the *motor nerves are fully myelinated* and the *cerebral cortex* is fully connected to the cerebellum, permitting better coordination and control of bowel, bladder, and fine muscle movements, such as tying shoelaces, cutting with scissors, or holding a pencil or crayon. However, muscle development and bone growth are still far from mature. Excessive activity and overexertion can injure delicate tissue. Internal organs can adjust to moderate change; at five years, the brain is at 90 percent of the weight of the adult brain and the eruption of deciduous teeth is complete.[56] Physical characteristics to assess in this child are listed in Table 9-2. Because each child is unique, the normative listings indicate only where most children of a given age are in the development of various characteristics. Characteristics are listed by age in all following tables for reasons of understanding sequence and making comparisons. Consideration of only the chronologic age is misleading as a basis for assessment and care. For example, opportunity for muscle movement and exercise and nutritional status, rather than gender, influences strength. Still, by using the norms for the child at a given age, you can assess how far the child has deviated from the norm. With certain types of parental guidance, the child might reach some norms ahead of age. Certain situations, such as prenatal alcohol or drug exposure, are likely to cause the child to be below the norms.[57]

**Developmental Assessment** The Denver II—Revision and Restandardization of the Denver Developmental Screening Test (DDST) evaluates four major categories of development: gross motor, fine motor–adaptive, language, and personal–social (see Figure 9-1). It is used to determine whether a child is within normal range for various behaviours. Like the original DDST, the Denver II is applicable to children from birth through six years of age. The age divisions are monthly until 24 months, and then every 6 months until 6 years of age.[58]

Although it is not the purpose of this discussion to describe the administration and interpretation of the Denver II, the following points should be noted. First, to avoid errors in administration and interpretation and hence invalid screening results, the examiner should carefully follow the protocol outlined by the test's authors. A manual and workbook, videotape, and proficiency test have been developed to

## Table 9-2 Assessment of Physical Characteristics: Motor Control

| Age 3 Years | Age 4 Years | Age 5 Years |
|---|---|---|
| Occasional accident in toileting when busy at play; responds to routine times; tells when going to bathroom | Independent toilet habits; manages clothes without difficulty<br>Insists on having door shut for self but wants to be in bathroom with others | Takes complete charge of self; does not tell when going to bathroom |
| Verbalizes difference between how male and female urinate<br>Needs help with back buttons and drying self<br>Night time control of bowel and bladder most of time | Asks many questions about defecation function | Self-conscious about exposing self<br>Boys and girls go to separate bathrooms<br>Voids four to six times during waking hours; occasional nighttime accident |
| Runs more smoothly than before, turns sharp corners, suddenly stops; trunk rotates with run | Runs easily with coordination<br>Skips clumsily<br>Hops on one leg<br>Legs, trunk, shoulder, arms move in unison<br>Aggressive physical activity | Runs with skill, speed, agility, and plays games simultaneously<br>Starts and stops abruptly when running<br>Increases strength and coordination in limbs |
| Walks backward<br>Climbs stairs with alternate feet<br>Jumps from low step | Heel-toe walk<br>Walks a plank<br>Climbs stairs without holding onto rail<br>Climbs and jumps without difficulty | May still be knock-kneed<br>Jumps from three to four steps |
| Tries to dance but has inadequate balance, although sense of balance improving<br>Pedals tricycle<br>Swings | Enjoys motor stunts and gross gesturing<br><br>Enjoys new activities rather than repeating same ones | Balances self on toes and on one leg; dances with some rhythm<br>Balances on one foot approximately 10 sec.<br>Jumps rope<br>Roller skates<br>Hops and skips on alternate feet<br>Enjoys jungle gym |
| Sitting equilibrium maintained but combined awkwardly with reaching activity | Sitting balance well maintained; leans forward with greater mobility and ease<br>Exaggerated use of arm extension and trunk twisting; touches end of nose with forefinger on direction | Maintains balance easily<br>Combines reaching and placing object in one continuous movement<br>Arm extension and trunk twisting coordinated<br>Tummy protrudes, but some adult curve to spine |
| Undresses self; helps dress self<br>Undoes buttons on side or front of clothing<br>Goes to toilet alone if clothes simple<br>Washes hands, feeds self<br>May brush own teeth | Dresses and undresses self except tying bows, closing zipper, putting on boots and snowsuit<br>Does buttons<br>Distinguishes front and back of self and clothes<br>Brushes teeth alone | Dresses self without assistance; ties shoelaces<br>Requires less supervision of personal duties<br>Washes self without wetting clothes |
| Catches ball with arms fully extended one out of two to three times<br>Hand movement becoming better coordinated<br>Increasing coordination in vertical direction | Greater flexion of elbow<br>Catches ball thrown at 1.5 m two to three times<br>Throws ball overhand<br>Judges where a ball will land<br>Helps dust objects<br>Likes water play | Uses hands more than arms in catching ball<br>Pours fluid from one container to another with few spills; bilateral coordination<br>Uses hammer to hit nail on head<br>Interest and competence in dusting |

*(continued)*

Table 9-2 (continued)

| Age 3 Years | Age 4 Years | Age 5 Years |
|---|---|---|
| Pours fluid from pitcher, occasional spills | | Likes water play |
| Hits large pegs on board with hammer | | |
| Builds tower of 9 to 10 blocks; builds three-block gate from model | Builds complicated structure extending vertically and laterally; builds five-block gate from model | Builds things out of large boxes<br>Builds complicated three-dimensional structure and may build several separate units |
| Imitates a bridge | Notices missing parts or broken objects; requests parents to fix | Able to disassemble and reassemble small object |
| Copies circle or cross; begins to use scissors; strings large beads | Copies a square or simple figure | Copies triangle or diamond from model |
| | Uses scissors without difficulty | Folds paper diagonally |
| Shows hand preference | Enjoys finer manipulation of play materials | Definite hand preference |
| Trial-and-error method with puzzle | Surveys puzzle before placing pieces | Does simple puzzles quickly and smoothly |
| | Matches simple geometric forms | Prints some letters correctly; prints first name |
| | Prefers symmetry | |
| | Poor space perception | |
| Scribbles | Less scribbling | Draws clearly recognized lifelike representatives; differentiates parts of drawing |
| Tries to draw a picture and name it | Form and meaning in drawing apparent to adults | |

Sources: Frankenburg, W., and J.B. Dobbs, *Denver II—Revision and Restandardization of the Denver Developmental Screening Test.* Denver: Denver Developmental Materials, 1990; Papalia, D., S. Olds, and R. Feldman, *Human Development,* 9th ed. Boston: McGraw-Hill, 2004; Seifert, K., R. Hoffnung, and M. Hoffnung, *Lifespan Development.* Boston: Houghton Mifflin, 1997; Wong, D., and M.J. Hockenberry, *Wong's Nursing Care of Infants and Children,* 7th ed. St. Louis: C.V. Mosby, 2003.

ensure accurate administration and interpretation by examiners. Second, before administering the test, explanations should be given to both the child and the parent(s). Parents should be advised that the Denver II is not an intelligence test but rather a means of assessing what the child can do at a particular age.[59] Children with advanced development and who are gifted can be identified.[60]

Because the Denver II is non-threatening, requires no painful or unfamiliar procedures, and relies on the child's natural activity of play, it is an excellent way to begin the health assessment. It is a general assessment tool that can help guide treatment and teaching. The Denver II form and instruction manual can be obtained from Denver Developmental Materials, Inc., P.O. Box 371079, Denver, CO 80237-5075; (303) 355-4729; www.denverii.com/order.html.

It is important to consider genetics, family factors, nutrition, and social environment when you assess and care for children who are *developmentally delayed*.[61] Occasionally, a child does not attain height within the norms for his or her age, although torso to leg proportions are normal. Such deviations are probably caused because the pituitary gland does not produce enough growth hormone.[62] **Growth hormone deficiency,** *which causes dwarfism in a preschool child,* can now be treated with a synthetic growth hormone. The person still remains short in stature, but is within a normal height range. The treatment is important because children who lag behind peers in growth are often teased, kept from participating in certain play activities, and may have difficulty finding clothes or play equipment, such as a bicycle, that is of correct size. The child may be regarded by others as being intellectually challenged. He or she may feel inferior, suffer a negative self-concept, lack initiative, and become withdrawn, depressed, or antisocial in later childhood or adult years.[63]

## Nutritional Needs

As stated in Chapter 8, *Eating Well with Canada's Food Guide* has been adapted for children by taking into account the smaller portions of food they eat. As a result, the guide has become a useful tool for everyone in the family over two years of age.[64] The dietary requirements of preschoolers are

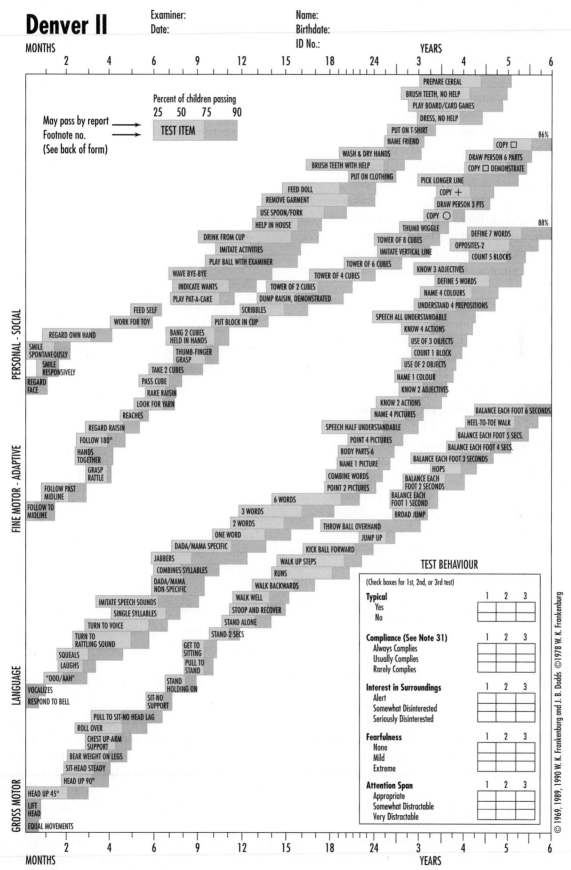

Source: Frankenberg, W.K., and J.B. Dobbs, Denver II—Revision and Standardization of the Denver Developmental Screening Test. *Denver Developmental Materials,* 1990.

similar to those of toddlers. Preschool children consume slightly more than toddlers, and nutrient density is more important than quantity.[65]

A slower growth rate and heightened interest in exploring the environment may lessen the child's interest in eating. Because preschoolers have relatively high needs for energy, in addition to small stomachs, they may need to eat small amounts of food frequently throughout the day. This need is best achieved by three meals with a nutritious snack between meals. The amount of food a preschooler needs depends on age, body size, activity level, growth rate, and appetite.[66] Refer back to Figure 8-2.

Children who are reared in *vegetarian families* may be shorter and weigh less, but by the end of the preschool era the child's growth rate approaches the norm. However, children who follow a vegetarian diet are especially at risk for protein and vitamin deficiencies, such as vitamin B deficiency.[67]

Eating assumes increasing social interaction for the preschooler, and it continues to be an emotional and physiologic experience. The family mealtime promotes socialization in relation to meal preparation, behaviour during mealtimes, language skills, and understanding of family rituals and situations. The learning experience is positive or negative, depending on the parents' example. Much valuable learning is missed if there is little or no family mealtime. Table manners need not be rigidly emphasized; accidents will happen, and parental example is the best teacher.

An interesting and critical study by Broughton and her researchers was conducted to measure household food security. One variable they considered was the relationship between household food insecurity and preschool children's nutritional status. They found that household food insecurity was associated with indicators of suboptimal health status in preschoolers. One recommendation advocated that parents gain practical skills in the preparation of nutrient-dense foods.[68]

Another study examined Aboriginal preschool children across Canada who were at an increased risk for Early Childhood Caries (ECC) when compared with their non-Aboriginal age cohorts. It appears that dental health programs fail to prevent ECC because intervention often arrives too late. Lawrence and her researchers evaluated the effectiveness of the dental-hygiene-coordinated prenatal nutrition program delivered by community-based nutrition educators on First Nations reserves located in northwestern Ontario on the following criteria: (1) parents/caregivers' beliefs and behavioural decisions related to dental preventative practices and feeding habits of young children; (2) oral health status and treatment needs of those children; and (3) early

childhood obesity. It was concluded that the prenatal nutrition program improved caregivers' knowledge of ECC. However, factors that place undue strain on the caregiver, such as overcrowding, which can lead to poor oral hygiene and poor dietary habits among children in Aboriginal communities, need to be addressed.[69]

The preschooler likes to eat one thing at a time. Of all food groups, vegetables tend to be least liked, whereas fruits are a favourite. The child usually prefers vegetables and fruits crisp, raw, and cut into finger-sized pieces. New foods can be introduced gradually; if a food is refused once, offer it again after a few days. It is important not to pressure the child to eat. By trusting their hunger cues, preschoolers can learn to choose amounts they can expect to eat.[70]

*A child may be eating insufficiently for the following reasons:*

- Eating too much between meals
- Experiencing unhappy mealtime atmosphere
- Seeking attention
- Mimicking parental eating habits
- Responding to excessive parental expectations
- Having inadequate variety and quantity
- Suffering tooth decay, which may cause nausea or toothache with chewing
- Feeling sibling rivalry
- Experiencing overfatigue or physical illness
- Experiencing emotional disturbance

Eating a variety of foods is one of the best ways to ensure an adequate intake of nutrients. If a child is eating according to the revised Canada Food Guide, is growing well, and is healthy, vitamin-mineral supplements are rarely necessary.

## CRITICAL THINKING

*What criteria should be taken into account for an accurate nutritional assessment of a preschooler?*

## Exercise

This is the developmental period when the child seems to have a surplus of energy and is constantly on the move. The child needs time and space for physical exercise through play. Clothing and shoes should be comfortable and allow for easy movement. Children of all ages can, and should, be involved in a variety of different activities. Of course, the kinds of activities in which they participate depend on their age and stage of development. Although children follow a basic developmental pattern, they grow and develop at different rates.[71] The following three types of physical activities should be combined when planning activities for preschoolers:

- Endurance activities that strengthen the heart and lungs, such as running, jumping, and swimming
- Flexibility activities that encourage a child to bend, stretch, and reach, such as gymnastics and dancing
- Strength-building activities that build strong muscles and bones, such as climbing[72]

For more information, see Canada's Physical Activity Guide for Children and Youth at www.phac-aspc.gc.ca/pau-uap/paguide/child_youth/partners/boiler3.html.[73]

---

### CRITICAL THINKING

*What are some suitable physical activities for the preschooler?*

---

## Sleep

Sleep patterns vary widely among preschool children; but the average preschooler sleeps approximately 12 hours a night and seldom takes daytime naps. Waking during the night is common. In fact, the preschool years are a prime time for sleep disturbances.[74]

Parents should help the restless child develop sleep strategies, such as cuddling a teddy bear or blanket or babbling to an imaginary friend. Parents should provide reassurance and set and stick to limits.

Sleep problems usually subside spontaneously, but the child and parents may need therapy if the problem persists several times weekly or over a long period.

## Health Promotion and Prevention

**Immunization Schedules**  For immunization schedules for children of this age group, refer to Table 7-6, which is from the seventh edition of the Canadian Immunization Guide.[75]

**Dental Care**  Because caries frequently begin at this age and spread rapidly, dental care is important. Deciduous teeth guide the permanent ones, and they should be kept in good repair. If deciduous teeth are lost too early, permanent teeth grow in abnormally. Teeth should be brushed after eating, using a method recommended by the dentist. The intake of refined sugars should be limited to help prevent tooth decay. The Canadian Dental Association advises against fluoride supplements in young children before permanent teeth erupt.[76]

Before entering school, the child is usually required to have a physical examination (including urinalysis) and a dental examination.

**Safety Promotion and Injury Control**  The preschooler has more freedom, independence, initiative, and desire to imitate adults than the toddler does, but still has an immature understanding of danger and illness. This combination is likely to get him or her into hazardous situations rather frequently.

A major responsibility of caretaking adults is safety promotion and injury control, as the child needs watchfulness and a safe play area. The adult serves as a supervisor while patiently teaching caution and keeping the environment as safe as possible. Siblings can take some, but not total, responsibility for the preschooler. An interesting Canadian study by Morrongiello and her researchers examined unintentional injuries and sibling supervision in the home. It seems that older siblings supervise younger ones about 11 percent of their mutual awake time, typically with children playing and parents usually doing other chores. The behaviour of the supervisee (the preschooler) contributed to risk more than the behaviour of the supervising sibling. That is, the supervisee seemed to pay less attention to the sibling supervisor then he/she did to the parent. This result occurred even though the sibling supervisor was using the same type of strategies as their mother or father use. Interestingly, poor compliance by the younger child when the older sibling was supervising predicted injury.[77]

As the child learns to protect self, he or she should be allowed to take added responsibility for personal safety and should be given appropriate verbal recognition and praise to reinforce safe behaviour. If the parent voices fear overly often, natural curiosity and the will to learn will tend to be dulled, and the child may come to fear every new situation.

*Explore information in this section with parents so that they and you can use these safety suggestions:*

- Begin safety teaching early. Good teaching during the toddler years frequently pays off later.
- Avoid constant threats and frequent physical punishment. Incessant "don'ts" should be avoided because the child will learn to ignore them, feel angry or resentful, and purposefully rebel or defy adults, thus failing to learn about real danger.
- When you must forbid, use simple command words in a firm voice without anger to convey the impression that you expect the child to obey—for example, "stop," "no."
- Phrase safety rules and their reasons in positive, rather than negative, terms when possible. For example, say: "Play in the yard, not the street, or you'll get hurt by cars"; "Sit quietly in the car to avoid being hurt"; "Put tiny things (coins, beads) that you find in here (jar, bowl, box)."
- Teach the child his or her full name, address (including postal code), and telephone number. Be sure to teach

the child how to use police or adults in service roles for help (e.g., 911, emergency services, fire department).

- Teach the child not to give out information over the telephone about him- or herself or the family.

- Encourage the child to share "secrets"; emphasize that he or she does not need to fear saying anything.

- Tell the child not to leave home alone, or with a stranger. He or she should use a "buddy" system when going somewhere.

- Never leave the child alone in public or unattended in a car.

- Teach the child escape techniques—for example, how to unlock home doors or car doors.

- Never leave the child home alone. Make sure that the babysitter is reliable.

- Never allow the child to play in or near a busy driveway or garage. Forbid street play if other play areas are available. Teach children to look carefully for, and to get away from, cars. A fenced yard or playground is ideal, although not always available.

- Teach the child how to cross streets safely.

- Teach the child to refuse gifts or rides from strangers, to avoid walking or playing alone on a deserted street, road, or similar area, and about the possibility of child molesters or abductors.

- Keep matches in containers and out of reach.

- Dispose of, or store out of reach and in a locked cabinet, all of the poisons you have in the house: rat and roach killer, insecticides, weed killer, kerosene, cleaning agents, furniture polish, and medicines. Suntan lotion, shampoo, deodorants, nail polish, and cosmetics remain potential hazards; the child should be taught their *correct* use. The child is less likely to pull them out of cabinets or swallow them than when he or she was a toddler. Brightly coloured containers or pills, powders, or liquids raise curiosity, and the desire for experimentation. Keep medications out of the child's reach. Bright-coloured pills can be mistaken for candy. Keep the Poison Control Centre telephone number readily visible.

- Observe your child continuously while he or she plays near water. Cover wells and cisterns. Be sure to fence ponds and swimming pools.

- Keep stairways and nighttime play areas well lit.

- Equip upstairs windows with sturdy screens and guards. Have handrails on stairways.

- Store knives, saws, other sharp objects, and lawn or power tools out of reach.

- Remove doors from abandoned appliances and cars; campaign for legislation for appropriate disposal of them and for mandatory door removal.

- Discourage playing with, or in the area of, appliances or power tools while they are in operation: a washing machine with a wringer, a lawn mower, a saw, or a clothes dryer.

- Use safety glass in glass doors or shower stalls; place decals on sliding doors at child's eye level (and adult's eye level, too) to prevent walking or running through them.

- Use adhesive strips in the bathtub.

- Avoid scatter rugs, debris, or toys cluttered on the floor in areas of traffic.

- Use seatbelts in the car that are appropriate for the weight and size of the child.

- Teach the child sun safety rules: cover up, find shade, and use sun-safe products and sunscreens.[78]

If the child continually fails to listen or obey, ask the following questions: Is the child able to hear? Is he or she intellectually able to understand? Are demands too numerous, or expectations too great? Are statements too lengthy or abstract? Is anger expressed with teaching and discipline to the point that it interferes emotionally with the child's perception and judgment? Perhaps most important, do the parents demonstrate safety-conscious behaviour with equipment, movements, or use of sun safety rules? Although imitation is a major way to learn, let us pay a brief visit to one recent and relevant Canadian research study.

Bruce and her colleagues examined the relationship between two groups of Canadian preschoolers (injured and non-injured) and their parents' risk perceptions, safety behaviours, parenting stress, and children's risk behaviours. They found significantly higher numbers of injury behaviour in the group of injured children. Contrary to the researchers' hypothesis, parents' perception of risk and hazard were not found to be significantly less among those parents of injured children. However, the parents of injured children had a higher score for perceived dangers for their children and less parent stress.[79] The researchers conclude that injury behaviour screening may provide a useful tool for health care professionals in practical environments to target injury prevention counselling for those children and families most at risk.[80]

Agricultural injuries are an important health concern for the pediatric population, particularly for preschool children. A study was conducted to estimate rates and determine patterns of fatal agricultural injury among young Canadian children exposed to farming hazards and to identify strategies to prevent such injuries. A notable result was that the annual rate of fatal agricultural injury of children was substantially higher than that of national all-cause, unintentional fatal injury among Canadian children aged one to six years. In addition, most injuries occurred in the agricultural worksite, and higher rates of injuries were attributed to boys. Brison and his researchers concluded that preschool children exposed to agricultural worksites are at a high risk of fatal injuries. The results indicated that prevention strategies should focus on restricting children's access to these worksites.[81]

## CRITICAL THINKING

*What elements should be included in an injury behaviour screening tool?*

*Head injury* is the major cause of bicycle-related fatalities. The single most important aspect is to encourage the child to wear a protective helmet.[82] Safe Kids Canada supports helmet legislation as a proven strategy, in conjunction with sustained education and enforcement programs designed to prevent head injuries and deaths.[83] In a survey of helmet wear, the Canada Safety Council found that most parents reported that their children wear a helmet: when bicycling (84 percent), in-line skating (79 percent), riding a scooter (73 percent), and skateboarding (13 percent).[84] Nurses must continually teach parents the importance of children wearing protective helmets.

**Minor lacerations** and *cuts* should be examined for dirt and foreign objects even after they have been cleaned with warm water and soap. The laceration should be covered with a loose bandage that will keep out dirt and protect the wound from additional trauma. The parent or caretaker should watch for signs of infection: redness, heat, swelling, and drainage. It is especially important for the parent to wash his or her hands before and after application of topical therapies. Topical applications are applied to the skin to ease discomfort, prevent further injury, and facilitate healing.[85]

**Burns** are *thermal injuries to the skin*. A **first-degree burn** *usually shows redness only*; a **second-degree burn** *causes blister formation*, sometimes with peeling and weeping. Scalds often produce this type of burn. A **third-degree burn** *chars the skin, causing a whitish appearance, and injured tissue under the skin*. It may cause anesthesia. Flame and hot metal often cause third-degree burns.[86]

For a first-degree burn, the affected area should be plunged into cold water for a few minutes. Gentle washing with soap and water should be sufficient. A second-degree burn should have the same initial treatment. Blisters that form should be left intact, and the burned area should be covered with non-adherent gauze and a bulky, dry, sterile dressing. Tetanus immunization should be up to date. A third-degree burn, any second-degree burn that covers an area greater than an adult's hand size, any facial burns, and any burn in which child maltreatment is suspected should be seen by the health care provider and physician.[87]

*Accidental ingestions and poisonings* may occur in children under the age of five, sometimes even when the preventive measures discussed in Chapter 8 are taken. Ingestions of these materials can cause a great variety of symptoms and signs. *The following guidelines should be taught to parents:*

1. Look for an empty container nearby if sudden unusual symptoms or abnormal odour to breath or clothes are observed.

2. Try to determine what and how much was ingested and how long ago.

3. Call the poison control centre for help.

4. If there are no contraindications to vomiting (either from reading the side of the container or from getting directions at the poison control centre), induce vomiting with syrup of ipecac. Mechanical stimulation of the posterior pharynx can be used to induce vomiting *except* with ingestion of corrosive agents, such as lye, gasoline, and kerosene.

5. Take the child to the nearest clinic that is set up to deal with these problems.[88]

The bite of any animal will probably have few symptoms other than pain at the site of puncture wounds or small lacerations. Dog bites are most common, although the child may have contact with other animals that bite or scratch. The chief concern is the possibility of rabies. It is essential to establish the vaccination status of the biting animal, if possible, for if the animal is properly vaccinated, there is little chance of acquiring and transmitting the disease to humans. Rabies prophylaxis will be determined by the physician. The wound should be washed with copious amounts of soap and water. Tetanus prophylaxis should be up to date.[89] Bites from other children can also occur.

Regarding *lead poisoning*, before legislation that prohibited the use of lead-based paint in the interior of homes, the ingestion of small chips of paint from dilapidated houses was the most common cause of lead poisoning in children. In most Canadian and American cities, a number of old houses, constructed before 1950, may still contain lead-based paint. Children at risk for lead poisoning include those living in impoverished and overcrowded homes, inhabitants of large urban cities, and recent immigrants from countries that have not enacted measures to decrease lead exposure among children.[90] Bailey states that the incidence of lead poisoning is scarce in Canada.[91]

Prevention lies in keeping the preschooler in a lead-free environment as much as possible. You may call the housing inspector, with the family's permission, to test paint for lead. In many cities, landlords are required to repaint the house interior when lead paint is found. Treatment for severe cases of lead poisoning involves hospitalization.

## Common Health Problems: Health Promotion, Prevention, and Treatment

Teach parents that scheduled health maintenance visits to the doctor, or nurse practitioner, are important for the early detection of problems. Table 9-3 summarizes a few common health problems.[92]

**Child Maltreatment** In Canada, child maltreatment is classified as physical abuse, sexual abuse, neglect, and emotional maltreatment.[93] The selection of best practices for the prevention and treatment of child maltreatment is critical. Canadian child abuse programs have been delineated into three levels: tertiary, secondary, and primary.[94] Tertiary programs are implemented in families where child abuse has occurred. Secondary prevention programs of child maltreatment consist of the early identification of parents who are at risk for abusing their children.

A parenting program called First Nations Parenting is available to First Nations communities served by the Awasis Agency of Northern Manitoba. Primary prevention programs are focused at the general population to address underlying causes and to decrease the incidence of maltreatment. The purpose of these programs is to reduce the risk for families under stress and to promote wellness in families that are functioning adequately.[95] The main intent of prevention and health promotion programs regarding child abuse should address the aspect of quality living with emphasis on wellness and primary prevention. Some children who are frequently or severely maltreated develop post-traumatic stress disorder (PTSD), which involves extreme levels of anxiety. Other symptoms

### Table 9-3 Common Health Problems of the Preschooler

| Problem | Definition | Signs/Symptoms | Prevention/Treatment |
|---|---|---|---|
| Strabismus | Eyes not straight or properly aligned | Double vision (diplopia), followed by irreversible loss of vision in suppressed eye (amblyopia) | Appropriate vision testing E chart or Allen cards Use toy to go through visual field testing Test for colour blindness Functional amblyopia remedied through corrective lens, contact lens, and prisms |
| Conjunctivitis | Inflammation of the eyelids or conjunctivae or both; caused by bacteria or virus | Redness of conjunctivae; mild irritation; excessive lacrimation; normal vision | Cool compresses Appropriate eye drops |
| Hearing loss | Hearing less than normal for age group | Inability to speak by age 2; failure to respond to out-of-sight noise; tilting the head while listening | Use play technique to evaluate hearing Use earphones to transmit sounds and have child put peg in board when hearing sound |
| Otitis media | Infection of middle ear with accumulation of serop-urulent fluid in middle ear cavity | Earache, fever, upper respiratory infection; decreased hearing; bulging tympanic membrane; disappearance of landmarks | Lymphatic tissue, tonsils, and adenoids more abundant now than later and, therefore, are often involved in the infectious process |

*(continued)*

Table 9.3 (continued)

| Problem | Definition | Signs/Symptoms | Prevention/Treatment |
|---------|-----------|----------------|---------------------|
| Acute cervical adenitis | Inflammation of one or more cervical nodes in response to an infection in the ear, nose or throat; group A streptococcal often the cause | Painful swelling of neck; possibly high fever; usually unilateral cervical nodes enlarged and tender | Appropriate antibiotic<br>Antipyretic<br>Warm compresses |
| Urinary tract infection | Bacterial infection of part or all of urinary tract, collecting system of kidneys, and bladder | May be asymptomatic; urgency and frequency of urination; dysuria; flank and suprapubic pain; foul-smelling urine; fever | Appropriate antibiotic<br>Increased water intake<br>Personal hygiene |
| Enuresis | Involuntary passage of urine; occurs at night in 10–15% of 5-year-olds | Bedwetting | Reduction of liquid intake in the evening<br>Maintaining appropriate attitude<br>Signal device sometimes helpful<br>Getting child up at specified times to urinate |
| Nonspecific vulvovaginitis | Inflammation of vulva and vagina; usually nonspecific organism responsible | Discharge; pruritus; erythema | Personal hygiene<br>Wearing cotton underwear<br>Avoidance of bubble baths and perfumed soaps<br>Cold compresses to vulva |
| Measles | Highly contagious viral disease with severe complications | Rash (beginning at face and descending down body); 3C's—coryza, cough, conjunctivitis; Koplik's spots (red) on buccal mucosa; fever | Prevention: immunization<br>*If disease: isolation*<br>No specific therapy<br>Symptomatic treatment |
| Diarrhea | Inflammation of gastrointestinal tract caused at this age by *Giardia lambdia* and *Salmonella* | Stools more frequent and liquid than usual; abdominal cramps; foul-smelling stool; weight loss | Sometimes antibiotics<br>Personal hygiene; safe drinking water<br>Staying out of wading pools |
| Postural problems | Deviation of normal posture and normal spinal curves | Deviation seen as child bends anteriorly, laterally, posteriorly | Exercises prescribed by knowledgeable health care practitioner |
| Juvenile hypertension | Child more than age 3 who has diastolic pressure greater than 90 mm Hg | Probably none other than blood pressure elevation | Referral for overall cardiovascular investigation |
| Hypochromic anemia | Prevalent nutritional problem in childhood, caused by inadequate intake of absorbable iron | Associated with poor hygiene, chronic disease; major part of diet is milk or milk products | Encourage parents to feed child eggs, meat, fish, fruits, cereals, and dark green leafy vegetables<br>Normal, not excessive, amounts of milk |

Sources: Wong, D., and M.J. Hockenberry, *Wong's Nursing Care of Infants and Children,* 7th ed. St. Louis, MO: C.V. Mosby, 2003; Rath Rentfro, A.R. *Preschool Child. In* C. Edelman, and C. Mandle (eds.), *Health Promotion throughout the Life Span,* 6th ed. St. Louis, MO: C.V. Mosby, 2006.

include nightmares, feelings of isolation, flashback memories of episodes of abuse, guilt feelings, and other sleep disturbances.[96] Also see the section entitled "Child Maltreatment" in Chapter 7.

## CRITICAL THINKING

*What steps are involved in designing a primary prevention program in the community on child maltreatment?*

**Reactions to Illness and Hospitalization** During the preschool stage, when the child has heightened feelings of sexuality, fears of dependency and separation, fantasies, feelings of narcissism, and rivalry with parents, he or she is particularly vulnerable to fears about body damage. The child perceives and fears dental, medical, and surgical procedures as mutilating, intrusive, punishing, or abandoning. Such persistently recurring conflicts, fears, guilt, anger, or excessive concern about the body can influence personality development into adulthood.

Teach parents that many of these negative reactions can be averted by introducing the child to medical facilities and health workers when he or she is well. The best teaching is by positive example. If the parent takes the child with him or her to the physician and dentist, and if the child observes courteous professionals, a procedure that does not hurt (or an explanation of why it will hurt), and a positive response from the parent, a great deal of teaching is accomplished. These visits can be reinforced with honest answers to the many questions the preschooler will have. Research also indicates that being away from mother on a daily basis, in some kind of alternative daycare experience, moderates the separation anxiety and negative reaction to hospitalization.[97]

Emphasize the importance of continued and ample contact with the child whenever either parent, or the child, is hospitalized. You should advise parents to:

1. Trust their intuition (they know the child best).
2. Shop for a doctor and hospital.
3. Prepare themselves so that they can prepare the child.
4. Prepare the child a few days before hospitalization.
5. Be present at important times.

You will be in a position to offset the negative effects of hospitalization through planning individualized care, the use of play or art therapy, and your involvement in decision-making and policy-making. The hospital personnel should make the ward as homelike as possible through cheerful decor and furnishings and provision for toys, a playroom, and a central dining area. The staff members usually wear pastel uniforms or smocks and provide for the child to remain in his or her own clothes, keep a favourite toy, eat uninterrupted by procedures, and follow normal living routines when possible. Flexible visiting hours are essential because the presence of the mother can dramatically revive a child's interest in getting well, and mother or father's visit can improve eating, sleeping, and general behaviour. The family should be seen as collaborators in care. If collaboration does not seem realistic, one nurse should consistently care for the child while involving the parent as much as possible.

Encourage the parent to talk about their feelings of fear, anxiety, guilt, shame, or sadness that may be present and related to the child's illness or hospitalization, or other children left at home. Help parents to talk about the unique aspects of their family life and their child so that care can be truly individualized. For example, a child may prefer to wear his shorts instead of pajamas in bed.

On admission, obtain a developmental history from the mother and use it to plan care to follow the child's usual living routine. Help the child displace aggression onto toys, rather than onto parents. Allow the child to be angry. Objective involvement is important to avoid accidental favouritism by attending to only certain children. Several authors describe practical ways to help the child prepare for, and cope with, painful procedures.[98] Be aware of cultural differences in the family. For example, the Filipino family provides primary support during illness, and many members of the extended family become involved in the care.[99]

## CRITICAL THINKING

*What constitutes a child's developmental history?*

# Psychosocial Concepts

Use the following information in assessment, teaching, and health promotion with the child and parent(s).

**Cognitive Development** In this stage, the child is perceptually bound, unable to reason logically about concepts that are discrepant from visual cues. The child learns by interacting with knowledgeable people, being confronted with others' opinions, and being actively involved with objects and processes. More important than the facts learned are the attitudes the child forms regarding knowledge, learning, people, and the environment. Cognition and learning, at least partly a result of language learning and perceptual ability, can be studied through the child's handling of the physical environment and in connection with the concepts of number, causality, and time, abstractions highly developed in Western civilization.[100]

By helping parents understand the cognitive development of their child, including concept formation, you will help them to stimulate intellectual growth realistically, without expecting too much. **Concepts** *come about by giving precepts (events, things, and experiences) a meaningful label.* The name or label implies a similarity to other things with the same name, and a difference from things having a different name. **Concept formation** *develops when perception progresses from being diffuse, to roughly differentiated, and finally to sharply differentiated awareness of stable and coordinated objects.* The first concept is formed when a simple word comes to designate a crudely defined area of experience. As the late toddler and early preschooler acquire a number of words, each representing a loosely defined notion or thing, the global meaning becomes a simple, concrete concept. As perceived characteristics of things and events become distinguished from each other, the child becomes aware of differences among words, objects, and experiences, such as dog and cat, baby and doll, men and daddy, approval and disapproval. However, the preschooler cannot yet define attributes; and he or she cannot make explicit comparisons of the objects. The attributes are an absolute part of the object, such as bark and dog. Hence the child is said to *think concretely*. What he or she sees or hears can be named, which is different from conceptual or abstract thinking about the object.[101]

Concrete concepts become true concepts when the late preschooler can compare, combine, and describe them, and they can think and talk about their attributes. At this point, the child can deal with differences between concepts, such as "dogs bark, people talk." But not until after age six or seven will he or she be able to deal with opposites and similarities together.[102] For further information, see the box entitled "Categories of Concepts that Develop in the Preschool Years."

Some of the influences on concept development include the following:

- The child's inability to distinguish between his or her own feelings and outside events
- The ability to be impressed by the external, obvious features of a situation or thing rather than its essential features
- Awareness of gaps in a situation
- Emotional or contextual significance of words

The concreteness typical of a preschooler's concepts is found in the rambling, loosely jointed circumstantial descriptions. Everything is equally important and must be included. One must listen closely to get the central theme because young children learn things in bunches, not in a systematic, organized way. They can memorize and recite many things, but they cannot paraphrase or summarize their learning.[103]

**Concepts of Relationships** These concepts involve time, space, number, and causation. They are more abstract than those based on the immediately observable properties of things, and are greatly determined by culture.[104] See Table 9-4 for the pattern of mental development.

**Time Concept** For the preschooler, time is beginning to move. The past is measured in hours, and the future is a myth. Initially, formal time concepts have nothing to do with personal time. Adults are seen as changeless, and the child believes that he or she can mature in a hurry. Therefore, the preschooler thinks that he or she can grow up fast and marry his or her parent. Time concepts are further described in Table 9-4.[105]

## Categories of Concepts That Develop in the Preschool Years

- **Life:** ascribes living qualities to inanimate objects
- **Death:** associates death with separation, lack of movement; thinks dead people capable of doing what living people do
- **Body functions:** has inaccurate understanding about body functions and birth process
- **Space:** judges short distances accurately; aware of direction and distance in relation to body
- **Weight:** estimates weight in terms of size; by age five can determine which of two objects feels heavier, notion of quantity—more than one, big, small
- **Numbers:** understands up to five
- **Time:** has gradually increasing sense of time; present-oriented; knows day of week, month, and year

- **Self:** knows own sex, full name, names of outer body parts by age three; self-concept begins to include facts about his or her abilities and race, but not socioeconomic class
- **Sex roles:** has general concept of sex, identity, and appropriate sex roles developed at age five or six
- **Social awareness:** is egocentric but forms definite opinions about others' behaviour as "nice" or "mean"; intuitive; concept of causality is magical, illogical
- **Beauty:** names major colours; prefers music with definite tune and rhythm
- **Comedy:** considers as comic funny faces made by self or others, socially inappropriate behaviour, and antics of pets

## Table 9-4 Assessment of Mental Development

| Age 3 Years | Age 4 Years | Age 5 Years |
|---|---|---|
| Knows he or she is a person separate from another<br>Knows own sex and some sex differences | Senses self one among many | Aware of cultural and other differences between people and the two sexes<br>Mature enough to fit into simple type of culture<br>Can tell full name and address<br>Remains calm if lost away from home |
| Resists commands but distractible and responsive to suggestions<br>Can ask for help<br>Desire to please<br>Friendly<br>Sense of humour | States alibis because more aware of attitude and opinions of others<br>Self-critical; appraises good and bad of self<br>Does not like to admit inabilities; excuses own behaviour<br>Praises self; bosses or criticizes others<br>Likes recognition for achievement<br>Heeds others' thoughts and feelings; expresses own | Dependable<br>Increasing independence<br>Can direct own behaviour; but fatigue, excessive demands, fantasy, and guilt interfere with assuming self-responsibility<br>Admits when needs help<br>Moves from direct to internalized action, from counting what he or she can touch to counting in thought; uses more clues |
| Use language rather than physical activity to communicate | Active use of language<br>Active learning<br>Likes to make rhymes, to hear stories with exaggeration and humour, dramatic songs<br>Knows nursery rhymes<br>Tells action implied in picture books | Improves use of symbol system, concept formation<br>Repeats long sentences accurately<br>Can carry plot in story<br>Defines objects in terms of use<br>States relationship between two events |
| Imaginative<br>Better able to organize thoughts<br><br>Can be bargained with<br><br>Sacrifices immediate pleasure for promise of future gain<br>Understands simple directions; follows normal routines of family life and does minor errands | Highly imaginative yet literal, concrete thinking<br>Can organize his or her experience<br>Increasing reasoning power and critical thinking capacity<br>Makes crude comparisons<br><br>Concept of 1, 2, 3; counts to 5; does some home chores<br>Generalizes | Less imaginative<br>Asks details<br>Can be reasoned with logically<br>More accurate, relevant, practical, sensible than 4-year-old<br>Asks to have words defined<br>Seeks reality<br><br>Begins to understand money<br>Does more home chores with increasing competence<br>Can determine which of two weights heavier<br>Idea in head precedes drawing on paper or physical activity<br>Interested in meaning of relatives |
| Know age<br>Meagre comprehension of past and future<br>Knows mostly today | Realizes birthday is one in a series and that birthday is measure of growth<br>Knows when next birthday is<br>Knows age<br>Birthdays and holidays significant because aware of units of time<br>Loves parties related to holiday<br>Conception of time<br>Knows day of week | Understands week as a unit of time<br>Knows day of week<br>Sense of time and duration increasing<br>Know how old will be on next birthday<br>Knows month and year<br>Adults seen as changeless<br>Memory surprisingly accurate |
| Has attention span of 10–15 minutes | Has attention span of 20 minutes | Has attention span of 30 minutes |

**Spatial Concepts** Spatial concepts differ markedly in children and adults. There are five major stages in the development of spatial concepts. First, there is **action space,** *consisting of the location or regions to which the child moves.* Second, **body space** refers to *the child's own awareness of directions and distances in relation to his or her own body.* Third, there is **object space,** *in which objects are located relative to each other and without reference to the child's body.* The fourth and fifth stages, **map space** and **abstract space,** are *interrelated and depend on knowing directions of east, west, south, and north; allocating space in visual images to nations, regions, towns, rooms; and the ability to deal with maps, geographic or astronomic ideas, and three-dimensional space that use symbolic (verbal or mathematical) relationships.*[106]

The preschool child has action space and moves along familiar locations and explores new terrain. He or she is beginning to orient self relative to body space and object space through play and exploration of his or her own body. He knows up and down, front and back, sideways, next to, near and far, and later left and right. The child is not able, until approximately age six, to understand object space as a unified whole. He or she will first see a number of unrelated routes or spaces. He or she is generally aware of specific objects and habitual routes. The child does not see self and objects as part of a larger integrated space with multiple possibilities for movement. Map space and abstract space are not understood until much later.

**Quantitative Concepts** *Notions of quantity* such as one and more than one, bigger, and smaller are developed in the early preschool years. Understanding of the quantity or amount represented by a number is not related to the child's ability to count to 10, 20, or higher, nor can he or she transfer numbers to notions of money value, although he or she may imitate adults and play store, passing money back and forth. Ordinal numbers, indicating successions rather than totals, develop crudely in "me first" or "me last." The concepts of second, third, and so on develop later. The preschooler cannot simultaneously take account of different dimensions such as one quart equals two pints nor equal volume in different-shaped containers (see Table 9-4).[107]

Klein and Bisanz, of the University of Alberta, presented a nonverbal form of arithmetic problems to facilitate performance by helping children create an appropriate mental model of the tasks. They used poker chips in lieu of numbers for counting. They concluded that for two-term problems (e.g., $a + b$), the maximum number of units that must be held in working memory at the same time during problem solution is a major constraint on preschoolers' success in solving addition and subtraction problems when a nonverbal format is used. Some children, in a three-term problem (e.g., $a + b - b$) indicated the spontaneous use of procedures based on the arithmetic principle of inversion. This principle arises from give and take (subtraction and addition), and it occurs in play with other children and adults when solving such a problem. These findings could help teachers to optimize the instructional process so that children can learn to link the knowledge they have gained prior to formal schooling with the instruction offered in school.[108]

**Concepts of Causality** The ability to perceive cause and effect in the preschooler is marginal. Things simply are. The child may be pleased or displeased with events, but does not understand what brought them about. He or she does pre-causal thinking, confusing physical and mechanical causation or natural phenomena with psychological, moral, or sequential causes. When the child asks "why?" he or she is probably looking for justification rather than causation. Most things are taken for granted. The child assumes that people, including self, or some motivated inanimate being is the cause of events. Perception of the environment is **animistic,** *endowing all things with the qualities of life that Westerners reserve for human beings.* There is little notion of accident or coincidence. It takes some time to learn that there are impersonal forces at work in the world. Thinking is also **egocentric:** *things and events are seen from a personal and narrow perspective and are happening because of self.*[109]

---

### CRITICAL THINKING

*What is an example of an egocentric verbalization from a preschooler?*

---

The late preschooler fluctuates between reality and fantasy and a materialistic and animistic view of the world. Most adults never completely leave behind the magical thinking that is typical of the preschooler. The child plays with strange ideas, such as a tree growing out of the head, what holes feel like to the ground, and growing up starting as an adult. The adult finds no meaning in music, art, literature, love, and possibly even science and mathematics without a heavy dependence on fantasy or magic.

**Preoperational Stage** According to Piaget, the preschooler is in the preoperational stage of cognitive development. The preoperational stage is divided into the pre-conceptual and intuitive phases.[110] During the **pre-conceptual phase,** *from two to four years of age,* the child gathers facts as they are encountered but can neither separate reality from fantasy, nor classify or define events in a systematic manner. The ability to define the properties of an object, or denote hierarchies or relationships among elements in a class, is lacking. He or she is beginning to develop mental strategies from concept formation. Concepts are constructed in a global way. He or she is capable of perceiving gross outward appearances, but sees only one aspect of an object or situation at a time. For example, if you say, "Pick up the yellow pill," he or she will focus on either yellow or pill but cannot focus on both aspects at once. The child is unable to use time, space, equivalence, and class inclusion in concept formation. During the **intuitive phase**, which *lasts from approximately four to seven years of age*, the child gains increasing, but still limited, ability to develop concepts. He or she defines one property at a time, has difficulty stating the definition, but knows how to use the object. The child uses **transductive logic**, *going from general to specific in explanation*, rather than deductive or inductive logic. He or she begins to label, classify in ascending or descending order, do seriation, and note cause–effect relationships, even though true cause–effect understanding does not occur.

In addition to the previously described characteristics of concept development, the preoperational stage is characterized by the following:[111]

- Egocentric thought: child believes that all individuals see the world as he does

- Centration: child focuses on one aspect of a problem or situation but ignores other aspects of the problem

- Appearance as reality: child assumes that an object is what it appears to be[112]

**Sociocultural Perspective** Another approach to understanding how people learn is Lev Vygotsky's sociocultural theory, which was not fully described because of his death at the age of 38. Vygotsky formulated the sociocultural perspective to cognitive and language development. His main theme was that cognitive growth occurs in a sociocultural context and evolves out of the child's social interactions.

He believed that what people knew, thought, and said was shaped by the culture and historical time in which they lived. Each culture has certain "tools of the mind," as well as knowledge that it passes on to its members: languages, problem-solving tactics, and memory strategies. Thereby, cognitive development differs among cultures and some do not have formal operational thinking. The child, with an adult's help at a new task, expands the zone of cognitive development as the adult questions, demonstrates, explains, and encourages independent thinking, or praises a decision or outcome.[113]

From a sociocultural view, language is the primary vehicle through which adults teach culturally valued ways of thinking and problem solving, as well as what is to be learned. Piaget believed that cognitive development influenced language development. Vygotsky believed just the opposite.[114] Refer to Table 9-5 for a summary of Piaget's and Vygotsky's theories.

In general, the preschooler has a consuming curiosity. Learning is vigorous, aggressive, and intrusive. The imagination creates many situations he or she wishes to explore. Judgment is overshadowed by curiosity and excitement. The preschooler has begun to develop such concepts as friend, aunt, uncle; accepting responsibility; independence; passage of time and spatial relationships; use of abstract words, numbers, and colours; and the meaning of cold, tired, and hungry. The attention span is lengthening.

The child's ability to grasp reality varies with individual intelligence and potential intelligence, the social milieu, and opportunities to explore the world, solve problems independently, ask questions, and get answers. Table 9-4 summarizes the major characteristics of mental development, which can help you in assessment.[115]

Table 9-5 **Comparison of Piaget's and Vygotsky's Theories of Cognitive Development**

| Piaget's Cognitive Theory | Vygotsky's Sociocultural Theory |
| --- | --- |
| 1. Cognitive development is mostly the same universally. | 1. Cognitive development differs from culture to culture and in different historical eras. |
| 2. Cognitive development results from the child's independent exploration of the world. | 2. Cognitive development results from guided participation or social interactions. |
| 3. Each child constructs knowledge on his or her own. | 3. Children and adults or more knowledgeable persons or peers co-construct knowledge. |
| 4. Individual egocentric processes and language become more social. | 4. Social processes or interactions with others become individual psychological processes. |
| 5. Peers are important because children must learn to take peer's perspectives. | 5. Adults are important because they know the culture's way and tools of thinking. |
| 6. Development precedes learning; children cannot master certain things until they have the requisite structures. | 6. Learning precedes development; tools learned with adult cognitive help are internalized. |

## The Family's Role in Teaching the Preschooler

Parents can enhance the child's development by realizing the importance of the following approaches and their work with the child. Share this information with them.

*The single most critical factor in the child's learning is a loving caretaker, because that is who the child imitates.* How the mothering person speaks to, touches, and plays with the child governs the potential for socialization and cognitive development. This is true even for the child who had a low birth weight and was at risk for developmental lag or disability.[116] A child's problem-solving abilities are shaped by the parents' method of coping with problems and by the richness of opportunities for problem solving. In families where everyone gets a chance to speak out and jointly explore a problem, the child learns to express him- or herself logically. Automatic obedience or the acceptance of parental commands or decisions will interfere with the child's ability to reason.[117] Also important are the opportunities made available to the child to learn, explore, ask questions, and play a variety of games. Teaching involves demonstration, listening, and talking about the situation in direct and understandable terms, and giving reasons. Cognitive development includes more than fluency with words, a good verbal memory, and information. It includes the ability to use imagination, form mental pictures, and engage in fantasy appropriately, along with art, music, and other creative activities. It includes expanding one's skills in logical thinking. Most importantly, it involves the increasing integration of many kinds of brain functions. Much integrated learning comes from the child's motor activity, play, and language games, including talking with adults and peers and paying attention to both trivial and important aspects of the environment.[118]

---

### CRITICAL THINKING

*What specific examples of play activities can stimulate cognitive development?*

---

The amount of prosocial behaviour displayed by children varies from one child to another. One type of prosocial behaviour is altruism. Eisenberg and her associates found that a prosocial personality disposition emerges early in childhood and is somewhat consistent over time.[119]

A group of Canadian researchers have been studying relations among emotional expressiveness, empathy, and prosocial behaviour in children. They conclude that boys' level of empathy is a strong predictor of prosocial behaviour, compared to that of girls. Girls' level of empathy, as related to prosocial behaviour, was modest. This finding may possibly be due to social norms that require girls to be prosocial

whether they feel empathetic or not.[120] Other Canadian researchers claim that as children grow they eventually find themselves in situations that offer to them opportunities to consider their own future well-being (prudent behaviour) and the well-being of others (altruistic behaviour). The results of the children's considerations may conflict, however, with what is desirable for them at the present moment. Thompson and her colleagues at Dalhousie University concluded that between three and four years of age, children acquire the ability to deal with future-oriented situations through the development of some common mechanism that affects both future-oriented prudence and altruism.[121] They state that the findings of similar, age-related changes in performance provide support for the claim that four-year-olds, but not three-year-olds, have the ability to imagine various mental states that conflict with the child's own current states and involve a non-current situation. This ability has been described as double imagination and appears only in four-year-olds. In addition, the resolution of conflicts between current and future desires may involve other processes as well.[122] Further research is needed to examine more closely the processes involved in dealing with these particular kinds of conflicts during age-four transition.

The influence of the media on the psychosocial development of children is profound.[123] Refer to Chapter 1 for a discussion on television and the Internet.

A conservative estimate is that preschoolers spend more than a third of their waking time watching television.[124] In fact, many young children spend more time watching television than they spend in conversation with adults or siblings. In today's world, if children watch prime-time television, what may be the effects of television violence on them?

Television has many roles. It can teach children about stereotypes and provide them with violent models of aggression. On the other hand, television can teach the child that it is better to behave in positive prosocial ways than in negative, antisocial ways.[125] However, it is essential that professionals concerned with the health and well-being of children include TV violence in their work with families in both rural and urban communities.[126]

---

### CRITICAL THINKING

*Develop a series of critical guidelines that you could provide to parents to assist them in making television a more positive influence in their children's lives.*

---

## Communication Patterns

People have three types of communication at their disposal: (1) somatic or physical symptoms such as flushed skin colour and increased respirations; (2) action such as play or movement; and (3) verbal expression. The preschool child uses all of them.

Learning to use verbal expression—language—to communicate is an ongoing developmental process that is affected directly by the child's interaction with others.

Vygotsky's sociocultural approach to language development helps us understand the preschooler as he or she learns. Preschoolers often talk to themselves as they play or go about daily activities. Two preschoolers together may be in a collective monologue rather than truly conversing. Instead of the egocentric speech of preoperational thought, such speech can be considered **private speech**, *speech that guides one's thoughts and behaviour*. Private speech is extensively used when the child is struggling to solve difficult problems.[127] It is a step toward mature thought and a forerunner of the silent thinking-in-words that adults use daily. Private speech is expanded by **social speech**, or *conversations with others*. Then the child develops **inner speech**, or *mutterings, lip movements, and silent verbal thoughts*. The use of private speech increases during preschool years, and then decreases during early elementary school years. **Guided participation**, or *learning in collaboration with knowledgeable adults, or with companions who are more knowledgeable*, helps the child incorporate the learned problem-solving strategies into his or her own thinking.[128]

The *child uses language for many reasons:*

- To maintain social rapport
- To gain attention
- To get information
- To seek meaning about his or her experience
- To note how others' answers fit personal thoughts
- To play with words
- To gain relief from anxiety
- To learn how to think and solve problems[129]

He or she asks why, what, when, where, how, and who repeatedly.

A child learns language from hearing it and using it. Words are at first empty shells until he or she has experiences to match with them. Parents should provide age-appropriate experiences so the child learns that words and actions go together. It is equally important that parents avoid saying one thing and doing another. Attaining trust in the utility and validity of verbal communication and learning that talking helps rather than hinders life are crucial concepts to promote the transition from infancy to school years. If talking does not gain a response from others, or help the child solve problems and relate to those he or she needs, or if the world is too troublesome, the child is likely to find refuge in fantasy. If he or she does so, they might neglect the social and communicative meanings of language.

Being able to direct his or her life depends on language and understanding the meanings of words and the logic with which they are used. When the child acquires language, he or she gradually becomes freed from tangible, concrete experiences. The child can then internalize visual symbols, develop memory and recall, fragment the past, project the future, and differentiate fantasy from reality.

Language is also learned from being read to, and from having printed material available to look at. Share the following suggestions with parents for choosing books for the preschooler. The book should be durable, have large print that does not fill the entire page, and be colourfully illustrated. The concepts should be expressed concretely in simple sentences and should tell a tale that fits the child's fantasy conception of the world, such as a story with animals and objects who can talk and think like people. Or, the story should tell about the situations the child ordinarily faces, such as problems with playmates, discovery of the preschooler's world, nightmares, and the arrival of a new baby.

Use and share with the significant adults in the child's life the effective ways of talking with the preschooler (see Table 9-6).

Table 9-7 is a guide for assessing the preschooler's language skills. During assessment, keep in mind that the ways in which the child's parents and other family members speak, and the language opportunities the child encounters, all considerably influence his or her language skills.

Gaines states that good interaction skills have been related to lifelong success in academic, social, and vocational spheres of life.[130] However, many children with communication and language disorders are usually not identified until three years of age or later. Early identification, including hearing testing, may prevent many difficulties related to, and resulting from, speech, language, and communication disorders. In fact, the earlier intervention begins, the better the outcome.

In 1997, the Ontario Ministry of Health provided funding to initiate First Words, the Preschool Speech and Language Program in the Ottawa region. This program was the result of a provincial initiative to give enhanced dollars to serve the preschool population. A system of services, including a screening clinic, was developed to prevent and identify early speech and language disabilities in children. Now a system of services, including the screening clinic, is accessible to the general public.

Community care nurses can play a vital role in efforts to improve early detection of speech-language difficulties in children.[131] In a special health promotion endeavour, nurses can provide assistance to families concerned about a child's communication skills.

## Table 9-6 Guidelines for Communication with a Preschooler

1. Be respectful as you talk with the child.

2. Do not discourage talking, questions, or the make-believe in the child's language; verbal explorations are essential to learn language. Answers to questions should meet needs and give him or her awareness of but not dependence on adult attitudes and feelings about the topics discussed.

3. Tell the truth to the best of your ability and on the child's level of understanding. Do not say that an injection "won't hurt." Instead, say, "It's like a pinprick that will hurt for a short time." Admit if the answer is unknown, and seek the answer with the child. A lie is eventually found out and causes a loss of trust in that adult and in others.

4. Do not make a promise unless you can keep it.

5. The child takes every word literally. Do not say, "She nearly died laughing," or "I laughed my head off." Do not describe surgery as putting you "to sleep."

6. Respond to the relationship or feelings in the child's experience rather than the actual object or event. Talk about the child's feelings instead of agreeing or disagreeing with what he or she says. Help the child understand what he or she feels, rather than why he or she feels it.

7. Precede statements of advice and instruction with a statement of understanding of the child's feelings. When the child is feeling upset emotionally, he or she cannot listen to instructions, advice, consolation, or constructive criticism.

8. Do not give undue attention to slang or curse words, and do not punish the child for using them. The child is demonstrating initiative and uses these words for shock value. Attention or punishment emphasizes the importance of the words. Remain relaxed and give the child a more difficult or different word to say. If he or she persists in using the unacceptable word, the adult may say, "I'm tired of hearing that word, say ___"; ask him or her not to say the word again since it may hurt others, or use distraction. Children learn unacceptable words as they learn all others, and parents would be wise to listen to their own vocabulary.

9. Sit down if possible when participating or talking with children. You are more approachable when at their physical and eye level.

10. Seek to have a warm, friendly relationship without thrusting yourself on the child. How you feel about the child is more important than what you say or do.

11. Through attentive listening and interested facial expression, convey a tell-me-more-about-it attitude to encourage the child to communicate.

12. Regard some speech difficulties as normal. Ignore stuttering or broken fluency that does not persist. Do not correct each speech error and do not punish. Often the child thinks faster than he or she can articulate speech. Give the child time when he or she speaks.

13. Talk in a relaxed manner. Do not bombard the child with verbal information.

## CRITICAL THINKING

*What communication limitations indicate that a child might have difficulties in talking and/or understanding?*

## Play Patterns

Play is the work of the child. It occupies most of the child's waking hours and serves to consolidate and enlarge his or her previous learning and promote adaptation. Play has elements of reality, and there is earnestness about it. Piaget described play as assimilation. Play behaviour involves taking in, moulding, and using objects for pleasure and learning.[132]

The preschooler is intrusive in play, bombarding others by purposeful or accidental physical attack. He or she gets into people's ears and minds by loud, assertive talking; into space by vigorous gross motor activities; into objects through exploration; and into the unknown by consuming curiosity.[133]

The preschool years are when the child progresses from solitary and parallel play to co-operating for a longer time in a larger group. He or she identifies somewhat with a play group, follows rules, is aware of the status of self compared with others, develops perception of social relationships, begins the capacity for self-criticism, and states traits and characteristics of others that he or she likes or dislikes. At first, the child spends brief, incidental periods of separation from the parents. The time away from them increases in length and frequency, and eventually the orientation shifts from family to peer group.[134]

A **peer** is *a person with approximately equal status, a companion, often of the same sex and age and with whom*

## Table 9-7 Assessment of Language Development

| Age 3 Years | Age 4 Years | Age 5 Years |
|---|---|---|
| Appearance of individual sounds *y, f, and v* in words | Appearance of individual sounds *s, z, th, r, ch, j* in words | Appearance of individual sounds *sh, zh, th* in words |
| Vocabulary of at least 900, up to 2000, words | Vocabulary of at least 1500, up to 3000, words | Vocabulary of at least 2100, up to 5000, words |
| Uses language understandably; uses same sounds experimentally | Uses language confidently | Uses language efficiently, correctly |
| Understands simple reasons | Concrete speech | No difficulty understanding other's spoken words |
| Uses some adjectives and adverbs | Increasing attention span | Meaningful sentences; uses future tense |
| | Uses "I" and other pronouns | Increasing skill with grammar |
| | Imitates and plays with words | Knows common opposites |
| | Defines a few simple words | |
| | Talks in sentences; uses past tense | |
| | Uses plurals frequently | |
| | Comprehends prepositions | |
| Talks in simple sentences about things | Talks incessantly while doing other activities | Talks constantly |
| Repeats sentence of six syllables | Asks many questions | No infantile articulation |
| Uses plurals in speech | Demands detailed explanations with "why" | Repeats sentences of 12 or more syllables |
| Collective monologue; does not appear to care whether another is listening | Carries on long involved conversation | Asks searching questions, meaning of words, how things work |
| Some random, inappropriate answers | Exaggerates; boasts; tattles; may use profanity for attention | Can tell a long story accurately, but may keep adding to reality to make story more fantastic |
| Intelligibility is 70–90% | Frequently uses "everything" | Intelligibility good; some distortion in articulation of *t, s* |
| Sings simple songs | Tells family faults outside of home without restraint | Sings relatively well |
| | Tells story combining reality and fantasy; appears to be lying | |
| | Intelligibility is 90%; articulation errors with *l, r, s, z, sh, ch, j, th* | |
| | Variations in volume from a yell to a whisper | |
| | Likes to sing | |
| Knows first and family name | Calls people names | Counts to 10 or further without help |
| Names figures in a picture | Names three objects he or she knows in succession | Repeats five digits |
| Repeats three digits | Counts to 5 without help | Names four colours, usually red, green, blue, yellow |
| Likes to name things | Repeats four digits | |
| | Knows which line is long | |
| | Names one or more colours | |
| Talks to self or imaginary playmate | Talks with imaginary playmate of same sex and age | Sense of social standards and limits seen in language use |
| Expresses own desires and limits frequently | Seeks reassurance | |
| | Interested in things being funny | |
| | Likes puns | |

one can share mutual concerns. The **peer group** is *a relatively informal association of equals who share common play experiences with emphasis on common rules and understanding the limits that the group places on the individual.* The preschool play group differs from later ones in that it is more loosely organized. The activity of the group may be continuous. Membership changes, though, as the child joins or leaves the group at will, and the choice of playmates is relatively restricted in kind and number. This is the first introduction to a group that assesses him or her as a child from a child's point of view. When he or she joins the group, the preschooler is learning about entering a new, different, very powerful world. Although social play is enjoyed, the child frequently feels a need for solitary play.[135]

**Purposes of Play** The natural mode of expression for the child is play. *Purposes of play include the following:*

- Develop and improve muscular strength, coordination, and balance; define body boundaries
- Work off excess physical energy; provide exercise
- Communicate with others, establish friendships, learn about interpersonal relations, and develop concern for others
- Learn co-operation, sharing, and healthy competition
- Express imagination, creativity, and initiative
- Imitate and learn about social activity, adult roles, and cultural norms
- Test and deal with reality, gain mastery over unpleasant experiences
- Explore, investigate, and manipulate features of the adult world; sharpen the senses and concentration
- Learn about rules of chance and probability, and rules of conduct, and that at times one loses but that it is all right
- Build self-esteem
- Feel a sense of power, make things happen, explore and experiment
- Provide for intellectual, sensory, and language development and dealing with concrete experiences in symbolic terms
- Assemble novel aspects of the environment
- Organize life's discrepancies privately and with others
- Learn about self and how others see him or her
- Practise leader and follower roles
- Have fun, express joy, and feel the pleasure of mastery
- Act out and symbolically work through a painful physical or emotional state by repetition in play so that it is more bearable and assimilated into the child's self-concept; master overwhelming stimuli
- Develop the capacity to gratify self and to delay gratification
- Formulate a bridge between concrete experiences and abstract thought

The boxes entitled "Types of Play Related to Social Characteristics" and "Common Themes in Children's Play" give more insight into children's play.[136]

**CRITICAL THINKING**

*A farm family has one preschool child. The child's parents are wondering how frequently they should take their child to town to play with a cousin. What advice would you give to the parents?*

**Play Materials** Play materials should be simple, sturdy, durable, and free from unnecessary hazards. They need not be expensive. The child should have adequate space and equipment in an area that is sufficiently unstructured to allow for creativity, imagination, and uninterrupted work. He or she will enjoy trips to parks and playgrounds. Often, creative, stimulating toys can be made from ordinary household articles: plastic pot cleaners, empty thread spools, a bell, yarn, or empty boxes covered with washable adhesive paper. The child may like the box more than the toy.

Increasing emphasis is being placed on high-technology, interactive, and weaponry toys. These toys actually stifle imagination and discovery, and weaponry toys may cause fears, heighten aggressive fantasies, and cause injury and sometimes death. Weaponry toys should be avoided as much as possible. Young children need to direct their games so they are in control of their play and their fantasies. They use play to work out problems, to practise skills, and to act out roles in preparation for later real-life experiences.

The play materials that are available will determine the play activities. Play materials are enjoyed for different reasons. For example, **physical activity**, which *facilitates the development of motor skills*, is provided through play with such

---

### Types of Play Related to Social Characteristics

- **Parallel play:** Child plays independently but next to other children; displays no group association.
- **Associative play:** Children play together in similar or identical play without organization, division of labour, leadership, or mutual goals.
- **Imaginative play:** The most characteristic and pervasive preschool activity. Children play with dolls, dress-up clothes, hand puppets, and medical kits for self-expression.
- **Co-operative play:** Play is organized in group with others. Planning and co-operation begin before play starts to form goals, division of labour, and leadership.[136]

*Sources:* Papalia, D., S. Olds, and R. Feldman, *Human Development*, 9th ed. Boston: McGraw-Hill, 2004; Seifert, K., R. Hoffnung, and M. Hoffnung, *Lifespan Development*. Boston: Houghton Mifflin, 1997; Monroe, R.A., Health Promotion of the Preschooler and Family. In M.J. Hockenberry and D. Wilson (eds.), *Wong's Nursing Care of Infants and Children*, 8th ed. St. Louis, MO: C.V. Mosby, 2007.

## Common Themes in Children's Play

Various issues in the child's life will be repeated four to five times in each play session. These issues are shown in different styles of play, but the theme is the thread that ties all of the different styles together, as the pieces of a quilt unite to form the pattern of the whole.

- Power/control
- Anger/sadness
- Trust/relationships/abandonment
- Nurturing/rejection/security
- Boundaries/intrusion

- Violation/protection
- Self-esteem
- Fears/anxiety (separation, monsters, ghosts, animals, the dark, noises, bad people, injury, death)
- Confusion
- Identity
- Loyalty/betrayal
- Loss/death
- Loneliness
- Adjustment/change

things as musical instruments and records for marching and rhythm, balls, shovel, broom, ladder, swing, trapeze, slide, boxes, climbing apparatus, boards, sled, wagon, tricycle, bicycle with training wheels, wheelbarrow, and blocks. Swimming, ice-skating, roller-skating, and skiing are being learned. **Dramatic or imaginative play**, which *is related to special skills such as the ability to classify objects correctly, taking another's perspective, and problem solving*, is afforded through large building blocks, sandbox and sand toys, dolls, housekeeping toys, nurse and doctor kits, farm or other occupational toys, cars and other vehicles, and worn-out adult clothes for dress-up. This is a predominant form of play in childhood, and it can also include some aspects of physical play. **Creative play-things** *promote constructive, non-social, cognitive, and emotional development*. They include blank sheets of paper, crayons, finger or water paints, chalk, various art supplies, clay, plasticine or other manipulative material, blunt scissors, paste, cartons, scraps of cloth, water-play equipment, and musical toys. **Symbolic play** is *play that enables the child to create new images or symbols to represent objects, people, and events*. It results from actually taking part in dramatic and creative play. **Quiet play**, which *promotes cognitive development and rest from physical exertion*, is carried out through books, puzzles, records, and table games. Children's songs, nursery rhymes, and fairy tales are good to absorb anxiety, entertain, soothe, reassure that life's problems can be solved, and support the child's superego.[138]

The *role of the adult in child's play* is to provide opportunity, equipment, and safety, and to avoid interference or structuring play. Mothers and fathers tend to play differently with the child. How fathers play with their children appears to be determined not just by biology but also by cultural influences. All cultures recognize the fathering role. The role may be carried out directly, or shared by someone other than the biological father—for example, by the mother's brother, as in Botswana, or by the grandfather, as in Vietnam.[139] Dubeau

states that because immigrants make up 17 percent of Canada's population, we need research on the impact of various cultural models on fatherhood.[140] Becoming and being a father are, together, a significant step in one's life; for the child, having a father is stimulating and enriching because each parent interacts with the child in different ways.

*Parents should be taught the following:*

1. Allow the child to try things and enjoy personal activities.
2. Assist only if he or she is in need of help.
3. The child is not natural in play when he or she thinks adults are watching. Avoid showing amusement, and never ridicule play behaviour or their conversations.
4. Allow playmates to work out their own differences.
5. Distract, redirect, or substitute a different activity if the children cannot share and work out their problems.
6. There are times to play with the child, but avoid over-stimulation, teasing, hurry, or talking about the child as if he or she were not present.
7. Avoid doing the activity for the child. Let him or her take the lead.
8. Try to enter the child's world. If he or she wants you to attend the teddy bear's hundredth birthday party, go.

Even when free time, space, and toys are limited, most children find a way to play. They use household objects such as pots, pans, and furniture, and outdoor items such as trees, sticks, rocks, sand, empty cans, and discarded equipment—all for dramatic and fantasy play.

Table 9-8 summarizes play characteristics as a further aid in assessment and teaching.[141]

Share the above information with parents and explore their feelings about child's play and their role with the child.

Table 9-8 Assessment of Play Characteristics

| Age 3 Years | Age 4 Years | Age 5 Years |
|---|---|---|
| Enjoys active and sedentary play | Increasing physical and social play | More varied activity<br>More graceful in play |
| Likes toys in orderly form<br>Puts away toys with supervision | Puts away toys when reminded | Puts away toys by self |
| Fantasy not yielding too much<br>to reality<br>Likes fairy tales, books | Much imaginative and dramatic play<br>Has complex ideas but unable to<br>carry out because of lack of skill<br>and time | More realistic in play<br>Less interested in fairy tales<br>More serious and ready to know reality<br>Restrained but creative |
| Likes solitary and parallel play with<br>increasing social play in shifting<br>groups of two or three | Plays in groups of two or three,<br>often companions of own sex<br>Imaginary playmates<br>Projects feelings and deeds onto<br>peers or imaginary playmates<br>May run away from home | Plays in groups of five or six<br>Friendships stronger and continue over<br>longer time<br>Chooses friends of like interests<br>Spurred on in activity by rivalry |
| Cooperates briefly<br>Willing to wait turn and share with<br>suggestion | Suggests and accepts turns but<br>often bossy in directing others<br>Acts out feelings spontaneously,<br>especially with music and arts | Generous with toys<br>Sympathetic, cooperative, but quarrels<br>and threatens by word or gesture<br>Acts out feelings<br>Wants rules to do things right; but<br>beginning to realize peers cheat, so<br>develops mild deceptions and<br>fabrications |
| Some dramatic play-house or family<br>games<br>Frequently changes activity<br>Likes to arrange, combine, transfer,<br>sort, and spread objects and toys | Dramatic and creative play at a peak<br>Likes to dress up and help with<br>household tasks; plays with dolls,<br>trucks<br>Does not sustain role in dramatic<br>play; moves from one role to<br>another incongruous role<br>No carry over in play from day<br>to day<br>Silly in play | Dramatic play about most life events,<br>but more realistic<br>Play continues from day to day<br>Interested in finishing what started, even<br>if it takes several days<br>More awareness of yesterday and<br>tomorrow |
| Able to listen longer to nursery rhymes<br>Dramatizes nursery rhymes and stories<br>Can match simple forms<br>Identifies primary colours<br>Enjoys cutting, pasting, block building | Concentration span longer<br>Sometimes so busy at play forgets<br>to go to toilet<br>Re-enacts stories and trips<br>Enjoys simple puzzles and models<br>with trial-and-error method<br>Poor space perception | Perceptive to order, form, and detail<br>Better eye–hand coordination<br>Rhythmic motion to music; enjoys<br>musical instruments<br>Likes excursions<br>Interested in world outside immediate<br>environment; enjoys books |
| Enjoys simple puzzles, hand puppets,<br>large ball<br>Enjoys sand and water play | Uses constructive and manipulative<br>play material increasingly<br>Enjoys sand and water play; cups,<br>containers, and buckets for<br>carrying and pouring | Interested in the many hues and shades<br>of colours<br>Enjoys cutting out pictures, pasting,<br>working on special projects, puzzles |
| Enjoys dumping and hauling toys<br>Rides tricycle | Identifies commonly seen colours<br>Enjoys crayons and paints, books<br>Enjoys swing, jungle gym, toy<br>hammer or other tools,<br>pegboards | Likes to run and jump, play with bicycle,<br>wagon, and sled<br>Enjoys sand and water play; dramatic<br>and elaborative in play<br>Enjoys using tools and equipment of adults |

## Guidance and Discipline

The child learns how to behave by imitating adults and by using the opportunities to develop self-control. The child needs consistent, fair, and kind limits to feel secure and to know that the parents care for and love him or her enough to provide protection—a security he or she does not have when allowed to do anything, regardless of ability. Limits should be set in a way that preserves the self-respect of the child and parent. Only when the child can predict the behaviour of others can he or she accept the need to inhibit or change some of his or her behaviour and work toward predictable and rational behaviour. The parent should be an ally to the child as he or she struggles for control over inner impulses and convey to the child that he or she need not fear impulses.

Children learn from other children how to strike out or hit others, and hitting can also be learned by imitating the parents. It is important that behaviour that hurts another is stopped immediately. Do so by holding the child's arm gently and quietly saying, "No." Explain the reason. Spanking should be avoided because it teaches the child it is all right to hit.[142]

Attention deficit hyperactivity disorder (ADHD) may be associated with a neurotransmitter difference. It is noteworthy to mention that Washbusch and his colleagues reviewed three cases in the assessment and treatment of ADHD. These case studies highlighted the importance of the need for systematic, comprehensive, and individualized treatments for children with ADHD. In fact, pharmacological intervention is the most common form of treatment for children with ADHD, along with behavioural interventions.[143]

### CRITICAL THINKING

*What types of support can you, as a health professional, provide to parents who have a child with ADHD?*

A behaviour modification technique useful to discipline an aggressively acting-out child is *time-out*. Time-out involves immediately placing the child, after a mean act, in a quiet, uninteresting place (hall, small room, or corner of a room) for 5 to 15 minutes for the purpose of removing the child from positive reinforcement. Time-out stops the misbehaviour and is unpleasant enough to increase the possibility that the child will not repeat the undesirable act. *The child should be helped to realize that time-out means it is his or her behaviour—not the child—that is rejected. Thus, the use of rewards to reinforce desired behaviour is necessary*, in conjunction with the time-out technique.[144]

Canadian child care advocates stress the point that the use of physical interventions to discipline a child is

## CASE SITUATION

### Preschooler Development

Kalisha is an active, 38-month-old girl. She weighs 15.45 kg (34 pounds) and is 95 cm (38 inches) tall. She is playing on the sidewalk in front of her parents' home with her brother Marvin, four years old, and her next-door neighbour Lori, aged five years.

Kalisha is riding her small, two-wheeled bicycle, which has training wheels. Marvin and Lori are riding their small bicycles or scooters. Kalisha rides for a while, and then stops to watch the others. Although involved in the same activity, she plays next to, rather than with, the older children. Several times, Kalisha rides her bicycle into the path of her brother's approaching bicycle. The preschooler is typically intrusive in play, bombarding others by either purposeful or accidental attack. Kalisha continues to ride and stop, always staying within her mother's view as she moves farther away and then nearer on her bicycle. She demonstrates the attachment behaviour typical of this age by maintaining proximity to her mother.

When Marvin and Lori ride down the street, leaving Kalisha, Kalisha asks her mother to go with her to join them. She pulls her mother's hand insistently several times, and they walk together down the street. When she approaches the other children, Kalisha runs to them, laughing, and then gives Lori a hug. Lori chases Kalisha up the street, and Kalisha laughs and runs to her mother, seeking protection, security, assurance, and approval. Through this behaviour she affirms that her mother is still the most important person in her life.

As the older children ride their bicycles on the sidewalk toward Kalisha, she laughs and shouts, then waves her arms, telling them, "I am the stop sign." She tells Lori to stop, but Lori rides by, laughing and saying, "You'll have to give me a ticket." On the return trip, Lori stops at Kalisha's command. Kalisha and Lori repeat this pattern several times, and each time Kalisha becomes more animated. She demonstrates autonomy and beginning initiative in these interactions, displaying the egocentrism typical of the preschooler as she commands events for her own needs and purposes and gains a sense of power through symbolic play.

1. What other images or symbols, besides "I am the stop sign," might Kalisha use to demonstrate symbolic play?

2. How do you interpret Kalisha's behaviour of riding her bicycle into the pathway of her brother? How should her mother react to this behaviour?

3. Project yourself, if you can, into Kalisha's mind and body to respond to this question. What is your interpretation of the "sense of power" Kalisha experiences as she plays out the part of the stop sign?

not appropriate. They advocate the use of minimal non-physical interventions within the context of a loving and supportive family relationship. They encourage parents to be proactive. In doing so they can improve their parenting skills and either anticipate or limit the occurrence of situations that require intervention.[145]

## Emotional Development

If the child has developed reasonably well and if he or she has mastered earlier developmental tasks, the preschooler is a source of extreme pleasure to adults. He or she is more like a companion than someone to care for. The various behaviours discussed under development of physical, mental, language, play, body image, and moral-spiritual aspects contribute to his or her emotional status and development. Tolerance of frustration is still limited, but flares of temper and frustrations over failure pass quickly. As the child is learning to master things and handle independence and dependence, so is he or she increasing mastery of self and others and learning to get along with most people, both children and adults. The preschooler attempts to behave like an adult in realistic activity and play, and in doing so is beginning to learn social roles, moral responsibility, and co-operation, although at times he or she still grabs, hits, and quarrels.[146] If the child has the opportunity to establish a sense of gender and to identify with mature adults, if the attitude about self is sound and positive, and if he or she has learned to trust and have some self-control, he or she is ready to take on the culture. The preschooler begins to decide what kind of person he or she is, and self-concept, ego strength, and superego will all continue to mature. Self is still very important, but he or she does not feel omnipotent.

## Developmental Crisis

The psychosexual crisis for this era is initiative versus guilt, and all of the aforementioned behaviours are part of achieving initiative.[147] **Initiative** is *enjoyment of energy displayed in action, assertiveness, learning, increasing dependability, and the ability to plan.* Natural initiative is desirable. It is important, however, for parents not to expect too much, or to push the child excessively. If the child does not achieve the developmental task of initiative, an overriding sense of guilt develops from the tension between the demands of the superego, or expectations, and actual performance.

**Guilt** is *a sense of defeatism. It is anger, feeling responsible for things that he or she is not really responsible for, feeling easily frightened away from what he or she wants to do, and feeling bad, shameful, and deserving of punishment.* A sense of guilt can develop from sibling rivalry, a lack of sufficient opportunity to try things, restriction or lack of guidance in response to fantasy, or when parents interfere with the child's activity. If the guilt feelings are too strong, the child is affected in a negative way. Excessive guilt does not enhance moral or superego development, although the child is expected to experience a realistic amount of guilt for wrong behaviour.[148]

Help parents understand that if the child is to develop a sense of initiative and a healthy personality, they and other significant adults must encourage the use of imagination, creativity, activity, and plans. Parents should encourage the child's efforts to co-operate and share in the decisions and responsibilities of family life. The child develops best when he or she is commended and recognized for accomplishments. Appropriate behaviour should be reinforced so that it will continue. Affirming a child's emotional experience is as important as affirming his or her physical development. The preschooler needs to learn to recognize feelings of love, hate, joy, and antagonism, and of equal importance is learning how to cope with and express them in ways other than physically. The child needs guidance toward mature behaviour.

---

### CRITICAL THINKING

*How can a child who has a chronic illness develop a sense of initiative?*

---

## Self-Concept: Body Image and Sexuality Development

Self-concept, along with body image and sex role behaviour, are gradually developing in these years.[149] Positive self-concept develops from parental love, effective relations with peers and others, success in play and other activities, and gaining skills and self-control in activities of daily living. Body boundaries and a sense of self become more definite to the preschooler because of developing sexual curiosity and the awareness of how he or she differs from others. Body image and sexual development are supported as well by increased motor skills with precision of movement and a maturing sense of balance, improved spatial orientation, maturing cognitive and language abilities, ongoing play activities, and relationship identification with his or her parents.

Learning about the body—where it begins and ends, what it looks like, and what it can do—is basic to the child's identity formation. Included in this aspect of growing self-awareness is the discovery of feelings and learning the names for them. The child is beginning to learn how he or she affects others, and what others feel in response to the child's behaviours. He or she is learning the rudiments of control over one's own feelings and behaviours. The concept of body is reflected in the way the child talks, draws pictures, and plays. The child with little frame of reference in relation to self tends to show increased anxiety and misperception of self and others.

Discuss with the parents the concept of body image and how they can help the child's formulation of self. The child needs opportunities to learn the correct names and basic functions of body parts and to discover his or her body with joy and pride. Mirrors; photographs of the child; drawings of self, parents, and siblings; weighing; and measuring height all help to enhance the formation of his or her mental picture. The child needs physical and mental activity, not only to learn body mastery and self-protection, but also to express feelings of helplessness, doubt, or pain when the body does not accomplish what he or she would like. Specific nursing measures after illness or injury help the child to reintegrate his or her body image, because during prolonged illness the child can lose part of this image.[150]

## Adaptive Mechanisms

The preschooler has gained language and conceptual ability, greater experience, and a greater imagination. Now, he or she can talk about, and play out the fears of, being alone, ghosts, masks, the dark, strange noises, strangers, dogs, tigers, spiders, bears, snakes, closed places, thunderstorms, and separation from loved ones. These fears decline by age five but some may persist until age seven or eight, or beyond.

The child encounters a variety of frustrations when he or she engages in new activities, when he or she expects more of self, and when others expect more of him or her. Disappointments arise. The child must learn to cope with frustrations, just as he or she learns to handle and overcome fears. *Teach parents that they can help by:*

1. Showing concern about and acceptance of the child's feelings.
2. Encouraging the child to talk about his or her feelings.
3. Exploring with the child possible causes for the feelings.
4. Helping the child to realize that emotions have causes, and that the child can discover the causes of his or her personal feelings.
5. Emphasizing that the child is not expected to be perfect and that he or she should not expect that everything will always go as desired.
6. Helping the child to make a decision about handling a frustrating situation. In doing so, the child learns about problem-solving strategies.

How the parent handles frustrations and problems sets many examples for the child.

Sibling conflict is one of the most frequently reported child management problems that occurs in families. Parents face enormously complex issues in deciding how to manage such conflict.[151] Perlman and Ross examined the impact of parental intervention on the quality of children's conflict behaviour. The data used were from 40 English-speaking Canadian families with two- and four-year-old children. The researchers concluded that parental interventions in sibling conflict actually have beneficial effects in terms of the quality of children's fighting.[152] Parental intervention seemed to both decrease the level of intensity of conflict and allow the children to behave in ways that are more sophisticated than what they were capable of on their own.

---

CRITICAL THINKING

*What are your thoughts about parental interventions in sibling conflict?*

---

## Moral–Spiritual Development

Two powerful influences on the child during these early years are: (1) the parents' attitude toward moral codes (the human as a creative being, spirituality, religion, nature, love of country, the economic system, and education), and (2) their behaviour in the presence of the child. Parents convey to the child what is considered good and bad, and what is worthy of respect, or unworthy. Along with the developing superego, which calls for imitation of and identification with adults, the child is absorbing a great deal of others' attitudes. Many of those attitudes will remain with the child throughout life. Amid all this, he or she is also beginning to consider how his or her actions affect others.[153]

Following are some general considerations you might find helpful pertaining to moral and religious education. *The child cannot be kept spiritually neutral. He or she hears about morals and religion from other people, and they will raise detailed questions about the basic issues of life.* Where did I come from? Why am I here? Why did the bird (or Grandpa) die? Why is it wrong to . . . ? Why can't I play with Joey? How come Billy goes to church on Saturday and we go to church on Sunday? What is God? What is heaven? Mommy, who do you like best: Santa Claus, the Easter Bunny, the Tooth Fairy, or Jesus? These questions, often considered irrelevant from the adult viewpoint, should not be brushed aside. A parent's tone in answering these questions can be more important than the information given.

EVIDENCE-BASED PRACTICE

# Mother's Resilience, Family Health Work, and Mother's Health-Promoting Lifestyle Practices in Families with Preschool Children

Hypotheses derived from the developmental model of health and nursing (DMHN) were tested by examining relationships among mother's resilience (health potential), family health-promoting activity (health work), and mother's health-promoting lifestyle practices (competence in health behaviour) in 67 southern Ontario families with at least one preschool child, three to five years of age. Mothers completed a mailed survey containing self-report measures of the study variables and a demographic form.

*Health work,* the central concept in the DMHN, reflects the process through which families develop healthy ways of living by learning how to cope with life events and by promoting the healthy development of the family unit and its members. *Coping* is viewed as a function of problem solving—a process of attempting to deal with, or solve, challenging health situations. *Development* relates to growth-seeking behaviour seen in the family's ability to mobilize strengths and resources to achieve health goals.

## Results

As hypothesized, both mother's resilience and family health work were positively related to mother's health-promoting lifestyle practices. Mother's resilience was also associated with health work.

## Practice Implications

1. According to the DMHN, nurses must identify and support factors that contribute to family health promotion efforts to assist families in developing healthy ways of living. Both mother's resilience and health work were positively related to mother's health-promoting lifestyle practices, suggesting that attention to the development and support of each of these qualities is a potentially important nursing role.

2. Personal and family efforts to promote health may be quite intertwined, suggesting that attention be paid to developing programs and services aimed at both mothers and groups of family members.

3. Supportive learning environments should also be established that provide mothers and their families with opportunities to develop and use coping and goal attainment processes and to further identify and develop their health potential, particularly internal resources or strengths.

4. Mothers, fathers, children who are developmentally ready to participate, and other people who are considered to be family could be involved in such activities.

5. Viewing the family as a system that is influenced by a multitude of internal and external factors should direct nurses to be open to identifying and supporting a range of factors that influence both health work and healthy lifestyle practices. The combination of many different aspects of health potential may have the most persuasive influence on health work.

6. Nurses may be able to foster the development of resilient qualities such as optimism, perseverance, and confidence in mothers, as means of supporting family health promotion processes and mother's lifestyle choices.

7. Nurses can help mothers to reframe positively difficult situations by pointing out successes, and by providing positive feedback for their efforts. Such efforts can contribute to a sense of confidence and optimism.

8. There is sufficient evidence to justify nurses' lobbying government bodies to promote adequate education and a level of income for all families that is sufficient to sustain, if not promote, health.

Source: Monteith, B., and M. Ford-Gilboe, The Relationships among Mother's Resilience, Family Health Work, and Mother's Health-Promoting Lifestyle Practices in Families with Preschool Children, Journal of Family Nursing, 8(4) (2002), 383–407. Reprinted by permission of Sage Publications, Inc.

Encourage parents to discuss religion and related practices with the child. The preschool child is old enough to go to Sunday school, vacation Bible school, or classes in religious education that are on an appropriate level for the child. Religious holidays raise questions, and the spirit of the holiday and ceremonies surrounding it should be explained.

## HEALTH PROMOTION IN NURSING PRACTICE

Your role with the preschooler and family has been discussed in each section throughout this chapter. As a nurse, you should be prepared to observe and listen to issues of the child and the parents, and to seek the strengths of each and healthy responses for all. *Interventions* include your role modelling of caring behaviour to the preschooler and family with regard to the child, parent, and family education, support, and counselling. Also needed is your direct care to meet the preschooler's physical, emotional, cognitive, social, and spiritual and moral needs.

## Abuse

If you suspect abuse, establish rapport and talk with the child alone. However, do not pry. If the child finds it difficult to talk, gently offer to draw some pictures or play with the child, to *gain information as follows:*

1. *What* has happened to you?
   a. Has anyone ever told you to take off your panties?
   b. Has anyone ever put his or her finger (or another object) between your legs?
   c. Does anyone ever get in bed with you at night?
2. *Who* did this to you? Explain.
3. *How* did it happen? Tell me what happened just before that.
4. *Where* did this happen?
5. *When* did this happen?
6. *Who* saw this happen to you?
7. *Who* else have you told?
   a. What did they say?
   b. What did they do?

The child may not answer because he or she: (1) thinks abuse is normal; (2) is terrified that parents will be more abusive if they know he or she told; (3) feels loyalty to the parents and fears abandonment; or (4) believes abuse is deserved.

When you talk with the parents about the subject of child abuse, be very cautious that you do not give the impression that you are criticizing them, trying to impart your own values, or acting as their judge. Putting them on the defensive will not make them co-operate, and it may keep them from accepting help from other health care professionals. Do your best to be tolerant and understanding. Try to determine how realistically the parents perceive the child, how they cope with the stresses of parenting, and to whom they turn for support. As you talk, *attempt to obtain answers from the parents to the following questions:*[154]

- What do you do when he or she cries too much? If that does not work, what do you do?
- Does the child sleep well? What do you do when he or she does not sleep?
- How do you discipline him or her?
- How do you feel after you have disciplined the child?
- Are you ever angry because the child takes up so much of your time?
- Does he or she take up more time than your other children, or does he or she require more disciplining? If yes, why is this so?
- Do you think he or she misbehaves on purpose?
- To whom do you usually talk when your child upsets you? Is that person available now?
- Does the child remind you of a relative or former spouse that is disliked? (Explore this possibility with gentle questions: "It must be really upsetting for you when he acts like his father. What goes through your mind then?" "In what ways is she like your mother? Do those characteristics irritate you?")

As you discuss these and other matters, try to determine what the situation is at home. Does one or both of the parents seem unduly distressed? Perhaps they are facing other stresses with which they cannot cope such as a job loss, loneliness, illness, or alcoholism.

If you suspect **sexual abuse**, *find out the following from the parents:*

- What words or names does the child use to describe various body parts?
- What are the names of family members and frequent visitors?
- Who babysits for the child?
- What are the family's sleeping arrangements?
- Does the child have behavioural problems such as excessive masturbation?
- Does the child have any phobias or excessive fears of any person or place? Does he or she have any nightmares?

Parents may not be involved in the sexual abuse, and they may be unaware of its occurrence. Work up gradually to the subject of their child's being abused. Inform them of your suspicions in private and without judgment. Do not bombard the parents with questions that they will interpret as accusatory. Offer your support, telling them of your concern for the child. Suggest counsellors who would be helpful for the child and parents. Give them ideas on how to help the child work through feelings about the trauma. Urge parents not to punish or scold the child when he or she works through emotions by using masturbation or by playing with dolls.[155]

## Intervention

You are a key factor in intervention. You are limited, however, in what you can do, although reporting to the appropriate professionals is a necessary action for intervention.[156]

If you are in a health care facility and suspect child abuse, report it to the doctor and appropriate health team members. Report your suspicions to the proper agency: the police, the Crown attorney's office, a child protective service, or a social service group.[157] *Carefully document all evidence of abuse*, your interview of and actions with parents and child, any agencies or persons contacted about the abuse, and any agencies to which the parents were referred. List the names of children who are repeatedly brought to the hospital with injuries. Make sure the notes on the chart include what the parents said, how they reacted, and how they explained the accident. Provide other hospitals in the area with the names on file. Urge them to do the same with their files. Take the time to check with other hospitals when you have a questionable case.[158]

A **neglected child** needs help as much as one who has been abused. Careful assessment and interviewing of child and parents are essential. Parents and caregivers who experience workplace stressors, financial worries, and other frustrations sometimes abuse a child.[159] Notify your community's child protection service, and thoroughly document your findings and interventions.[160] Many of the guidelines described above are applicable.

## SUMMARY

1. The preschooler grows at a steady pace. Motor coordination is increasing.

2. The preschooler makes considerable gains in neuromuscular, cognitive, emotional, and social, moral, and spiritual behaviours.

3. Parents' provision of consistent love, guidance, and new experiences is essential for holistic development.

4. The child develops the ability to carry out basic hygiene and routine activities.

5. The child begins to participate within the family, and to communicate and relate more effectively with adults and significant others in the community.

6. The child slowly reaches out from the family, establishes beginning peer relationships, and learns to follow rules of the play group.

7. The box entitled "Considerations for the Preschool Child and Family in Health Care" summarizes what you should consider in assessment and health promotion with the preschooler.

## Considerations for the Preschool Child and Family in Health Care

■ Family, cultural background and values, support systems, and community resources for the family

■ Parents as identification figures for the child, secondary identification of the preschool child with the parents

■ Behaviours that indicate gender identity and a sense of sexuality in the preschool child

■ Behaviours that indicate ability of the preschool child to relate to siblings, adults in the extended family, and other adults and authority figures in the environment

■ Parental behaviours that indicate difficulty with parenting, or the potential of actual abuse of the preschool child

■ Physical characteristics and patterns, such as neuromuscular development, nutrition, exercise, and rest or sleep, that indicate health and are within age norms for growth for the preschool child

■ Cognitive characteristics and behavioural patterns in the preschool child that demonstrate curiosity, increasingly realistic thought, expanding concept formation, and continuing mental development

■ Communication patterns—verbal, nonverbal, and action—and language development that demonstrate continuing learning and age-appropriate norms for the preschool child

■ Behaviours that indicate that the child can participate in, and enjoys, early childhood education experiences

■ Overall appearance, behaviour, and play patterns in the preschool child that indicate development of initiative

>

- rather than excessive guilt, positive self-concept, body image formation, and a sense of sexuality
- Use of adaptive mechanisms by the preschool child that promote a sense of security, control of anxiety, and age-appropriate emotional responses
- Behavioural patterns that indicate that the preschool child is continuing moral and spiritual development

- Behavioural patterns and characteristics that indicate that the preschool child has achieved developmental issues
- Parental behaviours that indicate knowledge about, and how to guide and discipline, the child, and how to assist the child in becoming more independent

## Interesting Websites

### Canadian Institutes of Health Research (CIHR)

www.cihr-irsc.gc.ca/e/7263.html

CIHR is the major federal agency responsible for funding health research in Canada. It aims to excel in the creation of new health knowledge, and to translate that knowledge from the research setting into real-world applications. The results are improved health for Canadians, more effective health services and products, and a strengthened Canadian health care system.

### Child & Family Canada

www.cfc-efc.ca/menu/childcare_en.htm

This site is a place to share news, information, and ideas; access resources; and connect with the family child care community across Canada and elsewhere.

### Healthy Start for Life

www.dieticians.ca/healthystart/index.asp

Healthy Start for Life is a collaboration between Dietitians of Canada and nine organizations whose shared goal is to promote healthy eating and physical activity among toddlers and preschool children. The program aims to help parents and child care providers learn more about the nutrition and physical activity needs of preschoolers; suggests activities that promote positive attitudes toward healthy eating and active living; provides strategies to help tackle common preschool feeding issues, plan meals, and keep preschoolers active; and helps prevent childhood obesity, diabetes, and other health problems in later life.

## Key Terms

abstract space (333)
action space (333)
animistic (333)
authoritarian (310)
authoritative (310)
body space (333)
burns (327)
child-centred kindergarten (318)
compensatory programs (318)
concept formation (331)
concepts (331)

creative playthings (340)
daycare (317)
dramatic or imaginative play (340)
dyads (313)
early school experiences (318)
egocentric (333)
family daycare (317)
first-degree burn (327)
growth hormone deficiency (322)
guided participation (336)
guilt (343)

home daycare (318)
initiative (343)
inner speech (336)
intuitive phase (334)
map space (333)
minor lacerations (327)
Montessori programs (318)
neglected child (347)
neglectful (310)
nursery school (318)
object space, (333)
peer (310, 337)
peer group (338)

permissive (310)
physical activity (339)
pre-conceptual phase (333)
preschool years (310)
private speech (336)
quiet play (340)
second-degree burn (327)
sexual abuse (346)
siblings (313)
social speech (336)
symbolic play (340)
third-degree burn (327)
transductive logic (334)

# Chapter 10

## Assessment and Health Promotion for the Schoolchild

*If you are concerned about yourself, plant rice. If you are concerned about your family, plant trees. If you are concerned about your nation, educate your children.*

**Chinese Proverb**

## Objectives

*Study of this chapter will enable you to:*

1. Examine second-order changes in family status required to proceed developmentally in the family life cycle stage: families with young children.

2. Discuss the family relationships of the schoolchild.

3. Examine the influence of the child's peers and of adults other than parents on the schoolchild.

4. Compare and assess the physical changes and needs, including nutrition, rest, exercise, safety, and health protection, for the juvenile and preadolescent.

5. Assess intellectual, communication, play, emotional, self-concept, sexuality, and moral–spiritual development in the juvenile and preadolescent, and consider influences on these areas of development.

6. Discuss the crisis of school entry and determine ways to help the child adapt to the experience of formal education, including latchkey care.

7. Analyze the physical and emotional adaptive mechanisms of the schoolchild.

8. Discuss the significance of peers and the buddy relationship on the psychosocial development of the child.

9. Explore with parents their role in communication with, and guidance of, the child to foster healthy development in a holistic way.

10. Describe the influence that the media can exert upon behaviour.

11. Work effectively with the schoolchild in the nursing setting.

As growth and development continue and the child leaves the confines of the home, he or she emerges into a world of yet another set of new experiences and responsibilities. If previous developmental tasks have been met and the child has developed a healthy personality, he or she will continue to acquire new knowledge and skills steadily. If previous developmental stages have not been completely formulated and the child's personality development is immature, he or she may experience difficulties mastering the developmental stages of the school-aged child. Peers, parents, and other adults will likely exert a positive, maturing influence if the child is adequately prepared for leaving home for part of the day.

The *school-aged* years can be divided into **middle childhood** (*6 to 8 years of age*) and **late childhood** (*8 to 12 years of age*). The school-aged years can also be divided into the juvenile and preadolescent periods. *At approximately age six, the* **juvenile period** *begins*, marked by a heightened need for peer associations. **Preadolescence** *usually begins at nine or ten years of age* and is marked by a new capacity to love, when the satisfaction and security of another person of the same sex is as important to the child as personal satisfaction and security. Preadolescence ends at approximately 12 years with the onset of puberty. Preadolescence is also called **prepubescence** and is *characterized by an increase in hormone production in both sexes*, which is preparatory to eventual physiologic maturity. Psychological and social changes also occur as the child slowly moves away from the family. This chapter discusses characteristics to assess and intervention measures for you to use related to promote health care for the child and family.

In today's world, many conditions influence the development of a child. One of them is poverty. As mentioned in Chapter 1, the 2006 Report Card on Child and Family Poverty in Canada states that close to 1.2 million Canadian children—almost one child in six—live in poverty. A report called Summoned to Stewardship: Make Poverty Reduction a Collective Legacy, released in September 2007 by Campaign 2000 Policy Perspectives,[1] states that poverty reduction has now become the focus of international and national attention. Poverty reduction is central to Canada's future. Campaign 2000 is a cross-Canada coalition of more than 120 groups working to end child and family poverty. The report claims that 11.7 percent of Canada's children lived in low-income homes in 2005—the same rate as in 1989, when all parties in the House of Commons voted to work to eliminate child poverty by the year 2000. Campaign 2000 calls for a 50 percent reduction in child poverty by the year 2017. It outlines a national policy framework to ensure an out-of-poverty living standard for any parent or adult who works full-time. This includes providing a full child benefit of $5100 a year and work tax credits of $2400 a year, as well as raising the minimum wage to $10 per hour. The report argues that such actions would reduce national poverty by 37 percent and cost approximately $5 billion annually.[2] Poverty reduction in Canada must be a joint commitment of both the federal and the provincial governments.

Given the importance of the early years to the long-term healthy growth and development of children, the high rate of poverty of families with young children is a cause of serious concern.[3] In fact, children from families with the lowest incomes are more likely to exhibit manifestations of conduct disorder, emotional problems, and hyperactivity, and they are more prone to engage in delinquent behaviours.[4] Poverty does mean hunger, and many Canadian families resort to food banks.

A group of Canadian researchers claim that few data exist to establish whether low income alone affects infant morbidity.[5] Few studies have involved Canadian children specifically, and almost all of the available information comes from American research. It is difficult to generalize the results of U.S. studies to the Canadian situation, however, partly because of the different health care systems in the two countries.[6]

Health care professionals can endeavour to combat the effects of poverty and violence on the health of children and families. Regardless, money, effort, and time are necessary to accomplish the following:

- Provide children who are at risk of dropping out of school with special tutoring so that academic performance and self-esteem can be strengthened.

- Counsel parents and children in homes where child maltreatment, abuse, and violence are present.

- Assist parents with child care. Support the efforts of parents who are trying to improve their incomes and life.

- Provide daycare or after-school care for children when parents cannot be in the home because of job demands.

- Advocate at federal, provincial, territorial, and local governmental levels for policies and programs that will assist children (such as healthy school lunches) as well as eliminate the causes of poverty (such as employment conditions) for families.

- Work at the community level to reduce violence in the neighbourhoods, community, school, and nation.

- Support families in their efforts to protect their children from violence through church, community, and school programs.

## CRITICAL THINKING

*What steps would you take in developing a health promotion program in a community to address the need for a food bank?*

## FAMILY DEVELOPMENT AND RELATIONSHIPS
## Family Life Cycle

Refer to Table 4-3, which illustrates the stages of the family life cycle, the emotional processes of transition (key principles), and the second-order changes in the family required to proceed developmentally.

Help parents to be cognizant of these changes. Encourage them to talk through their concerns and the issues related to fulfilling the changes. Refer them to the school counsellor or community agency if help is desired.

## Relationships with Parents

Although parents remain a vital part of the schoolchild's life, the child's position within the family is altered with his or her entry into school. Parents play a major role in socializing the child to the adult world. They contribute to the socialization process in at least five ways:

1. By assuming the role of love providers and caretakers
2. By serving as identification figures
3. By acting as active socialization agents
4. By determining the sorts of experiences the child will have
5. By participating in the development of the child's self-concept[7]

The schoolchild now channels energy into intellectual pursuits, widens social horizons, and becomes more familiar with the adult world. He or she has identified with the parent of the same sex and, through imitation and education, continues to learn social roles and the tasks and routines expected by the culture or social group. The family atmosphere has much impact on the child's emotional development and on future responses within the family when he or she becomes an adolescent. Research indicates that children can become positive in their behaviour whether they are reared in authoritarian or permissive homes, provided parents are consistent in their approach.

Although parental support is needed, the schoolchild tends to pull away from overt signs of parental affection. Yet during illness, or when threatened by his or her new status, the child quickly turns to parents for affection and protection. Parents become frustrated with behavioural changes, antics, and infractions of household rules.

The child frequently changes ideas about and behaviour toward parents and adults as he or she grows. See the box entitled "Schoolchild's View of Parents and Adults."[8]

As you work with families and children, realize that there is no "typical family" for school-aged children. In fact, Cloutier and Alain from Laval University state that the contemporary family is undergoing transformation with the emergence of a greater variety of profiles and trajectories.[9] This development in family mobility has been observed for several decades, and the trend it represents can be regarded as a lasting one. The population must accept the fact of changing families and adapt to the family's process of transition. As well as a series of transitions that are part of the normal cycle

### Schoolchild's View of Parents and Adults

**Ages 6 to 8**

- Is still primarily family-oriented
- Sees parents as good, powerful, and wise
- Seeks parental approval
- Becomes emotionally steadier and freer from parents

**Ages 9 to 12**

- Begins to question parental authority
- Tends to feel smarter than parents, teachers, and adults in general
- Sees parent of the same sex as the more harsh disciplinarian

of a family, including growth and the development of children (known as developmental transitions), a family can also be significantly affected by non-developmental transitions, such as the placement of a child in substitute care, a death in the family, and parental separation.[10]

---

### CRITICAL THINKING

*What resources are available in your community to help a family with school-aged children that is in transition?*

---

According to the 2001 Canadian Census, the proportion of "traditional" families continues to decline. Children are living with common-law parents, and more young adults are living with their parents. The size of the Canadian household is declining because living alone is on the rise. Regarding same-sex couples, male couples outnumber female couples. In addition, more seniors are living with a spouse, more are living alone, and fewer are living in health care institutions.[11] The Aboriginal population is much younger than the Canadian average, and Aboriginal children represent 5.6 percent of all children in Canada.[12]

However, whatever the family structure, a child's adjustment is associated with the quality of parenting and not the structure of the family. For example, with at least one positive, warm, and authoritative parent, children of divorce are likely to be competent and well adjusted.[13] The responsibility for family life, and for looking after children, must be shared by parents, caregivers, employers, and the community. Because of the time pressures that parents face nowadays, all children need caring adults in their lives. These significant adults can be drawn from grandparents, aunts and uncles, neighbours, teachers, coaches, and child care providers.[14] For more information regarding Canada's children and their families, see www.cfc-efc.ca.

*What can you, as a health professional, do to lobby the government for a decrease in child poverty?*

*Refer to Chapter 4 for more information about trends in family life.* Increasing numbers of studies are being reported on how parent(s) can better focus quality time on the child, the effects of both parents being employed, the effects of being in a single-parent or step-parent home, and how much the child needs the love and support of parents. Studies also focus on the feelings of parents as they try to juggle the demands of child care and work.

Health Canada's publication *Because Life Goes On . . . Helping Children and Youth Live with Separation and Divorce* is intended to reach out to Canadian families who are in need of information and resources to help their children live through the process of separation and divorce.[15] Many factors are important for the child as the separation or divorce occurs. Keep in mind that however an adult understands or experiences the situation, the children see it and experience it differently. Typically, younger children view divorce as the enemy, while preteens and teenagers tend to hold their parents accountable for the divorce.[16] It is critical to remember that the emotional experience of anger is common to all children, but they express it differently. Talking to the children about separation and divorce is often the most difficult step that parents must take in the process. Yet, the way in which parents handle this crucial step can often set the pattern for future discussions and influence the level of trust children feel.[17]

Many videos are available for parents, children, and youth. *Kids Talk about Divorce*, created by Families in Transition (Family Service Association of Toronto), is intended for therapeutic/educational use. Children age 6 to 14 describe their struggles and successes in coping with divorce. You can contact Families in Transition at FSAT, 420-A 700 Lawrence Avenue West, Toronto, Ontario M6A 3B4 or online at www.fsatoronto.com/programs/families.html. Review with families the tasks summarized in Table 10-1. These tasks must be resolved by children after divorce.[18]

Although the poor child frequently shares the helplessness of an unemployed parent, the higher-income child often feels the relentless pressure on the parent who is a high-powered corporate executive, lawyer, professor, or government official preoccupied with his or her own survival. Too often, the demands of the workplace encroach on the needs and happiness of the family.

You will care for families in which abuse, neglect, or maltreatment occur. Refer to Chapters 4, 6, 7, and 9 for background information about precipitating factors, characteristics of abusing parents, and signs, symptoms, and treatment of abuse. Table 10-2 summarizes risk factors for sexual abuse.

## Table 10-1 Psychological Tasks for Children after Divorce

### Task I: Understanding the Divorce

*Schoolchildren*

1. Understand the immediate changes.
2. Differentiate fantasy from reality.
3. Manage concerns regarding abandonment, placement in foster care, not seeing departed parent again.

*Adolescents and Young Adults*

1. Understand what led to marital failure.
2. Evaluate parents' actions.
3. Draw useful conclusions for their own lives.

### Task II: Strategic Withdrawal

1. Acknowledge concern and provide appropriate help to parents and siblings.
2. Avoid divorce as the total focus and get back to their own interests, pleasures, activities, peer relationships.
3. Children allowed to remain children.

### Task III: Dealing with Loss

1. Deal with loss of intact family and loss of presence of one parent, usually the father.
2. Deal with feelings of rejection and blame for making one parent leave.
3. Task is easier if child has good relationship with both parents; this may be most difficult task.

### Task IV: Dealing with Anger

1. Manage anger at parents for deciding to divorce.
2. Be aware of parents' needs, anxiety, and loneliness.
3. Diminish anger and forgive.

### Task V: Working Out Guilt

1. Deal with sense of guilt for causing marital difficulties and driving wedge between parents.
2. Separate guilty ties and get on with their lives.

### Task VI: Accepting Permanence of Divorce

1. Overcome early denial and fantasies of parents getting back together.
2. Task may not be completed until parent remarries or child mourns loss.

### Task VII: Taking a Chance on Love

1. Remain open to love, commitment, marriage, fidelity.
2. Able to turn away from parents' model.
3. Most important task for growing children, adolescents, and young adults.

| Table 10-2 Sexual Abuse of the Schoolchild |
|---|

**Risk Factors**

- Having a stepfather
- Poor relationship between child and parent
- Mothers who work outside the home or are emotionally distant
- Having a parent who does not live with the child
- Sex: 25 percent of all females and 10 percent of all males by age 18

**Family Characteristics**

- An emotionally dependent adult male in the home
- Sexual estrangement between the parents or parental figures
- Mother deserted the family (literally or figuratively)
- Sexual offender suffers a crisis, such as loss of job
- Daughter begins to mature sexually
- Parent has poor impulse control
- Problems such as substance abuse, personality disorders, psychoses, and mental retardation in parent(s)

The **latchkey child**, *the child who has the door key because no one is home when he or she returns from school,* is seen more frequently because increasing numbers of women with children under 18 work outside of the home. Children voice different feelings about the working mother and having no one at home to meet them after school. Some like it. They enjoy the solitude, privacy, and responsibility at day's end. Some hate it for the same reasons. Some tolerate it out of necessity, disliking the separation and lack of time together. Some are afraid for themselves and their mothers. Some are proud of mother and how the family is managing together. Some develop discipline problems. All understand the financial reasons and sometimes they understand the career and emotional reasons that are usually the basis for mother working. Canada Safety Council's advice to the parents includes:

- Set firm rules, with dos and don'ts
- Prepare the child to deal with events that may arise
- Specify how his or her time is to be spent
- Keep in touch—a cellphone or pager may be an asset
- Make certain the home is safe and secure
- Limit the time that the child is left alone[19]

**CRITICAL THINKING**

*If you were asked by the Canada Safety Council to add more pointers for parents, what would you add to the list?*

In Canada, the age at which children can legally be left home alone for short periods varies from province to province, but ranges from 10 to 12 years. Therein, the president of the Canada Safety Council urges parents not to consider letting a child stay at home alone before age 10—and then only if the child is mature enough. The maximum time to be spent alone is an hour or two—and then only if there is a responsible adult nearby to help out if needed.[20]

To prepare children for the responsibilities of self-care, the Canada Safety Council has prepared the booklet *At Home on My Own,* which focuses on how to prevent problems, handle real-life situations, and keep children safely and constructively occupied.[21]

As a health care professional, you care for the family and the individual child. As a community nurse, your assessment may be the key to a child's receiving necessary care. You can conduct many of the health promotion activities described throughout this chapter. You can counsel and teach both parents and children. Be aware of cultural beliefs and practices as you work with children and families. A family who has lived in this country for several generations may follow the same cultural patterns as the newly immigrated family.

## Relationships with Siblings

Although parental influence is of primary importance, the child's relationship with siblings can strongly influence personality formation. During middle childhood, sibling rivalry tends to increase.[22] However, the influence of siblings on the development of the school-aged child depends on a number of factors, including age and sex of the siblings, number of children in the family, proximity of their ages, and the type of parent–child interaction. See Chapter 9

**CONTROVERSY DEBATE**

# Home Alone

Your neighbours routinely allow their seven-year-old child to be alone in their home for several hours each day after school until they arrive home from work. You have seen the child come home from school, sometimes alone, and at other times with a small number of age mates. One day, after seeing the child and eight other children go into the house, you decide to phone the home to see how they are doing. The telephone is not answered—even after you check the number and redial.

1. What is your immediate responsibility as a neighbour?
2. How will you approach the parents?

regarding the findings of a Canadian study on how siblings rate their relationship quality.[23]

## CRITICAL THINKING

*The Smiths are a blended family. In what ways might their tasks be similar to, or different from, the ones listed above?*

## Relationships with Adoptive Parents

An issue for adoptive parents is how to help their adopted child or children feel part of the family, especially if adoption occurs at an age when the child remembers the process.

Table 10-3 describes the adopted child's perception of adoption during the school years and how adoptive parents may respond. Adoptive families need professionals who understand child development, behaviour management, and the psychological issues for children who have undergone separation and loss. Ongoing supports such as workshops and networks can also be of tremendous assistance to adoptive families.[24]

## Relationships outside the Family

As the child's social environment widens, other individuals begin to function as role models. The child strives for independence and establishes meaningful relationships with peers, teachers, and other significant adults. These relationships provide the child with new ideas, attitudes, perspectives, and modes of behaviour. Although the parents remain role models, the influence of the family and the time spent with family diminish. Through contacts with the peer group, the child acquires a basis for assessing the parents as individuals and learns that parents can make mistakes.

Schneider, a Canadian researcher, investigated the friendships of children considered socially withdrawn by their school peers. The videotaped data showed the withdrawn children to be somewhat restricted in their verbal communication with their friends. They were less competitive with their friends than were friends in a comparison group. In dyads consisting of one withdrawn and one non-withdrawn child, the withdrawn child perceived the relationship as characterized by greater closeness and helpfulness than did the non-withdrawn friend. Despite some signs of inhibited behaviour within the friendship context, withdrawn children seem to have access to close friendships of high quality.[25] It is important to point out that peer rejection was not a variable in this study. Children are adaptable to their environment and usually gravitate to an acceptable niche for themselves.

The schoolchild has a growing sense of community that changes with increased mobility and independence and added responsibility. His or her understanding broadens to include a sense of boundaries, distance, location, and spatial relationships of resources and organizations, demographic characteristics, and group identity.

*You are in a key position to listen to and explore with families* their concerns about being parents, achieving the expected developmental tasks, and adjusting to the growing and changing child as he or she interacts with parents, siblings, other relatives, peers, and other adults outside the home. At times you may validate their approach to a given situation. At other times you may help them to clarify their values so they can, in turn, better guide the child. Such practical suggestions as how to plan a nutritious meal more

## Table 10-3 Adopted Child's Perceptions and Suggested Parental Responses

| Age | Child's Perception | Suggested Parental Response |
|-----|--------------------|-----------------------------|
| 5–7 | ■ Begins to grasp full notion of adoption, that parents are not blood relatives, and that most children live with biological parent(s)<br>■ Feels sense of loss | ■ Emphasize that child is important to them and was chosen.<br>■ Answer questions comfortably and naturally. Explain that it is normal for child to have mixed emotions about adoption. |
| 8–11 | ■ Fantasizes and wonders about birth parents<br>■ Realizes he or she is different from non-adopted children<br>■ Wants to question parents about adoption but fears appearing disloyal or ungrateful<br>■ Feels grief and goes through mourning process<br>■ Frequently asks questions about why birth parents relinquished him or her, parents' appearance, and whether there are siblings | ■ Discuss the adoption openly, when appropriate, to help the child vent curiosity and feelings.<br>■ Help child accept fact that he or she is different and emphasize other differences as well.<br>■ Answer questions truthfully.<br>■ Do not criticize or overpraise birth parents.<br>■ Adjust depth of answer to age of child.<br>■ Realize that children who are not adopted also fantasize that they are. |

economically or handle sibling rivalry can help a distraught parent feel and become more effective.

Your ability to assess beyond the obvious and to help the family use community resources effectively to meet basic needs is often the first step in promotion of both physical and emotional health.

CRITICAL THINKING

*What are some criteria that children might use to choose their friends?*

# PHYSIOLOGIC CONCEPTS

The following information is pertinent to assessment and health promotion strategies. Share this information with families.

## Physical Characteristics

The *principles of growth* or *growth patterns* are generally comparable across cultures. For example, progression of the maturation of body organ systems is similar in all cultural groups. The child between 6 and 12 years of age exhibits considerable change in physical appearance. Growth during this stage of development is hypertrophic (cells increase in size) instead of hyperplasic (cells increase in number). The growth rate is usually slow and steady, characterized by periods of accelerations in the spring and fall and by rapid growth during preadolescence.[26]

**Weight, Height, and Girth** These measurements vary considerably among children and depend on genetic, environmental, and cultural influences.

Most Asian children born and raised in Canada or the U.S. are larger and taller than those children born and raised in Asian countries because of differences in diet, climate, and social milieu.[27]

The *average schoolchild grows* an average of 5 cm per year to gain 30 to 60 cm height by age 12. A *weight gain* of 2 to 3 kg occurs per year. The average weight for a six-year-old boy is 21.5 kg (48 pounds), and the average height is 117 cm (46 inches). By age 12, the average child weighs approximately 40 kg and is more than 150 cm tall. By that age, the child has usually attained 90 percent of adult height.

During the *juvenile* or *middle childhood period*, girls and boys may differ little in size. Their bodies are usually lean, with narrow hips and shoulders. Although the amount of muscle mass and adipose tissue is influenced by muscle use, diet, and activity, males usually have more muscle cells, while females have more adipose tissue. The muscles are changing in composition and are growing at a rapid rate, becoming more firmly attached to the bones. Muscles may be immature in regard to function, resulting in children's vulnerability to injury stemming from overuse, awkwardness, and inefficient movement. Muscle aches may accompany skeletal growth spurts as developing muscles attempt to keep pace with the enlarging skeletal structure. Ossification, the formation of bone, continues at a steady pace. The schoolchild loses the pot-bellied, swayback appearance of early childhood. Abdominal muscles become stronger and the pelvis tips backwards so the posture becomes straighter.[28]

**Neuromuscular Development** The brain of the child is very active. Studies reveal that from age four to puberty, glucose metabolism by brain cells is twice that of the adult brain. Thus, the child is capable of readily processing new information.[29]

By age seven, the brain has reached 90 percent of adult size. The growth rate of the brain is greatly slowed after age 7, but by age 12 the brain has virtually reached adult size. Memory has improved. The child can listen better and make associations with incoming stimuli.

Myelinization is complete. *Neuromuscular changes* are occurring along with skeletal development. Neuromuscular coordination is sufficient to permit the schoolchild to learn most of the skills he or she wishes.

Refer to Table 10-4 for a summary of neuromuscular development from 6 to 12 years of age.[30]

**Cardiovascular System** The *heart* grows slowly during this age period, while the left ventricle of the heart enlarges. After seven years of age, the apex of the heart lies at the interspace of the fifth rib at the midclavicle line. Before this age, the apex is palpated at the fourth interspace just to the left of the midclavicle line. By age nine, the heart weighs six times its birth weight. By puberty, it weighs ten times its birth weight. Even though cardiac growth does occur, the heart remains small in relation to the rest of the body. Because the heart is smaller proportionately to body size, the child may tire easily. Sustained physical activity is not desirable. The schoolchild should not be pushed to run, jog, or engage in excessively competitive sports such as football, hockey, and racquetball.[31]

CRITICAL THINKING

*What are several factors that promote cardiovascular fitness?*

**Vital Signs** Vital signs of the schoolchild are affected by size, sex, and activity. Temperature, pulse, and respiration gradually approach adult norms with an average *temperature* of 36.7°C to 37°C, *pulse rate* of 70 to 80 per minute, resting pulse rate of 60 to 76 per minute, and *respiratory rate* of 18 to 21 per minute. The average *systolic blood pressure* is 94 to 112, and average *diastolic blood pressure* is 56 to 60 mm Hg. As respiratory tissues achieve adult maturity, *lung capacity* becomes

## Table 10-4 Neuromuscular Development in the Schoolchild

| Age (Yr) | Characteristic |
| --- | --- |
| 6 | High activity level but clumsy<br>Moves constantly: skips, hops, runs, roller skates<br>Can do manipulative skills: hammer, cut, paste, tie shoes, and fasten clothes<br>Grasps pencil or crayon, makes large letters or figures<br>Can throw with proper weight shift and step<br>Walks chalk mark with balance<br>Tandem gait<br>Girls are superior in movement accuracy<br>Boys are superior in forceful, less complex activity |
| 7 | Lower activity level; enjoys quiet and active<br>Pedals a bicycle<br>Prints sentences, reverses letters less frequently<br>Spreads with a knife<br>Can balance on one foot without looking<br>Can walk 5-cm-wide balance beam<br>Can hop and jump accurately into small squares<br>Can do accurate jumping jack exercise |
| 8 | Moves energetically but with grace and balance<br>Enjoys vigorous activity<br>Improved coordination<br>Can engage in alternate rhythmic hopping in 2-2, 2-3, or 3-3 pattern<br>Faster reaction time<br>More skilful at throwing because of longer arm; girls can throw small ball 1.2 m<br>Better grasp of objects<br>Begins cursive writing rather than printing, better small muscle coordination<br>Has 5.5 kg (12 pounds) of pressure in grip strength |
| 9 | Less restless<br>Bathes self<br>Refined eye–hand coordination, skilled in manual activities<br>Draws a three-dimensional geometric figure<br>Enjoys models<br>Uses both hands independently<br>Spaces words and slants letters when writing<br>Strives to improve coordination and perfect physical skills, strength, and endurance<br>Boys can run 5 m (16.5 feet) per second<br>Boys can throw a small ball 25 m (70 feet) |
| 10 | More energetic, active, restless movements<br>Finger drumming or foot tapping<br>Balances on one foot for 15 seconds<br>Can judge and intercept pathway of small ball thrown from a distance<br>Girls can run 5.25 m (17 feet) per second |
| 11–12 | Standing broad jump of 1.5 m (5 feet) is possible for boys, 15 cm (6 inches) less for girls<br>Standing high jump of 1 m (3 feet) possible by age 12<br>Can catch a fly ball<br>Skilful manipulative movements nearly equal to those of adult<br>Physical changes preceding puberty begin to appear |

proportional to body size. Between the ages of five and ten, the respiratory rate slows as the amount of air exchanged with each breath doubles. Breathing becomes deeper and slower. By the end of middle childhood, the lung weight will have increased almost ten times. The ribs shift from a horizontal position to a more oblique orientation. The chest broadens and flattens to allow for this increased lung size and capacity.[32]

**Head** Facial proportions change as the face grows more rapidly in relation to the rest of the skull. The skull and brain grow very slowly during this period and increase little in size thereafter. The child loses the childish look as the face takes on features that will characterize him or her as an adult. Jaw bones grow longer and more prominent as the mandible extends forward, providing an extended chin and a place into which *permanent teeth* can erupt. Since all of the primary teeth are lost during this lifespan, the "tooth-less" appearance may produce embarrassment for the child. The first permanent teeth are six-year molars that erupt by age seven and are the key teeth for forming the permanent dental arch. Evaluation for braces should not be undertaken until all four six-year molars have appeared. The second permanent molars erupt by age 14, and the third molars (wisdom teeth) come in as late as age 30. Wisdom teeth for some people never erupt (see Figure 10-1). When the first permanent central incisors emerge, they appear too large for the mouth and face.[33]

Many governments and health organizations, including Health Canada, the Canadian Public Health Association, the Canadian Dental Association, the Canadian Medical Association, and the World Health Organization, endorse the fluoridation of drinking water to prevent tooth decay.[34] The Canadian Paediatric Society position statement on the Use of Fluoride in Infants and Children states that the ingestion of too much fluoride can result in varying degrees of fluorosis. In practice, the administration of fluoride should strike a balance between the two situations.[35] Health Canada works in collaboration with the provinces and the territories to maintain and to improve drinking water quality. Together, both levels of government have developed *Guidelines for Canadian Drinking Water Quality* (see Chapter 2). These guidelines are reviewed and revised periodically to take into account new scientific knowledge.[36]

Drinking water that meets quality guidelines does not usually need extra treatment. The following are several steps that parents can take to keep fluoride intake within safe limits:

■ Do not give fluoridated mouthwash or mouth rinses to children under six years of age, because they might swallow it.

■ Talk to the dentist before using a fluoride supplement or a fluoridated mouthwash.

**Figure 10-1** Normal tooth formation in the child

| Median Age of Eruption | | Median Age When Shed | | THE PRIMARY TEETH |
|---|---|---|---|---|
| 6–9 months | — | 6–7 years | — | Medial Incisor |
| 7–10 months | — | 7–8 years | — | Lateral Incisor |
| 16–18 months | — | 10–12 years | — | Cuspid |
| 12–14 months | — | 9–11 years | — | First Molar |
| 20–28 months | — | 9–11 years | — | Second Molar |

| Median Age of Eruption | | THE PERMANENT LOWER TEETH |
|---|---|---|
| 6–7 years* | — | Medial Incisor |
| 7–8 years* | — | Lateral Incisor |
| 9–12 years* | — | Cuspid |
| 10–12 years | — | First Premolar (Bicuspid) |
| 11–12 years | — | Second Premolar (Bicuspid) |
| 5½–7 years | — | First Molar |
| 11–13 years* | — | Second Molar |
| 16–21 years | — | Third Molar (Wisdom Tooth) |

*Note: These specific teeth for the upper jaw erupt on the average of 1 year later than do the lower teeth.

- Do not take fluoride supplements if the drinking water is already fluoridated.

- Be informed. The Canadian Dental Association and the Canadian Paediatric Society have made recommendations for the use of fluoride supplements in communities where the water is not fluoridated.

- Make certain that children use no more than a pea-sized amount of toothpaste on their toothbrush, and teach them not to swallow the toothpaste.

- Children under six years of age should be supervised while brushing, and children under the age of three should have their teeth brushed by an adult without using toothpaste.

## CRITICAL THINKING

*What evidence can you think of to support the notion of a gender difference about brushing teeth?*

**Vision** Most school-aged children have keener vision than when they were younger. The shape of the *eye* changes during growth, and the normal farsightedness of the preschool child is gradually converted to 20/20 vision. Binocular vision is well developed in most children at six years of age and peripheral vision is fully developed. Girls tend to have poorer visual acuity than boys, but their colour discrimination is superior. Large print is recommended for reading matter, and regular vision testing should be part of the school health program.[37]

**Gastrointestinal System** Secretion, digestion, absorption, and excretion become more efficient. The maturity of the gastrointestinal system is reflected in fewer stomach upsets, better maintenance of blood sugar levels, and an increased stomach capacity.[38]

**Urinary System** The urinary system becomes functionally mature during the school years. Between the ages of five and ten, the *kidneys* double in size to accommodate increased metabolic functions. Individual variations occur in frequency of urination and variations occur in the same child at times due to factors such as humidity, temperature, and the amounts of fluids ingested. Fluid and electrolyte balance becomes stabilized, and *bladder capacity* is increased, especially in girls. *Urinary constituents* and specific gravity become similar to those of an adult. However, 5 to 20 percent of school-aged children have small amounts of albuminuria.[39]

**Immune System** The body's ability to localize infection improves and produces an antibody-antigen response. Sore throats, upper respiratory infections, and ear infections are common because of frequent exposure to other children.[40]

**Prepubertal Sexual Development** During the *preadolescent* or *prepuberty period*, both males and females develop preliminary characteristics of sexual maturity. It is a period of rapid growth, especially for girls. The girl's growth spurt begins as early as eight years. The average start is 10, and maximum growth rate is reached around 12 years. The boy's growth spurt begins near 12 years. Maximum height velocity is reached by approximately 14 years. The male grows approximately 10 cm per year for 2.5 years and then begins a slower rate of growth. The female grows an average of 7.5 cm per year until menarche. This variability, especially in relation to the onset of secondary sex characteristics, is of utmost concern to the preadolescent. Either early or late appearance of these characteristics can be a source of embarrassment and uneasiness. Late-development boys often have a negative self-concept. Meanwhile, the early appearance of secondary sex characteristics may be associated with the dissatisfaction of physical appearance and lower self-esteem. Changes in secondary sex characteristics include breast development in girls, changing voice pitch and beard growth in boys, and the growth of body hair in both sexes.[41]

As sebaceous glands of the face, back, and chest become active, acne (pimples) may develop. Acne is further discussed in Chapter 11.

Teach parents about the physical and growth characteristics of the school-aged child and the importance of nutrition, rest, immunizations, healthful activity, and regular medical and dental care. The rest of the chapter refers to variables that influence physical health.

## CRITICAL THINKING

*What steps can you take to promote the emotional well-being of a child with acne?*

## Physical Assessment of the School-Aged Child

Information will be gained from the child, the parents or caretakers, or both when assessing the child.

A child may be better at drawing than at explaining what is wrong. For example, when asked to draw a big circle where it hurts, the child can normally identify the part, if given a simple outline drawing of a child.

The child over age ten may wish to talk to the health care provider without the parent present. Being alert to the child's chronologic and developmental stage and his or her relationship with parents or caretakers will guide you in interviewing. Where the child lives (house or apartment, rural or urban area), how much personal space he or she has (own room, own bed), parents' marital situation, presence or absence of siblings, what is usually eaten, the amounts of exercise and rest in 24 hours, who cares for the child after school if parents are working, and how he or she spends free time are all important in assessing the health status.

When doing a review of systems, remember to use words the child understands. For example, instead of asking whether the child has ever experienced any otitis problems, simply ask: *Do your ears ever ache?* or *Can you always hear when people talk to you?*

In assessing skin, remember that the school-aged child is subject to allergic contact dermatitis, warts, herpes type 1, ringworm, and lice. When seeing any rash, a thorough history is necessary to determine the diagnosis and treatment.[42]

Understanding that visual function is more than reading the *20/20* line on a Snellen chart will help you to suggest a more comprehensive visual examination when a child is experiencing difficulty with schoolwork. Children and their parents do not always react predictably when there is a need for corrective lenses. Some children may feel self-conscious with their peers when wearing glasses. Parents may react as if the child's visual problem were a flaw and will deny it (stating that they are sure the child will outgrow the problem), ignore the information, or even go from doctor to doctor in search of reassurance.

If you are able to provide accurate information, using the principles of therapeutic communication, it will be exceedingly valuable to a child and family who are having difficulty adjusting to the need for therapy for a visual impairment. (This also holds true when therapy or a corrective device is needed on another body area.)

When assessing a child's hearing and ears, remember that hearing should be fully developed by age five. By age seven, most children should speak clearly enough to be understood by adults. If either of these factors seems deficient, a thorough investigation into congenital or inherited disorders and how this deficiency affects daily activities and communication is in order.

In the young child, because the ear canal slants upward, pull the auricle down, but not back as you would in an adult, when using the otoscope. Remember, the ear canal is short in the young child, so take care not to insert the ear tip too far. The otoscope should be controlled so that if the young child moves suddenly, you can protect the eardrum from being contacted by the otoscope. The cone of light is more indistinct in a child than in an adult.[43]

Keep in mind the following as you continue assessment of the child's body systems: (1) if you think you hear fluid in the lungs, check the child's nose because sounds caused by nose fluid can be transmitted to the lungs; (2) an $S_3$ sound and sinus arrhythmia are fairly common in children's heart sounds; (3) a child's liver and spleen will usually enlarge more quickly than an adult's in response to disease; (4) the bladder

is normally found much higher in a child than in an adult, and the kidneys can more often be palpated; (5) the genitalia should be inspected for congenital abnormalities that may have been overlooked, and for irritation, inflammation, or swelling; and (6) developmental guidelines must be used to assess the nervous system, specifically language development, motor and sensory functions, and cerebral function.[44]

In the last decade, musculoskeletal and posture problems, especially scoliosis detection, have gained wide attention. **Scoliosis**, *lateral curvature of the spine*, is more common in girls than in boys and is of two types: functional and structural. Ask the child to bend over and touch the toes without bending the knees and keeping the palms of the hands together. If the child has functional scoliosis, the external curve will disappear with this exercise. If it is structural, the curve will remain and sometimes become more pronounced. Early diagnosis is extremely important to arrest this problem.[45] Refer the child and family to an orthopedic specialist. If scoliosis is not corrected early in life, it can result in mobility problems, obstructive pulmonary disease, and problems with body image later in life.

## CRITICAL THINKING

*What questions can you realistically ask the schoolchild about health conditions within the family?*

## Nutritional Needs

The school years are important regarding eating habits. Meeting the nutritional requirements of the school-aged child requires larger amounts of the same food needed by the preschool child. Growth during prepuberty is slow and steady, with gradual increases in height and weight.[46] With the introduction of school into one's routine, the child's meal pattern will likely change. Even though children may prepare their own breakfast, parents should try to eat breakfast with their children as with other meals. Stockmyer found that beneficial effects on nutritional intake occur when children eat dinner with their family.[47]

During the school years, children become more responsible in making their own choices about what they eat. Children have built-in cues—hunger, feeling full, thirst, and taste—to help them decide what and when to eat. Do you recall making your own snacks? Parents and significant caregivers struggle to make certain they help children to make good choices while respecting the child's ability to make his or her own decisions. Most children prefer meals and snacks on a regular basis and in familiar surroundings. The amount of food eaten at each meal and snack will vary from day to day depending on the child's appetite, activity level, and whether he or she is experiencing a growth spurt.[48]

*Eating Well with Canada's Food Guide* (www.hc-sc.gc.ca/fn-an/food-guide-aliment/index_e.html) encourages eating and enjoying different foods from each food group every day. This selection helps children to meet their nutrient needs every day. Children eat mainly from the following four food groups:

- Vegetables and fruit, especially dark green and orange vegetables as well as orange fruit, should be chosen more often.

- Grain products, such as whole-grain and enriched products, should be chosen most often.

- Milk products are important. Make sure to offer children a total of two cups of milk or fortified soy beverage every day. This will help meet their requirements for vitamin D.

- Meat and alternatives: for young children, nutritious foods that contain fat should not be restricted.

See Figure 10-2 for a sample one-day menu for a 12-year-old boy.[49]

Other foods—that is, foods that are not part of the four main food groups—can also add energy and some nourishment. To promote variety in foods, children can try food from other cultures. Doing so can help them to learn about their friends and the world around them. Children must be encouraged to drink water to quench their thirst. In fact, children need more water during hot weather and when they are playing hard. Most beverages (e.g., milk and juices) and many foods (such as fruit) are good sources of water.[50]

If children are healthy, growing well, and eating a variety of foods, they are not likely to need a vitamin-mineral supplement.[51]

*Nutritional assessment* is determined by obtaining a history of the child's food intake; looking at the general appearance and skin colour and turgor; correlating height and weight; measuring subcutaneous tissue; checking for dental caries, allergies, and chronic illness; testing hemoglobin and hematocrit levels; and determining physical, cognitive, emotional, and social well-being.

**Eating Patterns**  It is important to discuss the child's eating needs and patterns with parents so that they can provide a diet with adequate caloric intake and nutrients. Culture usually determines the type of foods eaten, when certain foods are to be eaten, and the manner in which they are consumed. The many dietary variations must be assessed for nutritional adequacy.[52] By age eight, children have increased appetites, and by age ten, their appetites are similar to those of adults. Despite increasing appetites, children seldom voluntarily interrupt activities for meals. Television, sports, and other activities compete with mealtimes.

Parents should be encouraged to establish a consistent schedule for meals, and to allow their school-aged child to participate in the meal planning. Schoolchildren of six or seven are capable of learning about healthful eating, and helping plan and prepare meals. Such activities develop a healthy sense of industry and independence in the child, if they are not overdone. Diet is influenced by a child's activities. If the child has been active all day, he or she will be hungry and ready to eat. On the other hand, if the child has had limited activity or emotional frustrations during the day, he or she may have little or have no appetite.

Research indicates that encouraging or pressuring children to consume more vegetables and fruits is associated with lower intakes of vegetables and fruits and higher intakes of dietary fats. In fact, rewarding a child for eating foods can lead to unintended consequences. With respect to parenting styles, an authoritarian style of feeding, in which eating demands placed on children are high and responsiveness to children's needs are low, promotes overeating, overweight, food rejection, and picky eating.[53]

Evidence is mounting that Canadian children are making unhealthy food choices. This national predicament is leading to both dietary inadequacies and excesses. Unhealthy eating patterns during childhood interfere with optimal growth and development and set the stage for poor eating habits during adolescence and adulthood.[54]

## CRITICAL THINKING

*How effective do you believe parental practices are regarding adequate nutrition?*

*Share the following suggestions with parents to improve nutrition and mealtime enjoyment:*[55]

1. Create an environment of respect, love, acceptance, and calm. Make time for healthy eating so that children don't feel rushed.

2. Make food attractive and manageable. Offer a variety of foods in relatively small amounts.

3. Establish basic rules regarding table etiquette and table language, topics of conversation, and behaviour. Sit down and eat with the children. Enjoy them.

4. Have a firm understanding with the child that play and television do not take precedence over eating properly. Keep the television turned off at mealtime.

5. Light between-meal snacks are necessary and enjoyable if they do not interfere with food intake at meals and are eaten an hour or longer before mealtime. Milk, cheese, fresh fruits and vegetables, peanut butter, and fruit juices are desirable snacks for both general nutritional needs and dental health.

**Figure 10-2** Sample one-day menu for Malcolm, a 12-year-old boy

| | Recommended Daily Food Guide Servings | | | |
|---|---|---|---|---|
| | **Vegetables and Fruit** | **Grain Products** | **Milk and Alternatives** | **Meat and Alternatives** |
| Boys 9 - 13 years | 6 | 6 | 3-4 | 1-2 |

| | Number of Food Guide Servings | | | | |
|---|---|---|---|---|---|
| **Foods** | **Vegetables and Fruit** | **Grain Products** | **Milk and Alternatives** | **Meat and Alternatives** | **Added Oils and Fats** |
| **Breakfast**<br>• 1 small slice of leftover cheese pizza on whole wheat crust<br>• 250 mL (1 cup) milk<br>• 125 mL (½ cup) orange juice | 1 | 1 - 1/2 | 1/2<br>1 | | |
| **Snack**<br>• 1 whole grain granola bar<br>• water | | 1 | | | |
| **Lunch**<br>• roast beef sandwich with 75g (2½ oz) beef and mayonnaise on 2 slices of whole grain bread<br>• 250 mL (1 cup) milk<br>• 1 nectarine | 1 | 2 | 1 | 1 | ✔ |
| **Snack**<br>• 125 mL (½ cup) cantaloupe cubes with low fat fruit yogurt dip<br>• water | 1 | | 1/2 | | |
| **Dinner**<br>• chicken stir-fry with 75g (2½ oz) chicken and 250 mL (1 cup) broccoli and red peppers cooked in canola oil<br>• 175 mL (¾ cup) whole wheat noodles<br>• 250 mL (1 cup) milk | 2 | 1 - 1/2 | 1 | 1 | ✔ |
| **Snack**<br>• 125 mL (½ cup) blueberries | 1 | | | | |
| **Total Food Guide Servings for the day** | 6 | 6 | 4 | 2 | |

Source: *Eating Well with Canada's Food Guide. A Resource for Educators and Communicators* © Adapted and Reproduced with the permission of the Minister of Public Works and Government Services Canada, 2008.

6. Breakfast is crucial for providing the child with sufficient calories to start the day. The child who attends school without breakfast frequently exhibits fatigue and poor attention.

7. Be a positive role model for children. With a comfortable environment and adults eating the food on the table, the intake is likely to be adequate for the child because the parents are providing good role models.

## Nutritional Hurdles

You have two school-aged children and an infant. Last week, your family orthodontist placed braces on the teeth of the older two children. The orthodontist instructed you and the children that they could not eat raw fruits or vegetables, but starches are acceptable provided the teeth are brushed immediately after eating. Brushing after lunch at school is easily arranged. However, you wish to prepare snacks for the children to take to school to have after school before hockey practice twice weekly, but brushing at that time is a problem for them.

1. List foods from each group of *Eating Well with Canada's Food Guide* that your children could take for their after-school snack.

2. How will you alter the snacks to maintain a variety?

Please see Chapter 8 for a discussion of malnutrition.

It is often surprising, and somewhat disappointing, to realize the effects of hunger on children in Canada. McIntyre and her colleagues examined the prevalence of hunger among Canadian children. In doing so, they studied the characteristics of, and coping strategies used by, families with children who were experiencing hunger.[56] The data originated from the first wave of data collection for the National Longitudinal Survey of Children and Youth conducted in 1994. The data included 13 439 randomly selected Canadian families with children aged 11 years or under. The researchers found that hunger was experienced by more than 1 percent (206) of the families in the survey. The survey sample represented a population of 57 000 Canadian families. In addition, they found that single-parent families, families relying on social assistance, and off-reserve Aboriginal families were overrepresented among those experiencing hunger. Hunger coexisted with the mother's poor health, activity limitation, and the poor health of children. Parents tend to offset the needs of their children by not taking food themselves.[57]

Obesity is sometimes defined as the condition of an *individual who is 20 percent or more above ideal weight.* The concept of body mass index (BMI), rather than weight alone, is currently used to determine whether an individual is obese.[58] Obesity is the most frequently occurring nutritional disorder of children in developed countries. Poor diet and inactivity during childhood have been implicated in the worrisome increase of childhood obesity, which is considered to be at epidemic proportions in Canada and other developed nations.[59] In fact, the World Health Organization (WHO) refers to the escalating global epidemic of obesity as "globesity."[60] In addition, childhood obesity often has serious physical, social, and emotional effects that carry over into adulthood.[61] Specifically, risk factors for cardiovascular disease and type 2 diabetes are known to develop early in life.[62] The prevention of childhood obesity, through early nutrition education and established exercise habits, is of utmost importance. Berry and her colleagues critically evaluated the evidence related to family-based interventions developed to treat childhood obesity. Thirteen studies were evaluated and all of the interventions used nutrition education, exercise, and behavioural interventions, including behavioural modification, behavioural therapy, or problem solving. The results indicated that behavioural modification interventions, which targeted children and parents either together or separately, were reported to be successful in improving weight-loss outcomes in both parents and children. Behavioural therapy interventions, which targeted children and parents together or the parents of children separately, improved weight outcomes. Problem-solving interventions that targeted parents of children showed improved weight outcomes for their children. However, when problem solving was used with both parents and children together or with children alone, weight outcomes did not improve.[63] The Weight Realities Division of the Society for Nutrition Education developed guidelines for obesity prevention programs that encourage a health-centred, rather than a weight-centred, approach. This approach focuses on the whole child, physically, mentally, and socially. The focus is on living actively, eating in normal and healthful ways, and developing a nurturing environment that helps children to recognize their own worth and to respect cultural footways and family traditions.[64]

*Malnutrition and obesity may have the same causative factors.* The child may be reflecting food habits of other family members. Both parents and child may displace unrelated anxieties onto food and mealtime, or eating may serve as a reward or punishment for both parents and child. In some cultures, being overweight is considered a sign of health and family affluence. In other cultures, obesity is considered unsightly and unhealthy.[65]

You can help parents to learn about adequate nutrition for their child, and what behaviour to expect at each age. You can also facilitate health promotion strategies at school or in the community. Several learning activities for the schoolchild could include visiting grocery stores, dairies, or farms, as well as taking part in tasting parties and playing store. They could plan menus, examine food labels, and cook various foods and taste them. Such activities are unlimited.

*What are the main consequences of obesity for the schoolchild? How can these consequences be overcome?*

## Rest and Exercise

Review the child's rest and exercise needs with parents. At the same time, you may have an opportunity to discuss with parents how they are meeting their own needs for rest and exercise and how the parents and child can engage in activities that are mutually interesting and healthful.

The number of hours of sleep needed depend on such variables as age, health status, and the day's activities. Schoolchildren usually do not need a nap. They do not use up as much energy in growth as they did earlier. A 6-year-old usually requires approximately 11 hours of sleep nightly, but an 11-year-old may need only 9 hours.[66] The schoolchild does not consciously fight sleep but may need firm discipline to go to bed at the prescribed hour. Sleep may be disturbed by dreams and nightmares, especially if he or she has considerable emotional stimulation before bedtime.

Exercise is essential for muscular development, refinement of coordination and balance, gaining strength, and enhancing other body functions such as circulation, aeration, and waste elimination. Regular physical activity at this age, and thereafter, helps to prevent coronary artery disease, hypertension, hypercholesterolemia, obesity, and type 2 diabetes in future years.[67]

More than half of Canadians aged 5 to 17 are not active enough for optimal growth and development. The term *active enough* is equivalent to an energy expenditure of at least 8 kilocalories per kilogram of body weight per day.[68] The most reported physical activity of children 5 to 12 is bicycling, followed by swimming, playing on swings, using playground equipment, and then walking. In this age group, the next most popular activities are winter activities such as tobogganing and skating. Athletic activity is attractive to both boys and girls and is becoming more accessible to girls than in the past.[69]

Health Canada recognized that the rapid increase in overweight and obesity, combined with low levels of physical activity, represent a serious threat to the health of Canadian children and youth.[70]

Health Canada and the Canadian Society for Exercise Physiology initiated the development of *Physical Activity Guides for Children and Youth* that were launched in 2002. To enable people to order the guides free of charge, Health Canada has set up a toll-free telephone service at 1-888-334-9769. The guides are also available at www.phac-aspc.gc.ca/pau-uap/paguide/child_youth/partners/boiler3.html.The guides recommend that inactive children and

1. Listen, evaluate, and categorize
2. Recognize legitimate concerns
3. Provide context
4. Refute misinformation
5. Provide valid information
6. Recognize that it is the parents' decision
7. Educate about potential consequences
8. Make a clear recommendation

youth increase the amount of time they currently spend being physically active by at least 30 minutes per day, and decrease the time they spend watching TV, playing computer games, and surfing the Internet by at least 30 minutes per day. This increase in physical activity should include a combination of moderate activity (skating, riding a bike) with vigorous activity (running, playing soccer). The guidelines recommend that inactive children and youth accumulate this increase in daily physical activity in periods of at least five to ten minutes each.[71]

*What criteria would you include in developing an exercise program for schoolchildren in the community?*

## Health Promotion and Health Prevention

**Immunizations** Immunization is one of the most significant measures for protecting children from serious illness and death resulting from vaccine-preventable diseases.[72] The seventh edition of the Canadian Immunization Guide can be viewed at www.phac-aspc.gc.ca/publicat/cig-gci/index-eng.php.[73] See Table 7-6 for routine immunization schedules for infants and children.

Bigham and Hoefer, researchers from British Columbia, conducted a population-based analysis using communicable disease and vaccine-associated adverse events (VAAEs) that are routinely collected in British Columbia and other provinces and territories.[74] They considered four universal childhood immunization programs in British Columbia: measles, rubella, paralytic poliomyelitis, and invasive Haemophilias influenza type b (Hib). They found that after implementing universal programs, the average incidence of reported cases decreased by 90 to 100 percent over a five-year period.[75] These benefits were sustained or strengthened over time. The rates of reported serious VAAEs were low. The researchers conclude that, overall, this study affirms the remarkable effectiveness of four universal childhood immunization programs and a high degree of safety associated with immunization.[76]

Some parents may have concerns about immunizations. A health professional has a responsibility to listen and try to understand the parent's concerns, fears, and beliefs about vaccination. Halperin indicates that an eight-step approach to addressing the issue is effective. See the box entitled "Eight-Step Approach to Respond to Parents Unsure about Immunization."[77] Many sources of information, such as the Canadian Immunization Guide, are available for parents.[78]

The Canadian Nurses Association has written an article for all nurses called "Nurses and Immunization—What You Need to Know." The Canadian Immunization Awareness Program (CIAP), a coalition of health care organizations that includes the Canadian Nurses Association (CNA), the Canadian Nursing Coalition for Immunization, and the Canadian Public Health Association (CPHA), has identified common misconceptions about immunizations. One such misconception is that of complacency. The fact is that immunization programs have been so successful at preventing serious disease that many people have become complacent. People believe that vaccine-preventable diseases have been eliminated from Canada. However, with an increasing number of people travelling the globe, diseases can easily be brought back to Canada.[79]

Nurses play a vital role in promoting and delivering immunization programs across Canada. Consider your own immunization. Are you up to date? What is the status of your family's immunization? These are important questions for you to consider and to act upon.

## CRITICAL THINKING

*How would you respond to an older person who questions you about the benefits of a flu shot?*

**Safety Promotion and Injury Control** Injuries are the leading cause of death and a major cause of morbidity among children aged 14 years and less in Canada.[80] For children over the age of four, injuries cause more deaths than all other causes of death combined.[81]

About 50 Canadian children and adolescents die each year from bicycle-related injuries, and 75 percent of all bicycle-related deaths are due to head injuries.[82] Leblanc and his colleagues conducted a study in which trained observers, who had a direct view of oncoming bicycle traffic, recorded helmet use, sex, and age group of cyclists in Halifax. They found that the rate of helmet use rose dramatically after legislation was enacted. Furthermore, the

proportion of cyclists with head injuries in 1998–99 was half that in 1995–96.[83] Traffic-related injuries are responsible for the vast majority of injury-related deaths and long-term disabilities of Canadian children.[84] Howard states that more Canadian children die of road traffic accidents than of any other cause. The non-use and misuse of child restraints is common and leads to preventable severe injuries or death.[85] Visit Transport Canada at www.tc.gc.ca for important notices about *child restraints* and *booster cushions*. Lapner and his colleagues found that proper seatbelt restraints reduce the morbidity involved in motor vehicles. Discussing safe travel with parents may be the health professional's most important child health promotion activity. In addition to counselling, health professionals could choose to be involved in advocacy, public education campaigns, legislation, research, and the treatment of injuries.[86]

In addition, injuries occurring in the home and those from sports and leisure activities are responsible for the bulk of younger and older children being taken to emergency departments and admitted to hospitals. Modifications to play equipment and to rules of play, such as regarding body checking in hockey, can make sports and leisure activities safer.[87]

Drkulec and Letts studied injury patterns of snowboarding trauma in children. They found that 79 percent of the injuries were to the upper extremity, whereas 7 percent were to the lower extremity. They concluded that the predominance of snowboarding injuries of the upper extremity seen in children differs significantly from those in adults in whom lower injuries are more common.[88] It is important that health professionals be aware of the types of injuries that occur and know the importance of instruction on the use of proper equipment, risk avoidance, and falling techniques for novice snowboarders.[89] Refer to *Planning Ski and Snowboarding Education Programs: A Reference Guide for Schools,* prepared by the Manitoba Association of School Trustees (www.mast.mb.ca/).[90] Wesner evaluated the impact that the Think First Saskatchewan school visit program had on students' knowledge of brain and spinal cord injury prevention. She found that the program statistically improved self-reported knowledge of the students receiving the *Think First* message.[91]

During the first 17 years of life, a major health concern for First Nations and Inuit people is injury. According to the First Nations and Inuit Regional Health Survey (FNIRHS), 13 percent of First Nations and Inuit individuals will have broken a bone by the time they are 17; 4 percent will have incurred a serious head injury; 3 percent will have been seriously burned; 2 percent will have experienced frostbite; and 3 percent will have almost drowned.[92] Bristow and her team of researchers analyzed the drowning data of the Manitoba Paediatric Death Review Committee to identify drowning risk factors and potential prevention strategies. Their results indicated that the highest mortality rates regarding drowning were found in First Nations children, followed by all boys, and then toddlers who are one to four years old.[93] In summary, the death rate for Aboriginal children as a result of injuries is much higher than that of the total population of Canadian children.[94]

Health care professionals are recognizing the importance of injury prevention efforts in preserving the health and well-being of children. Nurses should be aware of the General Injury Prevention Guidelines.[95] *Injury prevention* should be taught and enforced in school and at home. You must promote safety by helping parents and children to identify and avoid hazards. The school-aged child has increasing cognitive maturity, including improved ability to remember past experiences and anticipate probable outcomes of his or her actions. This makes the child a good candidate for safety instructions. Nurses can be politically active in activities such as legislative efforts, public awareness campaigns, group classes on injury prevention, and counselling with families and children.

## CRITICAL THINKING

*If you were asked to develop a community program on water safety to prevent drowning, what would be your first few steps?*

If there are chronically ill or disabled students in school, special preparation should be given to the teachers, the students, and the parents. You can promote a better understanding of the child and his or her condition, of the child's need to reach individual potential, and of a total rehabilitation program.[96]

In summary, the recognition of injuries as a leading cause of death in children has resulted in extensive research and, from that research, the generation of a considerable amount of comprehensive information on the issue.[97] Health professionals must be aware, not only of the statistics related to injuries in children but of health promotion strategies to prevent such injuries. Then they need to impart that vital information to parents and significant caretakers.

# Common Health Problems: Health Promotion and Prevention Strategies

Although the child should now remain basically healthy, health problems do exist. Teach parents about expected illnesses. School-aged children get sick about half as often as preschoolers and about twice as much as their parents.[98] Inform parents of the need to treat both acute and chronic conditions.

*Respiratory conditions* (colds, sore throats, and earaches) account for more than 50 percent of the reported acute illnesses among children in this age group. *Asthma*, a persistent congestion in the lungs, is increasing in incidence, possibly related to environmental conditions—and it is a major health problem in Canada.[99] Optimal management of asthma requires adequate evaluation of the client and his or her environment. Recent studies have confirmed that various methods of asthma education can improve symptoms, one's emotional state, communication patterns among family members, school absenteeism, activity restriction, self-management skills, and the need for oral corticosteroids.[100]

*Infective and parasitic diseases* (scabies, impetigo, ringworm, and head lice) are of concern because of their health threat to the child and others. *Diseases of the digestive tract* (stomach aches, peptic ulcers, colitis, diarrhea, and vomiting) may have both a psychosocial and a physiologic cause. Visual and hearing impairment, sickle cell anemia, asthma, hyperactivity, epilepsy, migraine headaches, hypertension, juvenile diabetes mellitus, and obesity are *chronic health problems* that may affect the school-aged child. The child may have been born with a congenital anomaly that can be only partially corrected, or with a disease such as hemophilia that needs continuing treatment. A considerable number of schoolchildren have *risk factors that in adults are predictive of coronary heart disease:* hypertension, increased serum cholesterol and triglycerides, and obesity. The elementary school population may be the main reservoir of *infectious hepatitis* because schoolchildren often have a mild undiagnosed disease that is spread from person to person.[101]

Because of the short urethra, girls are prone to *urinary infection*. This condition may be diagnosed by reddened genitals, a feeling of burning on urination, and abnormal appearance and chemical analysis of the urine. Normal urinary output from age 6 to 12 ranges from 500 mL to the adult output of 1500 mL daily. Pinworms accompany urinary tract infections in approximately 50 percent of the cases.[102]

The seven-year-old has relatively fewer illnesses but may complain of *fatigue* or *muscular pain*. It is common to call these "growing pains," but this is not accurate because growing is not painful. Tension, overactivity or exertion, bruising, or injury may cause the leg pains. Pains in the knees, with no physical signs of exertion, are also common in school-aged children. Such pains usually occur late in the day or night, and disappear by the morning. Children with persistent leg pains should be referred to a physician.

*Visual impairments* that occur in the younger child may go undetected and untreated until the child attends school. Visual acuity may not develop normally. For more information, see the box entitled "Signs and Symptoms Indicating Defective Vision in Schoolchildren."[103] It is essential that visual problems be corrected.

Table 10-5 summarizes other common health problems, their definitions, symptoms and signs, and prevention or treatment measures.[104]

**Rabies,** *an acute infectious disease characterized by involvement of the central nervous system, resulting in paralysis and finally death,* is fortunately not a common disease, but it comes from a common problem—the biting of a human by a mammal. The prevention of rabies is achieved by keeping the child away from unfamiliar animals, particularly ones that act agitated. One can also see that all pets are properly vaccinated, and get pre-exposure immunization for high-risk children—those living in or visiting countries where rabies is a constant threat.

Increasingly, the ill effects of *smoking* and *drug and alcohol abuse* are emerging as a regular health problem. These habits are influenced by the habits of parents, siblings, and peers. In addition to the ill effects caused by smoking, children in families with cigarette smokers have an increased rate of respiratory conditions and cancer from secondary smoke. These small children are experiencing increasing numbers of days per year when their activities are restricted because of illness.[105]

Emphasize to adults that more effective than organized educational attempts is the influence of significant adults, those who take a personal interest in the child and who set a good example. Good examples come from parents who neither smoke, drink, or use drugs nor give cigarettes, alcohol, or drugs to their children. Equally important, or more so, is the *peer group*. Leaders of the peer group who have positive health habits should be used as models. Peer communication is also effective for initiating hygienic habits. You may have a role in working with the peer group.

## CRITICAL THINKING

*If you were asked to teach a group of schoolchildren in a community centre about the hazards of substance abuse, what topics would you address?*

According to the Public Health Agency of Canada, several determinants are interrelated and influence population health. One key determinant is healthy child development. Recent evidence on the effects of early experiences on brain development, school readiness, and health in later life has initiated a growing consensus about early childhood development as a powerful determinant in its own right. All of the other determinants of health affect the physical, social, mental, emotional, and spiritual development of children

## Signs and Symptoms Indicating Defective Vision in Schoolchildren

**Behaviour**

- Attempts to brush away blur; rubs eyes frequently; frowns, squints
- Stumbles frequently or trips over small objects
- Blinks more than usual; cries often or is irritable when doing close work
- Holds books or small playthings close to eyes
- Shuts or covers one eye, tilting or thrusting head forward when looking at objects
- Has difficulty in reading or in other schoolwork requiring close use of the eyes; omits words or confuses similar words
- Exhibits poor performance in activities requiring visual concentration within arm's length (e.g., reading, colouring, drawing); unusually short attention span; persistent word reversals after second grade
- Disinterested in distant objects or fails to participate in games such as playing ball
- Engages in outdoor activity mostly (e.g., running, bicycling), avoiding activities requiring visual concentration within arm's length
- Sensitive to light

- Unable to distinguish colours
- Steps carefully over sidewalk cracks or around light or dark sections of block linoleum floors
- Trips at curbs or stairs
- Poor eye–hand coordination for age, excessively hard-to-read handwriting, difficulty with tying shoelaces or buttoning and unbuttoning

**Appearance**

- Crossed eyes (iris of one eye turned in or out and not symmetric with other eye)
- Red-rimmed, encrusted, or swollen eyelids
- Repeated sties
- Watery or red eyes

**Complaints**

- Cannot see blackboard from back of room
- Blurred or double vision after close eye work
- Dizziness, headaches, or nausea after close eye work
- Itching or burning eyes

Sources: Hoole, A., C. Pickard, R. Ouimette, J. Lohr, and W. Powell, *Patient Care Guidelines for Nurse Practitioners,* 5th ed. Philadelphia: J.B. Lippincott, 1999; Ball, J.W., and R.C. Bindler, *Pediatric Nursing Caring for Children,* 4th ed. Upper Saddle River, NJ: Pearson Education, 2008.

Table 10-5 Common Health Problems of Schoolchildren

| Problem | Definition | Symptoms/Signs | Prevention/Treatment |
|---|---|---|---|
| Accommodative esophoria | Eyes converge excessively in response to accommodation | Close work becomes exhausting and overwhelming | Eyeglasses and taking "eye breaks" recommended. |
| Otitis externa | Inflammation of the external auditory canal and auricle | Pain in ear aggravated by moving the auricle; exudate in ear canal | Prevention: Keep instruments out of ears. Keep dirty water out of ear. Use acetic acid (2%) solution in ear after swimming. After the fact, use antibiotic or steroid drops. |
| Serous otitis media | Accumulation of nonpurulent fluid in middle ear | Fullness and crackling in ear; decreased hearing | Administer decongestants (questionable help). |
| Allergic rhinitis | Allergic reaction affecting nasal mucosa (and sometimes conjunctiva) | Clear, thin nasal discharge; breathes through mouth; often does "allergic salute" (rubs nose upward) | Find offending irritant or antigen and try to eliminate. Administer antihistamines. Obtain workup by allergist if problem persists. |
| Asthma | Disease of lungs characterized by partially reversible airway obstruction, airway inflammation, and airway hyperresponsiveness; caused by hyperreactivity of the tracheobronchial tree to chemical mediators | Wheezing, cough, dyspnea, anxiety, restlessness | Try to stay away from allergens, if known. Avoid being around those with upper respiratory infections; avoid overexertion, rapid temperature or humidity changes, air pollutants, emotional upsets. Follow NAEP (National Asthma Education Program) step-care approach described by Boynton et al.[106] for appropriate timing of essential medications. |
| Herpes type I | Vesicular eruption of skin and mucous membranes above the umbilicus (usually mouth) | Soreness of mouth from eruption of mucosa; inflammation and swelling; sometimes fever and enlarged lymph glands (sub-mandibular) | Apply Zovirax ointment to slow down severity. Drink adequate fluids. Use saline solution mouthwash. Administer antipyretic. Isolate from susceptible persons. |
| Contact dermatitis | Vesicular formation on skin, usually from poison ivy or poison oak | Itching and formation of vesicles, sometimes on most body parts | Apply cold compresses and drying lotion. Sometimes administer cortisone-based oral medicine or injections. Teach how to avoid plants. |
| Tinea corporis (ringworm of non-hairy skin) | Superficial fungal infection involving face, trunk, or limbs | Red patch areas that scale and are oval in shape; usually asymptomatic or mildly itchy; no systemic signs | Apply a topical antifungal daily for 2 or 3 weeks. |
| Tinea capitis (ringworm of the head) | Fungal infection involving scalp | Same as Tinea corporis | Apply fungal cream persistently. Sometimes it is necessary to shave hair. |

(continued)

Table 10-5 (continued)

| Problem | Definition | Symptoms/Signs | Prevention/Treatment |
|---------|------------|----------------|----------------------|
| **Warts** | Intradermal papillomas | Usually appear as common (on hands or fingers) or plantar (on feet) | Dichloroacetic acid will often dissolve them. Other removal methods are available from dermatologist. |
| **Pediculus humanus capitis** (head lice) | Infestation of head, hair, scalp | Itching scalp; see nits or ova as little dots attached to base of hairs | Shampoo with approved medication. Apply antihistamine for itching. Comb out any remaining ova-nits. Boil all head care items. |
| **Mumps** | Viral disease characterized by acute swelling of salivary gland, especially the parotid | Anterior ear pain; headache; lethargy; anorexia; vomiting; complication orchitis (*inflammation of one or both testes*) | Prevention: obtain vaccine. Use only supportive treatment such as antipyretics (not Aspirin products) and encourage fluid intake. |
| **Diabetes mellitus type I** (formally called juvenile diabetes) | Inherited disease with metabolic component that causes elevated blood sugar and vascular component that causes effects on eyes and kidneys | Increased urination; increased thirst and hunger; weight loss and fatigue | Obtain workup by appropriate health care practitioner. Follow diabetic diet and exercise recommendations. Administer insulin. |
| **Fifth disease** (erythema infectiosum) | Mild viral illness caused by human parvovirus B19; no ongoing harm to child but maternal infection can cause spontaneous abortions and stillbirths | Three-stage exanthemas: (1) slapped cheek appearance; (2) maculopapulary rash on trunk and extremities; looks lacy; (3) rash has evanescence and recrudescence | If it is a school-related breakout, expect a 25% infection rate. Stay away from pregnant women. There is no specific treatment, only symptomatic, i.e., acetaminophen for aches. Stay away from sun, which can exacerbate rash. |
| **Hand-foot-and-mouth disease** | Contagious viral disease caused by Coxsackie virus A | Abrupt fever; vesicular lesions of the mouth, palms of the hands, and soles of feet; anorexia | As it is highly contagious, keep isolated until temperature is normal for 24 hours. Treat symptomatically; saline mouth rinse; acetaminophen for temperature elevation; fluids; tepid baths. |
| **Pityriasis rosea** | An acute, self-limited, presumably viral disease, which produces a characteristic rash | Classic lesion on trunk, looks like a Christmas tree; starts with "mother spot" that is scaly, salmon-coloured, and spreads peripherally | There is no need to isolate. Expect rash to last as long as 4 months. Use symptomatic treatment such as cool compress, calamine lotion, Benadryl (if pruritis). Exposure to sunlight will relieve itching and shorten duration of rash. |

and youth. For example, a school-aged child's development is greatly affected by family income, where he or she resides (housing and neighbourhood), the level of the parent's education, access to nutritious foods, physical recreation, genetic makeup, and access to dental and medical care.[107]

*You can promote healthy behaviour in children, and design and implement health promotion interventions.* In fact, many areas such as traditional sites (schools, clinics) and non-traditional sites (shelters, social service programs, shopping malls, recreational settings) in rural and urban areas are places to implement health promotion programs.

## PSYCHOSOCIAL CONCEPTS

To guide assessment and promote health, share with parents and teachers the following information about the schoolchild's cognitive, emotional, and moral-spiritual development.

## Cognitive Development

The schoolchild has a strong curiosity to learn, especially when motivation is strengthened by interested parents and opportunities for varied experiences in the home and school.

Learning, behaviour, and personality are complex issues that are not easily explained by one theory. This section uses information from a number of theorists. Refer to Chapter 5 for a review of how the major schools of theorists explain the development of learning, behaviour, and personality. See Table 10-6 for a summary of cognitive abilities of the child from ages 6 to 12.

At approximately age seven, the child enters the stage of concrete operations. **Concrete operations** *involve systematic reasoning about tangible or familiar situations, and the ability to use logical thought to analyze relationships and structure the environment into meaningful categories.* The child must have interactions with concrete materials to be able to build

---

**Table 10-6 Cognitive Characteristics of the School-Aged Child**

| Age | Cognitive Ability |
|---|---|
| 6 | Thinking is concrete and animistic |
| | Beginning to understand semi-abstract concepts and symbols |
| | Defines objects in relation to their use and effect on self |
| | May not be able to consider parts and wholes in words at the same time |
| | Likes to hear about his own past |
| | Knows numbers |
| | Can read |
| | Learning occurs frequently through imitation and incidental suggestion and also depends on opportunities |
| | May not be able to sound out words; may confuse words when reading, such as *was* and *saw* |
| | High correlation between ability to converse and beginning reading achievement; may have vocabulary of 8000 to 14 000 words when reading, if assisted with language |
| 7 | Learns best from interaction with actual materials or visible props |
| | Learning broad concepts and subconcepts (e.g., car identified as Ford or Chevrolet), based on memory, instruction, or experience |
| | A number of mental strategies or operations are learned |
| | Becoming less egocentric, less animistic |
| | Better able to do cause–effect and logical thinking |
| | More reflective; has deeper understanding of meanings and feelings |
| | Interested in conclusions and logical endings |
| | Attention span lengthened; may work several hours on activity of interest |
| | More aware of environment and people in it; also interested in magic and fantasy |
| | Understands length, area, or mass |
| | Sense of time practical, detailed; present focus; plans the day |
| | Knows months, seasons, years |
| | Serious in inventing, enjoys chemistry sets |
| 8 | Less animistic |
| | More aware of people and impersonal forces of nature |
| | Improvises simple activities |

*(continued)*

Table 10-6 (continued)

| Age | Cognitive Ability |
|-----|-------------------|
| | Likes to learn about history, own and other cultures, geography, science, and social science |
| | Intellectually expansive; inquiries about past and future |
| | Tolerant and accepting of others |
| | Understands logical reasoning and implications |
| | Learns from own experience |
| | Extremely punctual |
| | Improvises simple rules |
| | Can read a compass |
| 9 | Realistic in self-appraisal and tasks |
| | Reasonable, self-motivated, curious |
| | Needs minimal direction |
| | Competes with self |
| | Likes to be involved with activities and complex tasks |
| | May concentrate on project for two or three hours |
| | Plans in advance; wants successive steps explained and wants to perfect skills |
| | Focuses on details and believes in rules and laws (they can be flexible) as much as in luck or chance |
| | Enjoys history |
| | Tells time without difficulty |
| | Likes to know length of time for task |
| | Likes to classify, identify, list, make collections |
| | Understands weight |
| 10 | Is matter-of-fact |
| | Likes to participate in discussions about social problems and cause and effect |
| | Likes a challenge |
| | Likes to memorize and identify facts |
| | Locates sites on a map |
| | Makes lists |
| | Easily distracted; many interests and concentrates on each for a short time |
| | Greater interest in present than past |
| 11 | Curious but not reflective |
| | Concrete, specific thinking |
| | Likes action or experimentation in learning |
| | Likes to move around in the classroom |
| | Concentrates well when competing with one group against another |
| | Prefers routine |
| | Better at rote memorization than generalization |
| | Defines time as distance from one event to another |
| | Understands relationships of weight and size |
| 12 | Likes to consider all sides of a situation |
| | Enters self-chosen task with initiative |
| | Likes group work but more inner-motivated than competitive |
| | Able to classify, arrange, and generalize |
| | Likes to discuss and debate |
| | Beginning formal operations stage, or abstract thinking |
| | Verbal formal reasoning possible |
| | Understands moral of a story |
| | Defines time as duration, a measurement |
| | Plans ahead, so feels life is under own control |
| | Interested in present and future |
| | Understands abstractness of space |
| | Understands conservation of volume |

understanding that is basic for the next stage.[108] The mental operations of school-aged children work poorly with abstract ideas—ones not apparent in the real world.[109]

The following operations are characteristic of this stage:[110]

- **Classification**. *Sorting objects into groups according to specific and multiple attributes* such as length, size, shape, colour, class of animals, and trademark. Schoolchildren can identify which kind of car is approaching on the highway. Usually, a single characteristic is focused on first, then additional characteristics are considered.

- **Seriation**. *Ordering objects according to decreasing or increasing measure* such as height, weight, and strength. The child knows that A is longer than B, B is longer than C, and A is longer than C.

- **Nesting**. *Understanding how a subconcept fits into a larger concept*. For example, a German shepherd is one kind of dog, and a reclining chair and a dining room chair are both chairs.

- **Multiplication**. *Simultaneously classifying and seriating*, using two numbers together to come out with a greater amount.

- **Reversibility**. *Returning to the starting point, or performing opposite operations or actions with the same problem or situation*. The child can add and subtract, and multiply and divide the same problems. A longer row of clips can be squeezed together to form a shorter row and vice versa. The child realizes that the number of clips has not changed.

- **Transformation**. *Ability to see the shift from a dynamic to static or constant state, to understand the process of change, and to focus on the continuity and sequence, on the original and final states*. For example, the child realizes or anticipates how a shorter row of pennies was shifted to become a longer row. He or she understands the gradual shift in level of fluid in a container as it is poured into another container and the increasing level of fluid in the second container.

- **Conservation**. *Understanding transformation, and that a situation has not changed, where the sameness of a situation or object remains despite a change in some aspect, and that mass or quantity is the same even if it changes shape or position*. There is an order to conservation: number, followed by length, liquid, and mass, followed by weight.

- **Decentring**. *Coordination of two or more dimensions, or the ability to focus on several characteristics simultaneously*. For example, space and length dimensions can be considered, but the younger child would consider only one or the other. When 12 paper clips are changed

from a spread of 6 cm to one of 12 cm, the child realizes that the spreads are different and there are not more clips.

- **Combination**. *Ability to combine several tasks or operations at once, to see the regularities of the physical world and the principles that govern relationships among objects*. Perceptions alone are less convincing than a logical understanding of how the world operates. For example, a sunset on the ocean looks like the sun is sinking into the water. Science teaches that what we see is a result of the earth's rotation on its axis.[111]

---

## CRITICAL THINKING

*What specific school and home experiences are likely to influence children's performance on Piaget's concrete-operational tasks?*

---

These operations increase in complexity as the child matures from an empirical to a logical orientation. The child can look at a situation, analyze it, and come up with an answer without purposefully going through each step. For example, if two rows of coins have been spread out, the child does not have to count the coins. He or she realizes that nothing was added to or subtracted from the rows, so each row still has the same number.

The child learns and can recall associations between sequences and groupings of events. At first, he or she makes associations within a certain context or environment. Later, memory is used to transfer these associations to different contexts or environments. The child also rehearses. In the time between a learning experience and a memory test or application of learning, he or she mentally reviews what has been learned.[112]

Piaget's theory has not gone unchallenged, however. Many questions are raised about several of his concepts. One such concept is stages: Piaget conceived of stages as unitary structures of cognition. His theory assumes *developmental synchrony*. That is, various aspects of a stage should emerge at the same time. However, some concrete operational concepts do not appear in synchrony.[113] In today's Information Age, some children who are at one cognitive stage can be trained to reason at a higher level. In fact, culture and education can exert strong influences on children's development—more so than what Piaget thought possible. Further, some cognitive abilities actually emerge earlier than Piaget thought. For example, *conservation of number* has been demonstrated as early as age three, although Piaget claimed that it did not emerge until age seven.[114] Because adolescents have attained the formal operational stage, it does not mean that they will always reason at this level. Adolescents often fail to reason logically, even when they are capable of doing so.[115]

Due to such limitations of Piaget's theory, a need exists to re-examine other approaches to cognitive development. Greater emphasis should be placed on how children process information through attention, memory, and strategy use.[116] See the box entitled "Characteristics of Information Processing."

As children progress through the school years, they advance in their information processing skills. The ability to make efficient use of short-term memory capacity increases steadily with age—a change that most developmentalists see as the basis for cognitive development. The best evidence that cognitive processing becomes more efficient is that it gets steadily faster with age. One of the most important ways in which processing efficiency becomes faster is through the acquisition of automaticity, which is the ability to recall information from long-term memory without using short-term capacity. For example, children can respond to the question "How much is 5 times 5?" by giving the answer 25 without thinking. Automaticity is achieved primarily through practice.[117] Another change in information processing is that of metacognition, which is knowing about knowing.[118] Metacognition encompasses knowledge about one's own memory, such as the student's ability to know that attending to a story requires effort. Another example of metacognition is a student's ability to monitor whether he or she has studied sufficiently for a test that is approaching.[119] Much research exists to indicate that the amount of knowledge an individual possesses makes a great deal of difference in how efficiently his or her information processing system works. Children who know much about a topic (dinosaurs, hockey cards, or songs) have the ability to categorize information about the topic in highly complex and hierarchical ways.

Pressley states that the key to education is assisting students to learn a rich repertoire of strategies that result in solutions to problems. Good thinkers routinely use strategies and effective planning processes to solve problems in a critical way. Good thinkers know when and how to use strategies.[120]

You can discuss with parents the child's changing cognitive abilities and ways in which they can contribute to cognitive achievement. If parents do not understand that a certain cognitive behaviour is age-appropriate, their interactions with, and guidance of, the child may be less effective.

Cognitive development, and an increasing understanding of implications, consequences, and cause–effect relations, may be factors in the changing *fearfulness* of the child. As a nurse, remember that the school-aged child has great fear of body injury, disease, separation from loved ones, death, excess punishment (some diagnostic and treatment procedures seem like punishment), and doing wrong actions. In your practice, you can help offset the child's fears. Advise parents to take their child's fears

seriously, and not force their child to "be brave." A child who is scared is really scared. In fact, telling children that it is okay to be scared is actually quite comforting to them.[121]

## CRITICAL THINKING

*John is a school-aged child being admitted to hospital for the surgical removal of a brain tumour. His parents tell you that he fears the surgery. How can you help to alleviate a few of John's fears?*

**Concept of Time** The concept of time evolves during the early school period. See Table 10-7 for a summary of how the schoolchild develops a concept of time.[122]

You can help parents to understand that their school-aged children do not have adult concepts of time. The mother who is distraught because her six- or seven-year-old constantly dawdles in getting ready for school can be helped

| Table 10-7 | School-Aged Child's Concepts of Time |
|---|---|
| **Age** | **Conceptualization of Time** |
| 6 | Time counted by hours; minutes disregarded<br>Enjoys past as much as present; likes to hear about his or her babyhood<br>Future important in relation to holidays<br>Duration of episode has little meaning |
| 7 | Interested in present; enjoys a watch<br>Sense of time practical, sequential, detailed<br>Knows sequence of months, seasons, years<br>Plans days; understands passage of time |
| 8 | Extremely aware of punctuality, especially in relation to others<br>More responsible about time |
| 9 | Tells time without difficulty<br>Plans days with excess activities; driven by time<br>Wants to know how long a task will take to complete<br>Interested in ancient times |
| 10 | Less driven by time than the nine-year-old<br>Interested primarily in present<br>Able to get to places in time on own initiative |
| 11 | Feels time is relentlessly passing by or dragging<br>More adept at handling time<br>Defines time as distance from one event to another |
| 12 | Defines time as duration, a measurement<br>Plans ahead to feel in control<br>Interested in future as well as present |

if she understands more fully the child's concept of time. The mother must still provide firm direction, but not expect the impossible. She can look forward to improvement in the eight-year-old.

Understanding maturing time concepts will also aid you as you explain the sequence of a procedure to the schoolchild in the doctor's office, school, clinic, or hospital.

Spatial Concepts Spatial concepts also change as a result of increasing experience. The six-year-old is interested in specific places and in relationships with his or her home, neighbourhood, and expanding community. He or she knows some streets and major points of interest. By age seven, the sense of space is becoming more realistic. The child wants some space of his or her own, such as a room or portion of it. The heavens and various objects in space and on the earth are of keen interest.[123]

For the eight-year-old, personal space is expanding as the child ventures to more places. He or she knows the neighbourhood well and likes maps, geography, and trips. He or she understands the compass points and can distinguish right and left on others as well as self.

Space for the nine-year-old includes the whole earth. He or she enjoys pen pals from different lands, geography, and history. For the ten-year-old, space is rather specific, the place where things such as buildings are. The 11-year-old perceives space as nothingness that goes on forever, a distance between things. He or she is in good control of getting around in personal space.[124]

The 12-year-old understands that space is abstract and has difficulty defining it. Space is nothing, air. He or she can travel alone to more distant areas and understands how specific points relate to each other.[125]

Encourage the parents to discuss spatial concepts with the child to facilitate abstract reasoning. The box entitled "Categories of Concepts Developed during the School Years" summarizes other concepts formulated at this time.

*Multiple intelligences*, rather than one intelligence, exist. The **Triarchic Theory of Intelligence** proposed by Robert Sternberg *incorporates three realms of cognition*. This comprehensive theory views intelligence as a product of inner and outer forces.[126] The *first realm* includes how thinking occurs as well as the main components of thinking. Based on the information processing model, thinking includes skills at coding, representing, combining information, planning, and self-evaluation in problem solving. The *second realm* includes how individuals cope with experiences, how they respond to novelty in solving new problems, and how quickly they adjust to a new form of the task. *The third realm* of intelligence relates to the context of thinking—the extent to which children adapt to, alter, or select environments supportive of their abilities.[127] The **Theory of Multiple Intelligences** proposed by Howard Gardner *presents factors that reflect the influence of culture and society on intellectual ability.* It provides yet another view of how information processing skills underlie intelligent behaviour.[128] Multiple intelligences take the following forms:[129]

1. *Language skill.* The child speaks fluently, learns new words easily, and memorizes easily.

2. *Musical skill.* The child plays one or more musical instruments, sings, discerns subtle musical effects, and has a sense of timing or rhythm.

3. *Local skill.* The child organizes objects and concepts, and performs well at mathematics.

4. *Spatial skill.* The child can easily find his or her way around without getting lost, more so than other children of the same age.

5. *Kinesthetic or body balance skill.* The child is sensitive to the internal sensations created by body movements, and easily learns dancing and gymnastics.

6. *Intrapersonal and interpersonal skills.* The child has an understanding of self and others that is accurate and promotes empathy. The child relates easily to others and can handle social encounters.

Gardner's list of abilities has yet to be firmly grounded in research. However, his ideas have been challenging enough to reawaken the debate over a unitary versus multi-faceted human intelligence.[130]

## CRITICAL THINKING

*Compare and contrast "core knowledge," as explained in Sternberg's Triarchic Theory of Intelligence and in Gardner's Theory of Multiple Intelligence.*

**Irony** Because ironic remarks occur rather frequently in everyday interaction, the research into the child's understanding of verbal irony is both interesting and relevant. Irony is a manner of speaking in which the meaning literally expressed is opposite to the meaning intended and that aims either at ridicule, humour, or sarcasm.[131] However, the inferences involved in understanding a speaker's irony can be complex.[132]

In one research study to investigate how children develop the ability to understand verbal irony, 70 six- to

ten-year-old children experienced short puppet shows within a context of *ironic criticism* and *ironic compliments*.[133] Ironic criticisms are positive statements meant to convey a critical or negative attitude (e.g., saying "that was a great play" to someone who tried to kick a soccer ball and missed). Ironic compliments, on the other hand, are negative statements meant to convey a praising or positive attitude (e.g., saying "that was a terrible play" to someone who kicked a soccer ball and scored a goal). Several aspects of comprehension were assessed: appreciation of the speaker's belief, the speaker's intent to tease, and the speaker's attitude. The findings suggest the following developmental progression: for ironic criticisms, speaker's belief understanding emerges first, before understanding of speaker's intent to tease and speaker's attitude. These latter two components merge together. For ironic compliments, speaker's belief understanding emerges with understanding of the speaker's intent to tease, and an understanding of speaker attitude emerges later.[134] Another study conducted by Pexman and her researchers investigated whether providing information about a speaker's personality traits would influence children's interpretations and processing of verbal irony. Findings indicated that children's interpretations of ironic remarks were modulated by speaker personality traits, and processing data revealed that older children were more efficient than younger children at coordinating cues to verbal irony.[135]

The findings of this research are interesting for nurses who interact with children on a unit. Nurses must be aware that irony comprehension improves with age, but not rapidly. In addition, children tend to find ironic criticisms easier to understand than ironic compliments. This places ironic compliments at an interpretive disadvantage. At the same time, speakers use ironic criticisms more frequently than ironic compliments. It seems to follow that the nurse should not use ironic compliments because, generally speaking, children lack sufficient social experience with such remarks to understand them adequately. An example is provided from the researcher's study of both ironic criticisms and ironic compliments.[136]

Becoming able to understand verbal irony is an important aspect of social-cognitive development, which occurs over a long period between middle and late childhood. A child's ability to grasp the meaning of verbal irony will depend on his or her neural maturation, mental skills, and social learning.[137]

**Entering School** School entry is a crisis for the child and family because behaviour must be adapted to meet new situations. The school experience has considerable influence on the child because he or she is in formative years and spends much time in school. School is society's institution to help the child to do a number of things:

1. Develop the fullest intellectual potential and a sense of industry.
2. Learn to think critically and make judgments based on reason.
3. Accept criticism.
4. Develop social skills.
5. Co-operate with others.
6. Accept adult authority.
7. Be a leader and a follower.

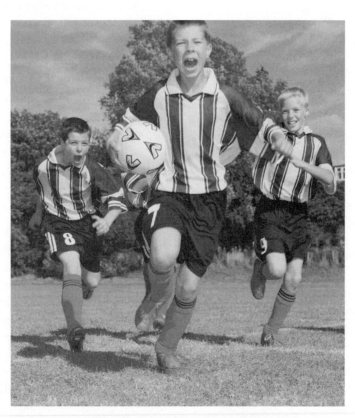

Exposure to a variety of peers and learning to work and play co-operatively are important for the school-aged child.

The child who attends a school with children from various ethnic or racial backgrounds, or with children who have immigrated, will learn not only about other cultures, but possibly several languages firsthand. The course of instruction should be such that every child has a sense of successful accomplishment in some area. Not only school promotes these cognitive and social skills, however. The home and other groups (e.g., peer or organized clubs) are important in their own way for intellectual and social development, and for promoting a sense of achievement and industry.

Various actions, such as teaching the child his or her address and full name, independence in self-care, and basic safety rules, help prepare the child for school. The parent or classroom teacher (and the nurse in the health care setting) can *stimulate the child's learning in the following ways:*

- Let each child's success be measured in terms of improved performance.

- Structure for individuation, not for convergence. Avoid having all learning activities structured so that there is only one right answer.

- Provide activities that are challenging, not overwhelming.

- Arrange for the child to accomplish individual activities in the company of peers, when appropriate, because peer interaction provides encouragement and assistance.

- Demonstrate problem solving and thinking behaviour to serve as a model for the child.

- Use a multisensory teaching approach.

- Include content and experiences that promote further understanding of various cultures.[138]

Research shows that certain skills are more easily learned at a certain age. Foreign languages and geometry can be more easily learned by younger children. In fact, a second language can be learned from age one. Introducing music in preschool, and continuing during the school years, helps to train the brain for higher forms of thinking and reasoning, including spatial intelligence. Children are capable of far more at a younger age than schools generally realize.

The *teacher–pupil relationship* is important, because it is somewhat similar to that of the parent–child relationship. The child needs from the teacher a wholesome friendliness, consideration, fairness, a sense of humour, and a philosophy that encourages his or her maturity. The teacher should have a thorough understanding of child development.

**Diversity** Most schools today have a culturally diverse student body. Canadian children and youth are ethnically, culturally, and linguistically diverse. In the last census, more than 200 ethnic origins were reported. Some children in Canada speak a variety of languages. Among the almost 1 million children whose mother tongue was neither English nor French, Chinese was the most commonly spoken language.[139] More than 5 percent of children in middle childhood are Aboriginal. The proportion of Aboriginal children and youth has been growing—and in 2001 they represented about one-third of all Aboriginal people.[140] Increasingly, Aboriginal children live in urban areas. According to the 2006 Census, the number of children aged less than 15 years could be outnumbered within ten years by the number of seniors aged 65 or over. The proportion of seniors in the Canadian population could nearly double in the next 25 years, but the proportion of children is expected to continue falling.[141] Students benefit when educators understand their unique culture. However, *there are many intracultural, socioeconomic, geographic, generational, religious, and individual differences among families and children.* Regardless, the structure of the family often shapes the rules, roles, and resources that exist within it.[142]

Teachers may *foster a personal understanding of one's cultural differences* through the following measures:

- Observing the behaviour, as well as listening to the words of the child.

- Emphasizing that each person is unique and worthy of respectful behaviour, regardless of perceived differences.

- Reading stories, books, and articles about the history, life patterns, and achievements of people from various cultures and religions.

- Having bulletin board displays that commemorate the special days and historical leaders for each cultural group represented in the classroom.

- Encouraging parents from various cultural groups to come to the classroom, bring artefacts that are important or representative, and discuss commonly held beliefs or practices for the specific cultural group.

- Encouraging children to find similarities, as well as differences, among the cultural and religious groups represented in the classroom.

Strengths, as well as problems, of the family and child are brought into sharp focus when the child enters school. The teacher can see many qualities in the child and family, as well as difficulties where they exist. Some of the strengths to be observed include the willingness of the child to learn, the attitudes of the child's family, and the closeness of the family. Another is the importance and value of the extended family in the child's life. On the other hand, a few of the difficulties may be the loneliness of an only child, the pain of the child dealing with divorce or death in the family, the negative self-image of the child who is not as physically coordinated or as intellectually sharp as his or her peers, the child with dyslexia or learning difficulties, the child with separation anxiety or **school phobia** (*fear of or refusal to attend school*). School phobia can be an indicator of a larger medical problem, or it can be nothing more than a normal child with a temporary conflict.[143]

Help parents to realize that the child's ability to learn and achieve in school is affected by factors other than intellectual ability. For example, at home, parents should maintain an atmosphere with ample praise and encouragement. Times for parent and children to play together should be frequent, and the provision of opportunities for stimulation and learning through hobbies, games, and outings to parks and libraries should be equally important and a part of family life. Parents should stress the importance of learning. They should monitor school assignments and stay in touch with the child's teachers.[144] Typically, Canadian parents are deeply involved in the education of their children. When parents attend parent–teacher conferences and become involved in helping at school events, children are more strongly motivated, their self-esteem is better, and they adapt and adjust more satisfactorily to the learning activities in school.[145]

In Canada, according to the National Longitudinal Survey of Children and Youth (NLSCY), although most children do well at school, girls are more likely than boys to do "very well." More research is needed to identify the specific reasons behind such gender differences among school-aged children.[146] Researchers and others are concerned about the education of Aboriginal children. Hamilton found that supporting culturally based curricula and sharing with non-Aboriginal students is important if negative stereotypes are to be erased and replaced with respectful knowledge and understanding.[147]

## CRITICAL THINKING

*As a health professional, what can you do to support the education needs of students with Aboriginal heritage?*

Too much pushing by parents for the child to be a success, perfect in physical skills, the most intellectual, or a hard worker can backfire. The pressure that is generated may be so intense that eventually the child stops trying at anything. Perfectionistic, highly successful, career-focused, or professionally focused parents are apt to push the child too much. Certain signs and symptoms provide clues. The *perfectionist child* manifests:[148]

- Extreme concern about his or her appearance.
- Avoidance of tasks, play, or school because of fear of failure
- Dawdling or procrastinating on easy tasks to avoid harder ones, or working so slowly on projects that creativity is lost

- Jealousy and envy of the apparent success and perfection of others
- Wanting to do something for which the child has little or no ability or talent
- Low tolerance for mistakes (e.g., the child who wins the race may feel unsuccessful because he or she did not set any records)

If these behaviours are present, teach the parents to work on relaxing both themselves and the child, and help them to develop a sense of tolerance and humour. You may be their counsellor, or you may refer them to counselling.

Education in Canada is the responsibility of the provinces and territories. In Canadian schools, the intellectual assessment of children, together with achievement test results, are no longer routinely used to assess students. Critics of achievement tests state that although these tests are viewed as indicators of what children learn in school, they are very similar to IQ tests.[149]

A relatively new concept in the field of interpersonal communication studies provides considerable insight into understanding one's own emotions and the emotional behaviour of others. Goleman's theory of emotional intelligence has added a considerable measure to researchers' understanding of intelligence and achievement.[150] Snow states that emotional intelligence is the ability to manage oneself and one's relationships effectively.[151] Emotional intelligence has three components: (1) awareness of one's own emotions; (2) the ability to share one's emotions in an appropriate manner; and (3) the capacity to channel emotions in the pursuit of one's worthwhile goals.[152] In essence, Snow indicates that with the effective application of one's emotional intelligence it is considerably more possible to achieve one's potential.[153]

## CRITICAL THINKING

*How can parents assist in the development of emotional intelligence in their school-aged children?*

A *classroom with diversity* in the children's intellectual ability, skills, and personality is a most helpful experience for the child because it is here that he or she learns about the real world. A small percentage of disabled or maladjusted children in a classroom will not adversely affect the educational process of the normal child. Placing the exceptional child in a normal classroom, however, may not make him or her feel normal because he or she still is perceived, and perceives self, as different. The exceptional child may need special classes to obtain the help needed. Teachers are not expected to be specialists in all areas of education, and large classrooms hamper teachers from spending all of the necessary time with the child who has learning disabilities.

The **gifted child** is *characterized by achieving a superior education, consuming vast amounts of information, and possessing an outstanding ability to produce information, concepts, and new forms, and to perform consistently at a higher level than most children of the same age.* The gifted child demonstrates to a greater extent than other children the many types of intelligence: logical-mathematical; linguistic; musical; spatial; body-kinesthetic; interpersonal; and intrapersonal. The child is adept at problem solving and problem finding. The gifted child is considered educationally exceptional. This child's full intellectual, creative, and leadership potential may be curtailed if:

1. Parents are not attuned to the child's abilities and needs
2. Parents or teachers are threatened by the gifted child, who grasps concepts more quickly than they do
3. Parents do not value cognitive, creative, or leadership abilities
4. The child is not given freedom to explore and be different
5. The school system does not have a program suited for the child's abilities

Often, the gifted child is misunderstood. Research indicates that gifted students have higher self-esteem than others, and that they are more popular with their peers than other children.[154]

Yet, the gifted child may not excel or be ahead of the norm in all dimensions. The child may be intellectually ahead of chronological age, but may be behind in physical growth and coordination, emotional development, or social skills. The inconsistency inherent in a lack of developmental synchrony may be difficult for parents, teachers, and peers to accept. You can be instrumental, first, in fostering empathy for the child and, second, in individualizing a program to enhance the child's development and competency.[155]

Encourage parents to respect the individual interests and talents of their child. If parents are not intimidated by the child's unusual interests and behaviour, they will not fear deviations from neighbourhood patterns. Consequently, they will be less likely to crush budding interests or creativity. That is perhaps the essence of raising a gifted child—to facilitate, provide opportunity, let alone, and not hold back or insist that something be done a certain way. *Home schooling* is conducted by some parents who believe that the public school system is insufficiently adequate to teach their children all of their needed skills. They are usually well-educated professionals who wish to teach their own children at home.

Provincial and territorial jurisdictions establish curricular plans for each grade level and academic year with subject content, suggestions for teaching, and evaluation methods. The parents have a choice, depending on cost factors and perceived needs and interests of the child. Often, all of the parents and children in a locale who are enrolled in home schooling gather periodically for social events to foster social skills in, and friendship among, the children. Parents, or groups of parents, may also plan field trips to enhance the child's education—for example, to museums, parks, and historical sites.

When you work with these parents, help them realize the importance of curricular integrity. When the child graduates from a home school program, he or she is expected to have achieved a certain standard. Emphasize the child's need for friendship and interaction with people from diverse backgrounds. Explore whether the child will have access to regular physical educational activity, to playing a musical instrument or choral singing, and to art classes. Explore whether the parents will be able to engage the child consistently in learning activities and monitor the necessary testing or evaluation. Several authors explore various facets of the home schooling movement.[156]

## CRITICAL THINKING
*What are the advantages and disadvantages of home schooling?*

The *chronically ill child* poses unique problems for the school and parents. Ray explains that acquiring the knowledge, skills, and organization necessary to raise a child with a chronic health condition presents many challenges. Beyond that, a heavy demand is placed on family resources as well. She presents a model—Parenting and Childhood Chronicity (PACC)—that was developed in an interpretive study with 43 parents of 34 children (aged 15 months to 16 years) with various chronic conditions.[157] Ray indicates that the care required for the child with a chronic condition, as described under three sections of the PACC model, includes medical care, parenting plus, and working the systems. The PACC model provides a comprehensive framework for assessing areas of responsibility and concern for families; and it can provide a visual aid for conveying the full scope of responsibilities faced by parents of children with chronic conditions.[158]

Chronic illnesses exact a heavy toll on children and their parents or significant caregivers. For example, a diagnosis of childhood cancer poses challenges to the stability and adaptive functioning of the entire family setting.[159] In fact, Woodgate states that childhood cancer is described by families as an extremely overwhelming experience and that both physical and mental suffering become part of their daily lives.[160] Hypertension is an under-recognized clinical entity in children that poses huge management concerns.[161]

Children with fetal alcohol syndrome or fetal alcohol effects present a particular national health concern.[162] The rates of FAS/FAE in some First Nations and Inuit communities are much higher than the national average. There, it exists in the context of the history of colonization and the devaluation endured by First Nations and Inuit, which has resulted in a loss of culture.[163] Awareness and strategies are emerging for affected children through identification, prevention, and intervention efforts. Federal, provincial, and territorial governments have agreed to work with Aboriginal peoples to find practical solutions to address the developmental needs of children.[164]

In a study, Harris and his team of researchers described disease patterns among children in an isolated community and compared them with patterns found among other Aboriginal and non-Aboriginal Canadian children.[165] They found that the illnesses most frequently seen in Aboriginal children are respiratory tract infections and skin conditions.

Because childhood obesity in Canada has become increasingly prevalent over the past two decades, the risk factors for cardiovascular disease and type 2 diabetes have been associated with increased levels of body fat in youth.[166]

In spite of chronic illnesses, the child's learning remains very important. Professionally, you should help parents to understand that it is they who are responsible for their child's behaviour and learning. The box entitled "Suggestions for Parents about Children's Homework" summarizes how parents can assist the child. The children must do their own growing and developing, and only through their own motivation.

**Intellectual Needs of the Hospitalized Child** You can help meet the hospitalized child's needs and educate the child and parents. A hospital tour, if it can be prearranged, helps the child feel acclimated during illness when his or her energy reserve is low. Because the child is beginning logical thought, he or she needs simple information about the illness to decrease the fear of the unknown and promote co-operation in the treatment plan. He or she needs to handle, and become familiar with, the equipment used.

Dealing with pain in children is difficult and complex, not only for the child, but also for the whole family.[167] Pain interferes with the child's schooling and social development. Children often lack the necessary coping mechanisms and the ability to communicate to others the type and degree of pain they experience. The box entitled "Ten Ways to Ease Pain in Children" offers some practical suggestions.[168]

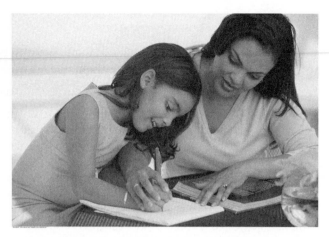

Parents nurture their children by providing support and encouraging their efforts and activities.

The child who must spend long periods in the hospital needs to learn about the outside world. Some hospitals take chronically ill children to the circus, athletic events, and restaurants. Teachers are also employed sometimes to work with the child in the hospital so that the child can continue with formal education.

## Communication Patterns

Many factors influence the child's communication pattern, vocabulary, and diction. Some of these factors have been referred to in previous chapters. Influences include:

1. Spoken, verbal, and nonverbal communication patterns of parents, siblings, other adults such as teachers, and peers
2. Attitudes of others toward the child's effort to speak and communicate
3. General environmental stimulation
4. Opportunity to communicate with a variety of people in a variety of situations
5. Intellectual development
6. Ability to hear and articulate
7. Vocabulary skills
8. Contact with television or other technology such as computers, the Internet, and video games[169]

Literacy, the ability to read and write, is the focus of education in the 6- to 12-year-old period. The skills that children develop during their early childhood experiences can profoundly influence their early reading development. The significant skills comprise the set known as phonological awareness, or sound-symbol connections. When children have mastered the basic reading processes, they are able to comprehend prefixes and suffixes, which

# Fathers' Experiences of Parenting a Child with Juvenile Rheumatoid Arthritis

Family life in Western society has undergone many changes over the past century, but the implications of these changes for men are not fully understood. Whereas men's roles and achievements in the public sphere have been well documented, their private lives, particularly their identities as husbands and fathers, have been far less studied. Although fathers are assumed to be an integral part of family life, they have emerged as a focus of interest from an academic perspective relatively recently.

One domain in which fathers' experiences are not well understood is in families of children who have a chronic health condition. Although a family-centred approach (i.e., family as primary unit of care) is advocated in pediatric health care literature, it has not translated into an understanding of the actual experience of fathers and the way they interpret their role.

The researcher examined the experience of fathers who have a child with juvenile rheumatoid arthritis (JRA). He used grounded theory methodology, in which 22 fathers participated in semi-structured interviews, and developed a substantive theory of fathers' experience that addresses the impact of their child's JRA, their responses of adaptation, and the meanings they associated with their experiences. Fathers were profoundly affected, perceived their child's condition as a catalyst for meaningful involvement, experienced many emotions, and sought to adopt a positive approach to making sense of their child's condition. Fathers' efforts to be strong for others resulted in an over-reliance on self-support strategies, particularly during periods of stress. Given the nature of fathers' experiences and the extent of their involvement, greater attention by health care practitioners to fathers' adaptation is indicated.

## Practice Implications

The findings from this study might be transferable in a manner consistent with qualitative research and used to sensitize clinicians about possible patterns of experience among fathers. Used in this way, the findings point to a number of potential considerations for clinicians:

1. Fathers are profoundly affected in multiple ways by their child's condition. Some fathers will welcome the opportunity to talk about their experience. This might be challenging for clinicians because fathers can be reluctant to disclose their more intense feelings in the presence of their partner, because doing so might be seen by them as undermining their ability to be a support for their partner. Fathers, therefore, might initially need some privacy to discuss their feelings.

2. The related finding that fathers attempted to be positive and pragmatic by addressing the things that could be changed to improve conditions for their child might mask their own underlying needs and be misinterpreted by clinicians as their not wanting or needing support for their feelings and reactions.

3. Fathers reported a willingness to be unpopular with the team if they feel a need to advocate for their child might bring them into greater conflict with the team. There was evidence that fathers perceived this responsibility as part of their protective role. Understanding this behaviour in the context of the couple relationship and the way partners co-construct their respective roles, rather than solely as an individual characteristic (e.g., unreasonable, difficult, hostile, angry), might provide a helpful vantage point.

4. Based on the many ways in which fathers are involved, consideration of their role should be part of any overall assessment plan. Increased efforts might be needed to ensure that service delivery strategies reach fathers and are truly accessible to them.

5. Providing quiet places for reflection and prayer might be particularly appreciated given the value that fathers in this study and elsewhere appear to place on prayer during stressful times.

6. Given that fathers' responses appear to be different from, but often related to, mothers' responses, it suggests the value of a family systems approach to understanding families as the unit of care.

Source: McNeill, T., Fathers' Experience of Parenting a Child with Juvenile Rheumatoid Arthritis, *Qualitative Health Research*, 14(4) (2004), 526–545. Used with permission.

are actually highly meaningful word parts. These skills enable them to become more efficient readers and to understand better what they have read. However, children need to be exposed to good literature, both in their own reading and in what parents and teachers read to them.[170] The acquisition of writing skill goes hand in hand with the development of reading. As children begin to translate words into speech, they learn that they can use written words to express their thoughts and feelings. Writing is difficult for young children because the child must keep in mind a variety of constraints: punctuation, spelling, grammar, and capitalization, as well as the

**Do:**

- Let your children know you believe they can do well. Encourage self-evaluation.
- Minimize time spent watching television.
- Help your children organize. Encourage them to do the most difficult tasks first.
- Talk and read to your children.
- Volunteer at your children's school.
- Encourage outside activities and having friends at home.
- Work with your children's teachers and let the teachers know you understand and are supportive.
- Insist on good eating habits.
- Plan activities with your children.
- Be a good example.

**Do not:**

- Dwell on the negative by criticizing.
- Allow the television to be your babysitter.
- Do homework for the children.
- Leave them to their own devices.
- Forget to encourage verbal exchange.
- Push them to have every minute scheduled.
- Criticize and interfere with everything you do not understand.
- Allow constant eating.
- Send them off without you to family functions (e.g., school plays, potluck dinners).
- Say, "Do as I say and not as I do."

physical task of forming a letter. Children who use computers write better, because they need not to contend with the mechanical demands of handwriting.[171] Language abilities continue to grow during middle childhood. In fact, the major area of linguistic growth during the school years is in pragmatics, the practical use of language to communicate. Pragmatics includes the skills of both communication and narration. For example, most six-year-olds can retell the plot of a short book, movie, or television show. By grade two, children's stories become longer and more complex. As the child shares ideas and feelings, he or she learns how someone else thinks and feels about similar matters. The child expresses himself or herself in a way that has meaning to others, at first to

a buddy and then to others. Thus, he or she is validating and expanding vocabulary, ideas, and feelings. The child learns that a friend's family has similar frustrations and life patterns, and demands on the child, as their own family has. He or she learns about self in the process of learning more about another. Older children recall what has happened in the past, realize how this has affected the present, and then consider what effect present acts will have on future events.[172]

Canada is a bilingual country where both English and French have equal status, rights, and privileges at the federal level.[173] Statistics Canada reports that in the 2002–2003 school year, nearly 2 million students took courses in French as a second language.[174] A large body of carefully conducted research shows that bilingualism has positive consequences for development. That is, children who are fluent in two languages are advanced in cognitive development. Bialystok states that bilingualism helps with reading achievement because the bilingual child is more conscious of more aspects of language sounds.[175] Many students taught in French immersion programs become functionally competent in both French and English, and as a result they gain a special appreciation of the French-Canadian culture.[176]

### CRITICAL THINKING

*If you attended a French immersion program, what did you learn?*

Convey love and caring, not rejection, when you talk with children. Love is communicated through nonverbal behaviour such as getting down to the child's eye level and through words that value feelings and indicate respect. Children better understand language that is directed at their feelings rather than at the overt action.

**Effects of Television and the Internet on the Child** According to the Vanier Institute of the Family, Canadian children between the ages of 2 and 11 watch approximately 18 hours of television per week, or 2.57 hours daily.[177] Video and computer games are becoming more popular for children and youth. In 2000, 4.7 million Canadian households were connected to the Internet, and 71 percent of households reported that at least one person in the home regularly used the Internet at least seven times daily.[178] To find out how the Internet is influencing the lives of Canadian children and the degree of awareness parents have regarding its influences, the Media Awareness Network (MNet) conducted two benchmark surveys, one in 2000 with parents and the other in 2001 with children and youth. The results indicated that Canadian children and youth are big users of the Internet and that 53 percent of parents believe they are on top of the situation. However,

1. Pain should not go untreated
   - Untreated pain causes stress and can sensitize a child's pain pathways making future bouts of pain worse.

2. First, assess the child's pain
   - Ask, "How much does it hurt? Small? Medium? A lot?"
   - Ask, "How much pain on a scale of 0 to 10? Zero is no pain and 10 is the worst pain you can imagine."

3. Remember the three Ps: pharmacological (medication), physical, and psychological
   - Sometimes, it is helpful to combine pain-relieving medication with physical strategies (apply heat or ice) and use psychological strategies (such as distraction and controlled breathing) for pain control.

4. Prevention is better than treatment
   - It is important to give pain medicines regularly to get on top of the pain and prevent it from becoming unmanageable.
   - Over-the-counter medications can be effective in treating mild to moderate pain.
   - Always be cautious in giving medications to children.
   - Ask the pharmacist to help select a medication and determine how and when to give it to the child.

5. Use of cold water and ice can be very helpful in reducing pain
   - Running cool water over a scrape or minor cut will help clean the wound and cool the burning pain.
   - A cool cloth on the child's forehead can help with a headache.
   - Ice is immediately effective in relieving pain caused by bruising, muscle spasms and pulls, sprains, and insect stings because it acts as a mild local anesthetic.
   - Alternating ice and heat can be an effective pain relief strategy for swelling, muscle spasms, and sore joints.

6. Warm baths, warm water bottles, and heating pads can be helpful
   - Applying heat increases blood flow and can be effective in relieving the child's stiff muscles and joints, bruising, and sprains.

7. Massage can be helpful with painful muscle spasms and pulls
   - The sense of touch itself, especially a mother touching an infant in pain, is helpful in reducing a child's anxiety and pain.

8. Gentle exercise can help protect muscles from injury and encourage healing in injured areas
   - A physiotherapist can provide education and instruction on the most appropriate techniques for the child.

9. Distraction is a simple and effective way to reduce pain for infants and children
   - Distraction tends to work best for mild pain, but how you distract the child will depend on his or her age.
   - Babies can be distracted with colourful mobiles and mirrors.
   - Younger children can be distracted by blowing bubbles, reading a favourite book, or playing with a musical toy.
   - Older children can choose what they wish to be distracted by, such as a hand-held video game.

10. Know when to seek medical advice
    - This can be difficult. Although the child feels the pain of an injury, the caregiver determines the seriousness of the problem.
    - If you are worried about the child's pain, it is reasonable to seek medical attention.

Source: The Hospital for Sick Children. *10 Ways to Ease Pain in Children*. Toronto. Adapted with permission.

according to Swift and Taylor, parents need to go online with their children and learn what they do there.[179]

Television and movies, video and computer games, and the Internet exert a powerful influence on a child's communication and behaviour patterns.

Parents must help children select educational programming because it can:[180]

1. Present information about specific topics that add to one's understanding of the world in general

2. Present positive images of people from various ethnic groups, or of people who are disabled

3. Depict positive social behaviour and cultural values such as work, sacrifice, and goal-setting

4. Convey positive ethical messages about the value of family life, friendship, and commitment to relationships

5. Feature women and men in positions of authority, or performing heroic acts

6. Present and reinforce techniques associated with various sports or exercise routines

7. Present information

Teach parents that, increasingly, research indicates that watching violent, sexually seductive programs or pornographic material on television or in movies has long-term negative effects on children. Review Table 10-8 with them.[181] Heavy television viewing is associated with lower school achievement. Teachers report that more children

## Table 10-8 Negative Effects of Television

1. Promotes passive rather than active learning
2. Increases passivity from continual overstimulation
3. Encourages low-level, non-conceptual thinking
4. Takes time away or distracts from more creative and stimulating activity; reduces creativity and creative fantasy of the child
5. Encourages short attention span and hyperactivity through its use of snappy attention-getting techniques
6. Causes lack of understanding or comprehension of what is seen or inability to grasp consequences of behaviour because of fast pace of programming
7. Causes loss of interest in less exciting but necessary classroom or home activities
8. Creates a desire for the superficial rather than depth of information; teaches superficial judgments
9. Creates uncertainty about what is real and unreal in life and family
10. Creates a confusion of values
11. Promotes a desire for unhealthy products such as high-sugar and high-salt snacks, other products not normally used by the family, or toys or other products that may be unhealthy or dangerous
12. Interferes with correct pronunciation of words, vocabulary use, reading comprehension, and spelling achievement
13. Promotes sedentary lifestyle and snacking rather than participation in play, sports, physical exercise, community events discussion, or activities with parents
14. Increases aggressive behaviour because of program content, loud music, fast pace, and camera tricks
15. Increases passive acceptance of aggressive behaviour toward people as a way to solve problems
16. Becomes a way to keep the child occupied—a passive babysitter
17. Increases suspicion of others, fears, and anxiety
18. Competes with parents, school, and peers as a socializing agent
19. Promotes passivity and withdrawal from direct involvement in real life
20. De-emphasizes complexity of life with simplistic plots, fast action, no lasting consequences, and no visual or cognitive depth
21. Conveys unrealistic and stereotyped view of men and women and sex roles; women usually portrayed as sex objects, ornamental, young, with limited speaking and/or problem-solving behaviours
22. Emphasizes overt sexual behaviour; portrays nudity, perversions, and sometimes pornographic content
23. Fosters increased incidence of aggressive and violent behaviour
24. Promotes excessive fears about war, about walking in one's own neighbourhood, about the "violent" world, and about the police who use only force
25. Increases emotional problems, including conduct disorders and post-traumatic stress disorder (nightmares, flashbacks, paranoia, poor concentration, impaired attachment to people)

are entering school with decreased imaginative play and creativity and increased aimless movement, low frustration level, poor persistence and concentration span, and confusion about reality and fantasy. Rapid speech and constantly changing visuals on television interfere with mental reflection. The child does not learn correct sentence structure, the use of tenses, or the ability to express thought or feeling effectively. The result may be a child who is unable to enunciate or use correct grammar and who is vague in the sense of time and history and cause-and-effect relationships.[182]

The violence in television programming is graphic, explicit, realistic, and intensely involving. It affects both children and adults, but children more so because they have less ego control. Children act out more directly based on what they see and hear.

Aggressive actions lead to a heightened level of arousal of the viewer's aggressive tendencies. As a result, these aroused aggressive tendencies bring thoughts, feelings, memories, and actions to vivid consciousness, causing outwardly aggressive behaviour. Even fast-paced programming arouses certain aggressive impulses.[183]

Many programs, either directly or indirectly, teach violent behaviour, showing specifically how to carry out violent acts. It is not unusual for arson, rape, hostage taking, suicide, or homicide to be described graphically on the evening news, either locally or nationally, or to have a number of such incidents repeated within a few days. The live and explicit portrayals of violence suggest that aggression and violence are normal, justified, and rewarded. Realistic or punitive consequences of violent behaviour are seldom shown. The viewer gets the idea and forms an attitude over time that aggressive or violent behaviour should be used to solve problems, that it is normal or courageous to be violent, that violence is rewarded or socially acceptable, and that the violent person is the hero with whom to identify. Aggressive behaviour is expected in interactions and is used as a response in peer interactions and when frustrated. The world is viewed as dangerous; aggressive behaviour is a way to protect self.[184] Finally, the repeated and continual viewing of violence tends to desensitize the person to violence in general; it no longer becomes a noteworthy act, either in the home or in society. Even worse, television violence shows inequality and domination; the most frequent victims are women, elders, and children.[185]

Discuss with parents the need *to limit the amount of television viewing* (two hours a day), do alternative activities with their children, screen what their children are viewing, and work to reduce the trend toward more violent and pornographic programming. Parents can be more vigilant about the programs their children watch. Television programming can be improved. Networks and advertisers, of course, hope that parents will disregard research findings that make-believe violence makes for real violence in many settings. As long as violence on television is profitable, programming will contain violence. Parents can rebel by writing letters to stations, writing letters to advertisers, and refusing to buy the products advertised. This is a significant area of life that affects the child's and the family's physical, emotional, cognitive, social, and spiritual health.

In essence, interaction with parents and others, and real experiences rather than passive observations, help the child learn to work through conflicts of development and to solve problems.

## CRITICAL THINKING

*What effects can television advertisements have on children's social behaviour?*

## Play Patterns

The following information can be used to educate parents and children and to plan health promotion programs.

**Peer Groups** Peer groups, including the gang and a close buddy, provide companionship, shared time, conversation, and activity with a widening circle of persons outside the home. Peer groups are extremely important to the school-aged child. Between the ages of seven and nine, children usually form close friendships with peers of the same sex and age. Later in this age group, peers are not necessarily of the same age. Functions of the peer group are listed in Table 10-9.

Children must earn their membership in the peer group. Being accepted by one's peers, and belonging to a peer group, are major concerns for this age group. Many factors determine a child's acceptance, including attractiveness and friendliness. Most children find acceptance with at least one or two peers, but rejection and loneliness are always a risk. Children may be rejected because they are either too aggressive or too passive. Being an outsider carries all of the risks that are implied if the peer group functions cannot be attained. The effects of not being a peer group member can be corrected by having a buddy. If a child does not have a peer group it might set the foundation for either a shy, withdrawn personality or an overtly assertive, aggressive personality that tries to manoeuvre into groups. Actually, these effects may still be evident in adulthood.[186]

### Table 10-9 Functions of the School-Aged Peer Group

- Reinforces gender role behaviour
- Accepts those who conform to social roles
- Provides an audience for developing self-concept, self-esteem, and unique personality characteristics
- Provides information about the world of school and neighbourhood, games, dress, and manners; decreases egocentrism
- Provides opportunity to compete and compare self to others of same age
- Develops a personal set of values and goals; conformity is expected
- Teaches rules and logical consequences; punishes members who disobey rules
- Provides opportunity to test mastery in a world parallel to adult society, with rules, organization, and purposes
- Provides emotional support during stressful or crisis points in a member's life
- Protects against other peers who may threaten, bully, or intimidate, or actually harm if the member were alone

**Play Activities** Play activities change with the child's development. From age six to eight, he or she is interested chiefly in the present and in the immediate surroundings. Because he or she knows more about family life than any other kind of living, the child plays house or takes the role of various occupational groups with which there is contact: mail carrier, firefighter, carpenter, nurse, occupational therapist, and teacher. Although the child is more interested in playing with peers than with parents, the six- or seven-year-old will occasionally enjoy having the parent as a "child" or "student." This allows the child to have imaginary control over the parent, and at the same time allows the parent to understand how the child is interpreting the parent, or how the child perceives the teacher.

Both sexes enjoy some activities in common, such as painting, cutting, pasting, reading, collecting items such as baseball cards or stamps, simple table games, television, digging, riding a bicycle, construction sets or models, puzzles, kites, running games, team sports, rough and tumble play, skating, and swimming. Again, the parent can sometimes enjoy these activities with the child, especially if the parent has a special talent the child wishes to learn. The child imitates the roles of his or her own sex and becomes increasingly realistic in play.

By age eight, collections, more advanced models, the radio, art materials, "how to" books, farm sets, and train sets are favourite pastimes, and loosely formed, short-lived clubs with fluctuating rules are formed.

The schoolchild, usually near eight or nine years of age, enjoys computerized and electronic games, which give a sense of control and power, of being a peer with or even superior to the adult, of challenge and inventiveness, and an enjoyment of complexity and expandability. The computer can be a tool for robot thinking or for development of thought, for passivity or for releasing aggressive impulses or creativity, for play or for learning. Computer and video toys can help the schoolchild understand the nature of systems and the control of information—skills needed in the adult world. Let the child take the lead in moving into computer games. Actually, many schoolchildren prefer reading, painting, playing an instrument, doing crafts, camping, or playing sports to working with computers. These skills and what these activities teach are as essential as the ability to operate a computer.

At approximately age ten, sex differences in play become pronounced. Each sex is developing through play the skills it will later need in society. The child's interest in faraway places is enhanced through a foreign pen pal and through travel.

From age 9 to 12, the child becomes more interested in active sports, but continues to enjoy quieter activity. He or she wants to improve motor skills. The child may enjoy carpentry or mechanic's tools, advanced models or puzzles, arts and crafts, science projects, music, dance, cameras and film, and camping. Adult-organized games of hockey, softball, football, or soccer lose their fun when parents place excessive emphasis on winning. The hug from a teammate after scoring a goal means more than just winning.

Throughout childhood, girls compare favourably with boys in strength, endurance, and motor skills, but in late childhood, girls are physically more mature than boys. At about age 12, girls begin to perform less well than boys on tests of physical skills; they run more slowly, jump less far, and lift less weight if they are given no physical training. The traditional poorer performance is probably the result of gender expectations about behaviour. Athletic activity is attractive to both boys and girls and is becoming more accessible to girls than in the past.[187]

**Bullying** Data from the National Longitudinal Survey of Children and Youth (NLSCY) indicate that a significant proportion of school-aged children in Canada are either bullies (14 percent) or victims (5 percent). A higher percentage of boys, compared to girls, are involved in bullying. Children who bully display other antisocial behaviours such as physical aggression, indirect aggression, and hyperactivity. Along with the immediate effects of bullying and victimization, this behaviour has long-term consequences for all those involved, both bullies and victims.[188] It is important to stop bullying at a young age, and strive to create a peaceful and safe environment for everyone.

Recent research has shown that school bullying (the repeated and systematic psychological abuse of power by peers) is a serious problem for students and educators alike.[189] An interesting Canadian study was conducted to examine the association between bullying behaviours (physical, verbal, relational) with overweight and obesity status in a representative sample of 5749 boys and girls (11 to 16 years old). The researchers found that overweight and obese schoolchildren are more likely to be victims and perpetrators of bullying behaviours than are their normal-weight peers.[190] Bosacki and her researchers from Brock University investigated children's understanding of school bullying and victimization as represented through drawing, narratives, and open-ended quality questions. The sample comprised 82 children from ages 8 to 12. The children's drawings and narrative accounts of bullying suggested that some of the bullies they have encountered seemed to enjoy inflicting harm on the peer. The narratives of the participants indicated that it may be crucial to create comprehensive anti-bullying interventions that include a component on moral values related to bullying and victimization.[191]

Nurses can teach parents how to promote safety for the child. Nurses can take the leadership role in communities and advocate for the responsibility of children's safety. See

## Bullying: How Adults Can Help

### General information

1. Bullying is not a problem that children can solve themselves.

2. It is a power struggle—difficult to change without the help of an adult.

3. It requires only a few minutes to stop the behaviour, especially if you act immediately and in a consistent manner.

4. If you witness the bullying:

   ▪ Talk to the children who are being aggressive

   ▪ Explain the hurt they are causing

   ▪ Have the aggressors make amends to the ones who were harmed.

5. Most bullying happens when adults are not watching. When told about it, take it seriously.

6. Children usually go to adults with these problems as a last resort.

7. Sometimes bullying behaviour is a chronic problem requiring the involvement of families and the assistance of a health professional.

If you are a parent, guardian or caregiver

▪ Listen and respond to all complaints from children about bullying, even the seemingly trivial ones such as name-calling.

▪ Talk to other adults who were in charge when the bullying occurred to determine ways to remedy the hurt and prevent future problems.

▪ Stop bullying behaviour that happens at home. Consistency matters!

▪ Consider how you treat others and how you allow others to treat you. As a role model, your actions and reactions can influence how children relate to each other.

If you are an adult responsible for children (e.g., teacher or coach)

▪ Listen and respond to all complaints from children and parents about bullying, even the seemingly trivial ones such as name calling. Consistency matters!

▪ Be aware of the social interactions among children in the group. Arrange groupings to separate children who tend to have negative interactions with others.

▪ Place children who tend to be left out of groups into groups where they will be accepted. Try to avoid situations that will victimize at-risk children (e.g., picking teams or group partners).

▪ Consider how you treat others and how you allow others to treat you. As a role model, your actions and reactions can influence how children relate to each other.

If you are a leader of an organization responsible for children (e.g., school principal or manager of a sports team or other children's program)

▪ Listen and respond to all complaints from children and parents about bullying, even the seemingly trivial ones such as name-calling. Consistency matters!

▪ Support the adults who work directly with children in their constructive approaches to end bullying, such as separating disruptive children, increasing supervision in bullying hotspots, and placing vulnerable children in positive groups.

▪ Create an effective anti-bullying policy in your organization that clearly sets the limits on acceptable behaviour. Include meaningful consequences in the policy to help teach the aggressive children healthier ways of interacting.

▪ Allow time for the policy to be reviewed and agreed upon by everyone (including the children).

▪ Ensure that the policy is consistently and universally applied by all involved.

Source: Adapted from Public Safety Canada. *Keeping Canadians Safe.* Website: http:www.publicsafety.gc.cza/

---

the box entitled "Bullying: How Adults Can Help" for some practical suggestions on reacting to bullying.[192]

### CRITICAL THINKING

*How might you help teachers reduce bullying during the school years?*

## Tools of Socialization

An increasing body of research indicates that experiences at school have a profound influence on the social and emotional development of children. In particular, children's health behaviours and their view of themselves have been shown to be directly related to their school life.[193]

## Guidance and Discipline

In guidance, parents should invite the confidence of the child as a parent, not as a buddy or a pal. The child will find pals among peers. In the adult, he or she needs a parent. The atmosphere should be open and inviting for the child to talk with the parents, but the child's privacy should not be invaded. Parents should see the child as he or she is, not as an idealized extension of themselves.

The schoolchild has a rather strict superego, and uses many rituals to maintain self-control. He or she prefers to initiate self-control rather than be given commands or overt discipline. The stability and routine in his or her life provide this opportunity. You can talk with parents about methods of guidance and the importance of not interfering too forcefully or too often with behaviour. The child needs some alternatives from which to choose so that he or she can learn different ways of behaving and coping and be better able to express self later. Research indicates that preadolescent girls perceive their mothers as more support-ive, but also more punitive, than their fathers. Boys, who are less warmly treated by their parents, are more responsive to social or peer influences than girls, which has implica-tions for later antisocial behaviour.[194]

Guidance at this age takes many other less dramatic forms. A mother can turn the often harried "buying back-to-school clothes" experience into a pleasant lesson in guidance. She can accompany the child on a special shopping trip in which he or she examines different textures of material, learns about colour coordination, understands what constitutes a good fit, and appreciates how much money must be spent for certain items. This principle can be carried into any parent–schoolchild guidance relationship

such as learning responsibility for some household task or for earning, handling, and saving money.

## Emotional Development

The schoolchild consolidates earlier psychosocial develop-ment and simultaneously reaches out to a number of identification figures, expands interests, and associates with more people. Behavioural characteristics change from year to year. Table 10-10 summarizes and compares basic behaviour patterns, although individual children will show a considerable range of behaviour. Cultural, health, and social conditions may also influence behaviour.[195]

### CRITICAL THINKING

*What health problems might affect emotional development in a child?*

**Developmental Crisis**  The psychosexual crisis for this period is industry versus inferiority. **Industry** is *an interest in doing the work of the world, the child's feeling that he or she can learn and solve problems, the formation of responsible work habits and attitudes, and the mastery of age-appropriate tasks.*[196] The child has greater body competence and applies self to skills and tasks that go beyond playful expression. The child

| Table 10-10 Assessment of Changing Behavioural Characteristics in the Schoolchild | | |
|---|---|---|
| **6 Years** | **7 Years** | **8 Years** |
| Self-centred | Self-care managed | Expansive personality but fluctuating behaviour |
| Body movement, temper outbursts release tension | Quiet, less impulsive, but assertive | Curious, robust, energetic |
| Behavioural extremes; impulsive or dawdles, loving or antagonistic | Fewer mood swings | Rapid movements and response; impatient |
| Difficulty making decisions; needs reminders | Self-absorbed without excluding others; may appear shy, sad, brooding | Affectionate to parents |
| Verbally aggressive but easily insulted | Attentive, sensitive listener | Hero worship of adult |
| Intense concentration for short time, then abruptly stops activity | Companionable; likes to do tasks for others | Suggestions followed better than commands |
| Security of routines and rituals essential; periodic separation anxiety | Good and bad behaviour in self and others noted | Adult responsibilities and characteris-tics imitated; wants to be considered important by adults |
| Series of three commands followed, but response depends on mood | High standards for self but minor infractions of rules: tattles, alibis, takes small objects from others | Approval and reconciliation sought, feelings easily hurt |
| Self-control and initiative in activity encouraged when adult uses count-ing to give child time ("I'll give you until the count of 10 to pick up those papers") | Concern about own behaviour, tries to win over others' approval | Sense of property; enjoys collections |
| Praise and recognition needed | Angry over others' failure to follow rules | Beginning sense of justice but makes alibis for own transgressions |
| | | Demanding and critical of others |
| | | Gradually accepts inhibitions and limits |

*(continued)*

Table 10-10 (continued)

**9 Years**

More independent and self-controlled
Dependable, responsible
Adult trust and more freedom without adult supervision sought
Loyal to home and parents; seeks their help at times
More self rather than environmentally motivated; not dependent on but benefits from praise
More involved with peers
Own interests subordinated to group demands and adult authority
Critical of own and others' behaviour
Loyal to group; chum important
Concerned about fairness and willing to take own share of blame
More aware of society

**10 Years**

More adult-like and poised, especially girls
More self-directive, independent
Organized and rapid in work; budgets time and energy
Suggestions followed better than requests, but obedient
Family activities and care of younger siblings, especially below school age, enjoyed
Aware of individual differences among people, but does not like to be singled out in a group
Hero worship of adult
Some idea of own assets and limits
Preoccupied with right and wrong
Better able to live by rules
Critical sense of justice; accepts immediate punishment for wrongdoing
Liberal ideas of social justice and welfare
Strong desire to help animals and people
Future career choices match parents' careers because of identification with parents
Sense of leadership

**11 Years**

Spontaneous, self-assertive, restless, curious, sociable
Short outbursts of anger and arguing
Mood swings
Challenges enjoyed
On best behaviour away from home
Quarrelsome with siblings; rebellious to parents
Critical of parents, although affectionate with them
Chum and same-sex peers important; warm reconciliation follows quarrels
Secrets freely shared with chum; secret language with peers
Unaware of effect of self on others
Strict superego; zeal for fairness
Future career choices fantasized on basis of possible fame
Modest with parents

**12 Years**

Considerable personality integration; self-contained, self-competent, tactful, kind, reasonable, less self-centred
Outgoing, eager to please, enthusiastic
Sense of humour; improved communication skills
More companionable than at 11; mutual understanding between parents and child
Increasingly sensitive to feelings of others; wish good things for family and friends; caught between the two
Others' approval sought
Childish lapses, but wishes to be treated like adult
Aware of assets and shortcomings
Tolerant of self and others
Peer group and chum important in shaping attitudes and interests
Ethical sense more realistic than idealistic
Decisions about ethical questions based on consequences
Less tempted to do wrong; basically truthful
Self-disciplined, accepts just discipline
Enthusiastic about community projects

gets tired of play, wants to participate in the real world, and seeks attention and recognition for effort and concentration on a task. He or she feels pride in doing something well, whether a physical or cognitive task. A sense of industry involves self-confidence, perseverance, diligence, self-control, co-operation, and compromise rather than only competition. There is a sense of loyalty, relating self to something positive beyond the moment and outside the self. Parents, teachers, and nurses may see this industry at times as restlessness, irritability, rebellion toward authority, and a lack of obedience.

The danger of this period is that the child may develop a sense of **inferiority**, *feeling inadequate, defeated, unable to learn or do tasks, lazy, and unable to compete, compromise, or* co-operate, regardless of his or her actual competence.[197] See the box entitled "Consequences of Inferiority Feelings" for a summary of behaviours and traits of the child, and later the adult, if this stage is not resolved. If the child feels excessively ashamed, self-doubting, guilty, and inferior from not having achieved the developmental tasks, physical, emotional, and behavioural problems may occur. Sometimes opposite behaviour may occur as the person tries to cope with feelings of being no good, inferior, or inadequate. The person might immerse self in tasks. If work is all the child can do at home and school, he or she will miss out on many friendships and opportunities in life, now and later, and eventually is liable to become the adult who cannot stop working.

*Stress* is experienced by the school-aged child. Often, stress response occurs from the demands placed on the child in relation to school achievement or extracurricular performance, or from the fear that violence during transportation, or at school, may predominate.

Table 10-11 lists signs of stress that can be observed in the classroom and at school.

There are sharp differences in how children bear up under stress such as that which arises from abuse or divorce. Some children are **vulnerable** to stressors, and *they are sensitive to, or drawn in by, the events around them. They become nervous and withdrawn, and they feel inferior. Some are illness-prone* and slow to develop. Other children are **resilient:** *they shrug off the stressors, thrive, and go on to be industrious, have high self-esteem, and as adults lead highly productive lives.* True, some children are born with an innate easygoing

## Consequences of Inferiority Feelings

- Does not want to try new activities, skills
- Is passive, excessively meek, too eager to please others
- Seeks attention; may be "teacher's pet"
- Is anxious, moody, depressed
- Does not persevere in tasks
- Is very fearful of bodily injury or illness
- Does not volunteer to do tasks alone, always works with another on tasks
- Isolates self from others, withdraws from peers
- Tries to prove personal worth, a "good worker" with directives or assistance
- Lacks self-esteem unless praised considerably
- Is overly competitive, bossy
- Insists on own way, experiences difficulty with co-operation or compromise
- May immerse self in tasks to prove self, gain attention
- Acts out to prove self; lying, stealing, fire setting
- Displays extreme antisocial behaviour, destructive or aggressive acts
- Manifests illnesses associated with emotional state: enuresis, complaints of fatigue
- In adulthood, is unable to pursue steady work or become involved in life tasks as expected
- May become "workaholic" in adulthood, is unable to engage in leisure

## Table 10-11 Signs of Stress Observed at School

### Physical Signs

1. Morning stomach aches, leg cramps
2. Frowning, squinting, clenched jaw, facial expressions reflecting misery
3. Mixes cursive and manuscript, lower- and upper-case letters when writing
4. May invert, omit, or substitute letters and words
5. Laborious writing, tiring easily when writing
6. Frequent erasures, hates writing activities
7. Negotiates to minimize writing assignments
8. Alert and attentive to noises and distractions not associated with learning task
9. Misunderstands teacher's instruction, directions
10. Needs directions repeated, instruction repeated
11. Reading is difficult
12. Falls asleep during the school day
13. Nail biting, throat-clearing, coughing, eye-blinking, incontinent of urine at school, bed-wetting at home
14. Exhaustion from performing school tasks
15. Low resistance to illness
16. Absenteeism
17. Relieves tension through constant physical activity

### Emotional Signs

1. Seeks adult approval and reassurance
2. Needs a lot of praise
3. Needs immediate feedback and response from teacher

*(continued)*

**Table 10-11** (continued)

4. Fear of making a mistake, does not volunteer

5. Lacks confidence

6. Fears getting hurt

7. Withdraws from touch

8. Does not seek to try new things, does not take risks

9. Cannot readily change activities

10. Loses place in lessons

11. Daydreams

12. Often gives the right answer to the wrong question

13. Fears getting hurt

14. Cries easily

15. Picked on by classmates

16. Behaviour at school is acceptable, but parents report bad behaviour at home

**Intellectual Signs**

1. Inconsistent performance

2. Trouble keeping up the pace

3. Trouble completing assignments within the time limit

4. Has potential, but does not apply self

5. Loses the "low-grade" papers

6. Parents blame teacher for not challenging the child

**Social Signs**

1. Favourite at-home activity is watching television

2. Passive, apathetic, no initiative at school

3. Does not fit in with peer group

4. Avoids other children, tries to remain anonymous

5. Tries to annoy other children

6. Has few friends, feels uncomfortable in social situations

7. Does not take responsibility for not having assignments, makes excuses

8. Feels hurt and left out, may become angry or jealous of classmates

9. Can be a class bully

10. May show off in one area

11. Seeks out younger children to play with

12. Afraid to take risks

13. Avoids competition

14. Prefers to play alone

temperament and handle stressors better than do children with a nervous, over-reactive disposition. Children who have robust, sunny personalities are lovable and readily win affection, which further builds self-esteem and an identity. Resilient children are likely to have a number of protective factors, but the key is a basic, consistent, lasting, trusting relationship with an adult who is supportive and who is a beacon presence from infancy onward.[198] Vulnerable children, if placed in the right environment, become productive and competent adults. They need help to find a solid relationship—neighbour, teacher, relative—until they find at least one such adult. Then they distance self at least emotionally from the conflictual or abusive home.[199] *Basic health, and social and educational programs must be provided* to assist the child to adapt to the extent possible, now and in future adult life.[200] When the child's environment is overwhelmingly stressful, extra support and love are especially important. If the child is facing multiple stressors, it is more difficult for outside intervention to help the child. The greater the risk factors, the worse the outcome for the child, regardless of the intervention.

*Teach parents* that they can contribute to a sense of industry and avoid inferiority feelings by not holding on to unrealistic expectations of the child, and by using the suggested guidance and discipline approaches. They can encourage peer activities and home responsibilities, help the child meet developmental crises, and give recognition to his or her accomplishments and unique talents.

---

**CRITICAL THINKING**

*What are some activities a parent can pursue with a child at home that could contribute to a sense of industry?*

---

## Self-Concept, Body Image, and Sexual Development

Self-concept and body image are affected by cultural, ethnic, or racial background, gender, grade level of the child, parents' education, history of illness, and type of illness. Until the child goes to school, self-perception is derived primarily from the parents' attitudes and reactions toward him or her. The child who is loved for what he or she is learns to love and accept self.

The child with a positive self-concept likes self and others. That child believes that what he or she thinks, says, and does makes a difference, that he or she can be successful and can solve problems, and can expresses feelings of happiness.

Younger children use mostly surface, or visible, characteristics to describe themselves. At about age eight the child describes the self with less focus on external characteristics and more on enduring internal qualities, and he or she is more realistic. Because of their concern with appearance or body image, children may try to lose weight, influenced by the ultra-thin models in the media. Mothers can exert a strong influence over their daughters' weight-control efforts.[201]

A negative self-image causes the child to feel defensive toward others and self and hinders adjustment to school and academic progress. Children with a low self-concept show more social withdrawal, academic difficulties, and inappropriate attention seeking than children with a high self-concept.[202]

At school the child compares self, and is compared, with peers in appearance and motor, cognitive, language, and social skills. If he or she cannot perform as well as other children, peers will perceive the child somewhat negatively, and eventually he or she will perceive self as incompetent or inferior because self-image is more dependent on peers than it was earlier in childhood.

Schoolchildren are frequently cruel in their honesty when they make derogatory remarks about peers with limitations or disabilities.

Parents, teachers, and health care professionals can contribute to a positive self-esteem and competence in performance by emphasizing the child's positive, healthy characteristics and by reinforcing the child's potential. You, too, can be instrumental in fostering a healthy relationship.

The teacher (or nurse) can intervene when derogatory remarks are made among classmates. He or she could move a child into another work or play group that is more appropriate for his or her ability, or explain to peers in simple language the importance of accepting another who is at a different developmental level. Meanwhile, the teacher or nurse should continue to encourage the child who has the difficulty. Thus, the school experience may either reinforce or weaken the child's feeling about self as a unique, important person with specific talents or abilities. If he or she is one of 30 children in a classroom, and receives little attention from the teacher, self-concept may be threatened.

The *child's body image* is very fluid. Schoolchildren are more aware of the internal body and external differences. They can label major organs with increasing accuracy. Heart, brain, and bones are most frequently mentioned, along with cardiovascular, gastrointestinal, and musculoskeletal systems. The younger child thinks that organs change position. Organ function, size, and position are poorly understood. Organs, such as the stomach, are frequently drawn at the wrong place (this may reflect the influence of television ads). Children generally believe that they must have all body parts to remain alive and that the skin holds in the body contents.

Consider the effect that injury or surgery might have on the child. This is an excellent age to teach about any of these inaccuracies.

Table 10-12 shows how aspects of the child's view of self change through the school years.[203]

*Self-concept, body image, and sexuality development are interrelated and are influenced by parental and societal expectations of, and reactions to, each gender.* You can assist parents in promoting a positive self-concept and body image. During latency, boys and girls are similar in many ways, but differences are taught. Girls reportedly are less physically active, but they have greater verbal, perceptual, and cognitive skills than boys. Girls supposedly respond to stimuli—interpersonal and physical, including pain—more quickly and accurately than boys. They seem better at analyzing and anticipating environmental demands. Therefore, their behaviour conforms more to adult expectations, and they are better at staying out of trouble. Innate physiologic differences become magnified as they are reinforced by cultural norms and specific parental behaviours. Stereotypes are changing, however. Girls can cope with aggression and competition just as boys can.[204]

Early physical education activities teach general coordination, eye–hand coordination, and balance, basic movements that carry over into all movement and sports. Rigorous conditioning activities such as gymnastics are suggested for achieving high levels of physical fitness for prepubertal girls. These activities will improve agility, appearance, endurance, strength, feelings of well-being, and self-concept.

## CRITICAL THINKING

*What initial steps could you take in the development of a community-based physical activity program for school-aged children?*

**Sexuality Education**  Sexual health is one major aspect of personal health that affects people at all ages and stages throughout their life. Canada focuses on enhancing sexual health and on reducing sexual problems encountered among various groups in our society.[205] Health Canada's *Canadian Guidelines for Sexual Health Education* emphasizes the importance of assisting youth with the information, motivation, and skills needed to make informed and responsible sexual decisions.[206]

Wackett and Evans describe the first reported evaluation of family life/sexual health education program for elementary school students in Canada.[207] The program, called Choices and Changes, was designed following the concepts in the *Canadian Guidelines for Sexual Health Education*, and was presented to students in grades four to seven in a school in Whitehorse, Yukon. They found that

## Table 10-12 Assessment of Changing Body Image Development in the Schoolchild

| 6 Years | 7 Years | 8 Years |
|---|---|---|
| Is self-centred | Is more modest and aware of self | Redefines sense of status with others |
| Likes to be in control of self, situations, and possessions | Wants own place at table, in car, and own room or part of room | Subtle changes in physical proportion; movements smoother |
| Gains physical and motor skills | Has lower-level physical activity than earlier | Assumes many roles consecutively |
| Knows right from left hand | Does not like to be touched | Is ready for physical contact in play and to be taught self-defence mechanisms |
| Regresses occasionally to baby talk or earlier behaviour | Protects self by withdrawing from unpleasant situation | Is more aware of differences between the sexes |
| Plays at being someone else to clarify sense of self and others | Dislikes physical combat | Is curious about another's body |
| Is interested in marriage and reproduction | Engages less in sex play | Asks questions about marriage and reproduction; strong interest in babies, especially for girls |
| Distinguishes organs of each sex but wonders about them | Understands pregnancy generally; excited about new baby in family | Plays more with own sex |
| May indulge in sex play | Concerned he or she does not really belong to parents | |
| Draws a man with hands, neck, clothing, and six identifiable parts | Tells parts missing from picture of incomplete man | |
| Distinguishes between attractive and ugly pictures of faces | | |

| 9 Years | 10 Years |
|---|---|
| Has well-developed eye–hand coordination | Is self-conscious about exposing body, including to younger siblings and opposite-sex parent |
| Enjoys displaying motor skills and strength | Is relatively content with and confident of self |
| Cares completely for body needs | Has perfected most basic small motor movements |
| Has more interest in own body and its functions than in other sexual matters | Wants privacy for self but peeks at other sex |
| Asks fewer questions about sexual matters if earlier questions answered satisfactorily | Asks some questions about sexual matters again |
| | Investigates own sexual organs |
| | Shows beginning prepubertal changes physically, especially girls |

| 11 Years | 12 Years |
|---|---|
| States self is in heart, head, face, or body part most actively expressing him or her | Growth spurt; changes in appearance |
| Feels more self-conscious with physical changes occurring | Muscular control almost equal to that of adult |
| Mimics adults; deepening self-understanding | Identifies self as being in total body or brain |
| Masturbates sometimes; erection occurs in boys | May feel like no part of body is his or hers alone but like someone else's because of close identity with group |
| Discusses sexual matters with parents with reticence | Begins to accept and find self as unique person |
| Likes movies on reproduction | |
| Feels joy of life with more mature understanding | |

the program increased the motivation and personal insights of students regarding sexuality.[208]

### CRITICAL THINKING

*You have been asked to address a grade six class on sexuality education. What issues would you be sure to include in your presentation?*

## Adaptive Mechanisms

The schoolchild is losing the protective mantle of home and early childhood and needs order and consistency to help cope with doubts, fears, unacceptable impulses, and unfamiliar experiences. Commonly used *adaptive mechanisms* include ritualistic behaviour, reaction formation, undoing, isolation, fantasy, identification, regression, malingering, rationalization, projection, and sublimation. Assess for these behaviours. Help parents understand the adaptive mechanisms used by the child and how to help the child use healthy coping mechanisms.

**Ritualistic behaviour,** *consistently repeating an act in a given situation,* wards off imagined harm and anxiety and provides a feeling of control. Examples include avoiding stepping on cracks in the sidewalk while chanting certain words (e.g., so as not to break mother's back), always putting the left leg through trousers before the right, having a certain place for an object, or doing homework at a specific time.

Reaction formation, undoing, and isolation are related to obsessive, ritualistic behaviour. **Reaction formation** is used frequently in dealing with feelings of hostility. The child may unconsciously hate a younger brother because he infringes on the schoolchild's freedom, but such impulses are unacceptable to the strict superego. To counter such unwanted feelings, the child may become the classic example of a caring, loving sibling.

**Undoing** is *unconsciously removing an idea, feeling, or act by performing certain forms of ritualistic behaviour.* For example, the gang must follow certain chants and movements before a member who broke a secret code can return. **Isolation** is *a mechanism of unconsciously separating emotion from an idea because the emotion would be unacceptable to the self.* The idea remains in the conscious, but its component feeling remains in the unconscious. A child uses isolation when he or she seems to talk very objectively about the puppy that has just been run over by a truck.

**Fantasy** *compensates for feelings of inadequacy, inferiority, and lack of success* encountered in school, the peer group, or home. Fantasy is necessary for eventual creativity and should not be discouraged if it is not used excessively to prevent realistic participation in the world. Fantasy saves the ego temporarily, but it also provides another way for the child to view self, thus helping him or her to aspire to new heights of behaviour.

**Identification** is seen in the *hero worship of teacher, scoutmaster, neighbour, or family friend,* someone whom the child respects and who has the qualities the child fantasizes as his or her own.

**Regression,** *returning to a less sophisticated pattern of behaviour,* is a defence against anxiety and helps the child avoid potentially painful situations. For example, he or she may revert to using the language or behaviour of a younger sibling if the child feels that the sibling is getting undue attention.

**Malingering,** *feigning illness to avoid unpleasant tasks,* is seen when the child stays home from school for a day, or says he or she is unable to do a home task because he or she does not feel well.

**Rationalization,** *providing excuses when the child is unable to achieve wishes,* is frequently seen in relation to schoolwork. For example, after a low test grade, the response is, "Oh well, grades don't make any difference anyway."

**Projection** is seen as the child says about a teacher, "She doesn't like me," when really the teacher is disliked for having reprimanded the child.

**Sublimation** is a major mechanism used during the school years. The child increasingly *channels sexual and aggressive impulses into socially acceptable tasks* at school and home. In the process, if all goes well, he or she develops the sense of industry.

The use of any and all of these mechanisms in various situations is normal, but overuse of any one can result in a constricted, immature personality. If constricted, the child will find it difficult to develop relationships outside the home, to succeed at home or school, or to balance work and play. Achieving a sense of identity and adult developmental tasks will be impaired.

## Child in Transition

The school-aged child is especially affected by a geographic move, especially if he or she is just entering, or is well settled into, the buddy stage. The child cannot understand why he or she cannot fit into the new group right away. Because routines are so important to the schoolchild, he or she is sometimes confused by the new and different ways of doing things. The parents will find it helpful to consult with the new school leaders about their child's adjustment.

*Share the following ideas with parents.*

1. If a family can include the schoolchild in the decision about where to move, the transition will be easier.

2. Ideally, the whole family should make at least one advance trip to the new community. If possible, the new home and town should be explored, and the child should visit the new school so that he or she can establish mentally where he or she is going.

3. Writing to one of the new classmates, after meeting briefly—say, on a walk—and before the actual move can enhance a feeling of friendship and belonging.

4. If the child has a special interest such as gymnastics or dancing, contact with the new program can form another transitional step.

5. When parents are packing, they are tempted to dispose of as many of the child's belongings as possible, especially if they seem babyish or worn. They *should not do this.* These items are part of the child, and they will help him or her feel more comfortable and at home during adjustment to a new home and community.

6. Sometimes parents in the new community are reticent about letting their children go to visit at the new child's house. The new parents should make every attempt to introduce themselves to the new playmates' parents, assuring them that the environment will be safe for play. Alternatively, parents can have a get-acquainted party for the few children who are especially desired as playmates.

7. Just as the family initiated some ties before they moved, similarly they should keep some ties from the previous neighbourhood. If possible, let the child play with old friends at times. If the move has been too far for frequent visits, allow the child to call old friends occasionally.

8. If possible, plan a trip back so that some old traditions can be revived and friends can be visited. The trip to the old neighbourhood will cement, in the child's mind, that "home" is no longer there but in the new location.

9. The parents must accept as natural some grieving for what is gone. Letting the child express his or her feelings, accepting these feelings, and continuing to work with the above suggestions will foster the adjustment.

Foster adjustment through noticing the new child, watching his or her behaviour, working with the teacher and peers, and contacting parents if necessary.

## Moral–Spiritual Development

You can assist parents in understanding the importance of their role and that of peers, school, and even literature and the media, in moral and spiritual development. The child is learning many particulars about his or her religion, such as Allah, God, Jesus, prayer, rites, ancestor worship, life after death, reincarnation, heaven, and hell, all of which are developed into a religious philosophy and used in making an interpretation of the world. These ideas are taught by family, friends, teachers, church, books, radio, and television.

The child of six can understand God as creator, expects prayers to be answered, and feels the forces of good and evil with the connotation of reward and punishment. The six-year-old believes in a creative being, a father figure who is responsible for many things such as thunder and lightning. The adult usually interjects the natural or scientific explanation. Somehow the child seems to hold this dual thinking without contradiction. The adult's ability to weave the supernatural with the natural will affect the child's later ability to do so.

The developing schoolchild has a great capacity for reverence and awe, continues to ask more appropriate questions about religious teaching and God, and can be taught through stories that emphasize moral traits. The child operates from a simple framework of ideas and will earnestly pray for recovery and protection from danger for self and others. In prepuberty, the child begins to comprehend disappointments more fully, and to realize that his or her answers to problems or desires to change the world quickly are not always possible. He or she realizes that self-centred prayers are not always answered and that no magic is involved.

The schoolchild can be in the conventional stage of moral development, according to Kohlberg.[209] Beliefs about right and wrong have less to do with the child's actual behaviour than with the likelihood of getting caught for transgression and the gains to derive from the transgression. Other factors that influence moral development include the child's intelligence, ability to delay gratification, and sense of self-esteem. The child with high self-esteem and a favourable self-concept is less likely to engage in immoral behaviour, possibly because he or she will feel guiltier with wrongdoing. Thus, moral behaviour may be more a matter of strength of will or ego than of strength of conscience or superego. Morality is not a fixed behavioural trait, but is rather a decision-making capacity. The child progresses from an initial premoral stage, in which he or she responds primarily to reward and punishment and believes that rules can be broken to meet personal needs, through a rule-based, highly conventional morality, and finally to the stage of self-accepted principles.[210]

Part of moral development is the ability to follow rules. Unlike the preschooler who initiates rules without understanding them, the seven- or eight-year-old begins to play in a genuinely social manner. Rules are mutually accepted by all players and are rigidly followed. They come from some external force such as God and are believed to be timeless. Not until the age of 11 or 12, when the formal operations level of cognition is reached, does the child understand the true nature of rules—that they exist to make the game possible and can be altered by mutual agreement.

Moral development is related to self-discipline and empathy, and how this is taught varies with the culture.

## HEALTH PROMOTION IN NURSING PRACTICE

Your role in caring for the school-aged child and family has been described in each section of this chapter. Please be sure to consider the issues of both the child and the parent, their strengths and healthy responses. Interventions may involve measures that promote health (e.g., immunization or the control of hazards), teaching, support, counselling, or spiritual care with the child or family. Or you might direct care measures to the ill child. Your understanding of the child, developmentally, will enable you to provide holistic care—care that includes physiologic, emotional, cognitive, social, and spiritual aspects of the person.

# SUMMARY

1. The schoolchild grows at a steady pace and continues physical growth and cognitive, emotional, social, and moral–spiritual development.

2. The growth spurt at prepuberty or preadolescence accelerates and influences development in all dimensions. Sexual identity is strengthened.

3. Relationships with parents, siblings, peers, and other adults change and influence development in all dimensions.

4. The child is learning to get along with a variety of people in diverse settings.

5. Family is especially important as a base, while the significance to the child of peer relations develops.

6. The buddy of the same sex is a major support, and he or she is vital in psychological, self-concept, and social development.

7. The child meets many challenges, faces and overcomes insecurities, and develops competence, all of which indicates industry and development of concrete operations.

8. School, home, and community provide the needed avenues for development in all dimensions.

9. The box entitled "Considerations for the Schoolchild and Family in Health Care" summarizes what you should consider in assessment and health promotion with the schoolchild. The family is included.

## Considerations for the Schoolchild and Family in Health Care

- Family and cultural background and values, the school, the support systems available, community resources
- Parents' ability to guide the child, to help the child develop coping skills and gain the necessary competencies
- Relationships among family members
- Behaviours that indicate a parent (or parents) or another significant adult, such as a relative or teacher, is perpetuating abuse, neglect, or maltreatment
- Relationships among the family, school, and other community organizations (church, clubs) and resources
- Physical growth patterns, characteristics and competencies, nutritional status, and rest/sleep and exercise patterns that indicate health and are within age norms for the school-aged child
- Growth spurt and secondary sex changes in prepubescence that indicate normal development in the boy or girl; self-concept and body image development related to physical growth
- Nutritional requirements are greater than those for the adult
- Immunizations, safety education, and other health promotion measures
- Cognitive characteristics and behavioural patterns in the preschool child that demonstrate curiosity and concrete operations (concept formation, realistic thinking, and beginning social and moral value formation)
- Educational/school programs, demonstration of development of co-operation, compromise, and collaboration as well as competition
- Communication patterns; effect of television, computer, or the other media on communication, learning, and behaviour
- Overall appearance and behavioural patterns at home, school, and in the community that indicate development of industry rather than inferiority
- Use of adaptive mechanisms that promote a sense of security, assist the child with relationships, promote realistic control of anxiety and age-appropriate emotional responses in the face of stressors
- Behavioural patterns that indicate ongoing superego development and continuing moral–spiritual development
- Behavioural patterns and characteristics that indicate the child has achieved developmental tasks
- Parental behaviours that indicate they are achieving their developmental tasks
- Learning basic adult concepts and knowledge to be able to reason and engage in tasks of everyday living

## Interesting Websites

### Child & Family Canada

www.cfc-efc.ca

This is a unique Canadian public education website. Fifty Canadian non-profit organizations have come together under the banner of Child & Family Canada to provide quality, credible resources on children and families on an easy-to-navigate website. The managing partner of the consortium is the Canadian Child Care Federation.

### Centre for Immunization and Respiratory Infectious Diseases (CIRID)

www.phac-aspc.gc.ca/irid-diir/index.html

CIRID's mandate is to prevent, reduce, or eliminate vaccine-preventable and infectious respiratory diseases; reduce the negative impact of emerging and re-emerging respiratory infections; and maintain public and professional confidence in immunization programs in Canada. This is carried out in collaboration with the provinces and territories, other federal departments, and other national and international stakeholders.

### Safe Kids Canada

www.sickkids.on.ca/safekidscanada/default.asp

As a national leader, Safe Kids Canada is committed to reducing unintentional injury—the leading cause of death for children. By building partnerships and using a comprehensive approach, it advances safety and reduces the burden of injuries to Canada's children and youth. It advocates for changes to policy, standards, and legislation to keep children and youth safe where they live, play, and learn, and as they travel.

### Healthy Active Living for Children and Youth

www.cps.ca/english/statements/HAL/HAL02-01.htm

Physical inactivity among children and youth is reaching epidemic proportions in Canada. More than half of children and youth are not active enough for optimal growth and development. To help combat the growing problem of physical inactivity among Canadian children and youth, the Canadian Paediatric Society has developed tools and resources to help pediatricians and other health care professionals educate parents and patients about the benefits of physical activity, good nutrition, and an active lifestyle.

## Key Terms

classification (371)

combination (371)

concrete operations (369)

conservation (371)

decentring (371)

fantasy (393)

gifted child (378)

identification (393)

industry (387)

inferiority (388)

isolation (393)

juvenile period (350)

latchkey child (353)

late childhood (350)

malingering (393)

middle childhood (350)

multiplication (371)

nesting (371)

preadolescence (350)

prepubescence (350)

projection (393)

rabies (366)

rationalization (393)

reaction formation (393)

regression (393)

resilient (389)

reversibility (371)

ritualistic behaviour (393)

school phobia (376)

scoliosis (359)

seriation (371)

sublimation (393)

Theory of Multiple Intelligences (374)

transformation (371)

Triarchic Theory of Intelligence (373)

undoing (393)

vulnerable (389)

# Chapter 11

## Assessment and Health Promotion for the Adolescent and Youth

*For some, adolescence is short; for others, adolescence extends many years.*

Ruth Beckmann Murray

## Objectives

*Study of this chapter will enable you to:*

1 Examine the impact of adolescence on family life and the influence of the family on the adolescent.

2 Examine second-order changes in family status required to proceed developmentally in the family life cycle stage: families with adolescents.

3 Describe the physiological changes, including nutrition, exercise, and rest, of the adolescent.

4 Dialogue with parents about the cognitive, self-concept, sexual, emotional, and moral–spiritual aspects of the development of the adolescent, including various ways in which the family can support their healthy progress.

5 Identify examples of adolescent peer-group dialect and their use of leisure time. Discuss how knowledge of these issues can be used in your health promotion activities and teaching.

6 Explore the developmental crisis of identity formation with the adolescent and the parents, the significance of achieving this crisis for ongoing maturity, and ways to counteract influences that interfere with identity formation.

8 Assess and work effectively with an adolescent in all types of settings.

9 Discuss the challenges of the transitional period to young adulthood and your role in facilitating the transition from late adolescence into young adulthood.

10 Identify common health problems of the adolescent, factors that contribute to them, and your role in contributing to the adolescent's health.

How can I best describe my son? He is 13 years old, but physically and mentally he could pass for 16. He has the physique of a football player and appears to grow taller each day. His general knowledge is superior because he watches television for at least two hours a day, scans the morning and evening papers, and listens to the radio periodically during the day. He is full of contradictions; for example, he talks about love, but a hug or sign of affection from his mother will send him running to his room.

## PERSPECTIVES ON ADOLESCENCE

Adolescence is a time of passage, signalling the end of childhood and the beginning of adulthood. Adolescence is a developmental stage that differs cross-culturally in various ways. In Canada, children are maturing physiologically at an earlier age than previously. The increase in adult height, and the change in age at which physical maturation occurs, are called *secular growth trends*. This trend is attributed to improved nutrition and health practices. Along with early maturation, the developmental period is being extended now because of social, economic, employment, industrial, technological, and family changes. During adolescence, relationships with parents are different than when the child was in middle childhood. Times with peers become more intimate. Dating occurs, and so does sexual exploration; even sexual intercourse occurs for many by the end of adolescence.[1]

## DEFINITIONS

In the past, many people equated puberty with adolescence. Now, they are considered separate components. Puberty is preceded by prepuberty, which is discussed in Chapter 10.

**Puberty** is *a period of rapid physical maturation involving hormonal and bodily changes that happen during early adolescence.*[2] *Sexual maturation* first becomes possible with the onset of **spermatogenesis** (*production of spermatozoa*) and **menstruation** (*onset of menses*). Second, bodily changes occur, which include a dramatic increase in weight and height, as well as changes in the fat and muscle content of the body.[3] **Adolescence** is *the period in life that begins with puberty, and extends for eight to ten years or longer*, until the person is physically and psychologically mature, ready to assume adult responsibilities and be self-sufficient—all because of changes in intellect, attitudes, and interests.[4]

## Timing and Variation in Puberty

Although puberty begins at about age 10 in the average girl, and at about age 12 in the average boy, for many children puberty begins months, or even years, before or after these norms.[5] For girls, menarche (first menstruation) is considered within the normal range if it appears between the ages of 8 and 16. It is possible for the girl to become pregnant shortly after menarche, but irregular menstrual cycles are the norm for some time. Full adult fertility develops over a period of time.[6] An early maturing boy might begin puberty at age 11, whereas a late maturing boy might start at 14 or 15.[7]

The recent questioning of pubertal effects, in terms of overall development and adjustment in the human lifespan, suggests that pubertal variations are less dramatic than was commonly thought a few years ago. Many changes occur in the adolescent's world. These include cognitive, social, and personality aspects. All of these important processes work together to produce the identity of the adolescent.[8]

## FAMILY DEVELOPMENT AND RELATIONSHIPS

### Family Life Cycle

Refer to Table 4-3, which illustrates the stages of the family life cycle, the emotional processes of transition (key principles), and the second-order changes in the family required to proceed developmentally. Stage 4, families with adolescents, is the appropriate stage for the family with an adolescent. The overall family goal at this time is to allow the adolescent increasing freedom and responsibility to prepare himself or herself for young adulthood. Another change that often occurs at this time is that the family must be observant of the beginning need to care for the grandparents.[9]

---

**CRITICAL THINKING**

*What family-related issues and activities can you expect to arise in a family with frail grandparents?*

---

### Family Relationships

Discuss with the parents the following information and the points in the box entitled "Communicating with Your Teen." The home should provide an accepting and emotionally stable environment for the adolescent.

During early adolescence (ages 13 to 14), the teen typically remains involved in family activities and functions. Gradually, family relationships change and the adolescent develops social ties and close relationships with peers outside the family. The family's beliefs, lifestyles, values, and patterns of interaction may influence the development of these relationships. It is an important fact to remember that adolescents have been found to be more likely to have higher self-esteem when their parents are affectionate and involved with them.[10]

It is during late adolescence (ages 15 to 18) that the most dramatic changes occur in the parent–child relationship (see the box entitled "Adolescent's View of Parents").[11] The relationship must evolve from a dependency status to mutual affection, equality, and autonomy. This growing independence means that teens spend less time with their parents, and often argue with them about matters of taste, style, and freedom.[12] Parents should gradually increase the teenager's responsibilities and allow privileges that formerly were denied. The adolescent strongly desires to make independent decisions and to have increased freedom of movement. At the same time, he or she needs financial support, food, and safe

## Communicating with Your Teen

- Make time for listening and talking.
- Create a beginning and an ending to the day.
- Respect the teen's privacy; do not insist on his or her disclosure.
- Do not judge or shame; state facts and recognition of differences.
- Say "thank you" and "please" as appropriate.
- Be generous with honest praise.
- Apologize when it is appropriate.
- Let the teen make choices and the inevitable mistakes.
- Talk about ways to cope with the consequences of unwise decisions.
- Avoid lectures, preaching, talking down, or sarcasm.
- Use open-ended questions, such as "How was your day?"
- Speak to feelings—"you look frustrated"—or reflect back feelings that are disclosed.
- Nurture mealtime conversation; turn off the television, radio, computer, and stereo.
- Plan family times that emphasize casual talk.
- Take advantage of driving time, especially when you are alone with the teen, to talk. The need for the parent who is driving to keep "eyes on the road," thereby avoiding eye contact, often helps exploration of sensitive issues.
- Welcome their friends; engage them in conversation, often through activity.
- Use "I" statements. If you have a plan, be open about it (e.g., a shopping trip).
- Keep the teen and self in perspective.
- Talk about the behaviour, not the person.
- Talk about one issue at a time; do not bring in past events or behaviour unrelated to the current topic.
- Make requests in a neutral, kind tone of voice, assertively but not commandingly.

## Adolescent's View of Parents

### Ages 13 to 14

- No longer sees parents as all-powerful
- Feels parents love him or her but do not necessarily understand him or her
- Continues dependence on parents and seeks their emotional support

### Ages 15 to 18

- Continues need for parental support in self-evaluation of power and worth
- Continues selective process of self-identity by choosing various aspects of parental behaviour, feelings, and values
- Tends to gain autonomy through respect and continued affection for parents rather than through rebellious behaviour

In contrast to popular stereotypes, the development of freedom most often does not involve rebellion, nor is it usually accompanied by tense relationships. In households where guidelines are clear and consistent, and changes in these guidelines are open to discussion in an atmosphere of warmth and trust, a smooth maturational process usually occurs during the adolescent years.[14]

### CRITICAL THINKING

*What is your view regarding the notion that adolescence is typically a time of bitter conflict between the parents and the adolescent?*

## Changing Directions in Family Relationships

For some teens, there is little family life, not even discord. Sixty-three percent of teens are in households where both parents work outside of the home. Many teens help care for younger siblings and juggle part-time work with school and home responsibilities. At least half have lived through their parents' divorce. Loneliness, isolation, and craving attention from parents are major issues. These situations create a vacuum in which they must survive an intense peer culture. If parents and adults abdicate power, teenagers come up with their own rules.

Although many teens use computers and other technologies to send instant messages, visit chat rooms, download songs, or do homework, some are increasingly in their own secret world. The computer, Internet, video games, and other demands are creating new worlds that are

sanctuary. Parents must resist granting instant adult status when the child reaches teen years. Instead, they should remember that the adolescent needs to be independent yet remain dependent. Although he or she protests, the teen actually values parental guidelines, especially if those guidelines are reasonable. The adolescent feels more self-confident in exploring the environment if reasonable limits are imposed. Parents should listen to their adolescent's viewpoints concerning restrictions. Those viewpoints may offer hints about the readiness for additional independence and freedom.[13]

essentially unknown to adults. New technologies and the entertainment industry, combined with changes in family structure, have tended to isolated parents and other adults from teens. Many teens live in a reality that excludes parents and adults. Teens have less access to parents, more access to potentially damaging information, and more opportunity to engage in damaging behaviour. Stresses that frequently produce family discord in North America grow out of conflicting value systems between the generations of parents and their children. Today's adolescents are a generation born with technology, which tends to require less emphasis on people skills. Technology has brought remote corners of the world into their homes and minds and has fostered an attitude of questioning instead of reliance on authority. Grant states that a growing concern exists about whether the exposure of teenagers to sexual content in the media has an effect on their sexual attitudes and behaviours.[15]

Parents need support to see that the adolescent is a product of his or her time, and that their teenager is reflecting what is happening socially. In some families, the teen may turn to some form of alternate sexual orientation.[16]

Some parents may adhere to rules and the status quo to bolster their own security or cultural traditions rather than change for the offspring's benefit; other parents may overprotect. If the adolescent has come from a family that has provided past opportunities to learn responsibility, self-reliance, skills, and self-respect, he or she will make a smoother transition from childhood dependency to adulthood independence. If parents have been too liberal, overly permissive, or uninterested, the adolescent will have more difficulty adjusting because the past lacked appropriate structure and a system of relevant standards or values. He or she has no point of reference, other than peers, to determine whether the behaviour is suitable and if decisions are appropriate.[17]

One family factor that may affect parent–adolescent communication and relationships is the *stepfamily*, the adoptive family, or the *foster family structure*. Often, adolescents in these families struggle with whether they really belong to the family (see Chapter 4). The adopted and foster child may search for the birth parent(s). If this occurs, adoptive parents should co-operate rather than feel threatened. Because of the proliferation of divorce, single parenting, and stepfamilies, these adolescents may display a puzzling variety of behaviours. In one study, Mahon and her colleagues examined differences in anger, anxiety, and depression between early adolescents from divorced families and early adolescents from intact families. They concluded that early adolescents from divorced families reported higher levels of anger compared to their counterparts from intact families.[18]

## Abuse, Neglect, and Maltreatment

*Careful screening* and *astute communication skills* are essential. You must establish a relationship, and interview the adolescent alone. If you do so, you are more likely to learn of physical, sexual, and psychological abuse (maltreatment) or neglect.

Abuse, neglect, and maltreatment occur to numerous adolescents. Unfortunately, health care professionals may not always be alert to the physical and psychological cues that signify such turmoil. The adolescent who has been physically abused may appear in the emergency room with some of the same types of injuries that are seen in the younger child.[19] See Chapters 4, 6, 7, and 9 for further insights into these situations.

Research conducted in Canada with 16 refugee children and 16 children of battered women (aged 10 to 17 years) revealed parallels and common themes in their stories: pain, suffering, feelings of betrayal, uncertainty about the enemy, lack of a sense of peace, and finding unexpected resources. Both groups of children used creative strategies to survive physical, emotional, social, and cultural violence.[20]

### CRITICAL THINKING

*As a health professional, how can you help reduce maltreatment of the adolescent?*

## PHYSIOLOGIC CONCEPTS
## Influences on Physical Growth

The precise physiologic causes for the characteristic physical changes of adolescence remain unknown. It appears that the hypothalamus, probably in some way related to brain maturation, initiates the pubertal process through secretion of neurohumoral releasing factors. These neurohumors stimulate the anterior pituitary gland to release gonadotropic hormones, somatotropic hormone (STH) or growth hormone (GH), thyroid-stimulating hormone (TSH), and adrenocorticotropic hormone (ACTH). The amygdala, in the limbic system, apparently changes function and is thought to promote hormonal production.[21]

Gonadotropic hormones (follicle-stimulating hormone [FSH] and luteinizing hormone [LH]) stimulate the gonads to mature and produce sex hormones. In females, FSH stimulates the ovaries to produce estrogen and LH stimulates the Leydig cells in the testes to produce testosterone. The growth and development of the adrenal cortex and the stimulation of the secretion of androgens are promoted by ACTH. These androgens are responsible for producing secondary sex characteristics. Deoxyribonucleic acid (DNA) synthesis and hyperplastic cell growth, particularly of the bones and cartilage, are stimulated by STH. Under the influence of STH, thyroxin secretion is slightly increased during the pubertal period. Thyroxin levels increase to meet body metabolic needs.[22]

Both male and female hormones are produced in varying amounts, in both sexes, throughout life. During the prepubescent years, the adrenal cortex secretes a small amount of sex hormones. It is the production of sex hormones, however, that accompanies maturation of the ovaries and testes that is responsible for the physiologic changes observed in puberty. Physiologic changes in the male are produced by androgens, whereas large amounts of estrogens are responsible for the production of changes in the female.[23]

## Physical Characteristics

Your understanding of growth and development provides a unique perspective for helping adolescents and their parents anticipate and cope with the stresses of adolescence. Primary health care activities such as education can promote healthy development.[24] You can be especially helpful in teaching the adolescent about these topics, and you can offer special opportunities for discussion. Additional information can be obtained from the local library, community health resource, or counsellor.

**Growth**   Adolescence is the second major period of accelerated growth (infancy was the first). The growth spurt refers to the general increase in the growth of the skeleton, muscles, and internal organs. The adolescent growth spurt occurs approximately two years earlier in the female than in the male. Genetic endowment is the most important determinant of the onset, rate, and duration of pubertal growth.[25]

Changes in appearance occur, and growth is likely to be asymmetrical (Asynchronous Principle of Development). The nose, lips, and ears often grow larger before the head increases in size. Weight is likely to be gained before height increases occur. The girl is likely to gain in cumulative volume of fat; the boy tends to drop fat tissue. There is a steady increase in strength. Late-maturing individuals tend to be taller than their peers during late adolescence.[26]

During adolescence, females grow 5 to 20 cm (2 to 8 inches) and gain 7 to 25 kg (15 to 55 pounds). Males grow an average of 10 to 30 cm (4 to 12 inches) and gain 7 to 30 kg (15 to 65 pounds). In the initial phase of the growth spurt, the increase in height is due to lengthening of the legs. Later, most of the increase is in the trunk length. The total process of change takes approximately three years in females and four years in males.[27] Between age 15 and 18, girls and most boys are approaching full adult size and appearance. The teen is more physically stable, and body equilibrium is being re-established. The person is less awkward and handles his or

her body more efficiently.[28] Every system of the body is growing rapidly, but physiologic changes occur unevenly within the person.

**Sexual Development**   Four physical characteristics define puberty for most adolescents.[29]

*Females*

- Height spurt: ages 8 to 17; peak age, 12
- Menarche: ages 10 to 16; average age, 12.5
- Breast development: ages 8 to 18
- Pubic and underarm hair: ages 11 to 14

*Males*

- Height spurt: ages 10 to 20; peak age, 14
- Penile development: ages 10 to 16
- Testicular development: ages 9 to 17
- Pubic, facial, underarm, and chest hair: ages 12 to 16

*Menarche* is the indicator of puberty and sexual maturity in the female. Ovulation and regular menstrual periods usually begin 6 to 14 months after menarche. The onset of menarche varies among population groups and is influenced by heredity, nutrition, health care, and other environmental factors.[30] In industrialized countries today, the average age of menarche onset is 12.5 to 13.5 years. Research on the onset of menarche has revealed conflicting results. Some research has shown a relationship between the height and weight of a girl, and menarche. Internationally, the recent decrease in the average age at first menses has not been seen in countries where individuals are more likely to be malnourished and suffer from chronic illnesses.[31]

*Secondary sex characteristics in the female* begin to develop in prepuberty (see Chapter 10) and may take two to eight years for completion. Breast enlargement and elevation occur; areola and papillae project to form a secondary mound. Axillary and pubic hair grows thicker, becomes darker, and spreads over the pubic area.[32]

*Spermatogenesis* (**sperm production**) and seminal emissions mark puberty and sexual maturity in the male. The first ejaculate of seminal fluid occurs approximately one year after the penis has begun its adolescent growth. **Nocturnal emissions**, *expulsion of seminal fluid during sleep*, occur at approximately age 14.[33] Little research exists on the boy's feelings about the *first ejaculation* (**spermarche**), which occurs at the average age of 13.[34]

*Secondary sex characteristics in the male* begin in prepuberty (see Chapter 10) and may take two to five years for completion. Changes in body shape, growth of body hair, muscle development, changes in voice and complexion, and stronger body odours may continue to develop until

19 or 20, or even until the late twenties. The penis, scrotum, and testes enlarge; the scrotum reddens and scrotal skin changes texture. Hair grows at the axilla and base of the penis and spreads over the pubis. Body hair, especially facial hair, generally increases. The voice continues to deepen.[35]

**Sex hormones** are *biochemical agents that primarily influence the structure and function of the sex organs, and initiate the appearance of specific sexual characteristics.* **Androgens** are *hormones that produce male-type physical characteristics and behaviours.* **Estrogens** are *hormones that produce feminine characteristics.* **Progesterones** are *female hormones that prepare the uterus to accept a fetus and maintain the pregnancy.* They may have other functions in the body as well. All three sex hormones occur in both sexes. Androgens are found in greater amounts in males; the other two hormones exist in greater amounts in females.[36] More information about the function of sex hormones can be obtained in any good physiology text.[37]

Normal menstrual patterns are averages based on observations and reports from large groups of women.[38] Generally, a woman's menstrual frequency stabilizes at 28 days within 1 to 2 years after puberty, with a range of 26 to 34 days.[39] In early adolescence, irregular bleeding, both in length of cycle and amount, is the rule rather than the exception. It takes approximately 15 months to complete the first 10 cycles, and an average of 20 cycles before ovulation occurs regularly.[40]

Customarily, the menstrual cycle is divided into four phases, named for the major events that occur in them.[41] These phases are briefly discussed:

- *Menses or menstrual period*: occurs on days 1 to 5 of a new cycle.

- *Postmenstrual phase*: occurs before the end of the menses and ovulation. In a 28-day cycle, it usually occurs during cycle days 6 to 13 or 14. This phase is also called the estrogenic phase, or the follicular phase, because of the high blood estrogen level resulting from secretion by the developing follicle.

- *Ovulation*: is the rupture of the mature follicle with the expulsion of its ovum into the pelvic cavity that occurs frequently on cycle day 14 in a 28-day cycle. However, ovulation occurs on different days in cycles of different lengths, depending on the length of the pre-ovulatory phase. Typically, there is a decrease in basal temperature just before ovulation, and a rise in temperature occurs at the time of ovulation.

- *Premenstrual phase*: occurs between ovulation and the onset of menses. This phase is also called the luteal phase, or the secretory phase, because the corpus luteum secretes only during this time. In addition, it is also called the progesterone phase because the corpus luteum secretes mainly progesterone. The length of the premenstrual phase is fairly constant, lasting usually 14 days—during cycle days 15 to 28 in a 28-day cycle. Differences in length of the total menstrual cycle exist mainly because of differences in the duration of the postmenstrual, rather than the premenstrual, cycle.[42]

**Primary dysmenorrhea**, a *condition associated with abnormally increased uterine activity,* is due to myometrium contractions induced by prostaglandins in the second half of the menstrual cycle.[43] Pain begins at the onset of menstrual flow and lasts from 8 to 48 hours. The release of most prostaglandins during menstruation occurs in the first 48 hours, which coincides with the greatest intensity of symptoms.[44] Primary dysmenorrhea is not caused by some underlying pathology; rather, it is the occurrence of a physiological alteration in some women. This problem is most common in women in their late teens and early twenties. Its incidence declines with age. Management of primary dysmenorrhea depends on the severity of the problem and on the individual woman's response to various treatments. Health care professionals, such as nurses, can correct myths and misinformation about menstruation and dysmenorrhea by providing facts about what is the norm. Recently, non-steroidal anti-inflammatory agents have been used with some success. Some women find that adherence to a certain diet, such as one with decreased intakes of salt and sugar, may result in reduced discomfort. Both increased water intake, which may serve as a natural diuretic, and exercise habits can decrease symptoms. Heat to the painful area may be palliative.[45]

The hormonal system for reproductive behaviour is much simpler in the male because there is no cyclical pattern. The male gonads, the testes, produce sperm continuously and secrete androgens. The major androgen is testosterone.[46]

Just as FSH promotes the development of the ovum in the female, testosterone promotes the development of sperm in the male. A continuous level of sperm production takes place in the seminiferous tubules inside the testes. The secretion of LH stimulates the Leydig cells to secrete the androgen.[47]

**Musculoskeletal System** Structural changes, growth in skeletal size, muscle mass, adipose tissue, and skin are significant during adolescence. The skeletal system grows faster than the supporting muscles, hands and feet grow out of proportion to the body, and large muscles develop faster than small muscles. Poor posture and decreased coordination result. Males and females differ in skeletal growth patterns. Males have greater length in arms and legs relative to trunk size, in part because of a prolonged prepubertal growth period in boys. Males tend to be clumsier than females. Males have a greater shoulder width—a difference that begins in pre-puberty. Ossification of the skeletal system occurs later for boys than girls. In boys, testosterone promotes the growth of skeletal muscles. Testosterone is responsible for greater male muscular development and strength, and the growth of bone.[48] In girls, estrogen influences ossification and early unity of the epiphyses with shafts of the long bones, resulting in shorter stature. Muscle growth continues in males during late adolescence because of androgen production. Muscle growth in females is proportionate to the growth of other tissue. Adipose tissue distribution over thighs, buttocks, and breasts occurs predominantly in females, and is related to estrogen production.[49]

**Skin** The skin texture changes noticeably during adolescence. Sebaceous glands become extremely active, and they increase in size. Eccrine sweat glands are fully developed. They are especially responsive to emotional stimuli, and are more active in males. Apocrine sweat glands also begin to secrete in response to emotional stimuli.[50] Because facial glands are more active, **acne** (*pimples*) emerges.

**Cardiovascular System** The size and strength of the heart, blood volume, and systolic blood pressure all increase. The heat rate, however, decreases. These changes appear earlier in girls, who establish a slightly higher pulse rate and a slightly lower systolic blood pressure than boys do. On the other hand, blood volume, which has increased steadily during childhood, reaches higher levels in boys than in girls, a fact that may be related to the increased muscle mass in pubertal boys. Adult values are reached for all formed elements in the blood. Interestingly, increases occur in serum iron, the number of red blood cells, hemoglobin, and hematocrit in boys, but not in girls.[51] Hypertension tends to increase in adolescents males, in obese persons, and in those with a family history of hypertension. Higher systolic pressure occurs in urban dwellers. Higher diastolic pressure has been seen in those who smoke and who lack regular exercise. *Routine screening for hypertension should be carried out.*

**Respiratory System** The lungs increase both in diameter and length during puberty. Respiratory rate averages 16 to 20 per minute. Respiratory volume, vital capacity, and other physiological properties related to respiratory function increase to a greater extent in boys than in girls. Males have a greater shoulder width and chest size, resulting in greater respiratory volume, greater vital capacity, and increased respiration.[52]

**Brain Development** Adolescence is a time of continued brain growth. Two major growth spurts occur in the brain during the teenage years. The first involves the cerebral cortex, which becomes thicker and whose neuronal pathways become more efficient. The second involves the frontal lobes of the cerebral cortex. This area controls logic and planning, and neural activity coincides with the more advanced cognitive capacities that occur in youth.[53]

**Cultural Differences** Genetic differences can impact physical development and should be considered by nurses. For example, children of certain African heritages may attain a greater proportion of their adult stature earlier, and their skeletal mass may be greater. Using European norms of measurement means that bone loss could go undetected. Because of the changing body, the adolescent needs, in addition to sex education, information about the normality of anatomic and physiological changes. Because sexual health is a major aspect of personal health, and because it affects people at all ages and stages of their lives regardless of culture, the publication *Canadian Guidelines for Sexual Health Education* provides a valuable source to unite and guide individuals and professionals working in the area of sexual health education.[54]

---

**CRITICAL THINKING**

*What are some beliefs of the adolescent in the Western culture, as compared to non-Western cultures, regarding their pubertal growth changes?*

---

## Physical Assessment of the Adolescent

Regular physical examinations should be encouraged. The examination is conducted in much the same manner as for the adult. However, it is crucial that the examiner knows and understands the special emotional needs, developmental changes, age and maturation level of the person, and physiologic differences specific to adolescence. Several authors have provided valuable information on how to promote physical and emotional comfort while gathering the necessary evidence during a pelvic examination, including after rape.[55]

Confidentiality and trust are key issues when working with the adolescent. Be sure to express honestly to the teen what parts of the interview and examination can be kept in strict confidence, and what parts may need to be shared. The specific age of the person and the nature of the findings determine these factors.

Physical complaints and emotional symptoms may relate to underlying problems of drug abuse, alcoholism, sexual uncertainties and stress, date rape, pregnancy or fear of pregnancy, fear of sexually transmitted disease, depression, family or peer adjustment problems, school problems, or concerns about future plans.

The blood pressure should be at adult levels. The athlete in training may have a pulse rate slower than that of his or her less athletic peers.

Pallor, especially in girls, should be a strong cue to check hemoglobin levels.

The teen needs frequent dental visits because most have caries. Many young adolescents have orthodontic work in progress, or completed.

Because myopia seems to increase during these years, reading and studying tend to promote eye strain. Encourage regular eye examinations.

Although breast neoplasms are not common to this age group, females should be taught breast self-examination. Use this opportunity to discuss the importance of routine breast self-examination so that it becomes a practised habit during later years.[56] It is important to note that girls should not be surprised to find some asymmetric breast development.

The heart should be found at the fifth left intercostal space, as in the adult. Most functional murmurs tend to be outgrown. However, evaluate heart sounds for the following:

- *Quality*: sounds should be clear and distinct
- *Intensity*: sounds should not be either weak or pounding
- *Rate*: sounds should be the same as the radial pulse
- *Rhythm*: sounds should be regular and even[57]

Serum cholesterol and triglyceride levels should be obtained if there is a family history of cardiovascular disease. Preventive dietary and exercise regimens should be discussed.

The size and shape of the abdomen can give some indication of general nutritional status and muscular development. During adolescence, the usual male and female contours of the pelvic cavity change the shape of the abdomen to form characteristic adult curves, especially in the female.

The examiner should be acutely aware not only of the pattern of sexual development of both males and females, but also of the concerns and questions that may be voiced. The presence of the testes in the scrotum is of primary importance because undescended testicles at this age can signal sterility. Health Canada recommends that women should have their first Papanicolaou (Pap) smears at age 18, or when the adolescent becomes sexually active, whichever comes first. Pelvic examinations are also important. These procedures, done for the first time and followed by explanations of the terms with as much gentleness as possible, can set a positive tone for future examinations. It is important to initiate discussion about these issues at any appointment, because the adolescent may be in need of counselling.[58]

---

### CRITICAL THINKING

*What do you need to consider as you address the personal hygiene habits of an adolescent?*

---

Improving the health habits and quality of life of adolescents is important for community health nurses.[59] In fact, developing health promotion programs that are attractive to teenagers can be a major challenge. For example, in a rural Nova Scotia school district the teens were brought into the design and implementation of the *Teens for Healthy Living Project*. One of the most important implications for nurses that arose from the program is that nurses who are involved in planning and delivering health promotion programs for youth need to do so in collaboration with the teens.[60] Based on the longitudinal *National Population Health Survey*, which included 1493 adolescents aged 12 to 19 years, Vingilis and her colleagues examined the factors that predict adolescents' concepts of their health. The study suggests that adolescents' appraisals of their heath are shaped by their overall sense of functioning, which includes physical health and non-physical health dimensions—such as lifestyle, behaviours, and personal and socioeconomic factors.[61]

## Nutritional Needs

Physical, emotional, and social change characterize the time of adolescence. Adolescent girls may be at risk for inadequate energy and nutrient intake, especially of calcium and iron.[62] Because of a desire to be thin, many adolescent girls may excessively restrict their energy food intake. That is, to achieve weight loss, adolescent girls may deliberately skip meals, eat on the run, and adopt other irregular eating behaviours, including disordered eating. McVey and her colleagues examined the prevalence of dieting and negative eating habits of 2279 females (aged 10 to 14 years) in southern Ontario. They found that those with elevated ChEAT (Children's version of the Eating Attitudes Test) scores of 20 or higher were significantly more likely than those with lower scores to be engaged in dieting and other extreme weight-control measures. They state that the results suggest that unhealthy dieting behaviours are reported in girls as young as ten years of age.[63] On the other hand, boys usually have large appetites and consume a lot of food.[64] A few practical considerations to use with adolescents include:

- Assess whether their eating patterns follow the revised *Eating Well with Canada's Food Guide* (see www.hc-sc.gc.ca/fn-an/food-guide-aliment/index_e.html).[65]
- Identify adolescent girls who may be restricting their food consumption in order to be thin. Advise them on healthy eating patterns that promote healthy growth and development.
- Teach an integrated approach to healthy eating, active living, and the building of a positive self-concept.

- Encourage a healthy eating pattern according to *Eating Well with Canada's Food Guide*, which emphasizes limiting foods high in calories, fat, sugar, or salt such as French fries, potato chips, nachos and other salty snacks, fruit-flavoured drinks, soft drinks, and sports and energy drinks.[66]

- Provide factual and realistic information about body size to counteract social pressures to attain an unrealistic body weight.

- If you suspect an adolescent has an eating disorder or a problem with substance abuse, refer him or her to appropriate agencies in your community.[67]

In the development of nutrition intervention programs for teens, it is important to consider their culture and ethnic backgrounds, recognizing that food habits may differ.[68]

Taylor and her associates conducted a review to outline the state of knowledge and identify research gaps in the issue of determinants of healthy eating among children and youth. They defined health as eating habits and behaviours that are consistent with improving, maintaining and/or enhancing health. Several collective factors stand out as significant influences on healthy eating among children and youth. Some of these are familial factors such as food exposure and availability, parenting style, and food socialization practices. Others include the nature of foods available in the physical environment, such as at home, at schools, and in fast-food establishments. The media, particularly television, exerts an enormous influence on food selection, and can overshadow familial factors. Individual factors identified include knowledge, attitudes, and food preferences. Food preferences have been identified as a strong determinant of healthy eating in both children and adolescents. The researchers concluded that although the results of the review identified the availability of a significant body of literature on the area of determinants of healthy eating in children and youth, very little of this research has taken place in Canada.[69]

In summary, adolescents need good nutrition both to grow to their full potential and to decrease the risk of obesity and chronic diseases that come in adolescence and later life. The Food Habits of Canadians Study provided data on the important food sources of energy and nutrients in a sample of Canadian teenagers. Results from the survey of 178 teenagers found that a high intake of nutrient-poor foods, particularly high-sugar beverages, was a major problem.[70] The food frequently consumed by teenagers included cakes, cookies, carbonated beverages, salty snacks, and other poor-nutrient foods. Some nutrient-dense foods such as eggs, fish, and organ meats were notable in their absence or low consumption.[71] This high intake of nutrient-poor foods and high-sugar beverages is a serious concern. Health promotion programs for girls that will avert disordered eating behaviours during the preadolescent phase are certainly needed.[72] *Underweight* and *overweight* are probably the two most common, but most overlooked, symptoms of malnutrition. Assess the adolescent, and teach both the adolescent and the parents to foster good health.

---

## CRITICAL THINKING

*Develop a nutritional program for presentation to a grade ten class that focuses on food groups and menu selection.*

---

**Underweight**  Underweight can be caused by an inadequate intake of calories or poor use of the energy. It is often accompanied by fatigue, irritability, anorexia, and digestive disturbances such as constipation or diarrhea. Poor muscular development, evidenced by posture and hypochromic anemia, may be observed. In children and adolescents, growth and development may be delayed. Even with the recommended dietary intakes, malabsorption of protein, fat, or carbohydrate can result in undernutrition. Underweight may be a symptom of an undiagnosed disease.[73]

The most severe form of underweight is seen in individuals with anorexia nervosa and bulimia. You may be the first person to assess these conditions in the adolescent.

A study by Jones and her colleagues examined disturbed eating attitudes and related behaviours of females, 12 to 18 years of age, from a large school-based population in Ontario. It was found that disordered eating attitudes and behaviours were present in more than 27 percent of girls in that age group, and such behaviours tended to increase gradually throughout adolescence.[74] In another study, early adolescent females seeking treatment for an eating disorder were compared with healthy age-matched controls on psychosocial variables relevant to this stage of development. The results indicated that the eating disorder group had significantly lower ratings of competence in physical appearance and higher ratings on the importance of physical appearance and self-oriented perfectionism when compared to the control group. There were no group differences on the parental or peer support variables, or on negative life event variables. The researchers concluded that helping adolescents with eating disorders to lower the importance they place on physical appearance (or to value other domains of self-concept where they feel more competent) as well as to reduce self-oriented perfectionistic tendencies could prove to be a helpful strategy in addition to existing eating disorder treatment programs for early adolescent females.[75]

**Anorexia nervosa** is a *syndrome*, occurring usually in females between the ages of 12 and 18. Onset may occur in the twenties and thirties, *during which the person*

## Signs and Symptoms of Anorexia Nervosa

- Refusal to eat or eating only small amounts yet feeling guilt about eating; excuses about not eating; inability to tolerate sight or smell of food
- Denial of hunger (hunger becomes a battle of wills) but preoccupation with food (plays with food when eating; collects recipes)
- Intense fear of becoming obese, even when underweight; refusal to maintain body weight; compulsive exercise and weighing
- Large (at least 20 to 25 percent) weight loss with no physical illness evident
- Abuse of laxatives or diuretics; frequent trips to bathroom, especially after meals
- Distorted body image; perception of self as fat even when below normal weight

- Vital sign changes: bradycardia, hypotension, hypothermia
- Interruption of normal reproductive system processes in females: at least three consecutive menses missed when otherwise expected to occur
- Malnutrition adversely affecting (1) the skeleton, causing decalcification, decreased bone mass, and osteoporosis; (2) muscular development; (3) cardiac and liver function, arrhythmia; and (4) body metabolic functions, which may decrease as a result of liver involvement
- Skin dry, pale, yellow-tinged; presence of lanugo; hair loss
- Enlargement of brain ventricles, with shrinkage of brain tissue surrounding them; depression, irritability
- Apathy, depression, low motivation, poor concentration
- Regular use of loose-fitting clothing

voluntarily refuses to eat, presumably because of lack of hunger, but actually because of a distorted image of her or his body and conflictual relationships. Refer to the box entitled "Signs and Symptoms of Anorexia Nervosa."[76]

Turrell and her researchers conducted a study to examine conditions that needed to be in place to help adolescents and their families gain the confidence needed to continue recovery at home following the adolescents' hospitalization for anorexia nervosa. They found that the examination of responses revealed four prevalent themes: medical stability, education, psychological changes, and community resource planning. The findings suggest that each group of respondents has unique discharge readiness needs and that nurses have an important role to play in helping clients and their families make the transition home as successful as possible.[77]

Men may also suffer from this disease but may be even more reticent than women to reveal symptoms or seek treatment.[78]

**Bulimia** may be associated with anorexia nervosa and is a *syndrome characterized by voluntary restriction of food intake followed by extreme overeating and self-induced purging, such as vomiting, laxative abuse, and excess exercise.* Refer to the box entitled "Signs and Symptoms of Bulimia."[79]

Anorexia nervosa is more common than bulimia among adolescents, although the latter is increasing in incidence. Often both syndromes exist together. Impaired physiological and psychological functioning, disturbed body image, confused or inaccurate perceptions about body functions, and a sense of incompetence, depression, anger, and helplessness are present in all anorectic and bulimic clients. There are several current theories about the causation and dynamics of anorexia nervosa.[80]

Individuals with anorexia nervosa are usually treated on an outpatient basis. The treatment and management involves three major aspects. First, normal nutrition is reinstituted, or a severe state of malnutrition is reversed. Second, ineffective patterns of family interaction are resolved. Third, individual psychotherapy is provided to manage distortions and deficits in psychological functioning. However, hospitalization may be required, especially for complications, which are treated symptomatically. The anorectic person should be hospitalized if there is electrolyte disturbance; depression with suicidal thoughts or attempts; substantial disorganization of the family; or failure of outpatient treatment. These criteria also apply to the bulimic person; the additional criterion is spontaneous induced purging after binges. Hospitalization may also be helpful in defusing parent–adolescent tensions and the resultant power struggle and in preventing suicide.[81]

The goals of treatment for the anorectic and bulimic client are to:

1. Maintain normal weight
2. Treat the hypokalemia and metabolic alkalosis
3. Prevent physiological complications
4. Change attitudes toward food
5. Develop more effective coping skills to overcome the underlying conflicts

The approach is holistic. *Treatment involves any of the following methods: behaviour modification and insight-oriented, supportive individual, group, or family therapy.*[82] A resource to be considered seriously is the National Eating Disorder Information Centre (NEDIC). This is a Toronto-based non-profit

## Signs and Symptoms of Bulimia

- Binge eating—consumption of excessively large amount of food—followed by self-induced vomiting or laxative and/or diuretic abuse (at least twice weekly); secretive eating; frequent trips to bathroom, especially after eating
- Fear of inability to stop eating voluntarily
- Feeling of lack of control over the eating behaviour during eating binges
- Preoccupation with food and guilt about eating
- Weight fluctuations and fluid and electrolyte imbalances due to binges, fasts, and vomiting/laxatives
- Use of crash diets to control weight
- Weakness, headaches, fatigue, depression, dizziness
- Orthostatic hypotension due to fluid depletion

- Scars on dorsum of hand from induced vomiting
- Loss of tooth enamel and esophageal and gastric bleeding in vomiters
- Chest pain from esophageal reflux or spasm
- Parotid gland enlargement in individuals who vomit; swollen or infected salivary glands
- Increased peristalsis, rectal bleeding, constipation if laxative abuser
- Menstrual irregularities
- Bursting blood vessels in eyes
- Red knuckles from forced vomiting
- More time alone or cooking

organization whose philosophy is to promote healthy lifestyles. It encourages clients to make informed choices based on accurate information. Its national toll-free number is 1-866-NEDIC-20 (1-866-633-4220). (Also see the Interesting Websites section at the end of this chapter.)

Both the family and the adolescent need therapy. *Goals of family therapy* include:

1. Reducing pathogenic conflict and anxiety within the family relationships
2. Becoming more aware of and better at meeting each other's emotional needs
3. Promoting more appropriate role behaviour for each sex and generation
4. Strengthening the capacity of the adolescent and family as a whole to cope with various problems[83]

## CRITICAL THINKING

*How can you help a friend who you realize is bulimic?*

**Overweight** The World Health Organization (WHO) states that obesity is a blatantly visible—yet much neglected—public health problem. Paradoxically, together with undernutrition, an escalating global epidemic of overweight and obesity—"globesity"—is becoming prevalent over many parts of the world. In Canada, the dramatic increase in overweight and obesity over the last 20 years has been deemed to constitute an epidemic and is seen as a major public health issue.[84] A leadership role for public health exists in addressing this local, regional, provincial, national, and global challenge. In fact, there is hope that the new Canadian

Obesity Network (www.obesitynetwork.ca) may help to contribute to solutions.[85] The prevalence of overweight and obesity is commonly assessed by using the body mass index (BMI). The BMI is defined as the weight in kilograms divided by the square of the height in metres ($kg/m^2$). A BMI greater than 25 $kg/m^2$ is defined as overweight, and a BMI over 30 $kg/m^2$ is defined as obese.[86]

## CRITICAL THINKING

*If an adolescent is 14 years old, weighs 55 kg, and is 160 cm tall, what is his or her BMI? Would the adolescent be classified as obese?*

Research indicates that obesity is not just a problem for Canadian adults, but is also having a serious impact on children's health. For example, obese children and adolescents have a greater occurrence of hypertension, and they show high cholesterol levels.[87] Fernandes and McCrindle of Toronto's Hospital for Sick Children reviewed the recent recommendations of the Task Force on Blood Pressure Control in Children. They restricted the search criteria to studies with a primary focus of blood pressure for subjects 18 years or younger and concluded that hypertension is under-recognized in children. Further, clinical management is directed toward secondary causes and, in general, cardiovascular risk reduction is aimed at dietary modification, increased exercise, and attainment and maintenance of ideal body weight.[88]

Katzmarzyk states that Canada has recently experienced a major epidemic of obesity; in fact, the population prevalence of obesity more than doubled between 1985 and 1998. In 1998, the problem was nationwide, meaning that it did not appear to be limited to one province or region.[89]

Hanley and his colleagues conducted a study to evaluate the prevalence of pediatric overweight and associated behavioural factors in a Native Canadian community with high rates of adult obesity and type 2 diabetes. They concluded that pediatric overweight is a harbinger of future diabetes risk and indicates a need for programs targeting primary prevention of obesity in children and adolescents.[90] A more recent study by Janssen and his researchers examined overweight and obesity prevalence rates of 11- to 16-year-old Canadian youth. In particular, they compared overweight and obesity to dietary habits and leisure-time physical activities. They found that 15 percent of 11- to 16-year-old Canadian youth were overweight and 4.6 percent were obese in 2002. These excessive weights were greater in boys than in girls. No clear associations were observed between dietary habits and measures of overweight and obesity. Interestingly, physical activities were lower and television viewing times were higher in overweight and obese boys and girls than they were in normal-weight youth.[91] In 2004, Sheilds described the prevalence of overweight and obesity among Canadian children and youth aged 2 to 17 based on direct measurements of their height and weight. The main results indicated that 26 percent of Canadian children and adolescents aged 2 to 17 were overweight or obese, and 8 percent were obese. Children who ate fruit and vegetables at least five times a day were substantially less likely to be overweight or obese than those who ate these foods less often. The likelihood of being overweight and obese also rose proportionally to watching television, playing video games, and using a computer.[92]

All of the research studies cited show similar findings. That is, overweight and obesity are serious problems in children and adolescents. In fact, over the past 25 years the prevalence of overweight and obesity combined has more than doubled among youth aged 12 to 17.[93]

Dr. Kim Raine, a professor at and the director of the Centre for Health Promotion Studies at the University of Alberta, wrote a report on overweight and obesity in Canada that was commissioned by the Canadian Population Health Initiative of the Canadian Institute for Health Information. The report concluded that we need precise knowledge of the determinants and the root causes of obesity.[94] The application of a population health perspective to the problem of obesity may provide timely insight into the potential means of addressing this critical issue. The aspects that are most clearly established are the behavioural determinants of obesity—excess energy intake via overconsumption of food coupled with decreased energy expenditure. However, what is less understood are the environmental and social determinants of those behaviours, and the best ways to change them. It is important to note that the lack of available Canadian data on the environmental determinants of food consumption and physical activity patterns poses limitations to providing evidence-based policy options.[95] However, a comprehensive school health program would help to manage weight among overweight children and adolescents. The prevention of obesity can begin at the individual and interpersonal levels. Health Canada's Vitality program is a strategy that promotes healthy eating, active living, and positive concept of both self and body image.[96]

---

## CRITICAL THINKING

*Which schools in your area have nutritional programs to initiate healthy eating patterns? What can you do as a health professional to support such a program?*

---

In caring for an obese adolescent, the nurse needs to obtain a thorough health history and have knowledge of the adolescent's health practices regarding nutrition. Nurses play a vital role in the adherence and maintenance phases of most weight reduction programs. They assess, manage, and evaluate the progress of overweight adolescents. They also play an important role in recognizing potential weight problems and in assisting parents and adolescents to prevent obesity.[97] Promoting good nutrition and dietary habits is essential to maintain good health for the adolescent. Interventions need to be based on goals of lifestyle change for the entire family. The goal is to modify the ways the family eats, exercises, and plans daily activities.[98] Several interventions for working with families are provided in the box entitled "Guidelines for Managing Obesity."

The key to successful treatment may be improving the adolescent's self-image. If emotional problems exist, you will need to counsel the adolescent or refer him or her to an appropriate source. Regardless of the methods of intervention used, parental understanding and co-operation are needed, and you are one member of the health team with whom both parents and the adolescent can discuss their concerns. Your ability to listen, discuss, teach, and refer, when necessary, can assist the adolescent in preventing or overcoming the health hazard of obesity. You can also work with the school system to establish daily physical exercise programs that stimulate the teen to remain physically active. You can provide dietary instructions, check weight, and suggest low-calorie refreshments or low-carbohydrate snacks.

## Exercise, Play, and Rest

Research studies indicate that more than half of Canadian children and youth are not sufficiently active for optimal growth and development. Plotnikoff and his researchers conducted a study to compare the prevalence of physical inactivity, smoking, and overweight/obesity among youth in

## Guidelines for Managing Obesity

- Set goals related to a healthy lifestyle.
- Keep objectives realistic and attainable.
- Modify family eating habits to include low-fat food choices. Serve calorie-dense foods that incorporate *Eating Well with Canada's Food Guide:* fruits and vegetables, whole grains, low-fat dairy products, and lean-protein foods.
- Encourage family members to stop eating when they are satisfied. Encourage recognizing hunger and satiation cues.
- Schedule regular times for meals and snacks. Include breakfast and do not skip meals.
- Have low-calorie, nutritious snacks ready and available. Avoid having empty-calorie junk foods in the home.
- Encourage the habit of maintaining food intake and activity diaries.

- Promote physical activity. Make daily exercise a priority. Encourage family participation. Find different ways to make the activity fun. Include peers.
- Limit television viewing and Internet activity. Do not allow snacking while watching television.
- Scale back computer time. Replace sedentary time with hobbies, activities, and chores.
- Recognize healthier food choices when eating out. Order broiled, roasted, grilled, or baked items. Split orders or take home "doggy bags."
- Praise and reward people for the progress they make in reaching nutrition and activity goals.
- Understand the genetic features of the adolescent's body type.

Source: Adapted from Stanhope, M., J. Lancaster, H. Jessup-Falcioni, and G.A. Viverais-Dresler. *Community Health Nursing in Canada,* 1st Canadian ed. Toronto: Elsevier Canada, 2008.

---

urban and rural schools. The results indicated that physical activity was low, with only 57 percent of youth achieving Canada's Physical Activity Guidelines. The researchers concluded that an urgent need exists to promote physical activity among Canadian youth.[99] Canadian girls are less active than boys, with only 38 percent of girls versus 48 percent of boys determined to be sufficiently active.[100] The Public Health Agency of Canada (PHAC) recognized that the rapid increase in overweight and obesity, combined with low levels of physical activity, presents a serious threat to Canada's children and youth. The PHAC, along with the Canadian Society for Exercise Physiology, initiated the development of guides such as *Canada's Physical Activity Guide for Youth*, an excellent online edition. The main thrust of the guide is that everyday physical activity equals better health, strength, and well-being. The goal is to get youth moving more. The guide helps youth increase their activity time by 30 minutes per day and reduce "non-active" time by 30 minutes per day.[101] Recommended are moderate activities such as walking or bike riding and vigorous activities such as soccer or supervised weight training.

Health professionals are advocating that all youth increase their physical activity by at least 30 minutes per day initially, and up to 90 minutes a day over a five-month period.[102] In addition, leading experts in health have concluded that schools are important agents for increasing physical activity among Canada's young people. Teachers can stimulate conversations about the importance of physical activity and urge youth to undertake activities that would make them more active.[103]

### CRITICAL THINKING

*In what ways, if any, do cultural influences affect exercise habits in the adolescent?*

**Exercise and Play Activities** Help parents and teens realize that competitive activities prepare young people to develop a process of self-appraisal that will last them throughout their lives. Learning to win and to lose can also be important in developing self-respect and concern for others. Physical activities provide a way for adolescents to enjoy the stimulation of conflict in a socially acceptable manner. Participation in sports training programs in high schools can help decrease the gap between biological and psychosocial maturation while providing exercise. Some form of physical activity should be encouraged to promote physical development, prevent overweight, formulate a realistic body image, and promote peer acceptance. Being an observer on the sidelines will not fulfill these needs.[104]

### CRITICAL THINKING

*What steps can you take to initiate a physically active program for an adolescent who is hospitalized for depression?*

**Rest and Sleep** During adolescence, bedtime becomes variable because the adolescent is busy with an active social life. The teen is expending large amounts of energy and is functioning at times with an inadequate oxygen supply because the heart and lungs do not enlarge rapidly enough at the time of the growth spurt. Both events contribute to fatigue and the need for additional rest.[105] In addition, protein synthesis occurs more readily during sleep. Because of the growth spurt during adolescence, protein synthesis needs are increased.[106] Increased rest may also be needed to prevent illness.

## PSYCHOSOCIAL CONCEPTS

The following information will guide assessment and teaching of the adolescent and the parents.

## Cognitive Development

Parents sometimes underestimate the cognitive abilities of the adolescent. Help them work with the adolescent from an intellectual and creative perspective. Parents can learn from adolescents, just as adolescents learn from parents. Help the adolescent learn how to use their cognitive skills effectively in all situations.

**Formal Operations Stage**  Tests of mental ability indicate that adolescence is the time when the mind has great ability to acquire and use knowledge. One of the adolescent's developmental tasks is to develop a workable philosophy of life, a task requiring time-consuming abstract and analytic thinking and inductive and deductive reasoning.

The adolescent uses available information to combine ideas into concepts and concepts into constructs, develop theories, and look for supporting facts; consider alternate solutions to problems; project his or her thinking into the future; and try to categorize thoughts into usable forms. He or she is capable of highly imaginative thinking, which, if not stifled, can evolve into significant contributions in many fields—science, art, and music. The adolescent's theories at this point may be oversimplified and lack originality, but he or she is setting up the structure for adult thinking patterns, typical of Piaget's period of formal operations. The adolescent can solve hypothetical, mental, and verbal problems; use scientific reasoning; deal with the past, present, and future; appreciate a wide range of meanings and complex issues; and understand causality and contrasting features. The formal operations period differs from concrete operations in that a much larger range of symbolic processes and imagination, along with memory and logic, are used.[107] A few of Piaget's ideas on formal operational thought are being challenged. There is much more individual variation in formal operational thought than Piaget envisioned.

In industrialized countries, the emphasis in education, as well as in the work world, is on logical, analytical, critical, and convergent thinking. The goals of these linear thinking processes are precision, exactness, consistency, sequence, and correctness of response. The source of such

thinking is the left hemisphere of the brain. Even so, original concepts do not necessarily arise from logical thinking. Thinking that is creative or novel is marked by exploration, intentional ambiguity, problem solving, and originality. Creativity is a multivariate mental process, which is divergent, intuitive, and holistic in nature. Its source is the right hemisphere of the brain. Creativity is an intellectual skill in which the person creates new ideas rather than imitating existing knowledge.

*Creativity, problem-solving ability, and cognitive competence can be encouraged when the educational process requires the following:*[108]

- Written assignments that necessitate original work, independent learning, self-initiation, and experimentation

- Reading assignments that emphasize questions of inquiry, synthesis, and evaluation, rather than factual recall

- Opportunity for females, as well as males, to gain skills in all facets of computer sciences and technology

- Group work to encourage brainstorming and exposure to the creative ideas of others

- Oral questions that are divergent, or that ask for viewpoints during class times

- Tests that include both divergent and convergent questions that engage the student in reflective, critical, and exploratory thought. Questions should become increasingly complex in nature. Ideally, questions should be worded so that there is not just one right answer. Rather, answers should be innovative and express thoughtfulness.

- A creative atmosphere is needed whereby the learner is autonomous, self-reliant, internally controlled, and self-evaluated. The curriculum emphasizes process, and the teacher provides a supportive atmosphere and recognizes creativity. In such an environment one might observe puzzlement and frustration, but also eagerness, humour, laughter, and enjoyment related to the task at hand.

In addition, students cannot learn unless they are assured of an environment that feels safe and supportive and is as free as possible from the threats of bullies or the fear of system violence. Several strategies can be implemented:[109]

- Collaboration between administrators, teachers, and parents

- Development of a school safety plan to ensure a weapon-free school

- Work with churches and other support groups or organizations in the community

- Establishment of a crisis management team to handle crises and their media coverage

The adolescent does not always develop intellectual potential by staying in school. Students drop out of school for a variety of reasons.[110] Dropping out has many negative consequences, including unemployment, social assistance dependency, and problems with the law. For example, providing special classrooms for the teen during pregnancy and after delivery so that she can bring the baby for daycare while she attends class is one way to prevent school dropouts in that population.

## Sexual Harassment and Adolescent Bullying in School and with Peers

Sexual harassment is prevalent in Canada, both in schools and in the workplace. Tutty and Bradshaw state that some sexual harassment prevention programs are available as early as grade five, but most such programs are offered to high school students. The goal of these programs is to increase knowledge about sexual harassment: how it affects individuals and the school community, what attitudes and dynamics support this problem, and what strategies can be used to cope with harassment.[111]

In our society, the occurrence of child and adolescent bullying has been a persistent concern over a number of decades. This concern has been especially spurred by the recent fatal shootings of students and teachers in secondary schools across North America. A growing consensus exists that acts of youth aggression are becoming more violent and unpredictable. The profile of the assailant is not limited to stereotypical youth from low socioeconomic status communities; an assailant can just as easily originate from a well-respected family and an affluent community.[112]

Bullying is recognized as a significant risk to all domains (physical, cognitive, social, and personality) of the adolescent's growth and development. According to the Canadian Adolescents at Risk Research Network Fact Sheet, bullying can be defined as a relationship problem characterized by a negative physical or verbal action that has hostile intent, causes distress to victims, is repetitive in nature, and involves a power differential between bullies and their victims. The victim of bullying is repeatedly exposed to aggression by a more dominant individual, the bully.[113] Three common categorizations of victimization are used: direct physical abuse, direct verbal abuse, and indirect verbal abuse (spreading rumours and/or social withdrawal). Other forms of victimization include ethnic stereotyping and sexual harassment. Many studies reveal that bullying is influenced by several risk factors that have strong links with adolescence. These risk factors either emerge (drug and alcohol use, mental health issues, pubertal development), or undergo dramatic changes during adolescence (which

might involve health, parents, peers, schools).[114] A study by Volk and his researchers at Brock and Queen's University in Ontario examined correlates of different types of bullying and victimization relevant to the adolescent context. Of particular interest in the adolescent was the importance of risk factors that either emerge or undergo significant changes in adolescence. They found that high levels of victimization (7.6 percent), bullying (6.1 percent), and bullying-victimization (0.9 percent) were quite prevalent among adolescents. Regarding risk factors, alcohol use, mental health, and peer behaviour were the only risk factors that significantly predicted victimization. Bullies were significantly more likely to be young and male. They were more likely to have peers who engaged in antisocial behaviour, showed increased likelihood of higher levels of alcohol consumption, and more frequently experienced problems with parents and the school atmosphere. Bullying victims showed a distinct pattern of risks associated with both bullying and victimization.[115]

Cyber-bullying has received considerable attention recently. It is the use of communication technologies (email, cellphones, text messages, Internet sites, and instant messaging) to physically threaten, verbally harass, or socially exclude an individual or group. Using these technologies to distribute damaging messages and pictures allows bullies to remain anonymous and the practice of bullying to become widespread.[116]

Those who bully are at risk of developing antisocial behaviour such as criminality in adulthood. The use of power and aggression early in life can form a basis for sexual harassment, dating aggression, domestic violence, and child or elder abuse. Adolescents vary in their involvement in bullying, and different levels of support and intervention are required. For example, bullying is a multi-faceted issue and treatment programs may benefit from a comprehensive approach that attempts to address many of the risk factors.[117]

Parental involvement is a key issue in addressing bullying in schools. The main goal of involving parents is to improve the lines of communication between schools and parents and to secure their support for the school's policy and programs on bullying. Community representatives such as police, health, and human resources should be involved in the school's initiative in implementing an anti-bullying program.[118] Often the community nurse can provide the teachers and parents with support in carrying out the program.

---

### CRITICAL THINKING

*What information would you deem necessary for developing an anti-bullying program for adolescents?*

## Peer-Group Influences

The **peer group**, or *friends of the same age*, influences the adolescent to a greater extent than do parents, teachers, popular heroes, religious leaders, or other adults. Because peer groups are so important, the adolescent has intense loyalty to them.[119] Social relationships take precedence over family and counteract feelings of emptiness, isolation, and loneliness. Significance is attached to activities deemed important by peers. Peers serve as models or instructors for skills not yet acquired. Usually, some peers are near the same cognitive level as the learner. Therefore, their explanations may be more understandable to the learner. When student peers of varying cognitive levels discuss problems, less advanced students may gain insights and correct inaccuracies in thinking. The more advanced students also profit. They must think through their own reasoning to explain a concept satisfactorily to a peer.

The *purposes* of the peer group include promoting:[120]

■ A sense of acceptance, prestige, belonging, approval

■ Opportunities for learning how to behave

■ A sense of immediacy, concentrating on the here-and-now, what happened last night, who is doing what today, what homework is due tomorrow

■ A reason for *being* today, a sense of *importance right now*, and not just dreams or fears about what he or she might become in some vague future time

■ Opportunities to learn behaviour related to later adult roles

■ Role models and relationships to help define personal identity as he or she adapts to a changing body image, more mature relationships with others, and heightened sexual feelings

**Dating Patterns** Dating is but one use of leisure time. It is greatly influenced, however, by the peer group, and it varies according to one's culture, social class, and religious and family beliefs. Dating prepares the adolescent for intimate bonds with others, marriage, and family life. The adolescent learns social skills in dealing with the opposite sex. They also learn which situations and with whom he or she feels least and most comfortable, and what is expected sexually.

Banister and her colleagues conducted an ethnographic study to explore the health-related concerns within dating relationships. Their sample consisted of 40 female adolescents aged 15 and 16.[121] The results, from a health care point of view, suggested that unequal power dynamics in their dating relationships place girls at a disadvantage with serious consequences for their health. Difficulty in expressing their needs and desires within the intimate relationship made the participants sensitive to social isolation, substance misuse, and individual and social tolerance of violence. These researchers conclude that nursing professionals should seriously consider the value of providing health information and care to female adolescents in a group format. That is, nurses seem particularly suited to be able to establish the type of group environments in which adolescents feel safe to expose the high level of vulnerability they experience in their everyday life.[122]

As you work with adolescents, assess the stage of peer-group development and dating patterns. A few years will make a considerable difference in attitudes toward the opposite sex. Build your teaching on current interests and attitudes. The same age groups in different localities may be in different stages of development. Adolescents from another culture may sharply contrast in pattern with Canadian adolescents. For example, in Egypt the male is not supposed to have any intimate physical contact with the female until marriage. In Canada, certain physical contact is expected.

**Leisure Activities** During the past decade, developmental psychologists have focused attention on understanding the context of leisure activities and its effect on positive and negative developmental outcomes.[123] Leisure activities may be critically important to adolescent development because adolescents have more autonomy and exert more voluntary control on these activities than on other daily activities. As adolescents begin the process of self-discovery, it becomes evident that they can readily identify a special class of activities that provide a greater fit with their interests and talents. Clearly, not all activities in which the adolescent participates will provide the subjective experiences related to identity discovery.[124] Campbell states that given the importance of leisure, as well as identity formation process during adolescence, relationships between the two may be anticipated. However, little attention has been given, as yet, to research in this area.[125]

Sports, dancing, hobbies, reading, listening to the radio or stereo, talking on the telephone, daydreaming, experimenting with hairstyles, cosmetics, or new clothes, and just loafing have been teenagers' favourite activities for decades. Riding the all-terrain vehicle or motorcycle, driving and working on cars, using the computer, watching television, playing video games, and attending movies and concerts are also popular. Political activism draws some youth; various causes rise and then fade in interest as the youth matures. "Everybody's doing it" is seemingly a strong influence on the adolescent's interests and activities. Others participate in activities, such as camera club, French club, or yearbook projects, because of personal talents or interests. The decrease in exercise frequency may explain the increased amount of time given to other leisure activities, especially playing computer games. Playing computer games is much more prevalent among males than females.[126] Significant technological advances in computer games have made them more interesting and challenging.

Many parents consider a party in the home for a group of teenagers a safe use of leisure time. This is undoubtedly true if parents and other adults are on the premises and can give guidance as needed and if the parents are not themselves supplying the teens with alcohol and drugs. The police in one community give the following guidelines to help parents and teens host and attend parties. You may wish to share these suggestions with parents:

■ Parents should set the ground rules before the party to express feelings and concerns about the party, ask who will attend and whether adults will be present, and learn what is expected of their adolescent. The address and phone number of the host should be known by the parents of the teens who are attending.

■ Notify neighbours that you will be hosting a party, and encourage your teen to call or send a note to close neighbours notifying them of the party and asking them to let the family know if there is too much noise.

■ Notify the police when planning a large party. They can protect you, your guests, and your neighbours. Discuss with the police an agreeable plan for guest parking.

■ Plan to have plenty of food and non-alcoholic beverages on hand.

■ Plan activities with your teenager before the party so that the party can end before guests become bored (three to four hours is suggested as sufficient party time).

■ Limit party attendance and times. Either send out invitations or have the teenager personally invite guests beforehand. Discourage crashers; ask them to leave. Open-house parties are difficult for parents and teenagers to control. Set time limits for the party that enable guests to be home at a reasonable time definitely before a legal curfew.

■ A parent should be at home during the entire time of the party. The parent's presence helps keep the party running smoothly; it also gives the parent an opportunity to meet the teenager's friends. Invite other adults to help supervise.

■ Decide what part of the house will be used for the party. Pick out where your guests will be most comfortable and you can maintain adequate supervision. Avoid having the bedroom area as part of the party area.

■ Do not offer alcohol to guests under the age of 18 or allow guests to use drugs in your home. Be alert to the signs of alcohol or drug use.

■ Do not allow any guest who leaves the party to return to discourage teenagers from leaving the party to drink or to use drugs elsewhere and then return to the party.

■ Guests who try to bring alcohol or drugs or who otherwise refuse to co-operate with your expectations should be asked to leave. Notify the parents of any teenager who arrives at the party drunk or under the influence of any drug to ensure his or her safe transportation home. Do not let anyone drive under the influence of alcohol or drugs.

■ Teenagers frequently have parties at homes when parents are away. Typically, the greatest problems occur when parents are not at home. Tell your neighbours when you are going to be out of town.

■ Many parties occur spontaneously. Parents and teens should understand before the party that these guidelines are in effect at all parties. If, despite your precautions, things get out of hand, do not hesitate to call the local police department for help.

■ Emphasize to parents the importance of their being role models through minimum drinking of alcoholic beverages or use of drugs.

The teenager may also feel more secure when the parent is actively interested in knowing where he or she will be and what he or she will be doing even though rebellion may ensue. Parents should be awake or have the teen awaken them when arriving home from a party. This is a good sharing time. Peers are important, but if peer activity and values are in opposition to what has been learned as acceptable, the adolescent feels conflict. Explore with parents the adolescent's need for constructive use of leisure time and the importance of participation in peer activities. You may be involved in implementing constructive leisure activities.

For some teenagers, there is little leisure time. They may have considerable home responsibility, such as occurs in rural communities, or may work to earn money to help support the family. Other youth are active in volunteer work.

## CRITICAL THINKING

*What health promoting activities would you suggest are suitable for the adolescent during leisure time?*

# Emotional Development

**Emotional Characteristics** Emotional characteristics of the personality cannot be separated from family, physical, intellectual, and social development. Emotionally, the adolescent is characterized by mood swings and extremes of behaviour (see Table 11-1). Refer to the box entitled "Major Concerns of Teenagers"; these concerns

## Table 11-1 Contrasting Emotional Responses of Adolescents

| Independent Behaviours | Dependent Behaviours |
|---|---|
| Happy, easygoing, angry, loving, gregarious, self-confident, sense of humour | Sad, irritable, unloving, withdrawn, fearful, worried |
| Energetic, self-assertive, independent | Apathetic, passive, dependent |
| Questioning, critical or cynical of others | Strong allegiance to or idolization of others |
| Exhibitionistic or at ease with self | Excessively modest or self-conscious |
| Interested in logical or intellectual pursuits | Daydreaming, fantasizing |
| Co-operative, seeking responsibility, impatient to be involved or finish project | Rebellious, evading work, dawdling, ritualistic behaviour, dropout from society |
| Suggestible to outside influences, including ideologies | Unaccepting of new ideas |
| Desirous for adult privileges | Apprehensive about adult responsibilities |

contribute to emotional lability and identity confusion.[127] Emotional development requires an interweaving and organization of opposing tendencies into a sense of unity and continuity. This process occurs during adolescence in a complex and truly impressive way to move the person toward psychological maturity.

Share this information with parents and the adolescent. By using principles of communication and crisis intervention and through your use of self as a role model you will be able to help the adolescent work through identity diffusion and achieve a sense of ego identity and an appropriate sense of independence.

Developmental Crisis  The psychosexual crisis of adolescence is identity formation versus identity diffusion: "Who am I?" "How do I feel?" "Where am I going?" "What meaning is there in life?" **Identity** means that an *individual believes he or she is a specific unique person;* he or she has emerged as an adult. **Identity formation** *results through synthesis of biopsychosocial characteristics from a number of sources*—for example, earlier sex identity, parents, friends, social class, ethnic, religious, and occupational groups.

A number of influences can interfere with identity formation:

- Telescoping of generations, with many adult privileges granted early so that the differences between adult and child are obscured and there is no ideal to which to aspire
- Contradictory value systems of individualism versus conformity in which both are highly valued and youth believe that adults advocate individualism but then conform
- Emphasis on sexual matters and encouragement to experiment without frank talking about sexuality with parents or significant caregivers
- Increasing emphasis on education for socioeconomic gain, which prolongs dependency on parents when the youth is physically mature
- Rapid changes in the adolescent subculture and all of society, with emphasis on conforming to peers.

### CRITICAL THINKING

*What may be other relevant influences that interfere with identity formation?*

According to a recent worldwide survey of parents, children throughout the world have similar behaviour problems. The random sample consisted of 13 000 children,

## Major Concerns of Teenagers

- Their appearance
- Divorce of parents
- Having good marriage and family life
- School performance
- Choosing a career; finding steady employment
- Being successful in life
- Having strong friendships; how others will treat them
- Paying for university or college
- Making a lot of money
- Finding purpose and meaning in life
- Contracting AIDS
- Drug and alcohol use by self, friends
- Hunger and poverty
- Societal violence

Sources: Bee, H., D. Boyd, and P. Johnson, *Lifespan Development*, 2nd Canadian ed. Toronto: Pearson EducationCanada, 2006; Papalia, D., S. Olds, and R. Feldman, *Human Development*, 9th ed. Boston: McGraw Hill, 2004.

aged 6 to 17 years, in 12 countries: Australia, Belgium, China, Germany, Greece, Israel, Jamaica, the Netherlands, Puerto Rico, Sweden, Thailand, and the United States. Overall, geographical and cultural differences accounted for only 8 to 11 percent of individual differences in the scores. Puerto Rican and Jamaican children were more likely to internalize problems with anxiety, depression, and social withdrawal. American, German, and Swedish children were more likely to externalize problems by showing aggression, delinquency, and hyperactivity. In all cultures, boys showed more externalizing and had higher problem behaviours than girls.[128]

By far the most comprehensive and provocative discussion of identity development has been by Erik Erikson.[129] **Identity formation** implies an *internal stability, sameness, or continuity, which resists extreme change and preserves itself from oblivion in the face of stress or contradictions*. It implies emerging from this era with a sense of wholeness, knowing the self as a unique person, feeling responsibility, loyalty, and commitment to a value system. There are three types of identity, which are closely interwoven: (1) **personal**, or **real, identity**—*what the person believes self to be*; (2) **ideal identity**—*what he or she would like to be*; and (3) **claimed identity**—*what he or she wants others to think he or she is*.

Identity formation is enhanced by having support not only from parents but also from another significant adult who has a stable identity and who upholds sociocultural and moral standards of behaviour. If the adolescent has successfully coped with the previous developmental crisis and feels comfortable with personal identity, he or she will be able to appreciate the parents on a fairly realistic basis, seeing and accepting both their strengths and their shortcomings. The values, beliefs, and guidelines they have given him or her are internalized. The adolescent needs parents less for direction and support; he or she must now decide what acceptable and unacceptable behaviours really are.[130]

Students from different ethnic and racial backgrounds have unique needs and ways of adapting to stressors and unique aspects of the developmental crisis of identity formation. Some may feel isolated and alienated in relation to mainstream culture values. Parents, teachers, and health care professionals can help these teens work through values and cognitive and emotional conflicts.

Canadian psychologist James Marcia has analyzed Erikson's theory of identity development and concluded that it is important to differentiate between crisis and commitment in adolescent identity formation. According to Marcia, a *crisis* is a period of decision making when old values and old choices are re-examined. The outcome of this re-evaluation is a *commitment* to some specific role, value, goal, or ideology.[131] The extent of an individual's crisis and commitment is used to classify the adolescent in one of the four identity statuses:

- **Identity achievement**: the person has been through a crisis and has reached a commitment to ideological, occupational, or other goals.[132]

- **Identity moratorium**: a time of making no decisions but a rethinking of values and goals; no commitment has been made.

- **Identity foreclosure:** the goals, values, and life tasks have been established by the parents and the group, and the individual is not allowed to question or examine them. He or she is expected to follow the pattern set by the elders; usually the roles are related to sex and socioeconomic or caste status.

## Negative Consequences of Identity Diffusion

- Feels she or he is losing grip on reality
- Feels fragmented; lacks unity, consistency, or predictability with self
- Feels impatient but is unable to initiate action
- Gives up easily on a task; feels defeated
- Vacillates in decision making; is unable to act on decisions
- Is unable to delay gratification
- Appears brazen or arrogant, sarcastic
- Is disorganized and inconsistent in behaviour; avoids tasks
- Fears losing uniqueness in entering adulthood; displays regressive behaviour; acts out behavioural extremes to attract attention

- Has low self-esteem, negative self-concept, low aspirations
- Is unable to pursue academic or career plans; may drop out of school
- Isolates self from peers; is unable to relate to former friends or significant adults
- Feels cynical, disillusioned, excessively angry or suspicious
- Engages in antisocial or illegal behaviour; acts out sexually
- Seeks association with gang, cult, or negative community or media leader

- **Identity diffusion** results if the adolescent fails to achieve a sense of identity. He or she feels self-conscious and has doubts and confusion about self as a human being and his or her roles in life. With identity diffusion, he or she feels impotent, insecure, disillusioned, and alienated. Identity diffusion is manifested in other ways as well, as listed in the box entitled "Negative Consequences of Identity Diffusion" (previous page). The real danger of identity diffusion looms when a youth finds a negative solution to the quest for identity.

*Help parents to work with the adolescent who feels identity diffusion. Emphasize that parents must never give up trying to form a loving bond* with offspring. Parents can provide attention and extend empathy to the teen, whether they are a dual, step-parent, or single-parent family. *Refer parents to counselling services* when needed so that they can understand and work thorough, together, the teen's behavioural vulnerability.

---

## CRITICAL THINKING

*Acne may cause an adolescent a considerable amount of stress. What are ways you can help an adolescent to maintain the quest for his or her identity until acne therapy is successful?*

---

## Self-Concept and Body Image Development

The development of the self-concept and body image is closely akin to the cognitive organization of experiences and identity formation. The adolescent cannot be viewed only in the context of the present. Many earlier experiences carry an impact on the adolescent that continues to affect him or her throughout life. The helpful earlier experiences enable the adolescent to feel good about the body and self. If the youngster enters adolescence feeling negative about self or the body, adolescence will be a difficult period.

Jungwee Park examined factors associated with the adolescent self-concept and the impact of adolescent self-concept on psychological and physical health and health behaviours in young adulthood.[133] The data came from the household cross-sectional (1994–1995) and longitudinal (1994–1995 to 2000–2001) components of Statistics Canada's National Population Health Survey. A portion of the results indicated that self-concept tends to be low among girls, compared with boys. A strong self-concept has a positive long-term effect on girls' perceived health. Is it surprising to you that in the cross-sectional portion of the same study, adolescent self-concepts were directly associated with household income and emotional support?

*Various factors influence the adolescent's self-concept, including:*[134]

1. Age of maturation
2. Degree of attractiveness
3. Name or nickname
4. Size and physique appropriate to sex
5. Degree of identification with the same-sex parent
6. Level of aspiration and ability to reach ideals
7. Peer relationships
8. Culture

In a Canadian study, adolescents with higher scores on self-esteem were found to have a positive attitude toward school, good relationships with their parents and their peers, and to feel self-confident. In addition, they were less likely to feel depressed or lonely or be victims of bullying.[135] In addition, several studies have concluded that that high self-esteem is correlated with positive developmental outcomes. For example, adolescents with high self-esteem are able to resist peer pressure and get higher grades at school.[136]

The rapid growth of the adolescent period is an important factor in body image revision. Girls and boys are sometimes described as "all legs." They are often clumsy and awkward. Because the growth changes cannot be denied, adolescents are forced to alter their mental picture of both their self and their capabilities. Physical changes in height, weight, and body build often cause profound changes to be made in the adolescent's self-perception. To many male adolescents, the last chance to get taller is very significant.

If the adolescent should actually have a disability or defect, peers and adults may react with fear, pity, revulsion, or curiosity. The adolescent may retain, and later reflect, these impressions because a person tends to perceive self as others perceive him or her. If the adolescent develops a negative self-image, then motivation, behaviour, and eventual lifestyle may also be, in some way, inharmonious or out of step with social expectations.

By late adolescence, self-esteem should be relatively high, and self-concept should have generally stabilized. The older adolescent no longer believes that everyone is watching or being critical of his or her physical or personality characteristics. Interactions with the opposite sex are more comfortable, although awareness of sex is keen.

Your understanding of the importance and the value that the adolescent places on self can help you greatly with your work with the adolescent, parents, teachers, and community leaders. Your goal is to help the adolescent to avoid building a false self-image of himself or herself. It is important to help the adolescent evaluate strengths and weaknesses, accept those weaknesses, and build on the strengths that are present. You should listen carefully to the adolescent's statements about self and his or her sense of future. You will need to determine the best time and place when you might effectively speak and work with him or her, and you will also need to be alert to know when silence is best. Share an understanding of influencing factors on body image and self-concept development with parents, teachers, and other adults so that they can positively influence adolescents.

## CRITICAL THINKING

*Observe adolescents at a movie theatre or shopping mall. What actions do you see that denote the adolescents are struggling to gain self-identity?*

# Sexual Development

Healthy sexual development in adolescence is the outgrowth of healthy development from infancy to childhood. Positive childhood experiences assist to develop the self-confidence, trust, and autonomy the adolescent needs to handle peer pressure and navigate the sexual feelings natural to the teenage years. On the other hand, health development may be inhibited by harmful sexual attitudes, media images, and emotional, physical, and sexual abuse or neglect that may occur at this age. Because of hormonal and physiologic changes and environmental stimuli, the adolescent is almost constantly preoccupied with feelings of developing sexuality.

Sexual desire is under the domination of the cerebral cortex. Differences in sexual desire prevail in young males and females. Sexual desire is somewhat influenced by cultural and family expectations for sexual performance. The female experiences a more generalized pleasurable response to erotic stimulation, but she does not necessarily desire coitus. The male experiences a stronger desire for coitus because of a localized genital sensation in response to erotic stimulation, which is accompanied by production of spermatozoa and secretions from accessory glands that build up pressure and excite the ejaculatory response. The male is stimulated to seek relief through ejaculation.[137]

Menarche is experienced by the girl as an affectively charged event related to her emerging identity as an adult woman with reproductive ability. Family and cultural traditions are needed to mark the menarche as a transition from childhood to adulthood. Menarche is anticipated as an important event, but in Canada no formal customs mark it, and no obvious change occurs in the girl's social status. Nocturnal emissions are often a great concern for boys, but they are also a sign of manhood.

Both sexes are concerned about their development and the appearance of secondary sex characteristics, their overall appearance, their awkwardness, and their sex appeal, or lack of it.

The most common form of sexual outlet for both sexes, but especially for males, is **masturbation**, which is *the manipulation of the genitals for sexual stimulation.*

A substantial number of Canadian adolescents are sexually active at a relatively young age. In a recent analysis of Canadian adolescents, Garriguet found that the percentages of boys and girls who had intercourse by age 14 or 15 were almost the same: 12 percent and 13 percent, respectively. However, the characteristics associated with such behaviour differed. Among girls, the onset of puberty, region of residence, weak self-concept, having tried smoking or drinking, and not being overweight were significantly associated with early sexual activity. For boys, poor relationships with parents, older age, low household income, and having tried smoking were significant.[138]

Premarital sexual activity is often used as a means to get close, sometimes with strangers, and may result in feelings of guilt, remorse, anxiety, and self-recrimination. Adolescent males and females often report that the initial coitus was not pleasurable. The number of pregnant teenage females who are not marrying is significantly increasing. This development has implications for the future care and well-being of the baby and implications for future intimate relations of the teenage girl. A wide variety of sexual experiences before marriage may cause the person to feel bored later with a single partner.[139]

Evans and her colleagues assessed 539 teens in one Ontario city to identify knowledge about and use of birth control, comfort in discussing sexual health, and preferred sites, providers, and methods of service delivery. They concluded that becoming sexually active and using birth control appears to be maturational. Since teens were not comfortable talking with teachers, mall-based clinics may provide an alternative service for teens that require information about sexual activity and birth control.[140]

Canada focuses on enhancing sexual health and reducing sexual problems among various groups, including adolescents. The *Canadian Guidelines for Sexual Health Education*, published by the authority of the Minister of Health, are intended to unite and guide individuals and professionals working in the area of sexual health education and health promotion.[141] These guidelines are grounded in evidence-based research within a Canadian context.

## CRITICAL THINKING

*A shy 14-year-old girl you are caring for in a hospital setting informs you that she is concerned because she has not menstruated yet. How would you counsel her?*

## Adaptive Mechanisms

The **ego** is the *sum total of those mental processes that maintain psychic cohesion and reality contact; it is the mediator between the inner impulses and outer world.* It is that part of the personality that becomes integrated and strengthened in adolescence and has the following functions:

- Associating concepts or situations that belong together but are historically remote or spatially separated
- Developing a realization that one's way of mastering experience is a variant of the group's way and is acceptable
- Subsuming contradictory values and attitudes
- Maintaining a sense of unity and centrality of self
- Testing perceptions and selecting memories
- Reasoning, judging, and planning
- Mediating among impulses, wishes, and actions and integrating feelings
- Choosing meaningful stimuli and useful conditions
- Maintaining reality

The adaptive mechanisms used in adolescence are the same ones used (and defined) in previous developmental eras, although they now may be used in a different way.

Teach parents that adaptive abilities of the adolescent are strongly influenced by inner resources built up through the years of parental love, esteem, and guidance. The parents' use of adaptive mechanisms and general mental health will influence the offspring. Are the parents living a double standard? Has the teenager seen the parents enjoy a job well done or is financial reward the key issue? Do the parents covertly wish the teenager to act out what they could never do?

Even with mature and nurturing parents, the adolescent will at times find personal adaptive abilities taxed. But the chances for channelling action-oriented energy and idealism through acceptable adaptive behaviour are much greater if parents set a positive example.

## Moral–Spiritual Development

According to Kohlberg,[142] the adolescent probably is in the conventional level most of the time; however, the adolescent may at times show behaviour appropriate to the second stage of the preconventional level or the first stage of the postconventional level.

The early adolescent typically is in the conformist stage; structure and order of society take on meaning for the person, and rules are followed because they exist (analogous to Kohlberg's conventional level). The late adolescent is in the conscientious stage, in which the person develops a set of principles for self that is used to guide personal ideals, actions, and achievements. Rational thought becomes important to personal growth (analogous to Kohlberg's postconventional level, stage 1). The young adolescent must examine parental moral and religious verbal standards against practice and decide if they are worth incorporating into his or her own life. He or she may appear to discard standards of behaviour previously accepted, although basic parental standards likely will be maintained. In addition, he or she must compare the religious versus the scientific views. Although moral–spiritual views of sensitivity, caring, and commitment may be prevalent in family teaching, the Canadian adolescent is also a part of the scientific, technologic, industrial society that emphasizes achievement, fragmentation, and regimentation. Often adolescents will identify with one of the two philosophies. These two views can be satisfactorily combined, but only with sufficient time and experience, which the adolescent has not had.

Gilligan has found a difference between adolescent males and females in moral reasoning. Males organize social relationships in a hierarchical order and subscribe to a morality of rights. Females value interpersonal connectedness, care, sensitivity, and responsibility to others. Thus, adolescent males and females view the dating relationship differently and approach aggressive or violent situations from a different perspective.[143]

If the adolescent matures in religious belief, he or she must comprehend abstractions. Often when he or she is capable of the first religious insights, the negativism tied with rebellion to authority prevents this experience.

Help parents and adolescents realize that the adolescent who does find strength in the supernatural, who can rely on a power greater than self, can find much consolation in this turbulent period of awkward physical and emotional growth. If he or she can pray for help, ask forgiveness, and believe that he or she receives both, a more positive self-image develops. In this period of clique and group dominance, the church is a place to meet friends, share recreation and fellowship, and sense a belonging difficult to find in some large high schools. Several authors discuss the importance of parents and teachers: their faith, prayers, and efforts to focus on spiritual and moral formation, not just physical and intellectual development.[144]

---

### CRITICAL THINKING

*How can you engage an adolescent to talk openly about his or her belief system?*

---

## Late Adolescence: Transition Period to Young Adulthood

In some cultures, parents select schooling, occupations, and the marriage partner for their offspring. Canadian adolescents, however, are usually free to make some or all of these decisions.

By the time the teen is in grade 11 or 12, he or she should be thinking about the future. There are many options: whether to pursue a mechanical or academic job; to attend some form of higher education; to live at home or elsewhere; to travel; to marry soon, later, or not at all; and to have children soon, later, or not at all. Answers to these questions will influence the adolescent's transition into young adulthood.

**Establishing a Separate Residence** This step is one marker of reaching young adulthood. The late adolescent often spends less time at home and prepares for separation from parents. If there is intense intrafamily conflict, if the adolescent feels unwanted, or if the adolescent is still struggling with dependence on parents or identity diffusion, a different mode of separation may occur.

You may have an opportunity to discuss residence situations with the adolescent. If you can get to the person before he or she walks or runs away, help him or her consider the intolerability of parental demands and the family situation. Discuss alternative ways of handling the problem. You may contact a high school counsellor or potential employer. The teen should be encouraged to report incest or abuse so that the teen's parents and other siblings can receive proper therapy and an appropriate, healthy living situation can be found for the teen.

Health care is a problem for adolescent runaways. Health concerns include pregnancy, sexually transmitted infections, prostitution, alcohol and other drug abuse, and child maltreatment and incest. The following intervention strategies should be instituted when these youth are in treatment:

1. Clarification of the health care provider's attitudes and values
2. Establishment of trust
3. Use of effective interviewing skills
4. Ability to provide maximum medical treatment and information when the client presents self for care
5. Establishment of foundations for future interactions and care

**Career Selection** Many important career decisions, such as whether to attend university or a trade school or enter the job force directly after high school, are made during adolescence. Code and Bernes conducted a study to assess the career needs of junior and senior high school students in southern Alberta. The results of this research revealed that adolescents experience a range of concerns that relate to their post–high school transition and future career. These career concerns include distinct transition and career adjustment difficulties related to training

and education concerns, security, failing, satisfaction, commitment, wrong occupational choice, and having to decide. The researchers conclude that an integrated career planning curriculum beginning at the junior high school level may be helpful to address students' unanswered questions and unaddressed career concerns. In addition, by involving adolescents' own perceptions of their career concerns, the career-planning process may become more relevant for them, and students may be better prepared for the post–high school transition.[145]

*Occupation* represents much more than a set of skills and functions; it is a way of life. Occupation provides and determines much of the physical and social environment in which a person lives, his or her status within the community, and a pattern for living. Occupational choice is usually a function or a reflection of the entire personality, but the occupation, in turn, plays a part in shaping the personality by providing associates, roles, goals, ideals, mores, lifestyle, and perhaps even a spouse.

You can be a key person in helping adolescents clarify values and attitudes related to occupational selection and in talking with parents about their concerns.

## HEALTH PROMOTION IN NURSING PRACTICE
## Scope of the Health Care and Nursing Role

Your role in caring for the adolescent may be multi-faceted. An assessment is needed; knowledge from this chapter and relationship and communication principles described in Chapter 5 may be useful in gaining information from a client or family. It is important that you observe and listen to the adolescent and family regarding issues, strengths, and healthy responses. Interventions that may involve direct care to the ill adolescent or that involve various health promotion measures are described in the previous or following sections.

Many adolescent girls become pregnant each year, and many adolescents will run away from home. A significant number of youths will die from motor vehicle and other accidents, unintended gunshot wounds, and homicide and suicide.[146] Other health problems abound, including sexually transmitted infections, substance abuse, chronic illness, and obesity and nutritional deficiency (the latter two previously discussed). Although the scope of this book does not allow discussion of needs assessment and intervention for adolescents with physical disabilities, you may wish to consult several authors for information.[147]

## Health Promotion and Health Prevention

**Immunizations** Immunization is an important preventative measure that needs to be started in infancy and continued throughout the lifespan as recommended for specific ages.[148] Immunizations are a part of health protection for the adolescent, although they may be overlooked during that time of life. Your actions and teaching in relation to immunizations are important for the teenager's health now and in the adult years.

The first priority is to *ensure that children receive the recommended series of doses*, including the school leaving dose at 14 to 16 years of age. See Table 7-6 for immunization schedules at different ages. Nurses and physicians play an extremely important role in the identification of individuals in need of immunization.

According to the Canadian Nurses Association (CNA), immunizations are a way of exercising our immune systems to trigger what is already in place to fight against disease. Within the primary health care approach to nursing, nurses know that disease prevention, coupled with health promotion practices, is the best way to achieve a healthy population.[149]

### CRITICAL THINKING

*Bob is an adolescent. He tells you that vaccines cause many harmful side effects, including illnesses and even death. How will you respond to Bob?*

Nurses do have opportunities to work with adolescents who are well.[150] It is necessary that wellness diagnoses be developed in order to guide care that focuses on strengths of the adolescent client rather than on problems only.

**Safety Promotion** In Canada, injuries are the biggest contributors to premature death among the on-reserve First Nations population, at a rate of four times that of the general Canadian population.[151] Injuries are one of the most prominent health problems that young people face during their school-aged years, and they are the leading cause of death among youth.[152] It is interesting to note that diverse activities are associated with injuries among youth. However, the results of a recent survey demonstrate clearly that sports are the main cause of injuries in all grades and for both genders. Team contact sports (such as hockey and football), non-contact sports (such as basketball), and individual sports (such as cycling) can all lead to serious injuries. Improving the safety of school and sports-related environments and enhancing first aid are necessary.[153]

### CRITICAL THINKING

*As a health professional, what can you do to advocate for the safety of sports-related environments?*

Injury is an important public health issues in Canada. It is the leading cause of death for Canadians between the ages of 1 and 44.[154] In fact, motor vehicle accidents, injuries, homicide, and suicide are responsible for approximately 75 percent of all deaths between the ages of 15 and 24 and the incidence is higher for males alone. It is clearly established now that motor vehicle accidents are more common among young drivers who use alcohol, marijuana, and other drugs while driving.[155]

The 2001–2002 Health Behaviour in School Aged Children (HBSC) survey used the population health framework and recognized the broad set of determinants of health and

---

### NARRATIVE VIGNETTE
## Strengths and Healthy Responses

In your class today, on health promotion through the lifespan, you are discussing the importance of strengths and healthy responses being incorporated into nursing care plans. During the lively discussion, the focus comes to centre on assessing a combination of the client's strengths, concerns, and lifestyle patterns because such an approach provides the nurse with a foundation upon which to develop a variety of interventions to enhance health and wellness. For your assignment, you are given a case study of Roland. You are asked to respond to the questions immediately.

### Case Study

You are the school nurse and are expected to see each student. Roland is a 16-year-old who is taking drama in high school. He wants to be an actor. One member of the small group of friends he socializes with frequently is a girl in whom he has a growing interest. Roland really wants to ask this girl for a date. He is becoming increasingly tidy in his personal hygiene and appearance. Roland knows a lot about computers and he is even thinking of becoming a computer programmer—until the right acting job comes up. He spends much time reading about different computers and software.

### Questions

1. What two assessment questions will you ask Roland?

2. State two of Roland's strengths.

health behaviours in children and youth. The purpose of the HBSC study was to examine patterns in the determinants of health of these age groups as well as in selected trends in their health behaviours and attitudes.[156] One of the main findings focused on injuries. Most injuries (50 percent) occurred in organized team sports, followed by non-organized individual sports activities (18 percent). Canadian sports that most often lead to serious injury include team contact sports such as hockey and football; team non-contact sports such as basketball, soccer, and baseball; and individual sports such as cycling and gymnastics.[157] Contusions, dislocations, sprains, strains, overuse syndromes, and stress fractures occur frequently.[158] In the adolescent, the epiphyses of the skeletal system have not yet closed, and the extremities are poorly protected by stabilizing musculature. These two physical factors, combined with poor coordination and imperfect sports skills, probably account for the numerous injuries.[159]

As a group, adolescents represent one of the nation's largest underserved populations. Characteristic feelings and behaviours contribute to many of the health problems and must be considered in assessment and care.

A review of the leading causes of mortality and morbidity among teens shows that nearly all contributory behaviours can be categorized into the following seven areas:[160]

1. Heightened sense of sensation-seeking and risk-taking
2. Behaviours that result in unintentional and intentional injuries
3. Drug and alcohol use
4. Tobacco use
5. Sexual behaviours that cause sexually transmitted diseases, including HIV infection, and unintended pregnancies
6. Inadequate physical activity
7. Dietary patterns that cause disease

**Injury Prevention** The CNA states that at the individual level, injury prevention is the practice of assessing and managing risk, which leads to injury preventing behaviours or to living in healthy ways that minimize the risk of injury. Injury prevention deals with making positive choices about minimizing risk at all levels of society while maintaining healthy, active, and safe communities and lifestyles.[161] A population health approach to promoting the prevention of injury considers the following factors that can influence policy and behaviour of groups:

- Knowledge of behaviours that will increase safety and well-being, such as driver education, knowledge of safety programs in the community, instruction in water safety, routine safety practices, and emergency care measures

- Skills to implement injury preventing behaviours and manage risk
- Motivation to sense a feeling of goodness about engaging in injury preventing behaviours
- Opportunity and success to implement injury preventing behaviours given varied life circumstances throughout the lifespan
- Supportive environments to facilitate the implementation of injury preventing behaviours with the minimum of risk.[162]

The CNA provides a brief discussion of the built environment related to the issue of injury prevention in their CNA Backgrounder, *The Built Environment, Injury Prevention and Nursing: A Summary of the Issues*. The built environment can exert a strong impact on the health of the public. It consists of any part of the physical environment that is constructed, assembled, or fabricated by people and used by individuals on a daily basis. The built environment is recognized as being significant because of the mortality and morbidity implications related to it.[163] The nurse's role in injury prevention is important. See the box entitled "Role of the Nurse in Injury Prevention."

Parents and youths should be informed about the risks, the exercise, and the prestige value involved with certain sports and privileges. Because of the sports activities in which adolescents are involved, they may sometimes experience musculoskeletal chest pain, minor strains or sprains to a joint, and minor ankle strain.

The importance of a physical examination before participation and knowledge about how to prevent sports injuries should be emphasized.[164]

**Musculoskeletal chest pain** *arises from the bony structures of the rib cage and upper-limb girdle, along with the related skeletal muscles.* Age does not automatically rule out heart-related problems. Although musculoskeletal pain is usually aggravated by activity that involves movement or pressure on the chest cage rather than by general exertion (such as stair climbing), a thorough lung and cardiac examination is merited. Applying heat to the area (unless it is a fresh injury) and resting the area can be recommended.[165]

**Minor strains and sprains** to a joint involve a *mild trauma that results in minimal stretching of involved ligaments and contusion of the surrounding tissues.* The treatment is known as RICE: rest, ice, compression, elevation of the affected joint. Use an ice pack for 24 to 36 hours; local heat can then be used if needed. Because of the risk of Reyes syndrome, Tylenol (acetaminophen), if tolerated, can be used for its analgesic and anti-inflammatory effects.[166]

A **minor ankle sprain** involving *stretching of the ligament without tearing* can be treated in the same way as minor strains and sprains with the addition of an elastic bandage and possibly keeping weight off the ankle longer than 24 to 36 hours through the use of crutches.[167]

## Common Health Problems: Prevention and Treatment

Health care for the adolescent includes attention to a schedule of health screening measures, immunizations, counselling, and high-risk categories. A few references describe how to conduct physical assessments at various ages, including the adolescent.[168]

In addition to the hazards of injuries, teenage pregnancy, and obesity, other health problems are apparent among adolescents. Table 11-2 summarizes definitions, symptoms and signs, and prevention and treatment for common conditions.[169] Discuss the prevention of these problems with adolescents and parents.

Cancer, at any age, is devastating not only to the individual but also to the family. In childhood, the most common bone cancer is osteogenic sarcoma. Its peak incidence is between 10 to 25 years of age. Optimum treatment of osteosarcoma is surgery and chemotherapy. The nursing care depends on the type of surgical approach. The adolescent and family may have more of a difficult time adjusting to an amputation than to a limb salvage procedure. Tumours of the testes are not a common condition. However, when manifested in the adolescent, they are generally malignant. Testicular cancer is the most common form of cancer in males ages 15 to 44. Treatment for testicular cancer consists of the surgical removal of the affected testicle (orchiectomy) and the adjacent lymph nodes.[170] Males should be taught testicular self-examination. For females, the various types of human papillomavirus (HPV) are often classified into low and high risk according to their association with cancer. In fact, the "high-risk" types are more likely to lead to the development

## Table 11-2 Common Health Problems of Adolescents

| Problem | Definition | Symptoms/Signs | Prevention/Treatment |
|---|---|---|---|
| Hordeolum (stye) | Localized infection of sebaceous gland on eyelid margin | Painful, reddened swelling on eyelid; sometimes drainage | Apply hot compresses.<br>Administer antibiotic drops. |
| Epistaxis (nose bleed) | Spontaneous bleeding from nose caused by ruptured blood vessel | Bleeding from nose | Prevent dry and cracking nasal mucosa by keeping humidity level sufficient.<br>If nose bleeds, sit with head slightly forward and pinch nostrils for at least 15 minutes.<br>Use cold compresses. |
| Acne vulgaris | Comedones, pimples, and cysts formed from increased activity of sebaceous glands | "Blackheads," "whiteheads," and additional lesions, especially on face, chest, back | Use good hygiene techniques and cleansing agents.<br>Apply topical preparations.<br>Administer oral medications. |
| Dental caries and gingivitis | Decay of teeth and disease of gums | Broken, dark teeth; bleeding, inflamed gums | Use good dental hygiene.<br>Check periodically with a dental hygienist for education and treatment. |
| Aphthous stomatitis | Recurrent small painful ulcers in the oral mucosa, "canker sores"; unknown etiology, *not* herpes simplex | Burning and tingling before eruption; recurrent painful lesions from 1 to 10 mm; oval, shallow, light yellow or grey with erythematous border | Prevention: None is known.<br>Use Kenalog in Orabase or other topical anaesthetic.<br>Use tetracycline/Benadryl mouthwash. |
| Tinea cruris | Ringworm of the groin, "jock itch," superficial | Rash and soreness on groin and inner aspects of | Eliminate sources of heat and friction. |

*(continued)*

Table 11-2 (continued)

| Problem | Definition | Symptoms/Signs | Prevention/Treatment |
|---|---|---|---|
| | fungal infection of the groin | thighs; may include scrotum, gluteal folds, buttocks | Bathe daily; dry thoroughly. Wear cotton underwear. Use antifungal cream and Domeboro solution compresses. |
| Tinea pedis (athlete's foot) | Fungal infection affecting feet, especially toe webs | Intense itching; cracking; peeling | Soak feet and dry well. Apply antifungal agent. Wear clean cotton socks. |
| Infectious mononucleosis | Condition caused by Epstein-Barr virus | Fever, sore throat, enlarged lymph nodes; general malaise; enlarged spleen; sometimes jaundice | Treat symptoms; use rest (mono), increased fluid intake, antipyretic, good nutrition. |
| Hepatitis A virus | Inflammation of hepatocytes of liver caused by viruses, bacteria, drugs, chemicals; transmitted via fecal contamination of food or water with subsequent close person-to-person contact (25% of hepatitis cases) | Fatigue, anorexia, swollen glands; aversion to smoking (if smokes); short incubation period: 15–45 days | Prevention: Stay in good physical condition, handwashing. If condition develops, prevent transfer. Treat symptoms. Vaccine available for occupational risks |
| Hepatitis B virus (HBV) infection | Transmitted via blood, primarily parentally, although person-to-person contact possible (50% of hepatitis cases) | Prodromal stage: 2–20 days; jaundice phase: 2–8 weeks; recovery phase: 2–24 weeks | Vaccine is available; take recommended precautions. Treat symptoms. Avoid complications. |
| Hepatitis C virus (HCV) | Diagnosed by deduction (25% of hepatitis cases) | Hepatitis symptoms; history of transfusion (HDV) | Treat symptoms. |
| Rocky Mountain spotted fever | Acute febrile disease caused by *Rickettsia rickettsii;* passed to human by bite of infected tick | Symptoms start in 2 days to 2 weeks: headache, fever, rash on hands and feet, pain in back and leg muscles | Prevention: Be aware of problem and appropriate removal of ticks. Treatment: Administer tetracycline. |
| Lyme disease | Tick-borne disease introduced by the spirochete *Borrelia burgdorferi* from animal host to human (ticks are only 1–2 mm) | Early (3 or 4 days after bite): ring-like rash at bite site (approximately 10 cm in diameter) then secondary lesion, flu-like symptoms, sometimes cardiac problems (10%); in 4 weeks, neurological problems (in 15%); in 6 weeks to 1 year, arthralgias and synovitis (in 50%) | Administer antibiotic (doxycycline). Provide rest and healthy diet. Treat symptoms. Prevent through education. |

## Role of the Nurse in Injury Prevention

### Primary Prevention

■ Advocate for safer design of products, automobiles, equipment and buildings. Speak from the experience of what you have seen with your patients and from research.

■ Teach home safety related to falls and fire prevention, especially to families with children and elderly members.

■ Help parents and caregivers to develop knowledge and skills that reduce in-home hazards, and that support effective supervision skills.

■ Work with parents, schools and recreational staff on such issues as safety in sports, safety on the streets (as pedestrians, or on bicycles), and safety in playgrounds.

■ Develop worksite health and safety programs. Advocate other policies and practices that contribute to healthy workplaces (e.g., opportunities for physical activity, healthy lunches and stress reduction).

■ Ensure that younger workers, who are more vulnerable to job hazards because of their inexperience, are well-informed about workplace hazards and safety measures.

■ Help older adults to understand the benefit of regular exercise as a strategy to strengthen the body, improve coordination and balance, and lessen risk of falls.

■ Winter poses an increased risk of falling, especially for seniors. Help older adults to use techniques to reduce their risk (for example, canes with picks or "grippers" that slip on over boots).

■ Work with the community to identify icy stretches of sidewalk and advocate more extensive snow clearing practices by the municipality.

### Secondary Prevention

■ Assess homes, schools, worksites and communities for environmental hazards.

■ Routinely obtain occupational health histories from individuals, counsel about hazard reduction, and refer for diagnosis and treatment.

■ Help community groups to take action with the local municipality to deal with hazardous roads and intersections.

■ Work with older adults to understand what parts of their homes may pose risks for falls. Help them to access modifications (e.g., hand-rails in the bathtub) that will reduce their risk.

### Tertiary Prevention

■ Provide appropriate nursing care at worksite or home for persons with injury-related disabilities.

Source: Canadian Nurses Association. *CNA Backgrounder, The Built Environment, Injury Prevention and Nursing: A Summary of the Issues.* Ottawa: Author, 2005.

---

of cancer. Four of the common types of HPV (types a6, 11, 16, and 18) can be prevented through vaccination. The vaccine has been approved for use in Canada for females 9 to 26 years of age. It requires three doses to be given over the course of six months (at zero, two, and six months). The vaccine is not recommended for pregnant women, females under nine years of age, or males. The nurse can teach adolescents and young women that the HPV vaccine does not protect against all types of HPV, but only against the four most common types of HPV that cause cervical cancer and anogential warts.[171] Sexually active females should receive annual Pap smears and be taught breast self-examination.

Allergic dermatitis, cysts, and keloid formation of the earlobes are seen with considerable frequency, as ear piercing has become popular. Inner ear damage from exposure to loud music is increasing and can be assessed by pure tone audiometry. The adolescent is subject to postural defects, fatigue, anemia, and respiratory problems.

**Chronic Illness in Adolescents** During adolescence, chronic illness may impose the additional burden of hospitalization, pain, extensive diagnostic testing, surgery, school absences, medications, and activity restrictions.[172] Woodgate

states that such stressors may provoke anxieties such as fears and grief reactions.[173] Adolescents have a particularly difficult time dealing emotionally with chronic illness because they feel different from and set apart from peers. They may have fewer peer relationships and activities in which they can participate; and thereby have a disruption of their social support system. Psychosocial problems can lead to social disabilities that far outweigh the effects of the physical illness. Positive coping in the ill adolescent is associated with independent behaviours, peer contact, school achievement, and participation in normalization activities. Negative coping centres on fear, withdrawal, regression, use of symptoms for secondary gain in various ways, and low self-esteem.[174]

A health promotion strategy for the chronically ill adolescent is to help the adolescent learn about the chronic condition. Other strategies include teaching the adolescent about the care needed to control or manage the condition, and how to problem solve and engage in self-care activities so that the adolescent can integrate good care management into his or her daily life. Parents need to be coached to support the adolescent to make healthy choices regarding care. The adolescent should be encouraged and supported to build a safety network of friends who know about the chronic condition and who can assist if a problem occurs. Examples of such problems include an asthma attack, insulin reactions, or seizures.

Discuss sexual maturation and the importance of protected sexual activity. Discourage taking risky behaviours relative to their condition.[175] Provide that adolescent with referrals to career counsellors for occupational planning.

Suicide Adolescence is a time of dramatic change. Young people often feel tremendous pressure to be successful at school, at home, and in social groups. At the same time, adolescents may lack the life experience that lets them know that difficult situations will not last indefinitely. Depression can also be a factor among young people. Fortunately, these factors, or a combination of them, may become such a source of pain that relief is sought through suicide. According to the Canadian Mental Health Association, suicide ranks as the second leading cause of death after motor vehicle accidents. Usually, adolescents are reluctant to discuss suicide, partly because of the related social stigma, guilt, or shame surrounding the issue.[176] Unfortunately, this tradition of silence perpetuates the belief in certain harmful myths and attitudes. See the box entitled "Some Myths about Suicide."

Suicide in adolescents is frequently reported as an accidental death. Motor vehicle accidents, drug and alcohol overdose, firearm accidents, and even homicides can be disguised suicides.[177] Dramatizations of teenage suicides on the nightly news or in movies appear to contribute to increased waves of teenage suicide attempts and successes.

Adolescents who attempt suicide often come from families who have non-productive communication patterns, inconsistent positive reinforcement behaviours, and a high level of conflict or child abuse. Suicides occur in rich and poor, urban and rural families. In Canada, the First Nations on-reserve population has double the rate of suicidal deaths compared to the general Canadian population. In Nunavut, where 85 percent of the population is Inuit, the rate of deaths by suicide is more than six times the Canadian rate.[178] Boothroyd and her colleagues carried out a case-control study comparison of 71 people who died by suicide, between 1982 and 1996, among the Inuit in northern Quebec and 71 population-based living control subjects matched for sex, community of residence, and age within one year. The results indicated that most of the case subjects were single males aged 15 to 24 years. The two principal means of suicide were hanging and gunshot. It is interesting to note that about

## Some Myths about Suicide

| Myth | Reality |
| --- | --- |
| Young people rarely think about suicide. | Teens and suicide are more closely linked than adults might expect. In a survey of 15 000 grade 7 to 12 students in British Columbia, 34 percent knew of someone who had attempted or died by suicide; 16 percent had seriously considered suicide; 14 percent had made a suicide plan; 7 percent had made an attempt; and 2 percent had required medical attention due to an attempt. |
| Talking about suicide will give a young person the idea, or permission, to consider suicide as a solution to his or her problems. | Talking calmly about suicide, without showing fear or making judgments, can bring relief to someone who is feeling terribly isolated. A willingness to listen shows sincere concern; encouraging someone to speak about their suicidal feelings can reduce the risk of an attempt. |
| Suicide is sudden and unpredictable. | Suicide is most often a process, not an event. Eight out of ten people who die by suicide gave some, or even many, indications of their intentions. |
| Suicidal youth are only seeking attention or trying to manipulate others. | Efforts to manipulate or grab attention are always a cause for concern. It is difficult to determine whether a youth is at risk of suicide. All suicide threats must be taken seriously. |
| Suicidal people are determined to die. | Suicidal youth are in pain. They don't necessarily want to die; they want their pain to end. If their ability to cope is stretched to the limit, or if problems occur together with a mental illness, it can seem that death is the only way to make the pain stop. |
| A suicidal person will always be at risk. | Most people feel suicidal at some time in their lives. The overwhelming desire to escape from pain can be relieved when the problem or pressure is relieved. Learning effective coping techniques to deal with stressful situations can help. |

Source: Canadian Mental Health Association, Youth and Suicide. Adapted and reproduced with the permission of Canadian Mental Health Association © 2007.

33 percent had been in contact with medical personnel in the month before their death.[179] Furthermore, the case subjects were significantly more likely than the control subjects to have received a lifetime psychiatric diagnosis and to have had a history of psychiatric symptoms.[180] Recently, Chandler and Proulx, in their investigation of the epidemiology of suicide in First Nations communities, found that those First Nations communities that have proven to be successful in preserving ties to their cultural past and in achieving a measure of local control over their present and future civic lives were characterized by significantly lower suicide rates. Meanwhile, bands and tribal councils that have so far failed to achieve similar measures of cultural continuity typically suffered youth suicides many hundreds of times their national average.[181]

Females are now using forms of suicide previously usually associated only with males. Males, however, are more successful, more violent, and less likely to give warning before a suicidal act. Pinhas and her colleagues examined whether gender-role conflicts influenced the suicidal behaviour of adolescent girls. Gender-role conflict is defined as psychological or social difficulty that arises when individuals have internalized characteristics other than those ascribed to their sex. They concluded that gender-role conflict plays an important role in the suicidal behaviour of girls.[182]

*Signs of suicide are often subtle to detect, but a composite of behaviours should be a clue* that the teen is experiencing severe stress. See the box entitled "Warning Signs for Suicide and Interventions in Adolescents" for a list of behaviours associated with or indicators of suicide attempts.[183] Do not be reluctant to ask whether the youth has thought of suicide. The stressed person welcomes this query, which emphasizes the fact that you are taking the statements and behaviour seriously.

The suicidal adolescent may be a loner at school and feel unable to meet scholastic expectations of parents. School performance often drops and there may be frequent absences. If peers state that a friend is suicidal, investigate their concerns. No threat should be ignored.[184]

*Screen for emotionally distressed adolescents.* Be available to listen, and ask about, their problems. Take a careful history to identify the underlying stresses.[185] If you believe you are unable to handle the situation, discuss it with the teen and refer him or her to a guidance counsellor, clergy, school psychologist, family therapist, family physician, or psychiatrist. Frequently, the adolescent will turn to an adult with whom he or she has had a personal relationship or who is an advocate for teens. This relationship may help the adolescent through the present crisis. You can accept, support, inform, and serve as an advocate for teens, working with parents and adolescents.[186]

## Warning Signs for Suicide and Interventions in Adolescents

### Loss of Someone or Something Important

(The greater the number of losses in a short period, the higher the risk)

- Death
- Divorce
- Move to new school or geographic location
- Job
- Self-esteem related to poor relationship or loss of status
- Prolonged family disruption
- Pet
- Health

### Feelings and Behaviours of Depression

- Change in daily habits
- Changed eating or sleeping patterns
- Lack of energy; fatigue; weakness; extreme lethargy
- Problems of concentration; slow speech or movements
- Drop in grades or work performance
- Neglecting appearance more than usual

- Lack of friends or interests
- Truancy at school or poor work attendance
- Increase in drug or alcohol use; excessive smoking
- Appearing sad, angry, sullen, irritable most of time; mood swings
- Accident proneness
- Increase in promiscuity
- Continuous acting out that masks other behaviour
- Negative self-concept; feeling unloved, rejected, guilty, hopeless

### Statements about Suicide

- Direct or indirect statements about a plan
- Thought + Action = Suicide Attempt or Success

### Behavioural Actions or Changes

- Subtle or abrupt, different than norm
- History of suicide attempts
- Giving away prized possessions
- Withdrawal from activities and friends

>

- Writing, artwork, or talking about suicide and death
- Accident proneness
- Crying for no apparent reason
- Depressed mood quickly lifts
- Vague physical complaints
- Listening only to music about death

## High-Risk Symptoms

- A clear plan with time and details, using a lethal method
- Intoxication with drugs or alcohol
- Anniversary of the death of a loved one by suicide
- Auditory hallucinations telling the teen to die
- Extreme isolation and no support systems

- Feelings of hopelessness, helplessness, and worthlessness
- A previous suicide attempt using a lethal method and continued suicide ideation

## Interventions

- Determine lethality
- Encourage communication with family, teachers, or other supportive adults
- Encourage appropriate expression of feeling, especially guilt and anger
- Use self-esteem building activities
- Encourage positive statements about self
- Assist the child to cope with the situation that is causing despair or sense of helplessness

Kidd's research group studied the interactive effects of parent, peer, and school social relations, all in the social context of adolescent suicide attempts. These issues were examined using data from the National Longitudinal Study of Adolescent Health (Add Health). Add Health is a large-scale longitudinal data set that includes information on health-related behaviours of a heterogeneous sample of adolescents.[187] According to the researchers, their findings have two clinical implications. The first is the importance of parents in protecting against progressively increased suicidal behaviour. This implication means that a need exists to evaluate and to facilitate the development of effective parent–adolescent relationships. Second, the interactive effects between social domains—that is, the supportive social relations with peers, parents, and school—have an interactive effect in mitigating risk of suicide attempts for one specific high-risk group: boys who had a history of attempting suicide as well as poor peer relations. For this group, the protective effects of parental support against suicide attempt seem to have been bolstered by positive school relations. It then becomes advantageous to explore ways in which different support elements could be integrated.[188]

*Follow-up care with the family and adolescent after suicidal gestures* is important. Some adolescents who attempt suicide ultimately do commit suicide. If the adolescent makes a suicide attempt, crisis intervention is essential after the necessary medical and physical care is given (see Chapter 5). The goals, once life is assured, are to help the person work through feelings that led to and resulted from the suicide attempt, feel hope, identify the problem, see alternative ways of handling it, and mobilize supportive others to continue caring contact with the client. The family needs your support and help in working through their feelings of anxiety, shame, guilt, and anger.

## CRITICAL THINKING

*If you suspect that an adolescent who lives in your neighbourhood is contemplating suicide, what resources can you use for referral?*

**Substance Abuse** Hotton and Haans conducted an analysis of the prevalence of substance use among young adolescents in Canada. They used data from the 1998–1999 National Longitudinal Survey of Children and Youth. Analysis is based on a cross-sectional file from 4296 respondents aged 12 to 15 years. The main results indicated that drinking to intoxication and drug use were more common among 14- and 15-year-olds than among 12- and 13-year-olds. The odds of drinking to intoxication and drug use were highest among adolescents whose friends used alcohol or drugs or were often in trouble, who reported low commitment to school, or whose parents had a hostile or ineffective parenting style.[189] Boyle and his colleagues used data from the Ontario Health Survey to examine within-family influences on the use of tobacco, alcohol, and marijuana in households with offspring aged 12 to 24 years. They concluded that the treatment and prevention of substance use (and abuse) among adolescents and young adults might be enhanced by including a family focus, especially where there are two or more siblings at home.[190] Williams and Chang from the Addiction Centre Adolescent Research Group in Calgary claim that for treatment, outpatient family therapy appears to be superior to other forms of outpatient treatment.[191]

Alcohol consumption has been linked to a multitude of adverse consequences with respect to health and social harm.[192] Recently, the Alcohol Use Disorder Identification Test (AUDIT) was developed by the World Health

Organization (WHO) to identify individuals with hazardous and harmful patterns of alcohol consumption and/or alcohol dependence.[193]

Rehm and his researchers examined the influence of volume of drinking and patterns of drinking on alcohol-related harm on students (grades 9 to 12). The results indicated that both the average volume of alcohol consumption and patterns of drinking influenced alcohol-related problems at the student level. These findings may imply that since the culture of school is important in influencing alcohol-related harm, policies for school events are needed as well as strict enforcement of rules in respect to alcohol in schools.[194] In fact, the drinking environment around schools may also be influenced by the availability of alcohol for students.[195]

In 2002, the cost of alcohol-related harm for all ages totalled $14.6 billion, or $463 per living Canadian. This included $7.1 billion for lost productivity due to illness and premature death, $3.3 billion in direct care costs, and $3.1 billion in direct law enforcement. Although alcohol consumption enjoys enormous popularity in Canada, it also figures prominently around special and cultural events. The monetary figures quoted above are staggering regarding alcohol and its contribution to health and social harm.[196] The notion of sensible alcohol use, or developing a culture in which moderation is the goal, underpins the National Alcohol Strategy. The Strategy identifies four strategic areas for action:

- *Health promotion, prevention and education*: aims to raise public awareness about responsible alcohol use. A key recommendation is the development of national alcohol drinking guidelines, which provide a benchmark for Canadians in evaluating their personal drinking practices.

- *Health impacts and treatment*: aims to reduce the negative health impacts of alcohol consumption and address its contribution to injury and chronic disease. A key recommendation is expansion for the various health professionals, such as nurses, to implement screening, initiate brief interventions, and recommend referrals for those who may be at risk of developing, or may have already developed, alcohol-related problems.

- *Availability of alcohol*: aims to implement and enforce effective measures that control alcohol availability. It recommends shoring up the social responsibility of government liquor control boards, reinforcing liquor licensing and enforcement regulations, and harmonizing minimum purchase ages across Canada.

- *Safer communities*: aims to create safer communities by reducing the number of harmful events that occur related to intoxication. It examines how communities can foster a culture of moderation and create safer drinking environments, especially in nightclubs.[197]

In summary, the Strategy provides a long-term vision of how to reduce alcohol-related harm in Canada. All relevant stakeholders, including nurses and other health care professionals, must share responsibility for addressing the harm caused by the misuse of alcohol.

The problem of drug abuse (both illicit and prescription) continues to intensify. It is an epidemic with serious consequences for future generations. A major problem is the increasing number of infants born with addiction to one or several drugs (see also Chapter 6). Every age group takes a certain amount of medication at one time or another.[198] For example, in Canada, the increasing use of Ritalin to control children and youth who are diagnosed as having attention deficit disorder results in much of the drug ending up on the street.[199] A few of the findings of the prevalence of alcohol and drug use from the Canadian Campus Survey are outlined as follows:

- Alcohol was used by 85 and 77 percent of students during the past year and past 30 days, respectively. About one in ten (9.9 percent) were lifetime abstainers.

- By far, the most commonly used illicit drug was cannabis, used by 51 percent of students during their lifetime, 32 percent during the past 12 months, and 16 percent during the 30 days before the survey.

- Following cannabis, the most commonly used illicit drugs were hallucinogens such as magic mushrooms, mescaline, phencyclidine (PCP), and opiates.

- Undergraduates displayed diverse drinking patterns.

- Type of drinking varied according to region, gender, and year of study. For example, in the Atlantic provinces, both heavy frequent and infrequent drinking were significantly higher than the Canadian average. Compared to women, men were more likely to be frequent drinkers.

- Thirty-two percent of undergraduates reported hazardous or harmful patterns of drinking according to the WHO's Alcohol Use Disorders Identification Test (AUDIT) screener.

- Gambling activity increased with the year of study and varied across regions, with more students reporting gambling during the past school year in the Atlantic provinces and the least in British Columbia.[200]

- *A brief note on gambling*: In several Canadian provinces, an expansion of legalized gambling has been associated with increased rates in gambling. Cox and his researchers conducted a national survey across the ten Canadian provinces. Their sample was composed of Canadian residents aged 15 and older in all ten provinces. A sample size of 43 770 was used for this investigation. They found that Manitoba and

Saskatchewan had the highest rates of gambling, and that the lowest rates of gambling were found in Quebec and New Brunswick.[201]

## CRITICAL THINKING

*What steps can you take to initiate help for an adolescent with a gambling problem?*

Substance abuse of alcohol and drugs occurs in children and adolescents of all socioeconomic levels and is a growing health problem.[202] **Substance abuse** is *a maladaptive pattern of substance use manifested by recurrent and significant adverse consequences related to the repeated use of the substance.*[203]

*Reasons for substance abuse* are many:

1. Curiosity
2. Peer pressure
3. Need to overcome feelings of insecurity and aloneness and to be a part of the group
4. Need for acceptance
5. Easy availability
6. Imitation of family
7. Rebellion, escape, or exhilaration
8. Need for a crutch
9. Unhappy home life
10. Sense of alienation or identity problem
11. Attempt at maturity or sophistication

Gradually, members of drug subcultures tend to replace interest in family, school, church, hobbies, or other organizational activity. The beliefs and attitudes of the drug subculture are learned from experienced drug users and are often fortified by certain types of music and tabloid coverage of stars and other famous people.[204]

Substance abuse and addiction affect all socioeconomic, ethnic, and racial groups. Entire communities are affected. In large cities much of the drug trade involves street gangs, which have become drug trafficking organizations. Even rural communities are affected. When substance abuse is the presenting problem, a somewhat perplexing scenario frequently presents itself. It is often found that several factors—the accessibility of and ability to buy drugs, acceptance of their use by a subculture, and at least some immunity from legal consequences—mean that motivation for behavioural change does not occur. Total community effort is needed to stop or prevent the problem.

Therapy is usually entered into as a result of family pressure, or a crisis event such as attempted suicide or arrest. The behaviour and illness of the young drug abuser tend to control the entire family and cause family disruption. Parents must regain control of their home and force the youth to face the illness by seeking treatment. Love and care in a family are essential, but those alone will not cure the drug abuse problem.

Professional treatment should be obtained in a centre that treats the whole person and family, using an interdisciplinary team approach that provides after-discharge care to the person and family. Intensive treatment over time to the entire family system creates the type of attitude change that is essential for remaining healthy and functional and for ongoing maturity. A modality of treatments is essential to reduce symptoms and work through the underlying character and interactional pathology.

The change in attitudes, self-concept, and body image must be sufficiently effective so that person feels like a new person and is strong enough in that identity so that the new self is maintained in the face of the inevitable stress from peers, school, and family. The ability to give up aspects of the old self and maintain a new identity begins with treatment, but it can be accomplished only with love, support, and encouragement from family and other loved ones. *The person must feel that he or she is gaining more than what is being lost to maintain the changes begun in treatment and to move forward in maturity.* To remain drug-free involves more than just "saying no" or completing a one-time seminar. Support groups in the school and community for teens who do not want to use alcohol or drugs are essential to prevent the loneliness and ostracism some teens feel when they go against the expectations of peers. Illicit drug trade can be stopped most effectively by community action that reduces the supply to individuals.

Accurate information on the nature and extent of substance use and associated problems is a critically important basis for prevention program development.[205] The Canadian Community Epidemiology Network on Drug Use supports a number of communities in developing a profile of drug use. Each community in the network brings together local experts, such as treatment specialists, to contribute quantitative and qualitative information relevant to local needs.[206]

Table 11-3 will assist you in assessing the short-term and long-term effects resulting from commonly abused drugs. Table 11-4 outlines the selected interdisciplinary interventions in treatment of substance abuse. More information on working with these adolescents is provided.

## CRITICAL THINKING

*What are a few health promoting strategies for adolescents who are using crack?*

## 1. Hallucinogens

| Name/Street name | Description | Origin/Medical Use | Short-Term Effects |
|---|---|---|---|
| **PCP** (phencyclidine) *angel dust, elephant, hog* | Sold as powder of any colour, in crystals, liquid, tablet, capsule or paste. Frequently passed off as LSD, THC, mescaline or other drugs. In samples analyzed at drug testing labs, content of a single dosage unit (e.g., tablet, capsule) has ranged from 1.3 to 81 mg; however, 1-5 mg is enough for a high in non-tolerant people. Can be sniffed, smoked, swallowed or injected. | Originally developed as an intravenous anaesthetic; now discarded for human use. Later used in veterinary medicine as general anaesthetic or tranquilizer for large animals, but is no longer used for this purpose. | Effects of low to moderate doses last 3 to 18 hours. Effects of high doses may last for several days. It can produce a state of pleasurable intoxication, a sense of separation from surroundings, perceptual distortions, difficulty in concentrating and communicating. People may become highly confused, paranoid, terrified, aggressive, or passive. Bad trips are more common with PCP than with other drugs. Overdose can cause seizures, coma and death. Accidental death can result from drug-induced confusion. |
| **LSD**, and any salts thereof (Lysergic acid diethylamide) acid, *blotter* | Sold on street as coloured drops on blotting paper, on gelatin sheets, as tablets, capsules, or liquid solution. Common dose is 15 to 50 micrograms (1,000 micrograms = 1 mg), usually taken orally. | Synthesized from lysergic acid, which is found in a fungus growing on various grains. Produced in labs specifically for illegal drug market. No current medical use. | Effects are felt within an hour, and last 2 to 12 hours. Perception intensifies, colours appear brighter, objects more sharply defined or distorted. Possible changes in the perception of time and distance. A person may feel the body as light, heavy or distorted. Thinking and concentration are difficult and short-term memory is impaired. Extreme mood swings, including joy, inspiration, depression, anxiety, terror, aggression can occur. There are no known deaths directly caused by overdose, but drug-induced confusion has caused accidental deaths. |
| MDMA (3,4-methylenedioxy-N-methylamphet-amine) (3,4-methyl-enedioxy-m ethamphetamine) *Ecstasy, Euphoria, X, XTC, Adam* | Usually sold as white or off-white tablets. Common dose is 50 to 200 mg usually taken orally. A similar chemical MMDA has been misrepresented as Ecstasy on the street. | Produced in labs specifically for illegal drug market. No currently accepted medical use. | A hallucinogen with stimulant properties which can produce feelings of euphoria, pleasure, empathy and sociability, as well as confusion, depression, sleep problems, anxiety, panic attacks, blurred vision, nausea, muscle tension, teeth-clenching, faintness, chills, sweating and increased heart rate and blood pressure. Higher doses produce distortions in perception, thinking and memory, hallucinations and, in some people, anxiety and depression. Deaths as a result of kidney and/or heart failure due to dehydration or hyperthermia have occurred in the context of raves or dances. |

| Long-Term Effects | Tolerance and Dependence | Legal Status |
| --- | --- | --- |
| Flashbacks may occur (see LSD below). Other effects include persistent speech problems, depression, anxiety or more severe psychological consequences, including toxic psychosis, similar to amphetamine psychosis or acute schizophrenia | Regular use may produce tolerance. Chronic users may become psychologically dependent. PCP does not cause physical dependence. | In Canada, phencyclidine and its derivatives are governed by the provisions of the Controlled Drugs and Substances Act. Unlawful possession is a criminal offence punishable on indictment by imprisonment for up to seven years and on summary conviction for a first offence to a fine of up to $1,000 or imprisonment for up to six months, or both. A subsequent offence is punishable on summary conviction by a fine of up to $2,000 or imprisonment for up to one year, or both. Trafficking, possession for the purpose of trafficking, possession for the purpose of exporting, production, import and export are indictable offences punishable by up to life imprisonment. |
| Decreased motivation and interest, or prolonged depression and anxiety. LSD high may spontaneously recur days, weeks or even months later (called "flashback"). Use during pregnancy may be related to increased incidence of spontaneous abortion or fetal abnormality. | After using LSD, user must abstain for several days to regain sensitivity. This tolerance crosses over to mescaline and psilocybin. Chronic users may become psychologically dependent. LSD does not cause physical dependence. | In Canada, these hallucinogens are governed by the provisions of the Controlled Drugs and Substances Act applicable to Schedule III. Possession is a criminal offence punishable on indictment by imprisonment for up to three years and on summary conviction to a fine of up to $1,000 or imprisonment for up to six months, or both. A subsequent offence is punishable on summary conviction by a fine of up to $2,000 or imprisonment for up to one year or both. Trafficking, possession for the purpose of trafficking, possession for the purpose of exporting, production, import and export offences are punishable on summary conviction by imprisonment for up to eighteen months or on indictment by imprisonment for up to ten years. |
| Regular use may result in hangovers, weight loss, exhaustion, flashbacks, paranoia, depression, psychosis and liver damage. Studies in animals have found evidence of brain damage with repeated or heavy use | With repeated use, tolerance may develop. Chronic users may become psychologically dependent. MDMA is not known to cause physical dependence. | |

(continued)

Table 11-3 (continued)

## 1. Hallucinogens

| Name/*Street name* | Description | Origin/Medical Use | Short-Term Effects |
|---|---|---|---|
| Psilocybin, and any salts thereof (occurs together with psilocin in some *mushrooms*) *magic mushrooms, shrooms* | Can be distributed as mushrooms or in capsules containing powder of any colour. Can be sniffed, smoked or injected. Powder mixed with fruit juice is common form of preparation. Common dose is anywhere from 1 mg to 20 mg, taken orally. What is sold as psilocybin usually turns out to be PCP or LSD. | Active ingredients in several species of mushroom and other fungi that grow throughout Canada; the most common belong to the genus *Psilocybe*. | Effects are felt after about half an hour, last several hours, and include sensations of relaxation or fatigue, separation from surroundings, heaviness or lightness. Larger doses produce perceptual distortions, dizziness, abdominal discomfort, numbness of the mouth, nausea, shivering, yawning, flushing and sweating. There are no known deaths directly caused by overdose, but drug-induced hazardous behaviours have occurred in some individuals. |

## 2. CNS Depressants (Alcohol and Solvents/Inhalers)

| | | | |
|---|---|---|---|
| Alcohol (ethyl alcohol or ethanol) | In Canada, a standard drink contains 13.6 g or 17 mL of absolute alcohol. This amount is contained in a 12-ounce (341 mL) bottle of regular (5%) beer, five ounces (142 mL) of (12%) table wine or 1.5 ounces (43 mL) of 80-proof liquor. Definitions of standards drinks are different in other countries | Can be synthesized or produced naturally by fermentation of fruits, vegetables or grains. Although some physicians may occasionally recommend alcohol in moderation, this is not common medical practice | Alcohol affects the central nervous system in proportion to the amount of alcohol in bloodstream. Usual effects of small doses are euphoria, drowsiness, dizziness, flushing, release of inhibitions and tensions. Larger doses produce slurred speech, staggering, double vision, stupor. Alcohol, even in fairly low doses, impairs driving or the operation of complex machinery. In combination with other drugs, small doses of alcohol may produce exaggerated effects. A "hangover" with headache, nausea, shakiness and vomiting may begin 8 to 12 hours after a period of excessive drinking. Very large doses can cause death by blocking the brain's control over respiration. |

| Long-Term Effects | Tolerance and Dependence | Legal Status |
|---|---|---|
| | Regular use induces tolerance, making increased doses necessary to produce the desired effect. Psychological and physical dependence can develop. Withdrawal symptoms include anxiety, depression, irritability, dizziness, tremors, nausea, abdominal pains and headaches. | |
| Regular consumption of more than two drinks a day may gradually bring about liver damage, brain damage, heart disease, certain types of cancer, blackouts (loss of memory), impotence, reproductive problems, ulcers, and disorders of the pancreas. Chronic heavy use may result in disruptions of the drinker's social, family and working life. Consumption of alcohol during pregnancy may result in babies with alcohol related pre and postnatal developmental and growth delays, learning and behavioural disorders, and other CNS problems and physical abnormalities. Since there is no definite information regarding a safe quantity of alcohol use during pregnancy, the prudent choice for women who are or may become pregnant is to abstain from alcohol. | Regular use induces tolerance, making increased doses necessary to produce desired effect. In the case of chronic use, people may drink steadily without appearing to get drunk. Their condition may go unrecognized, even by themselves for some time. Chronic drinkers are likely to become physically and psychologically dependent. Withdrawal symptoms may range from jumpiness, sleeplessness, sweating, nausea and vomiting, to tremors, seizures, hallucinations and even death. | Offences relating to underage drinking include possessing, consuming, purchasing, attempting to purchase or otherwise obtaining liquor outside of home. In some jurisdictions, parent or guardian may legally supply liquor at home to an underage person, but in others supplying liquor or selling liquor to a minor is an offence. The age at which young people are allowed to drink in Canada is regulated by legislation and enforcement policy in each province and territory. In the majority of provinces and territories, the drinking age was twenty-one until the early seventies. Currently, in all provinces and territories with the exception of Quebec, Manitoba and Alberta, the drinking age is 19 years. In Quebec, Manitoba and Alberta, the drinking age is eighteen years. Though the trend has been to lower the drinking age, several provinces/territories first lowered and then increased their drinking age from 18 years to 19 years, for example, Ontario, PEI, and Saskatchewan. It is an offence to drive with a blood alcohol level (BAL) of .08% or greater, and to drive while impaired even if one's BAL is less than .08%. Many provinces/territories have introduced 90-day administrative licence suspensions to take effect almost immediately after a driver registers a BAL over the statutory limit or fails to provide a breath sample. In most provinces/ territories, this limit is a BAL of .05%. |

*(continued)*

Table 11-3 (continued)

## 2. CNS Depressants (Alcohol and Solvents/Inhalers)

| Name | Description | Origin/Medical Use | Short-Term Effects |
|---|---|---|---|
| Solvents/Inhalants (volatile solvents) *sniff* | Inhalants are found in many household and commercial products such as cleaning fluids, fast-drying glues, aerosols, paint thinners and removers. Inhalants also include gasoline and other fuels, anaesthetic gases (e.g., nitrous oxide) and some vasodilating nitrites (e.g., amyl nitrite).<br><br>Most are poured into a bag and inhaled, or inhaled from a saturated cloth held over the nose. Aerosols are inhaled either directly from can or by spraying them into a plastic bag. | With few exceptions, these inhalants have no medical use. Rather, they are intended for commercial and household use | Effects include feelings of euphoria, light-headedness, exhilaration, vivid fantasies, and sometimes recklessness and feelings of invincibility. Depending on the type of inhalant and method of use, possibly irritation and watering of the eyes, sneezing, coughing and nasal inflammation may occur. Inhalants enter the bloodstream from the lungs and then go to other organs, particularly the brain and liver. Breathing, heart beat and other body functions are slowed down. If the person passes out with a plastic bag over the nose and mouth, death from suffocation can occur. Death can also occur if the person is startled or engages in strenuous activity while intoxicated. There are also situational hazards such as explosions, burns and aspiration of foreign particles or objects into the lungs. |

## 3. CNS Depressants (Benzodiazepines)

| Name | Description | Origin/Medical Use | Short-Term Effects |
|---|---|---|---|
| Flunitrazepam, and any salts or derivatives thereof Rohypnol® *roofies, rope, the forget pill* | Available as tablets (but tablets may be crushed to yield a powder which dissolves more rapidly in liquids). Often sold on the street in "bubble" packs. It is odourless, colourless and tasteless when added to alcoholic or non-alcoholic beverages. | Although not approved for general marketing as a therapeutic drug in Canada or the U.S., it is legally available in 64 countries in Europe, Latin America, Africa and the Middle East. México and other Latin American countries are the main illegal source of supply for North America. Quantities of smuggled Rohypnol have been seized by the police in Canada. Its use has been associated with "date rape" when it is added to the victim's drink to lower inhibitions and reduce memory of the sexual assault. | Rohypnol is an extremely potent benzodiazepine, which produces drowsiness, dizziness, memory loss, muscle relaxation, impaired thinking and motor coordination. It can also produce aggressive behaviour. It is absorbed very rapidly after oral administration with effects occurring after about 20 to 30 minutes. It has been associated with date rape because it produces sedation and memory loss. Also, because it is odourless and tasteless, the victim may have no idea that anything has been added to his/her drink. The amnesia produced by Rohypnol ("the forget pill") means a rape victim may not remember the circumstances of the sexual assault or how the drug was taken. Combined with alcohol or other CNS depressants, the effects of Rohypnol can be dangerously increased. |

## Long-Term Effects

Effects include pallor, fatigue, forgetfulness, inability to think clearly, tremors, poor coordination and difficulty walking, thirst, weight loss, depression, irritability, hostility, and paranoia. Kidney, liver and brain damage may occur. It is not known to what extent the damage is reversible. Simultaneous alcohol consumption may compound the damage. Elevated blood-lead levels and consequent brain damage have been found as a result of chronic sniffing of leaded gasoline

## Tolerance and Dependence

Regular use induces tolerance, making increased doses necessary to produce the desired effect. Psychological and physical dependence can develop. Withdrawal symptoms include anxiety, depression, irritability, dizziness, tremors, nausea, abdominal pains, and headaches.

## Legal Status

Inhalants are generally not controlled in Canada. Inhalant abuse may be a factor taken into account in dealing with young offenders and children found in need of protection under provincial legislation. In Alberta, inhaling or selling inhalants to inhalers is illegal.

---

Some benzodiazepines which are eliminated slowly (such as diazepam) accumulate in body tissues during sustained use. Chronic abuse of benzodiazepines may result in impairment in thinking, memory and judgement, confusion, disorientation, and impaired motor coordination. Prolonged use may also lead to increased, rather than reduced, aggressiveness in some people. When benzodiazepines are used by pregnant women, they cross the placenta and are distributed to the fetus. After birth, babies exposed to benzodiazepines in the uterus may show withdrawal symptoms. There is some research evidence indicating an increased risk of major malformations and cleft palate.

Tolerance to the sedative, but not anxiety-relieving effects of benzodiazepines can develop with regular use over a few months, as can psychological and physical dependence. Stopping use abruptly may result in symptoms such as sleep disturbances, headache, tension, difficulty concentrating, trembling, anxiety, and feeling tired. During withdrawal from very high doses, there is a risk of seizures, depression, paranoia, agitation and delirium. Withdrawal symptoms may be greater for benzodiazepines that are eliminated rapidly from the body.

Rohypnol is not approved for general marketing as a therapeutic drug in Canada. Flunitrazepam (Rohypnol) is governed by the provisions of the Controlled Drugs and Substances Act applicable to Schedule III. Possession of Rohypnol is a criminal offence punishable by imprisonment for up to three years on indictment or upon summary conviction to a fine of up to $1,000 or six months imprisonment, or both, for a first offence, and a fine of up to $2,000 or up to one year imprisonment, or both, for a subsequent offence. Offences of trafficking, possession for the purpose of trafficking, possession for the purpose of exporting, production, import and export of flunitrazepam are punishable upon indictment by imprisonment for up to 10 years and upon summary conviction by imprisonment for up to eighteen months.

*(continued)*

Table 11-3 (continued)

**4. Stimulants**

| Name | Description | Origin/Medical Use | Short-Term Effects |
|---|---|---|---|
| Cocaine<br>*C, coke, snow, nose candy, crack* | Fine white crystalline powder often diluted with sugar, cornstarch, talcum powder or with substances which imitate its numbing effects, such as benzocaine. Can be sniffed, smoked or injected. As well as being sniffed through the nose, it can also be absorbed through other mucous membranes such as the mouth. Typical dose levels are 30-100 mg when sniffed; injected doses may be lower or higher, depending on the tolerance of the person. "Crack" is a smokable, freebase form of cocaine which has become increasingly available in recent years. It is made by adding baking soda to a cocaine solution and allowing the mixture to dry. | Derived from leaves of South American coca bush. Practice of sniffing cocaine began around turn of the century, when it was also consumed in the form of tonics and beverages. By 1911, cocaine was legally restricted in Canada. It is still used as a local anaesthetic for some surgery, but has been largely replaced by less toxic substances. | Effects resemble those of amphetamines with a shorter duration. The person feels euphoric, energetic, alert; has a rapid heartbeat and breathing, dilated pupils, sweating, pallor, and decreased appetite. Large doses can cause severe agitation, paranoid thinking, erratic or violent behaviour, tremors, unco-ordination, twitching, hallucinations, headache, pain or pressure in the chest, nausea, blurred vision, fever, muscle spasms, convulsions and death. Impurities in street cocaine may produce a fatal allergic reaction. People may experience depression, extreme tiredness and stuffy nose as a "hangover" from cocaine. The use of "crack" produces immediate and very intense effects. |
| Tobacco (Nicotiana tabacum) | Shredded, cured (dried) leaves of the tobacco plant, which can be smoked in cigarettes, cigars or pipes, or chewed, or inhaled. New regulations will require manufacturers to display health warnings, health information and toxic constituent information on packages of all tobacco products. The health warnings will occupy 50 percent of the package and will include graphic images of the | Discovered among Northern and Central American tribes during 16th century. There is no current medical use for tobacco. However, nicotine, the main psychoactive component of tobacco, is an active ingredient in nicotine "gum" and nicotine "patches," used as aids to assist smokers to quit smoking. | Effects include increased heart rate and blood pressure, drop in skin temperature, faster breathing, and decreased appetite. First-time smokers may feel dizzy and energized and may experience diarrhoea and vomiting. Tar accumulates in the lungs. Inhaling smokers subject themselves to very high carbon monoxide levels. They also subject people around them to smoke effects. Two or three drops of pure nicotine, the plant's most potent ingredient, may rapidly kill an adult. A single cigarette puts about 1-2 mg of nicotine into the bloodstream of the 15-20 mg found in tobacco. When eaten, nicotine is absorbed slowly in stomach, which is why small children sometimes survive after eating cigarettes. |

| Long-Term Effects | Tolerance and Dependence | Legal Status |
|---|---|---|

High-dose, chronic users, who alternate cocaine "binges" with crashes (periods of abstinence) may show mood swings, restlessness, extreme excitability, restlessness, sleep disorders, suspiciousness, hallucinations and delusions, eating disorders, weight loss, constipation and impotence. Characteristic signs of chronic cocaine sniffing are stuffiness and runny nose, chapped nostrils, perforation of nasal septum. Cocaine abuse is also associated with cardiac arrhythmias, myocardial infarctions, strokes, seizures and sudden deaths. People who inject cocaine are at risk for HIV and hepatitis.

Heavy use of cocaine by pregnant women is associated with reduced fetal weight and an increased risk of miscarriage, stillbirth, premature birth and malformation. Newborns exposed to cocaine in the uterus may also experience abnormal sleep patterns, poor feeding and irritability for several days or weeks after birth.

Tar is a complex mixture of particles found in tobacco smoke. It has been identified as causing cancer in smokers. An average smoker who consumes 20 cigarettes per day can inhale between 1 and 140 gm per year, depending upon the cigarette smoked and how it is smoked. Much of this is coughed up in phlegm. Possible effects of smoking include cancer of the lungs, mouth and throat, respiratory disease, heart attack, stroke and stomach ulcers. Smoking increases blood pressure, depletes Vitamin C levels, causes skin wounds to heal more slowly, and reduces immunity to disease. Research indicates that each cigarette cuts 5.5 minutes from smoker's lifespan. The babies of women who smoke tend to

---

Chronic use results in tolerance. Cocaine can produce very powerful psychological dependence leading to extremely compulsive patterns of use. In particular, the dependency-producing properties of cocaine are believed to be more powerful than any other psychoactive drug. Physical dependence may also develop. Withdrawal symptoms may include fatigue, long but disturbed sleep, strong hunger, irritability, depression, violence.

Most smokers are physically and psychologically dependent. Those who quit early may achieve the same health levels as non-smokers after a few years, although some damage may not be completely reversible.

---

In Canada, cocaine is governed by the Controlled Drugs and Substances Act applicable to Schedule I. Unlawful possession is a criminal offence punishable on indictment by imprisonment for up to seven years and on summary conviction for a first offence to a fine of up to $1,000 or imprisonment for up to six months, or both. A subsequent offence is punishable upon summary conviction by a fine of up to $2,000 or imprisonment for up to one year, or both. Trafficking, possession for the purpose of trafficking, possession for the purpose of exporting, production (cultivation of Erythroxylon coca), import and export are indictable offences punishable by up to life imprisonment.

The Federal Tobacco Act sets 18 as the minimum age at which retailers may furnish tobacco products to youth. Some provinces, notably Nova Scotia, New Brunswick, Newfoundland, Ontario and British Columbia, have set this age limit at 19. In addition, because it can harm the non-smoker in a variety of ways, from irritation to death, many municipalities and provinces have enacted by-laws that restrict or ban smoking in public places, including restaurants and bars. At the federal level, the Non-Smokers' Health Act bans smoking in all federally-regulated workplaces and bans smoking on trains, planes, buses and ships.

(continued)

Table 11-3 (continued)

## 4. Stimulants

| Name | Description | Origin/Medical Use | Short-Term Effects |
|------|-------------|--------------------|--------------------|
| | consequences of tobacco use. New regulations will also require manufacturers to collect and report on 43 of the over 4,000 chemicals found in tobacco smoke. Of these, tar, nicotine, carbon monoxide, benzene, formaldehyde and hydrogen cyanide will be listed on the package with a range of emissions, depending upon smoking patterns. | | |

## 5. Cannabis

| Name | Description | Origin/Medical Use | Short-Term Effects |
|------|-------------|--------------------|--------------------|
| Marijuana (marihuana) cannabis, pot, grass, weed, reefer, ganja, joint | Flowering tops and leaves of the cannabis plant. Ranges in colour from grey-green to greenish-brown; in texture, it resembles oregano or coarse tea. It usually contains seeds and stems. It has a strong odour and is smoked in a pipe or hand-rolled cigarette. There are greater concentrations of the active ingredient, THC, now than in the past. | Obtained from the plant Cannabis sativa, which grows in almost any climate. In the past, most Cannabis products found in Canada were grown in South and Central America. Now much is grown locally, some under hydroponic conditions. THC (delta-9 tetrahydrocannabinol) and other cannabis constituents have been claimed in anecdotal reports to relieve symptoms associated with the following medical conditions: nausea and vomiting, wasting syndrome, multiple sclerosis, epilepsy and glaucoma. THC | Effects of smoking are felt within a few minutes and last two to four hours. Effects from ingestion (e.g., eaten in baked or cooked foods) appear more gradually and last longer, and the person may feel dull and sluggish for some time afterwards. The person feels calm, relaxed, talkative and sometimes drowsy. Concentration and short-term memory are markedly impaired, and sensory perception seems enhanced, colours are brighter, sounds are more distinct, and the sense of time and space is distorted. Appetite increases, especially for sweets. Some people withdraw, or experience fearfulness, anxiety, depression; a few experience panic, terror or paranoia, particularly with larger doses. Some experience hallucinations with larger doses and symptoms worsen in persons with psychiatric disorders, particularly schizophrenia.<br><br>Physical effects include impaired coordination and balance, rapid heartbeat, red eyes, dry mouth and throat. Usual doses impair motor skills; especially when used in combination with alcohol; cannabis use before driving is particularly dangerous. THC, the active ingredient, has been detected in many bodies of fatally-injured drivers and pedestrians in Canada and the United States. |

| Long-Term Effects | Tolerance and Dependence | Legal Status |
| --- | --- | --- |

weigh less at birth than those of non-smokers; the risk of prematurity, miscarriage and stillbirth is greater. Studies suggest that the mother's smoking can have a detrimental effect on the child's growth, intellectual development and behaviour.

Second-hand smoke (passive smoking) increases the risk of lung cancer and heart disease in non-smokers. Children whose parents smoke have more ear infections, more chest infections and other lung problems, such as asthma, than children of non-smokers. Second-hand smoke is a special problem for allergic people and those with heart or lung disease.

Signs of chronic, heavy use may include decreased motivation and interest, as well as difficulties with memory and concentration. These problems tend to clear when regular use stops. However, there is increasing research evidence of lasting harmful effects on mental function in some people. The respiratory system is damaged by smoking; a single joint of marijuana yields much more tar than a strong cigarette. Tar in cannabis smoke contains higher amounts of cancer-producing agents than tar in tobacco smoke. Studies suggest that developmental delays may occur in children whose mothers used drugs heavily during pregnancy.

There is some evidence that tolerance develops in regular high-dose users. Psychological and physical dependence on cannabis can occur in people who use heavily or regularly. Withdrawal symptoms include anxiety, irritability, sleeping problems, sweating and loss of appetite.

In Canada, cannabis, its preparations, derivatives and similar synthetic preparations are governed by the provisions of the Controlled Drugs and Substances Act applicable to Schedule II. Both non-viable cannabis seeds and mature cannabis stalks without attached leaves, flowers, seeds or branches, as well as the fibre derived from such stalks are excluded from the application of the Act. However, the derivatives of non-viable cannabis seeds are covered.

Unlawful possession is a criminal offence. A conviction for unlawful possession of 30 g or less of cannabis marijuana or 1 g or less of cannabis resin is an exclusively summary conviction offence punishable by a fine of up to $1,000 or imprisonment for up to six months, or both. Unlawful possession of more than 30 g of cannabis marijuana, more than 1 g of cannabis resin, or any quantity of cannabis plant, hash oil, or other constituent of the cannabis plant or other preparations, derivatives or similar synthetic preparations is punishable upon conviction on indictment to

(continued)

Table 11-3 (continued)

**5. Cannabis**

| Name | Description | Origin/Medical Use | Short-Term Effects |
|---|---|---|---|
| | | chemically synthesized is marketed as Marinol® (dronabinol) and Cesamet (nabilone), a synthetic cannabinoid, are both used orally to treat nausea and vomiting resulting from chemotherapy. The treatment of AIDS-related anorexia associated with weight loss is another approved use of Marinol (dronabinol). | |

| Long-Term Effects | Tolerance and Dependence | Legal Status |
| --- | --- | --- |
| | | imprisonment for up to five years less a day or upon summary conviction for a first offence to a fine of up to $1,000 or imprisonment for up to six months, or both. Upon summary conviction for a subsequent offence, to a fine of up to $2,000 or imprisonment for up to one year, or both. |
| | | Trafficking and possession for the purpose of trafficking in 3 kg. or less of cannabis marijuana or cannabis resin is an indictable offence punishable by imprisonment for up to five years less a day. Trafficking and possession for the purpose of trafficking in quantities of cannabis marijuana or cannabis resin over 3 kg., any quantity of cannabis plant, hash oil, or other constituent of the cannabis plant, or other preparation, derivative or similar synthetic preparations is an indictable offence punishable by up to life imprisonment. Production (cultivation) of cannabis marijuana is punishable by imprisonment for up to seven years. Possession for the purpose of export, import and export of any quantity of cannabis plant, cannabis marijuana, cannabis resin, hash oil, or other constituent of the cannabis plant or other preparations, derivatives or similar synthetic preparations is an indictable offence punishable by up to life imprisonment. |

Source: Health Canada. *Straight Facts about Drugs & Drug Abuse: The Charts*. Ottawa: Author, 2000. © Adapted and reproduced with the permission of the Minister of Public Works and Government Services Canada, 2007.

## Table 11-4 Selected Interdisciplinary Interventions in Treatment of Substance Abuse

| Intervention | Description and Techniques |
|---|---|
| Breaking through defences | Breakdown of pathologic defence mechanisms in the denial system is a gradual process. The care professional:<br>• Must recognize and understand the client's defensive manoeuvre<br>• Assist client to come face-to-face with the objective reality that is being denied<br>• Maintain a consistent, persistent approach with the client (This conveys the message that there never is a valid reason for the client to use drugs or alcohol.)<br>• Refocus the client on the substance dependence problem (Do not become sidetracked around other problems.) |
| Understanding and accepting the disorder | Assist the client who is dependent on substances to attain an intellectual comprehension of the disorder:<br>• Disorders are illnesses, not mental problems<br>• Provide educational materials and clarification of misinformation<br>• Understanding the disease in an intellectual, factual manner helps client to accept the fact that the disorder is chronic and cannot be cured<br>• The disorder must be accepted on an emotional level and recovery on a long-term, day-to-day basis<br>• Abstinence is a prerequisite to recovery Identification with peers Peer group identification and confrontation are powerful experiences in recovery.<br>• Assist clients to recognize and internalize that they are not alone in their suffering and that they can receive support and hope.<br>• Groups allow for confrontation by peers who attack pathologic defence mechanisms. By doing so they help each other in the process of obtaining insight into their behaviours. |
| Development of hope | Initial feelings of clients often include hopelessness, discouragement, and demoralization.<br>• The client needs to realize that it is possible to escape from what may be seen as a hopeless situation.<br>• Identifying with others who are going through recovery is significant in providing hope.<br>• Positive attitudes of caregivers also instill hope. |
| Resocialization | The pursuit of the addictive substance often causes the user's life to become drug-centred.<br>• Consequently, the client becomes self-centred.<br>• Assist the client to review and rebuild the capacity for establishing interpersonal relationships that the previously self-centred attitude has eroded. |
| Developing self-esteem and self-worth | Self-esteem and self-worth increase as the client is able to see the substance abuse problem as an illness.<br>• The client can help self by taking the responsibility for making changes in own attitudes and actions.<br>• The client often needs help in developing self-discipline, such as organizing and adhering to a daily routine.<br>• Encourage positive efforts to change.<br>• Motivation is enhanced as involvement in the program increases. |

Source: Cornwell, C.J., The Client Who Abuses Drugs and Alcohol. In W.K. Mohr (ed.), *Johnson's Psychiatric-Mental Health Nursing*, 5th ed. (pp. 575–606). Philadelphia: Lippincott Williams & Wilkins, 2003. Adapted and reproduced with the permission of Lippincott Williams & Wilkins Copyright © 2007.

## Working with the Substance Abuser

**Personal Attitudes** You must work through your own attitudes about drug use and abuse to be able to assess the person accurately, or intervene objectively. Why does a drug problem exist? Do you believe that drugs are the answer to problems? How frequently do you use drugs? Do you use amphetamines or barbiturates? Have you ever tried marijuana, LSD, or heroin? What are the multiple influences causing persons to seek answers through the use of illegal drugs? What are the moral, spiritual, emotional, and physical implications of excessive drug use, whether the drugs are illegal or prescribed? What treatment do drug abusers deserve? How does the alcoholic differ from the drug abuser?

An accepting attitude toward the drug abuser and alcoholic *as a person* is essential while your are helping him or her to become motivated and able to cope with stresses without relying on drugs or alcohol. You will need to use effective communication and assessment techniques. However, because these problems are complex, you will need to work with others as well. References at the end of this chapter, cited previously, provide detailed information to aid you in your care.

Members of society impose heavy responsibilities on the young adult. With your intervention, some adolescents, who could not otherwise meet these forthcoming demands, will exert a positive force in society.

**Knowledge** Knowledge about drugs—current ones available on the street, their symptoms and long-term effects, and legislation related to each—is necessary for assessment, realistic teaching, and counselling. Learn about the short-term and long-term effects of alcohol. Know local community agencies that do emergency or follow-up care and rehabilitation with drug abusers and alcoholics.

Help teenagers to understand that problems of substance abuse can be avoided in several ways. They must get accurate information and make decisions based on knowledge rather than on emotion. They must have the courage to say "no," and know and respect the law. They must also participate in worthwhile, satisfying activities, have constructive interactions with parents, and recognize that the healthy person does not need medication except when prescribed by a family physician. Help teens to realize the unanticipated consequences of drug and alcohol abuse: loss of friends; alienation from family; loss of scholastic, social, or career opportunities; economic difficulties; criminal activities; legal penalties; poor health; and the loss of personal identity rather than finding, promoting, and developing the self.

---

CRITICAL THINKING

*As a health professional, what recommendations would you offer for effective programming for the prevention and reduction of substance abuse among youth?*

---

**Sexual Activity** Healthy sexual development begins in childhood. This includes the development of gender identification and sexual orientation, positive experiences of sexual and sensual feelings, and the development of intimacy and trust. On the other hand, exposure to harmful attitudes about sexuality and experiences of emotional, physical, and sexual abuse may occur at this age. Decisions about sexual activity and reproduction are made during adolescence and young adulthood.[207]

In 2003, about 6 in 10 young people aged 15 to 24 reported having sexual intercourse at least once in their lives. The average age at first-time sexual intercourse was consistent for both sexes: 16.5 years. As expected, the likelihood of having sex rose as teens approached adulthood.[208]

Adolescents have many reasons for wanting to be sexually active, including to:

1. Enhance self-esteem
2. Have someone care about them
3. Experiment
4. Be accepted by peers
5. Feel grown up
6. Be close and touched by another
7. Feel pleasure or have fun
8. Seek revenge
9. Determine normality
10. Love and be loved
11. Gain control over another[209]

Some of the specific reasons for the increase of sexually transmitted infections (STIs) in recent years include changing sexual patterns, changing attitudes and cultural mores regarding sexual behaviour, lack of understanding about STIs, and the feeling of "it can't happen to me."

Today, sexual activity is almost completely regarded as an individual responsibility. The areas related to adolescent sexual activity that influence health are those involving STIs, the use of contraceptives, pregnancy, abortion, and incest. A careful history is essential when caring for the adolescent regarding sexual activity.

## SEXUALLY TRANSMITTED INFECTIONS

**Sexually transmitted infections (STIs)** are *infections grouped together because they spread by transfer of infectious organisms from person to person during sexual contact, through sexual intercourse, oral sex, or anal sex. While some are curable with medication, others have no known cure and can only be managed through treatment.*

STIs are an escalating public health concern and challenge in Canada.[210] Since 1997, reported rates of genital chlamydia and gonorrhea have been steadily increasing. Rates of infectious syphilis began to increase slowly in 1997, and then rose rapidly from 2000 onward. Since 2004, all three reportable bacterial STIs are continuing their upward climb of reported occurrences, and are affecting increasingly more Canadians.[211] Genital chlamydia remains the most commonly reported STI and notifiable disease in Canada. Rates of chlamydia and gonorrhea were projected for the years 2005 to 2010 to provide a concrete example of what STI rates in Canada may look like in the absence of a substantive shift in the epidemic. If the current trends persist, rates will reach even greater heights than were predicted for the end of the decade. Since co-infections with multiple viral or bacterial STIs are common, especially in high-risk populations, factors that cut across infections need to be taken into consideration when developing public health interventions.[212]

In Canada, reported rates of chlamydia and gonorrhea are highest among Aboriginal (First Nations, Inuit) adolescents; in some regions (Nunavut, Northwest Territories), chlamydia and gonorrhea rates were reported to be more than ten times that of the national average.[213] Recently, the prevention of STIs and their negative health, social, and economic consequences for Aboriginal adolescents has become a central goal for many community-based health programs.[214] Working together with Aboriginal youth to address the psychosocial issues affecting their health and STI prevention is one way for holistic health nurses to develop a health care system that is accountable to the community for the adolescents' health needs. Group discussions and communication about STIs with encouragement and support for youth members to suggest realistic solutions are both important and essential to realize a beginning to the solution of this national threat.[215]

Steenbeck and her associates state that in helping Inuit adolescents achieve healthier reproductive health, public health nurses must understand the historical and cultural issues surrounding STIs in the Inuit adolescent population. For example, until recently, contraceptives were unknown to most Inuit people.[216] Public health nurses must understand the differences and similarities between this culture and the rest of the country. They must then use this knowledge to provide culturally specific care. To ignore such cultural differences may seriously undermine the nurse's ability to assist such a client effectively. As well, such an oversight could prevent the client from achieving their personally defined health state.[217]

See Table 11-5 for an over view of bacterial STIs.

---

## CRITICAL THINKING

*Prepare a nursing care plan for an adolescent who has chlamydia.*

---

**Contraceptive Practices** In Canada, new advances in contraceptive methods are making it possible for Canadians to have access to a broad range of options. However, the new and comprehensive second edition of *Sex Sense,*written by the Society of Obstetricians and Gynaecologists of Canada, states that youth and adults are unaware of the dangers of unprotected sex.[218] This handy little book provides answers to questions about today's contraceptive methods and the best protection from STIs and HIV/AIDS.

According to the Canadian Contraceptive Study 2002 Report, among respondents aged 15 to 44, oral contraception, condoms, and sterilization were the contraceptive methods of choice. Oral contraception and condoms were the predominant methods as reported by unmarried women aged 15 to 17. Meanwhile, sterilization was the predominantly selected method among married couples aged 35 to 44, with male sterilization being more than twice as common as female sterilization.[219]

**Contraception**, or **birth control**, is *the use of various devices, chemicals, or abortion to prevent or terminate pregnancy.* The adolescent may choose contraception to avoid pregnancy while continuing sexual activity. A number of contraceptive options are available to Canadians. Hormonal methods of contraception used in Canada are summarized in Table 11-6. Additional information may be obtained from other references.[220] It is important to work with adolescent clients to determine which method will be most appropriate, while acknowledging the medical issues as well as safer sex.[221] Your approach and the structure of the health care environment are critical to the teenager's adherence to instructions about contraceptive practices or abstinence.

Some youth, however, do not use contraceptives for the following reasons:

1. Misconceptions or ignorance about them

2. Inability to secure appropriate contraceptives

---

## CONTROVERSY DEBATE

# You Tell Him, Please

Rebecca, a 15-year-old adolescent, comes to the Women's Health Clinic for her first visit. Her boyfriend, John, is with her. Rebecca informs the nurse that she has been having unprotected sex with John for a while now. She goes on to say that she loves John, but does not know if she could ever tell him that he must wear a condom. She thinks that John does not believe in using condoms, and she does not wish to offend him by mentioning the subject to him. She pleads with you to speak to him privately about contraceptive measures.

1. What will be your initial response to Rebecca?

2. How will you initiate a dialogue about sexual health education with the couple?

3. What objectives will you set for yourself to educate this couple in sexual matters?

## Table 11-5 Bacterial Sexually Transmitted Infections (STIs)

| Name of STI | How You Get It | How Long before You May Notice Symptoms | Where You May Notice Symptoms | What If You are Pregnant? | Long Term Effects of Repeat and Untreated Infections | How are You Tested? | How are You Treated? |
|---|---|---|---|---|---|---|---|
| Chlamydia | Unprotected Oral, vaginal, and anal sex | 2 to 6 weeks. Most do not have symptoms | Eyes, throat, rectum, vagina, and urethra | Baby can develop pneumonia or eye infections during birth | Pelvic Inflammatory Disease (PID). Infertility and ectopic pregnancy for women. Inflammation of the testes and epididymous in men, which may affect fertility | Urine or swab from the infected area | Curable with antibiotics. |
| Gonorrhea | Unprotected oral, vaginal, and anal sex | 2 to 7 weeks. Most do not have symptoms | Throat, rectum, vagina and urethra | Baby can develop eye infections during birth. | PID. Infertility and ectopic pregnancy for women. Inflammation of the testes and epididymous in men, which may affect fertility | Swab from the infected area. Urine testing is available in some areas | Curable with antibiotics |
| Syphilis | Unprotected oral, vaginal and, anal sex. Rarely through contact with blood. Can transmit it during primary, secondary and early latent phase (less than a year) | Symptoms appear in stages: primary, secondary, latent and tertiary. Symptoms of earlier stages appear from days to months after exposure. Late latent and tertiary can take up to and beyond 30 years | Mouth, genital, and anal region; as it progresses to later stages, symptoms can be found throughout the body, e.g. rash on feet and hands | Baby can be infected during pregnancy, during primary, secondary and latent stage, possibly leading to birth defects and death. Baby can also be infected at birth | With tertiary stage irreversible damage to internal organs, such as heart and brain | Swab of any sores and/or blood sample | Curable with antibiotics, length varies with stage of infection. Damage from late phase is not reversed with treatment |
| Lyphogranuloma Venereum / LGV | Unprotected oral, vaginal, and anal sex | 3 days to 2 months. Symptoms progress in stages: primary, secondary and tertiary | Throat, rectum, vagina, urethra and glands in the infected area | Baby can be infected during birth | Swelling and damage to glands in the groin and neck. Scarring and irreversible damage to genitals and rectum | Swab of any sores, blood sample or fluid sample from swollen glands | Curable with antibiotics. Damage from tertiary stage is not reversed with typical treatment. May require surgery |

Source: Society of Obstetricians and Gynaecologists of Canada, *Sex Sense: Canadian Contraception Guide*, 2nd, revised ed. Ottawa: Author, 2005. Reproduced with the permission of the Society of Obstetricians and Gynaecologists of Canada © 2005.

**Table 11-6 Hormonal Methods of Contraception**

| | Oral Contraceptive Pill | Transdermal Contraceptive Patch | Contraceptive Ring | Progestin-only Pill | Injectable Contraceptive | Implant | Intrauterine System (IUS) |
|---|---|---|---|---|---|---|---|
| Type of drug | Tablet to take daily for 3 weeks, placebo pill to take daily for 1 week* | Patch to be changed every week for 3 weeks. No patch for 1 week. | Ring to be inserted and left in for three weeks. | Tablet to take every day. No breaks | Injection in muscle of upper arm, buttocks or thigh every 10-13 weeks. No interruptions. | Implant under skin of upper arm every 3-5 years. | One injection every 5 years. |
| Name | Many different brands to choose from | Evra® | NuvaRing® | Micronor® | Depo-Provera® | Norplant® Implanon® | Mirena® |
| Type of hormone | estrogen + progestin | estrogen + progestin | estrogen + progestin | progestin only | progestin only | progestin only | progestin only |
| Prevents pregnancy primarily by... | stopping ovulation | stopping ovulation | stopping ovulation | changing lining of uterus, thickening mucus | stopping ovulation | changing lining of uterus, thickening mucus | changing lining of uterus |
| Your periods are likely to become | very regular | very regular | very regular | somewhat irregular | sparse | somewhat irregular | sparse |
| Absence of regular bleeding (amenorrhea) occurs | rarely | very rarely | very rarely | occasionally | very often | often | often |
| You can stop the method . . . | any time | any time | any time | any time | only after the 12-week interval is over | any time (appointment for removal necessary) | any time |
| You can have a baby afterwards | when you have your first period | when you have your first period | when you have your first period | when you have your first period | when you have your first period (up to 9 months after the last injection) | when you have your first period | when you have your first period |

*1 week of placebo pills are supplied only in 28-day packs. They are also referred to as "sugar pills".

Source: Society of Obstetricians and Gynaecologists of Canada. *Sex Sense: Canadian Contraception Guide*, 2nd revised ed. Ottawa: Author, 2005. Reproduced with the permission of the Society of Obstetricians and Gynaecologists of Canada © 2005.

3. Inability to plan ahead for their actions
4. Belief that using contraceptives marks them as promiscuous
5. Rebelliousness

Males are less likely to recognize the risk of pregnancy as a result of sexual activity, have less information about contraceptives, and are less supportive of contraceptive use than females.

## CRITICAL THINKING

*What are some ways health care professionals can promote a better understanding of, and compliance with, practices related to family planning?*

Adolescent Pregnancy  Available data on adolescent pregnancy in Canada suggest that, over time, sexually active teens have become more successful in avoiding pregnancy.[222] The birth control pill, a highly effective form of safe contraception, plays an important role in helping young Canadian women control their fertility. The increased use of oral contraception appears to have been a factor in contributing to the decline in pregnancy rates. When used correctly and consistently, the birth control pill is a female-controlled method of contraception that prevents pregnancy 99.9 percent of the time.[223] According to the Canadian Youth, Sexual Health and HIV/AIDS Study, adolescents were familiar with the morning-after pill, but were less aware of other methods of contraception. The sexually active teens surveyed did not use spermicidal methods or IUDs.[224]

Other determinants that have likely contributed to the decrease in teen pregnancy rates in Canada include socioeconomic factors, access to user-friendly reproductive health services, and access to high-quality sexual health education.[225] Wackett states that in the Yukon, teen pregnancy in the late 1990s was almost 40 percent lower than it was in the 1980s.[226]

Unintended pregnancy causes much human misery—for the pregnant teen and her family, and often for the offspring. Effects on the teen father are less well known.[227]

Other factors and combinations of factors may also contribute to the teenage girl's becoming pregnant; the box entitled "Factors Influencing Incidence of Adolescent Pregnancy" summarizes most of them.[228]

Neonatal risks associated with teenage maternity are not uniform, but are common. The risks vary by age of the adolescent mother, amount of prenatal care, and ethnic identification.

Risks are highest for 11- to 14-year-old teens. Early fertility implies early menarche, which is associated with short stature, a risk factor for poor neonatal outcome. The excessive rates of short gestation, low birth weight, and neonatal mortality may result from a variety of physiologic consequences of environmental or sociocultural disadvantage, not primarily from biological developmental limits.[229] When teenagers choose to continue their pregnancy to term, exemplary care should be provided before, during, and after delivery to help minimize the risk of negative outcomes that may occur.[230] Peterson and her researchers conducted a qualitative study to describe adolescent mothers' satisfactory and unsatisfactory inpatient postpartum nursing care experiences. Their findings indicated that those nursing care qualities that contribute most to satisfactory experiences include information shared by the nurse about themselves. Doing so helps to demonstrate the nurse's confidence in the mothers, that she can anticipate unstated needs and interact with the adolescent mothers in the same way that they interact with other adult mothers.[231]

Often, the adolescent parent expects behaviour beyond the developmental ability of the baby. Such an expectation creates intense frustration and anger in both mother and father and can often result in child abuse or neglect.[232] *You may be able to assess these behaviours and intervene to provide support, teaching, and counselling.*

A major problem in adolescent parenting is that many teenage girls who become mothers themselves have come from single-parent homes or homes in which active participation by the father is minimal or lacking. Further, the teenage father often provides no real support—emotional or financial. Often, the maternal grandmother is the one who is left to raise the child.

There are ways to help the teenage mother be an effective and loving mother and at the same time feel secure and comfortable with parenting. Several research studies have examined teen experiences in motherhood and childrearing. The studies identified the importance of support groups designed for pregnant adolescents and their parents or significant caregivers.[233]

Agencies that provide adolescent pregnancy programs should cater to both teen fathers and teen mothers with parenting classes and child development information. A drop-in centre where the teen can take her baby for a few hours to be free of child care for a while and to gain emotional support and information is also a useful community support. The teen parent needs multiple supports from family, school, peers, church, the media, the community, and the legal system. In Canada, many government-sponsored child and family programs are in place, such as parental-leave benefits and the Canada Child Tax Benefit—a tax-free monthly payment based on family income.

## Factors Influencing Incidence of Adolescent Pregnancy

### Developmental Factors

- Low self-esteem
- Need to be close to someone; to relieve loneliness
- Recent experience of significant loss or change
- School dropout, school underachiever
- Personal fable (feeling that "it won't happen to me")
- Responsiveness to peers' sexual behaviour
- Independence from family
- Need to prove own womanhood

### Societal Factors

- Variety of adult sexual behaviour values
- Implied acceptance of intercourse outside of marriage
- Importance of involvement in heterosexual relationships stressed by the media

### Family and Friends

- Difficult mother–daughter relationship
- Mother, sister, or close relative pregnant as teen
- Sexually permissive behaviour norms of the larger peer group
- Sexually permissive behaviour of close friends; immediate peer group sexually active
- Inadequate communication in heterosexual relationships
- History of sexual abuse or incest
- Few, if any, girlfriends
- Older boyfriend
- Substance abuse or use in family or peer group

**Care Related to Sexuality** One key component of adolescent health is a regular sexual health assessment. Nurses can use a question framework as provided in the box entitled "Routine Sexual Health Assessment."[234] Discussions about sexual health issues will not always be initiated by adolescents. Consequently, nurses must be proactive in initiating such enquiries. Nurses should encourage adolescents to discuss health concerns and, during such discussions, nurses can provide teaching for the issues that are important to this age group. Several elements, described below, are important for nurses to consider before such discussions can take place.

**Personal Attitudes** First, examine personal attitudes toward yourself as a sexual being, the sexuality of others, family, love, and changing mores regarding sexual intercourse before you do any sex education through formal or informal teaching, counselling, or discussion. The adolescent may be trying to understand another kind of sexual experience in his or her own family. For example, sometimes adolescents must deal with a formerly hidden primary sexual orientation of their parents. Either parent may, during this time, announce a same-sex preference. So, in addition to working out his or her own sexual identity, the adolescent must now face the new identity of the parent. Your astute assessment, case finding, and ability to refer the adolescent elsewhere are all major contributions toward helping him or her stay healthy. The rapport necessary to work with the adolescent in any area is something to which the teen is highly sensitive. If he or she has a low level of rapport with the family, your attitude is crucial.

**Promoting Education** You can promote education about sexuality, family, pregnancy, contraceptives, and sexually transmitted infections through your own intervention and by working with parents and school officials so that objective, accurate information can be provided in the schools. Most adults favour sex education in school as a way to reduce the problem of teenage pregnancy.

Perhaps most important, you can *encourage the teenager and family to talk together. You can teach the parents* how and what to teach, where to get information, and the significance of formal sex education beginning in the home.

**Care and Counselling** You may find yourself working directly either with a pregnant teenager or with one who has an STI. That person needs your acceptance, support, and confidentiality while you do careful interviewing to learn his or her history of sexual activity, symptoms, and contacts. Use effective interviewing, communication, and crisis intervention as discussed in Chapter 5 and by other authors.

Information is needed about the type of disease, symptoms, contagious nature, consequences of untreated disease, and where to get treatment. In all of these diseases, both male and female partners (along with any other person who has had sexual contact with these partners) should be treated—through the use of medication, the use of safe hygienic measures, and by counselling and teaching. You are in a key position to observe meaningful signs and symptoms, and to help make a differential diagnosis.

The girl wants to find out whether she is pregnant. She wants to talk about her personal feelings, her family reactions, and what to do next. You can explain what services are available and answer her questions about the consequences of remaining pregnant, keeping or placing the baby for adoption, or even whether to terminate the pregnancy.

1. Are you sexually active? By sexually active, I mean have you had sexual intercourse? Have you had oral sex? Have you had anal sex?

2. Have you had sex with females, with males, or with both?

3. How many sexual partners have you had? Did you always use condoms?

4. What are you and your current partner doing to prevent pregnancy?

5. What are you and your current partner doing to prevent sexually transmitted infections/HIV infection?

6. Has anyone ever forced you physically to do something sexual?

7. Has anyone ever put a lot of pressure on you to do something sexual that you did not want to do?

8. You are _____ years-old? How old is your partner?

9. Do you experience any pain or discomfort in the genital area? Any pain or discomfort during sexual activity?

10. Are there any questions about sex that you want to ask me?

Source: McKay, A. Adolescent Sexual and Reproductive Health in Canada: A Report Card in 2004, *The Canadian Journal of Human Sexuality*, 13(2) (2004), 67–81. Reproduced with the permission of Sex Information and Education Council of Canada © 2007.

An adolescent girl may want to know about methods of abortion and related services available. Reputable abortion clinics provide professional counselling before the abortion so that the girl does not regret her decision. You, however, can begin counselling. The questions you raise and the guidance you provide can help her make many of the necessary decisions and avoid needless complications.

## CRITICAL THINKING

*What resources are available in your community for a disabled adolescent?*

**Abortion** Although the teenage pregnancy rate has decreased, the abortion rate per 1000 women aged 15 to 19 was relatively stable in 1997.[235] However, abortion

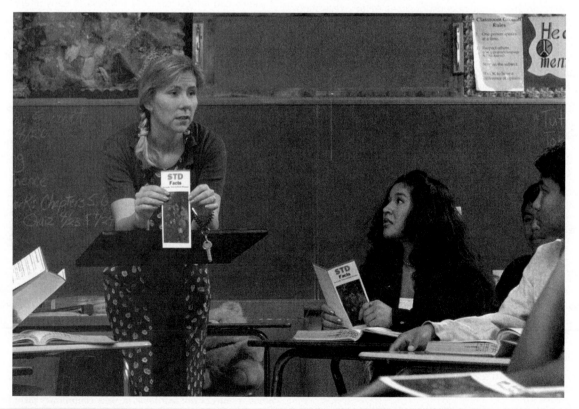

Nurses should encourage adolescents to discuss health concerns and provide teaching for the issues that are important to this age group.

## EVIDENCE-BASED PRACTICE

# The Home Environment of Métis, First Nations, and Caucasian Adolescent Mothers: An Examination of Quality and Influences

The purpose of this study was to compare maternal psychosocial, situational, and home-environment characteristics of Métis/First Nations and Caucasian adolescent mothers and to explore the role of psychosocial situational variables in shaping the home environment.

This longitudinal exploratory study compared maternal psychosocial, situational, and home-environment characteristics at four weeks and at 12 to 18 months after birth for a convenience sample of 71 Métis, First Nations, and Caucasian adolescent mothers.

The combined group of Métis/First Nations mothers had significantly higher infant-care emotionality scores than the Caucasian mothers at four weeks. The Caucasian mothers scored considerably higher on quality of the home environment; a refined multiple regression model containing infant-care emotionality, education level of the infant's maternal grandmother, ethnicity, and enacted social support explained 49 percent of the variance, with significant influences being infant-care emotionality and grandmother's education level.

The high number of infants born to Canadian adolescent mothers and the negative consequences of this parenting situation for the child underscore the need to better understand influences on adolescent mothering. Infants parented by adolescent mothers are at greater risk for negative parenting, health, and developmental outcomes than infants with mothers over 19 years of age. In 1994 alone, 24 700 infants were born to mothers between 15 and 19 years of age in Canada. The adverse social effects associated with adolescent parenting have been shown to endure even into adulthood.

An examination of the home environmental influences for Aboriginal adolescent mothers is especially critical, as this group is particularly likely to live in poverty. In fact, Canada's Aboriginal population scores well below the general population on the Human Developmental Index, at levels similar to those of developing countries. The development rating for Aboriginal people living off reserves is similar to that for residents of Trinidad and Tobago (ranked 35th globally), while those living on reserves are only marginally better off than Brazilians (ranked 63rd).

### Practice Implications

The findings from this study have implications for nurses caring for adolescent mothers and their infants in community, primary care, and acute care settings.

1. Economic factors have a greater effect than maternal age or ethnicity on the quality of cognitive stimulation in the home.

2. Nurses can assist adolescent mothers, especially those in low-income groups, to develop mothering practices that promote infant care.

3. Nurses who are aware that poverty is associated with numerous physical, social, cognitive, and emotional problems can refer adolescent mothers to early-intervention programs that focus on health promotion strategies and training in infant care.

4. Métis/First Nations adolescent mothers may be considered at special risk due to socioeconomic conditions and negative home environments.

5. The nurse may act as an advocate for health care and child care policies.

6. An appropriate goal for contemporary maternal-infant/child nurses is to develop a model of nursing care that helps mothers of various cultures to promote their infant's health.

Source: Secco, M.L., and M.E.K. Moffatt, The Home Environment of Métis, First Nations, and Caucasian Adolescent Mothers: An Examination of Quality and Influences, *Canadian Journal of Nursing Research, 35*(2) (2004), 106–126. Used with permission from CJNR.

became the most common outcome of teenage pregnancy. That is, the increasing proportion of teen pregnancies ending in abortion is a function of a pronounced decline in the birth rate. For example, between 1995 and 2000, the teen birth rate declined from 24.3 to 17.2 per 1000 whereas the abortion rate remained largely unchanged, declining from 21.1 in 1995 to 20.2 in 2000.[236]

Abortion carries risks to the physical and psychological health of the female. You may be involved in helping the pregnant female, the parents, and even the father of the baby to determine their values and feelings about continuing the pregnancy versus having an abortion. Provide full information, including the effects of abortion and alternatives, be non-judgmental, and listen.

### CRITICAL THINKING

*What resources are available in your community for a pregnant adolescent who is contemplating an abortion?*

## Nursing Role in Health Promotion

The adolescent period is between the periods of childhood and adulthood. Allow him or her to handle as much personal health care and business as possible, yet be aware of the psychosocial and physical problems with which he or she must cope alone. Watch for hidden fears that may be expressed in unconventional language. Today's adolescent, because of improved communications, knows more about life than did former generations. He or she is bombarded with information but does not have the maturity to handle it all effectively. Do not assume that because of apparent sophistication he or she understands the basis of health promotion.

Some teenagers, especially those with understanding and helpful families, go through adolescence with relative ease; it is a busy, happy period. But the increases in teenage suicide and in escape activities, such as drugs and alcohol, speak for those who do not have this experience. Adolescents are looking for adults who can be admired, trusted, and levelled with and who genuinely care. Parents are still important as figures with whom to identify, but teenagers now tend to look more outside the home—to teachers, community, and health professionals. As a nurse, you will be one of the community leaders with the opportunity, through living and teaching health promotion, to influence these impressionable minds.

---

### CASE SITUATION

#### Adolescent Drug Abuse

Jess, 17, was taken for treatment to an adolescent chemical abuse unit. "My parents, when they put me in (the hospital), they thought I was just drinking and using pot. When they got my tox screen back, my mom almost fainted."

The drug-screening analysis showed that marijuana, Valium, Demerol, Dilaudid, and codeine all had been ingested within a week. "All I did was live to get high—and, I guess you could say, get high to live," Jess said.

"I used to work at the home of a doctor who had a medicine cabinet full of everything anybody could dream of. He had a bunch of narcotics and stuff, and I thought I was in heaven. But I could go out right now and get drugs in about 15 minutes if I wanted. People, they're waiting for you to buy it. Around [age] 10, I started drinking a little bit—just tasting it, and getting that warm feeling. The first time I got high, I was 12, and I loved it. There wasn't no stopping me then. I got high all I could. I used to wake up and think, 'How can I get high today?'"

His friends put pressure on him to try other drugs. "I told myself I'd never do any pills, never drop any acid, but those

---

### CASE SITUATION (continued)

promises went by the wayside." He first took Quaaludes in the ninth grade and dropped acid that year at a concert. Soon he was drinking a lot and taking speed and Valium and other depressants.

"If I drank any beer, I'd want another one. If I got drunk, I'd want to get high; if I got high, I'd want to get pills. When I started out, I thought it was just cool, and that feeling was great. Instead of dealing with normal, everyday problems, I'd run off and get high. It got so I was picking fights just so I could stomp out of the house and get high."

He became a connoisseur. "I didn't buy dope at school. There's no good dope at school."

He also became more difficult to handle at home and at school. "I started fighting a lot with my parents. My grades dropped. I got into fistfights at school. I was real rebellious. I usually was high during class.

"I think it was real obvious to my teachers, because of the way I dressed and the way I acted in class. All the guys I hung around with had real long hair, moccasin boots, heavy metal T-shirts, and leather pants.

"I was pretty much an A student, and they [grades] dropped to low Cs and Ds. I was really withdrawing into myself.

"I wasn't myself when I was stoned. For years, I didn't even know how to feel (emotions). I've left home a few times.

"One time I was on LSD and I took a razor blade and cut my leg up. I still have the scars from that. I blanked out a lot. I'd come home beaten-up looking, and didn't know why."

Jess spent eight weeks in treatment and now says he's been clean for more than a year.

"It's a dependency," he said. "There's no way to eliminate it. You just try to control it. If I smoked a joint today or took a drink, I'd be right back."

Jess agrees with other former addicts: part of the problem is the naïveté of the parents.

"My parents, when I started getting in trouble, weren't going to admit it." Advice for parents who uncover a drug problem is simple: "Get some help. Not just for your kids, but for the parents and siblings also, because the whole family gets crazy. It's a family disease.

"I'll have to be on the lookout for the rest of my life to avoid falling back into drug use. I've learned just to be myself, and people will like me—and I never would have believed that before."

#### Questions

1. What could have been a motivating factor for Jess to go to the treatment centre?

2. What principles would you use as a guide for effective programming to prevent and reduce the harmful effects of substance abuse among youth?

## Counselling the Adolescent for Health Promotion

Help the teen and family to clarify values, beliefs, and attitudes that are important, to be more analytic in one's thinking. These are the first steps in bringing behaviour into congruence and, consequently, to reducing a sense of conflict. Value clarification exercises may be helpful.

Teach the adolescent effective critical thinking and decision-making skills so that he or she learns how to develop a plan of action toward a goal. The decision-making model involves (1) defining the problem; (2) gathering and processing information; (3) identifying possible solutions and alternatives of action; (4) making a decision about action; (5) trying out the decision; (6) evaluating whether the decision, actions, and consequences were effective or desirable; (7) rethinking other alternate solutions with new information; and (8) acting on these new decisions.

Promote warm, accepting, supportive non-judgmental feelings. Provide honest feedback as the adolescent struggles with decisions. Help him or her to make effective choices by fostering a sense of self-importance (he or she is a valuable and valued individual). Helping the person look ahead to the future in terms of values, goals, and consequences of behaviour can strengthen a sense of what is significant in life.

Both individual and group counselling are useful. In the group setting, the adolescent may be asked to bring a close friend or parent to share the experience. Some concerns and conflicts, however, are best worked through with the individual. Group sessions are effective for the following reasons:

- The person realizes concerns, feelings, and sense of confusion are not unique to him or her.
- Experiences and successful solutions to problems can be shared with others who are at different points of development.
- Ideas and roles can be tried out in the group before being tried in real life.
- Values can be clarified and decisions made with support and feedback from others.

## SUMMARY

1. Adolescence is the final period of rapid physical growth, as well as considerable cognitive and emotional change.

2. Relationships with the family remain basically important, but the peer group is dominant and exerts considerable influence on the adolescent's behaviour.

3. This is the time during which the individual works to develop his or her identity or sense of uniqueness, to become independent of and separate from parents while retaining basic ties and values.

4. Because of the many available options, determining one's identity, value systems, and career or life path can be difficult, take time, and sometimes be detoured by various societal forces of acquired habits, such as substance abuse.

5. A number of health problems may arise in the physical, psychological, or social dimensions.

6. The box entitled "Considerations for the Adolescent and Family in Health Care" summarizes what you should consider in assessment and health promotion.

7. The home situation affects emotional and physical health, adaptive ability, school performance, social skills, later job and marital adjustment, and the type of citizen and parent the adolescent will become.

## Considerations for the Adolescent and Family in Health Care

- Family, cultural background and values, support systems, and community resources for the adolescent and family
- Parents as identification figures, able to guide and to allow the adolescent to develop his or her own identity
- Relationship among family members or significant adults and its impact on the adolescent
- Behaviours that indicate abuse, neglect, or maltreatment by parents or other significant adults

- Physical growth patterns, characteristics and competencies, nutritional status, and rest, sleep, and exercise patterns that indicate health and are within age norms for the adolescent
- Completion of physical growth spurt and development of secondary sex characteristics that indicate normal development in the male or female; self-concept and body image development and integration related to physical growth

\>

- Nutritional requirements greater than for the adult
- Immunizations, safety education, and other health promotion measures
- Cognitive development into the stage of formal operations, related value formation, ongoing moral–spiritual development, and beginning development of philosophy of life
- Peer relationships, use of leisure time
- Overall appearance and behavioural patterns at home, school, and in the community that indicate positive identity formation, rather than role confusion or diffusion, or negative identity
- Use of effective adaptive mechanisms and coping skills in response to stressors
- Behavioural patterns in late adolescence that indicate integration of physical changes; cognitive, emotional, social, and moral–spiritual development, effective adaptive mechanisms
- Behavioural patterns and characteristics that indicate the adolescent is proceeding developmentally

## Interesting Websites

### "Talk to Me": Sexuality Education for Parents
www.phac-aspc.gc.ca/publicat/ttm-pm/contraception_e.html
"Talk To Me" is a sexual education program designed to help parents talk to their children about sexuality. It has been developed with emphasis on teenage perspectives. The intent of the program is to make parents more aware of adolescent needs and difficulties related to sexuality, to develop their communication skills, and to help them become more knowledgeable and more "askable" parents.

### Sexual Health and Sexually Transmitted Infections
www.phac-aspc.gc.ca/std-mts/index.html
This is a sexual health information centre that provides information on bacterial vaginosis, chlamydia, genital herpes, hepatitis B, human papillomavirus, gonorrhea, HIV/AIDS, pelvic inflammatory disease, syphilis, trichomoniasis, yeast infections, and more.

### National Eating Disorder Information Centre
www.nedic.ca
This Toronto-based, non-profit organization provides information and resources on eating disorders and weight preoccupation. NEDIC has a philosophy that promotes healthy lifestyles and encourages clients to make informed choices based on accurate information. It does not promote dieting or other behaviours that limit the full expression of our humanity.

### Canadian Adolescents at Risk Research Network
www.educ.queensu.ca/~caarrn
This is a Queen's University–led research program funded by the Canadian Population Health Initiative to study adolescent health. Find studies and national and international data on adolescent health in seven key areas: bullying, sexual health, injuries, school culture, disability and chronic conditions, social capital, and obesity and physical activity.

### Heart & Stroke Foundation of Canada
www.heartandstroke.ca
Unhealthy lifestyles threaten children's hearts. Overweight children could be three to five times more likely to suffer a heart attack or stroke before they reach the age of 65, warn the Heart & Stroke Foundation (HSF) and the Canadian Cardiovascular Society (CCS). This is just one example of the type of information available at this site.

## Key Terms

adolescence (398)
acne (403)
androgens (402)
anorexia nervosa (405)
birth control (444)
bulimia (406)
claimed identity (415)
contraception (444)
ego (418)
estrogens (402)

ideal identity (415)
identity (414)
identity achievement (415)
identity diffusion (416)
identity foreclosure (415)
identity formation (414, 415)
identity moratorium (415)
masturbation (417)
menstruation (398)

minor ankle sprain (421)
minor strains and sprains (421)
musculoskeletal chest pain (421)
nocturnal emissions (401)
peer group (412)
personal identity (415)
primary dysmenorrhea (402)

progesterones (402)
puberty (398)
real identity (415)
sex hormones (402)
sexually transmitted infections (STIs) (443)
sperm production (401)
spermarche (401)
spermatogenesis (398)
substance abuse (429)

# Part IV

## The Developing Person and Family: Young Adulthood through Death

# Chapter 12

## Assessment and Health Promotion for the Young Adult

*When I was a child I spoke as a child, I understood as a child, I thought as a child, but when I became a man, [an adult], I put away childish things.*

I Corinthians 13:11

*To keep the lamp burning, you have to keep putting oil in it.*

Mother Teresa

## Objectives

*Study of this chapter will enable you to:*

1. Discuss young adulthood as a developmental crisis and explain how the present young adult generation differs from earlier generations of young adults.

2. Explore, with middle-aged and older adults, ways to be helpful to young adults.

3. Examine second-order changes in family status required to proceed developmentally in the family life cycle stage: leaving home: single young adults.

4. Assess the physical development of a young adult.

5. Disclose findings from sex behaviour research when asked for information about sexuality.

6. Teach nutritional requirements to the young adult male and female, including the pregnant and lactating female.

7. Identify various body rhythms, and give examples of body rhythms that maintain adaptation.

8. Examine factors that influence biological rhythms and illness, and the non-synchrony that can result.

9. Discuss nursing measures to assist the person's maintenance of normal biological rhythms during illness.

10. Compare and contrast the stages of the sleep cycle, explain the effects that deprivation of the different stages of sleep cause, and account for different sleep disturbances that occur.

11. Discuss with the young adult his or her need for rest, sleep, exercise, and leisure.

12. Assess emotional characteristics, self-concept and body image, and the adaptive mechanisms of a young adult, and determine the nursing implications for each.

13. Examine the meaning of intimacy versus isolation.

14. Compare and contrast lifestyle options and their influence on the health status of the young adult, and explain your plans for his or her care.

15. Describe ways in which cognitive characteristics, social concerns, and moral, spiritual, and philosophical development influence the total behaviour and well-being of the young adult.

16. Assess a young adult who has one of the health problems described in this chapter, write a care plan, and work effectively with him or her to enhance health status.

Childhood and adolescence are the periods for growing up. Adulthood is the time for settling down. The changes in young adulthood relate more to sociocultural forces and expectations and to value and cognitive changes than to physical development. In most cases, the young adult of today has a greater number of contacts with people of different ages than young adults did previously in history. This experience tends to influence the young adult toward a more settled viewpoint.

The young adult is expected to enter new roles of responsibility at work, at home, and in society. They are also expected to develop values, attitudes, and interests in keeping with these roles. The young adult might experience difficulty in simultaneously handling work, school, marriage, home, and childrearing. He or she will probably work at one of these tasks at a time, neglecting the others, which then adds to the difficulties.

The definition, expectations, and stresses of young adulthood are influenced by socioeconomic status, urban or rural residence, ethnic and educational background, various life events, and the historical era. This generation of young adults is unique. Many have experienced economic growth and the related abundance of material goods and technology, rapid social changes, and sophisticated medical care. They have never known a world without the threat of nuclear war, pollution, overpopulation, and threatened loss of natural resources. Instant media coverage of events has made the world a small and familiar place. Changes in the role of women, the decreasing birth rate, and increasing longevity are modifying the timing of developmental milestones in many people.

The term *generation* refers to individuals born in the same general time span, who share many key life experiences including historic events, demographic trends, public heroes, entertainment pastimes, and early work experiences.[1] Generation X is a term used to describe a group of young adults in Canada who are now in their 30s and 40s. They are usually well educated and either have the means to achieve or already have achieved the upper-middle-class lifestyle; however, they differ from the dominant culture in some ways. They are assertive, self-directed, and comfortable with technology. They are concerned about the quality of family life and divorce rates, and they usually want the type of job that will accommodate their family values and create a satisfactory balance between work and time off. They speak of promoting social equality, preserving parks, and improving the environment. They adapt well to change, recognizing that the world is a rapidly changing place and that they will continuously need to learn and adjust to be successful.[2]

CRITICAL THINKING

*What are some characteristics that define Generation X?*

# FAMILY LIFE CYCLE AND RELATIONSHIPS

A major goal of families is to maintain unity as young adults grow and move into lives of their own. Most parents actively prepare their children to leave home.

Use the following information for assessment and health promotion with young adults and their family members. You can help parents understand that, although they are releasing their own children, new members are being drawn into the family circle through their offspring's marriage or close relationships. That the young adult is ready to leave home indicates the parents have done their job. Use the following knowledge to teach and counsel families as they work through concerns about family relationships.

## Family Life Cycle

Refer to Table 4-3, which illustrates the stages of the family life cycle, the emotional processes of transition (key principles), and second-order changes in the family required to proceed developmentally. Stage 1, leaving home: single young adult, is the appropriate stage for the young adult in the family.

CRITICAL THINKING

*What are a few second-order changes in family status required to proceed developmentally for the young adult who has been recently divorced?*

## Family Relationships

In Canada, the young adult is expected to be independent from the parents' home and care. If the person has elected to extend his or her education, he or she will often choose to remain living with the parents to save expenses. Sometimes the young adult does not leave the parents' home as early in life as the parents would like. With the increasing number of separations and divorces, the tight job market, and increasing apartment rental rates, the young adult child might choose to move back home—sometimes with children.

Often, the main source of conflict between parents and their young adult offspring is the difference in philosophy and lifestyle between the two generations. Sometimes parents, who sacrificed so their children would have a nice home, material things, education, leisure activities, and travel, may now be criticized for the way they look or act, and for what they believe. In fact, the young adult will often insist that he or she will *never* live like the parents.

Help parents to understand that they can take solace in knowing that usually the basic values they instilled within their children will remain their basic guidelines, although outward behaviour seems to suggest otherwise. This becomes evident as the person becomes middle-aged. The parents need help in providing a secure home base, both as a model for the young adult and to reduce feelings of threat in the younger children. The parents can help the younger children realize that there are many ways to live and that they will encourage each to find his or her own way when the time comes.

Gradually, the parents themselves must shift from a household with children to being a couple again as the last young adult establishes a home. Family structure, roles, and responsibilities change, and their use of space and other resources change as well.

## PHYSIOLOGIC CONCEPTS

Use the following information to teach the young adult, as well as in your assessment and health promotion intervention.

## Physical Development and Age

Although changes in body and mind continue throughout life, most physical and mental structures have completed growth when the person reaches young adulthood. Changes that occur during adult life are different from those in childhood. They occur more slowly and in smaller steps. Young adulthood is the life era when most people are in their peak of strength, energy, and endurance.[3] This peak of physical performance occurs not only for the average young adult, but for outstanding athletes as well.[4] Compared with older adults, adults in their twenties and thirties have more muscle tissue, more brain mass, and better eyesight, hearing, and sense of smell. They have maximum bone mass, greater oxygen capacity, and a more efficient immune system.[5] However, after this early peak, a gradual decline occurs in almost every measure of physical functioning through the years of adulthood.[6]

**Musculoskeletal System** Physical appearance is determined by genetic endowment, and structural differences are evident by familial genetic contributions. Full adult stature in men is reached at approximately age 21. In women, full growth occurs earlier, typically by age 17. Optimal muscular strength occurs between the ages 25 and 30, then gradually declines by approximately 10 percent from ages 30 to 60. Most of this decline occurs in the muscles of the back and legs, with less of a decline occurring in the arms. Manual dexterity peaks in young adulthood and declines into the mid thirties.[7]

**Cardiovascular and Respiratory Systems** Normative changes in the cardiovascular system that contribute to disease frequently begin by young adulthood. Regarding the respiratory system, the maximum amount of air inhaled in one breath drops 40 percent from age 25 to 85. This drop is mainly due to the stiffening of the rib cage and air passage reductions that occur with age.[8]

**Immune System** The two key organs in the immune system are the thymus gland and the bone marrow. Two types of cells (B cells and T cells) are created in these two organs. B cells fight external threats by producing antibodies against such disease organisms as viruses or bacteria. On the other hand, T cells defend against internal threats such as cancer cells. One of the key physical changes that occurs over the years of adulthood is an increasing susceptibility to disease. Research points out that life experiences that demand high levels of change or adaptation will affect the function of the immune system.[9]

**Nursing Goals** Nursing goals for this age group are oriented toward prolonging this optimal period of physical energy; developing emotional, cognitive, and social potential; encouraging proper health habits; anticipating the onset of chronic illness at an early stage; and treating disease when appropriate.[10]

---

### CRITICAL THINKING

*What types of resources are available in your community to assist young adults to maintain their maximum functioning?*

---

**Weight** Each person is an individual, and normal values cover a wide range of healthy individuals. Weight depends on many factors: heredity, sex, socioeconomic level, geographic area, food habits and preferences, level of activity, and emotional and physical environments.

In Canada, the concept of weight classification has a broader meaning than solely that of body weight.[11] The *Canadian Guidelines for Body Weight Classification in Adults* provides a scheme for classifying weight as measured by the body mass index (BMI), according to the level of health risk. The BMI is an index of weight to height ($kg/m^2$). It is considered to be the most useful indicator of health risks associated with being underweight, overweight, or obese. The waist circumference (WC) is positively correlated with abdominal fat, and it is an independent indicator of health risk associated with abdominal obesity. The BMI does not, however, provide an indication of the distribution of fat in the body. Research has shown that excess fat in the abdominal area is associated with an increased risk to health. The information derived from the application of the weight classification system can help to guide policy decisions as well as provide a tool for the evaluation of public health intervention programs.

The 2003 Canadian body weight classification system categorizes BMIs between 25.0 and 29.9 as "overweight," and consequently this range is associated with increased health risk. A BMI of 30 or more reflects obesity. Obesity is associated with a high to extremely high risk of developing health problems. These categories are set in accordance with the World Health Organization (WHO) weight classification system. The "obese" category was further subdivided by WHO into Obesity Class I (BMI of 30.0 to 34.9), Obesity Class II (35.0 to 39.9), and Obesity Class III (40.0 and over). This differentiation has been adopted in the 2003 Canadian body weight classification system.[12]

**Obesity**   Obesity is a mounting health issue in Canada. The identification of the determinants of obesity is particularly important for the development of health promotion and prevention strategies.[13] Brien and her researchers conducted a study using a sample of 459 adults, ranging upward from 18 years. This sample was taken from the 2002–2004 Canadian Physical Activity Longitudinal Study (PALS). They concluded that cardio-respiratory fitness, and one's previous basal metabolic index are important predictors of a person's future weight gain and obesity. These predictors should be incorporated into strategies used to identify those individuals at increased risk of obesity.[14] In another study, Chen and Mao hypothesized that the association between physical activity and obesity varies among different age and sex groups.[15] They concluded that obese Canadians (both men and women) are inactive. However, overweight men especially tend to be more active than either normal weight or obese men, particularly among those between 30 and 49 years of age. The prevalence of physical inactivity in women increased proportionately with increasing basal metabolic index. Chen and Mao concluded that older age, being female, and obesity were all associated with a lower level of leisure time physical activity in the Canadian population.[16]

Overweight and obesity are known risk factors for type 2 diabetes, stroke, heart disease, hypertension, gallbladder disease, and certain types of cancer, osteoarthritis, and sleep apnea. Psychological disorder is also a risk factor of obesity and must be taken into consideration.[17] Researchers have found that exercise benefits both physical and mental health.[18]

Nurses in all settings are called on to promote healthy lifestyle practices that create minimal disruptions in health patterns.

---

**CRITICAL THINKING**

*How do you account for Canada's "obesity epidemic"?*

---

You can calculate BMI as follows:

1. *Convert body weight to kilograms.*
   (1 kilogram = 2.2 pounds)
   Body weight (pounds) ÷ 2.2 = weight (kilograms)
   *Example: 132 pounds ÷ 2.2 = 60 kilograms*

2. *Convert height to metres.*
   (1 metre = 39.37 inches)
   Height (inches) ÷ 39.37 = height (metres)
   *Example: 65 inches ÷ 39.37 = 1.65 metres*

3. *Calculate BMI.*
   Weight (kg) ÷ height (m)$^2$ = BMI
   *Example: 60 kg ÷ (1.65 m × 1.65 m) = 22.04 BMI*

4. *Check BMI against risk for health problems related to body weight.*

---

**CRITICAL THINKING**

*What health promotion activities should someone who has abdominal obesity pursue?*

---

## Sexuality and Sexual Development

**Sexual–Reproductive Maturity**   In healthy women, by the time of young adulthood, menstruation is well established and regular. The normal duration of menses is 5 days, and the usual interval of each menstrual cycle is 25 to 32 days. The optimum period for reproduction is between 20 and 30 years of age. A male's capacity to impregnate does not appear to change over the years of early adulthood. Male fertility declines somewhat only after the age of 40.[19]

Sexual awareness, feelings, and expressions—as fundamental to health as rest, nutrition, and exercise—develop steadily over the lifespan.[20] **Sexuality** may be defined as a *deep, pervasive aspect of the total person, the sum total of one's feelings and behaviours, the expression of which goes beyond genital response.* Sexuality includes **sexual orientation**, the *sense of self as male, female, bisexual (feeling comfortable with both sexes), homosexual, or transsexual/transgendered.* Sex orientation also includes **sex roles**, *what the person does overtly to indicate sexual orientation to self and others.* Throughout the life cycle, physiologic, emotional, social, and cultural forces condition sexuality. Today's society offers many choices in sexual behaviour patterns.

During adulthood, a number of sexual patterns exist, ranging from heterosexuality, bisexuality, and homosexuality to masturbation and abstinence. Few people are totally homosexual or heterosexual; most people feel attracted or sexually responsive at some time to both sexes. No one knows exactly why some individuals are homosexual and others are heterosexual.[21] Within each of these patterns the person may achieve a full and satisfactory life or be plagued with a lack of interest, impotence, or guilt.

Changes in sexual interest and behaviour occur through the life cycle. These important changes can be a cause of serious conflict unless the partners involved talk about their feelings, needs, and desires. Many misunderstandings arise because of basic differences between the male and female in sexual interest and behaviour. The more each can learn about the other partner, the greater will be the chance of working out a compatible relationship for a successful partnership. No person should assume that the partner knows his or her wishes, or vice versa. Each must declare his or her needs.

## CRITICAL THINKING

*How does homophobia develop in society? What health promotion strategies could be used to prevent homophobia in a community?*

**Sexuality Education** Often, the popular literature promotes misinformation, and you should be prepared to provide accurate information. Because some people feel free to discuss sexual matters, you might be questioned by the person recuperating from an illness, by the partner after delivery, or by the healthy young adult who feels dissatisfied with his or her personal knowledge or sexual pattern. The following are facts that you can teach young adults based on current research:[22]

- Sexual mores and norms vary among ethnic and cultural groups, socioeconomic classes, and even from couple to couple. Sexual activity that is mutually satisfying to the couple and not harmful to themselves and others is acceptable.

- Sexual activity varies considerably among people in relation to sex drive, frequency of orgasm, and the need for rest after intercourse.

- Various factors and feelings are influential in determining sexual expression.

- Simultaneous orgasm of both partners may be highly desired, but it is an unrealistic goal and occurs only in the most ideal of circumstances. It does not determine sexual achievement or satisfaction.

- No single most accepted position for sexual activity exists. Any position is correct, normal, healthy, and proper if it satisfies both partners.

- Achievement of satisfactory sexual response is the result of interaction of many physical, emotional, developmental, and cultural influences. Primarily, however, it depends on the total relationship between the partners.

- Chronically ill or disabled persons learn to live with physical changes, and often they learn to adapt to the expression of their sexual interests.

- Decreased sexual desire can be related to physical or emotional illness, prescribed medications, the use of alcohol or other drugs, changed behaviour in the partner, or to fatigue from the stress and demands of employment or professional life.

## CRITICAL THINKING

*In what ways do you think attitudes about sexuality will change in the next 25 years?*

# WOMEN'S HEALTH

Women's health addresses health promotion and prevention, as well as health maintenance, in adult women. This term recognizes that the health of women is holistic and is related to the physical, psychosocial, cultural, and spiritual dimensions of women's lives. This broad emphasis on women's health is in contrast to the view of reproductive problems.[23] A women's health information site is provided by the Society of Obstetricians and Gynaecologists of Canada (SOGC).

Health care providers, such as nurses, are becoming increasingly more aware of health promotion and disease prevention. Nurses can assist women to make good lifestyle choices involving the following:

- Eating a nutritious balanced diet
- Maintaining weight for height
- Performing regular aerobic exercise
- Getting adequate sleep
- Avoiding or stopping smoking
- Managing stress effectively
- Developing enjoyable hobbies and leisure activities
- Developing an inner life in some form of spirituality, personal reflection, yoga
- Fostering bonds of affection from family and friends
- Obtaining regular health screenings and assessments
- Ensuring that immunizations are up to date[24]

## Premenstrual Phenomena

**Premenstrual syndrome (PMS)** *is a group of manifestations associated with the luteal phase of the menstrual cycle (two weeks before onset of menses).*[25] Erlick Robinson states that the PMS symptoms that most often bring women to their doctors for help are irritability, depression, and agitation.[26] The box entitled "Common Manifestations of Premenstrual Syndrome" lists physiologic manifestations and psychological reactions that are reported by some women. No simple cause has been identified, although

## Common Manifestations of Premenstrual Syndrome

**Physiologic Manifestations**

- Fatigue, increased need for sleep
- Appetite change, craving for salty or sweet foods
- Abdominal distension, swollen hands or feet, puffy eyes
- Headache or backache
- Breast tenderness, swelling, increased nodularity just before menstrual period
- Weight gain
- Nausea
- Constipation or diarrhea
- Acne or hives
- Dizziness
- Menstrual cramps
- Clumsiness
- Sex drive changes
- Thirst
- Proneness to infection
- Lower alcohol tolerance

**Psychological Reactions**

- Apprehension or anxiety
- Confusion
- Forgetfulness
- Frequent crying
- Indecisiveness
- Irritability
- Restlessness
- Mood swings
- Sadness or depression
- Suspiciousness
- Tension
- Withdrawal
- Difficulty with concentration

several theories have been put forth to explain it. These theories include hormone imbalance, nutritional deficiency, prostaglandin excess, and endorphin deficiency.[27] PMS is not the same as **dysmenorrhea**, *painful or severely uncomfortable menstruation.*

Treatment for PMS is frequently symptomatic. It is advisable to combine natural approaches with a healthy lifestyle. For example, dietary measures and aerobic exercise are suggested. In addition to vitamin supplements, pharmacological treatment for PMS includes diuretics, calcium supplementation, and prostaglandin inhibitors.[28] Help clients to reframe their attitude toward PMS.[29] Self-help literature can also help women believe that they have control over their bodies.

*Teach women that the following measures can offset PMS manifestations:*

- Consume less caffeine in beverages, colas, and over-the-counter drugs, and take less sugar, alcohol, and salt, especially during the premenstrual period.

- Eat four to six small meals a day rather than two or three heavy meals to minimize the risk of hypoglycemia that accompanies PMS.

- Snack on complex carbohydrates, such as fresh fruits, vegetable sticks, and whole wheat crackers, which provide energy without excessive sugar.

- Drink six to eight glasses of water daily to help prevent fluid retention by flushing excess salt from the body.

- Limit fat intake (especially in red meats). Fat increases levels of hormones that cause breast tenderness and fluid retention. Choose dairy products low in fat.

- Eat more whole grains, nuts, and raw greens, which are high in vitamin B, magnesium, and potassium. Add vitamin $B_6$ and calcium to reduce symptoms.

- Develop a variety of interests, including regular exercise routines, so that the focus is not on self and body symptoms during this period.

- Walk. Perform aerobic exercises.

- Get extra rest and use relaxation techniques, meditation, and massage. Treat yourself to a relaxing and creative activity.

- Discuss your feelings with family and friends so that they can be more understanding of your behaviour.

- Join a self-help group to hear ideas from others on how to cope effectively with symptoms.[30]

- An empathetic relationship with a health care professional to whom the women feels free to voice concerns is highly beneficial.[31]

Premenstrual syndrome is not the same as **premenstrual dysphoric disorder (PMDD)**. PMDD is rare (3 to 5 percent of menstruating women) and *involves a pattern of severe, recurrent symptoms of depression and other negative mood states in the last week of the menstrual cycle; it markedly interferes with daily living.* PMS occurs in 3 to 8 percent of women and is less disabling.[32]

## CRITICAL THINKING

*What is your knowledge of complementary therapies and/or homeopathic remedies in assisting women who are experiencing PMS?*

## Natural Family Planning

You can share the following information about ovulation, especially with couples who wish to follow **natural family planning**. Many of the rhythmic and recurring events, which women recognize on an almost monthly schedule during their reproductive years, are collectively called "fertility" signs. They are manifestations of the body changes that are required for functions of successful reproduction. These changes include certain cyclical changes in the ovaries and the amount and consistency of the cervical mucus produced during each cycle, the amount of gonadotropin secretion, body temperature, and even the "mood or emotional tone."[33]

Being able to predict accurately the time of ovulation in any given menstrual cycle as a result of being able to recognize one or more of these fertility signs would obviously be of considerable help, either in achieving or avoiding conception. However, knowing the length of a previous menstrual cycle, or series of cycles, cannot ensure with any degree of accuracy the time of appearance of fertility signs in the current, or any subsequent, cycle. Simply put, prior cycle length is not an accurate fertility sign.[34]

Sophisticated natural planning methods, which are not based on the knowledge of previous cycle lengths as predictors of the ovulation day, have been shown to be more reliable. Such natural methods base their judgment about fertility, at any point in a women's cycle, on other changes. Examples include the measurement of basal body temperature and the recognition of cyclical changes in the amount and consistency of cervical mucus (Billings Ovulation Method). Both of these events occur in response to changes in circulating hormones that control ovulation. The time of ovulation can be approximated by over-the-counter urine tests that detect high levels of luteinizing hormone (LH) associated with the ovulation (LH) surge.[35]

The nurse is encouraged to discuss the above methods with the client, and then assess the extent of learning experienced by the client by having her describe the selected

**Figure 12-1** Relationship of menstrual cycle method to the Billings Ovulation Method (natural family planning)

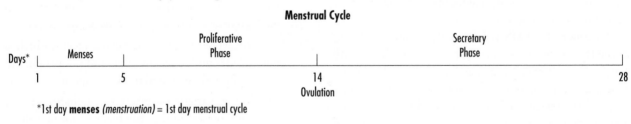

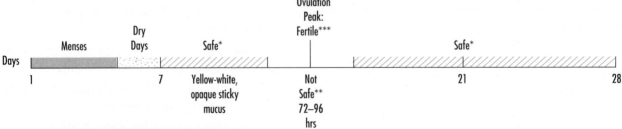

procedure in her own words. For example, before using the cervical mucus method, the woman abstains from intercourse for one entire menstrual cycle. During this time, she daily assesses her cervical mucus for the amount, feelings of wetness or slipperiness, colour, and clearness. Abstinence is essential during this time, not only so that the woman avoids pregnancy, but also because the presence of ejaculate in the vagina in the hours following intercourse could interfere with the woman's assessment of her cervical mucus. Women who feel uncomfortable testing their mucus should be encouraged to use an alternate method.[36]

## MEN'S HEALTH

The health of men is important, and the topic is steadily gaining interest in university courses in both nursing and medicine. Increasingly, the general public is inquiring about it as well. The website Men's Health Canada (www. menshealthcanada.com) is a comprehensive information centre that allows men to explore issues they have with their health. Topics such as obesity, birth control, depression, and cholesterol concerns that might lead to heart problems are addressed. The material is not intended to be used for self-diagnosis or self-treatment but rather for use in discussing health concerns with a medial practitioner. Details of a related website on andropause are provided at the end of the chapter.

## SEXUAL HEALTH

## Sexuality Health Assessment

Follow these guidelines when taking a sexual history:

- Ensure privacy and establish confidentiality of statements.

- Progress from topics that are easy to discuss to those that are more difficult to discuss. For example, ask questions such as: What does sexuality mean to you? Has your illness changed the way you see yourself?[37]

Sexuality assessment includes a history as well as a gynecologic examination, breast screening, Papanicolaou (Pap) smear in the female and a genital-rectal examination in the male.

Klingman discusses the following general assessment plan:[38]

1. Breast self-examination by the woman monthly after age 19 or 20. Clinical breast exam:
   a. Every three years for women aged 19 or 20 to 40.
   b. Annually for women over age 40.

2. Mammogram:
   a. Every other year for women between ages 40 and 50.
   b. Annually after age 50.

Klingman discusses in-depth examination of the female external genitalia and the internal genitalia, the Pap smear procedure and result categories, and the recto-vaginal examination.[39] She also discusses in-depth assessment of the male.[40] Her description covers the physical procedure, comfort and emotional considerations, and normal findings:

- Ask the person how he or she acquired sexual information before asking about sexual experience.

- Precede questions with informational statements about the generality of the experience, when appropriate, to reassure the person and reduce anxiety, shame, and evasiveness.

- Observe nonverbal behaviour while you listen to the person's statements.

- Do not ask questions simply to satisfy your curiosity.

The following are topics to include in the sexual history:

- How sex education was obtained
- Accuracy of sex education
- Menstrual history, if female, and nocturnal emission history, if male
- Past and present ideas on self as a sexual being, including ideas on body image, masturbation, coitus, childbirth, parenting
- Sexual experiences—with men, women, or both
- Number of partners in past year
- Use of condoms: when started, consistency of use
- Ability to communicate sexual needs and desires
- Partner's (if one exists) sexual values and behaviour
- Sexual partners who have AIDS
- History of sexually transmitted disease of self or partner(s)

If necessary, use several interviews to obtain information and be sure to include in the sexual assessment record any specific questions or concerns that the person voices. Respect the person's desire not to talk about sexual matters, or moral, spiritual, and aesthetic convictions. Your matter-of-fact attitude helps the adult to feel less embarrassed. Be aware of ways in which illness and drugs can affect sexual function. Do not assume that chronic or disabling disease or mutilating surgery ends the person's sexual life.

Provide accurate information and supportive counselling when the person or family asks questions or indicates concerns. You might decide to prepare instructional units for a specific teaching plan to share with clients with various conditions, especially chronic diseases. The same units could be shared with the families to help them better understand how to meet sexual needs. Provide information related to pursuit of sexual activity, rather than personal advice or judgment. Learn about available community resources that could be called on for consultation or referral when necessary.

## Variations in Sexual Behaviour

The identity crisis that occurs during adolescence will probably not be completely resolved by the time the person enters young adulthood chronologically. Identity confusion can lead to confusion over one's true sexual identity. Identity confusion can precipitate homosexual and heterosexual experimentation, with the related arousal of homosexual fears and curiosity.

**Homosexuality** Homosexuals are *people who are regularly aroused by, and who engage in sexual activity with, members of their own sex.* Being a **homosexual man** (*gay*), or a **homosexual woman** (*lesbian*) was accepted by many ancient cultures, and it is becoming more socially accepted in North America today. In Canada, a trend exists throughout the general population toward more accepting attitudes toward gays and lesbians.[41] Particularly among the religious, the less educated, and the older generations, a core of our society continues to remain opposed to same-sex marriage and same-sex family formation. Many are concerned with the abilities of lesbians and gays to parent, as well as with the effect on children of living with same-sex parents. Others contend that allowing same-sex couples to marry devalues the institution of marriage.[42]

The late 1900s and early 2000s saw dramatic shifts in the Canadian landscape regarding same-sex relationships and parenting rights.[43] For example, in 2000, the Canadian Parliament enacted the *Modernization of Benefits and Obligations Act*, which extended benefits and obligations to common-law couples, whether they are opposite or same sex. Furthermore, the definition of *spouse* was changed to include any two persons who have lived together in "marriage-like" relationships for at least two years.[44] The federal *Civil Marriage Act* has been changed to allow gay and lesbian couples to marry anywhere in Canada. The *Divorce Act* now applies to all married couples, whether the couples are same or opposite sex.[45]

Although more lesbians than gay men are in long-term unions, both value their unions. Lesbians often go out of their way to reduce power differences between partners. For example, they frequently share duties and decision making equally.[46]

According to Canadian sociologist Anne-Marie Ambert, from York University, most studies of same-sex parents have been conducted with small samples. Seldom have children been assessed against a wide range of developmental indicators, and few studies have followed children into adulthood. Any developmental problems that have been identified have been explained as adequately through the divorce or separation of their biological parents as through the sexual orientation of their mother or father.[47] However, the weight of evidence from the studies completed leads to the following tentative conclusions:

- lesbian and heterosexual mothers are similar regarding parenting
- children of homosexual partners usually develop heterosexual identities
- gay men are no more likely than heterosexuals to abuse children, and the same applies to lesbians[48]

Glossop assures readers that Ambert has reviewed the information provided by social science to this point in time.[49]

The process of **coming out** (*openly disclosing one's sexual orientation*) occurs in four stages, as follows:

1. *Recognition of being homosexual* can happen as early as age four, or as late as adolescence, or later. This time of trying to find oneself can be lonely, confusing, and painful.

2. *Getting to know other homosexuals* and establishing romantic and sexual relationships with them helps to diminish feelings of isolation and improves self-image.

3. *Telling family and friends* may not be accomplished at all, or at least not for a long time. This important revelation can bring disapproval, rejection, and conflict.

4. *Complete openness* involves telling colleagues, employers, and anyone else who has a relationship with the person. In this stage, there is a healthy acceptance of one's sexuality and the self.[50]

Parents, and the spouse, if the homosexual person was married, are likely to blame themselves when the person discloses his or her sexual orientation. The feelings of the parents are described by Blum in the article "What Made Troy Gay?"[51] Another interesting article, which explores the experience of disclosing HIV infection to family members, is by Anne Katz ("Mom, I Have Something to Tell You").[52]

Coming out, in the context of receiving health care, is regarded as an issue of paramount importance, and it is highly significant to the experience of health care services. For gay and lesbian individuals, achieving health and well-being is often a difficult task. Health care systems and health care providers must play an active role in combating prejudice and in reducing barriers to care in partnership, not only with gays and lesbians, but with bisexual and two-spirited people as well.[53]

Lesbians have not been studied as extensively as gay men. It is still more socially acceptable for two women to live together in one household than for two men to live together. Possibly, there is less societal fear of gay women than of gay men. As a result, less is known about lesbian feelings, reactions, lifestyles, or health problems. The Society of Obstetricians and Gynaecologists in Canada (SOGC) has developed a policy statement on Lesbian Health Guidelines.[54] This statement was reviewed and approved by the Social and Sexual Issues Committee and was also approved by the Council of the SOGC. The policy statement says that for the lesbian client to receive appropriate and quality care, her sexual orientation and lifestyle must be known and understood by her health care providers. Education is the first step toward improving care for lesbian clients; the final step is the enlightenment of attitudes toward sexuality among health care providers.[55]

An increase in sexually transmitted infections (STIs) has been reported in Canada.[56] However, specific information is generally unavailable regarding the sexual and reproductive health and the accessibility of services and information and health indicator trends of subpopulation groups, such as new Canadians, lesbian, gay, bisexual, and transgender individuals, as well as ethnic groups, the homeless, and disabled individuals.[57] However, O'Bryne and Holmes argue that with a record high of STI rates, one method to reduce such rates would be to institute anonymous testing. It should be remembered that high-risk individuals, such as men who are having sex with men, almost always refrain for confidentiality reasons from participating in testing within the current health care system. To reduce the number of partners between the time of infection and the time of testing, anonymous and non-judgmental services could provide treatment before the infection is spread to others. So that nurses working in sexual health centres are able to provide culturally sensitive care to groups whose sexuality defines a risk, a Canadian national standard might be implemented to ensure consistent STI surveillance, and that anonymous testing be mandated. With such a framework, nurses could re-instill the "care" in health care.[58]

## CRITICAL THINKING

*How do gays and lesbians develop their self-identity in today's society?*

**Cohabitation,** *a consensual informal union between two persons of the opposite sex who live together without being married,*
is not unusual. Sometimes people have had either no siblings or no siblings of the opposite sex. Sometimes such individuals want the experience of living with someone of the opposite sex who would be like a sibling. In such a situation, both people work to keep the relationship asexual. Research has shown that premarital cohabiters who eventually marry are more likely to divorce, or separate, than are persons who do not cohabit prior to marriage.[59]

Young adults sometimes live together in an effort to avoid some of the problems they saw in their parents' marriage, or they might wish to test the degree of the partner's commitment before actually becoming married. Those goals may be achieved for some, but the danger is that one partner may take the commitment very seriously, while the other may wish to use the situation only as a convenient living arrangement. Rather than replacing marriage, cohabitation is considered by many to be a stage before marriage.[60] The 2001 Canadian Census showed that an increasing proportion of couples choose to live common law, and the trend toward common-law relationships was strongest in Quebec.[61] Cohabitants have rights and legal obligations similar to those of married couples. These rights include property rights, eligibility and entitlements to health insurance, pension plans, and inheritances.[62]

Cohabitation varies from culture to culture, depending on traditional customs and socioeconomic pressures. In some cultures, cohabitation remains an acceptable alternative to marriage.[63]

## CRITICAL THINKING

*In what ways do you think that cohabitation, compared to a nuclear family, affects the health status of its members?*

# Personal Attitudes

Pangman and Seguire state that sexuality provides the opportunity to express affection, admiration, and affirmation of one's body and its functioning.[64] In fact, sexuality not only encompasses the whole individual, but also serves as a reference frame in relation to others. To incorporate human sexuality into health care and nursing practice, *you must accept your own sexuality and understand sexuality as a significant aspect of development.* Then you can acknowledge the concerns of your clients, recognize your own strengths and limits in working with people who have sexual concerns, help clients to cope with threats to sexuality, and counsel, inform, or refer them as your assessment indicates.

It is important for nurses to provide clients and their families with opportunities for open and genuine communication about sexuality. In doing so, a foundation of acceptance for the whole person is established, which

## How Do I Handle This Situation?

You are a clinical practitioner on a rehabilitation ward in a large hospital. One of your clients is a 16-year-old male who lost his legs below the knees in a train accident. Lately, he has been making lewd sexual comments and gestures at you when you provide basic care. Yesterday, you became so frustrated by him that you did not complete his basic care. You have been trying to cope by avoiding eye contact and ignoring his remarks. You are reluctant to confront the client directly because the doctor in charge is the client's uncle. To make matters worse, the client has informed you that he will report you to his uncle (the doctor) for not completing his basic care if you make a formal report of his behaviour to management. It is anticipated that this client will remain on your unit for at least several weeks while he becomes adapted to his prostheses.

1. If you had the opportunity to start over with this client, what would you do differently at the beginning of your interactions to avoid this situation?

2. Now that you are in the situation, however, how will you handle it from here on?

provides encouragement for clients to ask questions and seek assistance with sexuality issues.[65]

## PHYSICAL FITNESS AND EXERCISE

According to the 2004–2005 Canadian Community Health Survey, 49 percent of Canadians (20 years of age and older) are at least somewhat active during their leisure time, accumulating a daily average of at least 1.5 kilocalories per kilogram (KKD) of physical activity. This amount of physical activity could be achieved through walking a total of half an hour a day. Roughly 25 percent of adults are classified as moderately active, while 24 percent are classified as active.[66]

One group of Canadian researchers conducted a study to examine sociodemographic, geographic, and physical activity correlates of walking and cycling for non-leisure purposes (i.e., to work, to school, or on errands). Their results suggest that it is the young and the physically active who engage in such activities. Furthermore, this research points to a need to address barriers among those who could benefit the most from an increased use of both modes of travel. For example, what works for older Canadians might not work for the young. It appears that different approaches appear necessary for different regions, and for Canadians of different incomes.[67]

Health Canada, in partnership with the Canadian Society for Exercise Physiology, has developed *Canada's Physical Activity Guide to Healthy Active Living*.[68] Canadians wanted a valid and practical guide, similar to *Eating Well*

## Suggestions for an Exercise Program

- Obtain pre-exercise physical examination that includes the feet.
- Make exercise a part of your lifestyle: errands, stairs instead of elevator, parking at a distance.
- Start in small increments, keep it fun, and avoid injury.
- Avoid exercising for a period of two hours after a large meal, and refrain from eating for one hour after exercising.
- Avoid exercise in extremes of weather.
- Include at least ten minutes of warm-up and cool-down exercises in any exercise program.
- Use proper equipment, footwear, and clothing when exercising.
- Post goals, pictures of the ideal self, and notes of encouragement in a readily seen place for self-encouragement.
- Use visualization daily to picture successful attainment of exercise benefit (e.g., looking toned or graceful, ideal weight).

- Keep records of weekly measures of weight, blood pressure, and pulse.
- Focus on the rewards of exercise; keep a diary of feelings and compare differences in relaxation energy, concentration, and sleep patterns.
- Work with a peer or join a structured exercise class, running club, or fitness centre. Spend more time with people dedicated to wellness.
- Stop exercising, or at least slow down and consult with a practitioner, if any unusual, unexplainable symptoms occur.
- Reward self for working toward exercise goals and for attaining them. For example, after a month in an exercise program, buy a new pair of running shoes or treat yourself to a special wish.

with *Canada's Food Guide*, that would help them judge how much physical activity they need to achieve better health The guide addresses three types of activities: (1) endurance activities that help one's heart, lungs, and circulatory system to stay healthy; (2) flexibility activities that help one move easily, keeping muscles relaxed and joints mobile; and (3) strength activities that help one's muscles and bones stay strong, improve posture, and help to prevent diseases such as osteoporosis.[69] The guide also provides a wide variety of physical activities to help people have more energy, move more easily, and get stronger.

## CRITICAL THINKING

*How would you begin to develop a program of physical activity for a group of young adults who are physically disabled?*

As a matter of interest, jogging makes joints that are in good condition stronger. Jogging, however, as a regular form of exercise, can aggravate old injuries of the back, hips, knees, and ankles because it exerts as much as five times the normal body weight on lower joints and extremities. It can cause abnormal wear on joints and muscles. The person who jogs must also engage in exercise for the upper extremities and other muscles. Weight-lifting can strengthen. Aerobic exercise, brisk walking, jumping rope, and bicycling can actually be better exercise for the body than jogging. These activities promote bone building, thickness, and strength, and they increase circulation throughout the body.[70]

Swimming is probably the best overall activity because it increases strength and endurance and stimulates the heart and blood vessels, the lungs, and many other muscle groups, without putting excess stress on the person because of less gravity pull in the water. Further, swimming keeps joints supple, aids weight loss or weight control, and reduces hypertension. Perhaps more importantly, it is an enjoyable activity, either alone or with others.[71]

## Principles of Body Mechanics

- The wider the base of support and the lower the centre of gravity, the greater is the stability of the object.

- The equilibrium of an object is maintained as long as the line of gravity passes through its base of support.

- When the line of gravity shifts outside the base of support, the amount of energy required to maintain equilibrium is increased.

- Equilibrium is maintained with least effort when the base of support is broadened in the direction in which movement occurs.

- Stooping, with hips and knees flexed and the trunk in good alignment, distributes the work load among the largest and strongest muscle groups; stooping also helps to prevent back strain.

- The stronger the muscle group, the greater the work it can perform safely.

- Using a larger number of muscle groups for an activity distributes the work load.

- Keeping the centre of gravity of the body as close as possible to the centre of gravity of the work load to be moved prevents unnecessary reaching and strain on back muscles.

- Pulling an object directly toward (or pushing directly away from) the centre of gravity of the body prevents unnecessary strain on the back and abdominal muscles.

- Facing the direction of movement prevents undesirable twisting of the spine.

- Pushing, pulling, or sliding an object on a surface requires less force than lifting an object, because lifting involves moving the weight of the object against the pull of gravity.

- Moving an object by rolling, turning, or pivoting requires less effort than lifting the object, because momentum and leverage are used to advantage.

- Using a lever properly when lifting an object reduces the force required to lift the weight.

- The less friction between the object moved and the surface on which it is moved, the smaller the force required to move it.

- Moving an object on a level surface requires less effort than moving the same object on an upwardly inclined surface because the resistance due to gravity is less when moving horizontally than when moving upwardly.

- Working with materials that rest on a surface at a comfortable working level requires less effort than working on them above the comfortable working surface.

- Contraction of stabilizing muscles preparatory to activity helps to protect ligaments and joints from strain and injury during the activity.

- Dividing balanced activity between arms and legs protects the back from strain.

- Using a variety of positions and activity helps to maintain good muscle tone and prevent fatigue.

- Alternating periods of rest and activity helps to prevent fatigue.

Regular physical activity has been viewed as a natural tranquilizer because it reduces anxiety and muscular tension. Some studies show that regular physical exercise improves a number of personality characteristics that correlate with composure, extroversion, self-confidence, assertiveness, persistence, adventurousness, and superego strength.[72]

Regular exercise periods are frequently not planned by young adults. Some will get abundant exercise in their jobs; but many will not. Those who do not can check with the local YMCA or YWCA organizations, community recreation departments, recreational departments of community colleges or universities, or commercial gymnasiums and health salons for exercise programs appropriate to their lifestyles and physical conditions. Refer to the boxes entitled "Suggestions for an Exercise Program" and "Principles of Body Mechanics" (pages 466 and 467).

## Sex Differences

Women and men sometimes share the same physical exercise activities, but sometimes interests and energy levels are different, and partners engage in separate exercise activities. Women can have as much endurance as men, especially with training, but certain physiologic differences account for differences in performance in physical exercise activities or athletic events.

Men have greater upper-body strength, primarily because of their longer arms, broader shoulders, and higher muscle-fibre counts. Muscle can be conditioned by exercise, but muscle-fibre count cannot be increased. Whether men exercise or not, their muscle fibres gain bulk from the hormone testosterone. In men, the heart and lungs, which on average are 10 percent larger than those of women, provide more powerful and efficient circulation. The delivery of oxygen to men's muscles, a factor crucial to speed, is further enhanced by the higher concentration of hemoglobin in the blood. Finally, the longer limbs of men provide them with greater leverage and extension.

The aspects of female physiology that result in women's athletic advantages are not as self-evident as in males. A woman's body contains an average of 9 percent more adipose tissue than a man's body does. This tissue is deposited not only on the thighs, buttocks, and breasts, but in a subcutaneous layer that covers the entire body. It is this adipose tissue that makes women more buoyant and better insulated against cold, both of which are distinct advantages in long-distance swimming. Body adipose tissue may also be one of the reasons that few female runners report the pain and weakness that most male runners encounter. The body is conditioned to call on stored fats once its supply of glycogen, which fuels the muscles, has been exhausted. Because women have greater reserves of body fat, they are able to compete longer in an athletic event. Women, compared to men, perspire in smaller amounts and less quickly. Perspiring is the body's way of avoiding overheating. Yet women seem to be able to tolerate heat better than men can. Not only can body temperature rise in a woman several degrees higher before she begins to sweat, but women sweat more efficiently because of the even distribution of their sweat glands. In women, **vascularization**, *capacity for bringing blood to the surface for cooling*, is also more efficient. The woman has certain structural advantages for all types of running and swimming events. In swimming, narrower shoulders offer less resistance through water. Even at identical heights (and ideal weights), female bodies are lighter than male bodies, leaving them with less weight to carry while running.[73]

### CRITICAL THINKING

*How does physical activity aid women in the prevention of chronic disease?*

## Foot Care

Emphasize the importance of foot care in an exercise program. The feet, during walking, will meet the surface with a force one to two times the body weight, and at up to three times its weight when running. Proper shoe fit, which includes heel height, stability, and cushion, wedge support, and forefoot cushion, must be considered. Also, proper-fitting and absorbent socks are important, along with proper washing and careful drying of the feet after exercise. A foot care information sheet for seniors is available at the Public Health Agency of Canada website at www.phac-aspc.gc.ca/seniors-aines/pubs/info_sheets/foot_care/ index.htm. The info sheet has information on basic foot care that is applicable to individuals of all ages.[74]

## NUTRITION

*Eating Well with Canada's Food Guide* enables one to make wise food choices.[75] The guide is designed to assist individuals to make sure they get enough vitamins, minerals, and other nutrients from a healthy eating pattern. Many women who are young adults fit into the Women of Childbearing Age stage. Women who are trying to become pregnant, as well as those who are pregnant or breastfeeding, need a daily multivitamin containing folic acid. Pregnant women need multivitamins that contain iron to increase the maternal red blood count and nourish the growing fetus and placenta. In addition, pregnant and breastfeeding women need more calories during pregnancy to sustain an adequate weight gain to support the baby's growth and development.[76]

The recommended numbers of Food Guide servings for females and males are as follows:

- vegetables and fruits: females 7 to 8, males 8 to 10
- grain products: females 6 to 7, males 8
- milk and alternatives: females 2, males 2
- meat and alternatives: females 2, males 3

See Figure 12-2 for a sample one-day menu for James, a 45-year-old male.[77]

**Figure 12-2** Sample one-day menu for James, a 45-year-old male

| | Recommended Daily Food Guide Servings | | | |
|---|---|---|---|---|
| | Vegetables and Fruit | Grain Products | Milk and Alternatives | Meat and Alternatives |
| Male 19 – 50 years | 8-10 | 8 | 2 | 3 |

| | Number of Food Guide Servings | | | | |
|---|---|---|---|---|---|
| Foods | Vegetables and Fruit | Grain Products | Milk and Alternatives | Meat and Alternatives | Added Oils and Fats |
| Breakfast<br>• 1 large bowl of whole grain cereal (60 g) with 125 mL (½ cup) peaches and 30 mL (2 Tbsp) walnuts<br>• 250 mL (1 cup) 2% milk<br>• 1 coffee | 1 | 2 | 1 | 1/2 | |
| Snack<br>• 250 mL (1 cup) orange juice | 2 | | | | |
| Lunch<br>• Leftovers: marinated chicken breast (75 g or 2½ oz) with 250 mL (1 cup) whole wheat couscous and 125 mL (½ cup) cooked green beans with margarine<br>• 1 apple<br>• water | 1<br>1 | 2 | | 1 | ✔ |
| Dinner<br>• 110 g (3 ½ oz) roast pork<br>• 250 mL (1 cup) rice pilaf<br>• 125 mL (½ cup) steamed asparagus<br>• 250 mL (1 cup) romaine lettuce with 125 mL (½ cup) cut-up tomato, cucumber, celery and vinaigrette<br>• water | 1<br>1 | 2 | | 1 - 1/2 | ✔ |
| Snack<br>• 2 whole grain toast with margarine<br>• 1 banana<br>• 250 mL (1 cup) 2% milk | 1 | 2 | 1 | | ✔ |
| Total Food Guide Servings for the day | 9 | 8 | 2 | 3 | |

## Nutrition Assessment

Incorporate nutritional status into nursing assessment and the health history. Ask questions related to the following list to guide your assessment with the person or family:

- Knowledge of nutrients, food groups, balanced diet, and their relationship to health

- Knowledge of nutrient requirements at the person's present level of growth and development and knowledge of whether or not nutrient needs are being met

- Associations with food and how they influence food and eating patterns

- What increases or decreases one's appetite

- Cultural background, including religious beliefs, ethnic patterns, and geographic area, and how these beliefs influence food intake, likes, and dislikes

- Relationship of one's lifestyle and activity to food intake

- Income level and food buying power; the influence of income on dietary habits

- Knowledge of alternatives to high-cost foods

- Usual daily pattern of intake: times of day, types, amounts

- Which meal is the main meal of the day

- Eating environment

- Special diet requirements

- Food allergies

- Relationship of the eating patterns of family or significant other to the individual's habits and patterns of eating

- Medications and methods used to aid digestion and nutrition intake; the influence of other medications on nutritional intake

- Condition of the teeth and the person's chewing ability

- Use, condition, and fit of dentures

- Types of food the individual has difficulty chewing or swallowing

- Condition of the oral cavity and structures

- Disabilities that interfere with nutritional intake

- Assistance or special devices needed for feeding

## Nutrition and Disease Relationships

Your assistance will be sought when dietary problems occur during early pregnancy. These include the usual transitory nausea and vomiting, commonly called *morning sickness*.[78] Physiologic and psychological factors contribute to this condition. Small frequent meals of fairly dry, easily digested energy food, such as carbohydrates, are usually tolerated. Plain water will usually help. Constipation resulting from pressure of the expanding uterus on the lower portion of the intestine occurs in later pregnancy. Increased fluid intake and the use of dried fruits, fresh fruits and juices, and whole-grain cereals should induce regularity of elimination. Alcohol is to be avoided. Women should consider carefully the use of saccharin because it crosses the placenta and remains in fetal tissues owing to slow fetal clearance.[79]

CRITICAL THINKING

*A young woman informs you that to avoid morning sickness she has a diet cola for breakfast and a pizza for dinner. How should you respond to her?*

## Obesity

In Canada, obesity is a problem. We are a society that is preoccupied with losing weight and we spend billions of dollars a year on weight loss products and services. Strychar states that governmental and non-governmental organizations, as well as industry, need to join forces to ensure a safe and healthy environment for the Canadian population.[80]

## Vegetarianism

In addition to the political, philosophical, religious, and economic motivations for becoming vegetarian, the potential health benefits are attracting a growing a number of recruits, many of them being young adults. The Heart and Stroke Foundation of Canada recommends a balanced diet with emphasis on grains, fruits, and vegetables.[81] People who consider themselves vegetarians range from those who eat limited amounts of meat, milk products, or fish and animal products to vegans who eat only vegetables, fruits, legumes, nuts, and grains. Ovo-vegetarians consume eggs, and lacto-vegetarians consume milk products in addition to plant foods. It is generally considered that all vegetarians avoid all foods of animal origins.[82]

Gross nutrient deficiencies are rare among lacto-ovo-vegetarians, as they adapt to reduced intakes of certain nutrients, such as iron and calcium. Energy intake is generally lower among vegetarians than among omnivores, but it is usually adequate. Vegetarians frequently have a body mass index lower than that of omnivores, but it, too, is usually adequate.[83]

If animal proteins, eggs, or milk are inadequate in the diet, the person will need supplementary calcium, iron, zinc, and vitamins $B_2$ and $B_{12}$. Vegetarians are at a high risk of inadequate intake of vitamin $B_{12}$. In Canada, although vitamin $B_{12}$ fortification is permitted in meat analogues such as tofu burgers, these foods are often not fortified. It is very important to read food labels.[84] Soy milk fortified with vitamin D can supply that vitamin. Iron supplements are sometimes needed, even if enriched grain products are used.[85]

See Figure 12-3 for a sample one-day menu for Raj, a 20-year-old male vegetarian.

**Figure 12-3** Sample one-day menu for Raj, a 20-year-old male vegetarian

| | Recommended Daily Food Guide Servings | | | |
|---|---|---|---|---|
| | Vegetables and Fruit | Grain Products | Milk and Alternatives | Meat and Alternatives |
| Male 19 – 50 years | 8-10 | 8 | 2 | 3 |

| | Number of Food Guide Servings | | | | |
|---|---|---|---|---|---|
| Foods | Vegetables and Fruit | Grain Products | Milk and Alternatives | Meat and Alternatives | Added Oils and Fats |
| Breakfast<br>• smoothie: 250 mL (1 cup) fortified soy beverage; 125 mL (½ cup) frozen berries; 1 banana<br>• 2 scrambled eggs<br>• 2 whole wheat toast with margarine | 2 | 2 | 1 | 1 | ✔ |
| Snack<br>• 1 homemade muffin<br>• water | | 2 | | | |
| Lunch<br>• stir-fry: 175 mL (¾ cup) tofu; 125 mL (½ cup) orange pepper; 125 mL (½ cup) zucchini cooked with black bean sauce and canola oil<br>• 250 mL (1 cup) quinoa<br>• 1 apple | 1<br>1<br><br><br><br>1 | 2 | | 1 | ✔ |
| Dinner<br>• 175 mL (¾ cup) cooked red lentils (dahl)<br>• ½ naan<br>• 125 mL (½ cup) cooked spinach with margarine<br>• 250 mL (1 cup) orange juice | 1<br>2 | 2 | | 1 | ✔ |
| Snack<br>• 250 mL (1 cup) cantaloupe<br>• 250 mL (1 cup) fortified soy beverage | 2 | | 1 | | |
| **Total Food Guide Servings for the day** | 10 | 8 | 2 | 3 | |

## Cultural Influences on Nutrition

Cultural influences can have a significant impact on such health promoting factors as diet, exercise, and stress management.[86] Some cultural groups believe that certain foods maintain or promote health. Some foods are often restricted during illness, and there are "sick foods"—that is, special dishes, such as chicken soup, served to an ill person. Cultural preferences determine the style of food preparation and consumption, the frequency of eating, the time of eating, and even the type of eating utensils.[87]

Nurses who work with culturally unique clients must assess their dietary habits before they suggest foods. For example, milk is not always considered a suitable source of protein for blacks and some Asians because of their relatively high incidence of lactose intolerance.[88]

*Eating Well with Canada's Food Guide* is available for First Nations, Inuit, and Métis.[89] In addition to English and French, you can choose to print *My Food Guide* in the following languages: Arabic, Chinese (traditional or simplified), Farsi, Korean, Russian, Punjabi, Spanish, Tagalog, Tamil, or Urdu.[90]

### NARRATIVE VIGNETTE
## Cultural Patterns and Food

In your health promotion class on food habits and cultural patterns, you have been asked to select a person of a cultural background different from your own. You have selected a Filipino family to interview. Use the following questions as a beginning guideline for the interview. Record the family's responses and bring them to class.

1. What foods and preparation practices are used specifically by you?

2. What dietary practices do you use to promote health?

3. What, if any, food rituals are followed in your culture?

For assistance, check Purnell and Paulanka.[91]

## Nutrition Education

You might be called upon to advise young adults about nutrition in a variety of settings. Keep in mind the basic foods in *Eating Well with Canada's Food Guide* as you suggest a diet pattern. Be open to adjust your information to vegetarians, or to those who have allergies or specific ethnic or cultural preferences.[92]

# BIOLOGICAL RHYTHMS

Rhythms occur throughout the life cycle of every individual. In our brains, a biological clock governs the fluctuation of our hormone levels, urine volume, blood pressure, and even the responsiveness of brain cells to stimulation. Such physiological fluctuations are called biological rhythms. These rhythms are synchronized with external events, such as changes in clock time, temperature, and daylight—a process called *entrainment*.[93] However, many of these rhythms continue to occur even in the absence of external time cues; they are *endogenous*, or generated from within. These rhythms fall into three categories:

- Ultradian rhythms are regular fluctuations, shorter than 24 hours, that repeat more than once a day. An example is the 90-minute REM/non-REM sleep cycle. Other ultradian physiological responses and behaviours include stomach contractions, hormone levels, brain wave responses to cognitive tasks, and daydreaming.

- Infradian rhythms are regular fluctuations, longer than 24 hours. An example is the female menstrual cycle, which occurs on average every 28 days.[94]

- Circadian rhythms are regular fluctuations of a variety of physiological factors over 24 hours. These include adrenal, thyroid, and growth-secreting patterns, as well as sleep, arousal, temperature, energy, appetite, and motor activity patterns.[95]

Biological rhythms influence everything, from the effectiveness of medicine taken at different times during the day to alertness and performance on the job. Using this understanding of biological rhythms, we will eventually be able to design our days to take even greater advantage of the natural rhythms of our bodies.

## Circadian Rhythms

The most familiar biological rhythm is the circadian rhythm. Circadian rhythms, including daily sleep–wake cycles, are affected by light and temperature and external factors such as social activities and work routines.[96] These rather unique rhythms are controlled by a biological clock located in a tiny teardrop-cluster of cells in the hypothalamus called the *suprachiasmatic nucleus* (SCN). The SCN, for most circadian rhythms, is regarded as the master pacemaker.[97] One hormone regulated by the SCN is melatonin, which is secreted by the pineal gland. Both melatonin and the pineal gland serve as important components of the individual's biological clock—the timekeeping mechanism of the body.[98]

Sleep is a complex biological rhythm. When an individual's biological clock coincides with sleep–wake patterns and light–dark cycles, the person is said to be in *circadian synchronization*; that is, the person is awake when the physiological and psychological rhythms are most active, and is asleep when the physiological and psychological rhythms are most inactive.[99]

Researchers have theorized that many disasters have resulted from a failure to consider human biology as extensively as it should have. For example, at the nuclear accident at Three Mile Island, the three young men in the control area worked on a shift system called slow rotation—days for a week, evenings for a week, and late nights for a week. At the time of the disasters at Bhopal and Chernobyl, people were working unusual shifts. Work schedules that include changing shift rotations cause a *desynchronization* of circadian rhythms. The result is an altering of performance levels.

## CRITICAL THINKING

*How do you feel when you are "out of sync"? Under what conditions does this occur for you?*

Circadian rhythms vary extensively from individual to individual because of genetic differences. A variation in a single gene is possibly the reason why some people are early birds while others are night owls who love staying up late and cannot be pried out of bed until late in the morning![100]

Most health care facilities do not adapt care to a client's sleep–wake cycle preferences. Routines can either interrupt sleep or keep clients awake. In fact, changes to the sleep–wake cycle, such as falling asleep during the day, can indicate serious illness. Anxiety, irritability, restlessness, and impaired judgment are symptoms of disturbances in the sleep cycle.[101] In summary, a disruption to the usual sleep cycle can adversely influence overall health.

Circadian Rhythm Disorders  The circadian rhythm disorders are a distinct subgroup of sleep–wake disorders caused by a mismatch between an individual's sleep need and the timing of the signals from his or her circadian clock.[102] Conflicts arise from a variety of possible external pressures or lifestyle choices, and they result in fatigue, poor job or school performance, and sleep disturbances. A few of these disorders are as follows:

■ *Night shift work:* Individuals who work at night typically are performing their jobs at a time that conflicts with the sleep–wake regulating signals from their circadian clocks. This mismatch contributes to reduction in alertness and in job performance during the night shift and ultimately in inadequate daytime sleeps when they return home.

■ *Jet lag:* Each year, many travellers suffer from jet lag after a flight across multiple time zones. Jet leg causes a deterioration of their performance after arrival at their destination. These sleep–wake disturbances arise when travellers attempt to function immediately, while their internal clocks are synchronized to their original schedule and adapt only slowly to new local time cues.

■ *Delayed Sleep Phase Syndrome (DSPS):* This syndrome is characterized by a delay in the main sleep episode and an inability to fall asleep, or wake up, at the desired times. DSPS individuals are extreme "night owls," with bedtimes around 3 to 6 a.m. and wake times around noon to 3 p.m. Sleep quality and duration are normal, when individuals are allowed to sleep at the preferred biological times of their bodies. However, symptoms appear when individuals attempt to go to sleep earlier then they would otherwise choose, because of work or school demands. This syndrome often emerges after puberty and is relatively common among adolescents and young adults.[103]

Conflicts between the timing of the circadian rhythm and one's schedules of activities can lead to severe disturbances of sleep and waking. Careful control of exposure to light and dark, of sleep timing, and of other environmental factors can help many people with circadian rhythm disturbances to become better adjusted to the requirements of their jobs and social lives.[104]

## CRITICAL THINKING

*Over a period of a week to ten days, keep a daily log of your routines. What do you conclude from this log?*

An interrelationship exists between circadian rhythms and seasonal changes. Clinicians report that some individuals become depressed every winter, when periods of daylight are short. Then they improve again in mood each spring as daylight increases—a pattern that has come to be known as seasonal affective disorder (SAD). During the winter months, those affected report lethargy, sadness, drowsiness, increased appetite, and a craving for carbohydrates. To counteract these symptoms, some physicians and therapists have been treating SAD clients with phototherapy—having them sit in front of extremely bright lights at specific times of the day.[105]

Nurses can teach clients who have recurrent patterns of SAD to begin preparing for their symptoms by seeking light treatment in the early fall.[106]

## Nursing Assessment and Intervention

Nursing care should be planned with biological rhythms in mind. Because our cyclic functioning is synchronized with environmental stimuli, physiologic disequilibrium occurs whenever we are confronted with environmental or schedule changes. Episodes of disturbed mental and physical well-being, together with increased subjective fatigue, reflect the conflict that can exist between the internal time pattern and external events. Usually, several days are required before the person adapts to the environment and thereby begins to regain synchronization—normal biological rhythms.

Your *nursing history* should be directed toward obtaining information about the patient's pre-illness or pre-hospitalization patterns for sleep, rest, food and fluid intake, elimination, and personal hygiene. Once this information has been obtained, nursing actions can be initiated that support established patterns. Doing so can possibly prevent uncomfortable disruptions of body rhythms during hospitalization.

After the patient has been hospitalized for a few days, certain objective data are available that will assist you in determining a rough estimate of the person's circadian patterns. The routine graphic record supplies information about the patient's vital signs. Using this source, you might be able to identify peaks and lows in blood pressure, pulse, and temperature curves. An intake and output record that shows both the time and the amount voided will aid in determining the patient's daily urinary-excretory pattern. In addition to the post-admission nursing history, a daily log of sleep and waking hours, mealtimes, hunger periods, voiding and defecation patterns, diurnal moods, and other circadian rhythms recorded for 28 days before hospitalization can help determine the person's cyclic patterns.

**CRITICAL THINKING**

*What questions might researchers pose to individuals regarding the study of the internal clock?*

## Work Schedules

Work schedules should be developed with biological rhythms in mind. You can establish your own circadian patterns to help you gain insight into physical feelings and behaviours. Furthermore, you can use this information to plan your days to advantage. You might choose to cope with the most difficult patient assignment during your time of peak mental and physical performance, for example.

Nurses, and many industrial and law enforcement personnel, are frequently required to change shifts every week or month. Night shift and rotating shift workers are at excessive risk for accidents and injuries on the job because of disrupted circadian rhythms. Sleep cycles are interrupted. Difficulty is experienced in falling asleep. This disruption is made worse by a shorter duration of sleep, poorer quality of sleep, and persistent fatigue. Alertness and other physiologic processes suffer. Eating habits are altered, diets are less nourishing, and digestion is disrupted. Constipation, gastric and peptic ulcers, and gastritis are more common. Social activities and personal interactions, which are essential to good physical and mental health, are interrupted. Family life and relationships suffer and shift workers experience difficulty fulfilling family and parental roles. Rotating shift assignments are highly relevant to the worker's health and quality of work performance. Altering the sleep–wake sequence demands that time is allowed for the person to make adjustments and regain synchrony.

Thurston, Tanguay, and Fraser state that a common eight-hour nursing rotation is usually based on one week per shift, followed by a counter-clockwise rotation to the previous shift (day shift to night shift, night shift to evening shift, and evening shift to day shift). They claim that this type of shift change is the worst possible scenario. Just as the nurse is beginning to acclimate to the shift after one week, a second eight-hour phase shift is imposed. This change to a new shift is not unlike jet lag. It requires the nurse to be alert on the new shift at a time when alertness is at its lowest. A more preferred rotation is in a clockwise direction (day to evening, evening to night, night to day), because it is easier on the body to delay an internal clock than it is to advance it.[107] Unfortunately, this is not possible for the majority of nurses who work 12-hour shifts.

**CRITICAL THINKING**

*What safety concerns might be inherent in a rotating shift worker?*

## REST AND SLEEP

Rest restores an individual's energy and allows the person to resume optimal functioning.[108] Meanwhile, sleep is a *complex biological rhythm, intricately related to rest and other biological rhythms*. In essence, sleep is a basic human need necessary for normal everyday functioning.[109] To promote health, nurses must help young adults to realize that factors such as emotional and physical status, occupation, and the amount of physical activity one does determine the need for rest and sleep. For example, workers who alternate between day and night shifts frequently feel more exhausted and need more sleep than do people who keep regular hours. Surgery, illness, pregnancy, and the postpartum state all require the individual to obtain more sleep than usual.

Some young people find themselves caught in a whirlwind of activities. Jobs, social activities, family responsibilities, and educational pursuits occupy every minute.

The young adult can adjust to this pace and maintain it for a length of time without damaging physical or mental health. The person may think he or she is immune to the laws of nature, and that he or she can go for long periods without sleep. If the person finds that he or she is not functioning well on a certain amount of sleep, his or her schedule should be adjusted to allow for more hours of rest and sleep. He or she should be made cognizant of the biological rhythms for rest and activity. Setting aside certain periods for quiet activities such as reading, sewing, watching television, and various hobbies is restful, but time spent in these activities is not as beneficial as sleep.

Each person has his or her own sleep needs and cycle. Research is helping us to understand more clearly the different stages of sleep and the importance of sleep to well-being. The tradition that young adults should have seven to eight hours of sleep still seems valid, although some get along fine with less. When left to the body's natural pace, the person is likely to sleep every 25 hours.

## Physiology of Sleep

Sleep is a complex phenomenon. It involves a sequence of physiological states maintained by a highly integrated central nervous system (CNS) that is associated with changes in the activity of the cardiovascular, peripheral nervous, endocrine, respiratory, and muscular systems.[110] Current theory suggests that sleep is an active inhibitory process. The cyclic nature of sleep is controlled by centres located in the lower part of the brain. These centres inhibit wakefulness, thus causing sleep. In fact, the functional component of the brain stem that exerts influence on consciousness and the wake–sleep cycle is called the *reticular activating system (RAS)*. The RAS activates the state of consciousness and functions as a deactivation mechanism to decrease alertness and to produce sleep.[111]

**Electroencephalograms (EEGs)**, *recordings of brain wave activity*, vary with the awake and asleep states, and at different intra-sleep cycles (see Figure 12-4). When a person is wide awake and alert, the EEG recordings show rapid, irregular waves. High-frequency beta and alpha waves predominate. As he or she begins to rest, the wave pattern changes to an **alpha rhythm**, *a regular pattern of low voltage, with frequencies of 8 to 12 cycles per second*. During sleep, a **delta rhythm**, *a slow pattern of high voltage at a rate of one to two cycles per second*, occurs.[112]

## Stages of Sleep

Sleep is divided into **NREM** (*non–rapid eye movement*) and **REM** stages. NREM sleep is divided into four stages—light to deep. REM sleep, also known as stage V, follows the deepest NREM sleep as the person ascends to stage II sleep, and it occurs before repeated descent through stages II, III, and IV.

In **NREM stage I sleep**, the *person makes a transition from wakefulness to sleep* in approximately five minutes. The alpha rhythm is present, but the waves are more uneven and smaller than in later stages. The person is drowsy and relaxed, has fleeting thoughts, is somewhat aware of the environment, can be easily awakened, and may think that he or she has been awake. The pulse rate is decreased.

**NREM stage II sleep** is the *beginning of deeper sleep*. The person is more relaxed than in the prior stage, but can be easily awakened. It accounts for about 50 percent of total sleep.

**NREM stage III sleep** is a *period of progressively deeper sleep*. Muscles are more relaxed; vital signs and metabolic activity are lowered to basal rates; and the person is difficult to awaken.

**NREM stage IV sleep** is *very deep sleep*. It occurs approximately 40 minutes after stage I, and it rests and restores the body physically. This stage is as important as REM sleep, and it comprises 11 percent of sleep in healthy young adults. The person is very relaxed and seldom moves, is difficult to arouse, and responds slowly if awakened. Physiologic measures are below normal. After strenuous physical

**Figure 12-4** Changes in electroencephalogram tracing during sleep

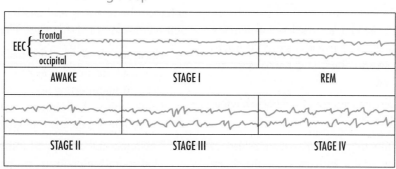

exercise, this stage is greatly needed. Deep sleep is less deep during the last half of the night.[113]

Stage V or **REM sleep** is called *active, or paradoxic, sleep* and is the *stage of rapid eye movements and dreaming that occurs before descending to the deeper sleep of stages II, III, and IV.* This stage is of great importance. In REM sleep, the EEG readings are active and similar to those of stage I sleep, but various physiologic differences from other sleep stages are present.[114]

Some of these differences include increase in heart rate, a rise in blood pressure, and faster and more irregular breathing. Small twitches in the face and fingers occur. In men, the penis becomes somewhat erect as the vascular tissue relaxes and blood fills the genital area faster than it exits. In women, the clitoris enlarges and vaginal lubrication increases. Most skeletal muscles go limp, preventing the aroused brain from producing physical movement.[115]

Dreams that occur during REM sleep allow for wish fulfillment and the release of potentially harmful thoughts, feelings, and impulses so that they do not affect the waking personality.

REM and non-REM sleep continue to alternate throughout the night, with Stages III and IV tending to become shorter or even to disappear. REM periods tend to get longer and closer together as the hours pass.[116]

REM sleep is essential for mental and emotional restoration. Loss of REM sleep impairs both memory and learning.[117]

---

### CRITICAL THINKING

*What is your understanding of dreams?*

---

## Sleep Disorders

Many people do not get normal sleep daily. They either sleep too much or not enough, suffer night terrors, or stop breathing for a minute or two during sleep. The cost of sleep disorders is enormous. Some people pay a great deal of money for pills and potions in endeavours to maintain normal sleep.

Sleep disorders are classified by their manifestations. The more common disorders fall into two groups:

■ *Primary sleep disorders* are characterized by insomnia or excessive sleepiness. These particular sleep disorders, such as insomnia, sleep apnea, and narcolepsy, are briefly discussed below.

■ *Secondary sleep disorders* are patterns of waking behaviour that appear during sleep.[118]

*Insomnia* is the inability to fall asleep, remain asleep, or go back to sleep. Young adults with this condition are usually highly distressed because they think they won't ever sleep again. Insomnia can result from physical discomfort; but more often it is a result of mental overstimulation due to anxiety.[119] It may occur as a result of illness, depression, acute stress, substance abuse, the side effects of medications, or poor sleep hygiene such as drinking beverages that contain caffeine before bedtime.[120]

*Sleep apnea* is a periodic disruption during sleep—an absence of air flow through the nose or mouth for at least ten seconds at a time. Episodes may occur several, or even hundreds, of times during the night and they can last for as long as one minute or more. Sleep apnea is seen most frequently in men over 50 years of age and in post-menopausal women.[121]

*Narcolepsy* is a sudden wave of sleepiness that occurs during the day. It is thought to be caused by a genetic defect of the central nervous system in which REM cannot be controlled. Falling asleep uncontrollably can be extremely troubling for the young adult. Strategies that can combat narcolepsy include eliminating the consumption of alcohol and avoiding heavy meals.[122]

## Sleep Deprivation

Sleep deprivation involves decreases in the quantity and quality of sleep, and the occurrence of inconsistency in the timing of sleep. Changes occur in the sequencing of the sleep cycle resulting in cumulative sleep deprivation. Causes include illnesses with symptoms of fever, difficulty breathing, or pain. Other symptoms include emotional stress, environmental disturbances, the side effects of medications, and variability in the timing of sleep due to shift work.[123]

A growing concern exists about the prevalence of chronic sleep deprivation in our busy 24-hour society. Sleep is an integral part of health and life, not only for young adults, but for all individuals across the lifespan.[124]

## Nursing Assessment and Intervention

Health promotion measures that nurses can implement to enhance the quantity and quality of sleep involve largely non-pharmacological strategies. They involve the following:

■ *Client and family teaching*: healthy individuals, such as young adults, need to learn the importance of rest and sleep in maintaining active and productive lives. In a family unit with an infant, strategies can developed for the couple to take turns in attending to the infant.

■ *Environmental control*: all individuals need a comfortable room temperature, proper ventilation, minimal noise, and a comfortable bed. People vary in their preferred need of a night light.

■ *Supporting bedtime routines*: most individuals are accustomed to bedtime rituals, or pre-sleep routines, that are conducive to sleep and relaxation. Common bedtime activities of adults include listening to relaxing music, praying, taking a soothing bath, or reading.[125]

## CRITICAL THINKING

*What other activities can you think of to promote sleep?*

Individuals, such as young adults, are the only ones who know whether their sleep problems have improved. As well as listening to the client, you can make comparisons with baseline sleep assessments to evaluate their sleep patterns.

# PSYCHOSOCIAL CONCEPTS

The following information is relevant for assessments, teaching, and health promotion interventions.

## Cognitive Development

Different learning abilities are required in different life stages. Youth is the time for acquisition; young adulthood is the time for achievement; middle age is the time for responsibility; and old age is the time for reintegration.

**Theories about Cognitive Development** Cognitive theories are described here. The reader is encouraged to refer also to Chapter 5. Erikson theorized that the basis for adult cognitive performance is laid during the school years when the child accomplishes the task of industry, learns how to learn and win recognition by producing and achieving, and learns to enjoy learning. The child learns one particular attitude that lasts into adulthood: how much effort a task takes, and how long and hard he or she should work for what is desired or expected. The sense of industry is useful in adult life, both in coping with new experiences and in functioning as a worker, family member, citizen, and lifelong learner.

Current researchers and theorists propose that learning continues throughout the adult years. The brain shows increasing myelinization through middle age, which permits the continuation and extension of integrated modes of social response, as well as the maintenance of stable, or increasing, intellectual functions.[126]

Becoming mature in young adulthood involves intellectual growth, becoming more adaptive and knowledgeable about self, forming values, and developing increasing depth in analytic and synthetic thinking, logical reasoning, and imagination. Multiple and different intelligences are found in young adulthood besides academic aptitude. They include leadership ability, creative and performing arts abilities, and the ability to manage self, others, and a career. In fact, developing social and interpersonal skills and personal friendships probably have a powerfully maturing effect on intellectual skills.

**Influences on Learning** Influences differ somewhat from childhood to adulthood; they include: (1) level of knowledge in society generally; (2) personal values and perceptions, and previously learned associations, (3) level of education; (4) available life opportunities; (5) interests; (6) participation by the person in the learning activity; (7) the learning environment; and (8) life experiences.[127] As a result of these influences, the person develops a preferred way of learning or cognitive style—a characteristic way of perceiving, organizing, and evaluating information.

**Formal Operations Stage** The young adult remains in the formal operations stage, according to Piaget. The adult is creative in thought. He or she begins at the abstract level and compares the idea, either mentally or verbally, with previous memories, knowledge, or experience. The person combines or integrates a number of steps of a task mentally, instead of thinking about or doing each step as a separate unit. He or she considers the multiplicity and relativism of issues and alternatives to a situation, synthesizing and integrating ideas or information into memory, beliefs, or solutions so that the end result is a unique product. Adult thought is different from adolescent thought. The adult can differentiate among many perspectives and the adult is objective, realistic, and less egocentric. Thinking and learning are problem-centred, not just subject-centred. Reality is considered only a part of all that is possible. The person can imagine and reason about events that are not occurring in reality, but that are possible or in which he or she does not even believe. Hypotheses are generated; conjectures are deduced from hypotheses, and observations are conducted to either confirm or independently disconfirm the expectations. The thought system works independently of its context, and it can be applied to diverse data. The person can evaluate the validity of a train of reasoning independently of its factual content. A concrete proposition can be replaced by an arbitrary sign of symbolic logic such as $p$ or $q$. Probability, proportionality, and the combining of thought systems occur.[128]

Arlin[129] proposed that some people continue to develop cognitively beyond the formal operations proposed by Piaget into a *fifth stage* of cognitive development that progresses through adulthood. The stage of formal operations describes strategies used in problem solving. The *problem-finding stage*, or post-formal thought, goes beyond the problem-solving stage. It is characterized by creative thought in the form of discovered problems, relativistic thinking, the formation of generic problems, the raising of general questions from ill-defined problems, the use of intuition, insight, and hunches, and the development of significant scientific thought.

Based on longitudinal and cross-sectional studies, researchers have concluded that the thinking process of young adults represents a qualitative change beyond formal operations.[130] Post-formal thought probably varies from situation to situation and solutions must be realistic to be reasonable, In addition, ambiguity and contradiction are the rule rather than the exception, and a most important realization is that feelings and subjective factors usually play a significant role in thinking.[131]

In adulthood, several research-based descriptions of the development of thinking have been offered. One of the best is the description of the development of reflective judgment.[132] This is a way in which adults reason through dilemmas that make current affairs, religion, science, personal relationships, and the like.[133]

## CRITICAL THINKING

*Compare and contrast adult and adolescent thought. What is distinctive about adult thought?*

There are *four criteria for post-formal thought*:

1. *Shifting gears*. Going from abstract reasoning to practical, real-world considerations.

2. *Multiple causality, multiple solutions*. Awareness that most problems have more than one cause and more than one solution and that some solutions are more likely to work than others.

3. *Pragmatism*. Ability to choose the best of several possible solutions and to recognize the criteria for making the choice.

4. *Paradox recognition awareness*. A problem or solution has inherent conflict.

Sternberg, in his Triarchic Theory of Intelligence, stated that IQ tests do not measure creative insight and practical intelligence. He proposed *three elements of adult intelligence*:[134]

1. *Componential or analytic*. How efficiently people process information, solve problems, monitor solutions, and evaluate results.

2. *Experiential, insightful*. How people approach novel and familiar tasks, compare new information to old, and think originally, while automatically performing familiar operations.

3. *Contextual, practical*. How people deal with the environment, size up a situation, adapt to or change a situation, or find a new, more suitable setting.

The person may use different types of thinking for scientific operations, business transactions, artistic activities, and intimate interpersonal interactions. Thus, mature thinkers can accept and live with contradictions and conflicts, and they can engage in a number of activities at the same time. At times, however, the adult will, of necessity, conduct thinking that is typical of concrete operations. At other times, the adult will regress to the preoperational stage (some never get beyond this period), as shown by superstitious, egocentric, or illogical thinking. Some adults simply do not have the ability to perform formal operations.

## CRITICAL THINKING

*In what kinds of situations in the health care delivery system would post-formal thought be most useful?*

Young adults continue to learn both formally and informally. As a result, they enhance their cognitive and job skills and self-knowledge. Learning may be pursued in "on-the-job training," job-sponsored orientation courses, vocational schools, university and college studies, or continuing education courses. Environmental stimulation is important in continued learning. Increasingly, young adults are changing their minds about what their life work will be. They change directions, sometimes after several years of study or work in the original field.

**Gender Differences** The confident young adult takes pride in being mentally astute, creative, progressive, and alert to events. He or she normally has the mental capacity to make impressive social and occupational contributions. They are self-directive and curious, and they like to match wits with others in productive dialogue.

Both men and women have similar basic needs. In each case, their own unique cognitive abilities and talents, and often unspoken ideas and feelings, long for self-expression. From young childhood on, both females and males should be considered cognitively capable to achieve their maximum potential, and they should have the opportunity, especially in the adult years, to meet that maximum potential.

## CRITICAL THINKING

*Give examples of the influence that culture has on the cognitive abilities of men and women.*

**Teaching the Adult** Information on cognitive development should be considered whenever you are teaching adults (see Table 12-1 for principles of the learning process). Schuster outlines four adult learning principles—teaching strategies that are especially appropriate for client and family education.[135]

■ *Build on previous experiences*: it is important to assess the client's and family's knowledge or understanding of the information you want them to learn. Adults learn by building on previous experiences.

■ *Focus on immediate concerns first*: adults are generally concerned with solving the immediate issues at hand. They want health professionals to tell them what they need to know, rather than what is nice to know.[136] Instead of detailed explanations, they want to know the basics of how to perform a prescribed regimen of health care, and they want to know how to adapt it into their current lifestyle.

■ *Adapt the teaching into the lifestyle*: teaching must meet the client's present activities and responsibilities. Include the family in your teaching on health promotion activities.[137]

■ *Make the client an active participant*: one successful key to teaching and learning is based on the active involvement of the adult in their learning process.[138] Teaching methods should include discussion and demonstrations that encourage clients to ask questions.

With young adults, emphasize a sharing of ideas and experiences, engage them in role play, and have them realize practical applications of the information. In some cases, you will be helping the person to unlearn old habits, attitudes, or information and to acquire new habits and attitudes.

---

## CRITICAL THINKING

*How would you modify your teaching strategy for a group of young adults who have learning deficits?*

---

**Gender** More women are enrolled in all major fields of study except for two: engineering/applied sciences, and mathematics/physical sciences.[139] Specific job selections, though, remain strongly affected by gender. Despite the women's movement and the vast increase in the proportion of women working, about 70 percent occupy traditional female occupations such as teaching, nursing, and clerical positions. However, the trend is shifting: Canadian women are increasing their presence in traditionally male-dominated jobs such as doctors, senior managers, and dentists. And they are doubling their ranks in manufacturing and agriculture.[140] It is not surprising that women's income has been increasing steadily—in 2002, it was slightly more than four-fifths of the man's wage overall.[141]

It is still very important to realize that academic skills (the ability to think critically), teamwork skills (the ability to respect others and collaborate effectively), and personal management skills (including positive attitudes) are all most critical in work situations, regardless of gender. The combination of these skills, attitudes, and behaviours provides the foundation to obtain the position, maintain the job, and progress within the organization to achieve the best possible results.[142]

## Work Options and Attitudes

Many work options and attitudes are available. There are people who work long hours and who are highly involved in their work, but who are not workaholics. They feel exhilarated about the flow of work, the challenge, their goals, and the use of skills involved, and they feel creative, active, and motivated. These feelings are more likely to come from

---

### Table 12-1 Principles of the Learning Process

1. Learning is an active, self-directed process.

2. Learning is central to ongoing development and behavioural changes.

3. Learning is influenced by readiness to learn, abilities, potential to learn, and emotional state.

4. Learning is facilitated when the content or behaviours to be learned are perceived as relevant.

5. Learning proceeds from simple to complex and from known to unknown.

6. Learning is facilitated when the learner has opportunities to take risks, test ideas, make mistakes, and be creative.

7. Learning is facilitated when the person has knowledge of his or her progress and receives feedback that serves as a measure for further learning.

8. Learning transfer occurs when the person can recognize similarities and differences between past experiences and the present situation.

9. Learning is most effective when it can be applied immediately.

10. Learning occurs best when the teaching methodology is relevant to the content to be learned.

11. Learning occurs best in an environment that is non-threatening, comfortable, and free of distractions.

12. Learning occurs best, and is continued, when the learner feels satisfied and successful.

work than from leisure. These people contribute a great deal generally to the advancement of their vocation or profession, and to the individuals they serve. However, work stress has been receiving increasing attention in the media and research journals. Shannon and his researchers conducted a study to determine changes in the levels of work stressors in a nationally representative sample of Canadian workers from 1994–1995 to 2000–2001. They found that the levels of work stressors did not increase over the period despite media reports to the contrary.[143]

A combination of the effects of changing economic conditions in Canada, especially in the agriculture industry, and changing demographics have forced many people out of their job. As a result, many young adults feel insecure about their jobs. A study examined coping strategies for comparable samples of laid-off and employed high-technology workers.[144] It discovered that although unemployed participants reported higher level of stress compared with employed participants, employment uncertainty mediated the association between employment status and perceived stress. That is, individuals who believed that their work was in jeopardy and they might lose it, even though this may be untrue, indicated levels of stress similar to unemployed participants. The stress levels were due to differences in coping strategies. Two of the more common ways of coping are emotion-focused coping and problem-focused coping. Individuals who used emotional coping as a strategy reported higher levels of stress, particularly under low uncertainty conditions. Others focused on the problem and examined strategies of how to solve it. In summary, individuals whose jobs are not really in jeopardy can report levels of stress if they tend to use emotion-focused strategies.[145]

## CRITICAL THINKING

*How do you find yourself coping with job uncertainty?*

Balancing work and family life responsibilities is often stressful for the woman, especially if she is a single parent, a divorced parent, or a member of a two-career family. There is never enough time and often too much to do.[146] Some employers, to attract and keep competent workers, offer flexible work schedules, job sharing, and on-site daycare. The following *suggestions can be shared with the parent who has highest responsibility for balancing home and work:*

- *Identify priorities.* Discuss with the spouse, or the children if they are old enough, what tasks must be done, what can be delegated (either on the job or to a service company for essential needs in the home), and who can take on which responsibilities to even the load.

- *Allocate tasks.* Design a system for assigning tasks, based on skill, age, availability, and fairness. Rotate tasks, if possible, or assign tasks that are especially requested.

- *Speak up for yourself at home and on the job.* Explore grievance channels if necessary.

- *Use a support network.* Family, friends, neighbours, and child care providers can be asked for assistance on a regular basis, or for help in emergencies.

- *Re-channel emotional investments.* Carrying multiple roles provides opportunities to excel in one realm if you have problems in another.

- *Assess progress.* Plan frequent review sessions to discuss the effectiveness of the plan, or to determine problem areas, in order to avoid resentments or rebellions.

Young adults can prepare for their future by keeping up with the occupational outlook in various fields, and by enhancing their knowledge and skills set accordingly.[147] An excellent source for such information is Canada WorkinfoNet, which is revised every two years.[148] A close relationship exists between occupational and family satisfaction. If the person is dissatisfied in either work or family life, he or she will try to compensate in the other.[149]

As an occupational nurse, you might be asked for professional advice by managers, executive-level employees, or employers to provide assistance to those employees who find it difficult to understand the young adult worker. Help them to understand that each generation of worker has a different value system, and that each responds to different values and different motivational stimuli.

## CRITICAL THINKING

*How do baby boomers and members of Generation X view the world of work?*

As a nurse, through your role as counsellor or educator, you can assist both the individual employee and administrative or management personnel to realize the importance of feelings of self-respect in relation to employment. Management consultants have learned that low self-esteem and feelings of stress in the worker definitely lower productivity, morale, and profits. You can be instrumental in helping the work system to promote feelings of self-esteem, and among the workers you can be instrumental in having them realize the importance of their work.

You may also become an advocate for the woman who is undergoing sexual harassment on the job. Increasingly, women workers are gaining the courage to talk publicly about, and to seek legal aid for, sexual harassment in workplaces such as factories, mines, offices, migrant farm fields, and health care facilities.[150]

Many Canadian workplace health programs offer educational, organizational, and behavioural interventions to support positive health maintenance behaviours that are conducive to the well-being of all employees in a workplace. These interactions can include such activities as stress management, fitness exercises, and health-promoting information, as well as supervised daycare.[151]

**Leisure** Many young adults are in pursuit of leisure.[152] **Leisure** is *freedom from obligations and formal duties of paid work, and includes the opportunity to pursue, at one's own pace, mental nourishment, enlivenment, pleasure, and relief from the fatigue of work.* Leisure may be as active as backpacking up a mountain or as quiet as fishing alone in a remote lake. Some people never know leisure; and others manage an attitude of leisure even as they work. Various factors influence the use of leisure time: sex; the extent of responsibilities of family, home, work, or community; mental status; income and socioeconomic class; and past interests.

Maintaining friendships is a particularly healthy use of leisure time. It takes time, self-disclosure, and the desire to share interests to form friendships. Gradually, a sense of reliability and confidentiality grows as a core to the friendship. Some conflict will surface, but this is natural as intimacy deepens. In a world in which women juggle career, love, and family, the availability of time can limit the size of the friendship circle. Several close friendships should be made and maintained. Successful friendship combines the freedom to depend on one another with the freedom to be independent.

Doing volunteer work with a favourite charity or community group is one way to use non-work time that can promote a sense of leisure and enjoyment, while simultaneously using skills and talents to improve life for others. The rewards are dual—to the self and to society. Help the client to realize the importance of leisure as a vital part of balanced living. The young adult needs to develop a variety of interests in preparation for the years ahead when they continue their efforts to maintain physical and mental health.

CRITICAL THINKING

*What are some of your leisure activities? What other activities would you like to develop?*

# Emotional Development

Emotional development in young adulthood is an ongoing, dynamic process, an extension of childhood and adolescent developmental influences and processes. Development is still influenced by the environment; but the environment is different. The fundamental developmental issues continue to be central aspects of adult life, but they do so in an altered form. Now, trust, autonomy, initiative, industry, and identity are all reworked and elaborated upon, based on current experiences. Young adulthood is a time when an increased clarity and consistency of personality is sought. At this time, the following receive high priority: stabilization of self and identity; established preferences of interests and activities; increased coping ability; less defensiveness; a decrease in youthful illusions, fantasy, and impulsiveness; more responsiveness to, and responsibility for, self and others; more giving than taking; and a greater appreciation of one's surroundings. It is a time to develop expanded resources for happiness.

In 1990, two psychologists, Salovey and Mayer, coined the term *emotional intelligence.* Emotional intelligence refers to the ability to recognize and deal with one's own feelings and the feelings of others.[153] Strickland states that, according to Daniel Goleman, who popularized the concept, there are five components of emotional intelligence: self-awareness, self-regulation, motivation, empathy, and social skills.[154] Health care delivery systems that wish to thrive need leaders in the health professions who have high emotional intelligence.[155]

CRITICAL THINKING

*In what kinds of situations would emotional intelligence be most appreciated?*

**Theories of Emotional Development** Various theorists discussed in Chapter 5 present research findings on which they base their beliefs about adult personality development. The findings of Levinson and Erikson are discussed in the following pages.

Levinson[156] studied only men in formulating a concept of adult developmental stages. He believes that the stages are age-linked and universal and, thus, should be applicable to women (see Table 12-2). In each period, various timetables, such as biological, psychodynamic, cultural, and social, operate in only partial synchronization. This situation makes for developmental difficulties. The organizing concept of **life structure** *refers to a pattern of the person's life at a specific time,* and it is used to focus on the boundary between the individual and society.[157] In its external aspects, life structure *refers to roles, memberships, interests, conditions or style of living, and long-term goals.* In its *internal aspects,* life structure includes the personal meanings of external patterns, inner identities, care values, fantasies, and psychodynamic qualities, all of which help shape the person.

## Table 12-2 Levinson's Theory of Early Adulthood

| Era | Age Range | Life Structure |
|---|---|---|
| **Pre-adulthood** | 0–22 | Preparing for adulthood |
| | 17–22 | Transition to early adulthood |
| | | Begin novice phase; person is guided out of adolescence |
| **Early adulthood** | 17–45 | Combine social and occupational roles that are adapted to personality and skills |
| | 22–28 | Enter young adulthood. Novice phase tasks: |
| | | a. Form dream for life |
| | | b. Establish or enter relationship |
| | | c. Select occupation |
| | | d. Establish love relationship |
| | 28–33 | Age 30 transition: reappraise life plan and modify it |
| | 33–40 | Culminating life plans and structure for early adulthood: seek to realize goals |
| | 40–45 | Transition to or preparation for midlife |

**Developmental Crisis** According to Erikson, the psychosexual crisis is in intimacy versus self-isolation situation. **Intimacy** is *reaching out and using the self to form a commitment to and an intense, lasting relationship with another person or even a cause, an institution, or a creative effort.*[158] In an intimate experience, one finds mutual trust, a sharing of feelings, and responsibility to and co-operation with each other. The physical satisfaction and psychological security of another person are more important than one's own satisfaction and security. The person is involved with people, work, hobbies, and community issues. He or she has poise and ease in the lifestyle because identity is firm. A steady conviction persists of who he or she is. It is a self-acceptance, and a unity of personality that will improve through life.

Intimacy is a situation involving two people that permits the acceptance of all aspects of the other. Intimacy demands self-disclosure and collaboration where one person adjusts his or her behaviour to the behaviour and needs of the other in pursuit of mutual satisfaction.[159]

A person's mental health depends on his or her ability to enter into a relationship and experience self-disclosure. In doing so, the support and maintenance gained in the relationship alleviates most of the feelings of loneliness.

Women, more so than men, are concerned with relationships. Women tend to be interested in the process, rather than the product, of something. They usually recognize their vulnerability, and they can acknowledge the need to change more readily than men. Women self-disclose more easily than men. If a healthy balance between dependence and independence exists, social relationships and intimacy are maintained more easily.

Consequently, the risk of experiencing loneliness and isolation decreases.

With the intimate person, the young adult is able to regulate cycles of work, recreation, and procreation (if chosen). They are able to work toward satisfactory stages of development for their children, and they are able to maintain the ongoing development of self and partner.[160]

### CRITICAL THINKING

*What factors within a relationship promote and maintain intimacy?*

**Love** Love is the feeling that accompanies intimacy. Love and intimacy change over time.[161] The young adult often has difficulty determining what love is. A classic description of love, as stated by the apostle Paul in I Corinthians 13:4–7, has been the basis for many statements on love by poets, novelists, humanists, philosophers, psychiatrists, theologians, and common people:

> Love is patient and kind; love is not jealous or boastful; it is not arrogant or rude. Love does not insist on its own way; it is not irritable or resentful; it does not rejoice at wrong, but rejoices in the right. Love bears all things, believes all things, hopes all things, and endures all things.

One of the most important things a person can learn within the family, as a child and as an adolescent, is to love. By the time the person reaches the mid-twenties, he or she should be experienced in the emotion of love. If there was deprivation or distortion of love in the home when he or she was young, the adult will find it difficult to achieve

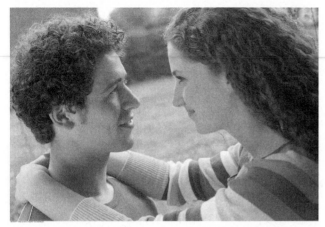

The principal developmental task of young adults is the formation of close relationships with significant others. When you help people to sort through their feelings about life and love, you are indirectly making a direct and powerful contribution to their health and stability and to their family.

mature love in an intimate relationship. By this time, the person should realize that one *does not fall* in love; one *learns* to love; one *grows into* love.

**Marriage** In Canada, as well as in other countries, marriage is a legal relationship, usually involving economic co-operation, sexual activity, and childbearing. For the 2006 Canadian Census, a married couple might be of opposite or the same sex.[162] Marriage is endorsed in some form by all cultures, in all periods of history, because it formalizes and symbolizes the importance of family.

The pattern and sequence of a person's life history together influence whom, when, and why he or she marries. Apparently, many people do not really know the person they are marrying, and they do not realize initially how greatly the partner's personality will come to influence their own personality.

Mates often choose each other on the basis of unconscious needs. They strive to meet these needs through a mate whose personality complements, rather than replicates, their own. Alternatively, they choose their mate out of fear and loneliness, or on the basis of physical attraction. The person chooses someone for an intimate relationship whose lifestyle and personality pattern they believe will strengthen and encourage his or her own personal development.

There are *four patterns of marriage*:[163]

1. *Traditional*: the male is provider; the female is homemaker and mother.

2. *Romantic*: sexual passion is the main focus.

3. *Rescue*: marriage makes up for previous painful experiences.

4. *Companionate*: the relationship is based on friendship and equal division of work and family roles.

---

## CRITICAL THINKING

*What are the benefits of marriage in today's society?*

---

Gottman has been studying married couples' lives since the early 1970s.[164] In his research, he found seven main principles that determine whether a marriage will work. They are as follows:

- *Establishing love maps:* People in a successful marriage have personal insights and detailed maps of each other's life and the world around them. They use these "love maps" to express their liking and understanding of each other.

- *Nurturing fondness and admiration:* In successful marriages, the partners sing glowing praises of each other.

- *Turning toward each other rather than away:* In good marriages, partners turn toward each other. They consider each other as good friends, and their friendship is a powerful shield against conflict.

- *Letting your partner influence you:* In successful marriages, the willingness to share power is a prerequisite to compromising.

- *Solving solvable conflicts:* Gottman found two types of problems in marriage: perpetual and solvable. Perpetual problems, such as whether to have a family, do not go away. However, marital therapists have discovered that couples do not need to solve their perpetual problems to make their marriage work. Gottman claims that a gentle approach works best to resolve conflicts, regulate emotions, and become tolerant of the other's faults. Among the typical areas of marital conflict are work, stress, in-laws, money, sex, housework, and a new baby.[165]

- *Overcoming gridlock:* Gridlock usually happens when, for example, one partner insists that the other attend church when that partner does not want to. Gottman believes that the key to ending gridlock is not to try to solve the problem, but to move from gridlock to dialogue, and to be patient.

- *Creating shared meaning:* The more the couple can speak gently and respectfully with another, the more likely they will create shared meaning in their marriage.

The most important aspect between partners is the role of interacting with one another—the willingness to see the other's point of view, and to be empathetic with each other.

You can ask certain valuable questions to ascertain readiness for marriage in a young adult, or in yourself. One such question is: Are you willing to take responsibility for your own behaviour? You can explore this question and other questions in premarital counselling or courses in family living.

## CRITICAL THINKING

*As a health professional, what would you ask a couple regarding their readiness for marriage?*

**Isolation**, or **self-absorption**, is *the inability to be intimate, spontaneous, or close with another, thus becoming withdrawn, lonely, and conceited and behaving in a stereotypical manner*. The isolated person is unable to sustain close friendships. This type of person often does not marry. There is an avoidance of the need to bond with another. If he or she does marry, the partner is likely to find personal emotional needs unmet while giving considerably of the self to the isolated, self-absorbed person.

You might have opportunities to counsel the self-absorbed person, and help him or her to achieve the characteristics of intimacy. You could also be a role model of commitment to serving others. Use the principles of communication and relationship described in Chapter 4.

## Moral–Spiritual Development

The young adult could be in either the conventional or the post-conventional level of moral development. In the post-conventional level, he or she follows the principles defined as appropriate for life. There are two stages in this level. In both stages, the person has passed beyond living a certain way just because the majority of people do. Yet in stage I of this level, the person adheres to the legal viewpoint of society. The person believes, however, that laws can be changed as people's needs change, and that he or she is able to transcend the thinking of a specific social order and develop universal principles about justice, equality, and human rights. In stage II, the person still operates as in stage I but is able to incorporate injustice, pain, and death as an integral part of existence.

Kohlberg[166] espouses that the reason for one's behaviour indicates the level of moral development attained, and that for a person to be at any level, the reasons for behaviour should be consistent to the stage at least 50 percent of the time. Therefore, it would appear difficult for the average young adult, concerned about family, achievement in a career, paying the bills, and so on, to be in the post-conventional level. Although the person might follow the principles some of the time, conflicting situations and demands arise. To be consistently in the post-conventional level requires considerable ego strength, a firm emotional and spiritual identity, and a willingness to stand up to societal forces. It may take years of maturing before the adult can be that courageous and consistent in Western society.

## CASE SITUATION

### Young Adult Development—Marriage and Commitment

James, 26 years old, received his bachelor's degree in nursing this year after combining full-time employment as an attendant at a local hospital and part-time school attendance for five years. He has recently accepted a position at the hospital as a nurse in the surgical intensive care unit. James and his wife, Mary, have been married for two years. Mary, 25 years old, is finishing her bachelor's degree in accounting while she continues employment with an insurance firm. James and Mary plan to wait a few years before starting a family because both realize the importance of graduate education in their fields. They would like to move from their apartment to a home with more space and a yard.

To save money to achieve their plans for the future, both James and Mary work extra hours when asked. This has frequently interfered with their studies. They find they have little time for leisure activities, and spend even less time together. Communication is sometimes in the form of memos posted on the refrigerator. Increasingly, the stresses of balancing school, work, and home demands have resulted in arguments, often over minor issues.

When a long-anticipated vacation must be cancelled because of unexpected expenses, James and Mary are disappointed and angry. They decide, however, to plan a week of inexpensive activities in the local area that will allow them to spend time together uninterrupted. They decide to tell no one that they have remained at home. The resulting vacation is truly restful and meaningful as they share favourite activities and explore their dreams and goals for the future.

### Questions

1. What do you think James and Mary could have done earlier to minimize, or avoid, the hardships they encountered?

2. To what extent do you agree, or disagree, that marital anger and conflict are necessary in an intimate relationship? What makes you think so?

3. What do you believe are the underlying strengths in each partner that enabled their conflict to be resolved? Was the resolution gender-based?

Today's young adults have grown up with the influence of science and technology. Although some young adults fit this description, and others are rejecting the institutional church, many have retained the desire and ability to apply spiritual and moral principles in this world. Increasingly, parents with young children are joining a church or synagogue, seeking religion and a way to instill societal values in their children.

In young adulthood, a humanizing of values and a trend toward relativism occurs as conflicts are encountered. The person increasingly discovers the meaning of values and their relation to the achievement of social purposes. He or she becomes increasingly more able to bring both personal experiences and motives to affirm and promote a value system. The person's values, whatever they are, become increasingly his or her own and become part of a unified lived philosophy of life. At the same time, these young adults show expanding empathy for others and their value systems.[167]

---

## CRITICAL THINKING

*What are some of the differences in moral principles held by young adults from cultures different from your own?*

---

## Adaptive Mechanisms

The young adult seeks stability while he or she is adapting to new or changing events. When the young adult is physically and emotionally healthy, total functioning is smooth. Adaptation to the environment, the satisfaction of needs, and social interaction all proceed relatively effortlessly and with minimum discomfort. The young adult behaves as though he or she is in full control of his or her impulses and drives; he or she appears to be in harmony with the superego's ideals and demands. He or she can tolerate frustrations created by his or her needs, and is capable of making choices that seem best for total equilibrium.

## Self-Concept and Body Image Development

The person's perception of self—physically, emotionally, and socially—is based on:

1. Internalized reactions of others
2. Self-expectations
3. Perceived abilities
4. Attitudes

5. Habits
6. Knowledge
7. Other characteristics

These factors influence one's self-concept, and the combined effects of the self-concept and these factors certainly affect the ways in which that person will handle situations and relate to others. How the person behaves depends on whether he or she feels positively or negatively about self, whether the person believes others view him or her positively or negatively, and how he or she believes that others expect him or her to behave in this situation. The reactions of the family members, including spouse and partner, and the employment situation, are strong influences on the young adult's self-concept. Additionally, the person discloses different aspects of self to various people and in various situations, depending on his or her needs at the time, what is considered socially acceptable, the reactions of others, and past experiences with self-disclosure.[168]

**Body image**, *a part of self-concept, is a mental picture of the body's appearance integrated into the parietotemporal area of the cortex.* Body image includes the surface, internal, and postural picture of the body. Body image also includes values, attitudes, emotions, and personality reactions of the person in relation to the body as an object in space, separate from others. This image is flexible. It is subject to constant revision, and it may not be reflective of the person's actual body structure. Body image shifts back and forth at different times of the day and at different times in the life cycle. Any disturbance to the body influences one's total self-concept.

**Contributing Influences** *Many factors contribute to the body image:*[169]

- Parental and social reaction to the person's body
- The person's interpretation of others' reactions to him or her
- The anatomic appearance and physiologic function of the body, including sex, age, kinesthetic and other sensorimotor stimuli, and especially illness or deformity
- Attitudes and emotions toward, and familiarity with, the body
- Internal drives, dependency needs, one's motivational state, and the ideals to which the person aspires
- Identification with the bodies of others who have been or are considered ideal (a little bit of each person who has been significant to the person is incorporated into the self-concept and personality)

- The perception one has of the space and objects immediately surrounding the body, such as an easy chair or car; the sense of body boundaries

- Objects attached to the body such as clothing, a wig, false eyelashes, a prosthesis, dentures, jewellery, makeup, or perfume

- Activities that the body performs in various roles, occupations, and recreations

## CRITICAL THINKING

*What are a few other psychosocial factors in the health care system that contribute to one's perception of body image?*

The combined messages the brain receives from kinesthetic receptors in the muscles, tendons, and joints and the labyrinth receptors in the inner ear inform the person about his or her position in space.

**Self-Knowledge** How do you visualize your body as you walk, run, stand, sit, or gesture? How do you feel about yourself as you go through various motions? What emotions are expressed by your movements? How do you think others visualize you at that time? The message you convey about yourself to another will always aid or hinder the establishment of a therapeutic relationship. You must be realistically aware of the posture and movement of your own body, and to the messages they convey to those around you.

Body image in the adult is a social creation. Self-concept continually influences and enlarges one's perception of the world, one's mastery of and interaction with it, and one's ability to respond to the many experiences the world offers. This integration, largely unconscious, is constantly evolving, and it can be identified in the person's values, attitudes, and feelings about self. One's experiences with the body are interpreted in terms of feelings, earlier views of the self, and group or cultural norms.[170] *In the adult, a close interdependence develops between one's body image and one's personality, self-concept, and identity. You need to remember and use information about self-concept and body image. Your feedback to others is important.* If you are to help another to elevate his or her self-esteem or feel positively about his or her body, you must provide repeated positive reinforcement to help that person overcome unrealistic guilt and shame.

## Body Image Change during Illness
A wide variety of messages about the body are constantly fed into the self-image for rejection, acceptance with integration, or revision. You will see disturbances in the person's body image after the loss of a body function, structure, or quality—teeth, hair, vision, hearing, breast, internal organs, or

youth—that necessitate adjustment of the person's body image. Because the body image provides a base for identity, almost any change in body structure or function, acute or chronic, is experienced as a threat, especially in our society, where wholeness, beauty, and health are highly valued.[171]

The person with limited adaptive abilities, who is easily made to feel helpless or powerless, will experience greater threat with a change in body structure or function.

## CRITICAL THINKING

*Discuss how gender and the effects of culture can affect the body image of a client who is physically disabled.*

## The Adult Undergoing Body Changes

**Assessment** Assessment during illness, injury, or disability that will eventually result in changes to the self-image is often difficult because of the abstractness of self-image.[172] If you listen closely to the person and validate their statements for less obvious meanings, and if you explore feelings with him or her, you can gain considerable information for worthwhile intervention. Assessment could include consideration of the person's responses to the following:[173]

- Feelings about the self before and since the condition occurred

- Values about personal hygiene

- Values on beauty, self-control, wholeness, and activity

- Value of others' reactions

- Relation to the body part affected

- Reactions to hospitalization, treatment, and care

- Awareness of the extent of the condition

- Effect of the condition on the person's roles, daily activities, family, and use of leisure time

- Perception of others' reactions to the person with this condition

- Problems in adjusting to the condition

- Mechanisms used in adapting to the condition and its implications

Any observation of the client must be combined with purposeful conversation. Observe movements, posture, gestures, and expressions as he or she answers your questions or talks about self to validate the consistency between what is said and what is meant.

**Nursing Intervention** Measures to help someone with a threat to, or change in, body image involve assisting the person to reintegrate the self-view and self-esteem in relation to his or her condition.[174] You can help the person in the following ways:

- Encourage the person to talk about their feelings in relation to the changed body function or structure. Talking about feelings is the first step to the reintegration of body image.
- Assist the client, without pressure, to become reacquainted with self by looking at the dressing or wound, feeling the cast, bandage, or injured part, prostheses, or looking at self in a mirror. The client who wants to "show the scar" should be allowed to do so. Reaction from you and the family can make a difference in how the person accepts the changed body.
- Provide the opportunity for the client to gain information about the body, both the intact and changed parts, and its strengths and limits.
- Provide the opportunity to learn mastery of the body, to resume activities of daily care and living routines as indicated, move about, become involved with others, resume roles, and handle equipment.
- Provide honest recognition to the person for what they can do. Avoid criticism, derogation, or any nonverbal reactions of impatience.
- Help him or her to see self as a whole person, despite losses or changes.
- Encourage talking about unresolved experiences, distortions, or fears in relation to body image.[175]

You will encounter many young adults with body image distortions or changes as a result of such events as accidental injuries, disease, weight gain or loss, pregnancy, or identity problems. You can make a significant contribution to the promotion of health of this person for the remainder of their life by providing assistance through physical care, listening, counselling, teaching, and working with family and significant people important to his or her life. Your efforts are important for your own positive self-concept so that you can provide unbiased care of each person.

### CRITICAL THINKING

*What are a few health promoting strategies for clients who are undergoing body changes?*

## Lifestyle Options

Despite recent technological development intended to make life easier, the resulting increased pace of life has brought people into an unparalleled degree of social alienation at all levels of society. Growing into a lifestyle is very different from one's childrearing experiences, which sometimes result in attempts to ward off alienation and organize one's life around meaning. The young adult has many options.

**Singlehood,** *remaining unmarried and following a specific lifestyle,* is not new. The single person can accomplish the task of intimacy through emotional investment of self in others. Many are extroverts. They have several very close friends with whom they share activities, they have a meaningful career, and they have a harmonious, rather than conflictual, relationship with their parents.[176]

Research consistently indicates that delaying marriage tends to increase the likelihood that a person will never marry. Findings from one Canadian study indicates that mature singles who do not intend to marry have rather unconventional views about the importance of love, marriage, and family—they don't value being part of a couple, or a family, as highly as do singles who expect to marry.[177]

The number of years a person has been single appears to be an important factor in the influence of singlehood on his or her development. Developmentalists have discovered that a transition time occurs during which long-term singles change from thinking of themselves as someone who will be married, or partnered, in the future to viewing themselves as single by choice.[178] In this event, singlehood becomes an important component of the person's self-identity. This type of self-affirmation can actually protect singles from negative health consequences associated with singlehood.[179]

## Family Planning: The Expectancy Phase and Parenthood

Parenthood is an option for either the couple or the single person. Today, the technological options of oral contraceptives for the female, and skilled vasectomy procedures for the male, make it possible for couples to say: "We don't want children now," "We don't want children ever," or "We want to try to have two children spaced three years apart."

Information presented in Table 11-6 summarizes contraceptives, and the various references provided at the end of this chapter will help you teach all aspects of family planning. Chapter 4 provides useful information for understanding the family with whom you are working.

**Reasons for Childbearing** *The couple may have a child for a variety of reasons:*

1. Extension of self
2. To offset loneliness
3. Sense of pride or joy
4. Psychological fulfillment of having a child

5. Having someone to love self

6. Attempt to hold a marriage together

7. Feeling of power, generated by the ability to create life

8. Representation of wealth

9. To secure replacements for the workforce

10. To have an heir for family name and wealth

11. Religious convictions

Whether the couple chooses to have only one child or more children is related to more than fertility and religious background. Lifestyle, finances, career, available support systems, and emotional maturity are some of the factors that determine if and when a couple will have children.

**Developmental Tasks for the Couple during the Expectant Stage** You are in an excellent position to assist the expectant couple to understand the changes that childbearing will create. The following developmental tasks for this stage of family life will be helpful to you:

- Rearrange the home to provide space, facilities, and supplies for the expected baby.

- Rework the budget to determine how to obtain, and spend, the income required to accommodate the new needs, and at the same time financially maintain the family unit.

- Evaluate the changing roles and the division of labour. Determine how the responsibilities of child care will be divided, who has the final authority, and whether the woman should continue working outside the home, if she has a career or profession.

- Adapt patterns of sexual relationships to the pregnancy.

- Have the couple assess the communication system between them. Help them to explore feelings about the pregnancy, share ideas about childrearing, and work to resolve any differences that are detected.

- Acquire knowledge about pregnancy, childbirth, and parenthood.

- Have the couple assess the communication system and relationships with family, friends, and community activities, based on the reality of the pregnancy and their reactions.

- Use family and community resources as needed.

- Examine and expand the philosophy of life to include responsibilities of childbearing and childrearing.

Developmental tasks that must be mastered during pregnancy and the intrapartum period to ensure readiness for the maternal role are:

1. *Pregnancy validation:* Accepting the reality of the pregnancy, working through feelings of ambivalence and/or doubt

2. *Fetal embodiment:* Incorporating the fact of the fetus and the enlarging body into the body image

3. *Fetal distinction:* Seeing the fetus as a separate entity, fantasizing about what the baby will be like

4. *Role transition:* After birth, an increasing readiness to take on the task of parenthood

A number of authors have researched transition to parenthood, feelings, symptoms, body image changes, and needs for social support during pregnancy. Events that occur during pregnancy profoundly affect family functioning and child care after birth.[180]

## CRITICAL THINKING

*What are some of the advantages and disadvantages in today's society of choosing not to have children?*

**Father's Response** Some research indicates that the attachment of the father to baby begins during pregnancy, rather than after the birth. It is believed that a strong marital relationship and vicariously experienced physical symptoms resembling pregnancy (and sometimes the couvade syndrome) actually strengthen attachment.[181]

Studies indicate that a characteristic pattern occurs among first-time expectant fathers in the development of a growing subjective emotional involvement in pregnancy. Three phases occur: the announcement phase, moratorium, and the focusing period.

The **announcement phase** occurs *when pregnancy is suspected and confirmed.* If the man desired the pregnancy, he shows desire and excitement. If he did not want the pregnancy, he shows pain and shock.

During the **moratorium period**, the *man suppresses thoughts about the pregnancy.* This period can last from a few days to months, and it usually ends when the pregnancy is obvious. This period is characterized by emotional distance, a feeling that the pregnancy is not real. It may result in the man showing extreme concentration on himself and other life concerns. Sometimes, he will leave home. Gradually, the man begins to face the financial and lifestyle implications of the pregnancy. If he feels financially insecure, or if he is unstable with his partner, or if he wishes to extend the childless period, then he resents the pregnancy and spends a longer than usual time in the moratorium stage. Most men eventually become enthusiastic about the pregnancy and the new baby, when they feel the baby move or hear the heartbeat. If the man does not become enthusiastic and supportive, the couple may then be at risk for marital and parenting problems.

The **focusing period** occurs *when the man perceives the pregnancy as real and important in his life*. The man redefines himself as father; he begins to feel more in tune with, and is more helpful to, his partner. He begins to read or talk about parenting and child development. He notices other children, and he is willing to participate in childbirth classes and in purchasing baby supplies. He will likely construct a mental image of the baby, sometimes different from the woman's mental image of the baby. Sometimes the circle of friends changes to those who have children. The man who participates in pregnancy and the birth process experiences an important closeness with the infant and his partner. He also experiences heightened self-esteem and esteem for the spouse. The man's readiness for pregnancy will significantly influence the emergence of his father involvement activities and interests.

**Mother's Response** Certainly one would expect that an even stronger attachment would occur in the woman as she physically experiences the fetus and the physical symptoms related to pregnancy. It is reasonable to expect that her feelings for the child will be stronger if she has a loving, supportive partner.

**Nursing Roles** An important decision for the expectant parents is whether to attend childbirth education classes. Encourage the pregnant woman and her partner to attend these classes during pregnancy. Insist that they be allowed to use during the labour and delivery process the techniques and practical suggestions they learned in childbirth classes. The woman who is well supported during pregnancy experiences fewer complications during labour and delivery. The woman who has taken childbirth education during pregnancy, and who can practise Lamaze techniques during labour, uses less medication and is more likely to choose rooming-in with the baby.

Your importance and value to the new parents is based on your support, acceptance, and flexibility in helping the couple to use what they learned and practised in prenatal classes. You will be valued for letting them assume responsibility for their decisions when possible, for your assistance to the new mother, and for your teaching during the postpartum period. All of these are crucial to family-centred care. Cultural considerations are important as well.[182]

The Health Surveillance and Epidemiology Division at Health Canada's Centre for Healthy Human Development has established the Canadian Perinatal Surveillance System (CPSS). The CPSS is guided by a steering committee composed of expert representatives of health professional organizations, consumer and advocacy groups, provincial and territorial governments, and Canadian and international specialists in perinatal health and epidemiology. The CPSS is part of Health Canada's efforts to strengthen Canada's national health surveillance capacity.[183]

The CPSS has identified that the proportion of pregnant women reporting physical abuse is an important health indicator.[184] During pregnancy, physical abuse has been associated with adverse maternal and fetal health outcomes. More extensive understanding of the epidemiology of physical abuse during pregnancy, including its frequency, risk factors, adverse maternal conditions, and birth outcomes, carry important clinical and public health implications. Improved methods of early identification followed by insightful interventions to prevent the abuse of pregnant women will go far to reduce the adverse outcomes of the abuse of women.[185]

---

### CRITICAL THINKING

*What health promotion strategies can you advocate for women who are victims of physical abuse during pregnancy?*

---

**Other Approaches to Parenthood** *Some couples delay childbearing* until they are in their thirties or early forties. The woman may wish to pursue her education, a career, or a profession. The couple may choose to travel, start a business, become financially established, or have a variety of experiences before they settle down with children. Maternal age does not affect maternal role behaviours. The sense of challenge, role strain, and self-image in the mother role is similar during the first year for childbearing women of all ages. *The single person might desire to be a parent.* The single woman may, through pregnancy or adoption, choose to have a child. A review of the literature reveals that much is being written about the single woman who decides to become a mother and remain single. Some single men who will not be biological fathers are also choosing to experience fatherhood through adoption. The woman might choose to remain single, but maintain a relationship with the biological father, or with a man who can act as father to the child. The man frequently has a close relationship with a woman who has agreed to assist in mothering. On the other hand, he can decide to nurture alone.

*You are in a key position to help the person as he or she thinks through the alternatives in deciding to have a child, but remain single.* Many considerations are necessary: Who will make up the support system? Who in a time of need can act in the father or mother role to the child? The responsibilities of a single mother or father to the child during school years and adolescence should be discussed. Finally, the social, familial, and economic consequences of single parenthood should be addressed. Implications related to the cultural and religious background of the person must also be considered.

Family planning is sometimes made difficult by infertility. **Infertility** is defined as *the inability to achieve* *pregnancy after one year of regular, unprotected intercourse, or the inability to carry a pregnancy to a term, live birth.* Canadians are turning to assisted human reproduction (AHR) procedures to help them build their families.[186]

# HEALTH PROMOTION IN NURSING PRACTICE

## Health Promotion and Health Prevention

Young adulthood is a time when a shift occurs from developing one's own personal identity to making attachments with others that result in intimate relationships. The need for human closeness and sexual fulfillment is paramount for many young adults. During the assessment phase, it is important that you listen to the young adult regarding their issues, strengths, and healthy responses. Include the family in your assessment with the client's consent.

Health promotion interventions to assist the young adult and the family to meet physical, cognitive, emotional, social, and spiritual needs are described further in the following section.

**Immunizations** The prevention of infection by immunization is a lifelong process. All adults should be counselled concerning their personal immunization status. Heath care professionals should regularly review the clients under their care to ensure not only that their immunization status is up to date but also that they have been made aware of new vaccines.[187] Practitioners should regularly audit their clients' immunization records during those clinical encounters that coincide with a mid-decade birthday (i.e., 15, 25, 35, 45, 55 years).

All adults should be immunized against diphtheria, tetanus, pertussis, measles, mumps, rubella, and varicella. In Canada, all adults require maintenance of immunity to tetanus and diphtheria, preferably with combined (Td) toxoids and a single dose of acelluar pertussis vaccine. For adults not previously immunized against pertussis, only one dose of Tdap is required because it is assumed that most adults have some degree of immunity due to prior pertussis infection. Combined measles, mumps, rubella vaccine (MMR) is preferred for vaccination of individuals not previously immunized against one of more of these viruses.[188]

Adults born before 1970 may be considered immune to measles. Adults born in 1970 and later who do not have documentation of adequate measles immunization or who are known to be seronegative should receive MMR vaccine. One additional dose of vaccine should be offered only to those adults born in 1970 or later who are at greatest risk of exposure and who have not already received two doses or demonstrated immunity to measles. That is, priority for a second dose should be given to health care workers, college students, and travellers to areas where measles are epidemic.[189]

A history of chicken pox infection is adequate evidence of varicella immunity. Serologic testing should be performed in adults without a history of disease because the majority of such adults will be immune, and they will not require the varicella vaccine.[190]

One of the new vaccines licensed in Canada since August 2006 is the human papillomavirus (HPV) vaccine.[191] HPV is transmitted mainly by sexual contact. The vaccine is made available to protect against infection that has occurred years before, but is associated with the appearance of cervical cancer. Vaccines against avian influenza, West Nile virus, and malaria are all in development.[192]

An adult immunization guide is provided by the Public Health Agency of Canada,[193] or you can visit the website at www.naci.gc.ca.

---

CRITICAL THINKING

*What protocol should be followed for the healthy management of a person after possible contact with rabies?*

---

## Common Health Problems: Prevention and Treatment

**Physical Problems** Typically, young adults in Canada are healthy. Many have no disease. For these individuals, health problems and risks, preventive behaviour, and the best response to illness are influenced by their sex and lifestyle, as well as by other factors. Table 12-3 summarizes the most common health problems encountered by the young adult.[194]

**Acquired Immunodeficiency Syndrome** AIDS was defined by the Centers for Disease Control and Prevention (CDC) in 1987 as *a disabling, or life-threatening, illness caused by human immunodeficiency virus (HIV), and characterized by HIV encephalopathy, HIV wasting syndrome, or certain diseases resulting from immunodeficiency in a person with laboratory evidence for HIV infection, or without certain other causes of immunodeficiency.*[195]

In Canada, AIDS was first identified in 1979 and became a reportable disease in 1982.[196] By 2003, an estimated 56 000 Canadians were living with HIV/AIDS, of whom 17 000 were not aware of their infection.[197] To date, no vaccine exists to prevent HIV infection, and no cure exists for the disease.

The federal government, as one of the partners in Canada's response to HIV/AIDS, elaborated its approach for 2005–2010 in the 2004 policy document called the *Federal Initiative to Address HIV/AIDS in Canada*. The action plan, Leading Together: Canada's HIV/AIDS Action

Table 12-3 Common Health Problems for Young Adults

| Problem | Definition | Symptom/Signs | Prevention/Treatment |
|---|---|---|---|
| **Upper respiratory infection** (URI) or common cold | Acute infection of the upper respiratory tract, lasting several days | General malaise; nasal stuffiness and discharge, mild sore throat, watery eyes; sometimes ear discomfort | If bacterial: antibiotic; otherwise, symptomatic treatment; antipyretic, antihistamine, decongestants |
| **Influenza** | Acute contagious viral illness often occurring in epidemics | Fever, malaise, myalgia, and respiratory symptoms; sometimes cough, rhinitis, and scattered rales | Prevention: immunization Treatment: antipyretic, increase fluid intake, rest; amantadine hydrochloride |
| **Hypertension, essential** (uncomplicated) | Persistent elevation of arterial blood pressure 150/100 but less than 200/110 present on three weekly determinations, without secondary cause found | Sometimes none; sometimes headache, dizziness, light-headedness | Appropriate lab workup along with other testing; diet; weight reduction; exercise; possibly medication |
| **Mitral value prolapse** | Insufficiency of valve to open and close appropriately | Usually in young adult female; chest pain, arrhythmias, palpitations, tachycardia, sense of fullness in neck and head, feeling faint, anxious | Medication, adequate rest; reduction of stress in life to extent possible |
| **Iron deficiency anemia** | Blood hemoglobin level ≤ 10 g/dL, compared with normal value of 12–16 g/dL (for women) | Usually caused by menses; sometimes no signs; fatigue, irritability, depression, weakness, dizziness, headache, pallor of skin and conjunctivae, brittle nails | Prevention: blood screen, iron-rich foods Treatment: iron preparation (ferrous sulphate) |
| **Atopic dermatitis** of adulthood | Dry, thickened skin, accentuating normal folds (different appearance than in infancy) | Hyperpigmentation, especially on flexor areas of extremities, eyelids, dorsi of hands and feet, and back of neck | Keeping skin dry in humid conditions; mild, non-drying soap; hydrocortisone cream |
| **Folliculitis** | Localized infection of hair follicle | Irritated area around hair follicle | Washing well; hot compresses |
| **Furuncle** (boil) | Infected area that has draining point | Raised red area with exudate | Hot compresses; antibiotics; sometimes incision and drainage |
| **Carbuncle** | Large group of furuncles with several draining points | Raised red area with multiple exudate areas | Hot compresses; antibiotics; incision and drainage |
| **Urticaria** (hives) | Allergic reaction, usually to drugs, food, inhalants, or insect bites | Itching, red raised welts, usually on trunk or extremities | Cool compresses; sometimes antihistamine or epinephrine; attempt to find offending agent |
| **Scabies** | Dermatitis caused by mite burrowing into skin and consequent allergic reaction | | Lindane (Kwell) treatment (all sexual and household contacts too) |

*(continued)*

Table 12-3 (continued)

| Problem | Definition | Symptom/Signs | Prevention/Treatment |
| --- | --- | --- | --- |
| **Simple diarrhea** of adulthood | Gastrointestinal upset by viral infection, caused psychological disturbance, dietary changes, laxatives | Frequent loose, watery stools that are not greasy, bloody, or purulent | Clear liquid diet; anti-diarrhea preparation (e.g., loperamide hydrochloride [Imodium]) |
| **Cystitis** | Inflammation of bladder (often seen in young adult women) | Dysuria, frequency, bladder spasms | Appropriate antibiotics after clean-catch urinalysis and culture; increased water intake (at least eight 8-oz [250 mL] glasses daily); sometimes antispasmodic medication |
| **Acute pyelonephritis** | Cystitis plus inflammation of kidneys and collection system | Dysuria, frequency, flank pain, chills, nausea, vomiting | Appropriate antibiotic treatment plus antipyretic and anti-nausea medicine if necessary |
| **Chronic fatigue syndrome (CFS)** | Debilitating fatigue that lasts at least 6 months | Eight of the following must persist or recur over 6 months: chills or low-grade fever; sore throat; tender lymph nodes; muscle pain and weakness; extreme fatigue; headaches; joint pain without swelling; neurological problems (confusion, memory loss); sleep disorders | Prevention: none known Treatment: adequate rest, nutritious diet, small amounts of exercise; rationing of energy; dealing emotionally with disease; possibly tricyclic antidepressants |
| **Hepatitis B** | Type of liver inflammation | Jaundice, malaise, may lead to liver cancer, cirrhosis, or death; some are carriers only | Immunization (series of 3 injections), rest, nutritious diet |
| **Dental caries and periodontal disease** | Tooth decay and bleeding, hypertrophied gums | Gradual receding of gums and bones and loss of teeth | Early dental checks and personal mouth care; proper diet |
| **Lactose intolerance or milk malabsorption syndrome** | Lactose (milk sugar) not hydrolyzed because of lack of appropriate amounts of the enzyme lactase | Severe abdominal discomfort and flatulence following direction of milk products | Products containing concentrated forms of the enzyme; also *Lacto-bacillus sp.* milk; avoid foods made with milk or milk products |
| **Anxiety** | Combination of fearfulness, nervousness, apprehension, and restlessness, often associated with family or personal crisis and sometimes with physical or mental illness | Loss of appetite, increased appetite, lack of sleeping ability; increased perspiration, "thumping of heart," headaches, weakness, fatigue, trembling | Supportive therapy, crisis intervention, some medicines for short term |
| **Tension headache** | Band-like pressure across forehead and around back of skull | Dull, aching pain with a feeling of tightness, tension in neck muscles | Reassurance, mild analgesics, occasionally a muscle relaxant, massage, manipulation, elimination of tension |

*(continued)*

Table 12-3 (continued)

| Problem | Definition | Symptom/Signs | Prevention/Treatment |
|---------|-----------|---------------|---------------------|
| **Migraine headache** | Vascular in origin: arterial spasm followed by dilation | Throbbing unilateral pain, sometimes preceded by **aura** (*inherent warning, usually visual*); sometimes nausea and vomiting | Try to rest when aura first appears; various medications, such as anti-inflammatory drugs and caffeine; rest in a dark room; nutrition; chiropractic care; biofeedback |
| **Lyme disease** | Infection caused by *Borrelia burgdorferi*, spirochete spread by bites of deer tick | Erythema migrans, red, raised circular rash that spreads and itches<br>Flu-like, vague symptoms<br>If untreated: Arthritic symptoms (with swollen, painful joints).<br>Neurological symptoms (paraesthesis, insomnia, lethargy)<br>Heart symptoms (irregular pulse, faint, dizzy, short of breath)<br>Psychological symptoms (mood changes, depression)<br>Pregnancy may result in miscarriage | In tick-infested areas: Walk along cleared surfaces, avoid tall grass and woods if possible<br>Avoid light-colour garments; wear long-sleeved shirts, long pants tucked into socks, closed shoes; use insect repellent<br>Shower as soon as possible after returning indoors from tick-infected area.<br>If bitten by tick, remove immediately by grasping it close to skin, tug gently<br>Use flea and tick collars on pets, brush them after being outdoors<br>Mow weeds and grass around house<br>Antibiotic treatment |

Plan 2005–2010, will guide the federal government's involvement to 2010.[198]

The decline in the annual number of AIDS cases that began in 1995 is continuing. The rate of decline, however, has slowed, and the curve is levelling off.[199] The number of annual deaths due to HIV/AIDS has also decreased.[200] It is interesting to note that the number of deaths has decreased more quickly than the incidence rate, indicating that people with HIV are progressing at a slower rate and that people with AIDS diagnoses are living longer.[201]

---

## CRITICAL THINKING

*What factors might contribute to the fact that people who have HIV, or AIDS, now tend to live longer?*

---

AIDS will be a major global cause of death, if not the biggest killer in some countries,[202] because it is occurring in epidemic rates in countries not previously affected. Africa, India, Thailand (and other countries in Southeast Asia), and countries in the former Soviet Union and the Middle East are now experiencing HIV epidemics.[203]

AIDS is a devastating disease. It is frequently found in the already disadvantaged, who are often carrying other sexually transmitted diseases, and who are often in the IV drug and crack-cocaine culture. These young adults have a resigned attitude about their diagnoses and a mistrust of the conventional medical system. Thus, they often will not take the medicine suggested, or they will not co-operate by informing about past or current sexual partners.[204]

---

## CRITICAL THINKING

*In what ways do you think the presence of AIDS will change sex and relationships?*

---

The human immunodeficiency virus attacks white blood cells (T-cells), and it weakens the immune system. AIDS occurs when an HIV-infected person develops a life-threatening condition, or if the number of T-cells becomes dangerously low. T-cells regulate the body's immune system. If they are destroyed, the capacity to fight disease is gone. *HIV is transmitted through:*

1. Body fluids containing blood, semen, and vaginal secretions during unprotected vaginal, oral, or anal sex with an infected person.

2. Contaminated needle-sharing among injection drug users, or the use of contaminated needles during tattooing or piercing body parts.

3. During pregnancy, birth, or breastfeeding, from the HIV-infected woman to the baby.

4. Transfusions of infected blood or blood products before 1985 (since then, all blood has been tested), or the use of blood-contaminated equipment.

5. Contact with open sores of an infected person.[205]

Diagnosis can be determined in a person by testing their blood, or oral mucus, for the presence of antibodies to the virus.[206] The person with a positive test result should not donate blood, plasma, sperm, organs, or tissue. Pregnancy should be postponed (see Chapter 6). *Abstinence from sexual intercourse is the only sure way to avoid infecting another.* If partners choose to have sex, a latex condom must be worn. The condom should not be used past the expiration date. Condoms are not foolproof, and they must be used as soon as the penis is erect. A water-based lubricant should be used for vaginal and anal sex. The condom must be carefully removed.[207]

HIV/AIDS can take up to ten years to manifest in signs and symptoms. The following symptoms of AIDS are also caused by other conditions. *The warning symptoms include:*[208]

1. Swollen lymph nodes

2. Weight loss

3. Fever

4. Cough, shortness of breath

5. Persistent diarrhea[209]

These symptoms can indicate early stages of the disease. By the time AIDS develops, one's immune system has been severely damaged, making the individual susceptible to opportunistic infections. The signs and symptoms of these infections include:

1. Soaking night sweats

2. Shaking chills or fever

3. Dry cough and shortness of breath

4. Chronic diarrhea

5. Persistent white spots or unusual lesions on tongue

6. Headaches

7. Blurred and distorted vision

8. Weight loss[210]

Anti-retroviral treatment has reduced mortality, hospitalizations, and the incidence of opportunistic infections for people with HIV infections. However, anti-retroviral regimens are complex, and they have major side effects. They pose difficulties with adherence, and they carry serious potential consequences from the development of viral resistance due to the lack of adherence to the drug regimen or suboptimal levels of anti-retroviral agents.[211]

*Health care professionals are not immune.* The Canadian Association of Nurses in AIDS Care (CANAC) is a national professional nursing organization committed to fostering excellence in HIV/AIDS nursing, to promoting the health, rights, and dignity of persons affected by HIV/AIDS, and to preventing the spread of HIV infection.[212] The Canadian AIDS Treatment Information Exchange (CATIE) has teamed up with CANAC to provide an extensive resource centre for HIV/AIDS-related nursing information.[213]

The Canadian Nurses Association endorses the implementation of policies and procedures requiring the use of standard precautions (previously called universal precautions).[214] The adherence to standard precautions is the appropriate and effective means to protect nurses, clients, and others from the spread of blood-borne pathogens. The adherence to standard precautions is ethically acceptable because it precludes the need to know the blood-borne pathogen status of nurses or clients, and further safeguards the rights of individuals for privacy and confidentiality of information. In caring for all clients, whether or not their status regarding blood-borne pathogens is known, the nurse is guided by the values of the Code of Ethics for Registered Nurses. Nurses have the professional responsibility to update regularly their knowledge of blood-borne pathogen practices. That is, all practices related to prevention, immediate exposure, testing, reporting, and the use and disposal of equipment are of particular importance. Nurses have a special responsibility, along with experts and other professionals, to develop clear policies and procedures based on current knowledge.

## CRITICAL THINKING

*What would you do if your friend found out that he or she had HIV?*

It is essential to have access to accurate, up-to-date information on HIV/AIDS. Information that is reliable enables people at risk to change their behaviours to avoid

HIV infection, and those living with HIV/AIDS can find help to learn about new treatments, to manage their health, and to improve their quality of life. The Canadian HIV/AIDS Information Centre is Canada's largest distributor of HIV/AIDS materials (see www.aidssida.cpha.ca).[215]

## CRITICAL THINKING

*What resources are available in your community regarding HIV/AIDS?*

**Tuberculosis** Whitney, Marchant-Short, and Yiu state that in the case of tuberculosis, it was anticipated in the late 1940s that with treatment protocols, the disease would be eradicated by 2000. However, it has re-emerged as an increased public health threat because of multi-drug-resistant strains, and in clients who are non-compliant with chemotherapy. It affects vulnerable populations such as the elderly, women, children, and those who are poverty stricken, homeless, or with immune deficiencies.[216] According to the Public Health Agency of Canada, in their report *Tuberculosis in Canada 2006 Pre-Release*, individuals between the ages of 35 and 44 made up the largest number of reported cases. The highest rate, of 156 per 100 000 population, was reported in Nunavut. The three most populous provinces (British Columbia, Ontario, and Quebec), which collectively made up 76 percent of Canada's population in 2006, accounted for 73 percent of the total number of reported cases.[217] After their first birthday, Aboriginal children are invited to clinics to be tested for tuberculosis. Meanwhile, screening is conducted at schools on reserves when children are in grade four.[218]

**Injuries** In Canada, injury mortality increases over the adolescent years, and peaks among 20- to 24-year-olds. First Nations and Inuit people are at particularly high risk of injury.[219] The mortality rates associated with major vehicle crashes are high across all age groups, but the highest rates are for youth between 15 and 24 years of age. Even though there has been a reduction in injury and deaths associated with motor vehicle crashes, automotive crashes still remain the leading cause of unintentional injury deaths among Canadians. It is interesting to note that when injury mortality rates are compared internationally, Canadian rates have been found to be higher than those for some other nations.[220]

## CRITICAL THINKING

*What job features are associated with higher rates of injury at work?*

**Malignancies** Cancer is the leading cause of premature death (early death) in Canada. In a given year in Canada 160 000 new cases of cancer are predicted, with 72 700 deaths.[221] Approximately 10 000 Canadians aged 20 to 44 were expected to be diagnosed with cancer in 2005 and 2000 of them were expected to die from it.[222]

Several important reasons exist to examine cancer patterns specifically in young adults. First, cancers occurring during young adulthood result from exposures relatively early in life. The developing tissues of children and adolescents are possibly more sensitive to some carcinogenetic events, which can manifest as a cancer diagnosed in early adulthood. Second, lifetime cancer risks tend to be shared to some extent by individuals who are born about the same time (a "birth cohort"). For example, adolescent boys today have a much lower prevalence of smoking than did their grandfathers. As they age, they will have lower rates of lung cancer compared to their grandfathers at comparable ages. The "cohort effect" will first be evident during young adulthood, when lung cancer begins to appear. Therefore, the incidence of lung cancer in today's young adults will be important for forecasting future lung cancer rates and for planning health promotion and preventative strategies and cancer services. Finally, cancers that occur in this age group could reflect a heightened genetic susceptibility to disease. Cancer patterns in young adults may, therefore, suggest directions for the investigation of genetic factors and the interactions between genetic factors and risk factor exposures.[223]

For cancers that occur in younger and older adults, individual risk modifiers may vary in their strength, or relative importance, at younger and older ages. Table 12-4 outlines the 18 cancers that are of two general cell types, epithelial and non-epithelial. Eight of the 18 cancers are non-epithelial, and they originate in such tissues as smooth muscles, melanocytes, stem cells, and lymphatic tissue. Two types, testis and Hodgkin lymphoma, both peak in the young adult age group, and then decline. Cancer of the testis peaks in the 30 to 34 age group and Hodgkin lymphoma peaks at ages 20 to 24. Epithelial cancers arise in the cells that line the internal and external surfaces of the body. Breast, colorectal, kidney, oral, bladder, lung, and thyroid cancers and cancers of the ovary, uterus, and cervix are the epithelial cancers important among young adults. Incidence in most of the epithelial cancers is very low in the 20 to 24 age group, but it rises abruptly across the young adult age range for some cancers.[224]

Risk modifiers are, to some extent, distributed in accordance with these cell types and age distributions, as Table 12-4 demonstrates. Some behaviours—physical inactivity, obesity, high alcohol consumption, various aspects of diet, and tobacco use—are established risk factors for epithelial cancers but not, in general, for non-epithelial cancers. Reproductive and hormonal factors and

# Table 12-4 Summary of Epithelial and Non-Epithelial Cancer Patterns in Young Adults: Risk Modifiers, Time Trends, Incidence across Age Range

| | | Physical inactivity | Obesity/ height | Diet | Alcohol | Tobacco smoke | Reproductive/ hormonal | Medical conditions | Radiation (ionizing/ ultraviolet) | Other occupational/ environmental | Viruses/ altered immunity | Incidence M | Incidence F | Mortality M | Mortality F |
|---|---|---|---|---|---|---|---|---|---|---|---|---|---|---|---|
| Epithelial | Breast | ✓ | ✓ | ✓ | ✓ | | ✓ | | | | | | ← | | → |
| | Colorectal | ✓ | ✓ | ✓ | ✓ | ✓ | | ✓ | | | | → | → | → | → |
| | Uterus | ✓ | ✓ | | | | ✓ | | | | | | | | |
| | Kidney | | ✓ | | | ✓ | | ✓ | ✓ | | | ← | ↕ | ↕ | |
| | Lip, etc. | | | ✓ | ✓ | ✓ | | | | | ✓ | ↕ | ↕ | ↕ | ↕ |
| | Bladder | | | ✓ | | ✓ | | ✓ | ✓ | ✓ | | → | ← | → | |
| | Lung | | | ✓ | | ✓ | | ✓ | ✓ | ✓ | | → | → | → | ← |
| | Thyroid | | | | | | ✓ | ✓ | ✓ | | | ← | ← | | |
| | Ovary | | | | | | ✓ | | ✓ | | | | → | | → |
| | Cervix | | | | | ✓ | ✓ | | | | ✓ | → | → | | → |
| Non-epithelial | Sarcoma | | | | | | ✓ | ✓ | ✓ | ✓ | | ↕ | ↕ | | |
| | Leukemia | | | | | ✓ | | | ✓ | ✓ | | ↕ | ↕ | ↕ | ↕ |
| | Brain | | | | | | | | ✓ | | | ↕ | ↕ | ↕ | ↕ |
| | Melanoma | | | | | | | | UV | | | → | ↕ | → | → |
| | NHL | | | | | | | | | | ✓ | ↕ | ← | ↕ | ↕ |
| | Hodgkin | | | | | | | | | | ✓ | ↕ | ← | | |
| | Testis | | | | | | ✓ | ✓ | | | | ← | | | |
| | Kaposi | | | | | | | | | | ✓ | → | | | |

Incidence low in young adults, rises exponentially across CYAC age range

Incidence rises gradually across young adult age range

Incidence rises, then flattens across CYAC age range (for females only, in thyroid cancer)

Incidence peaks in young adults, then falls

← / → Significant increase/decrease in average annual percent change in most recent trend within period 1983–1999

↕ Non-significant increase/decrease in average annual percent change in most recent trend within period 1983–1999

*Supporting references in risk modifier sections of text

Source: Public Health Agency of Canada, "Cancer in Young Adults in Canada," www.cancer.ca (accessed March 2008).

various medical conditions are associated more with epithelial than non-epithelial cancers. Radiation and other occupational or environmental exposure, and viruses and/or immunosuppression, are established risk factors for some cancers in both groups. There is strongly suggestive evidence that the three main risk reduction recommendations, namely *avoiding smoking, minimizing sun exposure,* and *regular Pap smear screening,* are being increasingly followed by young Canadians, and that these trends are paying off. Certain cancers, however, show increasing trends—testis, thyroid, and female lymphomas, in particular. The reasons for the increase are not yet understood.[225]

## CRITICAL THINKING

*What might be the cause of the increasing trend of cancer in testis, thyroid, and female lymphomas?*

**Breast cancer** is the most frequently diagnosed cancer in Canadian women and around the world.[226] In 2007, an estimated 22 300 women were diagnosed with breast cancer and 5300 were expected to die of it.[227] Age-specific incidence increases sharply with age. The incidence in each age group 25 to 29 through 40 to 44 increased by nearly 2.5 times the rate of the previous age group.[228] In a study conducted by Demers and his researchers, which reports a comprehensive array of breast cancer statistics in Manitoba for a 40-year period, it was concluded that the probability of being diagnosed with breast cancer in the next ten years increased most for women 60 years of age.[229] Due to mammographic screening, early detection of disease, and improved therapies, the rate of breast cancer mortality is steadily declining in Canada.[230]

Many women are alive and well today because their breast cancer was detected early. It is important to realize that no screening test is 100 percent accurate. For the group of women from 40 to 49, it is recommended that a clinical breast examination be performed by a trained health care professional at least every two years. In addition, consultation with one's physician regarding the benefits and risks of mammography is important.[231] Women can become familiar with their breasts by looking at and feeling them. Experts used to suggest that this should be done by following a particular method every month. Research has shown that this is not necessary. In essence, there really is not a right or wrong way for women to examine their breasts as long as they get to know the whole area of their breast tissue up to the collarbone, under the armpits, and including the nipples well enough to note any changes that occur.[232]

Organized screening for breast cancer in Canada began in 1988, and it has been implemented in all provinces and two of the three territories. Nunavut has not yet developed an organized screening program. Breast cancer screening consists of two-view mammography in all programs. However, the clinical breast examination is offered in only 4 of the 12 provincial/territorial programs. These provinces are Ontario, Nova Scotia, Prince Edward Island, and Newfoundland and Labrador. The results of Canadian performance indicators, such as participation rate, compare favourably with those of other well-established international screening programs. However, continued monitoring of performance with appropriate feedback and refinement of screening programs should further the continued decrease in morbidity and mortality from breast cancer—the goals of breast cancer screening programs.[233]

The use of complementary and alternative medicine (CAM) by women with breast cancer is often said to be increasing. However, data are scarce to confirm this belief. Boon and her researchers compared the overall patterns of CAM use as well as use of specific products and therapies at two different points in time (1998 and 2005) by women diagnosed with breast cancer. They found that in 1998, only 67 percent of women reported using CAM, as compared with 82 percent in 2005. The most commonly used products and practitioners for treating breast cancer, as reported in 2005, were green tea, vitamin E, flaxseed, vitamin C, massage therapists, and dieticians/nutritionists. The researchers state that CAM can no longer be regarded as an "alternative" or unusual approach to managing breast cancer. It is important to note that the rising popularity of CAM increases the urgency for research into the safety and efficacy of these products and therapies.[234]

## CRITICAL THINKING

*What are the risk factors of breast cancer?*

## CRITICAL THINKING

*How would you teach about breast cancer to women from culturally diverse backgrounds?*

Testicular cancer is one of the most common malignancies among young men between 15 and 35 years of age, and it accounts for approximately 1 percent of all male cancers. During young adulthood, the man should be taught how to perform testicular self-examination (TSE). This is a simple pain-free way to check what is normal for the man's testicles

# Women's Perceptions of Breast Cancer Screening and Education Opportunities in Canada

Breast cancer remains one of the leading causes of death among Canadian women. Early detection continues to provide women with increased treatment options and improved survival. A comprehensive breast assessment program to facilitate early detection includes breast self-examination (BSE), clinical breast examination (CBE), and mammography for selected population segments. While organized (government) screening opportunities exist in most provinces, especially for populations of high risk, participation rates have been lower than desired.

A large body of nursing literature has examined many aspects of breast screening and breast cancer. The vast majority of studies have been quantitative and have tended to focus on women who had already received a diagnosis of breast cancer, or represented particular ethnic populations.

The purpose of this study was to examine the perceptions of a random sample of Canadian women about breast health education and screening practices. The investigators wished to determine which opportunities for breast health education and screening women believed were available to them.

The participants were 63 women taken from a larger telephone survey involving 1224 women living in Canada. Questions in the follow-up interviews asked about knowledge of, and satisfaction with, specific breast education and screening opportunities in each woman's geographic area. Information was sought on factors that hindered or encouraged each woman's participation in breast screening.

## Nursing Implications

1. Examination of barriers to breast cancer screening identified in the study supports the notion that the meaning of the experience determines the motivation for participation in healthy behaviours. Cues to action, such as breast cancer in a family member or friend, acted as a barrier or a motivator, or both. Global cues, however, such as reminder cards, media attention, and marketing, were identified as motivating. Although barriers and motivators were mentioned by many women, it appeared that if the motivation was present, barriers were not a significant issue.

2. Teaching and attitudes of the nurses in the screening clinics were clearly a very positive aspect of the screening experience. While nurses may not always be readily identified as the first contact for health teaching, for these women, nurses were a credible and caring source of information.

3. Lack of information related to screening, or to the opportunities to participate, appeared to be a large issue.

4. Nurses may be so concerned about completing patient teaching that it is critical to the medical diagnosis that general health promotion topics such as breast health, may be far down on the priority list. Thus, nurses may inadvertently be guilty of contributing to the lack of cues to action related to breast cancer screening.

5. A cue to action need not be a major discussion or full-fledged teaching plan. Nurses have a unique opportunity to respond to people during informal "teachable moments." Such cues to action may pay large dividends in terms of increasing the motivators and raising the personal awareness of patients and clients.

Source: Leeseberg Stamler, L., B. Thomas, K. Lafreniere, and R. Charbonneau-Smith, Women's Perceptions of Breast Cancer Screening and Education Opportunities in Canada, *Canadian Nurse*, 97(9) (2001), 23–27. Used with permission.

so that changes can be detected. Table 12-5 describes the self-examination and procedure. Teach the information about the examination.[235]

Because testicular cancer may not always create a noticeable lump on the testicle, you should teach the client to look for the following

- A hard lump, like a pea, on the front or along the side of either testicle
- Any change in size, shape, tenderness, or sensation of testicles or scrotum
- A change in the consistency, or swelling, of the testicles or scrotum
- Pain in the testicles or scrotum

- A dull ache or heaviness in the lower abdomen
- Abnormal or persistent backache
- Unexplained weight loss
- Breast development

It is critical to inform the client that if any of these changes are noticed, he should see a physician immediately.[236]

Cheung and his Manitoba researchers conducted a three-year population-based review of testicular clients to evaluate management patterns. They concluded that deficiencies were evident in testicular cancer management in Manitoba from 1998 to 2000 and indicated the need for well-defined management guidelines and the improved education of caregivers. The researchers were hopeful that

| Table 12-5 Procedure for Examination of the Scrotum and Penis |
| --- |
| 1. Perform the examination immediately after a shower or warm bath. Both the scrotum and examiner's hands should be warm. |
| 2. Hold the scrotum in the palms of the hands and palpate with thumb and fingers of both hands. Examine in a mirror for swelling. |
| 3. Examine each testicle individually, using both hands. Gently roll testicle between thumbs and fingers. (One testicle should be larger.) |
| 4. Locate the epididymous (found on top of and extending down behind the testicle); it should be soft and slightly tender. |
| 5. Examine the spermatic cord next; it ascends from the epididymous and has a firm, smooth, tubular texture. |
| 6. Become familiar with the consistency of normal testicular structures so that changes can be detected. |

these results would prompt other clinicians to review similar parameters in other jurisdictions for purposes of quality assurance.[237]

## CRITICAL THINKING

*What educational strategies should be developed in a clinic for clients coming in with testicular cancer?*

There are three main types of skin cancer: basal cell carcinoma, squamous cell carcinoma, and malignant melanoma.[238] Melanoma is the most fatal type and is the second most common cancer among young adults.[239] The long-term rise in incidence is presumed to be related to increased sun exposure, based primarily on more time spent outdoors and inadequate use of protective clothing. Sunscreens have been widely available since the late 1960s, but no evidence exists that their use has reduced melanoma.[240] Improved sunscreen formulation with higher sun protection factor (SPF) and broad spectrum (UVA and UVB) protection have not been in use long enough to determine their effect on melanoma risk.[241]

Health Canada indicates that many studies of skin cancer show links between malignant melanomas and the intolerance of the individual to sun exposure. One of the main causes of skin cancer is exposure to ultraviolet radiation, or invisible UV rays. These rays are produced by the sun, and by tanning lamps.[242] Most individuals can prevent skin cancer by avoiding exposure to the sun and other sources of ultraviolet light. You can teach the client to heed the following health promotion strategies:

- Select a shaded area for outdoor activities
- Wear a broad-brimmed hat and clothing with a tight weave
- Use a sunscreen lotion with a sun protection factor (SPF) of at least 15. Make sure it has both UVA and UVB protection. Apply liberally to exposed skin 15 to 30 minutes before going out in the sun, and reapply 15 to 30 minutes after sun exposure begins.
- Avoid unprotected overexposure to the sun, especially between 11 a.m. and 4 p.m. during summer months
- Avoid tanning lamps
- Be aware that certain medications can make the skin sensitive to UV rays.[243]

The precautions listed above are especially important for babies and children, who are at a greater risk than adults because of their more sensitive skin.

In summary, the consequences for the young adult of a cancer diagnosis are dismal. These individuals have most of the potentially great years of life ahead of them, and they will either spend decades living with the effects of the cancer diagnosis or have tragically shortened lives, with major repercussions on their families.[244]

## CRITICAL THINKING

*What are the implications for a family when the father, who is a young adult, has cancer?*

**Hepatitis C** In Canada, hepatitis C virus (HCV) is a significant public health problem.[245] Although the precise number of cases of HCV infection is unknown, it is estimated that approximately 240 000 Canadians carry the virus; and many are unaware of their infection. Hepatitis C is transmitted through blood or body fluids contaminated with the virus.[246] The most important risk factor associated with the transmission of HCV is the sharing of drug injection equipment. Adornment practices, such as tattooing, body piercing, and the sharing of personal hygiene items are presumed to be risk factors if the instruments are contaminated with blood or body fluids. However, according to a public health sentinel, only 3 percent of new cases of hepatitis C (as presented in clinics in Calgary, Edmonton, Winnipeg, and Ottawa-Carleton) are associated with body piercing or tattooing.[247] The risk associated with blood transfusions and the use of blood products is markedly reduced as a result of the screening of blood donations.

Côté and his colleagues present a practical guide for treating HCV infection in people co-infected with HIV. They indicate that effective anti-retroviral therapies have prolonged survival rates for HIV-infected people over the past decade, which in turn have made latent complications of HCV major causes of morbidity and mortality in these clients. Advances in the treatment of HCV offer the possibility of eradicating HCV infection in co-infected persons.[248]

---

## CRITICAL THINKING

*What are other strategies to prevent hepatitis C?*

---

**Lifestyle and Physical Illness** Life is rooted in, and organized around, a person's changing culture and society, whether the changes are dramatic or subtle. Coping with extreme change taxes the person both physically and psychologically, and such coping can be responsible for physical disease. *Research shows the existence of relationships between physical adaptation and both illness and sociocultural experiences.* Death rates from cancer, diabetes, tuberculosis, heart disease, and multiple sclerosis, for urban populations, are inversely proportional to income. This realization implies that the stresses of poverty could be a cause of disease.[249]

*Homeless* individuals and families have similar health care needs and problems (refer to Chapter 1). Be attuned to cultural differences, including language difficulties, definitions of health and illness, food preferences, lines of authority, health practices, job-related diseases, and the general lifestyle of your clients.

**Emotional Health Problems** **Stress reactions** include *physiologic and psychological changes resulting in unusually or disturbed adaptive behaviour patterns* and depression, including postpartum.[250] Stress is often the result when the young adult is unable to cope with newly acquired tasks and responsibilities. Mate selection, marriage, childrearing, college, job demands, social expectations, and independent decision making are all potential stressors that carry threats of insecurity, and possibly some degree of failure. Some of these stress reactions take the form of physical illnesses just described. Others take the form of self-destructive behaviour such as suicide, alcoholism, drug abuse and addiction, eating disorders, and smoking. Other stress reactions include the abuse of one's spouse. **Self-destructive behaviour**, in the form of death by suicide, is increasing despite the many religious, cultural, and moral taboos. Thousands of people either take their own lives or attempt suicide yearly.

**Suicide** In Canadian Aboriginal communities, compared with the rest of the Canadian population, suicide and self-inflicted injuries are three times higher (six times higher for the 15 to 24 age group). Aboriginal people are exposed to severe environmental hazards; industrial and resource development have polluted their water and disrupted fish and game stock in many reserve communities. Although changes are occurring, disruptions in the

quality of life remain prevalent. Men are more likely than women to commit suicide. Women, however, are twice as likely as men to be depressed, and their depression lasts longer.[251]

The predisposition to suicidal behaviours has been linked to a number of risk factors, including sociodemographic, psychiatric, genetic, and relational ones.[252] Brezo and her researchers investigated the relationships of personality traits with two suicidal behaviours in a cohort (n = 1140) of 21- to 24-year-old adults, representative of the general population of Quebec. They concluded that personality traits probably make independent contributions to current suicidal ideation, as well as to previous suicide attempts, in certain subgroups of suicidal individuals.[253]

The goal of another Canadian study was to explore the gender differences in clinical and behavioural characteristics, as well as temperament and character variables, of a large sample of unselected suicides. The intent was to further refine the profile of female suicide completers. The researchers concluded that despite a lower prevalence among females, high levels of alcohol abuse and impulsivity appear to be valid risk factors for both sexes. They state that subsequent research should focus on females for the identification of other suicide mediators.[254]

Educate the public about the emotional needs of people, and then address the early signs of suicide so that high-risk persons can be more easily identified by family and friends. To compensate for the effects of separation from home, and thereby encountering a variety of stressors, a close and significant relationship should be established between the high-risk person and a caring person. The person needs opportunity to talk through frustration, anger, and despair and to formulate life plans. Finally, encourage young adults to participate in group and extracurricular activities that counter social isolation.

Nursing responsibility for the suicidal person extends to the industrial setting, the clinic, the general or psychiatric hospital, and the general community. You are in contact with, and in the position to identify, persons who may be potential candidates for suicide: unwed mothers, divorcees, widows and widowers, alcoholics, the terminally ill, and depressed people; of all these, the most difficult to identify is the latter.

Depression is a particularly serious problem for women. The World Health Organization (WHO) concluded that depression is the leading cause of disease burden for women, and it predicts a steady upward trend during the next two decades.[255] Risk factors for depression include being female, family history of depression, unemployment, and chronic disease.[256] The Public Health Agency of Canada (PHAC) report on mental illness in Canada is available through the Internet, and it provides statistics and information on various forms of mental illness.[257]

*Watch for the following signs of depression:*[258]

1. Expressions of overwhelming sadness, worthlessness, hopelessness, or emptiness

2. Complaints of sleep and gastrointestinal disturbances, lack of energy, or chronic illness

3. Decreased muscle tone with slumped shoulders, slowed gait, drooped faces

4. Decreased interest in work, personal appearance, religion, family and friends, or special events

5. Preference for being alone; self-occupied

6. Inability to carry out ordinary tasks or make simple decisions.

Once identified, these signs of depression must be communicated to others: friends, relatives, a physician, or other persons concerned with the potentially suicidal person. A recent publication from the Canadian Psychiatric Association outlines the clinical guidelines for the treatment of depressive disorders.[259]

One of the most important aspects in caring for a young adult who is depressed is to show the person, verbally and nonverbally, that someone—you—understands, respects, and cares about him or her.

## CRITICAL THINKING

*In working with a depressed client whom you suspect has suicidal ideation, and who seems overwhelmed by personal problems, how can you assist this client to cope?*

**Drinking Alcohol** Research has shown a connection between the rates of drinking across the general population and rates of alcohol-related problems.[260] According to the 2004 Canadian Addiction Survey, 9 percent of Canadians over the age of 15 are current drinkers. Young adults, and males generally, consume more alcohol than other groups. In fact, according to the Canadian Addiction Survey, past drinking rates peaked among those 18 to 24 years of age, with about 90 percent of individuals in that age range consuming alcohol during the course of the year.[261]

Alcoholism is viewed by most experts as a form of addiction. This means that alcoholic individuals demonstrate a physical dependence on alcohol, and they experience withdrawal symptoms when they do not drink.[262] According to the Canadian Community Health Survey, 2.6 percent of the total population is considered alcohol-dependent.[263]

Alcohol addiction occurs over time because drinking alcohol alters the balance of certain chemicals in the brain, causing a strong desire for more alcohol. These chemicals include gamma-aminobutyric acid (GABA), which inhibits impulsiveness; norepinephrine, which is released in response

to stress; and dopamine, serotonin, and opioid peptides, which are responsible for feelings of pleasure.[264] At low doses, alcohol acts as a central nervous system depressant, producing relaxation and a release of inhibitions. At higher doses, it can produce intoxication and impaired judgment and coordination, and in extreme cases coma and death.[265]

The most widely known treatment modality is Alcoholics Anonymous, a 12-step program based on spiritual principles. Other treatment options include in-patient and outpatient programs at treatment centres.[266]

Anyone can write away for the self-administration test for alcoholism that is available through the National Council for Alcoholism, or through Alcoholics Anonymous. A certain score indicates alcoholic tendencies.

**Substance Abuse** These are other forms of self-destructive behaviour. Drug abuse is increasing in the young adult, including all levels of workers. Abuse and addiction contribute to a number of other physical, emotional, and social health problems. Cannabis is the most widely used illicit drug in Canada. Other commonly used illicit drugs include hallucinogens, LSD, speed, heroin, and cocaine.[267] Although the overall consumption of illicit drugs is relatively low, compared with that of alcohol and tobacco, research reports indicate that the use of illicit drugs, other than cannabis, has risen during the past decade.[268]

Nearly five million Canadians use, appropriately and inappropriately, one or more illicit drugs, including sleeping pills, tranquilizers, antidepressants, and diet pills. During the assessment process, it is vital that you list all medications being taken by the young adult.

As with alcoholism, male addicts are more numerous than female ones. Symptoms sometimes differ for the young adult at work; see the box entitled "Signs and Symptoms of Drug Abuse in the Young Adult" for a list.

Health promotion strategies for drug abuse and addiction involve helping the person work through emotional problems, seeing that he or she has proper medical and nutritional regimens, helping him or her return to a community where the dangers of becoming addicted again are less risky, and helping him or her get involved in worthwhile work or activities.[269] It is important that the family be involved in the rehabilitation process to offer support and encouragement to the young adult. Environmental support helps to ensure healthy conditions; practices and policies make it easier for individuals to achieve and maintain their health.[270]

**Gambling** Gambling is a controversial topic in our society today. In recent years, provinces in Canada have expanded their gaming activities.[271] Cox and his researchers used a Canadian Problem Gambling Index to investigate the current 12-month prevalence of gambling problems in the Canadian Community Health Survey: Cycle 1.2—Mental

## Signs and Symptoms of Drug Abuse in the Young Adult

- Late to work frequently; late in producing assignments.
- Increased absenteeism (abusers miss twice as much work as non-abusing employees).
- Increased productivity in work for a short period (cocaine will cause some people to perform better than normal, or more creatively for a short time; over-achievement can be used to compensate for, or cover up, initial stages of abuse).
- Falling productivity, poorer quality work, disorganized thinking and work outcome, missed deadlines.
- Forgetfulness, failure to follow instructions properly and to carry out usual steps of a procedure.
- Personality change; increasing irritability, depression, suspicion.
- Chronic runny nose from cocaine inhalation, sniffing glue, or other chemicals that cause irritation of the nasal mucous membrane; regular complaints of a cold.
- Napping or sleeping on the job.
- Accident proneness, clumsiness at work, poor gross or fine motor coordination on the job, reports of accidents in the auto or at home.
- Clandestine meetings and discussions with other employees (users become dealers for fellow employees and withdraw from supervisory staff).

Health and Well Being. In this survey a random sample of 34 700 community-dwelling respondents, 15 years and older, were interviewed. They concluded that Manitoba (2.9 percent) and Saskatchewan (also 2.9 percent) had the highest prevalence of gambling problems. These two provinces had significantly higher levels than the two provinces with the lowest prevalence of gambling problems. The researchers conclude that these findings support earlier predictions that the rapid and prolific expansion of new forms of legalized gambling in many regions of the country would be associated with a considerably high public health cost.[272]

### CRITICAL THINKING

*What resources are available in your community for the problem gambler?*

**Smoking** Smoking is considered to be the single most serious health problem in Canada.[273] Smoking has declined substantially over the past decade. The most noticeable decline in daily smoking occurred among teenagers and young adults, who were the target of numerous federal, provincial, and municipal anti-smoking campaigns in recent years. However, these declines have accelerated in the past two years. One-third (33.2 percent) of young adults aged 20 to 24 smoked either daily or occasionally in 2003, the highest rate of any age group.[274] The smoking patterns vary from province to province.

Second-hand smoke, smoke exhaled or given off by a burning cigarette, is toxic. Second-hand smoke is referred to as environmental tobacco smoke, or sidestream smoke. Children exposed to second-hand smoke experience increased episodes of ear and upper respiratory tract infections. Children of smokers, it has been found, are more likely to take up smoking.[275]

Tobacco is the most important preventable risk factor for chronic respiratory diseases. Smoking cessation among adults will have the greatest impact on reducing respiratory diseases such as lung cancer and chronic obstructive pulmonary disease (COPD).[276] Many people, even some with serious respiratory and vascular disorders, continue to smoke heavily despite the warnings from their physicians about the harmful effects of smoking.

Lung cancer is becoming a major health issue for women. In fact, lung cancer is the second most common cause of death in young adults.[277]

More women than men now smoke cigarettes. Smoking in younger women has significantly increased the number of cardiac deaths and the incidence of lung cancer in women. Other health problems are also attributed to smoking. The effects of smoking during pregnancy are discussed in Chapter 6.

Various reasons are offered for smoking: smoking is relaxing; it prevents nervousness and overeating; and it gives the person something to do with his or her hands in social gatherings. All of these reasons probably stem from internal tensions and are likely the young person's way of dealing with stress.

Chemicals found in cigarette smoke are commonplace in many work environments. Thus, the person who smokes may suffer double jeopardy. Further, the person who smokes has more occupational accidents and injuries and uses more sick time and health benefits.

According to the Canadian Lung Association, quitting smoking is a process that requires careful planning, courage, discipline, and commitment.[278] It advocates four steps to quitting smoking:

- *Pick a quit day*: choose a date within the next two or three weeks to quit
- *Choose one or more proven quit-smoking methods*: combine various methods such as counselling, self-help guides, the patch, and other medicines. Write down things that can replace smoking

- *Work your plan:* go for a walk instead of smoking; be positive about your choice
- *Celebrate your successes:* believe in yourself and your plan

The Canadian Lung Association has a number of links that can be accessed to assist one to quit smoking.[279]

*Work with the young adult to reduce or stop cigarette smoking.* To achieve this goal, you will be required to do more than give information about the health effects and morbidity and mortality rates. Explore his or her ideas of health and personal vulnerability to the adverse effects from smoking. The social dynamics of smoking must also be considered. Realize that to give up smoking represents a loss. Help the person who is trying to stop smoking to acknowledge the normal feelings of loss and grief related to giving up a part of self and social lifestyles. Instead of emphasizing that the person is "giving up" smoking, help the person to verbalize his or her feelings and help him or her to identify what is being gained by a smoking cessation program.

## Family Violence
Domestic violence happens to children, women, men, same-sex partners, and older adults. It involves any form of real or threatened physical, emotional, or sexual maltreatment and harassment in any relationship that involves intimacy.[280] Based on a study that examined police documentation over a ten-year period, domestic violence data included the following:

- Most victims of spousal violence report the abuse to police only once.
- Women are twice as likely as men to report abuse. Aboriginals are more likely to report than non-Aboriginals.
- Those aged 15 to 24 were more likely to report spousal violence to the police, while those aged 35 and older were least likely to go to police.
- The violence is more likely to be reported if children are witnesses to it.[281]

Current knowledge indicates that, rather than a discrete incident, spousal violence frequently involves multiple violent incidents. This pattern of behaviour of repeated violence increases the potential for life-threatening harm.[282] Women who are abused are at heightened risk for physical injury, sexual and reproductive disorders, and homicide.[283] They often develop feelings of anxiety, depression, and low self-esteem.[284]

## CRITICAL THINKING

*What elements should be included in a safety plan for a woman who is being abused?*

In a study of family health promotion in the aftermath of intimate partner abuse, the researchers found that families strengthen their emotional health by purposefully replacing previously destructive patterns of interaction with predictable, supportive ways of getting along in a process called regenerating family. The researchers claim that these particular findings add to the knowledge of family development and of how families promote their health when they experienced intimate partner violence.[285]

Family violence, which can cause significant injury and death, takes the following three forms: sexual abuse, emotional abuse, and physical abuse. These three forms tend to occur together as part of a system of coercive control.[286] *It is a pattern of behaviour that seeks to establish power and control over another through fear and intimidation.* Further, attempts have been made to make the police and legal system more protective of the woman who has been treated violently, and more punitive toward the violent man. Emergency shelters and safe homes for abused women and their children are increasingly being established in urban areas so that the woman who seeks help does not have to return home, or be at home, when the man who was released shortly after arrest returns home even more violent than before. Crisis telephone lines have been established and publicized by the media, and many women have memorized these numbers. In some communities, rap sessions and referrals are available for abused women.[287]

## CRITICAL THINKING

*What resources are available in your community for the women and children who are being abused?*

You can work with other health and legal professionals to identify, and overcome, the problem of abused women. The *assessment of a family and a woman who is suffering adult abuse often reveals the following typical characteristics:*[288]

- The family and the woman are isolated socially, or physically, from neighbours, relatives, and friends.
- The woman feels increasing helplessness, guilt, isolation, and low self-esteem. She feels trapped and has been forced to be dependent on the man.
- The woman may range in age from teens to old age and may suffer violent injury for months or years.
- The woman's educational and occupational status is often higher than that of the man.
- Most beatings begin early in the partnership and increase in frequency and intensity over the decades.
- Most violence occurs in the evenings or on weekends.
- Generally, there are no witnesses.

- The woman is frequently unable to leave the home because of lack of money, transportation, a place to go, support people, or support agencies in the community. Further, she has learned helplessness behaviours and feels unable to try to escape.

- The injuries from abuse are probably not visible, but if abuse is present, the woman usually talks about the problem freely when asked directly if abuse is occurring.

- With an increasing incidence of abuse and the physical and emotional consequences of abuse, the woman becomes more passive, less flexible, less able to think logically, more apathetic, depressed, and possibly suicidal.

- Eventually the frustration, stress, and anger can be externalized into physical behaviour that is more than protective of the self or the children; she may in turn become violent to the point of killing the abusing partner.

The Canadian Nurses Association Position Statement on Violence clearly states that violence is recognized as a social act involving a serious misdirection of power.[289] Nurses alone cannot manage or eliminate violence. The approach must be multidisciplinary, multi-sectorial, and multifaceted. All professionals, including the private sector, unions, and governments, have strategic roles to play to ensure that legislation, education, research, administrative supports, and adequate resources are in play to deal with the impact of violence.[290]

The box entitled "Identification of Partner Abuse in the Health Care Setting" describes some "red flags" that can help you identify a battered adult in an emergency room or intensive care, occupational, or other medical setting.[291]

---

### CRITICAL THINKING

*What health promoting strategies could you offer a woman who informs you that her spouse is verbally abusive to her?*

---

**Sexual Assault** The term *rape* is no longer used in Canada. Instead, according to the Criminal Code of Canada, the term *sexual assault* is used. The law prescribes three levels of sexual assault: level 1, sexual assault (touching, kissing); level 2, sexual assault with a weapon resulting in bodily harm; and level 3, aggravated sexual assault (wounding, disfiguring, or endangering the life of the victim). Women are far more likely than men to be sexually victimized. The majority of sexual offenders are known to the victim. Sexual assault is a crime of violence, not a crime of passion. The underlying

---

## Identification of Partner Abuse in the Health Care Setting

### Multiple Injuries

- Multiple abrasions and contusions to different anatomic sites should alert health care providers. There are relatively few ways of sustaining such injuries.

### Body Map

- Many incidents of abuse involve injury to the face, neck, chest, breasts, or abdomen, whereas most accidents involve the extremities.

### Severity of Injury

- Severity varies among abused victims. The presentation of medically insignificant trauma to the emergency service should alert medical personnel that ongoing assault and impending danger constitute the real emergency for which the woman is seeking aid.

### Pregnancy

- Abused women are more likely to be beaten when pregnant. There is a higher rate of miscarriage among battered women.

### Trauma History

- Frequent visits to the emergency department or physician.

- A history of trauma can be the key indicator! Asking about previous injuries and looking at medical records are important. Records may indicate repeated visits with injuries to the same site.

### Suicide Attempts

- Studies indicate that battering is a frequent precipitant of female suicide attempts; conversely, women who attempt suicide are likely to have a history of domestic violence.

### Inconsistent Description of Injuries

- Injuries do not fit with the victim's description of the genesis of injury.

### Vague and Non-specific Complaints

- Complaints include, for example, anxiety, depression, and sleeplessness, and many indicate intrafamilial crisis.

### Heavy Use of Alcohol and Drugs

- Victims are more likely than non-victims to use alcohol and drugs. Partners are much more likely to use alcohol and drugs excessively.

issues are power and control, rather than sexual desire. The defining issue is the lack of consent by the victim. Counselling the victim should focus on the crisis and the fears, feelings, and issues involved. Many young adult victims need follow-up mental health services to help them cope with the short-term and long-term effects of the crisis.[292]

**Interventions for Children** Research shows that children (aged 2 to 12) of abused women have deep feelings of fear about safety and abandonment, anger, confusion, social isolation, and aggression. The play of these children reveals conflicts about overpowering adults, and an identification with the same-sex parent; children are learning abnormal behaviour and roles that could be carried into their adult relationships and lifestyle.[293] You can work with others to establish emergency centres or crisis phone lines for the woman, and you can exert pressure to reform the current legal and judicial system so it will be more equitable to women.

CRITICAL THINKING

*In assessing the family of a child who has been brought in with injuries, what behaviours by the parents might indicate possible child abuse?*

CRITICAL THINKING

*After reading the myths about battered women, take a moment to reflect on them. See if any other myth comes to mind. If it does, jot it down.*

Social support and the meaning a person attaches to stressful events can influence whether the person becomes ill or remains healthy—physically and emotionally—in a situation. The abused woman who extricates herself from her violent situation has strengthened her ability to survive, to

## Myths and Realities about Battered Women

**Myth 1: Battered Women Are a Small Percentage of the Overall Population.**

- **Fact:** Domestic violence is one of the most underreported crimes. In the United States, the Federal Bureau of Investigation estimates that 60 percent of all married women experience physical violence by their husbands at some time during their marriage. There are an estimated two to six million female victims of family violence each year.

**Myth 2: Battered Women Are Masochistic.**

- **Fact:** Battered women are *not* masochistic. The prevailing belief has always been that only women who "liked it and deserved it" were battered; that women experienced some pleasure, often akin to sexual pleasure, from being beaten by the man they love. Because this is such a prevailing stereotype, many battered women begin to wonder if they are indeed masochistic.

**Myth 3: Battered Women Are Crazy.**

- **Fact:** Battered women are not crazy, although battering may contribute to mental illness. This myth places the blame for battering on the woman's negative personality characteristics and takes the focus off the batterer. Further, being abused and beaten can result in what apparently is abnormal behaviour—the woman's attempt to adapt.

**Myth 4: Middle-Class Women Are Not Battered as Frequently, or as Violently, as Poorer Women.**

- **Fact:** Women from lower socioeconomic classes are more likely to come in contact with community agencies, so their

problems are more visible. Middle- and upper-class women often fear that disclosure will result in social embarrassment and harm to their own, or their husband's, career or that people will not believe them. This is often true when the husband is held in high esteem in the community.

**Myth 5: Women from Ethnic or Racial Minority Groups Are Battered More Frequently than Caucasian Women.**

- **Fact:** Studies show that battering crosses all ethnic lines, with no one group suffering more than another.

**Myth 6: Battered Women Are Uneducated and Have Few Job Skills.**

- **Fact:** Educational levels of battered women range from grade school through completion of professional and doctoral degrees. Many successful career women would be willing to give up their careers if to do so would eliminate battering. Changing jobs or staying home to ease the situation usually has no effect on the partner's behaviour, and sometimes battering worsens.

**Myth 7: Batterers Are Unsuccessful and Lack Resources to Cope with the World.**

- **Fact:** It has been suggested that men who feel less capable than women resort to violence. Contrary findings were reported in England, where the highest incidence of wife beating was among physicians, service professionals, and police. Affluent batterers include lawyers, professors, and salesmen. Many of these men donate a great deal of

>

their time to community activities, and they could not maintain their involvement in these projects without the visible support of their wives.

## Myth 8: Batterers Are People with Personality Disorders.

**Fact:** If batterers could simply be considered antisocial personalities, individual therapy could be used to differentiate batterers from other men. Unfortunately, it is not that simple. One trait they share is the ability to use charm as a manipulative technique. Manipulation, acting out of anger, exhilaration felt when they dominate and beat the woman, and denial of the behaviour are characteristic of people with personality disorders.

## Myth 9: Police Can Protect Battered Women.

**Fact:** At most, only 10 percent of battered women call the police. Of those who did, many believe the police officers were ineffective. When the police left, the men continued the assault with vigour. Several thousand women are murdered annually by male partners, often as a part of the battering act. At least one-half of the injuries presented by women at an emergency room are the result of battering. Battering may also be the basis for a suicide attempt.

## Myth 10: Batterers Are Violent in All of Their Relationships.

**Fact:** Most men who batter their wives are generally not violent in other aspects of their lives. Although being violent in public has definite, negative consequences, there are few consequences in domestic cases.

## Myth 11: The Batterer Is Not a Loving Partner.

**Fact:** Batterers are often described by women during the honeymoon phase of the cycle of violence as fun-loving, playful, attentive, sensitive, exciting, and affectionate. The woman may describe some very positive characteristics in the man that cause her truly to love him.

## Myth 12: Long-standing Battering Relationships Can Change for the Better.

**Fact:** Relationships that have rested on the man's having power over the woman are stubbornly resistant to an equal power-sharing arrangement. Even with the best of help, such relationships usually do not become battering-free.

## Myth 13: Once a Batterer, Always a Batterer.

**Fact:** Batterers can be taught to change their aggressive responses; however, very few batterers are willing to get help. If the batterer does not get treatment and if he is divorced and then remarries, he is likely to batter the next woman he marries.

## Myth 14: Battered Women Can Always Leave Home.

**Fact:** Many battered women have no place to go and no means of survival outside the framework of their marriage. They usually have small children to care for, whom they would not want to leave home alone with the father. Because battering weakens a woman's self-esteem, she believes she is incapable of managing on her own.

## Myth 15: Battered Women Are Weak and Come from a Bad Background.

**Fact:** Typically the battered women in Hoff's study had a warm, loving relationship as a child with the mother, and a negative, destructive relationship with the father. Not all battered women were abused as children. Women who experienced violence before they were battered by their mates showed resilience and strength. But long-standing abuse breeds self-degradation and despair so that a woman feels unworthy of the continued love of even her mother, and she feels unable to reach out for help. The battered woman should be considered a survivor type of person.

## Myth 16: Battering May Occur Only Once or Infrequently and Could Be Predicted, and thus Prevented, by the Woman.

**Fact:** For most of the battered women in several studies, the violence was frequent, extended over time, and often unexpected, and included many similar incidents. Often, violence occurred concomitantly with the man's rages, drunkenness, and/or financial insecurity, and during the woman's pregnancy. Often, each beating was worse than the previous one. Women consistently report doing everything possible to avoid violence; they try to second-guess the husband: "It's like walking on eggshells." Women have been socialized into the nurturing role, so they doggedly try to succeed in it as wife and mother, regardless of the circumstances. Further, society and medical and psychiatric services and professionals reinforce the belief that the woman's troubles are the result of her own inadequacies and failures (men are taught that the source of stress is other than self). Although the battered woman may think of hurting or killing the man as a punishment, the woman is often inhibited from such action by concern for the children, if they are present, and fear of consequences for self. Yet, there have been times that the women retaliated; in those cases, most women found that if they fought back, the man became even more violent.

resolve crisis, and to move forward. Each professional, as a citizen and health care provider, must work in whatever way possible to decrease violence, its cause, and its effects.[294] Check, also, with the resources in your area for information.

## Social Health Problems

**Divorce** Divorce is *the termination of marriage, preceded by a period of emotional distress in the marriage, separation, and legal procedures*. Divorce is a *crisis* for those involved, and it can affect the physical and emotional health of the persons involved.[295]

Divorce has greatly increased since 1968, when the divorce laws entered into effect; in fact, there has been a five-fold increase in divorce from 1968 to 1995. In 2005, the United Nations statistics gave the divorce rate per 1000 for selected Western countries. The United States has the highest divorce rate in the Western world. Canada's rate is modest, when compared to that of the United States, but it is still fairly high. As more young couples choose to cohabit before marriage and as the "children of divorce," who are at a higher risk of divorcing, enter into marriage themselves, there is good evidence that divorce rates could keep rising.[296]

Many researchers have tried to explain today's relatively high divorce rate.[297] The following are some of the hypotheses generated:

- *Individualism is on the rise:* today's family members spend less time together
- *Romantic love fades:* relationships tend to fail as sexual passion wanes
- *Women are less dependent on men:* women find it easier to leave unhappy marriages because many are in the workforce and can support themselves.
- *Many of today's marriages are stressful:* with both partners working, divorce is most common during the early years of marriage, when many couples have young children
- *Divorce is socially acceptable:* divorce no longer carries the powerful stigma it once did
- *Legally, a divorce is easier to obtain:* the Divorce Act 1968 allowed for divorce in circumstances beyond adultery[298]

Helping divorced women and men to identify and pursue personal goals is important. The primary needs of divorced women are economic independence, education, managing parenting, maintaining friendships, establishing a partner relationship, and obtaining adequate housing, school, and environment for self and children. Goals for divorced men are usually similar, although typically they experience less economic difficulty. Groups for children of divorcing and divorced parents can help the child work through feelings of loss, anger, guilt, and ambivalence about relationships with parents and often, eventually, step-parents and stepsiblings. The key is for the parents to continue showing love to their children and to maintain open communication between them about the offspring.

**Continuing Health Promotion** As a nurse, realize that the health state of the young adult, and the type of health care sought, are influenced by the person's background, knowledge, experience, philosophy, and lifestyle. Young adults with health problems might more readily seek care and information if they could find programs compatible with their expectations and lifestyles. You can initiate programs that are specifically aimed at young adults, as they seem to accept the treatment plan more readily when they understand the rationale and expected effects. Keep in mind the previously discussed health problems and unmet physiologic needs as you talk with young adults and plan and give care.

**Continuing Adjustments** One couple invited others to a celebration of their twenty-fifth wedding anniversary with the following words:

> We continue to adjust to each other, an adjustment that started 25 years ago, and will never stop because we each continue to grow and change. We will always be different. Don't mistake it for a solid marriage. There is no such thing. Marriage is more like an airplane than a rock. You have to commit the thing to flight, and then it creaks and groans, and keeping it airborne depends entirely on attitude. Working at it, though, we can fly forever. Only the two of us know how hard it has been or how worthwhile. Celebrate with us . . .

## SUMMARY

1. Young adulthood is a time of stabilization. Physical growth is completed.

2. The person has established independence from parents but maintains a friendly relationship with them.

3. The person is settling into a committed intimate relationship and friendships and into career or profession.

4. The couple may choose to become parents or remain childless.

5. The person may choose to live a single lifestyle.

6. Development continues in the cognitive, emotional, social, and moral–spiritual dimensions. The philosophy of life is being formulated.

7. Behaviours, whether at home, on the job, at leisure or with family, friends, or strangers, are adaptive in response to stressors.

8. Stress effects may result in unhealthy habits or physical or emotional illness.

9. The box entitled "Considerations for the Young Adult in Health Care" summarizes what you should consider in assessment and health promotion of the young adult.

## Considerations for the Young Adult in Health Care

- Cultural and family background, values, support systems, community resources
- Relationships with family of origin, extended family, family of friends or spouse
- Behaviours that indicate abuse by spouse or significant other
- Physical characteristics, nutritional status, and rest/sleep and exercise patterns that indicate health and are age-appropriate
- Integrated self-concept, body image, and sexuality
- Immunizations, safety education, and other health promotion measures used
- Demonstration of continued learning and use of formal operations and concrete operations competencies in cognitive ability
- Overall appearance and behavioural patterns that indicate intimacy rather than isolation
- Behavioural patterns that demonstrate a value system, continuing formation of philosophy of life, and moral–spiritual development
- Established employment, vocation, or profession, including homemaking and child care
- Behavioural patterns that reflect commitment to parenting, if there are children
- Relationships with work colleagues, coping skills for work stress
- Demonstration of integration of work and leisure and avoidance of physical or emotional illness
- Behavioural patterns and characteristics indicating the young adult has achieved developmental tasks

## Interesting Websites

### Canadian HIV/AIDS Information Centre
www.aidssida.cpha.ca
The mandate of the Canadian HIV/AIDS Information Centre is to provide information on HIV prevention, care, and treatment to community-based organizations, health and education professionals, resource centres, and others with HIV and AIDS information needs in Canada.

### Dietitians of Canada
www.dietitians.ca
This organization provides nutritional advice that is accurate, reliable, and trustworthy because it is based on science.

### EGALE Canada
www.egale.ca
This is a national organization dedicated to promoting the full acceptance of gay, lesbian, bisexual, and transgendered Canadians.

### Sex Information and Education Council of Canada
www.sieccan.org
This national non-profit organization was established in 1964 to foster public and professional education about human sexuality.

### Andropause Canada
www.andropausecanada.com/
This website provides information about andropause and explains the physical and psychological changes experienced. It provides different options to avoid or alleviate problems and describes the medical treatments that may be required.

## Key Terms

| | | | |
|---|---|---|---|
| **AIDS** (490) | **body image** (485) | **coming out** (464) | **dysmenorrhea** (461) |
| **alpha rhythm** (475) | **breast cancer** (497) | **delta rhythm** (475) | **electroencephalograms** |
| **announcement phase** (488) | **cohabitation** (465) | **divorce** (507) | **(EEGs)** (475) |

# Chapter 13

## Assessment and Health Promotion for the Middle-Aged Person

*Forty is the old age of youth. Fifty is the youth of old age.*

Victor Hugo

## Objectives

*Study of this chapter will enable you to:*

1 Explore with middle-aged persons ideas about their generation, lifestyle, and the conflict they see among generations.

2 Examine the second-order changes in family status required to proceed developmentally in the stage of the family life cycle: launching children and moving on.

3 Discuss the family relationships and sexual development of the middle-aged adult, conflicts that are to be resolved, and your role in helping the family work through issues and conflicts.

4 Discuss the emotional, social, economic, and lifestyle changes usually encountered by the widow(er).

5 Describe the hormonal changes of middle age and the resultant changes in physical appearance and body image.

6 Discuss the nutritional, rest, leisure, work, and exercise needs of the middle-aged adult, factors that interface with achieving those needs, and your role in promoting their health.

7 Describe how the middle-aged adult's cognitive skills and emotional and moral development influence your nursing care practice.

8 Debate both the authenticity of the mid-life crisis of this era and its significance to social well-being.

9 Compare and contrast the behaviour of generativity or maturity, and self-absorption or stagnation, and related adaptive mechanisms.

10 Describe the developmental tasks for the middle-aged person and your role in helping him or her accomplish these tasks.

11 Explore with a middle-aged adult strategies to promote health.

12 Assess the body image, physical, mental, and emotional characteristics, and family relationships of a middle-aged person.

13 Plan and implement effective care to a middle-aged person.

The period of middle age is becoming one of the most interesting areas to study due to the presence of the baby boom generation.

New concepts of adulthood involve changes in the definitions of gender and age roles. The concept of plasticity suggests that what people do, and how they live, have much to do with how they age.[1] Middle adulthood is a time of widening social interest in which the family becomes increasingly better oriented to its responsibility to the greater society.

Defining middle age is a nebulous task. Chronologically, **middle age** *covers the years of approximately 45 to 65 or even 70, but each person will consider as well the physiologic age condition of the body and one's psychological age—how old he or she acts and feels.*[2] People who were in their fifties at the millennium are called the baby boom generation. They have lived through an affluent era that has kept them young physically, and they perceive themselves as youthful and in control as they enter their second half of life.

Because of changing demographics, an increasing number of Canadians is considered middle-aged. They earn most of the money, pay a major portion of the bills and most of the taxes, and make many of the decisions. Thus, the power in government, politics, education, religion, science, business, industry, and communication is wielded not by the young or the old, but by the middle-aged.

Middle age is a time of relatively good health, both physical and mental. It is a time of new personal freedom, maximum command of self, and significant influence over the social environment. At work, the person has increasing ability to make decisions, hold high-status jobs, and earn a maximum income. The person enjoys expanding family networks and vast social roles.

## FAMILY DEVELOPMENT AND RELATIONSHIPS

The following information will assist you in understanding the middle-aged family system in the processes of assessing and promoting health.

## Family Life Cycle

Refer to Table 4-3, which illustrates the stages of the family life cycle, the emotional processes of transition (key principles), and the second-order changes in the family required

to proceed developmentally. Stage 5, families in later life, is the appropriate stage for the middle-aged adult.

## Relationship with Children

The **generation gap**, *the conflict between parents and adolescents,* has probably always existed to some degree. The experience of the parent generation, and therefore their values and expectations, differs from that of their offspring. Actually, the generation lines are blurring. The changing attitudes, values, behaviour, and dress of middle-aged persons reflect our current cultural emphasis on youth and beauty, rather than on tradition and wisdom. Yet, each generation is concerned about the other, although for different reasons. In fact, the younger and older generations can successfully combine their efforts to work for legislation, policy changes, and social justice.

**Social mobility**, *in which the child moves away from the social position, educational level, class, occupation, and ethnicity of the parents,* overtly causes offspring to forsake parental teaching and seek new models of behaviour. The mass media and societal trends help to set standards and expectations about behaviour that may be counter to parental teaching or wishes. Rapid social changes and the growing awareness that much about the future is unknown threaten established faiths, and they stimulate attraction to new ideologies and exceptional behaviour. This is a particularly difficult conundrum for immigrant and refugee families.[3]

Typically, the values of young adults are more similar to those of their parents than to those of other adults or peers. This is true in Canadian society as well as in other societies.[4] You can help youth to ask the questions that adults do not think of, but the youth must trust their parents enough to work on the answers together. Middle-aged parents can be encouraged to listen and exchange information and ideas honestly, and with a sense of humour. If the parent works to maintain open communication, the generation gap will be minimal. The middle-aged cohort of any family tends to have the most responsibility. They are "sandwiched" between their children and their aging parents.[5] Your work with families of this type can promote much appreciated harmony.

*Divorce of offspring* is a situation of increasing concern for middle-aged parents. The parents may feel shock (or relief if they did not like the child's spouse). They may believe that their efforts and help in moving the child "out of the nest" through marriage, or helping the couple set up a home, were to no avail. This feeling may be especially strong if the divorced family member decides to return to live again at the parents' home. The parents might blame their child or the in-laws, and they might criticize the couple for not working on their marital problems as effectively as the middle-aged parents have done.[6]

If the divorced son or daughter is in a financial crisis, the parents' savings might also go to help their child instead of being used as originally planned. If the divorcing couple has children, additional strain will be added.[7]

The divorce may not have a completely negative effect on the middle-aged parents. If the parents have a healthy self-esteem and an ability to proceed cautiously, they might help their offspring to gain the essential maturity that he or she was previously lacking. However, the crisis and stages of grief that accompany divorce and the loss of a family member are still keenly felt.[8]

*Young adults may return home to live with parents for reasons other than separation or divorce.* Some recent university graduates have been unable to find the job of their choice. Alternatively, they are finding that their first jobs do not pay enough for them to cover high rents, along with other costs of living. Consequently, they are living with their parents until they can accumulate more money, or until they can move to a higher-income job.[9]

This situation can cause stress because some middle-aged parents actually look forward to having their children leave the home—to create the so-called "empty nest."[10] The middle-aged adults seek space, time, and financial resources to pursue personal, organizational, and civic goals rather than continue with child care responsibilities. Prolonged dependence of young adult offspring can create conflict with grandparents, and with other children who are still at home.

The *grandparent role* has a different dimension if it occurs during middle age rather than in later maturity. Some people do become grandparents during middle age, or even in late young adulthood.[11] If the offspring has established his or her own home, and has a family, grandparenthood is usually a happy status and role. The relationship to the grandchild is informal and playful; the child is a source of fun, leisure activity, and self-indulgence. The emphasis is on mutual satisfaction, authority lines are irrelevant, and the child is seen as someone for whom to buy gifts.[12] Because of the recent increases in the number of baby boomers who are becoming grandparents, grandparent–grandchild relationships have begun to receive more research attention.[13] For example, research findings suggest that regular interactions with grandparents usually leave children with fewer prejudices about old people.[14]

The high rate of divorce in Canada has actually placed a severe strain on grandparents.[15] In the case of divorce, the middle-aged grandparents wonder what their future relationship will be with their grandchildren. Relations may be strained between the in-laws as each family wonders how to interact with the other. Currently, many grandparents are raising their grandchildren because their children have died, are divorced, or are incapacitated through drugs or other devastating problems.[16] The increase in the rate of divorce among Canadian families, and in the number of children affected by divorce, has resulted in the emergence of "grandparents' rights groups" across the country.[17] British Columbia, Alberta, Quebec, and New Brunswick have laws recognizing the rights of grandparents to have access to their grandchildren; other Canadian jurisdictions do not have such laws.[18]

Increasingly, you will be caring for middle-aged parents who are being threatened emotionally, or who are having social or financial problems because of their children's separation or divorce. Milan and Hamm state that, in some cases, grandparents are the financial maintainers of households containing not only the grandchild, but also at least one parent.[19] Some middle-aged grandparents need encouragement in securing visitation rights when divorce or death has severed the relationship. Help the middle-aged couple to regain a sense of self-esteem, a sense of confidence in setting limits so that they can pursue their own life goals, and a method of working through decisions and problems with the young adult offspring.[20] You, as a nurse, may suggest certain strategies for grandparents; see the box entitled "Tips for Today's Grandparents."[21]

Little Canadian research has been generated regarding such issues as the prevalence of grandparents providing primary care for their grandchildren, the reasons the grandchildren came to them, and the effects grandchildren have on the grandparents.[22] Inwood states that nurses practise in a variety of settings where they may encounter grandparents who are raising grandchildren. It is imperative that nurses be aware of the financial, household, and other issues that grandparents face. It is important, as well, that nurses conduct appropriate nursing assessment to promote the health of both grandparents and grandchildren. Nurses who are sensitive to the needs and responsibilities of grandparents and grandchildren can help to decrease the stress and increase the wellness of the family.[23]

Recent research has revealed that *skipped-generation households* (households that include only grandparents and grandchildren) are vastly overrepresented among Aboriginal Canadians. Using custom tabulation data from the 1996 Canadian Census, it was found that despite extremely high rates of poverty and disability, one-third of Aboriginal skipped-generation families were raising two or more grandchildren. In comparison to other grandparent caregivers, Aboriginal custodial caregivers were more likely to be caring for a senior (23 percent) and to be spending more than 30 hours a week on child care duties (46 percent) and on housework (41 percent).[24] The study shows Aboriginal grandparents in skipped-generation households as resilient caregivers who are often raising their grandchildren in the context of ill health and extreme poverty.[25] These findings have profound implications for nurses who are working with Aboriginal households. A thorough assessment of such families is warranted because even though the grandparents are resilient, as the study finds, they may be experiencing severe role conflict and role overload. It is critical that effective strategies to promote health in these families be developed.

## CRITICAL THINKING

*Talk to a few grandmothers and grandfathers. How do they see their role in grandparenting? From their statements, what do you conclude about grandparenting today?*

**Relationship with Spouse or Partner** Of equal importance to rearing children and establishing wholesome affectional ties with them, and later with the grandchildren, is the middle-aged adult's relationship with his or her own spouse or partner.

**Stable Marital Relationship** A *happy marriage or partnership* has security and stability, although there are also struggles. The couple knows each other well; they no longer have to pretend with each other. Children can be a source of pleasure rather than concern, because conflicts that arose between partners about rearing or disciplining children vanish when those children leave home. Each has become accustomed to the ways of the other. Increased shared activity is

now the norm, and the sexual relationship can be better than ever before. Because the middle-aged adult is likely to have roots firmly planted in the community of choice, he or she is able to cultivate warm friendships with members of his or her own generation, and with parents, the family of the spouse, and the families of any married children. In middle adulthood, security, loyalty, and mutual emotional interest become more important as relationships mature. Most married individuals in mid-life voice considerable satisfaction with being married.[26]

Although there has been much discussion in the literature about the crisis of menopause and the *"empty nest,"* menopause and middle age may bring both men and women an enriched sense of self and an enhanced capacity to cope with life. The timing of the "empty nest" in the family life cycle depends on the person's (or the couple's) age when the last child was born.[27] The "empty nest," in recent years, has become increasingly a *"cluttered nest."*[28] Adult children are remaining at home considerably longer, and some adult children are returning (sometimes several times) to the parental home. Therefore, rates of adult child–middle-aged parent(s) co-residency have increased in the last few decades. These young adult children returning to the parental home are sometimes referred to as boomerang kids.[29] Research indicates that the presence of boomerang kids does not necessarily cast negative effects upon the marriages of middle-aged parents.[30] Mothers, in particular, are often pleased to have their children back. However,

## Tips for Today's Grandparents

- Establish your role as a grandparent
  - Consult and negotiate with your adult children (parents of your grandchildren) regarding their and your expectations of your role as a grandparent.
  - Supporting the values and decisions of the parents will allow you to be more involved in the lives of your grandchildren.

- Mentor your grandchildren
  - Be prepared to talk about lively, interesting, and even difficult topics.
  - Introduce them to new things and places (museums, trips, etc.).
  - Teach them the rudimentary skills they are less likely to have acquired (woodworking, baking, gardening, fishing, sewing, etc.).

- Engage your grandchildren
  - Listen to them; tune in to their interests (TV shows, hobbies, books, heroes, etc.).

- Invite them to help plan family events and gatherings with you and decorate your home and garden.
- Seek their input on films to see, or on computer tips.

- Be there for your grandchildren
  - Being fair doesn't necessarily mean treating each grandchild the same.
  - Be fair by accepting each grandchild's uniqueness, family situation, and needs at different times in his or her life.

- Keep in touch with your grandchildren
  - While mail and phone calls are still a good means of communication, bear in mind that today's grandchildren often use email.
  - Keeping in touch with them (especially over long distances) has never been easier with the help of the Internet.
  - Learning to use these communication tools will show your grandchildren not only that you care but also that you are a modern grandparent.

Source: Adapted from *Seniors in Canada, 2006 Report Card*. Ottawa: Government of Canada, 2005.

boomerang kids can have a disruptive effect if they "bounce" back and forth several times. Fortunately, this pattern is not common.[31]

## CRITICAL THINKING

*Is the "cluttered empty nest" syndrome a fact, or fiction, among some family groups? State the rationale for your opinion.*

**Unstable Marital Relationship** *Negative, critical feelings can gradually erode what was once a happy relationship.* At some point, the husband and wife may feel that they are each living with a stranger, although the potential remains for a harmonious marriage. Their relationship is changing because they are changing. *Marital crisis may result from:*

1. Feelings of disappointment with self
2. Feeling emotionally depleted because of communication problems with the spouse
3. Seeking some type of rebirth, a change of direction
4. Seeking escape from reality and superego pressures[32]

Often, the woman and man overlook the fact that they still do really love each other. They simply need to become reacquainted. It may be difficult for the middle-aged man and woman to "tune in" to each other because both are encountering problems peculiar to their own personality and sex. The woman may equate her ability to bear children with her capacity to enjoy sexual relationships, although they have nothing to do with each other. Whereas the woman needs the man's support to reinforce her femininity, he too is undergoing a crisis; he believes that he is losing his vigour, virility, and self-esteem, which are all primarily products of psychological reactions rather than physiologic inabilities.

Physical changes in appearance, changes in energy levels, and the multiple stresses of daily living can together result in an increased desire for physical intimacy and the need for the reassurance of continuing sexual attractiveness and competency. The middle-aged person is an active sexual being. Intercourse is not valued for procreation but for body contact, to express love and trust, and to reaffirm an integral part of the self-concept. The person may fear loss of potency and rejection by the partner, but talking with the spouse about feelings and preferences related to sexual activity can promote increased closeness.

Men and women differ in their sexual behaviour. Males reach their peak in their late teens and early twenties. Females peak in desire in the late thirties or forties and maintain that level of desire and activity past menopause into late middle age. The enjoyment of the quality of sexual relations in younger years, rather than the frequency, is a key factor in the maintenance of desire and activity in women. It tends to be the frequency of the relations and their enjoyment that are the important factors for men.[33]

**Extramarital Relationship** Some married people seek sexual intimacy outside of marriage. It is difficult to know how common extramarital sex is because the authenticity of such reports can not be verified. However, the fear of AIDS and other sexually transmitted diseases may have curtailed extramarital sex since its reported peak in the late 1960s and early 1970s.[34] In the community health setting, you will have opportunities to work with troubled families who are in conflict, who are contemplating divorce, or who have experienced separation and divorce.

**Reducing Marital and Partnership Stress** Helping the couple to regain earlier levels of closeness and happiness is worth the effort because the mature years can be regarded as the payoff on an investment of many years together, many problems shared, and countless expressions of love exchanged. Each knows that his or her way of life and well-being depend on the other, so there is a willingness to change outlook, habits, and lovemaking, if necessary, to enhance the marriage and partnership. You can help to promote such changes.

You will have opportunities to teach or counsel the middle-aged adult who is having difficulty in relating to his or her spouse or partner. Help the person determine, and then live out, the values of continuing to love and being patient and forgiving when the spouse or partner has been unfaithful. Facilitate a desire to change behaviour so that two people can grow together rather than apart. Work with the couple or refer them to counselling.

## CRITICAL THINKING

*What are some possible ways of reducing economic stress in same-sex marriages or partnerships?*

**Marital Losses** Marital losses that occur during middle age could be caused by the death of a spouse, separation, divorce, and the choice between remaining single or remarrying. A widowed, separated, or divorced individual journeys through a process of grief and must learn to adjust to the change in marital status. The nurse should assess the coping abilities and strategies of the middle-aged adult to handle the grief and loss associated with these life changes.[35] The individual may need someone to listen to feelings of anger, sadness, or guilt. You may be better able to listen, support, and encourage than family or friends. You can gently test reactions to determine whether he or she is ready for the shock of death by offering to call a clergyperson, or by asking whether family members need to be prepared for rapid deterioration of the spouse's condition. After death, the person may linger on the nursing unit—a place of support—rather than leaving for home, a very empty place. You may inform the person that many support groups exist to help people with the grieving process.[36]

The person's reaction to the death of a spouse depends on his or her personality and emotional makeup, the relationship enjoyed by the couple (how long they have been married, how long the mate has been ill), and religious, cultural, and ethnic background. One's reaction to death will also be determined by other factors that existed in the relationship. For example, there may be less sorrow now, or even relief, if the deceased spouse was abusive, or severely or chronically disabled, either physically or mentally.

The *loss of a spouse can mean many things:*

1. Loss of a sexual partner and lover, friend, companion, caretaker.

2. Loss of an audience for unguarded spontaneous conversation.

3. Loss of a "handy man," helper, accountant, plumber, or gardener, depending on the roles performed by the mate.

4. Financial problems, especially for the widow.

5. Secondary losses involving reduced income, which frequently means a change in residence, environment, lifestyle, and social involvements.

6. Return to the workforce.

7. Giving up any number of activities and experiences previously taken for granted.

The *widow* might pose a threat to women with husbands. These women might perceive her as competition, and she is a reminder of what they might experience. Among many friends, the widow is the odd person in number, so social engagements become stressful and are a constant reminder of the lost partner. Yet in contrast to assumptions, most widows are quite competent in managing their lives.[37]

Although the *widower* is more accepted socially, he too will experience painful gaps in his life. If the wife concentrated on keeping an orderly house, cooking regular and nutritious meals, and keeping his wardrobe in order, he may suddenly realize that what he had taken for granted is gone. The loss is even more significant if his wife was a "sounding board" or confidante in business matters. Such a loss can be especially felt if she was actively involved in raising children who are still in the home.

Your contact with the widow(er) can help to resolve the crisis. The death of a husband in middle age is more common than that of a wife. Therefore, you will encounter more widows. You can assist the person in the following ways as you promote crisis resolution:

1. Encourage the bereaved to talk about feelings, and help the widow(er) to find a supportive relationship.

2. Build up confidence and self-esteem in the widow(er), especially if he or she has lived a protected life.

3. Help him or her identify people, other than the children, who can assist with various tasks to avoid feelings of burden in any helper.

4. Encourage him or her to try new experiences, expand interests, join community groups, do volunteer work, seek new friends, and become a person in her (or his) own right.

5. Encourage getting a medical checkup and following practices of health promotion. Encourage self-care.

6. Inform him or her that books and articles can be useful to the widow(er).[38]

Caserta, Lund, and Rice have developed a Pathfinder Program that teaches widows and widowers many skills and promotes good self-care behaviours.[39] Some of the important topics in this intervention include stress management, immunizations, health screenings, medication management, physical and social activities, meal planning and preparation, and housekeeping skills.[40] In fact, learning new skills is one of the best ways to build self-esteem—at any age.

## CRITICAL THINKING

*If you were asked to develop a program for bereaved widows and widowers in the community, how would you begin?*

# Relationship with Aging Parents and Children

According to Chappell, Gee, McDonald, and Stones, the "sandwich generation" refers to mid-life families, especially women, who are caught between the care demands of children and the care demands of aging parents. Caregiving to elderly parents tends to occur after the dependent children have left home. Martin-Matthews states that the notion of the sandwich generation is largely a myth. That is, very few families in Canada face competing intergenerational demands simultaneously.[41] Although daughters provide most of the care to their elderly parents and family members, sons are increasingly involved in providing care and assistance across generations.[42]

**Responsibility for Elderly Relatives** The following cultural trends affect the dilemma of caring for older dependent relatives:[43]

- Long-term societal emphasis on personal independence and social mobility of middle-aged and young adults,

## The Gay Widower and His Partner's Family

You have been providing care to John, a gay middle-aged client who has just lost his partner of 20 years to cancer. John informs you that he is unable to attend his partner's funeral because the family has told John that he is not invited. John confides to you that he is quite depressed and is worried about his own future—both personally and professionally. He states that this partner's family does not acknowledge that their son was gay, or that he was living with another man for the past 20 years. John is aware that you know his partner's family well, as he has often seen you interact with them. From your discussions with the family, you know that they are ashamed of their son's gay lifestyle. John pleads with you to intervene on his behalf in an attempt to allow him to attend the funeral.

1. How do you respond initially to John?

2. How would you assist John to help him to build his self-esteem?

3. What strategies will you employ with this family?

which creates physical separateness of generational households and new kinship patterns of intimacy at a distance

- Focusing on the dynamics of the marriage bond and socialization of young children, with the emphasis on affection, compatibility, and the personal growth of each person in the nuclear family as the most important aspects of family life

- Longer lifespans of older people and the problem of caring for the older generation when they become dependent

**Filial responsibility** is *an attitude of personal responsibility toward the parents that emphasizes duty, protection, care, and financial support*, which are all indicators of the family's traditional protective function. Families provide nurturance and companionship through:

1. Visits and telephone calls

2. Providing information

3. Assistance in decision making

4. Transportation

5. Assistance with shopping, laundry, and household chores

6. Immediate response to crisis

7. Being a buffer against bureaucracies

8. Help in searching out services

9. Facilitation for continuity of individual–bureaucracy relations

In many cultures, the structure and style for the younger generation(s) have evolved through an extended family system to provide support, assistance, protection, and mobility.

Middle-aged children of various racial and ethnic groups are more likely than Caucasians to provide a home for elderly parents or other relatives. Some differences can be seen within cultural groups. For example, elderly Japanese are more likely to live with spouse, or alone, than are other Asian groups. Family members who come to Canada from Asia and the Middle East indicate that it is the son, and not the daughter, who has the closer relationship with an elderly mother.[44] The amount of research conducted on Asian male caregivers is scant.[45] Fortunately, however, many possibilities present themselves for nurses to conduct research on male caregivers in diverse cultures.

### CRITICAL THINKING

*In recent decades, Canada has had an immigration policy of family reunification. What does that mean regarding caregiving obligations of family members from diverse cultures?*

**Caregiver Role** Many issues related to caregiving and social support are important to Canadians. Demographic changes (such as the aging population and the increasing life expectancy), family restructuring (such as delayed marriage and low fertility), and increased ethnic diversity and intermarriage between ethnic groups all continue to affect the proportion of Canadians requiring and providing care.[46] Between 1981 and 2005, the number of seniors increased from 2.4 to 4.2 million, and their portion of the total population increased from 9 to 13 percent. Consequently, older age groups are increasingly more represented in the total Canadian population.[47] Ward-Griffin and Marshall state that a shift away from institutionalization has left the bulk of caregiving duties to family members and friends.[48]

Hawranik and Strain conducted a study on the experiences of informal caregivers of older adults in which they explored whether employment, the use of home care services, or other factors influenced the health of caregivers and their ability to cope with their caregiving and other responsibilities. The sample comprised 24 females and 6 males. The median age was 59 years.[49] The researchers found that caregiving, coupled with other responsibilities, can have serious health effects. Many participants spoke of physical changes and mental stress, particularly when caregiving took place with other responsibilities and various life events at the same time.

These findings have particular implications for nurses, who must take the caregiving situation into consideration by assessing the physical, mental, emotional, and spiritual health of the caregivers. They must also take into account the other responsibilities of the caregivers, recognizing that employment can have both positive and negative effects. In regards to home care services, the researchers state that nurses should determine from caregivers the extent to which they would like to be involved in the decision-making process. In addition, the caregivers' assessment of the situation should be taken into consideration. The policies of community agencies may need to be modified to address the potential dual role of the caregiver as a client and a member of the planning team. Nurses, as advocates of clients and agents of health promotion, can play an important role in modifying the focus of the system. Nurses can help to modify agency policies to include greater input by caregivers and clients.[50]

An interesting study by Gahagan and her associates explored the perceptions and experiences associated with caregiving and leisure among a group of caregivers from Nova Scotia.[51] A major theme in the findings revealed that a potential for leisure exerts a mediating effect on the health of these caregivers. The need for caregivers to engage in leisure outside the home was reported as an important facet for them. It seems apparent that in working with unpaid caregivers, nurses must consider their diverse health needs by accepting the benefits and burdens of caregiving and by encouraging that leisure be scheduled into their lives. The researchers state that the health of unpaid caregivers needs to be a social priority because they provide an essential social service.[52]

Various *factors that influence the caregiving role* include the following:[53]

- Seriousness of the elder's health status
- The caregiver–care recipient relationship and living arrangement
- Duration of the caregiving experience
- Other roles and responsibilities of the caregiver
- Overall coping effectiveness of the caregiver
- Caregiver sex and age
- Number of generations needing care
- Help and support from others—family or social agencies
- Information needed to carry out tasks related to physical care of the parent

*Meeting the dependency needs of parents may have many diverse effects:*[54]

- Financial hardship
- Physical symptoms such as sleeplessness and a decline in physical health, especially in the primary caregiver

- Emotional changes and symptoms in the caregiver and other family members, including feelings of frustration, inadequacy, anxiety, helplessness, depression, guilt, resentment, lowered morale, and emotional distance
- Emotional exhaustion related to restrictions on time and freedom heightened by increasing responsibility
- A sense of isolation from social activities
- Conflict because of competing demands, often with diversion from care created by other family members
- Difficulty in setting priorities
- Reduced family privacy
- Inability to project future plans
- Sense of losing control over life events
- Interference with job responsibilities brought about by late arrivals, absenteeism, or early departures when needed to take care of emergencies or even routine tasks
- Interference with lifestyle and social and recreational activities

Schumacher and her research team conducted a study to develop systematically the concept of family caregiving skill by using a process of qualitative analysis of interviews with clients and their family caregivers. They determined that family caregiver skill is defined as the ability to engage effectively and smoothly in nine processes (outlined in Table 13-1).[55] These particular indicators make up a valuable tool for nurses as they assess family caregiving skills.

The *caregiver role* is a major one, especially for the woman.[56] In Canada, 14 percent of all women and 10 percent of all men provide informal care to family or friends.[57] It is interesting to note that men represent a substantial group of caregivers. However, relatively little is known about the characteristics of men as caregivers. Taylor and Kopot conducted one study to examine men's experiences based on two major considerations: (1) the conceptualization of male spouses and sons providing care to individuals with Alzheimer's disease or related dementia, and (2) participation in a male support group called the "Breakfast Club."[58] The researchers found that, as caregivers, men shared common perceptions of stress and burden. They learned from each other how to adapt to the ever-changing trajectory of Alzheimer's disease. Further, the support group was a successful intervention approach providing an opportunity for men to deal with their feelings in a safe, confidential, and supportive environment.[59]

## CRITICAL THINKING

*Compare and contrast the roles of formal and informal caregiving.*

## Table 13-1 Indicators of Skill in Family Caregiving Processes

| Skill | Indicators |
|---|---|
| Monitoring | Notices subtle changes |
| | Uses appropriate vigilance |
| | Makes accurate observations |
| | Keeps a written record when appropriate |
| Interpreting | Recognizes deviations from normal or expected clinical course |
| | Recognizes that something is "different" or "wrong" |
| | Judges the seriousness of a problem |
| | Asks detailed questions for the purpose of developing an explanation |
| Making decisions | Takes into account multiple illness care demands |
| | Weighs the importance of conflicting priorities |
| | Attends to multiple care issues at the same time |
| | Thinks ahead about the possible consequences of a given action |
| Taking action | Uses effective "reminders" to time actions |
| | Paces actions to correspond with the ill person's pace |
| | Takes own needs into account in timing actions |
| | Organizes multiple actions systematically |
| | Develops routines to manage complex tasks |
| | Has the ability to take action on multiple issues at the same time |
| Making adjustments | Modifies long-standing routines to accommodate the illness situation |
| | Modifies environment to accommodate the illness situation |
| | Searches for an alternative when one illness care strategy no longer works |
| | Uses creativity in problem-solving |
| Accessing resources | Seeks resources wisely; casts a broad net |
| | Uses advice judiciously |
| | Takes initiative in seeking resources |
| | Makes own needs known |
| Providing hands-on care | Performs procedures safely |
| | Performs procedures gently |
| | Pays attention to ill person's comfort |
| Working together with the ill person | Perceives when to take a more active role in illness care |
| | Perceives when to step back |
| | Provides care in a way that is meaningful in the context of the care receiver's personal history and identity |
| Negotiating the health care system | Evaluates care received in the health care system |
| | Advocates for patient and/or self when necessary |
| | Seeks assistance from health care providers in a timely way |

Source: Schumacher, K.L., B. J. Stewart, P.G. Archbold, M.J. Dodd, and S.L. Dibble, Family Caregiving Skill: Development of the Concep., *Research in Nursing & Health,* 23 (2000), 191. Adapted and reproduced with the permission of John Wiley & Sons, Inc., 2007.

Over several decades, the disciplines of social science and health care have explored the stresses and burdens of the major consequences of caregiving.[60] These scholarly articles and research studies have enriched the understanding of caregiving, but they did not yield a total picture of the process of becoming a caregiver.

Perry conducted a study on wives giving care to spouses with dementia. The grounded theory study describes the wives' experiences as a process of interpretive caring. Perry states that this process is neutral and allows for positive aspects of caring to be considered along with grief and frustration.[61] Another study, by Bar-David, described caregiver self-development through the caregiving journey.[62] Bar-David concludes that the caregiver's capacity for caring was found to be at the core. It unfolds in three phases: (1) development of caring capacity for the care recipient, (2) development of capacity for self-care, and (3) development of caring capacity for others. The four elements of caring capacity (perception, motivation, competency, and action) are expressed in relation to the care recipient, to the self, and to less familiar others.[63]

These studies reflect the positive aspects of caregiving. Health professionals need to focus on the strengths of the family in the caregiving situation. As well as assessing the burden of caregiving, it is necessary to explore the rewards that the caregiver is experiencing.

One of the most difficult decisions facing caregivers, when parents become aged and dependent, concerns the housing arrangement. The older daughter is usually the one to take the dependent parent into her home. Or, the unmarried adult child might move into the parent's home. When the parent(s) cannot manage living alone, the middle-aged person may not have the room to take the parent(s) into his or her home. Even if there is adequate space, if all members of the household are working or going to school, finding someone reliable to stay with the parent during the day could be difficult. Such an arrangement or the use of adult daycare is less cost prohibitive, however, than placing the parent who is in poor health in an institution. Most communities do not have adequate, or any, daycare facilities for elderly adults. Placing the parent(s) in an institution may be the only answer. Typically, though, it is considered as the last resort.

**Health Care Role** You are in a key position to help the middle-aged adult work through feelings of frustration, guilt, and anger about the increased responsibility and past conflicts or old hurts from parents or siblings.

The middle-aged adult who verbally expresses great irritation typically loves the older relative very much. Assist the middle-aged adult to gain a sense of satisfaction and reward from the help he or she gives, and from the greater understanding and (often unstated) appreciation of the person being helped. The generation gap and negative feelings that exist between the middle-aged adult and elderly person can be overcome with love, realistic expectations, a sense of forgiveness, and the realization that sometimes it is all right to say "no" to the demands of the elders. The rewards the caregiver experiences will assist her or him toward a desire to promote positive outcomes for the person being cared for.

One study indicated that teaching the caregiver stress management and time management techniques reduced the sense of burden more than did participation in a support group.[64] Encouraging the caregiver to maintain other roles, outside of caregiving and family roles, can also increase the sense of caregiver well-being and health. Refer to a counsellor or spiritual leader if necessary. Counselling can promote a resolution of feelings that in turn fosters a more harmonious relationship between the middle-aged adult and parents.

---

CRITICAL THINKING

*In what ways can you foster the creative abilities of family caregivers?*

---

Policy analysts have attempted to address the costs borne by the caregiver. In particular, the issue of financial compensation for family members providing informal care to elderly relatives has been debated for some time in Canada and around the world. One program that financially compensates family members for the care of an elderly relative is Nova Scotia Home Life Support.[65] The Canadian Caregiver Coalition's broad aim is to ensure the respect and support of family caregivers, and to emphasize that they are not a substitute for public responsibility in health and social care (see the Interesting Websites section at the end of the chapter).

# Death of Parents in Adulthood

A critical time for the adult is when each parent dies, regardless of whether the relationship between parent(s) and offspring was harmonious or conflictual. The first death of a parent signals finiteness and mortality of the self, of the other parent, and of other loved ones. When the other parent dies, the adult is an orphan. The person will probably feel forlorn and alone, especially if there are few other relatives or friends. Sometimes, no other living relatives are left and there are no sons, so that the adult offspring represents the last of the family line. The person may question who and what will be remembered and by whom. This is a time of spiritual and philosophical searching, whether the adult child is alone, has siblings, or has other relatives.

Throughout the period of parental loss, you may be a key person in helping the adult survivor relive, express, and sort out feelings. Accept that any close relationship will not always go smoothly. Achieve a balance between happy, sad, and angry memories and feelings in regard to the parent(s). Finally, through such counselling, the person can mature to accept and like the self and other significant persons better, and can change behaviour patterns so that future relationships are less thorny.

CRITICAL THINKING

*What are some second-order changes in family status required for the single middle-aged person to proceed developmentally?*

## PHYSIOLOGIC CONCEPTS

You are in a key position to help the middle-aged adult work through feelings about the meaning of mid-life changes and ways to prevent or minimize their effects.

## Physical Characteristics

The growth cycle continues with physical changes in the middle years, and different body parts age at different rates. One day, the person is suddenly aware of being "old," or middle-aged. Not all people decline alike. How quickly they decline depends on the stresses and strains they have undergone, and on the health promotion measures that were maintained. If the person has always been active, he or she will likely continue with little slowdown. People from lower socioeconomic groups often show signs of aging earlier than people from more affluent socioeconomic groups because of their years of hard physical labour, poorer nutritional status, and shortage of money for beauty aids to cover the signs of aging.[66]

Now, the person looks in the mirror and sees changes that others may have noticed some time ago. Grey, thinning hair, wrinkles, coarsening features, decreased muscular tone, weight gain, varicosities, and capillary breakage may be the first signs of impending age.

Because a number of your clients will be middle-aged, you are in a key position to help them, first, understand the physiologic changes that occur in middle age and, second, work through feelings about these changes, reintegrate the body image, and find specific ways to remain as healthy as possible. Use the following information to assist you in listening, teaching, reaffirming a positive self-concept, and counselling.

**Physical Changes**  Table 13-2 summarizes the physical changes that occur in middle age, the physiological reasons for the changes and characteristics that are commonly seen, and the implications for health promotion and client teaching.[67]

**Table 13-2  Physical Changes and Characteristics of Middle Age and Health Promotion Implications**

| Body System or Physical Parameter | Change/Characteristic | Implications for Health Promotion |
|---|---|---|
| *Endocrine and Reproductive Systems* | | |
| Women | Decline in production of neurotransmitters that stimulate hypothalamus to signal pituitary to release sex hormones | Reproductive cycle is ended; this may represent sexual liberation or loss of femininity. |
| | Less estrogen synthesized | Counsel about meaning of femininity. |
| | No estrogen produced by ovaries; menses stops | Support group may be helpful. |
| | Aging oocytes (eggs) destroy necessary genetic material for reproduction | Instruct in Kegel exercises. Hormone replacement therapy may be prescribed. |
| | Uterine changes make implantation of blastocyte unlikely | Artificial (water-soluble) lubrication can be used during intercourse to reduce |
| | Gradual atrophy of tissues: | discomfort. |
| | Uterus and cervix become smaller | Regular sexual intercourse maintains |
| | Vulvar epithelium thins | lubrication and elasticity of tissue. |
| | Labia majora and minora fatten | |
| | Vaginal mucosal lining thinner, drier, pale (20%–40% women; some never experience this) | |
| | Natural lubrication during intercourse decreases | |
| | Neuroendocrine symptoms, such as hot flashes and night sweats followed by | Avoid precipitating factors such as hot drinks, caffeine, alcohol, stress, and warm |

*(continued)*

Table 13-2 (continued)

| Body System or Physical Parameter | Change/Characteristic | Implications for Health Promotion |
|---|---|---|
| | chilling, fatigue, nausea, dizziness, headache, palpitations, and paresthesias may occur. | environment. Counsel to stop smoking. Hormone replacement therapy may reduce symptoms. |
| Men | Testosterone production gradually decreases, which eventually causes: Degeneration of cells in tubules Production of fewer sperm More time needed to achieve erection Less forceful ejaculation Testes less firm and smaller | Sperm production continues to death, so man is capable of producing children. Premature ejaculation is less likely, which may contribute to more enjoyable intercourse. Practise Kegel exercises for firmer erections. |
| *Basal Metabolism Rate (BMR)* | | |
| Minimum energy used in resting state | BMR declines 2% per decade<br><br>Gradually reduces as ratio of lean body mass to adipose tissue decreases (metabolic needs of fat are less than for lean tissue) | If eating pattern is maintained, 3 to 4 pounds are gained per decade<br>Fewer calories (2%) need to be consumed, even if the person exercises regularly, to avoid weight gain. |
| Weight | Gain should not occur; weight gain occurs if as many calories consumed as earlier: wider hips, thicker thighs, larger waist, and more abdominal mass | Overweight contributes to a number of health problems; crash diets should be avoided. |
| *Integumentary System* | | |
| *Sebaceous oil glands* | Produce less sebum secretions, skin drier and cracks more easily More pronounced in women after menopause than in men of same age | Protect and lubricate skin with lotion or moisturizer. Avoid excess soap and drying substances on skin. Avoid excessive strong sun and wind exposure. |
| *Sweat glands* | Decrease in size, number, and function | Ability to maintain even body temperature is affected; dress in layers to maintain comfort. |
| *Skin* | Skin wrinkles, tissue sags, and pouches under eyes form because: Epidermis flattens and thins with age, collagen in dermis becomes more fibrous, less gel-like Elastin loses elasticity, causing loss of skin turgor Loss of muscle tone causes sagging jowls | Wrinkles are less apparent with use of moisturizer or lotion. Wrinkled appearance of skin is made worse by excess exposure to sun or sunburn; use sunscreen. Skin is more prone to injury; healing is slower. Use humidifier in home. |
| Women | Estrogen decrease gradually causes skin and mucous membranes to lose thickness and fluids; skin and mucous membranes thinner, drier, and begin atrophy Estrogen decrease gradually causes breasts to sag and flatten | Avoid burns and bruises. Use lotions. Maintain support with correctly fitted brassiere. Maintain erect posture. |

*(continued)*

Table 13-2 (continued)

| Body System or Physical Parameter | Change/Characteristic | Implications for Health Promotion |
|---|---|---|
| *Hair* | Progressive loss of melanin from hair bulb causes grey hair in most adults by age 50; hair thins and growth slows; hair rest and growth cycles change | Slow hair loss by gentle brushing, avoiding excess heat from hair dryer, and avoiding chemical treatment. |
| Women | Estrogen decrease may gradually cause increased growth of facial hair<br>Hair loss not as pronounced as in male | Accept change.<br>Manage cosmetically. |
| Men | Testosterone decrease causes gradual loss of hair<br>Hereditary male-pattern baldness occurs with receding hairline and monk's spot area on back of head | Accept change.<br>Manage with styling, hairpiece, or hair transplant. |
| *Muscular System* | Slight decrease in number of muscle fibres; about 10% loss in muscle size from ages 30 to 60<br>Gradual loss of lean body mass<br>Muscle tissue gradually replaced by adipose unless exercise is maintained<br>Most loss of muscle occurs in back and legs<br>Grip strength decreases with age<br>Gradual increase in subcutaneous fat | Physical exercise and fitness, proper nutrition, and healthy lifestyle can improve or sustain muscle strength during middle age.<br>Variations in peak muscular activity depend on type of exercise. |
| *Skeletal System* | Gradual flattening of intervertebral disks and loss of height of individual vertebrae cause compression of spinal column | Maintain erect posture.<br>Maintain adequate calcium intake (1000–1500 mg daily).<br>Exercise maintains bone mass and joint flexibility, improves balance and agility, and reduces fatigue.<br>Loss of height occurs in later life. |
| Men and women | At age 70, osteoporosis risk equal in men and women unless vitamin D has been taken to increase bone density | Vitamin D decrease risk of fractures. |
| Women | Estrogen reduction increases decalcification of bones, bone resorption, decreased bone density, and gradual osteoporosis<br>Cultural differences: Caucasians and Asians more likely than Latinos and blacks to suffer bone porosity because their bones are less dense and they lose mass more quickly | Maintain exercise and calcium intake.<br>Maintain erect posture.<br>Maintain calcium and good nutrition intake.<br>Teach safety factors; forearms, hips and spinal vertebrae are most vulnerable to fractures.<br>Supplemental vitamin D and regular small amounts of exposure to sunlight improve calcium absorption.<br>Avoid smoking, high alcohol intake, and high caffeine intake, all of which interfere with nutrition. Caffeine causes calcium loss.<br>Women may eventually be 7.5 cm shorter if they have vertebral osteoporosis. |

*(continued)*

Table 13-2 (continued)

| Body System or Physical Parameter | Change/Characteristic | Implications for Health Promotion |
|---|---|---|
| | | Dowager's hump will form in cervical and upper thoracic area if osteoporosis occurs. Women who have taken oral contraceptives for 6 or more years have higher bone density in lumbar spine and femoral neck. |
| *Neurologic System* | Speed of nerve conduction, nerve impulse travelling from brain to muscle fibre, decreases 5% by age 50, and only 10% through life cycle Brain structural changes minimal; gradual loss of neurons does not affect cognition | Sensation to heat and cold and speed of reflexes may be impaired. Teach safety factors. Functional abilities are maintained, and learning from life experiences enhances functional abilities. |
| *Vision* | Average 60-year-old requires twice the illumination of 20-year-old to do close work Eyes begin to gradually change at about 40 or 50, causing **presbyopia** (*farsightedness*) Lens less elastic, loses accommodation Cornea increases in curvature and thickness, loses lustre Iris responds less well to light changes; pupils smaller Retina begins to lose rods and cones Optic nerve fibres begin to decrease | Wear brimmed hat and sunglasses that block UV rays to protect vision. Person eventually needs bifocals or trifocals to see small print or focus on near objects. Eyes do not adapt as quickly to darkness, bright lights or glare (implications for safety and night driving). More light is needed to see well. |
| *Hearing* | Auditory nerve and bones of inner ear gradually change Gradual decrease in ability to detect certain tones and certain consonants Loss of hearing from high-pitched sounds | Reduce exposure to loud work machinery or equipment; wear ear protectors. Reduce exposure to loud stereo, radio, or electronic music. Cross-cultural studies show our high-tech culture contributes to increasing and earlier impairment. Hearing aids, correctly chosen, or surgery may correct hearing impairment. |
| Voice | | |
| Women | Estrogen decrease gradually causes lower pitch of voice | |
| Men | Testosterone decrease gradually causes higher pitch of voice | |
| *Cardiovascular System* | Efficiency of heart may drop to 80% between 30 and 50 Decreased elasticity in muscles in heart and blood vessels Decreased cardiac output | Regular aerobic exercise maintains heart function and normal blood pressure. Inactivity affects system negatively. Quit smoking. Maintain healthy diet. |

(*continued*)

Table 13-2 (continued)

| Body System or Physical Parameter | Change/Characteristic | Implications for Health Promotion |
|---|---|---|
| | Cardiovascular disease risk for women equal to that of men by age 70 because reduced estrogen causes lipid changes, increase in low-density lipoproteins (LDLs), decrease in high-density lipoproteins (HDLs), and gradual increase in total serum cholesterol | Take regular low doses of Aspirin. Maintain low-cholesterol diet. |
| *Respiratory System* | | |
| | Gradual loss of lung elasticity Thorax shortens Chest cage stiffer Breathing capacity reduced to 75% Chest wall muscles gradually lose strength, reducing respiratory efficiency | Regular exercise enhances respiratory efficiency. Inactivity affects system negatively. |
| *Urinary System* | | |
| Women | Glomerular filtration rate gradually decreases Loss of bladder muscle tone and atrophy of supporting ligaments and tissue in late middle age causes urgent urination, possibly cystocele, rectocele, and urine prolapse | Maintain adequate fluid intake; drink 8 glasses of water daily. Instruct in Kegel exercises as follows: Draw in perivaginal muscles (pubococcygeus muscle) and anal sphincter as if to control urination, without contracting abdominal, buttock, or inner thigh muscles. Maintain contraction for 10 seconds. Follow with 10 seconds of relaxation. Perform exercises 30–80 times daily. |
| Men | Hypertrophy of prostate begins in late middle age; enlarging prostate around urethra causes frequent urination, dribbling, and nocturia | Urinary stasis may predispose to infections. Drink adequate amount of water. Surgery may be necessary. |

## Hormonal Changes

**Female Climacteric** This is the era of life known as *menopause* for the woman, or the *climacteric* for either sex. The terms are often used interchangeably. **Menopause** is *the permanent cessation of menstruation preceded by a gradually decreasing menstrual flow.* The term **perimenopausal years** denotes *a time of gradual diminution of ovarian function and a gradual change in endocrine status from before menopause through one year after menopause.* The **climacteric** is the *period in life when important physiologic changes occur, with the cessation of the woman's reproductive ability and the period of lessening sexual activity in the male.* Basic to the changing physiology of the middle years is the decline of hormonal production.[68]

Contrary to myth (see Table 13-3), depression or other symptomatology is neither inevitable nor clearly related to the perimenopausal or climacteric years.[69] Most women feel relieved, or neutral about menopause; only a small percentage view it negatively.[70]

Menopause is seen as a normal life event, although some of the physical changes can be problematic. In Canada, most women and men, and a growing number of scientists, realize the great number of roles and the enjoyable life that awaits one beyond menopause. A wellness approach is needed as a routine strategy for health promotion during this life event.

**Male Climacteric** This comes in the fifties or early sixties, although the symptoms may not be as pronounced as in the female climacteric. A man's "change of life" may be passed almost imperceptibly, but he usually notices it when he makes comparisons with past feelings and performances. Testosterone

**Table 13-3** Myths about Menopause

| Myth | Fact |
|------|------|
| 1. Menopause is a deficiency disease and catastrophe. | 1. Menopause is a normal developmental process. |
| 2. Most women have serious disability during menopause | 2. Most women pass through it with a minimum of distress. Some have no noticeable symptoms or reactions and simply stop menstruation. |
| 3. Menopause is the end of life. | 3. The average life expectancy for today's 50-year-old woman is many years; one-third of her life is post-menopausal. Postmenopause is a time of new zest. |
| 4. Menopausal women are more likely to be depressed than other people (older men are handsome, distinguished, and desirable; older women are worn out and useless). | 4. Menopausal depression in middle age is likely to be caused by social stressors:<br>a. The double standard of aging<br>b. Caregiver demands<br>c. Loss of loved ones<br>d. Loss of roles<br>e. Other health problems (the decreased level of estrogen affects neurotransmitters that regulate mood, appetite, sleep, and pain perception) |
| 5. Numerous symptoms accompany menopause. | 5. Predictable manifestations of menopause are:<br>a. Change in menstrual pattern<br>b. Transient warm sensations or vasomotor instability (hot flashes) to some degree (47 to 85 percent of women)<br>c. Vaginal dryness in some women |
| 6. Hot flashes are "in the woman's head." | 6. Vasomotor instability results from hemodynamic compensatory mechanisms. Until the body adjusts to less estrogen, hypothalamic instability causes dips in body's core temperature. The flash is the body's adaptive response to equalize peripheral and core temperatures through dermal heat loss. |
| 7. The woman may have a heart attack during a hot flash. | 7. The tachycardia that occurs during a flush is the body's adaptive response to skin temperature changes. |
| 8. The woman loses sexual desire during and after menopause. | 8. Vaginal changes may cause some discomfort, which would reduce libido. Psychosocial concerns about the empty nest, partner's loss of sexual capacity, or expectation of loss of libido are more likely the cause than reduced estrogen. |
| 9. The indicators of menopause are the various symptoms women experience. | 9. Women may have regular menstrual cycles with decreased estrogen levels; hot flashes may occur before menopause begins. |
| 10. Only women have to worry about osteoporosis. | 10. By age 70, osteoporosis risk is equal in men and women. |

production begins to decline about 1 percent a year during middle adulthood. Although the sperm count indicates a slow decline, this decline does not affect fertility. However, a drop in testosterone can reduce one's sexual drive.[71] Some men who experience an abnormally rapid decline in testosterone production report symptoms similar to those experienced by some menopausal women: hot flashes, chills, rapid heart rate, and nervousness. Some physicians label this drop *andropause*, and consider it as a parallel to menopause.[72]

**Sexual Dysfunction** The decline in testosterone production can be expected to reduce the sex drive of the middle-aged man. Erections are less frequent and full and require more stimulation. However, smoking, diabetes, elevated cholesterol levels, and hypertension are reasons for many erectile problems in men.[73] Some men have been prescribed medications such as Viagra, Cialis, and Levitra to treat impotence and erectile dysfunction. However, the manufacturers of these three drugs, in consultation with Health Canada, are advising individuals to consult their physicians and seek immediate attention if they experience vision loss or vision-related problems while taking these drugs.[74]

In doing an assessment, it is important for the nurse to ask the middle-aged adult male what medications they are taking and whether they are experiencing any visual problems.

The middle-aged person may subtly, hesitantly, or openly discuss problems of sexual function with you. Listen carefully. Let him or her know that such problems are not unusual. You may not know the answers, but your listening can help the person make a decision regarding seeking medical care or counselling. The person must realize the need to change behaviour. You can assist in attitude and value clarification about sexuality and sexual behaviour. Refer the person or couple to a counsellor who can help with physical and emotional problems. Sometimes a change in medication dosage, or a modification in treatment regimen, can reduce sexual dysfunction.

**Menopause** Menopause usually occurs when a woman is between her late forties and early fifties, and it can last until beyond age 55. By definition, menopause means the cessation of menstruation for a full year.[75] In women, the process of aging causes changed secretion of follicle-stimulating hormone (FSH), which brings about progressive and irreversible changes in the ovaries, leading to menopause and the loss of childbearing ability. The primordial follicles, which contain the ovum and grow into vesicular follicles with each menstrual cycle, become depleted, and their ability to mature declines. Finally, ovulation ceases because all ova have either degenerated or have been released. Thus, the cyclic production of progesterone and estrogen fails to occur and levels rapidly fall below the amount necessary to induce endometrial bleeding. (The adrenal glands continue to produce some estrogen.) The menstrual cycle becomes irregular; periods of heavy bleeding alternate with amenorrhea for one or two years, eventually ceasing altogether.[76] Consistent or regular excessive bleeding may be a sign of pathology, not of the approaching menopause.

The pituitary continues to produce FSH and luteinizing hormone (LH), but the aging ovary is incapable of responding to its stimulation. With the pituitary no longer under the normal cyclic or feedback influence of ovarian hormones, it becomes more active, producing excessive gonadotropins, especially FSH. A disturbed endocrine balance influences some of the symptoms of menopause. Although the ovaries are producing less estrogen and progesterone, the adrenals

continue to produce some hormones, thus helping to maintain younger feminine characteristics for some time.[77]

During the perimenopausal period (approximately five years), some discomforts occur in a small percentage of women. Vasomotor changes cause hot flashes associated with chilly sensations, dizziness, headaches, perspiration, palpitations, water retention, nausea, muscle cramps, fatigability, insomnia, and paresthesia of fingers and toes. Many symptoms, including irritability, depression, emotional lability, and palpitations, are frequently attributed to menopause. Some women experience *no* symptoms, only a decrease, then cessation, of menses. The great majority of women experience no effect in their sexual relationships from menopause. Most find menopause a time of integration, balance, liberation, confidence, and action.[78]

Difficulties experienced during menopause are associated with concurrent life change such as recent loss, or marital, psychological, or social stress. The cause of the symptoms is apparently more complex than simple estrogen deficit. Psychological factors such as anger, anxiety, and excitement are considered important in precipitating hot flashes in susceptible women. They give rise to excess heat production or retention such as a warm environment, muscular work, and hot food. The symptoms may arise, however, without any clear psychological or heat-stimulating mechanism.[79]

The Heart and Stroke Foundation provides a Menopause Checklist that women can complete online, print out, and take to the doctor (see the Interesting Websites section at the end of the chapter).

---

### CRITICAL THINKING

*What health teaching episodes could you implement for women experiencing hot flashes?*

---

**Hormone Replacement Therapy** For many years in Canada, women have been prescribed estrogen with or without progestin hormone replacement therapy (HRT) to relieve some of the symptoms of menopause.[80] Recent scientific studies have identified significant risks associated with this therapy.

In 1991, the U.S. National Institutes of Health launched the Women's Health Initiative (WHI), a set of studies involving healthy postmenopausal women that was carried out in 40 U.S. centres. The WHI included a clinical trial to evaluate the risks and benefits of the two types of HRT (in pill form) and to observe how they affected the incidence of heart disease, breast cancer, colorectal cancer, and fractures in postmenopausal women.[81] The trial was divided into two arms:

■ One arm involved more than 16 000 postmenopausal women aged 50 to 79 who had not had a hysterectomy. They took pills daily that were either a combination of estrogen and progestin or a placebo pill.

- The second arm involved more than 10 000 women who had received a hysterectomy and who took either estrogen pills alone or a placebo.[82]

The safety monitoring board of the WHI recommended premature cessation of the combination Premarin/Provera arm, and concluded that there were more risks than benefits among the group using the combined HRT.[83] That is, the risks of breast cancer and cardiovascular disease, although small, outweighed potential benefits (reduced incidence of osteoporotic fractures and the possibility of colorectal cancer) in these asymptomatic subjects.[84] The WHI estrogen-alone trial continued until March 2004, when it too was stopped because of lack of cardiovascular protection.[85]

The negative findings obtained in the WHI study are considered to be an important breakthrough for women's health. The extensive media coverage of the WHI study results was partially responsible for the resulting fear about the use of HRT in the postmenopausal population. Many additional studies have been conducted in order to confirm or refute those results. As a consequence, public opinion is now ambivalent. The medical community in general has come to the consensus that HRT is not indicated for the prevention of chronic disease.[86] Two benefits of the use of HRT, supported by the evidence, are symptom relief and the prevention of bone loss and fractures.[87]

In a study conducted at the University of Montreal and Université de Sherbrooke, the researchers examined the impact of the WHI on the rate of HRT prescription. They found that the trend in HRT dropped less than a year after the WHI publication.[88] In a related study, Wathen explored women's information-seeking behaviour and decision-making trends regarding menopause, HRT, and the use of complementary and alternative medicines (CAM) during menopause. She found that the vast majority of women in the study who had either stopped or were thinking about stopping HRT actively sought information to help them make the decision. Most frequently they went to their physicians to seek answers to their questions.[89] This particular finding has important implications for nurses who work with middle-aged women. Nurses should be equipped with resources to help these women make decisions regarding HRT.

Humphries and Gill conclude that the use of HRT should be individualized, with the risks and benefits of HRT for each woman being taken into consideration.[90]

## CRITICAL THINKING

*What health promoting strategies would you use to counsel a woman who is considering HRT?*

## Emotional Changes Related to Physical Changes

Depression, irritability, and a change in sexual desire may occur following certain physical changes, but they do not always occur. Some women fear the loss of sexual identity. Actually, earlier personality patterns and attitudes are more responsible for the symptoms than is the cessation of glandular activity. Women who had low self-esteem and unfulfilled life satisfaction are more likely to experience difficulties during menopause. Reactions to menopause are consistent with reactions to other life changes, including other reproductive turning points, such as puberty. Women with high motherliness scores and heavy investment in childbearing react more severely to menopause.

Postmenopausal women generally take a more positive view than premenopausal women, agreeing that menopause creates no major discontinuity in life, except for the underlying biological changes. Women, in fact, have a relative degree of control over their symptoms, and they need not inevitably have difficulties. In general, menopausal status is not reliably associated with measurable anxiety in any group.

Women in various cultures experience menopause differently. A study of Japanese, American, and Canadian women revealed that Japanese women experience menopause differently than Western women. Fewer than 10 percent reported hot flashes, with little or no physical or psychological discomfort. This was substantiated by physician survey. There is no Japanese term for "hot flash," although their language makes many subtle distinctions about body states. In Japan, menopause is regarded as a *normal* life event, *not* a medical condition requiring treatment, in contrast to beliefs in the United States and Canada. Hot flashes are rare among Mayan women, North African women in Israel, Navaho women, and Indonesian women.[91]

Cultural attitudes affect the ways in which women interpret the physical sensations of menopause, and their interpretation of menopause as a life event. Childbearing and nutritional practices can influence the experience of menopause. Mayan women, who are almost constantly pregnant or breastfeeding, look forward to menopause as the end of a burden. Asian dishes using tofu or other soybeans products have more phytoestrogens, an estrogen-like compound, which may lower premenopausal hormone levels. When natural estrogen levels fall, the phytoestrogens act like estrogen in inhibiting menopausal symptoms. Japanese women, the longest-lived women in the world, have a lower incidence of osteoporosis than Caucasian women in North America despite lower average bone mass. Japanese women are about one-fourth as likely as North American women to die of coronary heart disease or breast cancer. Besides phytoestrogens in the diet, Japanese women eat well-balanced diets, exercise throughout life, and seldom smoke or drink.[92]

## Nutritional Needs

In Canada, the revised *Eating Well with Canada's Food Guide* is recommended.[93] For the first time, a national food guide has been created that reflects the values, traditions, and food choices of First Nations, Inuit, and Métis. It can be an important tool for individuals, families, and communities to learn about and share ways of eating well, including the use of traditional as well as store-bought foods.

For middle-aged men and women over 50, the need for vitamin D increases significantly. Vitamin D needs increase because the skin has a reduced capacity to produce the vitamin. Vitamin D and calcium are important for bone strength and they help to reduce the risk of osteoporosis and fractures in older adults. Consuming 500 mL (2 cups) of milk each day will provide approximately 5 micrograms (200 IU) of vitamin D. Adding a supplement containing 10 micrograms (400 IU) of vitamin D will ensure that individuals over 50 meet the recommended intakes. Therefore, all adults over the age of 50 should take a daily vitamin D supplement of 10 micrograms (400 IU) in addition to following Canada's Food Guide.[94]

The recommended number of daily Food Guide servings for females and males are the following:

- Vegetables and fruits: females and males, 7 servings
- Grain products: females 6 servings and males 7 servings
- Milk and alternatives: females and males, 3 servings
- Meat and alternatives: females 2 servings and males 3 servings

See Figure 13-1 for a sample one-day menu for Isabelle, a 60-year-old female.[95]

The body mass index (BMI) is the most useful indicator, to date, of health risks associated with being overweight or underweight. In the body weight classification system, categories of BMI are used to identify levels of health risk. A BMI in the normal range has been shown in population-wide studies to be associated with the lowest relative risk of morbidity and mortality.[96]

Obesity is a growing health issue in Canada. In attempting to understand the dramatic increase in obesity, it has been learned that since the rate of increase is so severe and sudden, environmental factors and not genetic factors play the more causal role. It seems that caloric consumption has increased generally in Canada, and a lower amount of calories is being expended.[97] Brien and her researchers investigated the relationships that exist among physical activity, cardiorespiratory fitness, BMI, and the development of future obesity. The sample included 459 adults, 18 years and older, from the 2002–2004 Canadian Physical Activity Longitudinal Study (PALS). The results indicate that cardiorespiratory fitness and previous BMI are important predictors of future weight gain and obesity. Both of these predictors should be incorporated into strategies to identify individuals who are at increased risk of obesity.[98]

Teach people to limit their intake of carbohydrates and foods with high fat, saturated fat, and cholesterol content, including foods with "empty" calories such as rich desserts, candies, fatty foods, gravies, sauces, and alcoholic and non-diet cola beverages. Substitute sparkling waters or reduced-calorie wines or beers. The intake of salty food should be limited. Herbs, spices, and lemon juice can be used for flavouring. Obesity should be avoided because it is a factor in diabetes, cardiovascular and hypertensive disease, and problems with mobility, such as arthritis.[99]

Drinking too much coffee or tea can be a serious problem in middle age. Intake should be limited to one or two cups daily, including decaffeinated forms, and be drunk between meals. There may be a direct association between coffee and high blood cholesterol levels. Coffee and tea, other than green tea, should be avoided if there is a family history of heart disease, or if the person is overweight, eats a high-fat diet, and does not exercise.[100]

Joining self-help groups such as Weight Watchers or Take Off Pounds Sensibly (TOPS) is effective for many people. It is definitely possible to change overeating habits and to lose weight during middle age.

Teach the middle-aged person to avoid using extreme diets that decrease weight quickly. In such diets, large weight losses are often quickly followed by rapid weight gains. Each gain–lose cycle reduces the total muscle mass results in weight loss and increases body fat, because regained weight appears in the form of adipose tissue. Adipose tissue burns fewer calories than muscle, so each round of dieting makes it more difficult to lose weight and maintain weight loss. Extreme low-calorie diets should also be avoided because, with them, the basic metabolic rate becomes lower so that, even with restricted calories, little weight is lost.

The promotion of healthy eating in Canada carries significant implications for improving the health of populations—not only at a local level, but globally as well. Raine, in her article, applies a population health perspective to examine the complex set of interactions among the determinants of healthy eating. For example, she states that the social environment, social status (income, education, and gender), and cultural milieu are determinants of healthy eating that may affect food choice. Collective determinants could include the interpersonal environment created by family and peers, the physical environment that determines food availability and accessibility, and the economic environment in which food becomes a commodity

**Figure 13-1** Sample one-day menu for Isabelle, a 60-year-old female

| | Recommended Daily Food Guide Servings | | | |
|---|---|---|---|---|
| | Vegetables and Fruit | Grain Products | Milk and Alternatives | Meat and Alternatives |
| Female 51+ years | 7 | 6 | 3 | 2 |

| | Number of Food Guide Servings | | | | |
|---|---|---|---|---|---|
| Foods | Vegetables and Fruit | Grain Products | Milk and Alternatives | Meat and Alternatives | Added Oils and Fats |
| Breakfast<br>• 175 mL (¾ cup) oatmeal<br>• 125 mL (½ cup) 1% milk<br>• 1 pear | 1 | 1 | 1/2 | | |
| Snack<br>• 30 mL (2 Tbsp) almonds<br>• 3 graham crackers<br>• Tea with lemon | | 1 | | 1/2 | |
| Lunch<br>• Pasta salad: 250 mL (1 cup) whole wheat pasta; 125 mL (½ cup) roasted red peppers and corn; 125 mL (½ cup) broccoli florets and parsley; 1 hard boiled egg vinaigrette<br>• 125 mL (½ cup) blueberries<br>• 125 mL (½ cup) 1% milk | 1<br>1<br>1 | 2 | 1/2 | 1/2 | ✔ |
| Snack<br>• 175 mL (¾ cup) low fat yogurt<br>• 125 mL (½ cup) fruit salad | 1 | | 1 | | |
| Dinner<br>• Moroccan stew: 175 mL (¾ cup) chick peas; 125 mL (½ cup) green peas and sweet potato; cooked with olive oil<br>• 125 mL (½ cup) basmati rice<br>• 125 mL (½ cup) 1% milk | 1 | 1 | 1/2 | 1 | ✔ |
| Snack<br>• bowl of whole grain cereal (30 g)<br>• 125 mL (½ cup) milk<br>• 1 small banana sliced | 1 | 1 | 1/2 | | |
| **Total Food Guide Servings for the day** | **7** | **6** | **3** | **2** | |

Source: *Eating Well with Canada's Food Guide. A Resource for Educators and Communicators,* Health Canada, 2008. © Adapted and reproduced with permission from the Minister of Public Works and Government Services Canada, 2007.

to be marketed for profit. Finally, individual determinants could include food preferences, nutritional knowledge, perceptions of healthy eating, and psychological factors. Understanding the complex interactions among these multiple determinants is essential to guide efforts to promote and support healthy eating.[101]

CRITICAL THINKING

*Plan a daily menu, for a week, for a middle-aged person who lives alone.*

## Physical Activity

Physical activity is one of the most important things we can do as we get older to maintain our physical and mental health and quality of life. Walking, stretching, and keeping our muscles in good condition may not increase longevity, but these actions do enhance our quality of life by keeping us healthy and independent.[102]

The Public Health Agency of Canada (www.phac-aspc.gc.ca/) has published a pamphlet called *Physical Activity Guide to Healthy Living for Older Adults*.[103] The guide helps one make wise choices about physical activity. It serves as a road map, explaining why physical activity is important, and it offers tips and simple ways to increase physical activity. The guide states that accumulating 30 to 60 minutes daily of moderate physical activity is important. Sessions of ten minutes at a time can be accomplished easily. The guide recommends that if one is not sure about physical activity, a consultation with a health care professional is imperative.

Tannenbaum and Shatenstein examined age differences regarding the extent to which older Canadian women exercise effectively and eat nutritiously. The study

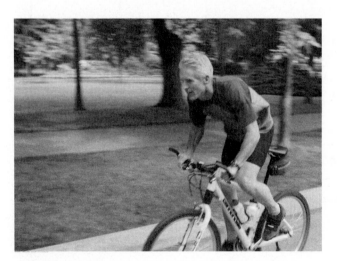

Middle-aged adults should be encouraged to participate in healthy behaviours such as exercising.

identified the interventions women prefer to help them commit to maintaining physical and nutritional fitness. The findings indicated that 62 percent of women aged 55 to 74, versus 56 percent of those over age 75, reported exercising 3 times a week for 20 minutes or longer. In addition, 33 percent in both age groups were eating nutritiously, and 24 percent compared to 21 percent were both exercising and eating nutritiously. Thirty-five percent of women aged 55 to 74, who were not exercising or eating nutritiously, desired the availability of low-cost, suitable health promotion programs and additional written materials to improve these habits, whereas only 25 percent did so in the 75 year and older age group. Sedentary women, and those at higher nutritional risk, were two to three times more likely to seek encouragement from health professionals as well as from family and friends. The researchers concluded that women aged 55 to 74 who do not exercise and eat nutritiously are most receptive to a variety of health promoting community interventions.[104] These findings have specific implications for nurses who work with middle-aged women in the community.

Nurses can teach that although physical changes do occur, adopting sedentary habits will not maintain health. Physical activity must be balanced with rest and sleep to maintain optimum body posture and function. The capacity for intense and sustained effort diminishes, especially if engaged in irregularly, but judicious exercise can modify and retard the aging process. In addition to the physical benefits, regular and vigorous exertion is an excellent outlet for emotional tensions.

Teach about the value and precautions of exercise. The type of exercise does not matter, especially if the person likes it and engages in it regularly, and it is suitable for personal strength and physical condition. *The middle-aged person should take certain precautions however:* (1) gradually increase the exercise until it is moderate in strenuousness; (2) exercise consistently; and (3) avoid overexertion. Ten minutes after strenuous exercise, the heart should be beating normally again, respirations should be normal, and there should be no sense of fatigue. If the person is overweight, has a personal or family history of cardiovascular disease, or has led a sedentary life, new exercise routines should not be started until after a thorough physical checkup.[105] Using exercise as an overcompensation to prove youthfulness, health status, or prevent old age is pointless. The person may benefit greatly by enrolling in an exercise program that is directed by a health professional or trained fitness person.

CRITICAL THINKING

*What activities would you include in an exercise program for a middle-aged adult?*

**Foot balance**, *the ability to alter one's position so that body weight is carried through the foot with minimum effort*, is essential to prevent strain, foot aches, and pain during exercise as well as when walking or standing. Foot imbalance may result from contracted toes, improper position, size or shape of one or more bones of the foot, weak or rotating ankles, muscle strain, weak ligaments, poor body posture, overweight, arthritis, injuries, and improperly fitted or shaped shoes. Treatment by a podiatrist consists of the careful assessment of the posture and the provision of balance inlays for insertion into the shoes.[106]

*Foot problems* may occur in middle age. Teach the person to watch for the following common signs of the need for diagnostic evaluation and possible treatment:[107]

- Swelling of the feet and ankles
- Cramps in the feet and the calf while walking or at night
- Inability to keep the feet warm
- Loss of the fat tissue on the padded surfaces of the feet
- Chronic ulcers on the feet that fail to respond to treatment
- Absence of or bounding pulse in the arteries of the feet
- Showing of arteries in the foot on routine x-ray film
- Burning in the soles of the feet

*Foot care should include the following:*

- Clean the feet with soap and water at least once daily; dust with foot powder or cornstarch.
- Exercise the feet, extend the toes, and then flex rapidly for one or two minutes. Rotate the feet in circles at the ankles. Try picking up a pencil or marble with toes.
- Walk barefoot on uneven surfaces, thick grass, or sandy beach.
- Walk daily and properly. Keep toes pointed ahead and lift rather than push the foot, letting it come down flat on the ground, placing little weight on the heel.
- Massage the feet to rest them after a tiring day.
- Lie down with feet higher than head for approximately a half-hour daily.
- Avoid wearing poorly fitted shoes or shoes with high heels and pointed toes.

Teach that the callus or other foot problems should be treated by a podiatrist. If the person scrapes or cuts a callus, there is risk of infection.

## Sleep

Sleep is a vital physiological process with important restorative functions.[108] Most middle-aged adults sleep without difficulty; seven to eight hours of sleep constitute a normal pattern. Insomnia may be a sign of a more serious underlying medical condition—for example, cardiac or thyroid disease or depression. Some medications interfere with sleep, such as some antidepressants, antihypertensives, thyroid medication, and corticosteroids. See the box entitled "Sleep Hygiene Recommendations" to promote better sleep.[109]

Sleep apnea occurs in two main forms: *obstructive sleep apnea*, the more common form that occurs when throat muscles relax, and *central sleep apnea*, which occurs when the brain fails to send proper signals to the muscles that control breathing. Additionally, some people have *complex sleep apnea*, which is a combination of both obstructive and central sleep apneas.[110] Obstructive sleep apnea occurs two or three times more often in older adults, and it is twice as common in men as it is in women. The manifestations of obstructive and central sleep apnea overlap, which makes the type of sleep apnea more difficult to determine. The most common signs and symptoms of obstructive and central sleep apnea include:

- Excessive daytime sleepiness
- Loud snoring
- Observed episodes of breathing cessation during sleep
- Abrupt awakenings accompanied by shortness of breath
- Awakening with a dry mouth or sore throat
- Morning headache
- Difficulty staying asleep

### Sleep Hygiene Recommendations

- Establish pre-sleep routines, e.g., a warm bath or reading.
- Maintain a regular time for sleep and awakening. Use the bed only for sleeping.
- Go to bed when feeling sleepy, or do something boring to become drowsy.
- Get regular exercise, but avoid doing exercise during the hours just before bedtime.
- Avoid caffeine (coffee, tea, cola, and chocolate) within six hours of bedtime.
- Avoid alcohol within several hours of bedtime.
- Avoid daytime naps.
- Avoid sleep medications, if possible, since they interfere with deep sleep and have a detrimental effect if taken for too long.

Disruptive snoring may be a more prominent characteristic of obstructive sleep apnea, while awakening with shortness of breath may be more common with central sleep apnea.[111] Clients with obstructive sleep apnea are more often male and are frequently, but not necessarily, obese. They may deny having any problems with sleep, and they come to medical attention only because a bed partner has noted loud snoring punctuated by silences (with no breathing) of varying length.[112]

Epidemiological studies have suggested a relation of obstructive sleep apnea to hypertension, stroke, and ischemic heart disease.[113] An important concept, especially for health professionals such as nurses who care for elderly people, is the notion that obstructive sleep apnea can contribute to cognitive impairment.[114]

---

**CRITICAL THINKING**

*How do you respond to a middle-aged adult who tells you she is planning to take herbal remedies to enhance sleep?*

---

# Health Promotion and Health Prevention

**Immunizations**  All Canadian adults require maintenance of immunity to tetanus and diphtheria, preferably with combined (Td) toxoids and a single dose of acellular pertussis vaccine. All adults should receive adequate doses of all routinely recommended vaccines, and other vaccinations should be given under certain circumstances when appropriate. Hepatitis B vaccine is recommended for health care workers and others who may be exposed to blood and blood products, or who may be at increased risk of sharps, bites, or penetrating injuries. In addition, annual influenza immunization is recommended for all health care personnel who have contact with individuals in high-risk groups.[115]

---

**CRITICAL THINKING**

*What are some methods of identification for the use of vaccines for adults in community centres?*

---

**Injury and Accidents**  A person's gradually changing physical characteristics and a preoccupation with responsibilities may contribute to the middle-aged person's risk of having accidents. Accidents are the fourth leading cause of death in middle age.

Fractures and dislocations are the leading cause of injuries for both sexes, with more men affected than women, probably because of occupational differences. Because of the middle-aged adult's changing physical abilities, motor vehicle accidents are the most common cause of accidental deaths in the later years, especially for men. Occupation-related accidents rank second and falls in the home rank third, as causes of death. However, women suffer less than one-third as frequently as men from fatal falls during the middle years.[116]

You can teach about safety as it relates to remodelling a home, maintaining a yard, or establishing a work centre. Handrails for stairways; a handgrip at the bathtub; conveniently located electric outlets; indirect, no-glare, and thorough lighting; and tools, equipment, and home or yard machines kept in proper working condition all provide ways to avoid an accident, especially in later middle age. Sensible middle-aged people plan for the gradual failing of their physical abilities by making the home as safe, convenient, and comfortable as possible as they rethink homemaking functions for the coming decades. Fortunately, you can be instrumental in initiating or strengthening a safety program in an occupational or school setting, or even in someone's home.

---

**CRITICAL THINKING**

*You have been asked to develop an exercise program for middle-aged adults in a community centre. How will you begin?*

---

**Illness Prevention**  Middle age is not automatically a period of physical or psychological hazard or disease. No single disease or mental condition is necessarily related to the passage of time, although the middle-aged person should be carefully assessed for signs of illness. Major health problems of this era include: cardiovascular disease, cancer, pulmonary disease, diabetes, obesity, alcoholism, anxiety, depression, and glaucoma.[117]

You can help the person maintain energy and improve health by teaching the information presented in this section and the chapter. The person can learn moderate eating, drinking, or smoking habits, and how he or she can learn to use only medically prescribed drugs. *Many measures promote health:*

1. Regular physical examinations
2. Pursuit of leisure activity
3. Use of relaxation techniques
4. Working through the emotional and family concerns related to middle age
5. Affirming the worth of self as a middle-aged person
6. Preparing for the later years
7. Confronting developmental tasks

The person also needs to prepare for possible accidents or illness.

Teach that the mounting statistical, experimental, and autopsy findings point to cigarette smoking and second-hand smoke as a causative factor in breast and lung cancer, cardiovascular disease, and chronic obstructive pulmonary disease.[118] For the person who feels trapped, depressed, frustrated, or isolated, easily accessible escapes include alcoholism, drugs, and excess food intake. Assist the person in finding other ways to cope with stressors.

Because nursing care is holistic, you can meet the emotional and spiritual needs of the person while giving physical care and doing health teaching related to the common health problems discussed in the following pages.

## Common Health Problems: Prevention and Treatment

A variety of health problems occur, although most middle-aged adults remain healthy. Table 13-4 lists a summary of diseases that are frequently experienced, and texts provide for more information on the diseases summarized in the table.

Common health problems in middle age, in addition to those listed in Table 13-4, are cardiovascular disease, asthma, impaired vision and hearing, AIDS, arthritis, osteoporosis, various kinds of cancer, and obesity (BMI of 25.0 to 29.9).[119]

**Obesity** Most adults with a high BMI (overweight or obese) have a high percentage of body fat. Extra body fat is associated with increased risk of health problems such as diabetes, heart disease, high blood pressure, gallbladder disease, and some forms of cancer. The waist circumference provides an indicator of abdominal fat. Excess fat around the waist and upper body—"*apple body shape*"—is associated with greater health risk than fat located more in the hip and thigh area—"*pear body shape*."[120]

**Cancer** In men, the primary sites for cancer are the prostate, lung, colon, rectum, and bladder. In women, the common sites are breast, lung, colon, rectum, and cervix.[121] The primary site for cancer in women is the breast followed by the lung.[122] The greatest risk for women is after age 50. Exposure of the breast tissue to estrogen increases cancer risk because of cell proliferation. Early menarche, late menopause, and long-term use of oral contraceptives increase risk. Adipose tissue stores estrogen, so obesity is a risk factor. Other *gynecologic cancers* also affect the middle-aged woman:[123]

1. *Cervical.* Highly curable if diagnosed and treated early. A history of human papillomas virus (HPV) infection, a prevalent sexually transmitted disease, carries an 80 percent risk of cervical cancer. Other risk factors include first intercourse before age 18, multiple sexual partners, large number of children,

and history of smoking. In Canada, even though the mortality and morbidity rates have fallen significantly since screening began, cervical cancer kills about 370 women annually; another 1350 or so are diagnosed with it each year.[124] Health Canada has approved a vaccine that protects against HPV, which is responsible for most cases of cervical cancer. The vaccine Gardasil offers a new prevention method and is expected to at least complement and augment the prevention of cervical cancer through the existing screening program in Canada.[125]

2. *Endometrial.* In Canada, endometrial cancer is the most common gynecological malignancy. Approximately 3900 new cases are reported each year, the majority of which present early as stage I or II disease.[126] Risk factors include irregular menses (especially postmenopausal), estrogen therapy without added progestin, polycystic ovary disease, diabetes, and hypertension.

3. *Ovarian.* Higher mortality exists because of the absence of early symptoms. Risk factors include the presence of the BRCA-1 gene mutation; a history of breast, colon, or endometrial cancer; and having ovulated for more than 40 years. Epithelial ovarian cancer remains the most common cause of death from tumours of the pelvis, and it ranks fifth among causes of death from cancer overall in Canada.[127]

The colorectal area (the colon and rectum combined) is now the third most common site of new cancer cases and deaths in Canada. *Colorectal* cancer usually grows slowly and in a predictable way. It is curable, however, when diagnosed at an early stage.[128] A variety of screening tests can detect the precancerous polyps. Surgical removal in the early stages is curative.

The Canadian Cancer Society recommends that men and women aged 50 and over have a fecal occult blood test (FOBT) at least every two years. The FOBT helps to identify polyps early, before they become cancerous.[129] Regular screening for colorectal cancer should begin at age 50. The prognosis for colorectal cancer is good if diagnosed and treated in the precancerous or early stages.

The rate of death from prostate cancer has recently declined in many areas of the world. Over the past 15 years, prostate-specific antigen (PSA) screening has increased in popularity, which has resulted in increases in the incidence of prostate cancer.[130] Over the same period, changes have emerged in the management of the disease. Pickles states that all men older than 45 with at least a ten-year life expectancy should be informed of the potential benefits and drawbacks of PSA screening so they can make an informed decision about whether to have the test.[131]

Table 13-4 Common Health Problems in Middle Age

| Problem | Definition | Symptom/Signs | Prevention/Treatment |
|---|---|---|---|
| **Sinusitis,** nonbacterial and bacterial | Inflammation of mucous membrane lining parnasal sinuses; may be caused by bacteria, viruses, irritants, or allergies | Normal sinus drainage prohibited<br>Usually clear drainage in nonbacterial type<br>Purulent drainage in bacterial type, with fever (headache and tenderness of frontal and maxillary sinus to palpation frequent with bacterial involvement) | Oral antihistamine and decongestant for nonbacterial type<br>Addition of antibiotic for bacterial type |
| **Hiatal hernia** with esophagitis | Herniation of stomach through diaphragm with reflux of acid into esophagus | Substernal pain, usually worse when bending over or lying down<br>Sometimes nausea and vomiting | Maintenance of ideal weight<br>Avoidance of tight clothing<br>Eat frequently in small amounts<br>Elevation of head of bed |
| **Duodenal peptic ulcer disease** | Ulceration of duodenal mucosa | Pain in the epigastrum or right upper quadrant usually 1–2 hours after meals | Antacids or prescription drugs (e.g., cimetidine [Tagamet] or omeprazole [Prilosec])<br>Small frequent meals<br>Avoidance of caffeine, alcohol, and spices |
| **Angina pectoris** | Imbalance between oxygen needed by myocardium and oxygen supplied | Pain in substernal region but sometimes in neck, back, and arms | Workup to determine accurate diagnosis<br>Nitroglycerine |
| **Secondary hypertension** | High blood pressure based on specific cause | Blood pressure >150/100<br>More common in men, but after 55 years, women likely to be affected | Following treatment plan based on cause of high blood pressure<br>Reduction of sodium and cholesterol in diet<br>Reduction of weight as needed<br>Relaxation techniques |
| **Hyperthyroidism** (Grave's disease) | Too much secretion of thyroid hormone | Can mimic heart problems with accelerated or irregular heartbeat<br>Feeling of agitation | Antithyroid medications or radioactive iodine therapy |
| **Hyperuricemia, or gout** | High uric acid level, causing acute inflammatory arthritis (can also be chronic) | Usually red, hot tender joint; often in great toe but can be in other joints | Specific drugs<br>Rest<br>Elevation of joint(s)<br>Cold compresses |
| **Diabetes mellitus (type 2)** | Glucose intolerance corrected by means other than insulin | High blood sugar<br>Thirsty<br>Weight loss<br>Frequent urination | Diet<br>Exercise<br>Oral medication |
| **Prostatitis, acute** | Acute infection of prostate gland; often caused by *Escherichia coli* | Low back and perineal pain referred sometimes to inguinal region and testes<br>Extremely tender prostate | Sitz baths<br>Appropriate antibiotics |

*(continued)*

Table 13-4 (continued)

| Problem | Definition | Symptom/Signs | Prevention/Treatment |
|---|---|---|---|
| **Prostatitis, chronic** | Prolonged inflammation of prostate | Only slightly tender and enlarged prostate | Prostatic massage<br>Sitz baths<br>Increased sexual activity |
| **Lubosacral strain,** mild | Strain and inflammation of ligaments and musculature in Lubosacral region | Muscle spasm over region but no radiation<br>No flank pain<br>No pain on straight leg raising | Cold packs<br>Muscle relaxant<br>Analgesic<br>Bed rest<br>Chiropractic treatment<br>Education in bending and lifting techniques<br>Use of firm mattress |
| **Foot callus** | Thickness of the outer layers of the skin on the sole of the foot | Pain when congestion and swelling press nerve endings, and underlying bursa | Avoid shoes that put excess pressure and friction on the sole of the foot |

## CRITICAL THINKING

*What are some drawbacks of PSA testing for middle-aged men?*

**Cardiovascular Disease** Cardiovascular disease is the underlying cause of death in 33 percent of Canadians.[132] Males are more likely to die from ischemic heart disease and acute myocardial infarction, while women die from congestive heart failure and cerebrovascular disease. Risk factors are increasing despite the knowledge that many of these hazards are preventable. Approximately 80 percent have at least one risk factor (smoking, physical inactivity, overweight, hypertension, or diabetes), while 10 percent have three or more risk factors.[133]

According to Tanuseputro and his colleagues, even though a high prevalence of potentially modifiable cardiovascular factors and a large variation exists between subgroups in the Canadian population, the burden of cardiovascular disease could be reduced through risk factor modification.[134]

## CRITICAL THINKING

*How can you encourage men to become more physically active?*

**Respiratory Conditions** Acute, as well as chronic, pulmonary diseases are a frequent cause for days absent from work. Generally, middle-aged women have more disability days from work because of respiratory and other acute disorders, but men have more disability days from injuries.

**Hypothyroidism** *Hypothyroidism* can cause weight loss, heat intolerance, insomnia, and restlessness or irritability. All individuals over 50, especially women, should have an annual thyroid test, even if there are no apparent symptoms. Either hyperthyroid or hypothyroid disease is easily treated with drugs.[135]

**Chronic Illness** The middle-ager might experience chronic illness in self or a family member. A number of references give information about reactions to, as well as coping with, chronic illness in this era.[136]

Chronic illness of any kind represents multiple losses, including threatened self-concept and low self-esteem; unpredictability, fear of the future, and feelings of loss of support; abandonment by family, friends, and health care workers; and reduced function and spontaneity.[137] Chronic sorrow is experienced with chronic illness.[138]

Help the person to:

1. Work through feelings and practical problems
2. Formulate new meanings and understandings
3. Discover personal strengths and new support systems
4. Deepen a sense of hope and faith and a personal belief system
5. Develop a sense of humour and broaden perspective as the illness is acknowledged
6. Make choices; take control where possible
7. Share insights and solutions with others in similar situation
8. Learn how to manage the situation

Sometimes the chronic disease osteoporosis is not preventable in women. The article by Dowd and Cavalieri gives practical suggestions to help the person stay as comfortable, safe, and healthy as possible.[139]

In Canada and abroad, researchers have identified the high national costs of diabetes. Jacobs and his colleagues obtained data from the Manitoba Medicare database and the Manitoba diabetes database. They concluded that the prevalence and use of the health care system were considerably higher for the Aboriginal population.[140]

---

**CRITICAL THINKING**

*What are some of the ways that our society can combat the escalating incidence of diabetes?*

---

## PSYCHOSOCIAL CONCEPTS

The following information is relevant to understand, assess, and intervene with the middle-ager. Health promotion strategies, physical as well as psychosocial, to aid mental and emotional functioning, may be used.

## Factors That Influence Research Findings on Cognitive Ability

Because most studies on adult cognition have been cross-sectional, caution is necessary in interpreting the results because many factors are influential. For the middle-aged person especially, the *following can negatively influence test scores:*

1. Amount of education
2. Experiential differences
3. Fixed attitudes
4. Number of years since formal schooling was completed
5. General health status

The gradual neuron loss that occurs over the lifetime does not affect cognitive function. Because most intelligence tests are developed for children and adolescents, the kind of test used can influence the scores. The middle-aged adult scores relatively high on tests that require general information or vocabulary abilities. At age 60, intelligence quotient (IQ) test results are equal to, or better than, those of young adults. Only arithmetic reasoning shows a plateau through the adult years. Speed requirements of the test may mitigate against the IQ test scores; adults show a peak in speed of performance in the twenties and a gradual decrease in one's overall speed of performance sets in through the years. Adults usually value accuracy and thoroughness more than speed.[141] In fact, IQ tests may be irrelevant. What should be tested is how people identify problems and use reason and intuition to solve problems.

In various studies, physically fit and active men were found to have a higher IQ score than men who engaged in little physical activity.[142]

In the past decade, more middle-aged women have returned to university for baccalaureate, graduate, doctoral, and postdoctoral degrees. They have shown themselves to be as capable as men both scholastically and in applying intellectual ability in the workplace.

---

**CRITICAL THINKING**

*What motivates women to achieve academic success in our society?*

---

## Cognitive Development

Cognitive processes in adulthood include reaction time, perception, memory, learning and problem solving, and creativity. These skills are performed through the characteristics of both concrete and formal operations, depending on the situation.[143]

*Reaction time or speed of performance* is individual and generally stays the same, or diminishes, during late middle age. The speed of response is important primarily in test situations because much of the problem-solving skills necessary in adulthood require deliberation and accuracy rather than speed. Reaction time is related to the complexity of the task, the habitual pattern of response to stimuli, and familiarity with the task. Time required for new learning increases with age, but adults in their forties and fifties have the same ability to learn as they did in their twenties and thirties.[144]

*Memory* is maintained through young and middle adulthood, and no major age differences are evident. Some quantitative changes do occur. For example, a person in early adulthood who could recite a ten-digit span of numbers as a series of discrete units may only be able to recite eight grouped or categorized digits in late middle age. The ability to categorize or group information, to sharpen observational skills and give more attention to the phenomenon, to relate meaning to what is to be remembered, and to use interactive imagery—imagining events in a story form with self in the interaction—are all ways to strengthen memory and aid learning.[145] The middle-aged adult has greater difficulty in memorizing material that is not well organized. This same person also seems to retain less from the oral presentation of information than younger students do.[146]

There are three different types of memory. *Sensory memory*, information stored in a sense organ, is transitory and lasts only a few seconds. *Short-term memory* is based on recall and can last for days or weeks. *Long-term memory* can last a lifetime. Memory is not reliable in the adult years, or at any age. Most people forget or ignore episodes that do not fit the self-image, or that are considered unimportant.

People who think they remember an event from childhood, or from a number of years previously, may be making up plausible scenarios, fantasies, or confabulations based on earlier reports or stories. The middle-aged adult who continues to use their memory will retain a keen memory.[147]

*Learning* occurs in adults of all ages. The highly intelligent person becomes even more learned. The capacity for intellectual growth is unimpaired and is enhanced by interest, motivation, flexibility, a sense of humour, confidence, and maturity attained through experience. A reluctance to learn occurs if the new material does not appear to be relevant, or if it does not serve the person as well as current information.[148]

*Problem-solving abilities* remain keen throughout adulthood. No significant differences have been found among 20-, 40-, and 60-year-olds in learning a task. Generally, better-educated people perform better than less well educated people in any age group. When there is no time limitation, no task differences are found in complex task solutions because young and middle-aged adults use different strategies. Young adults, knowing they can function quickly, may be more likely to use less efficient reasoning strategies, such as trial and error. In late middle age, because people know they are becoming slower, they tend to think a problem through first so they can solve it in fewer tries. Thus, they appear to be slower in grasping and solving a problem, but the fact is, though, that wider life experiences prompt recognition of more variables in a situation and thus enhance problem solving.[149]

The middle-aged adult is able to do all the cognitive strategies of *Piaget's stage of formal operations* described in Chapters 11 and 12. Sometimes, the practicality of a situation will call forth the use of concrete operations. Because not all problems in life can be solved by abstract reasoning, the middle-aged adult does both operations realistically in problem solving. He or she also uses the fifth stage of cognitive development, problem finding, described in Chapter 11. Societal, occupational, and general life experiences are crucial to the cognitive operations of the middle-aged person. Thus, perceptions about the same situation, problem, or task can vary considerably within a group of middle-aged adults.[150]

Cognitive characteristics that are developed in the young adult are used throughout middle age. Various patterns mark the development of *intellectual skills*. The mature adult can symbolize experiences, and he or she will frequently behave in ways that show organization, integration, stability, and unity in the cognitive process. The person can recall past defeats and triumphs, and frequently monitors ongoing thoughts for consistency and logic. Because the mature adult is more imaginatively productive, he or she is capable of producing abundant images, thoughts, and combinations of ideas, is able to use reflection to gain perspectives about life, and is aware of personal beliefs, values, motives, and powers.

The mature person is increasingly interested in other persons, and in warm, enduring relationships. He or she is adaptable, independent, self-driven, conscientious, enthusiastic, and purposeful. The person can reflect about personal relationships, the ups and downs or contradictions in relationships, and their sources of strain and satisfaction. Concomitantly they will undoubtedly be able to understand why other persons feel and act as they do.[151]

---

## CRITICAL THINKING

*What are some ways that our society can foster the learning of adult citizens?*

---

**Creativity** Simonton examined the lifetime creativity and productivity of thousands of notable scientists from the nineteenth century and earlier. In every scientific discipline represented, the thinkers produced their best work at about age 40, on average.[152] However, many of them were publishing their first significant work, even outstanding work, through their forties and into their fifties. Among musicians and other artists, peak creativity can occur later and be maintained far longer.

Streufert, Pogash, Piasecki, and Post examined adult creativity beyond the realm of scientific research. They created 45 teams. On 15 of the teams, the participants were between ages 28 and 35. Members of another 15 teams were middle-aged, between 45 and 55. The last 15 teams included only older adults aged 65 to 75. Each team was given a complex simulated task. The younger teams asked for additional information to the point of creating information overload. The middle-aged teams asked for the right amount of information, enough to make decisions and use the information correctly. The oldest teams performed less well than the middle-aged and younger teams. These findings suggest that the ability to apply creative thinking efficiently to complex problems may indeed be at its peak during the middle-aged years.[153]

You can encourage the middle-aged adult to pursue creative ideas and activities and to approach roles, responsibilities, and tasks in a creative way. Help the middle-aged adult to overcome any self-consciousness he or she may have about some unique cognitive response he or she may favour regarding some situation.

**Continued Learning** When it comes to acquiring new knowledge, middle-aged adults seem to be just as capable as younger adults at learning and remembering new information.[154] With increasing emphasis on continued learning, the middle-aged person frequently enrolls in special interest courses, continuing education courses, or workshops related to their occupation or profession. He or she takes college

# Learning to Live with Early Dementia

Much of the literature on early dementia is focused on care-giver perspectives, while little is known about the perspectives of persons with early-stage dementia, such as what it is like to live with this syndrome. This study was conducted to explore the process of learning to live with early-stage dementia. Interviews were conducted with six early-stage participants (three men and three women) ranging in age from 61 to 79 years. A preliminary theoretical framework was developed from the data, which outlines a five-stage process of "learning to live with dementia" that begins with various *antecedents* and proceeds through the stages of *anticipation*, *appearance*, *assimilation*, and *acceptance*. This process evolved as participants' awareness of themselves and their outer world changed. Ultimately, the findings of this study have several implications for clinicians working with persons in early-stage dementia.

The term *dementia* refers to a clinical syndrome comprising a wide range of neurological diseases that typically occur with increasing age and are distinguished by progressive memory loss, impaired judgment, and decreased capacity for abstract reasoning. The most common cause of dementia is Alzheimer's disease.

Each participant was interviewed twice. Once transcripts from the first interviews were coded and analyzed, a preliminary theory comprising six categories was identified. A second interview was conducted with each participant for the purpose of verifying and clarifying emerging theory. During the second interview (one to three months later), the interview process evolved and became more unstructured and open-ended as clarification was sought on issues that emerged in the previous interview.

## Practice Implications

1. Nurse-clinicians and researchers should be cognizant of the emotional strain endured by dementia sufferers and seek to minimize any further emotional distress that may result from the interview process during a nursing assessment or research study. One means of minimizing distress may be to conduct assessments or interviews in the dementia sufferer's home.

2. Denial has been identified as a common coping method used among individuals with early memory loss. In this study, however, evidence of denial did not surface. On the contrary, participants demonstrated a striking openness and willingness to talk about their memory impairment and its effects on their lives. Intellectualizing the disease (e.g., by educating oneself about it) was another conscious means used by participants to assimilate it into their lives.

3. One of the factors participants saw as instrumental in the assimilation process was connecting with, and learning from, other dementia sufferers in support groups. The participants in this study who attended a support group identified (many) benefits. These findings clearly indicate that more support groups should be established for persons with early-stage dementia. Research into the design, function, and efficiency of such groups, once established, could serve to ensure maximum benefit for participants and to secure funding to staff them with educated personnel such as nurses.

4. Supportive family and friends played a key role in enabling participants to come to terms with their memory loss. Based on this finding, it seems reasonable to conclude that nurses can play a role in educating family members and others on the importance of learning to understand and support persons in the early stages of the disease.

5. The clinical approach of health care professionals who work with people with early-stage dementia is important. One participant, for example, explained that the insensitivity of her physician in blurting out to her the news that she had Alzheimer's disease had discouraged her from asking the physician questions about the diagnosis. These findings suggest that nurse clinicians and researchers must be aware of the impact of their verbal and nonverbal communication on early-stage sufferers. Adopt an individualized, unhurried approach in working with early-stage sufferers, and demonstrate the recognition of, and respect for, the unique difficulties and concerns of these persons.

6. Because people are being diagnosed earlier in the disease process, it is becoming increasingly important to identify the coping methods that early-stage sufferers employ and determine whether these methods facilitate or hinder adaptation to early dementia.

*Source:* Werezak, L., and N. Stewart, Learning to Live with Early Dementia, *Canadian Journal of Nursing Research,* 34(1) (2002), 67–85. Adapted with permission.

credit and non-credit courses to learn interesting content; to find an academic program that is necessary for changing a profession or occupation; to gain personal satisfaction; to relieve boredom, loneliness, or an unhappy situation; or to broaden the mind and learn for the sake of learning. Rapid technologic changes in business or the professions cause obsolescence of knowledge and skills, which can also entice middle-aged persons to want to continue learning.

When you are teaching, *use methods that capitalize on the learning strengths of mature adults*, including:

1. Active discussion and role-play
2. De-emphasis on memorization
3. Presentation of large amounts of new information
4. Suggestions to develop cognitive strategies that will help them synthesize, analyze, integrate, interpret, and apply knowledge
5. Validate them, and others, that they are highly capable learners, and that myths to the contrary are prevalent
6. Provide a conducive environment, one that considers sensory changes
7. Consideration of the sensory changes discussed previously

## Work and Leisure Activities

**Work** Work will be viewed differently by different middle-agers. Consider that the older middle-aged person grew up under the influence of the Great Depression and with the Protestant work ethic. Both stressed the economic and moral importance of work. Thus, work became respected and sought. Being without a job or idle was a harbinger of problems and meant being lazy and worthless. How has this middle-aged adult adjusted to mechanization, waning of the work ethic, and the demise of a full day's work for a full day's pay? For the young middle-ager, what was a promising career or lifetime employment may have ended in being laid off permanently by the company, forced early retirement, or forced job hunting. Finding work might have been difficult.[155] If the person is unemployed and job hunting, see the box entitled "Suggestions for Someone Who Is Unemployed,"[156] or you

### Career Track Options in Late Middle Age

**Coast into Retirement**
- Do the job but no more; collect the paycheque; enjoy the final years.

**Go for Last Promotion**
- Campaign to obtain final reward for all that was contributed to receive public acknowledgment of the importance of work done.

**Try for Great Achievement**
- Work to outdo the present record and others' records so that others will see you saved the best for last.

**Survive Difficult Period**
- Recognize the company's difficult period; learn to survive and even prosper in the challenging time.

**Retire Early**
- Take the attractive package being offered by the company so that the years of later maturity can be enjoyed.

**Start Your Own Business**
- If tired of working for others, go into business for self (e.g., consulting in work arena, turning hobby into business).

may want to explore career options described in the box entitled "Career Track Options in Late Middle Age."

### CRITICAL THINKING

*What strategies might you use with a middle-aged unemployed Asian adult?*

### Suggestions for Someone Who Is Unemployed

- Offer hope and encouragement, but guard against sounding "spiritually superior." This is a dark valley, emotionally, economically, philosophically, and spiritually.
- Remind the person that unemployment is a reflection of current economic conditions, not of personal worth.
- Seek opportunities to affirm the person's talents and positive attributes.
- Help him or her consider all options, including launching a business from home, changing careers, and working part-time.
- Allow the person to express feelings, but do not encourage self-pity. Your time with the person should leave him or her

feeling uplifted and hopeful. Pray with the person if he or she desires.
- Offer to hold him or her accountable to a specific job-hunting schedule. It is often hard to stay motivated and organized without a friendly nudge.
- Talk about subjects other than unemployment.
- Encourage the person and family to relax and have fun. If you are a friend, invite them to your home or give them a gift certificate for dinner and a movie.
- If the person is a friend or relative, provide practical but discreet help, including food, clothing, and finances.

The person may be fortunate enough to be in a business or profession in which he or she works successfully for self or is allowed freedom within a specialized area of work. He or she will experience the dignity of being productive and will enjoy increasing self-esteem, autonomy, and sense of achievement. Most middle-aged adults, however, are employed in a system in which the value is on production, not the person. Often, in contrast to union-set rules, whereby no more than a specified amount can be done within a specified time, ever-greater output is demanded on the job.

There are several categories of workers that are different from the past. They have been described as follows:

1. *Free agents*. They seek and find professional and financial independence in a variety of entrepreneurial occupations. Many work alone, out of a home office, and are involved in community services as well as business ventures. They know how to market talents to the highest and most interesting bidder.

2. *Nomads*. They have no real loyalty to the job or the boss as they move from one geographic area and job to another. They spot the next trend, find a job at a company, and are ready to move with it. In their job-hopping and hunting, they develop great contacts and a variety of skills. They take advantage of job opportunities as they arise.

3. *Globalists*. They travel from time zone to time zone around the world as they work in a borderless economy with their laptop computers. They constantly network, scout out opportunities, and improvise as necessary.

4. *Niche-finders*. They spot new markets emerging from recent social and economic trends and build, market, and manage a company to capitalize in it. They are the leaders in the new industry.

5. *Retreads*. They relish learning and stay abreast of technological change. Because of their maturity and experience, they'll never be without a job. Self-improvement, helping peers adapt, and reminding younger workers that computer skills are only one facet of the job guarantee that they will never become obsolete.

6. *Corporate leaders*. New-age bosses redesign jobs to incorporate new skills and ventures. They give workers freedom to manoeuvre as needed to hang on to valuable employees. They expand responsibilities for self and others as they dream up new projects.

But whatever the category, for employed Canadians, the biggest chunk of time goes to working for a living. The time spent at the full-time job has increased over the past two decades. There is a decline in leisure. Many feel that they are overworked and have insufficient time for family. For some, the ideal playground is the workplace. All sorts of workers carry cellphones or pagers; business-related calls come in constantly. It can be difficult in some jobs to keep up with voice mail and email, let alone the necessary reading. Baby boomers declared their contempt for "the man in the grey flannel suit"—the company-oriented worker. However, they have done more than any other generation to erase the line between work and private life in many professions, managerial jobs, or careers. Work is considered the way of such fulfillment. Work has forced the middle-ager to develop and expand skills beyond what was considered possible to accomplish.[157]

## CRITICAL THINKING

*What would life be like in today's society for a middle-aged person without technology?*

Many middle-aged women work outside of the home. Consequently, whether they desire it or not, they are especially in the middle in terms of the demands of various roles on their time and energy. The middle-aged woman is wife, mother, homemaker, grandmother, worker, and organization member. Women who are caregivers also have child care responsibility, and some may have quit their jobs or have work conflicts. The middle-aged woman is often in the middle in terms of two competing values: (1) traditional care of elders is a family responsibility, and (2) women should be free to work outside the home if they wish. Each family member feels the repercussions as the balance of roles and responsibilities changes. Most middle-aged women are working today for a variety of reasons:[158]

- Inflation and the rising cost of living
- Changes in attitudes about sex-appropriate roles as a result of the woman's movement
- The rising divorce rate that forces the woman to become economically independent
- Increasing educational levels that stimulate career interests or the desire to remain in the profession
- Expectancy of a higher standard of living
- Assistance with costs of sending children to university

Determine the degree of work stability, extent to which work is satisfying, and emotional factors that have operated in the person's concept of work and in the self-concept. Assess how well the middle-aged person can function as a mentally and physically healthy person. As a professional person, you will be called on to resolve conflicts related to your own work role. Hence, you are in a valuable position to assist the middle-aged person in talking about and resolving feelings and values related to work and other activity.

Because the demands on middle-aged adults are often overwhelming—work, home, family, church, and social and civic organizations—teach steps for effective *time management* (see the box entitled "Guidelines for Time Management").

CRITICAL THINKING

*What other strategies can you use to manage time more effectively?*

**Retirement** Settling into retirement involves changes in many aspects of a person's life. Certainly, financial adjustments are involved as employment income and spending patterns are altered. Individuals often must make psychological and social adjustments as well. Social contacts are likely to be realigned now that time is mainly spent with family and friends, rather than with co-workers and business associates.[159] The process of retiring, as well as bringing bliss to the marital relationships, can produce a temporary increase in marital conflict as couples settle into a new routine.[160]

The retirement preparations of the baby boom cohort, who are now middle-aged, are quite different from those of their parents. Baby boomers believe that they need higher retirement incomes than those of their parents. Most have enjoyed a comfortable standard of living compared with earlier generations due to the income earned in the dual-earner family. They expect some decline in income after retirement, but also expect little change in their standard of living.[161]

Because of the extent of retirement wealth that baby boomers have accumulated, and because of their intentions to continue working after they retire, economic analyses predict that, as a group, they are likely to enjoy levels of affluence in retirement that far exceed those of their parents.

The most recent evidence suggests that the average age of retirement is rising in Canada, as well as in the United States and the United Kingdom. That is, the likelihood that individuals will work past age 65 is increasing.[162] A Canadian study investigated the differences in how people allocate time among productive and other activities pre- and post-retirement. They found that people remain engaged in productive activities even as they move out of the labour force and begin to substitute unpaid work for paid work.[163]

CRITICAL THINKING

*How can you assist a middle-aged individual plan for retirement?*

**Leadership Role** The middle-aged adult's cognitive stage is supportive of the notion of being a leader, either informally or formally designated. (Usually middle-aged leaders have developed necessary qualities from childhood on, but occasionally a person does not believe that he or she has this ability until there is a measure of success in the life work.)

The *leader* usually has the *following characteristics*:[164]

■ Adequate socioeconomic resources

■ Higher level of education or success than the majority of the group to be led

■ Realistic self-concept

■ Realistic goals and the ability to encourage others toward those goals

■ High frustration tolerance

■ Ability to express negative thoughts tactfully

■ Ability to accept success or failure gracefully

■ Ability to delegate authority

■ Understanding of group needs

■ Flexibility in meeting group needs

The middle-aged person may demonstrate this leadership ability on the job, in the community, or in church organizations. Women who are most successful in leadership careers are those who have little conflict in the multiple

---

## Guidelines for Time Management

■ Establish priorities; maintain a log if necessary. *Write goals.*

■ *Do it now.* Do not procrastinate with small tasks; schedule large projects.

■ Recognize *unpleasant tasks; work on them first.*

■ *Clear the decks and desks.* Eliminate clutter; organize the workplace for efficiency.

■ *Stick to the job.* Avoid distractions.

■ *Do one thing at a time.* Finish one major task before beginning another; however, *there are times you can do two things at once,* e.g., planning while waiting in line.

■ *Plan ahead.* Assemble what is needed for a task before initiating it; set aside relaxation time.

■ *Consider limitations—your own,* equipment not available for a project, and other responsibilities that will interfere.

■ *Learn to say "no" and suggest someone else* who would be able to handle the situation. Delegate low-priority jobs to others.

■ *Anticipate delays* that are inevitable in every task; plan for interruptions and unforeseen events.

■ *Plan on alternative way* to do the job; have backup activity if a selected task cannot be done as scheduled.

■ *Use odd times.* Shop when stores are not crowded; carry a notebook to jot down ideas while you wait.

roles of career woman, mother, and wife. Their husbands' support and encouragement are major assets, but women are becoming more assertive on their own behalf about their roles outside the home.

You can encourage and reaffirm the middle-aged person in his or her leadership roles. You can also assist him or her in working through any ill feelings or conflicts related to the work setting or the job itself.

**Leisure** The middle-aged person, taught little about how to enjoy free time, will now be faced with greater amounts of leisure because of retirement. The average middle-aged adult has moved up the pay scale, their children will have grown, and now they will have more time to take trips or try new hobbies. Yet, *various factors hinder the use of these new opportunities:*[165]

- Value of work learned in younger years
- Cultural emphasis on intellectual pursuits so that play is considered childish and a poor use of time and talents
- Conditioning to at least appear busy
- Fears of regression and not wanting to return to work
- Lack of previous opportunities to learn creative pursuits or hobbies
- Reluctance to try something new because of fear of failure

Help that person to avoid the feelings of alienation that result from an inability to use leisure time fully. Use the suggestions in the box entitled "Teaching Use of Leisure in the Daily Schedule" with your middle-aged clients.

---

### CRITICAL THINKING

*What are some other strategies you might use to teach a client and his or her family about the effective use of leisure time?*

---

### CRITICAL THINKING

*What are some leisure activities you may pursue for yourself?*

---

## Emotional Development

The middle years, the climacteric, are a period of self-assessment, and greater introspection—a transitional period. In middle age (and beyond), the person perceives life as time left to live rather than time since birth. Time is seen as finite; death is a possibility. Middle-aged adults clock themselves by their positions in different life contexts—changes in body, family, career—rather than by chronologic age. Time is seen in two ways: (1) time to finish what the person wants to do, and (2) how much meaning and pleasure can be obtained in the time that is left. He or she realizes that the choices of the past present

### Teaching Use of Leisure in the Daily Schedule

- Emphasize that both play and recreation are essential to a healthy life.
- Stress the indispensability of leisure as a part of many activities, whether work or creative endeavours. Leisure is both a state of mind and the satisfying use of time away from work. Have the person analyze their leisure activities, whether they bring pleasure, work off frustration, make up deficits in life, or create a sense of thrill or competition.
- Help the person to recognize the interplay of physical and intellectual endeavours and their contribution to mental health.
- Differentiate compulsive, competitive, and aggressive work and play from healthy, natural work and play. Intrinsic in play are spontaneity, flexibility, creativity, zest, and joy.
- Recognize the person's creative efforts to encourage further involvement in leisure activities.
- Educate the person about the importance of preparing for retirement.
- Inform the person of places, courses, or workshops at which he or she can learn new creative skills and use their current talents.
- Encourage the person to enjoy change, to participate in organizations, and to initiate stimulating contacts with others.
- Encourage the person to stop the activity when it no longer meets personal needs.

only a number of limited choices now. He or she can no longer dream of infinite possibilities. Some goals have been reached, others have not. Aspirations need to be modified. The possibility for advancement is more remote. The person will go on, and there will be ever-brighter, ever-younger men and women crowding into the competitive economic, political, and social arena.

**Developmental Crisis** According to Erikson, the psychosexual crisis of middle age is generativity versus self-absorption and stagnation.[166] **Generativity** is *a concern about providing for others, equal in strength to the concern of providing for the self.* If other developmental stages were managed successfully, the person has a sense of parenthood and creativity, of being vital in establishing and guiding the next generation, the arts, or a profession, and of feeling needed and being important to the welfare of humankind. The person can assume the responsibility of parenthood.

As a husband or wife, or as partners, each can see the strengths and weaknesses of the other and will combine their energies toward common goals.

A biological parent does not necessarily get to the psychosocial stage of generativity, but the unmarried person, or the person without children, can be very generative.

The middle-aged person who is generative takes on the major work of providing for others, either directly or indirectly. There is a sense of enterprise, productivity, mastery, charity, altruism, and perseverance. The greatest bulk of social problems and needs falls on this person who can handle the responsibilities because of personal strengths, vigour, and experience. A strong feeling of care and concern emerges for that which has been produced by love, necessity, or accident. He or she can collaborate with others to do the necessary work. Ideas that one generates in life about personal needs and goals eventually tend to converge with a resulting deep understanding of the social community. These are the very ideas that guide the actions that people take on behalf of future generations

The generative middle-aged adult can be a mentor to a young adult. A **mentor** is *an adult with experience, wisdom, patience, and understanding who befriends, guides, and counsels a less experienced and younger adult in the work world, or in a social or educational situation.*

Mentoring differs from coaching. The mentor has the following roles:

- Adviser
- Guide
- Sponsor
- Tutor
- Advocate
- Coach
- Role model
- Protector
- Friend

Mentoring involves developing a long-term relationship and carrying out many roles. Coaching is performance-oriented. The mentor is usually about ten years older, is confident, warm, and flexible, enjoys sharing knowledge and skills, is trustworthy, and promotes the psychosocial development and success of the younger person. The mentor is found in business, management, nursing, or other careers or professions, sponsoring the younger person as an associate, creating a social heir, teaching him or her as much as possible for promotion into a position, or recommending the one being mentored for advancement. Several authors present further, interesting information on mentoring.[167]

CRITICAL THINKING
*What is your conceptual understanding of the process of mentoring?*

With approaching middle age and the image of one's finite existence faintly in view, the person consciously reappraises and uses self. With introspection, the self seems less important, and the words *service, love of others*, and *compassion* gain new meaning. These concepts motivate action. In church work, social work, community fund drives, cultural or artistic efforts, a profession, or political work, the person is active and often the leader. The person's goal is to leave the world a better place in which to live. A critical problem, however, is that of coming to terms with one's accomplishments, and of accepting the responsibility that comes with achievement.

The generative person feels a sense of comfort or ease in their lifestyle. Realistic gratification emerges from a job well done, and from what has been given to others. He or she accepts self and their body, realizing that although acceptance of self was originally based on acceptance from others, unless he or she accepts self, he or she cannot really expect acceptance from others.

The mature middle-aged person has tested many ways of doing things during his or her lifetime. He or she can draw on a great wealth of experience. He or she will likely have deep sincerity, mature judgment, and a sense of empathy. He or she has a sense of values, and a philosophy underlying life, that enable a sense of stability. The person recognizes that one of the most generative things he or she can give to society is the life he or she has led, and the way he or she is living it. Consider the following statement by a 50-year-old man:

> Those were full years—raising the kids with all its joy and frustration. I'm glad they're on their own now. This is a new stage of life. I can go fishing; Mary can go out to lunch. We have more time together for fun, and now we have more time for working at the election polls and in volunteer activities.

CRITICAL THINKING
*What do you believe is the main message of this 50-year-old man?*

The middle years can be wise and felicitous, or they can be foolish and frantic, fraught with doubts and despair.

If the developmental task of generativity is not achieved, a sense of **stagnation**, or **self-absorption**, tends to enshroud the person. Thus, *he or she regresses to adolescent, or younger, behaviour, characterized by physical and psychological invalidism.*[168] This person hates his or her aging body and feels neither secure nor adept at handling self, either

## Consequences of Self-Absorption

- Denial of signs of normal aging
- Unhappiness with advancing age, desire to stay young, fear of growing old
- Regression to inappropriate youthfulness in dress or behaviour, rebelliousness, foolish behaviour
- Preoccupation with self, self-indulgence
- Physical, emotional, social, and interpersonal insecurity
- Attempts to prove youthfulness with infidelity to spouse
- Resignation, passivity, non-involvement with societal or life issues
- Isolation or withdrawal from others
- Despair about signs of aging (considers self old, life is over)
- Either overcompliance or excessive rigidity in behaviour
- Intolerance, cynicism, ruthless attitude
- Lack of stamina, chronic health problems that are not coped with
- Chronic defeatism, depression

physically or interpersonally. He or she has little to offer even if so inclined. He or she operates on a slim margin and soon burns out (see the box entitled "Consequences of Self-Absorption"). Consider the following statement by a 50-year-old woman:

> I spent all those years raising the kids and doing housework while Bob moved up the professional ladder. We talked less and less about each other, only about the kids or his job. Now the kids are gone. I should be happy, but I'm lost. I can't carry on a decent conversation with Bob. I don't have any training for a job. And I look terrible! I sit around and eat too much. I wear high collars to hide my wrinkled neck, and no cosmetics will hide the dark circles under my eyes.

Immature adults have impaired and less socially organized intellectual skills and value systems. Their intellectual skills are fused by personal emotions, and those skills are coordinated in strange and unrealistic ways. The immature person seeks private self-absorption and vicarious immersion in subjective problems of others. Yet the characteristics of the self-absorbed person are actually health-endeavouring attempts, and they are reparative efforts to cope or adapt. These characteristics may or may not work well, depending on the intensity of the personality and the social and physical environment.

## CRITICAL THINKING

*What strategies could you develop to help the middle-aged person who is highly self-absorbed?*

**Maturity**  Because **maturity**, *being fully developed as a person*, is not a quality of life reached at any one age or time, the characteristics described as generativity are general guidelines. Emotional intelligence, described elsewhere in this text and in other excellent sources, is an important concept in the middle-aged individual. It encompasses interpersonal skills, partnership building, networking, and critical thinking skills.[169]

Realize that if the person is doing what is appropriate for his or her age, situation, and culture, he or she is acting maturely. As the person grows older, the ideal level of maturity and autonomy can recede further into the future and never be fully achieved. Maturity is rather formally defined as the achievement of efficiently organized psychic growth predicated on the integration of experiences of solving environmentally stimulated conflicts. The external environment is a potent force on the person, and conflicts are primarily socially incurred. The psychosocial organization in maturity shows a cultural direction. As one ages, the psychic interests broaden and are less selfish. In adulthood, there is no one set of appropriate personality characteristics. You will work with many personality types as you promote health. Each of us leads a particular life at a particular time, place, and circumstance, and with a particularly unique personal history. Success in leading that life depends on a *pattern* of qualities appropriate to that life.

The mature person is reflective, restructures and processes information in the light of experience, and uses knowledge and expertise in a directed way to achieve desired ends. No one will reach the highest ideal of self-actualization described by Maslow (Chapter 5). Yet, each of us can reach his or her own ideal and peak of well-being and function relatively free of anxieties, cognitive distortions, and rigid habits and with a sense of the individuality and uniqueness of the self and others.[170]

## CRITICAL THINKING

*What is your understanding of emotional intelligence?*

## Body Image Development

The gradually occurring physical changes described earlier eventually confront the person and are mirrored by others. The climacteric causes a realignment of attitudes about the self that cut into the personality and its definition. Life stresses cause the person to view self and body differently.

The person realizes that he or she not only is looking older but subjectively feels older as well. Work can bring a sense of stress if he or she feels insufficient stamina and vigour to cope with the task at hand. Illnesses or the deaths of loved ones can create a concern about one's own personal health, sometimes to excess, and thoughts about one's own death tend to occur more frequently. The person begins to believe that he or she is coming out second-best to youth. Depression, irritability, and sometimes anxiety about femininity and masculinity can result.

Whether a man or a woman, the person who lacks self-confidence and who cannot accept the changing body sometimes has a compulsion to try cosmetics, clothes, hairstyles, and the other trappings of youth in the hope that the physical attributes of youth will be attained. The person tries to regain a youthful figure and face, perhaps through surgery. Some will tint the hair to cover signs of grey, or will turn to hormone creams to restore the skin. Healthy signs are that he or she prefers this age and has no desire to relive the youthful years.

You can promote the integration of a positive body image through your communication skills and teaching. Reaffirm to the client the strengths of being middle-aged by using the information presented in this chapter and by emphasizing the specific strengths of the person.

## Adaptive Mechanisms

The adult may use any of the adaptive mechanisms described in this or in previous chapters. **Adult socialization** is defined as *the processes through which an adult learns to perform the roles and behaviours expected of self and by others and to remain adaptive in a variety of situations*. The middle-aged adult is expected, and normally considers self, to be adaptive. The emphasis is on the active, reciprocal participation of the person with little preparation directed toward anticipating, accepting, or coping with failure. The ability to shift emotional investments from one activity to another, to remain open-minded, and to use past experience as a guide rather than as the rule, is closely related to adaptive ability.

The adult, having been rewarded over the years for certain behaviours, has established a wide variety of role-related behaviours, problem-solving techniques, adaptations to stress, and methods for making role transitions. These behaviours, however, may not be adaptive to current demands or crises, or to increasing role diffusion. There is a continuous need for socialization in adulthood, for a future-related orientation, for being able to anticipate events, and for learning to respond to new unexpected demands.[171]

Coping or adaptive mechanisms, or the ego defences used in response to emotional stress in the middle years, depend on the person's capacity to adapt and satisfy personal needs, sense of identity, sense of usefulness, and interest in the outside world, and the nature of interactions with others.

You can help the middle-aged adult prevent or overcome many of the maladaptive mechanisms they have established. As you extend empathy and reinforce a sense of emotional maturity and health, the person will feel more able to cope with life stressors and perceived failures. If you feel unable to listen to or work with the problems of someone who may be twice your age, refer the person to a counsellor. Be mindful, however, that being able to refer such a person to a counsellor requires thoughtful insight, patience, tact, and consideration to enable the person to retain his or her composure.

### CRITICAL THINKING

*What are some other ways that you can help a middle-aged adult from another culture to overcome maladaptive mechanisms?*

## Mid-life Transition/Crisis

Middle age can be seen as a transition or a crisis. The **mid-life crisis** is *a major and revolutionary turning point in one's life, involving changes in commitments to career or spouse and children and accompanied by significant and ongoing emotional turmoil for both the individual and others*. The term **mid-life transition** has a different meaning. It includes *aspects of crisis, process, change, and alternating periods of stability and transition*.[172]

For many, mid-life is one of the better periods of life. It is a *transition* from youth to later maturity. Life expectancy is longer, both psychologically and physically. Mid-life is healthier than ever in history; and parental responsibilities are decreasing. Most people are in their late forties or early fifties when the last child leaves home. This leaves a couple of decades for the spouses to be together without the obligations of childrearing. The couple often realizes that the myth of decreasing sexual powers at this age is not true. Women in mid-life often begin or continue their education, or extend their career. Men see mid-life as a time of continuing achievement. Experience, assurance, substance, skill, success, and good judgment more than compensate for the disappearance of youthful looks and physical abilities.

It is healthier in the long run for the person to acknowledge the disruptive feelings and the diffusion of identity, and to work through them rather than to deny them, and to seek a healthy and constructive outlet for these feelings.

You can be instrumental in assisting such a person in working through his or her crisis. You will be called upon to use principles of good communication and crisis intervention (see Chapter 5). Refer the person to a counsellor who can work with the individual and family. *The following*

### Mid-life Crisis

Louise, a 48-year-old architect, had an uneasy feeling about her relationship with her teacher husband, Charles, age 49. The feeling had been there for some time, and she had tried a time or two to talk about it but had been rebuffed by Charles.

Louise believed that she and Charles were slowly drifting apart, each into his or her own profession. Yet, the pronouncement by Charles seemed so sudden. As she joined him in the family room after dinner, he quietly looked at her and said, "I have something to tell you. I'm leaving. There's nothing here for me anymore. I'm almost 50. I've got to get on with things."

Louise was overcome with shock, grief, guilt, disbelief, helplessness, and worry. They had been married for 22 years! She had often thought about all of the things they could do together when they retired. Because they were childless, they would be free to travel. She panicked as she thought of life and aging without him. For days, she slept and ate little but managed to go to work.

In the following months, Louise and Charles met several times to talk. She hoped they would see a marriage counsellor and work out their differences. As Charles continued to move his clothes, belongings, and favourite items from the home, he revealed that he would be living with another woman, a colleague from his work, and that they would marry as soon as both divorces were finalized.

The divorce proceedings took more than a year. During that time, Louise sought counselling for herself. Gradually, she revealed her situation to her family, other relatives, and friends. She often blamed herself for Charles's leaving and talked frequently of what a wonderful person he was. She maintained a hectic pace, caring for the home and yard and handling the responsibilities of her job. However, in the months after the initial separation, Louise re-established a daily exercise routine, which she had interrupted after Charles left home. She contacted a number of friends she had seen only occasionally in the past few years and began to attend the church of her childhood faith. She was pulling herself together—physically, emotionally, mentally, socially, and spiritually.

After the divorce was finalized, Louise continued to blame herself for several years. She worked hard and achieved considerable recognition at the architectural firm where she was employed. She maintained her home and neighbourhood ties and became active in her church.

After ten years, Charles, who is remarried, still visits Louise occasionally and calls every few weeks. Louise has resolved the events of Charles's mid-life crisis but has cast aside opportunities to date or remarry. She believes the struggles and crises of the past decade, including various illnesses and the death of

her parents, have prepared her for adaptation to her eventual retirement, aging, and dying. She still believes that she and Charles could re-establish a marriage and that it would be more love-filled and happy than before. Yet, she remains fully committed to caring for a number of older friends, to the responsibilities of her profession, home, and church membership, and to continuing to deepen her spiritual and emotional maturity.

1. In your assessment, you note that Louise has avoided opportunities to enlarge her social network on an intimate level. How can you assist Louise to work through her grief?

2. Discuss the psychosocial implications of Louise's belief system.

3. List, with your rationale for each, several health promotion strategies you would employ with Louise.

*guidelines may help the person who feels that he or she is in mid-life crisis. Share and use them as you work with others*, or use them in your own life.

- Face your feelings and your goals realistically. If you feel confused, see a counsellor who can help you sort through your feelings and goals.

- See your age as a positive asset. Acknowledge your strengths and the benefits of middle age. Take steps to adjust to your liabilities, or to correct them if you can. If a change in hairstyle or clothes makes you feel better, make that change.

- Reconcile yourself to the fact that some, or many, of your hopes and dreams may never be realized and may not be attainable. Remain open to the opportunities that are available to you. They might actually exceed your dreams.

- If the job is not satisfying, consider another job or another field after appraising yourself realistically. Be willing to relinquish some responsibility at work.

- If you dread retirement, plan for it financially, along with leisure and other activities.

- If job pressures are great, seek outlets through recreational activities or other diversions. Become involved in community service, and renew spiritual study and religious affiliations.

- Renew old friendships and initiate new ones. Invest in others and, in the process, enhance their personal self-esteem and emotional well-being.

- If you are concerned about sexual potency, realize that typically the problem is transient. The more you worry, the worse it gets. Talk with your spouse about your sexual feelings and concerns. The love and concern you have for each other can probably overcome any feelings of impotency. It is important for the woman to perceive sexuality apart from childbearing and menstruation. And for men it is important to perceive sexuality apart from having children and love affairs. If you are so inclined, read some how-to sex manuals together. Seek a marriage counsellor if you are unable to work out problems of sexual dysfunction together.

■ Examine your attitudes as a parent. Strike a balance between care and the protection of offspring. Realize their normal need for independence.

■ Obtain a physical examination to ensure that persistent physical symptoms are not indicators of physical illness. Do not think that vitamins or health foods alone will cause you to feel differently.

■ Seek counselling for psychological symptoms. The counsellor may be a nurse, religious leader, mental health therapist, social worker, marriage counsellor, psychologist, or psychiatrist.

*Following are some specific suggestions to the spouse of the man in mid-life crisis:*

■ Make it easier for him to talk about his feelings and fears by listening to verbal and nonverbal messages. Avoid telling him how he should feel, dress, or behave.

■ Try not to make him feel guilty by hurling your fears or anger at him. His guilt about your fears will only cause him to withdraw and refuse to discuss his problems with you.

■ Emphasize to him that he does not have to leave to find what he is looking for. Try to find new joint interests, friends, or hobbies. Be willing to see a marriage counsellor with him.

■ Focus on changing yourself. Become more alive by taking care of your appearance, keeping informed, and broadening your interests.

■ Try to re-establish the intimacy and closeness that you once shared. Be willing to compromise and change your own attitudes and behaviour.

■ Try to maintain spontaneity in your sexual life. Allow a sense of adventure to rekindle the relationship. If you can re-establish an active and satisfying sexual life at this point, you can both be certain that it will continue for many more years.

■ If he is coping with a mid-life crisis symptom, focus on his strengths. But do not hand out empty praise. Instead, find a real reason to praise him.

Assist individuals considering mid-life career or work changes to assess their current job skills and applicability of them to new careers, to explore alternatives within their current job position and external counselling services, and to examine personal values.

Some of the benefits available from a mid-life crisis include personality growth and a deepening maturity because of personal introspection and the desire to change behaviour to feel better and improve one's life. The concern about mortality can motivate the person to take better care of their health and to take time to pursue new interests or reinitiate old relationships. The person can experience an invigorating rebirth, generating new energies and new commitments.

## Moral–Spiritual Development

The middle-aged person continues to integrate new concepts obtained from a widened variety of sources into a form of religious philosophy, if he or she has gained spiritual maturity. Faith and trust in God, or another source of spiritual strength, are increased. Religion offers comfort and happiness. The person is able to deal effectively with the religious aspects of upcoming surgery and its possible effects, illness, death of parents, or unexpected tragedy.

Spiritual beliefs and religion take on added importance. The middle-aged adult who becomes revived spiritually is likely to remain devout and active in his or her faith throughout life. If the person does not deepen spiritual insights, a sense of meaninglessness and despair is likely to come upon him or her in old age.

Moral development is advanced whenever the person has an experience of sustained responsibility for the welfare of others. Middle age, if it is lived generatively, provides such an experience. Although the cognitive awareness of higher principles of living develops in adolescence, consistent commitment to their ethical applications continues to develop in adulthood, after the person has had the time and opportunity to meet personal needs and to establish self in the family and community. Further, the level of cognitive development attained sets the upper limits for moral potential. If the adult remains in the state of concrete operations, he or she is unlikely to move beyond the conventional level of moral development (law-and-order reasoning), because the post-conventional level requires a deep and broad understanding of events and a critical reasoning ability.[173]

Although Kohlberg's work on moral development was conducted on men, women generally come out at stage 3 of the conventional level (refer to Table 5-9), which emphasizes an interpersonal definition of morality rather than a societal definition of morality or an orientation to law and order.[174] Perhaps the stage of moral development often seen in women, with concern for the well-being of others and a

## Table 13-5 Moral Development in Women

| Level | Characteristics |
|---|---|
| I. Orientation of individual survival | Concentrates on what is practical and best for self |
| Transition 1: from selfishness to responsibility | Realizes connection to others; thinks of responsible choice in terms of another as well as self |
| II. Goodness as self-sacrifice | Sacrifices personal wishes and needs to fulfill others' wants and to have others think well of her; feels responsible for others' actions; holds others responsible for her choices, dependent position; indirect efforts to control others often turn into manipulation through use of guilt |
| Transition 2: from goodness to truth | Makes decisions on personal intentions and consequences of actions rather than on how she thinks others will react; takes into account needs of self and others; wants to be good to others but also honest by being responsible to self |
| III. Morality of non-violence | Establishes moral equality between self and others; assumes responsibility for choice in moral dilemmas; follows injunction to hurt no one, including self, in all situations |

Source: Gilligan, C., In a Different Voice: Women's Conceptions of Self and of Mortality, *Harvard Educational Review,* 4(4) (1977), 481–517.

willingness to sacrifice self for others' well-being, is an aspect of stage 5 of the post-conventional level.

Gilligan, whose research centred on moral development in women, found that women define morality in terms of selfishness versus responsibility.[175] Women subjects with high morality scores emphasized the importance of being responsible in behaviour and of exercising care, and avoiding hurt, to others. Men think more in terms of general justice and fairness; women think in terms of the needs of specific individuals. Gilligan's view of moral development is outlined in Table 13-5. It is based on three levels and the transition points between levels I and II, and between levels II and III.

## HEALTH PROMOTION IN NURSING PRACTICE

The role of the caregiver for the middle-aged person and family has been described throughout this chapter. When working with the middle-aged person and his or her family, it is important to assess whether there are any issues that are important for them. Please be certain to consider the client's strengths and healthy responses during your assessment.

Interventions may involve the health promotion or direct care measures described throughout the chapter. These interventions are intended to assist the person and family in meeting physical, emotional, cognitive, spiritual, and social needs. Stolte states that, generally, middle adulthood is productive with much energy placed on career development,

family responsibilities, and community concerns.[176] Nurses often have contact with middle-aged adults either in hospitals or community settings. A wellness diagnosis would be helpful to enhance the person's life.

The middle-aged adult has developed a sense of the life cycle. Through introspection, he or she has gained a heightened sensitivity to his or her personal position within a complex social environment. Life is no longer seen as an infinite stretch of time into the future. The person now anticipates and accepts the inevitable sequence of events that occur as the

---

### NARRATIVE VIGNETTE
### Caretaker's Role

Mrs. L, age 60, has breast cancer, which has metastasized to the bone and brain. Her husband, age 75, is somewhat fragile, and her 40-year-old daughter resides with her own family about one hour away from their home. During your visit to Mr. and Mrs. L's home, you note that Mrs. L appears calm and comfortable, and she informs you that the medication is effectively controlling her pain. You observe that Mr. L is sitting at her bedside, holding his wife's hand. In a soft and loving tone of voice, Mr. L informs his wife not to worry and that "everything's going to be okay," adding that their daughter and family will be in later for a visit.

1. List several strengths that this family displays.

2. List several possible interventions, with rationales, for the strengths.

human matures, ages, and dies. The middle-aged adult realizes that the course of his or her life will be quite similar to the lives of others. Sex differences between men and women diminish, both in reality and in perception. Turning points affect all and are inescapable. Personal mortality, achievements, and failures, along with personal strengths and limits, must be faced if the person is to prepare him- or herself emotionally and developmentally for later maturity and the personal aging process. The person realizes that his or her direction in life has been set by decisions made related to occupation, marriage, family life, and having or not having children. Although occupations and lifestyles can be changed, at least to some extent, the results of decisions made earlier cannot be changed. The current and future consequences must be faced and resolved. The middle-aged person realizes that he or she will not achieve all of his or her dreams, but remaining open to life's opportunities from then on will enable the person to achieve accomplishments never before contemplated.

The person in late mid-life realizes that life's developmental markers and crises call forth changes in self-concept and sense of identity, necessitate the incorporation of new social roles and behaviours, and precipitate new adaptations. But they do not destroy the sense of continuity within the person that reaches from youth to old age. This adaptability, and a sense of continuity, are essential for the achievement of ego integrity in the final years of life.

## SUMMARY

1. The middle-age years are filled with challenges, pleasures, and demands.

2. The middle-ager is in the "sandwich generation," caring for children and grandchildren, aging parents, and other relatives.

3. This is the prime of life, although some physical changes occur that require adaptation.

4. The middle-ager continues to learn and, in turn, is a mentor and leader in the community.

5. This is a time of generativity, of wanting to leave the world a better place.

6. The middle-ager relies on experience, resolves value conflicts, and initiates action that is relevant to the situation.

7. For some, middle age is a time of struggle, crisis, loss, or illness.

8. The box entitled "Considerations for the Middle-Aged Client in Health Care" summarizes what you should consider in assessment and intervention with the middle-aged client and family.

9. Health promotion behaviours are important for present and future well-being.

## Considerations for the Middle-Aged Client in Health Care

1. Family and cultural history
2. Personal history
3. Pre-existing illness
4. Risk factors for disease in family (e.g., cardiovascular disease, cancer, osteoporosis, developmental disability, mental illness)
5. Psychosocial evaluation (age-related stresses, distress with partner, mid-life crisis issues)
6. Caregiver responsibilities
7. Knowledge of normal changes in middle age and coping strategies—adaptive capacity
8. Nutrition history—weekly diet intake

9. Complete physical examination
10. For women:
    a. Menstrual history (age onset, pattern, current pattern)
    b. History of estrogen administration
    c. Reproductive history (number of pregnancies, at what age, miscarriages or abortions)
    d. Perimenstrual history (beginning of menopausal symptoms, response, whether menopause has occurred)
    e. Interest in or current administration of hormone replacement therapy; any side effects
11. For other members of the household, review items 1–9 above with each member in mind

## Interesting Websites

## Key Terms

adult socialization (545)

climacteric (524)

filial responsibility (516)

foot balance (531)

generation gap (511)

generativity (542)

maturity (544)

menopause (524)

mentor (543)

middle age (511)

mid-life crisis (545)

mid-life transition (545)

perimenopausal years (524)

self-absorption (543)

social mobility (511)

stagnation (543)

# Chapter 14

## Assessment and Health Promotion for the Person in Later Adulthood

*Old age, to the unlearned, is winter: to the learned, it is harvest time.*

*Yiddish Proverb*

## Objectives

*Study of this chapter will enable you to:*

1  Define terms and theories of aging related to understanding of the person in later maturity.

2  Explore personal and societal attitudes about growing old and your role in promoting positive attitudes in the community.

3  Examine the second-order changes in family status required to proceed developmentally in the stage of the family life cycle: families in later life.

4  Compare and contrast relationships in the late years with those of other developmental eras, including with spouse, offspring, grandchildren, other family members, friends, pets, and other networks.

5  Compare and contrast the status of either singlehood or widow(er)hood in later adulthood to that status in early and middle adulthood.

6  Describe signs of and factors contributing to elder abuse.

7  Examine physiologic adaptive mechanisms of aging and influences on sexuality, related health problems, and assessment and intervention to promote and maintain health, comfort, and safety.

8  Discuss the cognitive, emotional, body image, and spiritual development and characteristics of the aged person, their interrelationship, and your role in promoting health and a positive self-concept.

9  Compare and contrast the adaptive mechanisms used by the person in this period with those used in other periods of life.

10  Identify changing home, family, social, and work or leisure situations of this person and your responsibility in helping the person face retirement, loss of loved ones, and changes in roles and living arrangements. Discuss selection of an adequate personal care home or residence for seniors.

11  Describe major federal, provincial/territorial, and local programs to assist the elderly financially, socially, and in health care, and describe your professional and personal responsibility in this regard.

12  Define remotivation and reminiscence; discuss the value, purpose, and use of these and other group processes with the elderly.

13  Assess the needs of the elderly and design health promotion strategies to assist in meeting their needs.

14  Assess and work effectively with a person in later adulthood, using the information presented in this chapter and showing empathy and genuine interest.

15  Assess and work effectively with a person in later adulthood, using the information presented in this chapter and showing empathy and genuine interest.

I really don't like being labelled a golden-ager. I acknowledge my age and my limits, but I certainly didn't turn incompetent at 65.

When does later adulthood begin? Historically, it was designation of an eligible age for receipt of Old Age Pension benefits that established 65 as the beginning age for this period in the life cycle. In reality, the age span for this period is continually changing. The chronologic age of 65 no longer determines or predicts behaviours, life events, health status, work status, family status, interests, preoccupations, or needs. Individuals undergo aging at different rates, and their view of the aging process is influenced by many factors: culture, generation, and occupation. Some individuals, especially members of ethnic minorities and lower socioeconomic levels, view the onset of old age as taking place earlier than age 65.[1] Younger generations sometimes misperceive how the old view themselves.

The predicted rapid increase in the number of older adults up to 2030 reflects the aging of the baby boom generation.[2] As mothers of the post–Second World War baby boom reach old age, the current trend of elderly women living alone will increase, according to a study conducted in 21 European and North American countries. Four-generation families will be the norm, and five-generation families will increase in number.

Recently, the elderly population has been growing faster among non-whites than Caucasians. By 2025, 15 percent of the elderly population is projected to be non-white, in contrast to 10 percent in 1980. This continued aging trend in the population requires changes in all aspects of our social structure—employment, housing, education, leisure activities, transportation, industrial development, and health care.

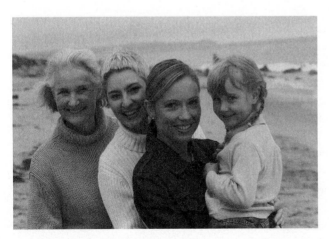

Four-generation families, once unusual, will become the norm as the population ages.

## DEFINITIONS

Because the terms describing this age group are not clearly defined by the general public or by health care professionals, it is important to clarify some of the terms used in this chapter.[3] **Aging**, which begins at conception and ends at death, is *a process of growing older, regardless of chronologic age.*

**Biological age** is *the person's present position with respect to the potential lifespan, which may be younger or older than chronologic age;* it encompasses measures of the functional capacities of vital organ systems.

**Social age**, which results from the person's life course through various social institutions, refers to *roles and habits of the person with respect to other members of society.* Social age may be age appropriate, older, or younger than that of most people in the social group. Social age includes such aspects as the person's type of dress, language usage, and social deference to people in leadership positions.

**Psychological age** refers to *the behavioural capacity of the person to adapt to changing environmental demands. It includes the capacities of memory, learning, intelligence, skills, feelings, and motivation for exercising behavioural control or self-regulation.*

**Cognitive age** includes *the age the person feels and looks to self, plus the fit of behaviour and interests to his or her chronologic age.* The person says, "I do most things as if I were ___ years old."

**Senescence** is *the mental and physical decline associated with the aging process.* The term describes a group of effects that lead to a decrease in efficient function.

**Later maturity** is *the last major segment of the lifespan. This stage begins at age 65 or 70.* The World Health Organization (WHO) divides this segment of life into the elderly (65 to 75), the old (76 to 90), and the very old (over 90). Some authors divide this group into **young-old**, *ages 65 to 74;* **mid-old**, *75 to 84;* and **old-old**, *80 or 85 and older.* The term *frail-old* is sometimes used instead of *old-old* or *very old.*

---

### CRITICAL THINKING

*Differentiate between social and psychological age in your own terms.*

---

**Gerontology** is *the scientific study of the individual in later maturity, and it includes the aging process from physiologic, pathologic, psychological, sociologic, and economic points of view.*

**Geriatrics** is *a medical specialty concerned with the physiologic and pathologic changes of the individual in later maturity.* It includes the study and treatment of the health problems of this age group.

Later maturity is divided into three sequential segments. The first segment is regarded as *a sociopolitical or cultural-organizational perspective.* The older person becomes concerned with the creation, ordering, and maintenance of a larger society. The second segment is characterized by *a reaffirmation of social, moral, and ethical standards.* The judgmental functions of the mind are most highly developed at this time, having been created out of actual and vicarious experiences with conflict situations and from cultural learning and values. The last segment of psychic maturity involves *retrospective examination,* the need to correlate the present with the past to determine the true nature of one's accomplishments, errors, and rediscoveries. Cultural vision is at its broadest possible development, embracing one nearly complete life cycle and its interrelatedness with a multitude of other life cycles. The person compares and contrasts his or her values with cultural values and, through reasoning and intuition, evaluates meaning and purpose and has an increased interest in the history of human development.

## SOCIETAL PERSPECTIVES ON AGING

I may be old and wrinkled on the outside but I'm young and vulnerable on the inside.

**Ageism** refers to *any attitude, action, or institutional structure that discriminates against individuals on the basis of their age, or that infers that elderly people are inferior to those who are younger.*

Your attitude, teaching, and advocacy can diminish ageism, stereotypes, and myths. Your teaching and practice need to consider cultural differences among the elderly. Ageist attitudes toward older adults are not new in Canada. Generally, older women are judged more harshly than older men. Children appear most positive in their perceptions of elderly persons.[4] Elsner and colleagues give an account of when health care providers were unethical and demonstrated ageism.[5]

In Canada, old age is frequently characterized as a time of dependence and disease. Negative presentations of older adults, especially women, in movies, television shows, books, magazines, and jokes contribute to negative beliefs and attitudes.[6] Society's fear of the changes associated with aging, such as grey hair, hearing loss, wrinkles, loss of muscle tone, slowness, and approaching death, also contributes to negative attitudes. However, Kaufert and Lock examined visual images of menopausal women portrayed in pharmaceutical ads. They found a shift from a negative image in the 1970s to a positive image in the 1990s. The new ads showed women with healthy teeth, hair, and skin.[7]

In the twenty-first century, as women assume positions of power in the political and corporate world, the view of women is changing radically. Industrialization and the development of computer technology have made the lives of women and men more alike than ever before. Because gender is deeply rooted in our way of life, change will be gradual, but efforts to increase gender equality will continue.[8]

When it comes to old age, both positive and negative stereotypes are held by many.[9] A research study conducted in Newfoundland asked 240 men and women, aged 18 to 86, about how they thought an older person would respond to a set of attitude questions. Younger people in the study thought that the elderly would give socially and politically conservative answers. People in the study thought that liberal views would decrease with age. The researchers concluded that both young and old people hold traditional age stereotypes.[10] Some of these myths and the contrasting realities are listed in the box entitled "Myths and Misconceptions and Their Realities for the Elderly Person."[11]

### CRITICAL THINKING

*What are some other prevalent myths about elderly people in our society? What fact goes furthest to dispel such myths?*

## Myths and Misconceptions and Their Realities for the Elderly Person

### Myth 1: Age 65 Is a Good Marker for Old Age

**Fact:** Factors other than chronologic age cause the person to be old. Many people are more youthful than their parents were at age 65. With increased longevity, perhaps 70 or 75 should be the chronologic marker.[12]

### Myth 2: Most Old People Are in Bed or in Institutions and Are Ill Physically and Mentally

**Fact:** In 2001, 7 percent of seniors and only about 3 percent of those aged 85 and over were living in health care institutions. Due to increasing health problems as they age, seniors are more limited in their activities than younger Canadians. Still, the vast majority of seniors who reside at home are independent. In 2005, only 7 percent of seniors reported needing help with activities of daily living (ADL) such as bathing or moving from room to room. In 2005, 22.4 percent of seniors needed help with instrumental activities of daily living, a slight increase over the rate of 19.5 percent observed in 1998–1999.[13]

>

## Myth 3: All Old People Are Alike

**Fact:** Each older adult is unique and *quite diverse*. This segment of the lifespan covers more years than any other segment—sometimes more than 35 years. The older people are, the more varied are their physical capabilities, personal style, economic status, and lifestyle preferences. From birth, physical and mental elaboration continues through life to make people more and more unlike one another.[14]

## Myth 4: The Next Generation of Older Adults Will Be the Same as This Generation

**Fact:** The next generation will be better educated, healthier, more mobile, more youthful in appearance, more accustomed to lifestyle change and technology, and more outspoken. The world is changing so quickly that each successive generation is vastly different from the ones that arrived before.[15]

## Myth 5: Old Age Brings Mental Deterioration

**Fact:** The older the person, the greater the neural decay and the slower the processing time. More work on brain function is needed to describe the neural sources of memory changes that come with age.[16]

## Myth 6: Old People Cannot Learn and Are Less Intelligent

**Fact:** Older adults *can* and *do* learn; however, they may need a longer period in which to respond to questions and stimuli. When learning problems occur, they are usually associated with a disease process.[17]

## Myth 7: Most Older Adults Are Incompetent

**Fact:** Older people may have a slower reaction time and take longer to do psychomotor tasks. However, they have more consistent output, less job turnover, greater job satisfaction, fewer accidents, and less absenteeism.[18]

## Myth 8: Most Older Adults Are Unhappy and Dissatisfied with Life

**Fact:** There are many positive aspects: life expectancy at age 65 has improved, and progress has been made in terms of functional health. Seniors assess their own physical and mental health in largely positive terms.[19]

## Myth 9: The Elderly Are Self-Pitying, Apathetic, Irritable, and Hard to Live With

**Fact:** Research shows that mood is related to the present situation and past personality. The older person is as likely as a younger one to have an interesting and pleasant personality.[20]

## Myth 10: The Elderly Are Inactive and Unproductive

**Fact:** Grandparenthood is a common experience for Canadians.[21] In 2001, there were about 5.7 million grandparents in Canada.[22] Some grandparents involve themselves in the daily lives and care of their grandchildren. Grandparents often care for their grandchildren because their own children cannot provide the care. This type of situation can occur because of separation, mental health difficulties, substance abuse, gambling addiction, or the death of an adult child.[23]

## Myth 11: The Elderly Do Not Desire and Do Not Participate in Sexual Activity

**Fact:** Recent research refutes this assertion. Sexual activity may decline because of the lack of a partner, or misinformation about sexuality in late life. The person who has been sexually active all along is able to continue sexual activity; sexual activity involves more than intercourse between the partners.[24]

## Myth 12: The Elderly Are Isolated, Abandoned, and Lonely, and They Are Unlikely to Participate in Activities

**Fact:** One of the most dramatic changes in living arrangements over the past several decades in Canada has been the increase in the proportion of older persons, especially women, who live alone.[25] Between 1971 and 2001, the 85 and over group showed the greatest increase in the tendency to live alone.[26] They enjoy caring for themselves and feel it is their turn now to do more as they wish because they have spent many years caring for others. Increasing numbers of single older people living alone will increase the demand for suitable apartment housing and better transportation.[27] Other elderly live in institutions or residences for the aged where they make friends and enjoy the facilities.

## Myth 13: Retirement Is Disliked by All Old People and Causes Illness and Less Life Satisfaction

**Fact:** Although this may be true for some people, many older people look forward to retirement and are retiring before 65 so that they can continue other pursuits. Most do not become sick from idleness nor do they experience a sense of worthlessness. More than three-fourths of them have satisfying lives.[28]

## Myth 14: Special Health Services for the Aged Are Useless Because the Aged Cannot Benefit Anyway

**Fact:** At age 65, the average person can look forward to 15 more years of life. The elderly have relatively few acute illnesses and accidental injuries, and these conditions are correctable, although older people take longer to recover than younger people do. Common chronic conditions are cardiovascular disease, cancer, arthritis, diabetes, sensory impairments, and depression, which can be treated so that the person can achieve maximum potential and comfort.[29]

Many of the myths and stereotypes associated with aging are culturally determined. The older adult in Canada lives in a culture oriented to youth, productivity, and rapid pace. Because of this orientation, older people often feel that they are not respected, valued, or needed.

As more people live longer, are healthy, and are aging successfully, attitudes are becoming more positive. The elderly are more frequently perceived, recently, as powerful, admired, healthy, active, sexy, and affluent.[30] Culture, ethnicity, and one's socioeconomic level influence the role of the older adult in family relationships, and they determine health practices. Differences exist among cultural populations in how they esteem and care for the elderly, how the elderly stay involved in family matters, and the types of health care services used.[31] Differences also exist between urban and rural families of the elderly.[32] Many older adults continue to follow health practices that are linked to their cultural heritage. Respect must be shown for these cultural aspects of aging, and for cultural influences on health practices and healing methods.[33]

---

### CRITICAL THINKING

*What changes have you noticed that occur in people in later life?*

## THEORIES OF AGING

There is no single model of longevity. Centenarians reach that milestone because of a unique mix of environmental, behavioural, and genetic factors. The older adult experiences

aging in many ways: physiologically, psychologically, sociologically, and spiritually. Physiological changes occur in all body systems with the passing of time. However, individual variation exists as well as the degree of aging within the various body systems in any one individual.[34] Risks for heart disease, cancer, and stroke can be reduced by eating a healthy diet, exercising, and avoiding carcinogens such as cigarettes.[35]

Theories make sense of phenomena; they provide order and a perspective from which to view facts. Contemporary gerontologists are interested in trying to determine how we can improve the quality of life, as well as extend the quantity of life.[36] Knowledge of these theories can be useful as you help the elder and the family to understand the aging process.

## Biological Theories

Biological theories address questions about the basic aging processes that affect all living organisms.[37] These age-related changes occur independently of any external or pathological influence.[38] See Table 14-1 for definitions or explanations and limitations related to these theories.[39]

Nurses need to be aware that although biological theories do not provide all of the answers, they can certainly explain some of the changes seen in the individual. Aging and disease do not necessarily go hand in hand, and the nurse caring for older adults needs to have a clear understanding of the difference between age-related changes and those that may be pathological.[40]

**Table 14-1 Theories of Physical Aging**

| Theory | Definition/Explanation | Applications/Limitations |
|---|---|---|
| *Wear and Tear Theory* | *Body systems wear out because of accumulation of stress of life and effects of metabolism.* Most general and obvious explanation of aging compares body to a machine. | Little scientific evidence. Theory does not consider self-repair mechanisms of body or differences of life span within the human species. |
| *Cross-linkage or Faulty DNA Repair Theory* | *Bonds or cross-linkages develop between molecules or peptides: these bonds change the molecules' properties physically and chemically. Thus collagen in intracellular or extracellular material is chemically altered and function affected.* When collagen is cross-linked with other molecules, changes range from wrinkling, to atherosclerosis, to inelasticity of tissue. When cross-linkages occur with DNA molecules that carry genetic program, DNA is damaged and repairs slowly; mutation or death of cell occurs. | A viable theory. |

*(continued)*

Table 14-1 (continued)

| Theory | Definition/Explanation | Applications/Limitations |
|---|---|---|
| Free Radical (or Oxidative Damage) Theory | Oxygen-free radicals (charged or unstable molecules) or chemicals that contain oxygen in a highly activated state and react with other molecules during normal metabolism cause damage to cells and aging. Exposure to radiation and certain enzymes may interfere with life activities. | Oxidation, as explained by theory, implicated in atherosclerosis, cancer, neurologic disease, and reduced immune function. |
| Biological Clock or Aging by Program Theory | Each organism contains genes or evolutionary processes that govern or control speed at which metabolic processes are performed. These genes or processes act as a genetic clock dictating occurrence of aging and dying. Cells are genetically programmed to reproduce only a certain amount of time; human limit may be 100 to 120 years. Hypothalamus may be the timer that keeps track of age of cells and determines how long they will keep reproducing. Reproduced older cells do not appear to pass on information accurately through the DNA, which weakens functioning ability of older cells. | Humans may be able to outlive inner governing processes because of medical technology and improvements in lifestyle. Cells in nervous system and muscles do not reproduce themselves; all other cells do, at least to some extent.<br><br>Cells are more likely to reproduce imperfectly as they get older. |
| Neuroendocrine Theory | Hormonal changes produce free radicals, cross-linkages, and autoimmunity. | Free radicals may be a special form of cross-linkage; may cause free radicals. |
| Genetic Gene Theory | Aging is programmed; the program exists in certain harmful genes. Genes that direct many cellular activities in early life may become altered in later years, which alters function and may be responsible for functional decline and structural changes associated with aging. | Genetic basis exists for longevity, although environmental factors such as vaccines, nutrition, pollutants, safety factors, and medical care and technology can alter life span. |

## CRITICAL THINKING

*What is the most outstanding contribution to the aging process made by the study of genetics?*

## Psychosocial Theories

Just as one single biological theory does not adequately address biological aging, one single psychosocial theory of aging is not adequate to explain psychological or social aging. The **Continuity Theory** proposes that *an individual's patterns of behaviour are the result of a lifetime of experiences, and aging is the continuation of these lifelong adjustments or personality patterns.* Personality traits remain stable, and early personality function is a guide for the retirement years.[41] Continuity Theory, as first proposed by Brim and Kagan, assumes neither a necessary reduction in

activity levels (*Disengagement Theory*) nor the necessity of maintaining high activity levels (*Activity Theory*). They associated successful aging with the ability of the person to maintain patterns of behaviour that existed before old age. Continuity in behavioural patterns and lifestyle exists over time, regardless of the actual level of activity present. Each of us has a powerful drive to maintain the sense of identity or continuity that allays fears of changing too fast or being changed against one's will by external forces. There is a simultaneous drive to develop and mature further, which fosters continuing change in at least small ways. Adult development is not in the genes, but it does lie in the intricacies of life experiences.

In recent decades, a number of theories of aging, particularly those that centre on lifespan perspectives, have focused on relationships between gender and aging.[42] A few of the studies have addressed diverse populations, such as lesbians, gay men, and transgendered individuals. One purpose of the gender-related psychological theories of aging has been to study gender role differences, and social roles and power.[43] It is important to keep in mind that this is a new area of research and findings will undoubtedly change during this century.

It is important for nurses to remember that almost all older adults continue be active, engage or disengage as they wish, and remain valued members of society.

## Developmental Theories

Several developmental theories have addressed psychosocial aging. **Erikson's Epigenetic Theory**[44] suggests that *successful personality development in later life depends on the ability to resolve the psychosocial crisis known as integrity versus despair.* Erikson's theory is psychodynamic and is part of a life cycle approach that emphasizes that the developmental tasks of each stage must be met before the person can work through the next tasks. The theory is discussed in detail later in this chapter.

**Peck's Theory**[45] *expanded Erikson's original theory and divided the right stage—ego integrity versus despair—into additional stages occurring during middle age and old age.* The stages described by Peck as specific to old age are *ego differentiation versus work-role preoccupation, body transcendence versus body preoccupation, and ego transcendence versus ego preoccupation.*[46] According to all developmental theories, the older adult's behaviour and response depend on how earlier developmental crises were handled.

When interacting with the older adult, these theories enable the nurse to understand the phases of the lifespan and how the older adults respond as they continue to grow with advancing years. In planning activities for elders, nurses need to understand that all older adults enjoy feeling valued and being considered contributing members of society.

## Sociologic Theories

**Disengagement Theory** suggests that *individuals in a society undergo a self-disengagement process during the middle and later years of life.* This process is characterized by a reduction in general energy levels, a reduction in societal involvement, and an increased preoccupation with one's own needs and desires.[47] Cross-cultural studies show that *disengagement* is not inevitable, and it is generally not applicable to family relationships.

### CRITICAL THINKING

*Which of the following theories would researchers use to direct their research in gerontology?*

Some theories claim that physical and mental declines in old age are actually part of the dying process. The **terminal drop hypothesis** asserts that *all adults retain excellent physical and mental function until just a few years before death, at which time significant declines occur in all functions.* Longitudinal research suggests that declines in most functions are gradual and only changes in IQ scores seem to fit the terminal drop pattern.[48]

**Activity Theory** implies that *the older adult has essentially the same psychological and social needs as do middle-aged people.* According to this theory, the older adult must compensate for the loss of roles experienced in later maturity. The older adult does not disengage, but does need to maintain a moderately active lifestyle.[49] This theory sees activity as necessary to maintain a person's life satisfaction and positive concept. By remaining active, the older person stays young and alive and does not withdraw from society because of an age parameter.[50]

It is important for the nurse to assist older adults to adapt to various limitations and secure appropriate living arrangements. In fact, helping adults to adjust to limitations, while accentuating their strengths, will often enable them to remain independent and perpetuate a high quality of life during later years.[51]

### CRITICAL THINKING

*What do you aspire to be like when you are elderly? Describe your profile.*

## FAMILY DEVELOPMENT AND RELATIONSHIPS

The changing demographic profile of developed countries has been associated with an increased number of four- and five-generation families. In such families, it is common to have two generations at or near old age, with the oldest person over 75 years. The "generation in the middle" can extend into retirement years in many families. Thus, the "young-old," who could be facing diminished personal resources, may be the group increasingly called on to provide additional support to aged kin—the old-old and the very old or frail-old.

Refer to Table 4-3, which illustrates the stages of the family life cycle, the emotional processes of transition (key principles), and the second-order changes in the family required to proceed developmentally. Stage 6, families in later life, is the appropriate stage for the older adult.

Assist the client and family to be cognizant of these changes. Establish a rapport with them and encourage the sharing of concerns, issues, feelings, and practical aspects related to fulfilling these changes. Refer them to a counsellor or community agency if help is desired.

## Relationship with Spouse

In later life, the responsibilities of parenthood and employment diminish, with few formal responsibilities to take their place. Usually, a corresponding decline occurs in social contacts and related activities. Most factors that affect the social life of the elderly are found in personal social skills. Marital status remains a major organizing force for personal life. With children gone, and being without the daily contact of co-workers provided by employment, the elderly begin to lose the basis for social integration. Declining health, limited income, and fewer daily responsibilities tend to create greater needs for social support. Thus, having a spouse provides the opportunity for needed companionship.

Although women, more than men, provide the greater amount of support to their spouses, husbands play a significant role in caring for their wives in later life.[52] Husbands make up about 40 percent of spousal caregivers. Although some men are not comfortable with giving care that involves "traditionally female" tasks, such as domestic work and personal care, many men feel a sense of accomplishment when they do provide care to their spouse.[53] However, a longitudinal study conducted with 232 older husband caregivers found that husbands vary in their response to caregiving over time. The findings support previous study results indicating that subjective stressors, such as fatigue, rather than objective stressors, such as family conflict and caregiver resources, are significant predictors of caregiving outcomes.[54] Possibly, men will take a more active role in caregiving in the future. For example, demographic changes, changes in family structure and size, and women's increased employment outside the home all tend to increase the probability that a man will provide care to an aging parent or spouse.[55]

## Relationships with Offspring and Other Family Members

Relatively recent developments such as trends toward smaller families, longer lifespans, increasingly long-term employment of women, and increasingly high mobility of both young and old carry important implications for children being a primary resource in old age.

Adult children tend to stay in touch with their older parents. Among adult children 25 to 54 years of age, seven out of ten contact their mothers at least once a week.[56] Daughters, compared to sons, have more frequent contacts with their mothers. Interestingly, both daughters and sons have more frequent contact with mothers than with their fathers.[57] Adult children provide much of the support needed by their parents. Research findings indicate that even older adults who reside in long-term care facilities receive informal help from their children.[58] Others report that strong feelings of attachment to a parent, and the recognition of past help and support from parents, lead to caregiving.[59] Geographic proximity is a stable predictor of older parent–child interaction, more than offspring gender or the health status of the parent.[60]

Older parents receive and perceive their children's help in several ways. Younger parents receive more help with automobile maintenance and help in the form of gifts. Older parents receive help with shopping and transportation. Parents who most strongly valued family are most desirous of, and most satisfied with, family support. Parents tend to expect less help from their children when they live at a distance or when they work outside the home. Parents appreciate most the help that keeps them self-reliant or autonomous, maintains social integration, maximizes choice and expressive interactions, and forestalls reliance on more extensive services.[61]

It is interesting to note that today individuals spend more years as an adult child of living parents than as parents of young children. This trend is expected to continue in the future. In some cases, child caregivers of older parents will, themselves, need support as they grow older.[62]

Some elderly people have a limited number of family members and some couples have no children. The childless couple will probably have adapted to childlessness psychologically, but they are especially vulnerable at crisis points, such as episodes of poor health, or the death of their spouse or housing companion. If those persons or couples cannot drive, and do not have transportation, they will have a greater need for help and will often hesitate to ask for help.

Your teaching and referrals might be particularly instrumental to enable the elderly person with few relatives or resources to manage more effectively.

## Grandparenthood and Great-Grandparenthood

Grandparenthood has multiple meanings for the person, depending in part on one's age at the initial time of grandparenthood, and the accomplishments of the grandchildren are probably a source of status.[63] The increasing divorce rate adds to the complexity of grandparent relationships. The grandparents may be the main caretakers for the children, or there may be a part-time commitment, sharing child care with their adult children. Likewise, grandchildren have a special tie to grandparents.[64] Research indicates that even when there was divorce in the family, adult children from divorced families continued their relationships with grandparents.[65] A Canadian researcher examined the subjective meanings of grandparent–adult grandchild relationships, and studied the experience of being grandparents and adult grandchildren. She found that these relationships grow more profound and meaningful as grandparents and grandchildren age, move through the life course, and experience life events.[66]

Grandparents are becoming the main caretakers of some children, often in the custodial role, although legal custody is unlikely even if the children have a permanent home. Sometimes the grandparents serve as babysitter or a daycare service. When mothers live in the home with grandparents, the grandmother as main caregiver frequently has a negative impact on both the mother's and grandmother's parenting practices.[67] Grandparents are often happy with their role in that they can enjoy the young person and enter into a playful, informal, companionable, and confiding relationship. The grandchild is seen as a source of enjoyable activity, someone for whom to buy things that are enjoyed together by the grandparent and the child. The number of *great-grandparents* and *great-great-grandparents* is increasing as more people live longer.

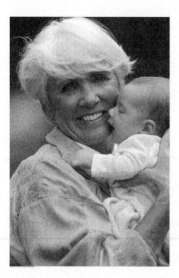

Grandparents often look forward to their role.

Source: Sherwen, L.N., M.A. Scoovena, and C.T. Weingarten. *Nursing Care of the Childbearing Family.* Stamford, CT: Appleton & Lange, 1991, p. 764.

**CRITICAL THINKING**

*What tips for grandparents would you provide when they are caring for preschool grandchildren?*

## Social Relationships

Social networks of family, friends, and neighbours provide instrumental and expressive support. They contribute to the well-being of the senior by promoting socialization and companionship, elevating morale and life satisfaction, buffering the effects of stressful events, providing a confidant, and facilitating the mastery of coping skills. For example, social supports buffer the effects of stressful life events. The components of informal support networks—spouses, children, close relatives, distant kin (cousins, aunts, uncles, nieces, nephews), co-workers, close friends, neighbours, members of volunteer community support services, and acquaintances—have a variety of functions, and they vary in importance to the senior. Some members of the community act as lay gatekeepers. Mail carriers, veterinarians, utility workers, grain dealers, and other business people provide informal social support and help look out for the rural elders.[68] Instrumental help is given in the form of advice, information, financial aid, and assistance with tasks. Socioemotional aid is given in the form of affection, sympathy, understanding, acceptance, esteem, and referral to services.[69] Planning for arranged contact between the generations (e.g., with preschoolers or adolescents) also contributes to meaningful social interactions for both generations.[70]

Formal health-related support services include services from both government and private agencies. Examples include home maintenance services, chore services, home-delivered meals, assistance from home health aides, home visits by professional therapists or nurses, and home care services. Formal support services that are available to elderly adults but that do not always come to the home include medical and social services, daycare, respite care, and the church.[71]

The frequency of use of social networks is not directly related to physical health. As income decreases, visiting with neighbours declines but visits to close friends or relatives increase, as does the tendency to talk to family members about feelings and talk with friends about events. The elderly rate the helpfulness of children and other family members as important. Lower income increases the senior's reliance on friends and relatives and the value placed on their help. A higher frequency of social contacts and greater intensity of kin and friend relationships have been found for women in comparison to men. Apparently intimacy or close friendship ties and having a confidant are less important to the male.[72]

Supportive ties become smaller and more unstable in old age. Social support sometimes provides burdens for those who provide support to the senior. Burdens and costs can result in being less willing or able to help, physical or psychological distancing, increasing the social isolation of the dependent senior, or becoming enmeshed in the caregiver role to the exclusion of other relationships or roles. Ideally, informal networks are integrated with formal support services.[73]

A system of informal assistance through family, friends, and neighbours is the major source of help for the elderly. For seniors, there are three types of neighbourhood exchange types:

1. High helpers, who exhibit a rather formal, quasi-professional style of helping without the expectation of payback.

2. Mutual helpers, who show an interdependent style of give and take.

3. Neighbourhood isolates, whose social ties and help sources are primarily outside the neighbourhood.

High helpers with neighbours are those who do volunteer work or who are active in self-help groups. Mutual helpers have more neighbourhood contact and are generally quite outgoing. Isolates have little contact with others and view themselves as quiet people. They are often in poor health and in need of help themselves.[74]

Many of the events of later life are exit events, involving continuous threat, stress, and loss, such as widow(er)hood, chronic or poor health, retirement, change in residence, and low income. Socialization contributes to well-being by lending continuity and structure to the transitions encountered by people.

Often you will be able to assist the elderly by asking for and accepting help from others, and in becoming familiar with community resources.

## Caregiver Role

The role of the middle-aged offspring in caring for the elderly parent was described in Chapter 13. Even as elders are being cared for, they are also a source of support—emotionally, socially, and financially (by providing living arrangement)—for the adult child.[75]

The caregiver in an elderly couple is most frequently the wife, primarily because women live longer than men, and they are usually younger than their spouses. If the woman is impaired, the husband is often the caregiver. The spouse is the primary source of help for married elderly with impaired capacity, and adult daughters are the major helpers when a spouse is not present or not able to help. In some cultures, the grandchild or great-grandchild becomes the

primary caregiver, especially if he or she was raised by the now-frail great-grandparent. This type of situation is discussed in Burton's research.[76] The practice of relying on friends is highest among unmarried impaired elderly who have few family members living within an hour's travel. The more frail the person, the more likely it is that a family member will be the primary caregiver, rather than formal care systems or non-related people.[77] The majority of non-institutionalized elderly are self-sufficient.

Be aware of personal feelings of the middle-aged or elderly caregiver and the family. In addition, you need to be aware of the needs and feelings of the elderly person, issues and conflicts within family, and ways to help families manage the caregiving experience. The family caregiver for the non-institutionalized elder is almost always in need of help from supportive services.[78] Education and support group programs appear to hold great promise as a means for assisting the family caregivers of older relatives. You will have an important role in implementing both of those interventions. A number of strategies can be helpful to the caregiver, both in preventing decline in the caregiver and in administering care to the elder.[79] *Various programs can be effective for reducing stress in the caregivers of elderly family members who are either emotionally or physically disabled:*

- Support groups, especially for caregivers of patients with Alzheimer's or other dementias, which offer practical solutions to problems and provide emotional support

- Respite care programs based at the person's home or in agencies, to care for the ill person when the caregiver needs time off (a day, weekend, or week)

- Education about stress management techniques that enhance one's abilities to care for the self as well as the family member

- Telephone crisis counselling services available to elders and their caregivers; the availability and use of telecommunication services are expected to become more increasingly available.[80]

## Widowhood

Because widowhood can occur before late life, the feelings, problems, and issues pertinent to the widow were discussed in Chapter 13.

For older couples, the death of a spouse is inevitable. The probability is greater that women will be bereaved rather than the man. In fact, when widowhood occurs, several consequences follow, including the loss of one's sexual partner, loss of companionship and intimacy, and increased dependency on others.[81] When marriage has lasted for many decades, as is common among individuals in their seventies and eighties, the impact of the loss can be tremendous and the feelings of grief, loneliness, and emptiness are often overwhelming. The findings of a study of grief responses among older widows concluded that being lonely and alone were the most troubling and most frequently cited problems.[82] However, widowhood, especially after a period of caregiving, will often introduce both a measure of freedom to make new contacts and a stimulus to do so. The widowed person may have greater intimacy with friends than those who are married, most likely because married people interact more with their spouses.[83]

Widowed women more than bereaved men are more likely to visit with close friends and relatives. They tend to talk to family about their worries and to their children about crises. Loss of a spouse allows for the expansion or addition of new roles. The frequency of contacts increases with widowhood. Widowhood results in greater involvement with informal social relationships than was the case during marriage. Chipperfield and Havens state that while life satisfaction declines for both men and women following the death of a spouse, men show a greater decline.[84]

Your teaching, emotional support, referral to services, and encouragement to continue as active a life as possible are important to the widow as she adjusts to losses and new roles.

## Divorce and the Elderly

There appears to be an increasing number of divorces occurring among older people.[85] Being divorced in old age, or at any age, can negatively affect a person's economic position, and it can increase one's demands for social welfare support. Typically, for women, divorce is associated with some deterioration in their standard of living, although divorce has little effect in that regard for men.[86] Family and kinship relationships are always affected by divorce. The children, or other relatives, who would provide physical help and psychosocial support will likely not be available to one of the parents in his or her old age.

Novak and Campbell report that researchers predict a higher divorce rate and a greater number of divorced older people in the future. This will make the economic well-being, mental health, and family life of divorced older people more important in the future.[87]

### CRITICAL THINKING

*Undertake a content analysis of several academic journals focusing on the consequences of divorce between elderly couples. What trends do you observe?*

## Singlehood

A small percentage of the elderly population remains single and never marries. They have no spouse or children. Singles have made unique adaptations to aging. They play vital and supportive roles in the lives of siblings, older parents, and others. They also form friendships and other social relationships to provide themselves with supporters, confidants, and companions. To date, little research exists on the lives and social relationships of lifelong single older individuals.[88]

Psychological integrity and social independence are somewhat unique features of the single personality. The single person views *fluidity and variety in social relationships*, rather than the exclusivity of marriage, as a distinct advantage in promoting his or her own opportunities for personal growth while still protecting autonomy. Lifestyle is geared to preserving personal independence and the development of self, with privacy, self-expression through work, freedom of movement, and preoccupation with expanding experiences, philosophic insights, and imaginative conceptions of life as goals for the person. Overall, never-married older people report that they lead active lives and that they feel happy, are in good health, and are satisfied with their standards of living. Many singles feel they have greater freedom and control over their lives.

Researchers project an increase in the proportion of older single people as baby boomers enter later life. These aging singles will play a significant role in helping to change societal attitudes about permanent singlehood. Researchers say that future studies should consider the coping strategies that older people use to maintain their high quality of life and their attitudes about singlehood.[89]

*Friends* are important. Friendship is a process that occurs throughout life. Although older adults rarely terminate friendships, acquaintances often fade away because of lifestyle changes, geographic moves, or illness. Friends often act as family and promote healing—emotionally, physically, and socially. Positive social interaction lowers the stress hormone levels, helps to preserve cognitive functions, and prevents depression. Sharing ideas, talking, and listening are the main components of friendships. Men talk more about past careers, politics, and sports. Women talk more about relationships and feelings.

Be alert to the special emotional and social needs of the single elderly, to their reticence at times to ask for help, and to their need for information about community resources. You could become a significant confidant.

### CRITICAL THINKING

*Compare and contrast the health promotion strategies required by the single elderly person and those required by the married elderly couple.*

## Elders and Pets

Pets are great companions for older people. They are therapeutic, whether they are in the home, or in the centre or institution for the elderly. Pets offer companionship and unconditional love. They soothe and lift the spirits, and a specially trained dog can offer assistance and security. Pets have a beneficial effect on one's physical health because their presence tends to lower the stress response. Touches from the pet and stroking the pet provide physiologic release, and they tend to lower anxiety. Pets can promote verbal communication skills; birds have been said to "talk" back. Although animals and birds do carry diseases, healthy pets can be obtained from well-run shelters and shops or the Humane Society. Volunteers regularly take their animals to visit residents in hospitals, personal care homes, and other institutions across Canada. Katz states that pet facilitated therapy (PFT), which has emerged during the past few decades, is refreshingly simple, low-tech, and effective.[90]

Explore accessible pet services. You can be instrumental in promoting pet therapy.

## Elder Abuse and Neglect

The abuse and neglect of older adults is not a new problem.[91] The 65-and-older age group comprises one of the fastest-growing segments of the Canadian population. According to Hawranik and McKean, this changing profile has heightened concern about the possible increase in the incidence of abuse and neglect among seniors.[92] Most Canadian research on elder abuse has used convenience samples, which at times produce low response rates. Consequently, generalizations from these results are uncertain.[93]

---

### CRITICAL THINKING

*What are your attitudes and beliefs about elder abuse?*

---

Usually, the abuser is a relative (spouse more often than offspring) residing with the victim. However, abusers are not always blood relatives, or even family members. The abuse can occur either in the home or in community programs, such as recreation centres and adult day programs.[94] Refer to the box entitled "Types and Manifestations of Elder Abuse" for further description.[95]

Hypotheses about the causes of elder abuse are listed in the box entitled "Causes of Elder Maltreatment, Abuse, or Neglect."[96]

Ways to prevent or reduce abuse are listed in the box entitled "Tips for the Older Person for Preventing or Reducing Abuse."

---

## Types and Manifestations of Elder Abuse

### Physical Abuse

- Neglect of physical care (food, eyeglasses, hearing aid, or information withheld)
- Slap, bruise, push
- Beating
- Burns, broken bones
- Brandishing a knife, cutting, stabbing
- Restraint (chain to toilet or tie to bed), resulting in skin breakdown or decubitus ulcers as well as fractures
- Sexual molestation, rape

### Psychological Abuse

- Verbal abuse (curse, scream, insult, demean, treat like a child)
- Verbal threats, name calling
- Decision making, voting denied
- Exclusion from family activities, isolation
- Placement in nursing home without consent or knowledge

### Financial Abuse

- Confiscation of pension or other income cheques
- Person forced to sign over property or assets
- Other financial exploitation
- Theft of property and personal items for sale
- Takeover of trust, guardianship
- Exploitation of resources for profit

### Social Abuse

- Forced isolation from family, friends
- Constant switching of doctors
- Refusal of home health care or other community resources (daycare, home health aide, Meals on Wheels)
- Inability to accept help or acknowledge difficulty with care
- Geographic isolation, e.g., rural, inner-city ghetto
- Caregiver or client minimize injuries or situation

- Elder becomes more dependent or disabled
- Elder is cognitively impaired or has Alzheimer's disease
- Family is under economic stress
- Caregiver is exhausted or loses control; unable to cope
- Adult offspring is unemployed, lives in parent's home, and expects to be cared for
- Adult offspring is mentally ill or alcohol- or drug-addicted
- Family interaction pattern of screaming, hitting, and violence has existed through lifetime of marriage or childrearing
- Retirement and lack of role clarity for both spouses result in much frustration in retired man
- Man who was abusive to co-workers now abuses most available person, the wife
- Woman is financially dependent on spouse
- Elder is abandoned or seldom visited by children
- Victim is unwilling or unable to report the problem

*Signs and symptoms of the abused or neglected elder* include the following:

- Bruises, fractures, malnourished status
- Undue confusion not attributable to physiologic consequences of aging
- Conflicting explanation about the senior's condition
- Unusual fear exhibited by the senior in a presumed safe environment, in the home, or in the presence of the caregiver
- A report of the daily routine that has considerable gaps in the sequence
- Apparent impaired functioning or abnormal behaviour in the caregiver
- Indifference or hostility displayed by caregiver in response to questions

During the assessment of potential abuse or neglect, show a willingness to listen to the caregiver's perspective. Solicit the caregiver's early memories of relationships with the senior to learn of any long-term conflicts. Most abused seniors are reluctant and ashamed to report abuse or neglect because of (1) fear of retaliation; (2) exposure of offspring to community censure or legal punishment; and (3) fear of potential removal from their home.

*Three questions help detect partner violence.* These questions are applicable to spouse abuse at any age:

1. Have you been hit, kicked, punched, or otherwise hurt by someone within the past year? If so, when?
2. Do you feel safe in your current relationship?
3. Is there a partner from a previous relationship who is making you feel unsafe now?

Based on the answers given, ask related questions in order to gain full information. Be gentle and allow the person time to give what may be painful answers.

### CRITICAL THINKING

*What nursing interventions can be developed in working with the abused elderly?*

In Canada, it is the older adult's right to make his or her own decisions. It is critical to note that if the older adult who is being abused is considered mentally competent, then he or she is supported in the decision to report or not to report. Some service providers believe that criminal prosecution is of little assistance to the older victim because the focus is on punishing the offender rather than on helping the victim.[97] However, anyone (victim, family member or friend, a witness to the

- Remain sociable and stay active in the community; enlarge your circle of friends; join a community group
- Plan for possible disability by completing an advance medical directive and arranging for power-of-attorney
- Familiarize yourself with community resources that help older people remain as independent as possible
- Do not share a household with anyone who has a history of violent behaviour or substance abuse
- Do not move in with a child or relative if your relationship is troubled
- Avoid taking into your home new or unknown people in a live-in arrangement
- Ask for help when you need it from a lawyer, physician, or trusted family member
- Check the *Directory of Services and Programs Addressing the Needs of Older Adult Victims of Violence in Canada*.[98] For example, residents in Nova Scotia may call the Health and Community Service Office, the Public Health Nurse, or the RCMP.

# Elder Abuse

Robert and Sarah Hughes have been married to each other for almost 50 years. Robert ran his own gasoline and automobile service station with two or three auto mechanics. Five years ago, he sold the business and seemed to become a changed person when he stopped spending long hours each day at work. Sarah had been a cashier in a large local grocery store. Robert insisted she stop work when he sold the business—so they could "do things together." Reluctantly, she gave up her job when she was 68 years old. Because of Sarah's memory loss in recent years, Robert has allowed home care workers into the home to help her with eating and personal care. The workers report that Robert yells at Sarah when she forgets things. They have even seen him attempting to force feed her when she

could not finish eating her entire meal. He sometimes swears at her and calls her names. Recently, they have seen bruises on Sarah's arms and welts on her legs. You are the home care coordinator to whom the home care workers report.

1. What intervention options are open to you to address the elder abuse that seems clearly evident here?
2. What is the role of the home care nurse in introducing and implementing interventions?
3. What barriers should you expect to encounter when the interventions are applied?
4. How will you address these barriers?

abuse, or a service provider) can report a suspected occurrence to the police. Reports can be made anonymously, if desired. In provinces and territories with mandatory reporting legislation, service providers who know of, or suspect, abuse are required to report the incident to the authorities.[99] Victim assistance programs can be most helpful in supporting older adults and their families as they proceed through the criminal justice system. Examples of victim assistance programs include law information lines, seniors' advocacy centres, and legal aid services. In Manitoba, for example, a Senior Abuse Line is available, which is a confidential information service aimed at providing seniors, family members, professionals, and others with a one-stop information resource on elder abuse.[100] Other provinces and territories have similar sources of assistance. The Department of Justice Canada supports the efforts of Aboriginal communities in developing culturally appropriate approaches to addressing violence and abuse.[101] Without appropriate interventions, the mistreatment of elders in community and institutional settings will assume epidemic proportions.[102]

## PHYSIOLOGIC CONCEPTS

*Use this information to assess, teach, and implement health promotion measures.*

## Physical Characteristics

When we are born, regardless of our genetic background or external influences, we all have one thing in common: the element of aging. From the day of birth, we begin the aging

process in our unique way. A great deal of diversity occurs from person to person in this process.

The rate and manifestations of aging in each individual depend on heredity, past illnesses, lifestyle, patterns of eating and exercise, the presence of chronic illnesses, and the extent of lifetime stress. Some generalized types of physiologic changes do occur, however. They include degenerative joint changes, decrease in the secretion of digestive juices, decreased elasticity, and calcification of the heart valves.[103]

Changes in organic and systemic functioning are highly variable, both among and within individuals. Aging, together with chronic stress, can depress immune function, which makes older people more susceptible to colds, pneumonia, and other respiratory infections.[104] Another important change that affects health is a decline in reserve capacity (or organ reserve). **Organ reserve** is *the extra capacity of the organs that is drawn upon in times of stress or illness.* With age, reserve levels tend to drop, and many older people cannot respond as quickly or as efficiently to extra physical demands as they could earlier in life.[105]

**General Appearance** The general appearance of the older adult is determined in part by the changes that occur in the skin, hair, and posture.

**Skin** The overall appearance of the skin changes dramatically with age (see Table 14-2).[106] Wrinkles on the face become pronounced, first, because of the decrease of elastin and, second, by pigmentation changes that result in the accumulation of discoloration. Decreases in eccrine,

## Table 14-2 Alterations in Integumentary System Related to Aging

| Tissue/Organ | Alteration and Rationale | Implications for Health Promotion |
|---|---|---|
| **Epidermis** | Skin manufactures less collagen, elastin, and other proteins. Cellular division decreases; thus, skin cells are replaced more slowly. (Skin cells live an average of 46 days in 70-year-old, compared with 100 days in 30-year-old.)<br>Elastin fibres are more brittle.<br>Loss of collagen fibres causes decreased turgor and loss of elasticity, wrinkles, and creases.<br>Permeability increases and cells are thinner.<br>Ability to retain fluids decreases, causes skin to become drier, less flexible.<br>Fair-skinned persons lose pink tones, become paler.<br>**Lentigo senilis**, *irregular areas of dark pigmentation on dorsum of hands, arms, and face* and uneven pigmentation occur.<br>Capillaries and small arteries on exposed skin surface become dilated.<br>Decreased response to pain sensation and temperature changes may cause accidents or burns. | Wounds heal more slowly.<br>Maintain nutrition and hygiene.<br>Use emollients and lotion to maintain moisture on skin.<br>Avoid hot water baths, excessive soap.<br>Rinse skin well; pat dry.<br>Some medications make skin more fragile and susceptible to bruising: Aspirin, prednisone, steroid topical creams.<br>Cosmetics may be used.<br>Protect from direct sun. Use sunscreen, protective factor of 15 or higher, with UVA and UVB protection.<br>Assist person in accepting appearance changes.<br>Teach safety factors.<br>Care with heating pads or hot water bottles and ice packs. |
| **Subcutaneous tissue (hypodermic)** | Loss of fat cells, especially in face and limbs, causes sagging and wrinkles.<br>Lack of tissue over bony prominences contributes to decubitus ulcers.<br>Lower cutaneous blood flow and loss of fat contribute to decreased insulation and susceptibility to chilling. | Assist adjustment to appearance and changes.<br>Protect bony prominences from pressure, abrasions, injury, and decubitus ulcers.<br>Provide adequate clothing and heat control for comfort. |
| **Dermis** | Decreased fat, water, and matrix content cause translucent appearance of skin.<br>Larger and coarser collagen fibres decrease flexibility of collagen, reduce elasticity, and cause sags and wrinkles.<br>Decreased number of fibroblasts and fibres cause thinning tissue. | Emollients, lotions, and cosmetics may be used.<br>Assist person in accepting appearance changes.<br>Avoid bumps, scrapes, and lacerations of skin.<br>Wear protective clothing. |
| **Hair** | Reduced melanin production causes greying. Thinning, stiffness, and loss of lustre are due to change in germ centre that produces hair follicles. Baldness is genetic.<br>In women, increased facial hair on upper lip and chin result from diminished estrogen. | Use hair colouring or cosmetic techniques if desired.<br><br><br><br><br>Assist person in integrating appearance changes into body image. |

*(continued)*

Table 14-2 (continued)

| Tissue/Organ | Alteration and Rationale | Implications for Health Promotion |
|---|---|---|
| Sebaceous oil glands | Decreased lubrication with oil causes skin to be drier, rougher, and scaly. | Use emollients/lotions. Avoid hot water, use minimal soap, rinse well. Pat dry. Use room humidifiers. |
| Sweat glands | Reduced number interferes with ability to sweat freely and regulate body temperature. | Prevent heat stroke. Drink adequate water. Dress in garments that allow heat transmission from body. Use fan or air conditioner as needed in hot weather. |
| Nails | Growth is slower. Increased calcium deposition causes ridges and thickening. | Encourage visit to podiatrist for care of toenails and cosmetologist for care of fingernails. |

apocrine, and the reduced activity of the sebaceous glands cause the skin to dry.[107]

**Hair** The hair of the older person looks grey or white because of the decrease in the number of functioning melanocytes and the replacement of pigmented strands of hair with non-pigmented ones. The texture and thickness of the hair also changes as it becomes coarse and thin.[108] The loss of hair, which occurs on the scalp, in the pubic and axillary areas, and on the extremities, is due to hormonal decline.[109]

**Posture** The posture of the older adult is one of general flexion. The head is tilted forward, and the hips and knees become slightly flexed. Muscles in the torso are held rigidly. The older adult stands with the feet apart to provide a wide base of support. He or she takes shorter steps, which usually produces a shuffling gait. A shift in the centre of gravity occurs as well, which affects movement and balance.[110]

## CRITICAL THINKING

*What other changes in general appearance can you think of that can be attributed to the aging process in late adulthood?*

## Neurologic System

**Nervous System Changes** With aging, there are major changes in the nervous system that occur normally; they tend to alter the individual's sensory response:[111]

- Loss of nerve cells
- Decrease in neurotransmitters
- Slower nerve impulse transmission
- Decrease in nerve conduction velocity
- Decline in electric activity
- Increase in sensory threshold
- Decline in integration of sensory and motor function

All of these neurologic changes create certain problems for the older adult. Because of these particular neurologic changes, older adults do not respond as quickly to changes in their external environment. This slower response affects many facets of their life (e.g., there is greater risk to overall safety, and drivers over 65 years of age are involved in a higher percentage of automobile accidents per kilometre driven than are drivers aged 25 to 54 years). The older adult's increase in sensory threshold affects pain and tactile perception and responses to stimuli, resulting in an increased susceptibility to burns or other injuries.[112]

**Brain** By age 90, the weight of the brain has decreased 10 percent from its maximum, and this reduction in size is not uniform throughout the brain. This particular weight loss is accompanied by a reduction of neurons (nerve cells) in the cerebral cortex, the part of the brain that handles most cognitive tasks. However, research suggests that the cause is not a widespread reduction in the number of neurons, but rather a shrinkage in the neuronal size due to the loss of connective tissue: axons, dendrites, and synapses.[113] The most significant of these changes is the loss of dendritic density. Research suggests that experience, as well as aging, is involved in the loss of dendritic density. Dendritic loss results in a gradual slowing of synaptic speed, with a consequent increase in reaction time for many everyday tasks.[114] Although a loss of grey matter occurs, the white matter is not significantly different than in young people. Certain brain structures, including the cerebral cortex, shrink more rapidly in men than in women. Aerobic exercise can slow the loss of brain tissue.[115]

**Vision** Normal age-related changes in vision occur gradually. Over time, however, these changes can limit the functional ability of the older adult. The number of fibres composing the optic nerve decreases over time. Lacrimal glands produce fewer tears, causing the cornea to become dry and irritated. The lens of the eye thickens and yellows. Objects take on a yellowish hue, and the cells within the lens lose water and shrink. The diameter of the pupil decreases and the pupil is less able to accommodate to light changes. The lack of pupillary response, increased lens opacity, and an irregular corneal surface, which causes light to scatter, together result in a reduced tolerance to glare and difficulty in adjusting from brightly lit to dim areas, or vice versa. Visual contrast sensitivity decreases for both size and light. These changes interfere with the ability of the eye to transmit and refract light. Because of the loss of elasticity in the lens, and slower response in accommodation, **presbyopia,** *inability to change lens shape for near vision*, is present in most adults after age 45 or 50. Even with corrective lenses, the individual might need longer to focus on near objects.[116] Visual impairment can lead to a loss of independence, social isolation, depression, and a decreased quality of life.[117]

Colour vision tends to be altered after age 60, because of retinal changes (rods and cones), a loss of sensitivity in the photoreceptors, and slower transmission of visual impulses to the nervous system. The reception of short wavelengths (blue) is affected first, followed by middle-wavelength hues (green, greenish yellow), and last by the long wavelengths (red). Thus, for the older adult, colours such as green, blue, and violet are more difficult to see than are red, orange, and yellow. Pastels fade so that they become indistinguishable from each other. Monotones, whites, and dark colours also become difficult to see. Brighter colours compensate for the decline in colour discrimination caused by the yellowing and opacity of the lens.[118]

Cataract development and glaucoma frequently occur in this age group. With **cataracts,** the *lens becomes opaque.* The result is diminished vision and increased sensitivity to glare. **Glaucoma** is *caused by damage to the optic nerve from increased intraocular pressure.*[119] **Age-related macular degeneration (AMD)**, a common, often slow-to-be-detected, eye disease in elders, *occurs when the macula, the most light-sensitive portion of the retina, begins to deteriorate.* An intact macula is necessary for good central vision and the discrimination of fine details. One-fourth of people over age 65 and one-third over age 80 experience some AMD. See Table 14-3 for health promotion implications related to visual changes, as well as the box entitled "Guidelines for Helping the Blind Person."[120]

**Table 14-3** Neurological Changes in the Eye—Implications for Health Promotion

| Change | Health Promotion Measure |
| --- | --- |
| **Dry cornea lens changes**<br>Presbyopia<br>Spatial-depth vision changes | Use artificial tears if needed.<br>Wear glasses to protect eyes from dust and flying debris.<br>Wear corrective glasses or contact lenses.<br>Use hard lens to magnify print for reading. |
| **Pupillary and lens changes**<br>Decreased tolerance to glare or light changes | Obtain books and periodicals in large print, or use pre-recorded materials.<br>Teach safety considerations; take time to focus for vision.<br>Teach safety factors related to doorways, space, and objects.<br>It is important that institutions: place colour guards on stair steps, clearly mark doorways, avoid having carpet, furniture, walls, and drapes all of same or similar colour. Walls, floor, doors, door frames, and furniture should be clearly delineated. |
| **Retinal changes**<br>Colour-vision altered | Wear tinted glass or brimmed hat to reduce glare or bright light.<br>Turn on light in dark room before entering.<br>Stand in doorway or at stairwell briefly to adjust to light changes from either bright light or dark.<br>Teach the need for more *indirect,* but adequate, illumination to perceive stimuli, do visual work. Avoid white or glossy surfaces.<br>It is important for institutions to cover windows and avoid putting shiny wax on the floor.<br>Avoid glare on floors in bedrooms, dining areas, lounges, and hallways.<br>Teach safety considerations, especially with driving in bright sunlight or at night.<br>Use a nightlight to provide low-lighted visibility. |

*(continued)*

Table 14-3 (continued)

| Change | Health Promotion Measure |
|---|---|
| | Teach implications for personal grooming and dress, the enjoyment of colours in nature, interior decoration, and the design of living environment. Brighter colours are enjoyed more than dull ones. |
| | Teach the family members implications for selecting greeting cards and gifts. |
| | Adapt to yellowed vision. Teach the relevant implications for selecting clothing, cosmetics, or interior decor. |
| | It is important for institutions to use colours in interior decor that can be seen readily, enjoyed, and not misinterpreted by the elderly. Use sharp contrasting colours on doors, strips of a contrasting colour on the bottom of the wall, with a coloured or white strip at the edge of each step to assist in distinguishing colours, space, and specific areas. |
| | Teach the safety considerations needed to avoid misinterpretation of colours, or of not seeing objects that are pale or light in colour. |

## CRITICAL THINKING

*What are the resources in your community to assist the blind older adult?*

**Hearing** With age, the pinna (external ear) becomes longer, wider, and less flexible, but this change does not appear to affect hearing. As cerumen production diminishes and the wax becomes drier, blockage of the ear canal can occur. The presence of dried, packed wax can interfere with sound transmission. Any auditory changes that occurred in middle age tend to continue through later life. Men are twice as likely as women to experience hearing loss. The tympanic membrane becomes thinner and less resilient, and it will sometimes show some sclerotic changes. In some older adults, calcification of the ossicles occurs. Changes occur in the organ of Corti.

## Guidelines for Helping the Blind Person

- Talk to the blind person in a normal tone of voice. The fact that he or she cannot see is no indication that hearing is impaired.

- Be natural when talking with a blind person.

- Accept the normal things that a blind person might do, such as consulting the watch for the correct time, dialling a telephone, or writing his or her name in longhand, without calling attention to them.

- When you offer assistance to a blind person, do so directly. Ask, "May I be of help?" Speak in a normal, friendly tone.

- In guiding a blind person, permit him or her to take your arm. Never grab the blind person's arm, for he or she cannot anticipate your movements.

- In walking with a blind person, proceed at a normal pace. You may hesitate slightly before stepping up or down.

- Be explicit in giving verbal directions to a blind person.

- There is no need to avoid the use of the word *see* when talking with a blind person.

- When assisting a blind person to a chair, simply place his or her hand on the back or arm of the chair. This is enough to give location.

- When leaving the blind person abruptly after conversing with him or her in a crowd or where there is a noise that may obstruct hearing, quietly advise that you are leaving so that he she will not be embarrassed by talking when no one is present.

- Never leave a blind person in an open area. Instead, lead him or her to the side of a room, to a chair, or to some landmark from which he or she can obtain direction.

- A half-open door is one of the most dangerous obstacles that blind people encounter.

- When serving food to a blind person who is eating without a sighted companion, offer to read the menu, including the price of each item. As you place each item on the table, call attention to food placement by using the numbers of an imaginary clock. ("The green beans are at 2 o'clock.") If he or she wants you to cut up the food, he or she will tell you.

- Be sure to tell a blind person who the other guests are so that he or she may know of their presence.

The changes include a loss of nerve cells in the eighth cranial nerve, and an increased rate of time required for the passage of impulses in the auditory nerve. Because of the changes to the inner ear and cochlea, a hearing aid or corrective surgery often improves hearing, but adjustment to them is often difficult. If there is sensorineural deafness (damage to the auditory nerve or the hearing centre of the brain caused by bacterial or viral infections), head injuries, or prolonged exposure to loud noise, a hearing aid will not improve hearing.[121]

Of all individuals over 65, 43 percent suffer severe **presbycusis**, *progressive loss of hearing and sound discrimination*. The consonants, especially *s*, *sh*, *ch*, *th*, *dg*, *z*, and *f*, and high-frequency sounds produce problems for the individual with presbycusis. The ability to locate the direction from which sound is coming diminishes, and older people have difficulty hearing individuals who speak rapidly or in high tones.[122] For some helpful suggestions, see the box entitled "Guidelines for Communicating with the Hearing-Impaired Person."[123]

## CRITICAL THINKING

*Why do some seniors reject hearing aids?*

**Tactile Acuity** The decreased number of nerve cells innervating the skin results in a decreased response or sensitivity to touch. Even the soles of the feet come to have fewer sensory receptors, and therefore are less responsive. Age-related deterioration of tactile acuity, like visual and hearing changes, begins in late middle age. Acuity of touch, however, varies

## Guidelines for Communicating with the Hearing-Impaired Person

- When you meet a person who seems inattentive or slow to understand you, consider the possibility that hearing, rather than manners or intellect, may be at fault. Some hard-of-hearing persons refuse to wear a hearing aid. Others wear aids that are so inconspicuous, or so clearly camouflaged, that you might not spot them at first glance.

- Remember, the hard-of-hearing often depend to a considerable extent on reading your lips. They do this even though they are wearing a hearing aid because no hearing aid can completely restore one's hearing. You can help by trying *always to speak in good light,* and by facing the person and the light as you speak.

- When in a group that includes a hard-of-hearing person, try to carry on your conversation with others in such a way that he or she can watch your lips. Never take advantage of the disability by carrying on a private conversation in his or her presence in low tones that cannot be heard.

- Speak distinctly but naturally. Shouting does not clarify speech sounds, and mouthing or exaggerating your words or speaking at a snail's pace makes it harder for you to be understood. On the other hand, try not to speak too rapidly.

- Do not start to speak to a hard-of-hearing person abruptly. Attract his or her attention first by facing the person and looking straight into the eyes. If necessary, touch the hand or shoulder lightly. Help him or her grasp what you are talking about right away by starting with a key word or phrase, for example, "Let's plan our weekend now," "Speaking of teenagers. . . . " *If he or she does not understand you, do*

*not repeat the same words.* Substitute synonyms: "It's time to make plans for Saturday," and so on.

- If the person to whom you are speaking has one "good" ear, always stand or sit on that side when you address him or her. Do not be afraid to ask a person with an obvious hearing loss whether he or she has a good ear and, if so, which one it is. The person will be grateful that you care enough to find out.

- Facial expressions are important clues to meaning. Remember that an affectionate or amused tone of voice may be lost on a hard-of-hearing person.

- In conversation with a person who is especially hard-of-hearing, do not be afraid occasionally to jot down key words on paper. If he or she is really having difficulty understanding you, the person will be grateful for the courtesy.

- Many hard-of-hearing persons, especially teenagers who hate to be different, are unduly sensitive about their disability and will pretend to understand you even when they do not. When you detect this situation, tactfully repeat your meaning in different words until it gets across.

- Teach the family to avoid the use of candles. Electric light will give the person a better chance to join the conversation because he or she can see the lips during conversation. Similarly, in choosing a restaurant, remember that *dim lighting can make lip-reading difficult.*

- Teach family members that they should not exclude the hard-of-hearing person from all forms of entertainment involving speech or music. Concerts and operas may present problems, but movies, plays, ballets, and dances are often just as enjoyable to people with a hearing loss as to those with normal hearing. (Even profoundly deaf

>

persons can usually feel rhythm, and many are good and eager dancers.) For children, magic shows, pantomimes, and the circus are good choices.

- When sending a telegram to someone who does not hear well, instruct the telegraph company to deliver your message, not telephone it.

- The speech of a person who has been hard-of-hearing for years can be difficult to understand because natural pitch and inflection are the result of imitating the speech of others. To catch such a person's meaning more easily, watch the face while he or she talks.

- Do not say such things as "Why don't you get a hearing aid?" or "Why don't you see a specialist?" to a person who is hard-of-hearing. Chances are that he or she has already explored these possibilities, and there is no need to emphasize the disability.

- *Use common sense* and tact in determining which of these suggestions apply to the particular hard-of-hearing person you meet. Some persons with only a slight loss might feel embarrassed by any special attention directed to them. Others, whose loss is greater, will be profoundly grateful for your attention.

with different body regions. The fingertip has more acuity in old age than the forearm for both texture and temperature. Acuity is also related to the space between different stimuli. For example, the fingertip, which is sensitive to a single nodule, will not be as sensitive to the dots of Braille, to the glucose testing monitor used by the diabetic, or to other tactile aids used by the sensory handicapped.[124] See Table 14-4 for health promotion implications related to tactile changes.

**Taste and Smell** With aging, a general decrease in taste perception occurs because of a decline in the actual number of taste buds (about half as many as in young adulthood, but women retain more than men). Diminished taste perception is linked to the changes in the processing of taste sensations in the central nervous system. Taste perception will also be affected by the diminished salivation that occurs in older persons. Taste deficits can lead to weight loss, malnutrition,

and impaired immunity.[125] Usually, older adults experience an increased preference for more sugar, salt, spices, and highly seasoned foods.

The sense of smell begins to decline in most people by middle age and continues a gradual decline into old age because both the number and sensitivity of receptors decrease, especially after age 80. It is believed that the sense of smell decreases because the olfactory nerves come to have fewer cells. This diminished sense of smell, combined with the decline in taste sensation, can often be used to account for the loss of appetite experienced by many older adults. The reduced ability to smell presents certain hazards for the individual in that he or she cannot quickly detect the odour of leaking gas, spoiled food, smoke, or burning food.

See Table 14-4 for health promotion implications related to changes in taste and smell.[126]

**Table 14-4 Health Promotion Implications for Other Neurologic Changes**

| Change | Health Promotion Implication |
|---|---|
| Tactile | Use firm but gentle pressure on hand, arm, or shoulder to indicate your presence or soothe with touch. |
| | Teach safety factors: |
| | 1. Walk more slowly to allow the feet to touch the surface fully and be cognizant of foot placement (e.g., on stairs, uneven surfaces, or outdoors). |
| | 2. Monitor the use of hot water bottles, heating pads, or ice bags to avoid burns or frostbite. |
| | 3. Teach ways to avoid bumps or abrasions. Bed-ridden or chair-bound person *must* have position changed frequently to prevent decubitus ulcer. |
| Taste and smell | Teach the need for more seasoning, preferably spices and herbs rather than sugar or salt, to enjoy food and to discriminate tastes. |
| | Encourage adequate nutrition. |
| | Teach safety factors related to reduced smell (e.g., how to monitor for burning food or gas leaks). |

Cardiovascular System   Although the cardiovascular system undergoes considerable changes with aging, in the absence of heart disease it is usually able to maintain the daily cardiac and circulatory functions of the older adult. However, the cardiovascular system might not be able to meet the needs of the body when a disease process is present, or when excess demands, caused by stress or excessive exercise, are placed on it. Obesity, physical inactivity, and abdominal fat distribution also reduce physiologic function. See Table 14-5 for cardiovascular changes and implications for health promotion.[127]

Respiratory System   Changes produced by aging affect both internal and external respiration. The older adult has difficulty taking oxygen from the atmosphere and delivering it to

**Table 14-5** Cardiovascular Changes with Aging and Health Promotion Implications

| Organ/Tissue | Change and Rationale | Implication for Health Promotion |
|---|---|---|
| **Heart**<br>Internal | At age 70, cardiac output at rest is 70% of that at age 30. | Medication may be needed to maintain adequate function. |
| | Number and size of cardiac muscle cells decrease, causing loss of cardiac muscle strength, reduction in stroke volume, and less efficient pumping and cardiac output. | Exercise routine should be maintained. Assess for myocardial damage, muscle damage, and congestive heart failure. |
| | Thickening of collagen in heart valves reduces efficiency of closure because of rigidity.<br>Calcification of valves increases. | Assess for aortic and mitral murmurs, valve stenosis or insufficiency, and endocarditis. |
| | Thickness of left ventricle wall increases; left ventricle is unable to pump volume of blood in cardiac cycle. | Cognitive, visceral, and muscular functions may not be adequately maintained with less cardiac output and inadequate blood supply. |
| | Blood flow is maintained to brain and coronary arteries to greater extent than other body parts. | |
| | Pacemaker cells in sinoatrial node and atrioventricular nodes are replaced by fibrous and connective tissue, causing delay in nerve transmission and more time to complete the cardiac cycle. | Assess for ectopic activity, arrhythmias, and conduction defects. |
| External | Increased amount and stiffening of collagen surrounding heart, causing inelasticity. Increased fat deposits on surface of heart, reducing oxygen supply to body. | Maintain fluid balance and adequate aeration; avoid standing too long or constipation to reduce strain on heart. Straining to defecate strains right side of heart as blood suddenly pours through vena cava after pressure is decreased. |
| **Blood vessels** | Reduced elastin content and increased collagenous connective tissue in arterial walls reduce elasticity of walls of peripheral vessels, aorta, and other arteries. | Assess for increased systolic and diastolic blood pressure, abdominal pulsation, bruits, and aneurysms. |
| | | Orthostatic hypotension may occur; blood pressure falls sharply on standing. Instruct person to rise to sitting position from lying position and stand slowly to allow for adjustment. |

*(continued)*

Table 14-5 (continued)

| Organ/Tissue | Change and Rationale | Implication for Health Promotion |
|---|---|---|
| **Blood vessels (Continued)** | **Atherosclerosis**, *increased accumulation and calcification in arterial walls,* makes smaller lumen diameter; vessel walls harder, thicker, and resistant to blood flow; and less rebound to vessel after being stretched. Blood flow is reduced to vital organs; cerebrovascular accidents (strokes) and multifarct dementia may occur. | Low-cholesterol diet should begin in early life, as these changes may occur in early life. Lifestyle: exercise, weight loss, no smoking, low-salt diet (under 3 g/day) can reduce blood pressure by 10/mm/Hg. Moderately elevated blood pressure may have protective effect on brain. Assess for hypertension and other circulatory problems. |
| | Walls of veins are thicker due to increased connective tissue and calcium deposits, decreasing elasticity. Valves in large veins may become incompetent; varicose veins are common. | Wear support hose to reduce varicose veins, which begin in early life. Sit with feet and lower legs elevated to enhance blood return to heart. Avoid prolonged standing. |

internal organs and tissues. See Table 14-6 for physiological changes and implications for health promotion.[128]

**Musculoskeletal System** The major age-related change in the skeletal system is the loss of calcium from bone. Bone loss is accelerated with the loss of gonadal function at menopause. Therefore, bone loss is greater in females than in males, and also in older rather than younger females. The decreased synthesis of bone and the increased decalcification, or osteoporosis in vertebrae, cause collapse; the resultant loss of collagen and atrophy in intervertebral disks cause the spinal column to compress and the posture to become curved

**Table 14-6** Respiratory System Changes and Health Promotion Implications

| Organ | Change and Rationale | Implication for Health Promotion |
|---|---|---|
| **Nose** | Reduced number and activity of cilia cause reduced bronchoelimination. | Less effective clearing of respiratory tract predisposes to infections. Avoid smoke-filled environment. Wear mask if air pollution exists. Avoid allergens. Maintain health status and avoid crowds in winter to prevent respiratory infections and pneumonia. |
| **Throat** | Cough reflex decreased. Sensitivity to stimuli decreased. | Teach safety factors, especially when eating (cut food into small portions, chew well, eat slowly). |
| **Trachea** | Flexibility is decreased; size of structure is increased. | |
| **Rib cage and respiratory muscles** | Calcification of chest wall causes rib cage to be less mobile. Decreased strength of intercostal and other respiratory muscles and diaphragm impairs breathing. | Maintain exercise, deep breathing, and erect posture to enhance respiratory muscle function. |

*(continued)*

Table 14-6 (continued)

| Organ | Change and Rationale | Implication for Health Promotion |
|---|---|---|
| | Osteoporosis of ribs and vertebrae weakens chest wall and respiratory function. | Avoid pressure to ribs to prevent rib fracture (e.g., leaning chest on edge of bathtub). |
| | Calcification of vertebral cartilage and kyphosis stiffen chest wall and impair respiratory movements. | |
| Lungs | Capacity to inhale, hold, and exhale breath decreases with age. Vital capacity at 85 is 50%–65% of capacity at 30. | Encourage deep breathing, full exhalation, and erect posture throughout life. Maintain exercise to enhance lung function. |
| | Elastin and collagen changes cause loss of elasticity of lung tissue; lungs remain hyperinflated even on exhalation, and proportion of dead space increases. Decreased elasticity and increased size of alveoli. Increased diffusion and surface area across alveolar-capillary membrane. | Activity should be adjusted to respiratory efficiency and ventilation-perfusion ratio. |

or stooped, and shorter. In addition to the decrease in height, bone strength is progressively lost because of the loss of bone mineral content. Osteoporosis is seen as the extreme version of the universal process of adult bone loss.[129]

The older adult experiences a gradual loss of muscular strength and endurance. Muscle cells atrophy, and lean muscle mass is lost. Adults generally lose about 10 to 20 percent of their strength up to age 70, especially in the muscles of the lower body, and more after that.[130] In controlled studies with individuals in their sixties and nineties, weight training, power training, or resistance training programs lasting eight weeks to two years increased muscle strength, size, and mobility; speed, endurance, and leg muscle power; and spontaneous physical activity.[131]

The musculoskeletal changes that have the most effect on function are related to the ligaments, tendons, and joints. Over time, these areas become dry, hardened, more rigid, and less flexible. In joints that have been subjected to trauma earlier in life (injuries), these changes can be seen earlier. As joint space becomes reduced, arthritis is diagnosed more frequently. Statistically, arthritis is the number one cause of disability in persons over the age of 65.[132] Changes in body weight also occur in the older adult. Interestingly, these changes follow definite patterns. Men usually exhibit an increase in weight until their middle fifties and then gradually lose weight. Women continue to gain weight until their sixties before beginning a gradual reduction in

weight. The most significant weight loss occurs near 70 years of age and is probably due to a decreased number of body cells, changes in cell composition, and decreased amounts of body tissue. See Table 14-7 for health promotion implications related to aging changes in the musculoskeletal system.[133]

**Urinary System** As with the other body systems, major changes in structure and function of the urinary system are associated with aging. The kidneys, bladder, and ureters are all affected by the aging process.[134]

**Kidney** The aging kidney suffers a decrease in renal function as one ages. By age 80, up to 50 percent of the nephrons are lost. Although large numbers of nephrons are gone, each kidney requires only one-quarter of its nephrons to maintain normal function. The narrowing of blood vessels and vasoconstriction, often due to arteriosclerosis and hypertension, produce a decreased total volume of renal blood flow. With age, the kidney has decreased ability to concentrate urine because of the decreased number of nephrons. Electrolyte imbalance occurs more rapidly in the elderly. These changes in kidney function can alter the renal excretion of drugs.[135] See Table 14-7 for health promotion implications.[136]

**Bladder** With age, the smooth muscle and elastic tissue of the bladder are replaced with fibrous tissue.[137] Coupled with a delayed desire to void, the elderly often have

## Table 14-7 Aging Changes and Health Promotion Implications

| System/Organ | Implications for Health Promotion |
|---|---|
| **Musculoskeletal** | Maintain calcium intake, normal nutrition, and exercise to slow degradation of bone or osteoporosis, to overcome stiffness, and to maintain strength, endurance, and joint mobility.<br>Teach safety measures related to reduced coordination and strength, postural and structural changes, and slower reaction times to avoid falls and fractures.<br>Teach ways to arrange the home environment and needed supplies to avoid the need for excessive reach or climbing.<br>Use devices to extend arm reach to obtain objects or supplies. |
| **Renal** | |
| Kidney | Avoid polypharmacy or excessive medication intake.<br>Assess for drug side effects and toxicity because kidneys are the major route of excretion.<br>Assess for renal insufficiency if the person is dehydrated, hypotensive, feverish, or using diuretics. |
| Bladder | Maintain adequate fluid intake and frequent toileting.<br>Avoid diuretic use in the afternoon, and before long travel.<br>Pads may be worn in underpants, or lined pants can be worn as a precaution.<br>Assess for urinary tract infections.<br>Explore self-esteem issues related to incontinence.<br>Engage in bladder retraining. |
| **Gastrointestinal** | |
| Mouth | Encourage drinking eight glasses of water daily to avoid dry mouth and dehydration.<br>Maintain dental hygiene and care to prevent periodontal disease and loss of teeth.<br>Teach the current brushing techniques, daily flossing, and the use of toothpaste with fluoride additive.<br>Teach safety factors related to the prevention of choking, and use of the Heimlich manoeuvre. |
| Stomach | Encourage adequate nutritional intake, adjusting food texture and taste as necessary, and with vitamin-mineral supplements if necessary.<br>Promote nutrition through programs like senior nutrition sites or Meals on Wheels, as needed. |
| Liver/gallbladder | Encourage adequate protein intake to overcome hepatic synthesis.<br>Avoid high-fat foods.<br>Avoid polypharmacy because of reduced metabolism and excretion. |
| Bowel | Encourage bulk, vegetables, fruits, and cereals; water; exercise; and regular toileting patterns to prevent constipation.<br>Avoid daily laxatives if at all possible, but if self-administered for years, it will need to be continued. Mild stool softener is preferred. |
| **Immune** | Maintain nutrition, hygiene, and health status to overcome delayed immune response and trend to infections.<br>Observe for masked signs of inflammation or infection (e.g., temperature or white blood cell count may not be as elevated as in middle age).<br>Teach safety measures and stress management strategies to overcome delayed or inadequate body response to stress.<br>Treat symptomatically for comfort if autoimmune processes occur. |

problems with frequent urination and a severe urgency to void. Aged women are especially prone to incontinence as the pelvic muscles become more flaccid. The pelvic diaphragm is the muscle mass that helps maintain bladder tone and proper closure of the bladder outlet. Weakening of the pelvic diaphragm leads to stress incontinence.[138]

Measures to combat urinary incontinence include regulation of fluid intake, pelvic muscle exercises (Kegel exercises), a regular pattern of voiding, and the use of drugs that block the hyperactivity of voiding. Teach the woman to control pelvic muscles and do the *Kegel exercise* as follows:

1. Tighten the muscles at least five times each day to help strengthen the pelvic floor muscles.
2. Don't tighten other muscles such as your hips or legs, during the pelvic floor exercises.
3. Sit, lie down, or stand during practice.
4. Practise this important exercise without anyone knowing.[139]

Nurses can help immeasurably by establishing routines for toileting, and by reinforcing the patient with a positive attitude, helping to foster self-esteem and independence.

## CRITICAL THINKING

*Look at media advertisements for products used for incontinence. What type of message is sent to the older adult?*

Hypertrophy of the prostate in the older man is very common and can begin as early as age 40. Irregular changes in the smooth muscle fibres and the prostate tissue occur with age. The problem consists of frequency, especially at night, difficulty starting the stream, dribbling, and retention with overflow. Cancer of the prostate is the most prevalent malignancy in men. Therefore, regular physical examinations should be encouraged to screen out the possibility of a malignancy. Some men are concerned about their sexual potency if surgery is to be performed.[140] Care should be taken to explain that although external ejaculation will be absent, erection and orgasm are likely to be unaffected.

See Table 14-7 for health promotion implications.[141]

**Gastrointestinal System** Changes occur throughout the gastrointestinal system.

**Mouth** The oral mucosa atrophies, the connective tissue becomes less elastic, vascular tissue becomes calcified and fibrotic, and nerve cells diminish in number. Tooth decay, loss of teeth, degeneration of the jawbone, progressive gum recession, and increased resorption of the dental arch all interfere with the older adult's ability to chew food. Saliva flow decreases and becomes more alkaline as the salivary glands secrete less ptyalin and amylase. Thirst sensation decreases. All of these changes alter the digestive process at the onset.[142] See Table 14-7 for health promotion implications.[143]

**Gastrointestinal Tract** Age-related changes in the gastrointestinal system begin before age 50 and continue gradually throughout life.[144] Because of decreased stimuli from the autonomic nervous system, peristalsis is slowed along the entire length of the gastrointestinal tract. Emptying of the esophagus and stomach are delayed. The gastric mucosa shrinks, causing decreased secretion of pepsinogen and hydrochloric acid, which delays digestion. Digestion is decreased further by the reduction in secretion of hydrochloric acid and pancreatic enzymes. Bile tends to be thicker, and the gallbladder empties more slowly. Hepatic synthesis is reduced. These changes result in a decreased absorption of nutrients and drugs by the gastrointestinal tract. In addition, some older adults do not have enough intrinsic factor and develop pernicious anemia.[145]

*Elimination of waste products* is of equal importance to gastrointestinal function in the aged. The changes in the cell, and therefore in tissue structure, and the loss of muscle tone tend to decrease intestinal mobility. Elimination depends on fluid intake, muscle tone, regularity of habits, culture, state of health, and adequate nutrition—all of which interrelate. Variations in many of these areas occur with aging. Poor nutrition and the lack of sufficient exercise add to the problem.

See Table 14-7 for health promotion implications.[146]

**Endocrine System** During aging, the ability of endocrine glands to synthesize hormones appears to remain within normal limits. Most hormones operate on the basis of a feedback system that maintains an optimal internal environment, or homeostasis, within the body.[147] Two major endocrine problems of importance are diabetes mellitus and thyroid disease.[148]

Diabetes mellitus (DM) is a syndrome of disorders of glucose metabolism resulting in hyperglycemia, either from the inadequate secretion of insulin (type 1) or from inadequate secretion and the development of resistance of tissues to insulin (type 2). Individuals with diabetes often have other health problems as well, including problems with the metabolism of lipids and proteins. Diabetes is the leading cause of end-stage renal disease and blindness.[149]

Elderly persons undergoing the stress of surgery, illness, injury, or emotional stress often manifest diabetic symptoms. The elevated blood and urinary glucose levels usually return to normal, however, when the stressor subsides.[150]

Thyroid disease is common, often undiagnosed, and easily treated in people of all ages. Hypothyroidism is much more common in women than in men at all ages, and is higher in older persons living in institutions than in older community-residing individuals.[151] On the other hand, hypothyroidism is characterized by a generalized reduction in metabolic function that most often manifests as a slowing of physical and mental activity.[152]

## CRITICAL THINKING

*What services are available for the community-living diabetic elderly person?*

**Immune System**  Multiple factors affect the person's immune system. First, the internal characteristics of the individual, such as age, gender, and the inherited genetic sequence, cannot be modified. Other factors, such as one's nutritional status and the existence of underlying disease, are potentially modifiable. External factors, such as environmental pollutants, radiation, ultraviolet light, and drugs, can have a substantial effect on the individual's immune system.[153] The immune system becomes less efficient with aging because of the reduced production and function of T and B cells. Hypersensitivity is either an excessive response to antigen stimulation or an overly extensive but normal response. A complex interrelationship exists between some hypersensitivity reactions and several of the autoimmune disease processes. For example, rheumatoid arthritis is believed to be an example of type III hypersensitivity that affects older women in particular.[154] See Table 14-7 for health promotion implications.[155]

**Hematologic System**  Most of the age-related changes in the hematologic system are the result of the reduced capacity of the bone marrow to reproduce red blood cells quickly when disease or blood loss occurs. At about age 70, the amount of bone marrow in the long bones begins to decline steadily. Minor, non-significant changes in the blood components of the older adult occur in the hemoglobin level, red blood cell count, and circulatory blood volume. Most of the changes that do occur are related to specific pathologic conditions rather than to normal aging.[156]

**Reproductive System and Changes That Influence Sexual Function**  Men and women experience some common changes as a result of aging. The gonads are the ovaries in the female and the testes in the male. Menopause, or the cessation of menstruation, occurs in approximately 95 percent of women by age 55. Estrogen production decreases; after menopause, progesterone secretion by the ovaries also decreases. As the estrogen level decreases, changes occur in the reproductive organs, including a decrease in the size of the ovaries, uterus, cervix, and fallopian tubes. There is also a decrease in the number of mammary ducts. The vaginal canal shortens and becomes drier. In the male, sperm production declines, but this does not prevent reproduction. Testosterone secretion decreases in the male. The ability to have a penile erection is slowed and is less intense than in the younger male.[157] In addition, the prostate gland enlarges, contractions weaken, the force of ejaculation decreases, and the volume and viscosity of the seminal fluid are reduced.

**Sexuality**  In the literature, sexuality has been described as one of the most natural and basic aspects of life that affects an individual's identity as a human being.[158] Sexuality can give an embellished meaning to life for the older adult. Regardless of age, every individual has a need for love, intimacy, and companionship. In a youth-oriented culture, sexuality is attributed to the young, healthy, and beautiful; the myth that the elderly are asexual beings predominates. Consequently, the sexual needs of the elderly are frequently overlooked or ignored.[159] The general view toward sexuality is likely to change as the baby boomers enter middle age. One's needs for intimacy can change over time. However, sexual activity often continues well into older adulthood. Nurses must take a proactive approach and openly discuss sexuality and sexual concerns with older adults.[160] The *PLISSIT model* has been used to assess and manage the sexuality of adults.[161] The *PLISSIT model* stands for:

- Obtaining **P**ermission from the client to initiate sexual discussion
- Providing the **L**imited **I**nformation needed to function sexually
- Giving **S**pecific **S**uggestions for the individual to proceed with sexual relations
- Providing **I**ntensive **T**herapy surrounding the issues of sexuality for that client.

*Questions to guide sexuality assessment among older adults include:*

1. Can you tell me how you express your sexuality?
2. What concerns or questions do you have about fulfilling your continuing sexual needs?
3. In what ways has your sexual relationship with your partner changed as you have aged?
4. What interventions or information can I provide to help you to fulfill your sexuality?[162]

## Nutritional Needs

Nutrition is the fundamental element of healthy human development, and it is an essential contributor to the overall health of older adults. The revised *Eating Well with Canada's Food Guide* was developed in the Canadian context and promotes a pattern of eating that meets nutrient needs, promotes health, and reduces the risk of nutrition-related chronic disease.[163] The recommended number of Food Guide servings per day for the adult over 51 years of age is as follows:

- Vegetables and Fruits: seven servings
- Grain Products: seven servings

- Milk and Alternatives: three servings
- Meat and Alternatives: three servings

It has been recommended that in addition to following the Food Guide, all adults over the age of 50 should take a daily vitamin supplement of 10 micrograms (400 IU).[164]

Special problems exist in the nutrition of older people. Factors that affect nutrition and its clinical manifestations are described in Table 14-7 and Table 14-8.[165]

It is important to note that determinants of healthy eating come from individual and collective factors. Individual components include age, sex, education, physiological and health issues, psychological attributes, lifestyle practices, knowledge, attitudes, and behaviours. Meanwhile, collective determinants include accessible food labels, an appropriate food shopping environment, marketing of the "healthy eating" message, adequate social support, and provision of an effective community-meal delivery service. It is necessary to study contributors to healthy eating in order to permit the development and evaluation of programs and services designed to encourage and facilitate healthy eating in older Canadians.[166]

Use *Eating Well with Canada's Food Guide* to assist older adults in planning meals for themselves.[167]

## CRITICAL THINKING

*Outline a general teaching plan you would use to instruct an older adult about dietary needs.*

## Table 14-8 Factors that May Affect Nutrition in Later Maturity

| Factor and Process | Effect | Clinical Manifestation |
|---|---|---|
| **Ingestion** | | |
| Loss of teeth; poor dentures; atrophy of jaws | Improper mastication; deletion of important foods from diet | Irritable bowel syndrome; constipation; malnutrition |
| Dietary habits | Overeating; eccentric diets | Obesity; malnutrition |
| Psychological losses and changes; changes in social environment; lack of socialization | Poor appetite | Anorexia; weight loss |
| Reduced income; difficulty with food preparation and ingestion | Excessive ingestion of carbohydrates | Obesity; malnutrition |
| Decreased fluid intake | Dry feces | Impacted stools |
| **Digestion and Absorption** | | |
| Decreased secretion of hydrochloric acid and digestive enzymes | Interference with digestion | Dietary deficiencies |
| Hepatic and biliary insufficiency | Poor absorption of fats | Fat-soluble vitamin deficiency; flatulence |
| Atrophy of intestinal mucosa and musculature | Poor absorption; slower movement of food through intestine | Vitamin and mineral deficiencies; constipation |
| Decreased secretion of intestinal mucus | Decreased lubrication of intestine | Constipation |
| **Metabolism** | | |
| Impaired glucose metabolism and use | Diabetic-like response to glucose | Hyperglycemia; hypoglycemia |
| Decrease in renal function | Inability to excrete excess alkali | Alkalosis |
| Impaired response to salt restriction | Salt depletion | Low-salt syndrome |
| Decline in basal metabolic rate | Lower caloric requirements but same amount of food eaten | Obesity |
| Changes in iron and calcium (phosphorus, magnesium) metabolism | Iron deficiency; increased requirements for calcium | Anemia; demineralization of bone; osteoporosis |
| Changes in vitamin metabolism | Deficiency in vitamins K and C, especially | Peripheral neuropathy, sensorimotor changes; easy bruising and bleeding tendencies |

*Sufficient water or other fluid intake is essential.* Fluid intake is often reduced in seniors for several reasons:

- The aging process reduces the thirst sensation.
- The senior who has incontinence problems limits fluid intake to reduce output.
- Fewer meals are eaten. Therefore, the opportunity for fluid intake is less apparent.
- The senior who takes a diuretic often wrongly assumes that fluid intake should be reduced.

At least six or seven glasses (250 mL or 8 ounces) of water should be ingested daily to: (1) soften stools; (2) maintain kidney function; (3) aid expectoration; (4) moisturize dry skin; and (5) aid the absorption of medications, bulk laxatives, and high-fibre foods.

*You can help make mealtime pleasant for the older person:*

- Encourage the person to prepare menus that are economical and easy to shop for, prepare, and consume.
- Encourage the person to do meal preparation to the extent possible.
- The environment should be a comfortable temperature and well lighted so that food can be seen easily.
- Place food where the person can smell, see, and reach it.
- If needed, open cartons and food packets of various sorts and help season the food.
- Keep the tray attractive, neat, and uncluttered to ensure an appetizing appearance.
- Use foods that can be easily chewed and digested.
- Ensure that dentures and eyeglasses are clean and in place on the person at mealtime, instead of in the drawer or on the bedside table.
- Oral hygiene is important and contributes to greater enjoyment of food. Mouth care also promotes healthy tissues in the mouth, thereby keeping the beginning of the alimentary canal intact and functional.
- Do not give medications with meals if it can be avoided, especially if the medication has an unpleasant taste.
- Offer foods when the person is hungry rather than only at set meal or snack times.
- If necessary, use adaptive feeding devices to help the person feed self.

Keller and McKenzie conducted a Canadian study to measure nutritional risk in a sample of vulnerable community-living seniors, and endeavoured to determine patterns of nutritional risk in these seniors.[168] The majority of the sample was female and the average age was 79 years. Common nutritional risk factors were weight change; restricting food; low fruit and vegetable intake; difficulty with chewing, cooking, or

shopping; and poor appetite. The principal components analysis identified four independent components within the Seniors in the Community: Risk Evaluation for Eating and Nutrition questionnaire. These components were low food intake, poor appetite, physical and external challenges, and instrumental activity challenges. The pattern of nutritional risks identified in this vulnerable population may help providers identify useful strategies for eliminating risks.[169]

## Rest and Sleep

*Rest* is important. Though older adults may not sleep as many hours as they once did, frequent rest periods and sensible pacing of activities provide the added energy for a full and active life. Rest can consist of listening to soft music, reading, and thinking of happy experiences, napping, or merely lying with eyes closed. Some older adults have several 15- to 60-minute naps during the daylight hours.

With so much diversity among individuals in this age group, it is difficult to state how many hours of *sleep* are recommended. Older adults who are in reasonably good health probably do not require any more sleep than was required during their middle adulthood.

Aging affects the process of sleep in three aspects: duration of sleep, distribution of sleep during the 24-hour day, and sleep stage patterns. The older adult requires a somewhat longer period to fall asleep, and sleep is lighter, with more frequent awakenings. The total amount of daily sleep declines as the frequency of instances of the spontaneous interruption of sleep increases. The older adult may actually spend more time in bed, but sleep less, with the result of waking with the feeling of inadequate sleep. The time spent in stage IV, the deepest sleep period, and REM sleep decreases. This development also contributes to feelings of fatigue.[170]

Insomnia is a common problem in the older adult and many factors contribute to it. Determine the person's usual sleeping patterns, the amount and type of daily activity, and the existence of any disturbing environmental conditions, such as the construction of a nearby high-rise. Assess the presence of pain, fear, anxiety, lack of exercise, or depression.

---

**CRITICAL THINKING**

*What health promotion strategies could you suggest to an older adult to combat insomnia?*

---

## Exercise and Activity

According to a substantial body of scientific evidence, regular physical activity can bring significant health benefits to people of all ages and abilities.[171] According to *Canada's Physical Activity Guide to Healthy Active Living for Older Adults*, 60 percent of older adults are not sufficiently active to achieve optimal health benefits. The guide serves as a road map to promote physical activity in an aging society. Being active is safe for most people. The guide recommends that an older adult begin exercise slowly and build up slowly, listening to the body. You might need to teach them what listening to the body means. The guide advocates a period of 30 to 60 minutes of moderate physical activity most days. One can even exercise 10 minutes at a time, adding up the time to the 30 to 60 minutes.[172]

See Table 14-9 for the physical, psychological, and social benefits of exercise.[173]

## Table 14-9 Benefits of Regular Exercise

**Physical**

- Helps slow the aging process, regardless of age
- Maintains good health and energy
- Improves general strength and body agility and balance
- Improves respiration and circulation
- Promotes muscle mass, strength, and endurance
- Protects against ligament injuries
- Promotes bone mass formation and slows the loss of bone tissue
- Induces better sleep patterns
- Normalizes blood cholesterol and triglyceride levels
- Controls blood glucose levels
- Normalizes blood pressure
- Improves appetite, digestive processes, and bowel function
- Promotes weight control (moderate exercise burns 240 to 420 calories/hour)
- Reduces the risk of heart disease

**Psychological**

- Reduces age-related decline in the oxidative capacity of the brain and helps to improve memory and information processing
- Promotes faster reaction time
- Contributes to improved mood and morale
- Improves cognition
- Enhances self-confidence
- Maintains interest in life and alertness
- Contributes to a sense of control
- Helps to prevent depression

**Social**

- Promotes socialization when exercise is included in group activity
- Maintains independence

## Table 14-10 Consequences of Not Exercising and Being Sedentary

- Decline in all body systems
- General weakness
- Lower energy level
- Stooped posture
- Muscle tissue replaced by adipose tissue
- Atrophy of tissues and functions
- Higher blood cholesterol and triglyceride levels
- Greater risk for heart disease
- Weight gain
- Lower self-concept, self-esteem
- Depressive mood

Even if the individual has a decreased exercise tolerance, with supervision a plan can be developed to help him or her achieve higher levels of physical fitness.[174] It is important, however, that the older adult consult a physician prior to starting a walking exercise program to identify any required limitations.[175]

Table 14-10 lists the consequences of not having sufficient exercise.[176]

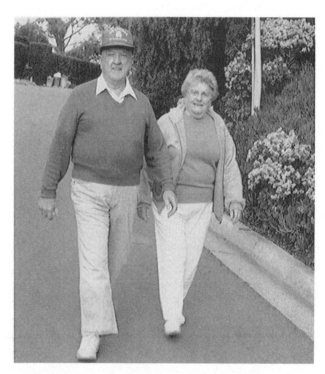

Older adults can maintain health and prevent illness by participating in regular exercise.
Source: Berger, K.J., and M.B. Williams. *Fundamentals of Nursing: Collaborating for Optimal Health.* Stamford, CT: Appleton & Lange, 1992, p. 1317.

For the individual who is not especially interested in planned exercise programs, you can suggest bowling, golf, swimming, dancing, and games such as shuffleboard and horseshoes, as well as home and garden chores. All of these activities can improve the well-being of the older adult. Also, see the box entitled "Guidelines for Walking Exercise."[177]

An exercise program regularly followed will bring a dimension of dynamic fitness to life that helps him or her move vigorously and live energetically. Histories of vigorous persons in their eighties and nineties, and even over age 100, show that the majority have been physically and mentally active throughout their earlier lives.[178] Movement therapy programs such as tai chi and other movement patterns contribute to improved morale, self-esteem, and favourable attitudes toward aging.

Carter and his research group from the University of British Columbia, called the Bone Health Research Group, found that women aged 65 to 75 who had been diagnosed with osteoporosis and who participated in an exercise program experienced improvements in dynamic balance and strength. Both are important determinants of risk for falls, especially in this sample of older women.[179]

## CRITICAL THINKING

*What information would you include in a health education plan on osteoporosis?*

**Devices to Assist Mobility** When we see persons using canes, walkers, wheelchairs, or electric scooters, we tend to think of them as not being an active part of the community. Actually, various assistive devices, when used correctly, can be a means of promoting mobility and independence. Often, the person who refuses to use a cane or walker develops a shuffling gait, characterized by short steps. In cases such as these, over time leg muscles become flaccid, the back tends to weaken, and posture suffers.

Electric scooters are another means of providing mobility for many people. They encourage more participation in social activities and promote the ability to get around in a retirement complex or a nearby store. They can be transported by car to outside events as well: going to the zoo, the shopping mall, or concerts where handicapped access is provided. The theory held by some that an electric cart keeps people from walking is not a valid one. If the client is able to walk at all, he or she should be given an appropriate walking and exercise program by the physician or therapist. Combining the use of cane, walker, and electric cart with an exercise program is the ideal arrangement.

In Canada, the guide *Go for It: A Guide to Choosing and Using Assistive Devices* was developed to assist seniors, veterans, and individuals with disabilities and their caregivers with

## Guidelines for Walking Exercise

1. No single program will work for all elders. Determine first the meaning and perceived value of exercise among sedentary elders before developing the following plan.

2. Begin, if previously sedentary, by walking slightly above a stroll for 15 to 30 minutes.

3. Aim to walk one kilometre in 15 to 20 minutes. Then build to two kilometres in 30 minutes.

4. A "training heart rate" is 60 to 90 percent of your fastest pulse rate per minute.
   - Subtract age from 220.
   - Multiply the result by 0.6 and 0.9 to get the bottom and top of target zone for aerobic training.

5. Walk three to five times a week, with a heart rate in the target zone for 15 to 60 minutes.

6. Develop a strategy to ensure a commitment to walking.

7. Wear shoes with a firm heel cup for stability, a rocker sole for smooth heel-to-toe motion, and plenty of toe room for push-off. Wear loose, comfortable clothing.

8. Maintain an erect posture. Lean forward from the ankles, not the waist. Keep the head level and the chin up.

9. Keep elbows bent at a 90-degree angle and swing arms at the shoulder. The hand should end its forward swing at breastbone height. On the backswing, the upper arm should be parallel to the ground.

10. Stretch before and during the walk. Maintain a long, smooth stride during the walk.

issues before starting the process of obtaining an assistive device. The guide provides comprehensive information about available assistive devices, and includes relevant contact information.[180]

## CRITICAL THINKING

*Describe your plans for a fall-prevention program for the older adult.*

## Health Promotion and Health Prevention

Male and female differences in longevity result from hormones, genetic makeup, natural immunity, and lifestyle behaviour. Because of the immunity effects of estrogen, women statistically develop heart disease ten years later than men do. In the past, the lifestyle choices of women gave them a biological advantage—less drinking of alcoholic beverages, less cigarette smoking, more attention to personal health care, and less exposure to risks at work and play. As women change their lifestyles, however, the gap between the sexes in health status and longevity is narrowing.[181]

Today's elders, overall, are healthier, better educated, more politically astute, more mobile and youthful in appearance, and more accustomed to changing lifestyles than were their counterparts of yesteryear. In one study of people aged 57 to 83, age was not related to differences in healthy behaviours. Many reported no digestive or sleep difficulties. All were active, kept in touch with family and friends, were confident that the environment was safe, and managed stress well. All but one attributed their health, quality of life, and zest to remaining active, eating healthily, exercising, pacing self, doing preferred activities, and reading the Bible or feeding the mind.[182]

Five conditions shorten life expectancy: coronary artery disease, stroke, cancer, diabetes, and confusion. Arthritis decreases functional ability. Decreasing the prevalence of arthritis would reduce functional limitation. Advances against common non-fatal disabling conditions would be more effective than advances against fatal conditions in reducing the anticipated increase in the functionally limited older population anticipated in the twenty-first century.[183]

Menec, Chipperfield, and Perry conducted a four-year study of 1406 older adults, ages 65 to 74, 75 to 84, and over 85, who lived in rural and urban communities (not in institutions). It was found that persons who had high perceptions of self-control and used active coping strategies had better perception of their health. Self-perception of health is an important indicator of mortality. Older adults who rated their health as "bad or poor" and "fair" were more than twice as likely to die in three to five years, compared to those who rated their health positively. Older adults who experienced some functional impairment were three times more likely to die than those who were unimpaired. Being hospitalized during the year doubles the risk of dying. More research is needed on factors that contribute to health as we age.[184]

Overall, about 25 percent of today's elders want to live to be 100 years old. Most would prefer to live to be 90 to 91. The main criteria for deserving longevity are to be able to care for self, to be able to do what fulfills contentment, and to be without intense pain.[185]

The focus of health care for individuals in this period of life should be on the *prevention of disease and the promotion of health*. Although numerous body changes occur with aging, many older adults live active, productive lives. Thorough assessment is essential. Several references are useful.[186]

**Immunizations** All Canadian adults require the maintenance of immunity to tetanus and diphtheria, preferably with combined (Td) toxoid and a single dose of acellular pertussis vaccine.[187] Adults who are 65 and over, and those with conditions that increase their chances of complications, should receive one dose of pneumococcal vaccine and yearly influenza vaccine. Vaccination against influenza lasts four to six months and is routinely given on an annual basis at the outset of the influenza season, typically starting in October in the northern hemisphere.[188] Each year, the influenza vaccine consists of three new influenza strains predicted by the World Health Organization (WHO) to be the most common, to give protection from circulating viruses.

---

## CASE SITUATION

Mrs. B, an 85-year-old resident of a life-care facility, is an example of someone who uses mechanical means to help maintain her participation in the life around her, to do volunteer work, to enhance her ability to walk long distances, and to promote a normal posture while walking.

Mrs. B has had both knees replaced as a result of arthritis. She has osteoarthritis of the spine and rheumatoid arthritis in both hands. She uses a cane for short distances, such as from car to church, shops, or private homes. However, her greatest help is that afforded by one of the newly designed four-wheel walkers. It has rack-and-pinion steering, 12 cm wheels with hand brakes, a seat to sit on when tired or waiting in line, and a basket for purse or packages. This type of walker is the first to have handles that adjust to allow the person to stand upright, supporting the back in a normal posture. Thus, she can stride forward without having to lift or turn the walker, because of the ease of steering.

Mrs. B finds that she uses her walker most of the time, thereby being able to maintain a normal gait and an erect posture and therefore uses the electric cart less often. She is able to use the shopping carts in supermarkets as she would a walker, and because her walker can be folded, it can go with her on more extensive shopping trips by car or bus. Her electric cart takes her to the swimming pool six days a week, where she does water aerobics. Her exercise program, combined with the use of assistive devices, has given Mrs. B an enriched life in her elder years.

1. What are the specific benefits to a client like Mrs. B of the type of exercise she does?
2. What safety concerns should you be aware of regarding walkers?
3. What other health promotion strategies do you need to consider for clients like Mrs. B?

## Safety Promotion and Injury Prevention

**Falls**  Older people experience a disproportionate share of accidents that cause body injury or death. This is especially true for injuries that occur in the home. Many of these accidents are directly related to physiologic changes that result from normal aging.

Teach that falls in the elderly occur for a number of reasons:

- Improper use of, or incorrectly fitted, assistive devices
- Lower-extremity disability
- A decrease in the functional base of support
- Vision and hearing impairment
- Arrhythmias, cardiovascular disease, strokes
- Kinesthetic changes, changes in postural reflexes, sway
- Vertigo and syncopal (fainting) episodes
- Peripheral neuropathy
- Inadequate swing foot clearance, tripping
- Depression, inattention
- Excess ingestion of alcohol
- Use of certain medications, such as diuretics, sedatives, antibiotics, antidepressants, and antipsychotics
- Excessive cigarette smoking or osteoporosis, which reduce bone mineral density and can cause fractures resulting in falls[189]

**Skin and Other Injuries**  *Teach the following safety measures to be used by the elderly to avoid injury to the skin or other injury:*

- Place padding on hard edges of wheelchairs and over rough or sharp corners or surfaces of furniture, tables, or countertops.
- Pad the wooden or metal arms of chairs used by elders.

- Wear gloves to wash dishes, or when working in the garden to protect the hands.
- Wear long sleeves to protect the arms.
- Wear long pants to protect the legs.
- Work and walk more slowly to avoid collisions with objects or falls.
- Wear flat, rubber-soled, well-fitted shoes. Avoid walking in socks, stockings, or loose slippers. Grip handrails (and place feet on the diagonal if the foot is long) when going up and down steps. Put non-skid treads on stairs.
- Use non-slip mats; remove throw rugs; tack rugs to the floor if not wall-to-wall.
- Use seat and grab bars in the bathtub or shower.
- Maintain exercise to improve gait and mobility. Tai chi and yoga also help to steady movements and improve posture and balance.
- Make sure the house is well lit, and that lights are easy to reach; motion-sensitive lights are useful.
- Remove or repair unstable furniture.
- Have vision and hearing checked annually.
- Review with the physician any medications that could increase the risk of falling.

**Scams**  Older adults are particularly vulnerable to fraudulent sales pitches and seemingly honest requests for help by strangers. Use the box entitled "Safety in the Home: Do Not Be a Victim of the Con Game" to teach elders to avoid fraud, scams, or unethical or illegal schemes. Encourage them to report such incidents promptly.

## CRITICAL THINKING

*Use the Internet to find more information about safety in the home.*

---

### Safety in the Home: Do Not Be a Victim of the Con Game

- **Carpet cleaner:** Ad offers very low price to clean carpeting in one or more rooms of your house. Workers flood room, ruin carpet, and scheme to charge more than quoted to replace damaged material, which may not be replaced.
- **City inspector:** "Inspector" knocks at the door to check plumbing, furnace, heater, wiring, trees, or whatever. Once inside, he or she might rob you or insist that something needs repair and charge excessively for the job.

- **Home repair:** "Contractor" offers to repair or remodel your home, exterminate pests, or check for radon. Some do work with leftover materials from another job in the area. The person will find "work" that is unnecessary, resulting in unnecessary expense.
- **Product demonstration:** Agent offers to describe only (not sell) new product if you will sign paper "for my boss" proving he or she did it. Once inside the house, anything can happen.

>

- **Contest winner:** You are told you have won a vacation, auto, or other prize but must send $5 for postage or registration or call an 800 number for details. Cost for anything will exceed its worth.

- **Lottery:** Person offers to sell you winning lottery ticket he or she cannot cash because "I'm an illegal immigrant," or "I'm behind in my child-support payments." Or "law firm" says anonymous donor has bequeathed a winning lottery ticket to you, but first you must send $20 for a computer search to verify your identity.

- **Land sale:** You are promised cheap land or complete retirement and recreational facilities in sunny, gorgeous site. The land may not exist, even if you paid for it.

- **Credit or phone card:** Person asks for your credit or phone card number to send you a product, check unauthorized charges, verify insurance, and so on. They can then use your number to charge items.

- **Governmental service:** Official-sounding firm offers governmental service that is "required" (e.g., plastic-coated identification cards), "critically needed" (e.g., to help keep agency solvent), or useful. The money sent obtains no service.

- **Mail-order health care or laboratory tests:** You are promised medical care by mail or laboratory screening for AIDS, cholesterol, cancer, hair loss, and so on. The results are likely to be phony if received at all for the money you sent.

- **Medical products:** You buy health, beauty care, or "cure" product by mail, or you are sent newspaper clipping extolling magic diet with note scribbled across it, "It works—try it!" signed "J." Avoid such products.

- **Obituary:** You are recently widowed; COD box arrives for product "your husband (or wife) ordered." Return unless actually ordered.

- **Pigeon drop:** Person offers to share "found" money with you if you will put some of your own money with it "to show good faith."

- **Need help:** Man says his wife is sick, his car has been impounded, he has run out of gas, or some such tale; he needs just $10 or $20, promises to pay it back, and shows extensive identification. The money will not likely be repaid.

- **Unknown callers:** Woman with child knocks on door and asks for some favour requiring entrance.

- **Travel club:** Firm offers bargain airfare or hotel package in glamorous foreign locale. You may never get anything that was promised.

- **Telemarketing:** You find yourself involved in a fraud that comes in many forms but usually implicates merchandise or investment scams.

Source: Modified from Marklein, M., Con Games Proliferate: New Threats Haunt City Folks, *AARP Bulletin, 32(2)* (1991), 1, 16–17.[190]

---

**Thermoregulation.** Changes in *temperature regulation* and the inability to feel pain also produce safety problems. Use Table 14-3 for teaching and implementing health promotion.

**Hypothermia.** The elderly usually feel cold more easily, and they often may require more covering when in bed. A room temperature somewhat higher than usual is often desirable.

Assess for *hypothermia risk or presence*, as follows:

- Medications to treat anxiety or depression, hypothyroidism, vascular disease, alcoholism, and immobility reduce the body's response to cold.

- Living alone or anything that increases nighttime accidents can increase risk, as do poverty and poor housing.

- The elder may insist he or she is comfortable in a cool environment; the person is probably unaware of the temperature of the surroundings.

- The person is not thinking clearly, or is acting as usual when they are clearly cold.

- Low body temperature, irregular or slow pulse, slurred speech, shallow respirations, hypotension, drowsiness, lack of coordination, and sluggishness may be present, singly or in combination.

- Environmental temperatures below 18°C may cause a serious drop in core body temperature to 35°C or less.

- Severe hypothermia can cause complications of the kidney, liver, or pancreas, ventricular fibrillation, and even death. Recovery depends on the severity and length of exposure, previous health, and the rewarming treatment.[191]

*Teach the elderly person the following measures to prevent hypothermia in cold weather:*[192]

1. Stay indoors as much as possible, especially on windy, wet, and cold days.

2. Wear layered clothing, and cover the head when outdoors.

3. Eat hot, high-protein meals and bedtime snacks daily.

4. Keep at least one room warm at 20°C or above.

5. Use extra blankets, caps, socks, and layered clothing in bed.

6. Have contact with someone daily.

7. Avoid drinking alcoholic beverages.

**Hyperthermia** Hyperthermia must also be prevented. Assess for the three types of heat-related illnesses that can affect any age, especially the older adult. The older adult is especially vulnerable if he or she has circulatory impairment or is taking psychotropic or beta-blocker medications, which interfere with heat regulation.[193]

Heat stroke is a life-threatening problem that must be treated immediately for maximum recovery. It is a temperature-related disease and is classified as a medical emergency. Increased sweating depletes sodium, but high humidity interferes with the ability of the body to lower its core temperature. Several physiological mechanisms operate to maintain normal body temperature. Thyroid function decreases and aldosterone and the antidiuretic hormone (ADH) production increases to conserve body water and sodium. If these mechanisms are overwhelmed, peripheral vasoconstriction conserves central circulatory volume, but the core body temperature rises dramatically. *Signs and symptoms* include:[194]

a. Fever

b. Headache

c. Vertigo

d. Faintness

e. Confusion

f. Hyperpnea

g. Abdominal distress

At the higher body temperature, skin is hot and dry, respirations are weak, and tachycardia, agitation, delirium, hallucinations, and convulsions often occur.

*Complications*, especially for heat stroke, include:[195]

1. Cerebral edema, brain damage

2. Pulmonary edema

3. Liver necrosis

4. Acute renal failure

5. Myocardial necrosis or infarction

6. Gastrointestinal bleeding or ulceration

Prompt recognition and treatment of heat-related illness is essential to prevent organ damage or death. *Teach prevention*, including staying in a cool environment, increasing fluid intake, applying a sunblock outdoors, wearing loose, light clothing, and sponging off or taking cooling showers. *Health promotion strategies* include removing the person to a cool place, applying cool clothes, loosening clothing, and giving fluids. Emergency department care could be necessary, to assess for and prevent complications, when the body temperature continues to rise.[196]

**Pain** Pain perception and the appropriate reaction to it often decrease with age. A thorough evaluation is needed to determine the cause of the client's pain, and to determine whether or not disease-modifying interventions can treat pain.[197] That is, more accurate assessment of the physical signs and symptoms are necessary to alleviate the conditions underlying complaints of pain such as abdominal discomfort and chest pain. These conditions may be more serious than the older person's perception indicates. A few of the reasons for undertreatment of pain in older adults is the underreporting of pain by clients, a concern by clients of the additional costs of medications, and a belief by clients and physicians that older adults experience less pain.[198]

Understand that some of the changed behaviour, discussed later under the heading "Psychological Concepts," is directly related to physical changes in nerve and sensory tissue. These behaviours can often influence your nursing practice, whether you are giving physical care, establishing a relationship, providing a safe environment, or planning recreational needs. The whole area of client teaching is also affected, because you must understand the altered responses and the changing needs of the elderly before beginning their health education.

---

**CRITICAL THINKING**

*Outline the content of your health promotion program on hypothermia and hyperthermia.*

---

## Special Considerations in the Physical Examination of Older Clients[199]

The *health history* of the elder should include:

1. Current problems

2. Complete history of past medical problems

3. Smoking, alcohol, and drug history

4. Medication list

5. Psychosocial history and mental status

6. Nutritional patterns

7. Review of body systems focusing on functional abilities

8. Exercise patterns

9. History of immunizations

10. Support systems

11. Caregiver roles, caregiver stress, possible neglect or abuse

12. Advance directives

*Physical examination* should include:

1. Vital signs and weight

2. Mobility screening

3. Hypertension and vascular disease screening

4. Cancer screening

5. Hearing and vision screening

6. Breast examination: mammography for women up to age 75 (and perhaps to age 85)

7. Papanicolaou smear, if inadequately screened at a younger age, or if there is a history of abnormalities

In carrying out any particular physical assessment in the older adult, the nurse might need to modify certain procedures to glean the maximum information. Even helping the patient undress gives the nurse a good opportunity to observe the patient's ability to perform the task, and to note anything unusual. For example, the condition of clothing, personal hygiene, or clothing that may be inappropriate for the season or temperature (e.g., thermal underwear in August) can provide relevant cues.

---

### CRITICAL THINKING

*State the questions you would ask and the observations you would make to assess the skin, exercise patterns, and medication list of an 85-year-old person.*

---

The following are specific ways to *increase patient comfort prior to and during the examination:*

■ Warm the examining room sufficiently

■ Use chairs that are high enough to make rising easy.

■ Provide a footstool for getting on and off the table.

■ Place a pillow under the head and perhaps under the knees, because many elders feel a strain on the back when lying supine.

■ Place grab bars near the scale.

■ Minimize positional changes during the examination.

Other important areas of exploration in the elderly include hearing and vision acuity; the condition of the dentures; suspicious lesions under the tongue; jugular venous pulse; carotid arteries for bruits; and breast examination, including the skin under pendulous breasts.

Suspected urinary incontinence can be tested by having the patient hold a small pad over the urethral area and coughing three times in a standing position. Cystocele, rectocele, or uterine prolapse should be ruled out. For men, a digital rectal examination should be done to check the prostate.

Examination of the elder patient's feet is most important. Have the patient sit up and hang the feet down to check the venous flow. Are the patient's shoes appropriate for good balance and the prevention of falls? The patient's gait can offer significant clues. For example, the Parkinsonian gait is shown by short, shuffling steps, short or absent arm swing, and a stooped trunk.[200]

## Common Health Problems for the Older Adult

The health problems of the older adult are possibly associated with the aging process, a disease state, or both. Yet, more than 90 percent of elders need no help with the activities of daily living. Consider all of the aspects of aging before deciding on a course of action. Refer to a medical-surgical nursing text for in-depth information on health problems. Other references will also be useful.[201]

Table 14-11 summarizes common neurologic and respiratory diseases: blood dyscrasias; genitourinary, skeletal, and cardiovascular diseases; and tuberculosis. Sexual function diseases and substance abuse are also presented in overview.[202] Use the information provided in these references in assessment, teaching, health promotion, and illness prevention.

With advancing age, the heart and blood vessels undergo both structural and functional changes.[203] The most significant risk factors that contribute to cardiovascular disease are the same for both younger and older adults, but the cumulative effects of these risks are likely to cause more serious consequences for older adults.[204] Gender-related differences in risk factors can significantly affect women beginning at menopause, while factors that increase the risk for hypertension begin affecting all older adults after the age of 70 to 75 years.[205] Physical deconditioning significantly influences many aspects of cardiovascular functioning, including blood pressure, heart rate, and oxygen consumption.[206]

Cardiovascular disease is the leading cause of death in the elderly population. Evidence of heart disease is found in approximately 50 percent of those between 65 and 74 years of age, and in 60 percent of individuals older than age 75. With more of the population reaching advanced age, cardiovascular disease will continue to be a significant threat to the health and well-being of the elderly population.[207]

Cancer is primarily a disease of older Canadians: 44 percent of new cancer cases and 60 percent of cancer deaths will occur among those who are at least 70 years old.[208] Tobacco use, unhealthy diet, excess body weight, physical

Table 14-11 Common Health Problems in Later Maturity

| Problem | Definition | Symptom/Signs | Prevention/Treatment |
|---|---|---|---|
| **Neurologic diseases** | | | |
| Herpes zoster (shingles) | Caused by same virus that causes chicken-pox | Unilateral vesicular eruption that follows dermatomes of affected nerve root | Analgesics; cool soaks; acyclovir (Zovirax) |
| | Involves dorsal root ganglia | Severe pain; rash that progresses from macules to crusting pustules | Investigation of underlying immunologic problems |
| Parkinson's disease | Slowly progressive degenerative disorder of nervous system | Resting tremor; masklike face; shuffling gait, forward flexion; muscle weakness; rigidity | Symptomatic, medicine to correct depleted dopamine and rid excessive acetylcholine |
| Alzheimer's disease | Presenile dementia or neural atrophy | Cognitive, physical, and emotional deterioration | Treatment extremely varied, depending on areas affected |
| | | | Much support and understanding needed from families and caretakers; in turn, families and caretakers need support |
| **Respiratory diseases** | | | |
| Chronic obstructive pulmonary disease | Consists of three components: bronchitis, bronchoconstriction, and emphysema | Three components: (1) bronchitis—excessive mucus and sputum production with inflammation of the bronchi; (2) bronchoconstriction—narrowing airways; (3) emphysema—irreversible destruction of distal air space | Smoking cessation; increased fluids; yearly influenza vaccine; one-time pneumonia vaccine; bronchodilator; expectorants as necessary; avoidance of sedatives and cold, wet weather, postural drainage; antibiotics if infection |
| | | Shortness of breath, sputum production, wheezing, tachypnea, hyperinflation | General attention to proper nutrition, rest, and hygiene |
| **Blood dyscrasias** | | | |
| Pernicious anemia | Progressive megaloblastic microcytic anemia that results from lack of intrinsic factor essential for absorption or vitamin $B_{12}$ | Weakness, numbness, tingling of extremities; fever, pallor; anorexia, weight loss | Vitamin $B_{12}$ injections; folic acid and iron medications |
| Secondary anemia | Reduced hemoglobin level, hematocrit, and red blood cells counts, resulting from nutritional deficiency, blood loss, and primary problem | Fatigue, shortness of breath, light-headedness, skin pallor; sometimes arrhythmia | Iron preparation or perhaps blood transfusion; maintenance or stable activities of daily living; attention to primary issue |

*(continued)*

Table 14-11 (continued)

| Problem | Definition | Symptom/Signs | Prevention/Treatment |
|---|---|---|---|
| Chronic lymph-ocytic leukemia | Neoplasm of blood-forming tissue | Characterized by small, long-lived lymphocytes, chiefly B cells in bone marrow, blood, liver, and lymphoid tissue | Complexity of disease dictates seeking medical-surgical text or physician |
| Hodgkin's disease | Malignant disorder | Characterized by painless progressive enlargement of lymphoid tissue | Complexity of disease necessitates seeking medical-surgical text or physician |

## Genitourinary diseases

| | | | |
|---|---|---|---|
| Benign prostatic hypertrophy (BPH) | Overall enlargement of prostate gland via enlargement of fibrous and muscular tissue | Difficulty in stopping and starting urinary flow; voiding frequent small amounts  Diffuse enlargement of prostate; landmarks preserved | Medication such as Hytrin; possible surgical inter-vention; rule out cancer |

## Skeletal diseases

| | | | |
|---|---|---|---|
| Osteoporosis | Absence of normal quantity of bone  Predisposes to fracture | Loss of normal cortical thickness; increased porosity in cortical bone; thinning, fragmentation, and loss of trabeculae in can-cellous bone | Prevention: diet in earlier years containing ade-quate calcium, vitamin D, phosphorus, protein, and fluoride |
| Osteoarthritis | Degeneration of articular cartilage and hypertrophy of bone | Pain and stiffness, mainly in weight-bearing joints and dorsal interphalangeal joints of fingers | Exercise to improve stiff-ness; rest to help pain; heat, antiphyretic, ade-quate nutrition, physi-cal therapy, Fosamat or other stabilizer |

## Cardiovascular diseases

| | | | |
|---|---|---|---|
| Congestive heart failure | Cardiac function altered so that there is not enough cardiac output to meet demands of tissue meta-bolism; consequently sodium and body water are retained | Arteriosclerotic heart disease and hypertension precursors; depressed breathing (unless sitting or standing); ankle swelling; frequent nighttime voiding; weight gain; distended neck veins; rales in lungs; heart with "gallop rhythm" | Low-sodium diet; correct high blood pressure with angiotensin-converting enzyme (ACE) inhibitors, nitrates, and other vasodilators, chemical trials being done with calcium channel blockers, prostacycline analogues, and oral inotropes; rate and rhythm regulated with digitalis preparation; urinary output increased with diuretics |
| Chronic occlusive arterial disease of the extremities | Because of partial or complete occlusion of one or more peripheral blood vessels, decreased blood flow to one or more extremities | Diabetes often a precursor; cramping pain in the muscles during exercise that is relieved by rest; sometimes nighttime cramping; extremity may feel cool; pulses may be decreased; skin may lose hair and appear shiny | Evaluate for revasculariza-tion; practise good skincare; avoid excess heat or cold; avoid tobacco and caffeine; drugs not effective |

*(continued)*

Table 14-11 (continued)

| Problem | Definition | Symptom/Signs | Prevention/Treatment |
|---------|-----------|---------------|---------------------|
| Stasis ulcer of the lower extremity | Chronic ulcerative skin lesion caused by venous stasis and consequent poor circulation | Peripheral pulses intact; **pitting edema** *(induration remains after pushing in skin and tissue with a finger)* or **brawny edema** *(thickened and hardened skin)* around ulcer site | Rest and elevation of involved leg; once or twice daily cleaning with povidone iodine (Betadine) or hydrogen peroxide solution; occasionally application of moist heat or Unna boot; watch for widening of lesion and cellulitis |
| **Infectious diseases** | | | |
| Tuberculosis (not yet common, but re-emerging) | Infectious disease transmitted by airborne route and caused by ***Mycobacterium tuberculosis;*** infection refers to successful colonization in a host; active disease indicates pathogenic process | Chronic flulike cough, decreased appetite, weakness, weight loss, continued slightly elevated temperature, night sweats, dyspnea on exertion, pain with respiratory movements if pleura involved, rales over apex of lung, hoarseness if larynx involved, dysphagia if pharynx involved | TB skin testing, x-ray if indicated, sputum testing, multiple-drug therapies (isoniazid, rifampin, pyrazinamide, and ethambutol or strepto mycin); appropriate infection control techniques for both patient and those in contact with patient |

inactivity, alcohol consumption, and overexposure to the sun are well-documented modifiable risk factors for several common forms of cancer. It is these factors that account for a substantial number of cancer diagnoses each year.[209] Other prevalent disorders are arthritis, diabetes, hypertension, and osteoporosis.[210] Older adults consistently have the highest rates of suicide in most societies. Despite the scarcity of research, recent studies have indicated that suicide in later life is best understood as a multidimensional event. Leenaars states that a need exists for greater study and theory building into the suicides of the elderly, including those who are terminally ill.[211]

Health and social factors are important predictors of social isolation and loneliness, and sensitivity to these factors can go far to improve the experiences of older adults.[212]

## CRITICAL THINKING

*Describe your suicide assessment plan.*

**Pharmacotherapy of Older Adults** Increased longevity has been the outcome of an improved quality of life and the ability to treat many chronic diseases effectively. As people age, many physiological changes occur. The age-related changes in older adults influence the client's response to drugs, which alter both the therapeutic and the adverse effects and create special needs and risks. As a consequence of aging, clients experience an increasing number of chronic health disorders. As a result, more drugs are needed to treat such disorders. The taking of multiple drugs is known as *polypharmacy*. It increases the risk for drug interactions and side effects.[213]

A number of drugs are excreted through the kidneys. Consequently, the altered physiology of the aging renal and urinary systems requires adjustments in both dosages and dosage intervals. For example, certain medications contribute to hyperkalemia in older adults by inhibiting the excretion of potassium in the kidney. Potassium supplements and potassium-containing salt substitutes have identified as causes of hyperkalemia in older people. Hypokalemia has been found in older people with fecal impactions or who abuse laxatives and have lost potassium in the stool. Diuretics increase urine volume. The resultant voiding frequency can cause or worsen incontinence, especially in women. Alcohol inhibits the perceived need to void, and it is a mild diuretic as well. Alcohol can also cause drowsiness.[214]

Normal physiological changes that affect pharmacotherapy include the following:

- *Absorption:* The absorption of drugs is slower due to diminished gastric motility and the decreased blood flow to digestive organs.

- *Distribution:* Increased body fat in the older adult provides a larger storage compartment for lipid-soluble drugs and vitamins. Plasma levels are reduced, and the therapeutic response is diminished. Older adults have less body water. This makes the effects of dehydration more dramatic, which increase the risk for drug toxicity.

- *Metabolism:* The liver's production of enzymes decreases, liver mass decreases, and the splanchnic blood flow is diminished resulting in reduced hepatic drug response.

- *Excretion:* Older adults experience reduction in renal blood flow, glomerular filtration rate, acute tubular secretion, and nephron function. When excretion is reduced, both serum drug levels and the potential for toxicity increase markedly.[215]

When administering medications to older adults, the nurse should offer the client the same degree of independence and dignity that would be afforded to middle-aged adults, unless otherwise indicated. Careful assessment is always necessary. Accommodations must be made for older adults who have certain impairments. Visual and auditory changes make it important for the nurse to provide drug instructions in large type. The nurse should obtain client feedback to be certain that medication instructions have been understood.[216] Elderly clients with cognitive impairment can benefit from aids such as medicine management boxes and clearly written instructions. The use of both prescription and over-the-counter medication should be assessed and monitored by the nurse.[217]

The goal is to develop individualized health promotion strategies. Doing so helps to promote optimal quality of life because, for many clients, cure as a result of medications may not be a realistic goal.

Table 14-12 presents medication–food interactions that may occur.[218]

## CRITICAL THINKING

*What tips would you give a group of older adults about taking medications?*

**Polypharmacy and Adverse Drug Reactions** In Canada, Gill, Misiaszed, and Brymer conducted a study to determine the prevalence and predictors of the potentially inappropriate prescription of medications in long-term settings. They found that a total of 69 potentially inappropriate

| Table 14-12 Common Medication–Nutrient Interactions in the Elderly | |
|---|---|
| **Drug** | **Interaction** |
| Methyldopa | Should be taken at times of day when high-protein foods are not being consumed, since absorption is competitive between this drug and amino acids in foods. |
| Antihypertensive drugs | May influence potassium and magnesium status. |
| Antibiotics | Influence intestinal absorption. |
| Aspirin | Can increase gastric acidity and cause anorexia. May require increased need for folic acid and vitamin C. May cause GI bleeding and subsequent iron deficiency. |
| Laxatives | Can cause gas, cramps, and anorexia. Can affect vitamin D absorption and in turn worsen calcium balance. Mineral oil can interfere with the absorption of vitamins A, D, E, and K. |
| Tetracycline | Calcium in dairy products makes the drug less effective. |
| Anticoagulants | Can be adversely affected when liver, green leafy vegetables, and other foods high in vitamin K are eaten in excess. |
| Monoamine oxidase inhibitors | Foods high in tyramine such as aged cheese, Chianti wine, pickled herring, salami, pepperoni, yogurt, sour cream, raisins, meat prepared with tenderizers, and chicken livers can increase blood pressure and may cause severe headaches, brain hemorrhage, and even death. Cola beverages, coffee, and chocolate should be taken in moderation. |

*(continued)*

Table 14-12 (continued)

| Drug | Interaction |
|------|-------------|
| Alcohol | Certain drugs may increase intoxication. Consumed with depressants, alcohol can compound the depressant effect; can cause anticonvulsants and anticoagulants to be metabolized more quickly, causing exaggerated responses; can raise blood sugar levels and interfere with medication prescribed for diabetes; can increase blood pressure when taken with MAO inhibitors; can reduce blood pressure when take with diuretics; with antibiotics, it can cause cramps, nausea, and vomiting. Alcohol may destroy the coating of time-release capsules, causing more rapid absorption of a drug. Can increase requirements for nutrients, such as folic acid, thiamine, vitamin $B_6$, zinc, and magnesium. |
| Diuretics | Can promote loss of potassium; can increase calcium excretion. |
| Antacids | Some contain aluminium hydroxide, which can contribute to phosphate deficiency. As a result, blood phosphate may be high but only at the expense of phosphorus released from the bone. |

prescriptions were found in 65 of 355 long-term care patients.[219] The most common types of potentially inappropriate prescriptions were anticholinergic drugs to manage antipsychotic cases (17 cases), tricyclic antidepressants with active metabolites (916 cases), and long-acting benzodiazepines (14 cases). The researchers concluded that potentially inappropriate prescribing in the long-term care setting is common and can be improved by providing a follow-up letter that suggests improving the alternatives.[220]

Health Canada developed a kit called *Medication Matters: How You Can Help Seniors Use Medications Safely*. It was designed to help health professionals give older adults information they need to use medication safely.[221]

*Teach elders and family members the following:*

1. To learn as much as possible about the medication being taken and the disease process.

2. How to keep track of medications, prescribed and over-the-counter, as well as vitamin-mineral supplements and herbs: the doses, times consumed, and any unusual reactions.

3. To inform each of the physicians about all of the prescribed and over-the-counter medications taken daily.

4. To follow the directions for taking the medications, such as drinking a tall glass of water to reduce side effects.

5. Consult a physician or pharmacist about any questions or symptoms. Report problems promptly.

## CRITICAL THINKING

*You are asked to give a 30-minute presentation to a local senior citizen group on "Medications and the Older Adult." What educational materials would you use?*

**Substance Abuse** Canadian estimates indicate that between 6 and 10 percent of older adults who drink alcohol have alcohol-related problems.[222] When medication issues are included, it is believed that up to 20 percent of older adults experience difficulties due to alcohol and/or medication misuse.[223] Older adults are at even greater risk for a number of adverse consequences of substance use because of changes in their body composition (less body water and more fat stores) and function (reduced organ efficiency, greater sensitivity of the central nervous system to substances).[224]

Alcohol interacts with various drugs through either potentiation of or interference with medication action. This situation is shown in Table 14-13. (Alcohol interacts adversely with at least 50 percent of the commonly used over-the-counter drugs.) Other effects, such as the loss of coordination, slower reflex reaction time, and slower mental responses, cause the person to be accident prone. Such can, in turn, result in injury, fractures, or death.[225]

While seniors can and do misuse/abuse substances, a general reluctance exists among families and caregivers to acknowledge these problems.[226] Some of the reasons are as follows:

- Health care providers are hindered by insufficient knowledge, hurried office visits, and limited research data

- The diagnosis of substance abuse causing dependence can be complicated by an atypical symptom that mimics other behavioural or medical problems

- The current generation of older adults tends to be reluctant to reveal such problems due to anticipated shame about what they regard as a private matter

| Table 14-13 | Alcohol Interactions with Medications | |
| --- | --- |
| **Medication Taken with Alcohol** | **Effect on Person** |
| Antidiabetic agents | Increased hypoglycemia; increased effects of alcohol |
| Anticoagulants | Increased effect; possible hemorrhage |
| Barbiturates | Increased central nervous system depression, oversedation Inhibition of antimicrobial action |
| Tranquilizers | |
| Narcotics | |
| Antidepressants | |
| Antihistamines | |
| Anaesthetics | |
| Antibiotics | |

- The ageist attitudes of younger adults can lead to unconsciously assigning different quality of life standards to older adults. It is then assumed that it is not worth the effort to treat these older adults with substance abuse problems

To help Canadian seniors with substance abuse problems, most special treatment programs are geared to use a "harm reduction" approach to reach and work with older adults. The term *harm reduction* refers to strategies to help a person avoid harm associated with his or her alcohol use. The goal is to work toward less problematic alcohol use or abstinence. It is a non-confrontational and non-judgmental approach that helps the person to deal with the problems that he or she finds most troublesome in his or her life. In summary, harm reduction attempts to minimize the potential hazards associated with alcohol use, rather then focusing exclusively on the alcohol use itself.[227] A useful booklet called *Responding to Older Adults with Substance Use, Mental Health and Gambling Challenges* is available.[228] A reproducible copy of this publication can be found on the Internet at www.camh.net/Publications/Resources_for_Professionals/Older_Adults/index.html.

---

**CRITICAL THINKING**

*Outline a plan for teaching older adults about substance abuse.*

## PSYCHOLOGICAL CONCEPTS

The psychological and socioeconomic concepts about aging are significant for all who work with the aged, and you will find older people concerned and needing to talk about the many changes to which they must adjust.

## Cognitive Development

One universal truth that concerns the process of aging is that its onset, rate, and pattern are singularly unique for each person. Within the individual, the cognitive functions neither change nor decline at the same pace. Some functions will not decrease at all. For example, the memorization of facts can be difficult, but one's wisdom will be evident. This is especially true of psychological and mental changes, which generally have a later and more gradual onset than physical aging. Unless the person develops Alzheimer's or another dementia or a vascular disease, age alone does not ruin memory. Although changes in one's processing abilities often reflect neurological deterioration, much individual variation exists, suggesting that declines in functioning are not inevitable and might be preventable.[229]

*Many factors must be considered when assessing the intellectual functioning of older people:*

- Physical health can affect the level of psychological distress, life satisfaction, and cognitive ability. (That is, anemia, lung disease, poor circulation, blood pressure or blood sugar changes, hypothyroidism, and fluid or nutritional imbalance can profoundly affect one's mental status).

- Medications either prescribed or over-the-counter that are being taken. Some drugs are acting slowly or they interfere with cognitive processes because of toxicity related to slower elimination from the body. Drug overdose or **polypharmacy**, *taking excess and unneeded combinations of drugs*, can cause drug interactions, toxicity, confusion, or depression, and must be avoided with careful monitoring and adjustments.

- Sensory impairments (vision, hearing) that interfere with the integration of sensory input into proper perception, consequent learning, and appropriate behaviours

- Sociocultural influences

- Motivation

- Interest

- Educational level

- Isolation from others

- Deliberate caution

- Using more time to do something, which others may interpret as not knowing

- Adaptive mechanism of conserving time and emotional energy rather than showing assertion

The elder demonstrates **crystallized intelligence**, *knowledge and cognitive ability maintained over the lifetime, dependent on sociocultural influences, life experiences, and broad education, that involve the ability to perceive relationships, engage in formal operations, and understand the intellectual and* *cultural heritage.* Crystallized intelligence is measured by one's facility with numbers, verbal comprehension, general information, and integrative and interpretive ability. It is influenced by the amount the person has learned, the diversity and complexity of the environment, the person's openness to new information, and the extent of earlier formal learning opportunities. Both self-directed learning opportunities and the availability of educational opportunities to gain additional information have been shown to increase crystallized intelligence after 60 years of age.[230]

A decline in mental ability occurs in many people after the late seventies. The loss of biological potential is offset by one's acquired wisdom, experience, and knowledge. In contrast, **fluid intelligence**, which is *independent of instruction, social or environmental influences, or acculturation, and is dependent on genetic endowment,* is less apparent. *Fluid intelligence consists of ability to perceive complex relationships, use short-term or rote memory, create concepts, and reason abstractly.* Fluid intelligence is measured by the ability to perform tasks of memory span, inductive reasoning, and figural relations. There is, however, no uniform pattern of age-related changes for all intellectual abilities, nor is there a consistent decline in all elders.[231]

**Intellectual plasticity** refers to the fact that *the person's performance or ability can vary a great deal, depending on social, environmental, and physical conditions.* For example, the time one takes to do a task, one's anxiety about evaluation, the attention to or motivation for a task, the amount of environmental stimulation needed, or the cognitive training or education needed for the task—all vary immeasurably from one older adult to another.[232]

The *senior performs certain cognitive tasks more slowly for several reasons:*

- Decreased visual and auditory acuity
- Slower motor response to sensory stimulation

- Loss of recent memory
- Divided attention
- Greater amount of prior accumulated knowledge and learning that must be scanned and appropriately placed mentally
- Perceived meaningfulness of the task
- Current motivation

He or she may be entirely disinterested in competing in timed intellectual tests. Reaction times are slower when the person suffers significant environmental or social losses, is unable to engage in social contact, and is unable to plan daily routines. The person who is ill often endures environmental and social losses by virtue of being in the client role. Thus, he or she will be inclined to respond more slowly to your questions or requests. Low self-esteem contributes significantly to poor cognitive function.[233]

Studies indicate that elderly adults are equivalent to young adults in cue use, encoding, specificity, decision-making speed, design recognition, and spatial memory or awareness of location, especially when distinctive cues are available. Other studies indicate that cognitive performances of young and older adults are comparable, when the task is divided or attention has not been interrupted, on assessing the contents and products of memory, and on the recall and recognition of factual information.[234]

Table 14-14 summarizes the types of cognitive functions, characteristics of the elderly, and health promotion implications.[235]

Both cognition and intellectual development are part of maturity. In the last half of life, the person draws best on their cumulative experiences to establish social, moral, and ethical standards; render decisions; assist in planning; and erect social guideposts. The judgmental functions of the mind are most highly developed after mid-life.[236]

## Table 14-14 Cognitive Development in Person

| Characteristic | Change during Aging | Implication for Health Care |
|---|---|---|
| **Sensory memory** | | |
| | Large amount of information enters nervous system through the senses; selective attention occurs. Some information is sent to short-term memory for further processing; some is lost because nervous system cannot process. | Avoid sensory overload. Assist hearing, visual, and tactile functions. |
| | | Recognize that person may be inattentive to your teaching or to their symptoms or situation. |
| | | Use variety of teaching methods, include visual aids. |
| | First step of memory process involves recall that lasts a few minutes. | Teach importance of health maintenance, as healthy elders maintain general intellectual function. |

*(continued)*

Table 14-14 (continued)

| Characteristic | Change during Aging | Implication for Health Care |
|---|---|---|
| **Short-term memory** | Brain holds information for immediate use: conceptualization, rehearsal, memorization, association with long-term memory. Deals with current activities or recent past of minutes to hours. Remains consistent with earlier abilities. Older person can repeat string of digits as well as younger person unless asked to repeat them backward; information about digits fades in about a minute unless person rehearses it. Overall mental status is poorly correlated with short-term memory. Recall is better for logically grouped, chunked, or sequenced information. | Give attention for memory abilities. Teach importance of continuing to use memory, memory retrieval tricks, or cues. Teach person to use variety of associative and memory strategies to enhance recall. Teach relaxation methods to reduce anxiety about memory and enhance attention, rehearsal, motivation, and general function. Teach cognitive tricks or use of lists or ways to organize information to improve memory or remember essential information. Teach person to overcome interferences. Let person set own pace to enhance learning and memory. |
| **Long-term memory** | Use of information acquired, transferred for storage, and stored over years. Unlimited, permanent storehouse of memories, which may not have to pass through short-term memory. Involves images (mental pictures) and verbalization. Three encoding systems are used: visual-spatial, verbal sequential, and abstraction. | Give attention for memory abilities. Recognize that dysfunctions in short- and long-term memories occur independently. Encourage person to use memories and associations in tasks. |
| **Declarative (episodic)** | Conscious memory of specific persons, places, events, or facts that is acquired quickly, but may not be accurately or easily recalled. Requires intact hippocampus. Older person stores long-term memories, but does not retrieve as quickly as younger person unless he or she uses memory tricks. | Give person adequate time for recall. Encourage use of memory tricks and associations. |
| **Recognition** | Involves selecting correct response from incoming information rather than recall or retrieval. Ability is retained with age for words, background, familiar objects. | Give support and recognition for ability to recognize and use information. |
| **Implicit (reflexive)** | Unconscious learning of information or skill through experience or practice (e.g., playing piano, riding bicycle). Requires intact cerebellum. Ideas, concepts, or ability to perform readily remembered. Does not weaken with age in absence of pathology, as person can demonstrate if not discuss. | Use practice in learning new skills for self-care. Reinforce use of habits. Encourage reminiscence or life review. Use habits and well-practised skills when possible in teaching or assisting them. Encourage continued practice of implicitly learned tasks or information. |

*(continued)*

Table 14-14 (continued)

| Characteristic | Change during Aging | Implication for Health Care |
|---|---|---|
| **Reaction time (RT)** | Speed of response slows during life, and is more obvious after age 60 because of central nervous system changes; shorter duration of alpha rhythm in brain wave (RT fastest between ages 20 and 30). RT remains faster in males than females. Reaction time remains accurate even if slower in both sexes in older adult. | If the person is hurried, response quality and quantity will be reduced. Allow person to proceed at own pace in learning, making decisions, or doing tasks. Do not consider slower response the same as confusion or dementia. |
| **Attentional selectivity** | Gradual reduced ability in focusing on a specific idea or event, especially as the information processing demands of the task increase. As capable as younger people in correcting unanticipated errors. | Call attention to specific tasks or ideas that the person must focus on when teaching or counselling. Recognize and reinforce capabilities. |
| **Problem solving** | Skills increase steadily into old age; performance unrelated to IQ test scores or formal education. Person adopts simpler judgmental strategies and relies on pre-existing knowledge more so than young adult. In low-memory–demand tasks, elder is more efficient than young adult. Is better at complex judgmental strategies than young adult. | Teach importance of continuing cognitive function. Engage person in goal setting and problem solving. |
| **Dialectical thinking** | Older people better able to see all sides of a situation and come to conclusion that integrates different viewpoints and contradictory ideas when given time and when experience rather than memory is required. Is better at solving conditional-probability problems than young adult. Is better at telling integrated story than young adult. | Listen to what may appear to be rambling or loose associations as ideas are likely to be related and pertinent. |
| **Social awareness** | Increased knowledge and empathy related to culture, living, value systems, or application of ethical and moral principles. Social responsibility traits remain stable or increase in older adult. | Recognize and reinforce capabilities. Use older people as consultants and teachers of the culture. |
| **Higher mental functions: calculations, abstract reasoning** | Involves integrity of several cognitive functions and exercising values and judgment in decision making and problem solving, logical thinking, future planning, comparison and evaluation of alternatives in context of | Encourage person to remain active in situations or roles that require use of cognitive abilities, e.g., volunteer, mentor, teaching aide, organizational committees, political activities. |

*(continued)*

Table 14-14 (continued)

| Characteristic | Change during Aging | Implication for Health Care |
|---|---|---|
| | reality and social responsibility, considering consequences of action. These functions are vulnerable to neurologic pathology; loss of abstraction ability may be first sign of disease or dementia. | |
| Creativity | Productivity continues into old age. Aesthetic sense and appreciation of beauty continue to develop. | Provide pleasing environment and opportunities for creativity. Teach family and elder that intellectual and creative mastery of the world exists in many forms and manifests itself daily. |
| General knowledge | Maintains or improves into old age, especially in vocabulary, verbal abilities, and verbal comprehension. General task-specific skills remain equal to those of young adult. | Encourage person to remain active in family and community; participation is a predictor of ability. Reinforce knowledge and wisdom and combat ageism. Teach health promotion as physical health can affect mental function. |
| Academic performance | Elderly students in college perform as well as younger students, tend to have fewer problems, and are able to use new technology and equipment. | Encourage elder to participate in classes, continue learning in credit or non-credit courses or in elder hostel. |
| Spatial discrimination | High-level cortical function related to (1) visual and kinesthetic senses; (2) frontal lobe (motor skill) and parietal lobe (association) functions; (3) ability to produce accurate representations of the way in which objects or parts of objects relate to each other in space; (4) interpretation of directions and top/bottom and visual and spatial cues. Loss of impairment occurs independent of altered sensory function, language dysfunction, or position sense. Older adult tends to need more time and be less accurate in case of maps or finding directions. | Teach spatial cues. Recognize impact on rehabilitation. Test for constructional ability (copy geometric figure or draw face of clock) and general orientation to determine early brain dysfunction. Observe for unilateral neglect of body, inattention to objects or people in left half of sensory field. Assist with and teach family about self-care and safety implications. |
| Wisdom | Superior knowledge and judgment with extraordinary scope, depth, and balance applicable to specific situations and the general life condition. Increases because of empathy and understanding developed over the years. Depends on cognitive and personality factors as well as virtue (character). | Acknowledge the elder's wisdom, creative ability, and productivity. Encourage family to use elder as confidant and consultant. |

*Creativity* is evident during the later years. The following are important points to remember as you teach, assist, and advocate for the elderly:[237]

- People at any age are not identical to others in creative output. The expected age decrement in creativity varies across disciplines; in some, there is scarcely any decline.

- Creative output of the person in her or his sixties or seventies will most often exceed that produced during the twenties, as long as the person is healthy.

- Creative output changes occur in relation to role changes during one's career or profession, rather than in relation to age.

- The person with a late start in career or profession usually reaches a later peak with higher output during the later years.

- Reduced creative output does not mean there will be a corresponding loss of intellectual or motivational capabilities.

- Some factors such as health and reduced vigour can interfere with one's creative output, but theses barriers can be overcome with individual motivation and supportive assistance provided to the person.

- Creativity can resurge in life's last years.

In your care of the older person, and in teaching about cognitive characteristics of later maturity, recognize that the normal aging brain, free of disease, can function as effectively and efficiently as the normal young adult brain, except for speed and accuracy of recent memory. Significant cognitive impairment is related to disease, not to normal aging.[238]

Minor memory loss, or "forgetfulness," can be due to "normal" aging changes. However, more than a minor loss, if it occurs, may be due to some disease processes. New cognitive theories of aging are developing, and the current debate is on whether intellectual skills, such as memory games and other forms of memory training, can enhance cognitive functioning, and perhaps even prevent cognitive deterioration.[239] A significant memory loss in older adults is likely to be caused by one or more of the three Ds of cognitive impairment:

- Dementia (progressive intellectual impairment)
- Depression (mood disorder)
- Delirium (acute confusion)[240]

Delirium and dementia are often referred to as cognitive impairment. A comprehensive assessment of the client is necessary. The administration of one basic tool, such as the Mini-Mental State Exam (MMSE), is important. The tool yields a considerable amount of valuable data regarding cognitive functioning. The MMSE is a 30-item instrument used to screen for cognitive deficiencies, and the information it provides is one of the factors used in the determination of a diagnosis of dementia and delirium.[241]

Alzheimer's disease is a severe form of dementia. The early stages become evident slowly, beginning with repetitive conversations, subtle memory difficulties, and disorientation to familiar settings. Although reports of studies vary about the rates of Alzheimer's disease at specific ages, gerontologists agree that the chance of having Alzheimer's disease increases with increasing age. The presence of neuritic plaques and neurofibrillary tangles are the hallmark pathologic criteria for the disease. In addition to studying genetic factors, researchers are investigating numerous other factors thought to be associated with Alzheimer's disease.[242]

A major goal of ongoing assessment is to identify factors that interfere with the older adult's level of functioning, or quality of life, so that intervention can be initiated to alleviate these contributing factors. Another goal is to identify the strengths and limitations in the individual's abilities so that individualized interventions can be planned to improve the person's functioning and quality of life.[243]

The elder can be taught to remember essential information (use suggestions in the box entitled "Effective Memory Strategies").

## CRITICAL THINKING

*You have been asked to present an in-service program on the medications used to treat dementia and to manage dementia-related behaviours. What information will you present?*

Use the following suggestions when you teach:

- Always approach the teaching situation in a way that enhances the person's self-concept and self-confidence.

- Keep in mind and assess the elder's experiences, current knowledge, needs, interests, questions, health status, and developmental level as you plan and implement teaching.

- Minimize distracting noise; select a comfortable setting.

- Tell the person that you are planning a teaching session, state the general topic, and emphasize importance. Get the person's attention and increase anticipation.

- Arrange for the person to be near the teacher, teaching aids, or demonstration.

- Consider the aged person's difficulty with fine movement and failing vision when you are using visual aids.

- Provide adequate lighting without glare; do not have the person face outdoor or indirect light.

- Use sharp colours with a natural background and large print to offset visual difficulties.

- Explain procedures and directions with the person's possible hearing loss and slowed responses in mind.
- Use a low-pitched, clear speaking voice; face the person so he or she can lip read if necessary.
- Teach slowly and patiently, with sessions not too long or widely spaced and with repetition and reinforcement.
- Mentally "walk through" or imagine a task through verbal explanation before it is to be done to enhance recall.
- Material should be short, concise, and concrete; present material in a logical sequence; summarize often.
- Break complex tasks or content into smaller and simpler units known as chunking; focus on a single topic to promote concentration.[244]
- Match your vocabulary to the learner's ability and define terms clearly and as frequently as needed.

## Effective Memory Strategies

### Selective Encoding (getting information into memory)
- Actively and creatively try to find meaning in facts
- Underline selectively; outline
- Distinguish between important and unimportant points and facts
- Summarize main points
- Reconstruct facts; test self

### Elaboration
- Use imagery, visualization of content
- Use metaphor
- Use analogy
- Paraphrase in own words
- Encode more than one strategy

### Organization
- Understand how information is organized
- Choose appropriate and effective retrieval cues
- Be aware that related items may cue memory
- Reorganize information so new material better relates to previous knowledge

### External Representation
- Take notes; outline
- Make charts, diagrams, tables, or graphs
- Make a conceptual map

### Monitoring
- Test self
- Check where errors are made; correct errors

- Give the aged person time to perceive and respond to stimuli, to learn, to move, and to act.
- Help the person make associations between prior and new information and emphasize abilities that remain constant to enhance recall and application.
- Have the person actively use several sensory modalities to make motions and repeat the content aloud verbally while seeing or hearing it.
- Plan extra sessions for feedback and return demonstrations and extra time for these sessions.
- Whenever possible, include a significant other in the teaching session to ensure further interpretation and support in using the information.

Two forms of recall serve as therapeutic interventions: reminiscence and life review.[245] Reminiscence and life review differ, but they share certain characteristics: (1) both use memory and recall for enjoyment, or to cope with difficulties and consider accomplishments; (2) both can be structured, or free-flowing; (3) both are integrative and can involve happy or sad feelings; (4) both serve a therapeutic function; and (5) both are implemented primarily with the elderly but can be used with middle-agers and young adults, especially in terminal illness.

**Reminiscence** involves *the informal sharing of bits and pieces of the past that surface to the consciousness*. Reminiscence is important because it involves the feelings related to memories. Thus, this memory process includes affective and cognitive functions. It is an oral history.

Goals for use of reminiscence include the following:

- Provide pleasure and comfort (but allow sad and angry feelings and memories to come forth)
- Improve self-confidence, self-esteem, and mood
- Improve communication skills and cognitive function; stay oriented
- Increase socialization, decrease isolation
- Improve alertness, connectedness with others
- Increase deeper friendships; put relationships in order
- Promote the role of confidant
- Promote ego integrity and satisfaction with life. Find meaning in the life cycle
- Provide strength to face new life challenges
- Obtain data
- Facilitate grieving for losses

During reminiscence therapy, your role is to:

- Encourage informal, spontaneous discussion
- Be supportive. Provide a positive atmosphere

- Avoid probing or pushing for insight
- Allow repetition in the person's discussion
- Encourage the person to integrate the happy and sad memories
- Allow the person to evaluate implications or prior outcomes as memories are recalled, if they desire to do so.
- Validate and support the meaningful contributions and activities of past life
- Use themes or props to stimulate discussion, especially in a group
- Avoid focusing on issues, or on the judgment of memories

Reminiscence may be done with individuals, with family and clients, or with a group of clients. You have a role in all of these.

## CRITICAL THINKING

*You are asked to give an in-service talk to a group of nurses in a personal care home on "Reminiscence Therapy." What are your goals?*

**Life review** involves *deliberately recalling memories—both positive and negative—about life events*. It is the life history or story recalled in a structured autobiographical way. It is a guided, or directed, cognitive process, used with a goal in mind. It can include both reminiscence and affective functions.[246]

Goals for the use of life review include the following:

- Increase one's self-esteem
- Increase life satisfaction or well-being
- Increase one's sense of wisdom, validate one's wisdom
- Increase one's sense of peace about life
- Decrease depression
- Integrate painful memories, crises, unmet needs, unfulfilled aspirations
- Promote ego integrity and resolve self-despair
- Work through prior crises, events, traumas, and relationships

During life review therapy, your role is to:

- Accept the story and accompanying photographs or memorabilia, but encourage a lifespan approach
- Convey empathy for experiences and feelings (happy and sad)
- Validate and support the values being expressed
- Allow repetition to promote necessary catharsis
- Discuss issues that arise so they can be resolved

- Reframe events if the person cannot do so
- Encourage the person to evaluate prior responses, achievements, or ways of handling a situation
- Allow the focus to remain on the person's own self
- Validate that which has been meaningful to the person in life
- Recognize that the person may not ever really resolve or accept the multiple losses that have occurred (sadness may remain)

These measures, combined as necessary, allow for one's comprehension and enable the appropriate response, and compensate for perceptual and memory limitations and for the slower formation of associations and concepts.

## Emotional Development

Erikson,[247] describing the eight stages of man, states: the developmental or psychosexual task of the mature years is ego integrity versus despair. A complex set of factors combines to make the attainment of this task difficult for the elderly person.

**Ego integrity** is the *coming together of all previous phases of the life cycle*.[248] Having accomplished the earlier tasks, the person accepts life as his or her own and as the only life for the self. He or she would wish for none other and would defend the meaning and the dignity of the lifestyle. The person has further refined the characteristics of maturity described for the middle-aged adult, achieving both wisdom and an enriched perspective about life and people (see the box entitled "Wisdom: Expert Knowledge"). Historical situation, family environment, marital status, and individual development all influence the integrity achievement.[249]

Ask for the person's counsel to you about various situations that relate to him or her personally or to ideas about politics, religion, or activities current in the residence or institution. Having the person reminisce also promotes ego integrity, and the reintegration and recasting of life events places traumatic events into perspective.

The person who has achieved ego integrity remains creative. Decrements in achievement are rarely so substantial at life's end that the person becomes devoid of creativity. Even an octogenarian can expect to produce notable contributions in their personal creative activity, as has been witnessed with artists, composers, politicians, and others. Creativity in the late years depends on one's initial creative potential, but creativity can often lie dormant during the demanding young adult years. The older adult possesses most of the necessary qualities for creativity: time, accumulated experience, knowledge, skills, and wisdom. Often, the changes mandated by retirement and late life trigger new creative levels, including those in ordinary people.[250]

- Knowledge that is both factual and strategic in the fundamental aspects of life.
  - Knowledge that considers the context of life and social changes.
  - Knowledge that considers the relatedness of values and life goals.
  - Knowledge that considers the uncertainties of life.
  - Knowledge that reflects good judgment in important and uncertain matters of life.

## CRITICAL THINKING

*In what ways can you promote creative expression?*

Without a sense of ego integrity, the person feels a sense of **despair**. *Life, he or she feels, has been too short and futile. The person wants another chance to redo life.* Refer to the box entitled "Consequences of Self-Despair" for a list of feelings and behaviours that are part of self-despair. Feelings of despair about self are compounded by the relationship losses suffered and the consequent feelings of loneliness and hopelessness that frequently occur. Not having a confidant or companion and being somewhat deprived in physical health status are both situations that relate closely to one's

## Consequences of Self-Despair

- Discuss unresolved conflicts related to people or life situations
- Wishes to relive life, redo their life course; fears death
- Suspicious or overly critical of others; angry toward others, especially significant others
- Has a sense of overwhelming guilt, shame, self-doubt, or inadequacy
- Disengages from others; withdraws from people, or life's interests
- Feels worthless, a burden
- Demonstrates decreasing cognitive competence
- Discusses their feelings of their lack of accomplishments in life or unfinished endeavours
- Is lonely, has had few relationships
- Describes their desire for relationships, a confidant, companion
- Feels hopeless, helpless, sad, depressed
- Has suicidal thoughts, or shows suicide-related behaviours

emotional status. Suicidal thoughts, or attempts at suicide can result. This is a growing problem.[251]

Nursing care for the person in despair involves the use of therapeutic communication and counselling principles, the use of touch and relaxation techniques, and being a confidant so that the person can work through their feelings, both from the past and the present—especially feelings of sadness and loneliness. *The maintenance phase of the nurse–client relationship* is particularly important because the person needs time to resolve old conflicts and learn new patterns of thinking and relating. The person can usually move to a sense of ego integrity if he or she has the ongoing relatedness and attention of at least one caring person—a person who listens; meets physical needs when the person cannot; nurtures and encourages emotionally; brings in spiritual insights; validates the senior's realistic concerns, fears, or points of anguish; and listens to the review of life, patching together life's experiences.[252]

# Personality Development and Characteristics

Encourage the uniqueness of the individual. Realize and explain to others that the earlier personality traits are maintained.[253]

It is widely agreed that older adults who are engaged in active interaction with supportive social networks have better mental and physical health than older adults who do not maintain meaningful ties with others. Components of emotional support include information that leads a person to believe that he or she is loved, cared for, esteemed and valued, and belongs to a network of mutual interactions.[254]

## CRITICAL THINKING

*What communication skills can a nurse use with an older adult who is rigid in his or her ways?*

**Personality and Lifestyle** Personality problems in old age are related to problems encountered in early life. However, even when the younger years have been too narrowly lived, or have been painfully overburdened, the later years can offer new opportunities. Different ways of living can be developed with an improved social environment as the person changes. Later maturity can provide a second and better chance at life.

Although researchers agree that personality in later life is characterized by both change and stability, many questions remained unanswered about the extent and variations of change and stability across the lifespan.[255]

*What cultural variations would you expect to find in the emotionality of the older adult?*

Self-concept is a component of personality that can be viewed as an attitude toward the self. An older person's self-concept can be eroded or enhanced over time as a result of circumstances and life experiences. Actually, an older adult's personality strongly influences self-concept and adaptation to role transitions, such as widowhood or retirement. Research related to personality traits and self-concept indicates that individuals can maintain continuity and coherence in the course of life. Individuals do not necessarily become depressed, isolated, and rigid with older age, and well-adjusted and happy individuals are likely to remain so in later life. Those who are less happy with themselves can be encouraged to take steps such as counselling or engaging in empowerment groups to improve their self-concept and change their lives.[256]

One study found that older adults tend to cling, or become more committed, to highly valued roles when they encounter stress in their role or in life generally. If the person gains a strong sense of self-esteem from the role (e.g., caregiving, community volunteer), the self-concept is less likely to be devalued, regardless of how high the associated stress. However, there may be a time when the person gives up the role in a sense of relief if stress is ongoing and deleterious to well-being. Further, the context of the role situation must be considered when determining how the senior values the role (e.g., great-grandparenthood or grandparenthood).[257]

CRITICAL THINKING

*What approaches would you use to identify an older adult's self-concept?*

## Adaptive Mechanisms

Nurses, and all health care professionals, need a strong commitment to assist the elderly in maintaining adaptive mechanisms appropriate to this period of life. It is generally agreed, however, that each person will accomplish them in his or her unique way, and they will be pertinent to the person's life experiences and cultural background.

People in their older years are capable of making changes in their behaviour, but they find changing difficult. As new crises develop from social, economic, or family restructuring, new types of ego defences will be needed. At the same time, the need to change might interfere with developing a sense of ego integrity.

Changing adaptive mechanisms must be developed for successful emotional transition in these later years. They help the person to maintain a sense of self-worth and control over external forces, which in turn promote a higher level of function.[258]

CRITICAL THINKING

*How can you encourage the older adult to use adaptive mechanisms to enhance his or her health?*

Peck[259] lists three developmental tasks related to adaptation. These tasks show the steps involved and the mechanisms that are undergoing change as the older personality strives to become integrated.[260] **Differentiation** *versus work-role preoccupation is involved in the adaptation to retirement. Its success depends on the ability to see self as worthwhile, not just because of a job, but because of the basic person he or she is.* **Body transcendence** *versus body preoccupation requires that happiness and comfort as concepts be redefined to overcome the changes in body structure and function* and, consequently, in body image and the decline of physical strength. The third task is **ego transcendence** *versus ego preoccupation, the task of accepting inevitable death.* Mechanisms for adapting to the task of facing death are those that protect against loss of inner contentment and help to develop a constructive impact on surrounding persons.[261]

CRITICAL THINKING

*What are other adaptive mechanisms of the older adult?*

**Successful Aging Paradigm** In recent years, one of the dominant themes in gerontology has been the concept of successful aging.[262] As defined by Rowe and Kahn, successful aging has three components: good physical health, the retention of cognitive abilities, and continuing engagement in social and productive activities.[263]

The box entitled "Characteristics of Successful Aging" summarizes a holistic perspective about successful aging.[264] Holistic care will contribute to these characteristics.

Acute illness at any age influences behaviour, affective responses, and cognitive function. These aspects of the person are also affected by chronic illness, but their effects and adaptive mechanisms are less well known.

Your approach during care can either increase or decrease the person's motivation to participate in treatment or rehabilitation, even when the person already feels self-motivated. Helpful approaches include the following:

- Set a definite goal with the client.
- Reinforce and support the basic drives or character/personality structure of the client. Do not label the

preoccupation with achieving, or the persistence in practice, as obsession or compulsion. Realize that the former "toughness" or "survival traits" of the person can now be an asset to them.

- Convey caring, be kind, and share "power" or control with the client rather than trying to be the boss. In turn, the client will feel, and be, more "co-operative."

- Encourage or reinforce with attention to the attempts as well as achievements.

- Use humour gently and appropriately to release tension or encourage. Do not use sarcastic humour.

- Convey a positive attitude that the person can achieve the goal, at least to the extent possible. Avoid negative comments, or an attitude that "puts down" the client, or nonverbal behaviour that conveys the suggestion that you do not perceive their capability.

- Avoid power struggles and insistence on the client doing an activity your way. Don't try to dominate the client. Let the person go at his or her own pace and in a way that is safe, and will achieve results.

---

## CRITICAL THINKING

*What does successful aging mean to you?*

---

## Characteristics of Successful Aging

### High Degree of Life Satisfaction

- Feels life has been rewarding; has met goals
- Has few regrets
- Has positive attitude about past and future
- Feels life is stimulating, interesting; sets new goal
- Is able to relax; has good health habits

### Harmonious Integration of Personality

- Has developed ego strength, unity, and maturity over the years
- Demonstrates self-actualization, satisfaction, individuation, authenticity
- Makes use of potentials and capabilities throughout life
- Has an accurate self-concept and body image
- Has meaningful value system and spiritual fulfillment

### Maintenance of Meaningful Social System

- Keeps involved with their caring network of family and friends
- Maintains interest in life through social attachments
- Feels affection both for, and from, others and has a sense of belonging

### Personal Control over Life

- Feels independent and autonomous
- Makes their own decisions, and is in charge of self to the extent possible
- Maintains a sense of dignity and self-worth with a positive self-concept

### Establishment of Financial Security

- Has made careful and effective financial plans
- Uses community resources to the extent necessary

## Body Image Development

The loss of skin tone, although not serious in itself, causes the aged in a society devoted to youth and beauty to feel stigmatized. Changing body contours accentuate sagging breasts, bulging abdomen, and the dowager's hump caused by osteoporosis. These changes all produce a marked negative effect. The loss of sensory acuity causes alienation from the environment. Full sensory status cannot be regained once it is lost through aging. Although eyeglasses and better illumination are of great help in fading vision, the elderly recognize their inability to read fine print and to do handwork requiring good vision. The danger of injury caused by the failure to see obstacles in their path because of cataracts, glaucoma, or senile macular degeneration makes the elderly even more insecure about the relationship of their body to their environment. They often seek medical help too late because they do not understand the implications of the diagnosis or the chances for successful correction.[265]

Hearing loss, the result of degeneration of the central and peripheral auditory mechanism and increased rigidity of the basilar membrane, is likely to cause even more negative personality changes in the older person than loss of sight. Behaviour such as suspiciousness, irritability and impatience, and paranoid tendencies often develop simply because hearing is impaired. Again, the person might be reluctant to admit the problem or to seek treatment, especially if he or she is unaware of the possibilities of help, through either hearing aids or corrective surgery.[266]

Often, the elderly person views the hearing aid as another threat to their body image. Eyeglasses are worn by all age groups and hence are more socially acceptable, but a hearing aid is conceived as overt evidence of advanced age. Adjustment to the hearing aid is often difficult for many people; if their motivation is low, the idea may be rejected.[267]

Encourage the senior to talk about their feelings related to their changing body appearance, structure, and function. Provide a mirror so that he or she can look at self to integrate the overt changes into his or her mental image. Photographs can also be useful in reintegrating a changing appearance. Help the senior to stay well groomed and attractively dressed, and compliment their efforts in that direction. Touch and tactile sensations are important modalities to use to help the person continue to define their body boundaries, and integrate the structural changes that are occurring to their bodies.

## CRITICAL THINKING

*What nursing responsibilities can you implement with an older adult who has a hearing impairment?*

## Moral–Spiritual Development

The elderly person with a mature religious outlook and philosophy will continue to strive to incorporate broadened views of theology and religious action into their thinking.[268] Because the elderly person is a good listener, he or she is usually liked and respected by all ages. Although not adopting inappropriate aspects of a younger lifestyle, he or she can contemplate the fresh religious and philosophic views of adolescent thinking, thus trying to understand ideas previously missed or interpreted differently. Similarly, others listen to him or her. The elderly person feels a sense of worth while sharing experienced views. He or she is likely to be concerned about moral dilemmas and conflict, and offers suggestions on ways to handle them. Basically, he or she is satisfied with living personal beliefs, which can serve as a great comfort when he or she becomes temporarily despondent over life changes or changes in the family's life, or when confronting the idea of personal death.[269]

Spiritual beliefs enable the older person to cope with painful or unexpected events and to be more productive and adaptive in a threatening environment. The spirit can be considered the primary locus of healing, since it is the basic characteristic of humanness. Spiritual health is necessary for physical, emotional, and mental well-being, satisfaction with life, happiness, and a sense of energy. Isaia, Parker, and Murrow, in their study of 37 people in a senior centre, found that these elders, regardless of age, perceived themselves to be highly spiritual. Women had higher scores for spirituality and well-being than did men.[270]

A study of life satisfaction in 166 black seniors ranging in age from 65 to 88 years (87 males and 79 females) revealed that men and women differed. High life satisfaction in women and men was related to church participation, religious faith, and family role involvements (often associated with their religious roles). High life satisfaction in men was related to income and education levels.[271]

Meaningful life experience has a spiritual quality. *Four themes give life meaning and promote spiritual well-being:*

1. Concern for the welfare of others
2. Opportunity to be helpful or useful as needed
3. Becoming involved in activity that is useful to someone else
4. Maintaining positive feelings about self and others

Religious belief and participation are important for most elders, regardless of ethnicity; however, different ethnic groups vary in how they participate, and they differ in the role that religion plays in providing a resource to them for coping with the adversities of aging. Non-organizational religious participation includes reading religious materials, watching or listening to religious programs, prayer, and requests for prayer. Demographics, religious denomination, and health disability factors influence one's participation in these and organizational activities.[272]

## CRITICAL THINKING

*What special coping mechanism would you like to develop to prepare yourself for older adulthood?*

**Nursing Care to Meet Spiritual Needs** The care and attention to clients' spiritual needs is an essential part of holistic care. This includes talking with the elderly, listening to their statements that indicate religious beliefs or spiritual needs, and reading scriptures or praying with the person when indicated or requested. Giving spiritual care to the elderly person can often involve providing prompt physical care and conversing about spiritual concerns.[273] Quoting or reading favourite scripture verses, saying a prayer, providing religious music, or joining with the person in a religious song often go far to calm inner storms. Acknowledging realistic losses and feelings with those who weep can provide a positive focus and hope. Helping the aged person to remain an active participant in church, religious programs, or Bible study in the nursing home can help to maintain his or her self-esteem and sense of usefulness. Finally, in dying and near death, the religious person might want to practise beloved rituals and say, or have quoted for them, familiar religious or scriptural verses.

# SOCIOECONOMIC CONCEPTS
## Retirement

Age, sex, health status, family background, ethnicity, type of job or profession, lifetime work experience, and economic incentives all influence when the person voluntarily or

## Later Maturity

Mrs. Bertini, 78 years old, has been a widow for 20 years. She and her husband had no children, but two nieces and a nephew who live in another city visit occasionally. Mrs. Bertini has coped with arthritis for many years and, with the help of a home health agency and friends, has been able to remain in her home after suffering a broken hip. She has taken medication for cardiac disease and hypertension since experiencing a mild heart attack ten years ago.

Despite increasing physical disability, Mrs. Bertini has maintained close ties with three female friends, two of whom had worked with her in a hat factory when they were young. These friends and their husbands were also friends of her husband. The four couples often played cards and attended social functions together.

Mrs. Bertini has begun to find it increasingly difficult to do her housework and to shop. Although the neighbourhood pharmacy still delivers medication, the family-owned grocery on the block where she has lived for 20 years recently closed, and she cannot manage the four-block walk to the bus stop. She has admitted to her friends that she needs assistance, but on her limited income of a small pension from her husband and the minimum amount from the Old Age Security pension, she cannot afford to hire help.

Although Mrs. Bertini has occasionally considered entering a nursing home, the decision is forced when her landlord announces a rent increase of $90 monthly. With great reluctance, she asks her closest friends to take her to several nursing homes in her area of the city. As a devout Catholic, her decision is immediate; she feels most comfortable with the home operated by Little Sisters of the Poor. It is accredited, looks homey, and is clean. The sisters and other workers are friendly and kind. Her friends help her sell her furniture and move to the nursing home. She takes her television and stand, her favourite chair and footstool, and her most treasured mementos and clothes with her.

The first few days in the nursing home are eventful as Mrs. Bertini meets new people and attends the planned activities. Then she begins to feel confined by having only a small room. She misses her independence and occasionally feels lonely. In her own home she could sleep until 9 a.m., but now if she wants breakfast, she must be in the dining room no later than 8 a.m. Although mobility is painful, slow, and possible only with the aid of a walker, Mrs. Bertini makes a point to attend the activities given in the home and accepts invitations from her friends to go out to eat at favourite restaurants. She looks forward to the letters, gifts, and holiday visits from her nieces and nephew and writes short notes to keep in touch with them. She also attends chapel services weekly.

She tells her visitors that she is not afraid of death; her only wish is that she does not suffer long.

1. Suppose that one of Mrs. Bertini's friends had contacted you, a health care professional, at the time when her rent increase had just been announced. The friend asked for your assistance for Mrs. Bertini. What steps would you have taken?

2. What municipal and provincial agencies are available for you to call upon for help and direction for Mrs. Bertini, should this situation have presented itself to you in the area where you now live?

3. If you were a health care professional working in the Little Sisters of the Poor home on Mrs. Bertini's ward, how would you deal with her thoughts about death and suffering?

involuntarily ceases the career or job. These variables all influence the retirement experience.[274] By 2030, there will be more grandparents than grandchildren. However, many of the baby boomers say they will continue to work part-time rather than retire completely.[275] With possible shortages in the labour market looming, policy-makers and employers are searching for new ways to retain older workers on the job.[276]

Retirement is influenced by each of the positions the person has held, and by the relationships they have had with others. Older adults who adjust best to retirement are healthy, have adequate incomes, are active, are better educated, have an extended social network that includes both friends and family, and usually were satisfied with their lives before they retired.[277] Meanwhile, for many people, retirement will mean a reduction in income. For financial reasons the person might seek a new job, either part-time or full-time. On the other hand, the search for a new job may be for emotional or social reasons. The inability to keep up with one's former activities in an organization or group will undoubtedly occur in retirement. Such a change in status can trigger a significant rift in one's social life.[278] See the box entitled "Phases of Retirement" for more understanding of the experience.

In Canada, the median age for retirement in 2005 for men was 62.6 years, higher than the 60.0 years for women.[279] Depending on educational attainment and gender, the average retirement age of a person may be as low as 57 or as high as 65. Self-employed individuals continue to retire at approximately age 65.[280] There is evidence to suggest that in the future there may be pressure on people of both genders to delay their retirement. The smaller "baby bust" generation (a term used interchangeably with "Generation X" and "13th Generation") will be the source of labour within the economy, and production in the economy may slow due to the decreased labour force, resulting in price inflation. This may force some potential retirees to postpone retirement, since the value of their assets will have decreased.[281] Health promotion at retirement is of considerable importance to retirees. In fact, Canadian researchers Wilson and Palha conducted a comprehensive search for published research articles that focused on health promotion immediately before or following retirement. It was concluded that in addition to being relevant to retirees, the data were valuable as well to the political, social, and health care leaders responsible for drafting policies and programs to help improve health and wellness in older adults.[282]

In Canada, more women than men retire.[283] Tompa states that a number of personal conditions lead people to choose retirement. These conditions include health, unemployment, the spouse's decision to retire, and attitudes toward work.[284]

Health professionals who work with the elderly need to be sensitive to the wishes of elders regarding retirement. Plans and dreams for retirement should be supported and encouraged.

## CRITICAL THINKING

*How old do you expect to be when you retire?*

Retirement as an experience and the tasks achieved differ among people in Canada, the United States, and other countries.[285]

**Retirement Planning** You are often with persons nearing retirement and may be asked directly or through nonverbal cues and disguised statements to help them sort out their feelings as they face retirement. Planning will help in the transition from worker to retiree. Although some persons who disliked their jobs, have an adequate income, and participate in a variety of activities eagerly look forward to a pleasurable retirement, many seniors would prefer and are able to work past age 65.[286]

Despite much work in recent years at both the national and the local levels to develop comprehensive programs for elders, few business organizations have recognized the many ways in which they might assist the potential retiree. Private organizations with large numbers of employees are, for the most part, the only ones offering effective retirement preplanning programs. The retiree might be faced with these questions:

1. Can I face the loss of job satisfaction?
2. Will I feel the separation from people close to me at work?
3. If I need continued employment on a part-time basis to supplement pension payments, will the old organization provide it, or must I adjust to a new job?

## Phases of Retirement

### Pre-Retirement

*Remote*
Adult works intensely and enjoys fruits of labour, job or professional status, financial security, and competence. Little thought or preparation for retirement.

*Near Retirement*
Adult begins thinking about and planning time for end of job, structured work, or professional position. Duties and obligations are gradually given up. Active planning for retirement.

*Retirement*
Leaving paid employment, its structure, and its stresses.

### Post-Retirement

*Honeymoon*
Adult is enthusiastic and feels euphoric about change immediately following retirement. Feels enthusiasm and excitement of self-initiated activities. Feels frustrated, angry, and anxious about the future, if forced to retire because of company policy, health, or some other life situation.

*Disenchantment*
Retiree's plans are beyond financial means, health status interferes, or plans are not as satisfying as anticipated. Feels disappointed, let down, depressed, cynical, or angry.

*Reorientation*
Retiree comes to grips with reality of retirement, reorients self to the future, and re-evaluates goals and strategies for their potential for achievement.

*Stability*
Retiree determines and implements long-term choices or goals. This stage may occur after the honeymoon; some people do not experience disenchantment and reorientation. Achieves long-term goals with contentment.

*Terminal*
The person becomes ill, disabled, or is facing death. Retirement, and the associated lifestyle, has lost its significance or meaning. Or the person may be dissatisfied with retirement goals, activities, and leisure and re-enter employment, usually part-time. Becomes a worker again, sometimes in a field unrelated to earlier career(s).

4. Shall I remain in my present home or seek a different one because of easier maintenance or reduced cost of upkeep?

5. Might a different climate be better and, if so, will I miss my relatives and neighbours?

Whatever the elderly person's need, your role will be a supportive one. Advocate retirement planning. Recommend agencies that will be useful in making plans and can provide current information.

## CRITICAL THINKING

*What coping mechanisms would you like to develop to prepare yourself for retirement?*

**Use of Leisure** The constructive use of free time is often a problem of aging. What a person does when he or she no longer works is related to past lifestyle, continuous core activities, accumulated experiences, and the way in which he or she perceives and reacts to the environment.

**Leisure time,** *having opportunity to pursue activities of interest without a sense of obligation, demand, or urgency,* is an important aspect of life satisfaction, the expression of self, and emotional and social development. Leisure activity is chosen for its own sake and for the meaning it gives to life, but it involves both physical or mental activity and participation. It is a way to cope with change. Adults value most the leisure activity that involves interaction with others or a pet, promotes development, or is expressive and maintains contact with the broader community. Most people have a core of activities that they enjoy. Reading and viewing television are popular pastimes; interestingly, television preferences are similar for older and younger adults, but reading preferences vary strongly with age and sex.

A Canadian study found that physically active leisure contributes directly to higher levels of physical health and well-being and lower levels of ill health among Canadians.[287]

*Elders can contribute in many ways to the community and society after their retirement:*

- Through volunteer or part-time work with hospital, community agency, or social, welfare, or conservation organization of choice

- Through a friendly visitor program to other old or homebound people

- Through a telephone reassurance program (calling the same person at the same time each day to determine his or her status)

- Through foster grandparent programs in nurseries, with failure-to-thrive children, and in preschool or daycare settings, homes for abused or orphaned children, or juvenile detention centres

- To homes for battered women or children, providing mothering or fathering skills

- To shelters for the homeless, and providing counselling

- To churches and church-related organizations in many capacities

- To Habitat for Humanity, an organization that builds or remodels homes for poor people in various rural and urban areas

- As a volunteer for a crisis hotline (e.g., suicide, drug use, child care, prayer line)

- Through collaboration with police, clergy, or community leaders, working to create drug-free and gun-free neighbourhoods and schools

The box entitled "Questions to Consider before Volunteering" lists questions to consider before assuming the volunteer role. Similarly, they are questions the senior should ask key people in an agency when he or she is thinking of being a volunteer. Explore these questions with the person.

As population shifts occur and society becomes more technologically complex, causing earlier retirement for some workers, the definition of productivity must be changed from

## Questions to Consider before Volunteering

- Do you have the time to give?
- Do you make punctuality a habit?
- Do you take responsibility seriously?
- Can you give reasonable advance notice if you must cancel plans or appointments?
- Do you consistently follow through on projects?
- Do you work well with others?
- Do you adhere to an organization's policies and procedures?
- Do you accomplish tasks that have been assigned?
- Would you receive orientation or training that you want or need?
- Do you understand and agree with the details of the position and the demands it will place on you?
- Would you have enough responsibility or authority to challenge you if you desired the challenge?
- Is the organization respected in your community?
- Does the organization respect its volunteers' time?
- Are the current volunteers dedicated to the organization or cause?
- Would you be able to use your experience or educational background?

that which involves the exchange of money. Family roles are likely to change, with an older family adopting or nurturing a younger family, giving assistance with child care or other tasks. The elderly will be needed as caregivers across family lines as home care becomes an important aspect of the health care system. The caregiving role can give added meaning to life. In Canada, preliminary estimates indicate that between 7 and 9 percent of older Canadians retire to caregive, and about 3 percent quit work to provide care.[288] McDonald states that studies rarely examine what happens to the older adults when the caregiving is over.[289]

---

### CRITICAL THINKING

*What are some of the Canadian research findings on retirement?*

---

## Federal Planning for the Aged in Canada

The 2004 Liberal Task Report states that all Canadians have the right to receive equal and accessible universal health care, either at home or in a public institution. It recommends that the federal, provincial, and territorial governments collaborate to develop a set of national home care objectives.[290] Many other recommendations were also developed to present a unique perspective on the experience of aging.

Regarding health status, the *2006 Report Card on Seniors in Canada* has indicated that life expectancy at age 65 has improved and progress has been made in terms of functional health (such as sight, hearing, and mobility). Seniors assess their own physical and mental health in largely positive terms. Rates of chronic pain and problems of being underweight are in decline. Negative developments include increasing obesity among seniors and increasing rates of chronic disease.[291] It is important to note that the prevalence of hypertension has increased significantly during the past five years, rising from 39 percent to 45 percent between 2000–01 and 2005. There have been no satisfactory improvements in certain areas such as physical inactivity, injuries, and falls (with the exception of hospitalizations for hip fractures). Suicide rates among seniors remain high. It is interesting to note that the positive trends at the national level with respect to life expectancy, dependence-free life expectancy, and perceived health status actually mask significant discrepancies. For example, in Nunavut and the Northwest Territories, which have a high Aboriginal population, life expectancy at age 65 was almost four years lower than the national average in 2003.[292]

### Old Age Security/Guaranteed Income Supplement
Old Age Security (OAS) provides basic income to Canadian citizens and residents who meet age, residence, and legal status requirements.[293] The foundation of the Canadian governmental system is to assure income for the elderly. It is provided by the Old Age Security (OAS) pension, the Guaranteed Income Supplement (GIS), and the Spouse's Allowance (SPA), as well as several provincial and territorial programs that augment the federal benefits.

**Canada Pension Plan** The Canada Pension Plan (CPP) is a contributory, earnings-related social insurance program that applies throughout Canada, except in the province of Quebec. In 1997, following a year of public comment, substantial reforms were implemented to the CPP. From 5.8 percent in 1997, the contribution rate rose to 9.9 percent in 2003 and beyond. The Quebec Pension Plan (QPP) covers workers in Quebec. Like the CPP, the QPP is compulsory and covers almost all workers. Almost all of today's seniors receive income from the CPP or QPP.[294]

## Community Planning

Planning and policy and program development must not be bound by ageism and myths about people in later maturity. Increasing numbers of very old people are taking care of themselves in their own home and should be allowed to remain independent to the extent possible. Elsner and colleagues give vivid accounts of ethical and policy considerations—and abuses by health care providers when they did not assess accurately, or when they intervened inappropriately.[295]

As people become older, infirm, and less mobile, a battery of community services is needed, not only to provide social activities and a reason to remain interested in life, but also to enable them to live independently. Most older adults require health care that is specific to their aging-related and disease-related needs, including their need to be cared for in a holistic way with diverse experiences, perspectives, and resourcefulness.[296]

---

### CRITICAL THINKING

*What will the future of health care be like for the older adult?*

---

**Community Services** Discuss available and needed services with the elder and family. Refer as appropriate. Advocate for needed services. Supportive services include the following:

- Referral services
- Visiting and telephone reassurance programs, sometimes offered through churches or private organizations
- Services that provide shopping aides
- Portable meals, sometimes from an agency such as Meals on Wheels, for those who cannot shop or prepare their own food

- Transportation and handy-person services, including home upkeep

- Daycare or foster home placement for the elderly (patterned after services for young children but modified for older adults)

- Recreation facilities geared to the older person

- Senior citizen centres that provide recreation and a place for the lonely to meet

- Respite services so that the family can get relief from care-giving while the elderly person receives needed care.[297]

All of these services can be used to promote health, prevent dysfunction, enhance a sense of independence, and aid family caregivers. *Adult daycare services* allow the person to remain at home and avoid institutionalization; the elder has daytime supervision and care, and the family member can continue employment. Help clients use the box entitled "Criteria for Selecting Personal Daycare." *Home care* prevents lengthy hospitalization, assists families and the elder with the tasks of care, and permits respite for the family. You could provide care in either setting.

Another helpful community service for elders is the senior centre. Senior centres are found in almost all communities and are based in a variety of settings. Some are operating in buildings built for this purpose, but most are housed in facilities originally planned for other purposes: church halls, community buildings, old schools, and mobile home park clubhouses. A small staff is maintained, and most of the help with programs, maintenance, and materials comes from volunteers among the older persons who attend the centre. Programs include activities such as crafts, social events from cards to dancing, exercise classes, and a full meal served at noon most weekdays. Other services include daily telephone calls to homebound elderly, information and referral services, home-delivered meals, minor profit-making endeavours, and discount programs in co-operation with local merchants.

Group work among the aged has been conducted with considerable success in a number of communities and in a variety of settings.

Some of this work has been initiated in centres operated for the elderly and has been used to encourage the individual to participate in a group activity, and to carry out health teaching. Many types of groups can be developed for the elderly. An abundance of information on older adults' health is available to both older adults and health care providers. Two excellent Web sources are Seniors Canada Online at www.seniors.gc.ca, provided by the Government of Canada,[298] and Seniors Health at www.phac-aspc.gc.ca/sh-sa-eng.php, provided by the Public Health Agency Canada.[299] As a citizen of the community, you can be active in initiating and supporting effective local programs.

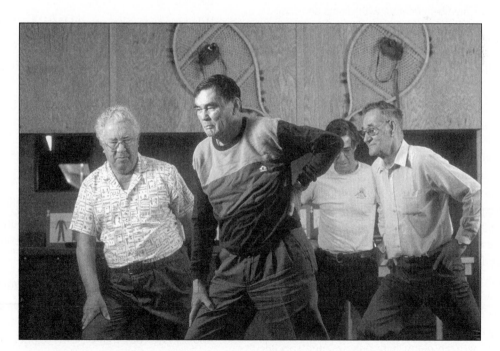

Adult daycare centres offer meals, nutritional counselling, mental health services, exercise classes, physical therapy, and social activities to elders.

Source: Berger, K.J., and M.B. Williams. *Fundamentals of Nursing: Collaborating for Optimal Health.* Stamford, CT: Appleton and Lange, 1992, p. 1717.

## Criteria for Selecting Personal Daycare

- Is the agency accredited?

- Is the agency designed well in space, furniture, decor and colour, equipment, and safety features for the elderly, including frail but ambulatory elderly and the cognitively impaired?

- What meals are served? Are special diets served? Ask the attendees about food.

- Are nurses and social workers employed? Physical therapists? Occupational therapists? Are attendants certified? Professionals should be available to the extent that the agency enrols elders with physical or cognitive problems.

- Is transportation provided? Some agencies have van service to pick up and deliver the senior home—within a certain radius and at certain hours—for a nominal fee.

- How do staff members handle medical or psychiatric emergencies? What is the policy if the elder becomes ill during the day?

- What is the schedule for the day? Are a variety of activities available? Are trips taken to the community? Are there activities of interest to and for participation by individuals and groups?

- What is the cost per day? Are there extra fees for activities? For clients with special physical or cognitive problems?

- How do staff members interact with clients and families?

- How do the clients interact? Do they appear to be satisfied with the care? Talk with them.

**Extended-Care Facility** The concept of long-term care for the elderly has broadened to be less custodial, more homelike, more holistic, and community focused. The names for the institutions vary: extended-care facility, or campus, or senior health care centre. The term *nursing home* is used less frequently. The facility must be approved for skilled nursing, although it may have both skilled and intermediate care levels for residents.

The extended-care facility serves as a transitional stop between hospital and home (generally for those over 65); in some cases, however, the stay is permanent.

The goals of the modern-day facility are to provide supervision by a physician, 24-hour nursing services, hospital affiliation, written client care policies, and specialized services in dietary, restorative, pharmaceutical, diagnostic, and social services. Unfortunately, these are sometimes hollow goals, even though the physical plant is new, licensing is current, and government funds are being used. Often the homes are operated for profit by those outside the nursing or medical profession. The residents are not always physically or mentally able to protest if care is poor, and often families of the residents do not monitor the care. Exposure of blatant neglect in some of the facilities has awakened public and government consciousness. Perhaps this exposure will correct the most glaring problems and alert other facilities of their obligation to follow prescribed goals. If standards are met, the nursing home provides an excellent and needed service to society because the elderly must be discharged from expensive acute care hospital beds as soon as possible. Prolonged hospitalization can foster confusion, helplessness, and the hazards of immobility. Further, some elderly persons cannot care for themselves. There are ways to individualize care, provide holistic care, and prevent the neglect or abuse of residents in long-term care settings.[300]

**Selecting a Care Facility** When you help the family or senior select a nursing home, the following questions should be asked:

- What type of home is it, and what is its licensure status?

- What are the total costs, and what is included for the money?

- Is the physical plant adequate, clean, and pleasant? How much space and furniture are allowed for each person?

- What safety features are evident? Are fire drills held?

- What types of care are offered (both acute and chronic)?

- What is the staff-to-resident ratio? What are the qualifications of the staff? What are staff attitudes toward the elderly?

- What are the physician services? Is a complete physical examination given periodically?

- What therapies are available?

- Are pharmacy services available?

- Are meals nutritionally sound and the food tasty?

- Is food refrigerated, prepared, distributed, and served under sanitary conditions? Is eating supervised or assisted?

- Are visitors welcomed warmly?

- Are residents aware of their Bill of Rights?[301]

- Do residents appear content and appropriately occupied? (Observe on successive days and at different hours.) Are they treated with dignity and warmth by staff? Is privacy afforded during personal care?

- Has the local Better Business Bureau received any complaints about this facility?

- Does the administrator have a current licence?

- Is the home certified to participate in government or other programs that provide financial assistance when needed?

- Is an ombudsman available to investigate complaints of residents or family?

**Bill of Rights for Residents of Extended-Care Facilities** The Bill of Rights is available for people who live in Ontario long-term care facilities.

**Assisted Living** **Assisted living** is *a residential and social model that is an alternative to the medical model of institutionalization.* The living arrangement is for people who are frail or who have physical limitations that necessitate help with care beyond the home health care model. The elder who lives alone, needs help with care, is lonely, and feels isolated may choose this option. Assisted living is staffed with a registered nurse (RN) and other levels of care providers.

The services typically offered in a nursing home are offered in a residential setting, at a lower cost. A comprehensive social, functional, and Medicare assessment is obtained. The RN starts the flow of resources, delegating care to professionals from various disciplines. The resident is to have independence, individuality, choice, privacy, dignity, and greater control over life than would be possible in long-term care. Confinement to one room is not acceptable practice. There is a choice of activities. Transportation is available to outside events and shopping. This setting, like the long-term care setting, requires an ombudsman or consumer protection advocate to assure that the original intent is maintained.[302]

**Life Lease** Life lease is a unique housing option for mature adults and seniors. A life lease project provides an opportunity to purchase an interest in the project and to "share" in any appreciated value of the building and property.[303]

**Translocation** The elderly person who is moved to a nursing home or long-term care facility (often rest-of-the-lifetime care facility), or who is moved from one room to another within the same facility, undergoes a crisis called **translocation syndrome**, *physical and emotional deterioration as a result of changes or movement.* Moves are made because of changes in health, in staffing, or in the residents, or because families desire it. Such a move can, at times, be life threatening, however.

People at greater risk are those who are depressed, highly anxious, severely ill, intermittently confused, or over 85 years of age. People who need structure, who cannot tolerate changes, or who deny problems or feelings, are also more likely to experience difficulty.

Reducing the impact of relocation begins with enlisting the resident's understanding of the need for the move, and then requesting their participation. The person should be prepared for the move. When he or she can make decisions about the move and can predict what will happen, the person maintains a sense of control, which diminishes the impact of the move. Moving to a similar environment helps to reduce the problems. The opportunity to express fears, concerns, and anger helps. If the person to be moved to an institution is relatively young, has good morale, and has an opportunity to select and then feel satisfied with the new surroundings, the translocation syndrome can be minimal.

One way to reduce the crisis of admission to a nursing home or long-term care centre, or to reduce translocation shock, is to have preschool or schoolchildren visit in the home. Both generations benefit from the exchange of affection. The youngsters bring stimulation to the elderly generation; the older generation can demonstrate stability, wisdom, and coping with adversities, and the qualities of ego integrity.

Taking one's frail loved one to a nursing home is not easy at that point in life when he or she can no longer care for self and home, at that point when the person has lost almost all that was precious and that gave life meaning.

---

### NARRATIVE VIGNETTE
## New Horizons

Mr. and Mrs. S are now 75 and 73 years old, respectively. They have moved to an assisted-living facility where you are the nurse. Their health conditions have not changed significantly in the last two years, except that Mrs. S. now has more difficulty walking because of her arthritis. Mr. and Mrs. S recently moved to the facility because they needed help with transportation, and wanted to live in a place where they had fewer responsibilities and more time to enjoy life. Mrs. S has become tearful and says she has been disappointed in their move from their own home. She says, "Now we have the time to enjoy our life together, but we seem to be in each other's way all the time. When we lived in our own home, we were so busy with yard and housekeeping and all the daily chores, we never had time to think about what we really enjoy together. Now I don't have to cook meals nor worry about getting to the grocery store; but we aren't enjoying the time we have together."

1. How do you respond to Mrs. S. when she shares this concern with you?

2. What activities will you suggest for her?

3. What are the strengths of this family?

4. What health promotion strategies can you develop based on those strengths?

5. Is there a problem here that needs your help, or will it just "go away"?

Many family members have provided poignant accounts of the pain they experienced for the elder and for the family, and they describe how the elder works to retain personal integrity and dignity despite the emotional assault.

**Group Action among Older Citizens** Interest in civic, social, political, and economic issues is shown in various action groups that have been organized among older citizens through community projects.

Older persons can help isolated elderly persons in their community. A survey of community services can determine which services are most and least used, which are inadequate, what changes are needed, and what sort of problems the elderly in the area must face. In one community, a one-to-one visiting service was needed; it brought joy and met needs of the isolated elderly. It also provided the elderly visitors with a sense of independence, social acceptability, recognition, status, and a sense of meaning in their lives at a time when losses of one sort or another had left them vulnerable.

Action groups have been formed in many major cities in recent years. Their members are elderly persons who are concerned about the needs of their peers and who believe that group action is effective in bringing about legislative change, especially in the area of financial assistance to meet rising costs. Many of these groups have exerted a considerable influence on federal and local planning. Such issues as tax relief, transportation, health care, and nutrition are of vital interest to many concerned elderly citizens who still feel responsible for themselves and their community.

You may have the opportunity to work with action groups in either an advisory, consultative, or direct participation role.

**Retirement Communities** Retirement brings many changes, and these situations are discussed by several authors.[304] Along with our increased lifespan and the development of social planning for retirement has come the emergence of a distinct social phenomenon: the retirement apartment complex community.

Apartment complexes are financed privately, or by the government. The senior must be able to maintain self, although visiting nurse services are acceptable. These complexes often include a central dining room, a nurse and doctor on call, planned social events, transportation services, and religious services. Essentially, all living needs are within easy access. Additionally, the seniors have the company of each other if they so desire.

In many cities, hotels have been converted to residence facilities for the elderly. Reminiscent of old-style rooming houses, they provide extended supervision and services, such as meals, laundry facilities, and shopping. In most of these residences, each person is responsible for his or her own room, laundry, and breakfast.

Many couples opt for continuous care facilities. One- or two-bedroom apartments or cottages are available for a one-time endowment and a monthly fee for two persons. Services include one meal a day, maid service, all utilities including local telephone, full maintenance, a full recreational and social program, and many extras. The residents have at their disposal a fully equipped health centre with 24-hour nursing care service as long as needed in the intermediate or long-term care sections of the nursing home facility.

In many regions of the United States, especially in Florida, the desert Southwest, and California, planned communities have been built that are specifically designed for and restricted to those persons over 55. Some are carefully planned miniature cities of low cost with simply designed homes built around clubhouse activities, golf courses, and swimming and therapy pools. Activities such as bingo games, dance instruction, foreign-language study, crafts, and bridge lessons are offered. Other communities are mobile home parks where elaborate bus-like motor coaches, which cost as much as a house, are set up as permanent homes. Many Canadians are taking advantage of residing in these communities during the winter months.

Discuss the information in the box entitled "Guidelines for Selecting a Retirement Community" with elders and their families.

**Effect of the Able Elderly** The emergence of a population group identified as the well elderly is the result of social and demographic progress in the industrial world. More people are living longer. Poverty, frailty, and dependence are no longer the common characteristics of most of these older people. In the future there will be more healthy elderly who are well educated and who are physically and emotionally capable. Our society can already use the elderly population's capabilities; in the future, we shall have a rich human resource in larger numbers.

The elderly often provide financial support and other kinds of assistance to their younger family members; most old people are not a drain on the family. An aging society offers expanding opportunities for family life. Four types of new potentials are available because of recent demographic changes: (1) increased complexity of social networks, (2) increased duration of relationships, (3) prolonged opportunities to accumulate experience, and (4) new opportunities to complete, or change, role assignments.

The elder's accumulated shared experience builds family bonds, but it also helps others to deal with a changing historical context. As the elder leaves certain roles behind, he or she can pick up new ones: as a grandparent; in a second career; as an activist in the political, social, or community arena; as a decision maker; as an advocate for ethical and moral actions; or as a participant in policy making or creative

## Guidelines for Selecting a Retirement Community

- Check climate, cultural, and recreational facilities in relation to your preferences and lifestyle.
- Visit the facility; talk with residents; eat a meal. Is it an active, lively community?
- Call regulators, Chamber of Commerce, and Better Business Bureau to check the track record of the developer or owner(s).
- Ask what insurance or bonding instruments will protect you in case the facility experiences financial difficulty. Get copies.
- Review all documents you are asked to sign and seek competent legal advice before signing.
- Ask about lease termination policies. How much notice must the owner give? What are the refund policies?
- Get terms of the deposit in writing. If it is refundable, how and at what percentage? Will interest be applied; if so, at what rate?
- Determine whether monthly fees are tied to an index. If so, which one? Ask for a history of increases to date, and check the index at a library.
- If it is a lifetime or continuing care community, are nursing home costs prepaid? If not, what are the additional costs?
- Ask about restrictions and policies about visitors (overnight, allowable duration), parking a recreational vehicle, parking more than one car, and the use of facilities by visitors.
- Take your time to decide. Visit different facilities.

pursuits in the arts. Well elderly are, and will be in the future, making valuable contributions to society; it is important to perceive the well older person as a contributing resource.

**Outlook for the Future** The current generation of older persons is where we shall all be one day. Therefore, planning for them is planning for all of us. Matters such as health care delivery, the distribution of income over a long lifespan, sustaining adequate social involvement, coping with organizational systems, and the use of leisure time are all problems for now and the future. Intervention that seems costly now could be, in the long run, the most economical in terms of tax dollars.

In the face of increasing costs of production that raise the cost of living, and the continuing change in age and sex distribution, future planning for the elderly will include employment and the general problems usually associated with younger persons. Our society will need the experience and wisdom of the senior generation. If persons are employed

as late as age 75, health maintenance programs, industrial planning, and the awareness of safety needs are only a few of the necessary considerations.

It will be you, the professional of the future, who will be challenged to be the innovator. You will be called on to devise and use new treatment methods so that the elderly will be able to function more effectively in society. It is your goal to help them:

1. Use the potential they have developed throughout life.
2. Pass through the years of late maturity with ego intact and satisfying memories.
3. Leave something of their philosophy for posterity.

## HEALTH PROMOTION IN NURSING PRACTICE

### Assessment

Your role in caring for the elderly person or couple has been described throughout this chapter. Assessment is very important because it serves for a detailed plan of care.

---

### CRITICAL THINKING

*What criteria will you use for an older client who seeks to change locations from a home environment to a condominium unit?*

---

### Interventions

Interventions often involve direct care, the use of verbal and nonverbal skills, the availability of self and therapeutic relationship, support, counselling, education, spiritual care, or referral, as you assist the person in later maturity to meet physical, emotional, cognitive, spiritual, and social needs.

You represent a large cluster of psychological potentials for the elderly person. You should expect to become the supportive figure, interpreter of the unknown, symbol of the people close to him or her, and possessor of important secrets or privileged information. You become a guide and a companion. All of this occurs if an empathic regard for the elderly person is reflected in your attitude and actions, even though your initial image of him or her has been different. Of prime importance is your willingness to listen, explain, orient, reassure, and comfort the elderly person. Your role is crucial because you are the one who is most likely to maintain personal contact with the client, either in an institutional setting or in a community agency.

Involve the person's family as much as possible. The interest of a family member does much to increase motivation on the part of the elderly. Determine family attitudes, and evaluate relationships during teaching-learning or during visiting sessions at which the family is present. This procedure helps the family members alter their attitudes to a more realistic acceptance of their relative's health needs. The social support of family and friends is critical for maintaining lifestyle behaviours, emotional and physical health, and coping skills, especially for the frail elderly.[305]

The *cognitive and emotional needs of the elderly person can be met in many ways:*

1. Ensure adequate environmental conditions to help overcome sensory impairment.

2. Use clear communication, including explanations of procedures and the necessity for them.

3. Use demonstration and written instructions along with the verbal message, divided into small units, for teaching skills related to self-care.

4. Combine explanations with practice sessions.

5. Organize information so that content is logically grouped and sequential, especially when a larger amount of data is given.

6. Indicate how, and when, the essential information is relevant to the person's needs, interests, and life experience. He or she is likely to recall this information when necessary.

7. Plan for a new task to overlap with the execution of a previous one, and allow the older person to work slowly and with care.

8. Simulate the real situation as much as possible so that essential steps of the task can be clearly perceived and the teaching can be adapted to the individual's pattern and ability.

9. Allow the person ample time to respond to a task.

10. Convey an understanding attitude to prevent discouragement and depression.

The display of genuine interest and a receptive attitude will show the older person that he or she is not alone, and it will help immeasurably in allaying fear. Candour helps to decrease anxiety. The person's fear of death, the dark, or the unknown can be overcome to a great degree through your presence, care, and attention.

Encourage the senior to *reminisce and engage in life review,* through discussion or the use of photographs, music, or literature. Ask questions about his or her early years, work experience, family, special events, travel, hobbies, and treasured objects. Listen as the person shares his or her life philosophy and gives you counsel.

*Loneliness* in the elderly is an outgrowth of age-related losses and psychological changes. It implies the need to assess carefully all situations to determine the signs of loneliness.

*Help the elderly person to remain in contact with the environment* by providing devices such as clocks, watches, and calendars. Let him or her be the one who winds the clock and turns the calendar page each day. If a hearing aid is worn, check its effectiveness. Sudden room moves, even within the same institution, increase mortality rates and psychological and physical deterioration. The person should be permitted to remain in familiar territory and with the desired clutter. If a move is essential, he or she should have some choice in the decision, an opportunity to keep valued possessions, and time to adjust to the idea. The person needs to have a personal lounging chair or specific place in the dining room. Room furniture should be arranged for physical safety and emotional security. Privacy must be respected.

Night-lights should be left on, and the call bell, tissues, and water all placed within easy reach. In the hospital room, contact should be available to the client through frequent, quietly conducted rounds at night. Sometimes a client remains oriented more easily if the room door is open so that he or she can see the nurses' station and be reassured that he or she is not alone.

## SUMMARY

1. Later adulthood spans many years; thus, the era is divided into young-old, mid-old, and old-old (or frail-old). Certainly the person at age 90 or 100 is different from the 70-year-old.

2. No theory of aging fully explains older adulthood.

3. Numerous changes occur over the lifespan, yet the person maintains many characteristics and abilities typical of the younger years.

4. Generally, the older person is more adaptive and able than is expressed in attitudes of ageism and stereotypes.

5. There are more well elders and more older adults who are living longer.

6. Older adults will continue to contribute to society; and their contributions will be needed.

# Positive Aspects of Caregiving: Rounding Out the Caregiving Experience

The negative consequences of caregiving have been clearly documented, and they include caregiver depression, poorly perceived health, and the increased risk of mortality. Recent research has endeavoured to elaborate the meaning of caregiving by examining the negative consequences of caregiving, and those seen as positive by the caregivers themselves. Four reasons have been emphasized for exploring these positive psychological factors: (1) caregivers want to talk about them; (2) clinicians will be assisted in knowing what works most effectively; (3) knowing these positive and negative consequences will be an important determinant of quality care provided to older adults; and (4) the need to enhance the theory in this area. The "satisfactions of caregiving" have been conceptualized into three dimensions: (1) satisfactions derived mainly from the interpersonal dynamic between carer and cared-for persons; (2) satisfactions derived mainly from the intrapersonal or intrapsychic orientation of the caregiver; and (3) satisfactions deriving mainly from a desire to promote a positive, or avoid a negative, outcome for the recipient. The study focused on 289 caregivers who were caring for someone residing in the community.

## Results

The majority of caregivers were women (68 percent). Spouses comprised 34 percent of the sample. The mean age of the recipients was 84.4 years, with a range of 71 to 100. The caregivers' ages ranged from 29 to 96, with a mean age of 64 years. Almost half (49 percent) were offspring of the care recipient, and 46 percent lived with the recipient.

Two hundred and eleven (73 percent) of the caregivers said they could find one positive aspect of caregiving, and an additional 7 percent could identify more than one. In terms of specific positive aspects of caregiving, 65 (23 percent) mentioned companionship; 63 (22 percent) fulfilling/rewarding; 37 (13 percent) enjoyment; 30 (10 percent) duty/obligations; 21 (7 percent) provide quality of life; 17 (6 percent) meaningful/important; 16 (6 percent) love people; 1 (less than 1 percent) likes making decisions; and 3 (1 percent) other. On a seven-point scale rating overall feelings of caring, 88 (30 percent) gave the happiest rating and 210 (73 percent) rated within the top three ratings.

## Practice Implications

1. Because positive feelings about caretaking were significantly related to the negative consequences of caregiving (caregiver depression, burden, and self-assessed health), clinicians should be asking about positive aspects of caring if they want to understand the caregiver experience and assist caregivers.

2. Satisfactions can be used as a quality control measure or indicator to determine whether services are meeting carer needs.

3. When caregivers feel that only they can provide the appropriate care, or that companionship is very important to them, they may refuse to allow others to assist with care. Therefore, asking more specifically about the satisfactions of caring may help to identify carers who will be more difficult to link to services, and who may be helpful in clarifying which services will be most acceptable to caregivers.

4. Satisfaction with caring may be helpful as a "risk" indicator. Caregivers who cannot identify any positive aspects of caring could be at a particular risk for depression and poor health outcomes. They could also be more at risk of institutionalizing their care recipient earlier than others.

5. Clinicians should consider incorporating the "feelings about caring" measure used in this study as a quick screen in their caregiver assessments. By doing so they are more likely to improve their understanding of the caregiving experience and target interventions more appropriately.

Source: Cohen, C. A., A. Colantonio, and L. Vernich, Positive Aspects of Caregiving: Rounding Out the Caregiver Experience, *International Journal of Geriatric Psychiatry*, 17 (2002), 184–188. Reproduced by permission of John Wiley & Sons Limited.

7. Well elders will have an increasing influence on their communities, as well as on local, provincial, and national legislation.

8. Because of the increasing number of older adults, a wider variety of resources will be needed soon, and they will be implemented.

9. Some changes that occur to the elder are the result of disease rather than the aging process, and these diseases need to be prevented or treated.

10. The box entitled "Considerations for the Elderly Client in Health Care" summarizes what you should consider in the assessment and health promotion of the elderly.

## Considerations for the Elderly Client in Health Care

- Personal history
- Family ties; family history; widow(er)
- Cultural history
- Current responsibilities with a spouse or other family members
- Impact of physiologic changes on the functional status and activities of daily living
- Behaviours or appearance that indicate that the person is being abused or neglected
- Implementation of safety measures, immunizations, and health practices
- Pre-existing illness
- Risk factors, past or current measures used to reduce or prevent them

- Current illness
- Behaviours that indicate age-appropriate cognitive status; the ability to manage one's own affairs
- Behaviours that indicate age-appropriate emotional status, including ego integrity instead of self-despair, and moral–spiritual development
- Behaviours that indicate that retirement and the losses that occur in late life have been grieved and integrated into the self-concept and life patterns
- Satisfactory living arrangements
- Involvement in the community to the extent possible
- Behavioural patterns that indicate that the adult has achieved the expected development tasks

## Interesting Websites

### Canada's Physical Activity Guide to Healthy Active Living for Older Adults

www.phac-aspc.gc.ca/pau-uap/paguide/older/
This guide serves as a road map for older adults—explaining why physical activity is important, offering tips and easy ways to increase their physical activity, and stating how much is needed to maintain good health and improved quality of living later in life.

### National Clearinghouse on Family Violence (NCFV)

www.phac-aspc.gc.ca/ncfv-cnivf/familyviolence/index.html
On behalf of the Government of Canada and its Family Violence Initiative, the Public Health Agency of Canada operates the NCFV. The NCFV is Canada's resource centre for information on violence within relationships of kinship, intimacy, dependency, or trust.

### Seniors Canada

www.seniors.gc.ca/home.jsp?lang=en
The Seniors Canada site is Canada's premier information source for seniors, caregivers, families, and service providers.

### National Framework on Aging (Nfa)

www.phac-aspc.gc.ca/seniors-aines/nfa-cnv/index_e.htm
The NFA is a conceptual tool useful in guiding current and future policy and program development. Designed to address the priorities of seniors and to assist policy-makers in reviewing proposed policy changes, the NFA reflects the changing demographic reality of a maturing Canadian society.

## Key Terms

**Activity Theory** (557)
**ageism** (553)
**age-related macular degeneration (AMD)** (567)
**aging** (552)
**assisted living** (609)
**biological age** (552)
**body transcendence** (600)
**cataracts** (567)
**cognitive age** (552)
**Continuity Theory** (556)

**crystallized intelligence** (591)
**despair** (599)
**differentiation** (600)
**Disengagement Theory** (557)
**ego integrity** (592)
**ego transcendence** (600)
**Erikson's Epigenetic Theory** (557)
**fluid intelligence** (592)
**geriatrics** (552)

**gerontology** (552)
**glaucoma** (567)
**intellectual plasticity** (592)
**later maturity** (552)
**leisure time** (605)
**life review** (598)
**mid-old** (552)
**old-old** (552)
**organ reserve** (564)
**Peck's Theory** (557)
**polypharmacy** (591)

**presbyopia** (567)
**psychological age** (552)
**reminiscence** (597)
**senescence** (552)
**social age** (552)
**terminal drop hypothesis** (557)
**translocation syndrome** (609)
**young-old** (552)

# Chapter 15

## Death: The Last Developmental Stage

*Death is universal, but there is no universal meaning to death. Meaning comes from a merging of philosophical, spiritual, emotional, sociocultural, historical, and geographical factors.*

Ruth Beckmann Murray

## Objectives

*Study of this chapter will enable you to:*

1 Explore personal reactions and ethical issues associated with active and passive euthanasia and the right-to-die movement versus extraordinary measures to prolong life.

2 Compare and contrast the concept of death held by the child, the adolescent, and the adult.

3 Examine personal feelings about death and the dying person.

4 Discuss the stages of awareness and related behaviour as the person adapts to the crisis of approaching death.

5 Describe the sequence of reactions that occur when the person and family become aware of terminal illness.

6 Dialogue with another about how to plan for eventual death.

7 Determine response options to the wishes and needs of a dying client and family members.

8 Plan and administer care to a client, based on a firm professional understanding of his or her awareness of eventual death. The administration of care should include the consideration of behavioural and emotional reactions and physical needs.

9 Intervene appropriately and in a professional manner, to meet the needs of the family members of the dying person.

10 Compare and contrast home or hospice care with hospital or nursing home care.

11 Evaluate the effectiveness of care given.

# ISSUES RELATED TO DYING AND DEATH

## Definitions of Death

Death has been avoided in name and understanding. There is no harm in saying "he passed" instead of "he died." However, there is harm in suddenly confronting a client about his or her death without sufficient emotional preparation.

The aged differ from persons in other life areas in that their concept of future is realistically limited. The younger person may not live many years into the future, but generally he or she thinks of many years of life ahead. The older person knows that, despite medical and technical advances, life is limited.

Death is the last developmental stage of the life cycle. It is more than simply an end process. It can be viewed as a goal and as fulfillment. If the person has spent his or her years unfettered by fear, if he or she has lived richly and productively, and if he or she has achieved the developmental task of ego integrity, he or she can accept the realization that the self will cease to be and that dying has an onset long before the actual death. If death is considered the last developmental phase, it is worth the kind of preparation that goes into any developmental phase, perhaps physically and certainly emotionally, socially, philosophically, or spiritually.[1]

---

### CRITICAL THINKING

*How do you personally view death?*

---

Most people want to die at home surrounded by their loved ones. However, Canadian research indicates that in some provinces, up to 75 percent die in hospitals or long-term facilities.[2] Wilson and her researchers conducted an interdisciplinary historical investigation of twentieth-century influences on the location of death in Canada.[3] The findings revealed two key influences on the location of death: (1) health care and health system developments that have amalgamated health care in hospitals, while at the same time increasing and sustaining public expectancies about curative, or least beneficial hospital care. The increase in the hospital death rate throughout much of the twentieth century may be considered due largely to the shift in illness care from home to the hospital; and (2) the decreased availability of home-based formal and informal caregivers for the dying family member. Regarding caregivers, Stajduhar examined the social context of home-based palliative caregiving. The results indicated a need for interventions to improve the amount of support for caregivers at home, and to examine how assumptions influence, and at times drive, the provision of home health care.[4] In fact, a need exists to examine closely the type and intensity of services required to provide care to clients and their families in the final stage of a terminal illness. In 2004, in the 10-Year Plan to Strengthen Health Care, the federal, provincial, and territorial governments recognized the need for hospice palliative care services in the home.[5]

Many terminally ill clients would like to die at home for reasons that would benefit both themselves and their families. One benefit that clients experience within their home is a sense of security and freedom of control. Benefits experienced by the family while caring for their loved one are primarily feelings of satisfaction and gratitude.

Because of technologic advances, the determination of **death** is *changing from the traditional concept that death occurs when the heart stops beating*. Medically accepted standards for *brain death* include the following neurological criteria:[6]

- Underlying cause of the condition, or brain injury, must be known and diagnosed as irreversible.

- Declaration of death can be made only if the patient is not suffering from hypothermia (32.2°C), nor receiving central nervous system depressants, either of which may present the appearance of brain death.

- The person must manifest cerebral unresponsiveness and no brain stem reflexes.

- Apnea testing must not produce spontaneous respiration.

Institutions have other criteria for their policies and procedures for pronouncing brain death. Most institutions require an electroencephalogram (EEG) to confirm the absence of brain activity. Some require a cerebral radionuclide scan or four-vessel arteriogram to verify the absence of blood flow.

Shemie, Doig, and Belitsky claim that, in Canada, brain death is legally defined as "according to accepted medical practice," and that procedures associated with neurological death are determined individually by each hospital setting.[7] The Canadian Neurocritical Care Group recently published Guidelines for the Diagnosis of Brain Death. These guidelines closely resemble those of the American Academy of Neurology.[8] In fact, the guidelines established by the Canadian Congress Committee on Brain Death in 1988, as well as the guidelines developed by the Canadian Neurocritical Care Group in 1999, began to clarify a set criteria, but the work has not yet led to any standardization of diagnostic criteria or uniform practice.[9] It is interesting to note that, according to Wijdicks, national and international variability and inconsistency exists in the "accepted medical practices" for determining neurological death.

Brain death is differentiated from **coma**, *a persistent vegetative state* in which the person, not assistive devices, maintains basic vital homeostatic functions and therefore is not dead, even though he or she does not respond either verbally or nonverbally. In brain death, the appearance of life continues when the ventilator is used to deliver enough oxygen to keep the heart beating and the skin warm. Many experience a certain discomfort when they view a person who is brain dead but who appears to be alive because the body is being sustained by life support.[10] The ventilation is maintained until there is a decision about tissue or organ donation. If there is no organ procurement, the ventilator is discontinued.

The Canadian Association of Critical Care Nurses (CACCN) firmly attests to the fact that critical care nurses play a significant role in how decision-making processes regarding the withholding, or withdrawing, of life support occur for the critically ill.[11] The position presented in the CACCN statement is based on the following beliefs and principles:

- Patients have a right to autonomy in decision-making regarding their own health care
- Patients' health decisions must be made on an individual basis
- Health care professionals should behave in ways that best benefit the patient
- *Life support* refers to the provision of taking into account any or all of the following: assisted ventilation, inotropic support, and all or any of the mechanisms used to maintain and/or support the life of the patient who is deteriorating. The removal of fluids and/or nutrition may be examined and discussed on an individual basis.

The CACCN believes that all health care institutions and provincial associations have a responsibility in managing and directing the process of withdrawing or withholding life support treatments.

To address the ethical issues affecting the practice of registered nurses, the Canadian Nurses Association (CNA), in collaboration with other national health-related organizations, has prepared a Joint Statement on Resuscitative Interventions. The Canadian Bar Association also played a part in the development of this Joint Statement. The statement includes the following: guiding principles for health care facilities when developing cardiopulmonary-resuscitation (CPR) policy; CPR as a treatment option; competence; the treatment decision and its communication, implementation, and review; palliative care; and other treatment.[12] Finally, the CNA Code of Ethics for Registered Nurses (2002) provides an ethical framework for the practice of nursing.[13] It reflects changes in Canadian social values and conditions that affect the health care delivery system and create challenges and opportunities for nurses in their practice setting. Nurses

must discover and honour an individual's wish regarding the manner in which they want to live the remainder of their life. In fact, decisions about life-sustaining treatments are guided by such considerations. Nurses must advocate for health and well-being as well as for social conditions that allow individuals to live and to die with dignity. Nurses must intervene if other individuals fail to respect the dignity of persons in care.

---

## CRITICAL THINKING

*Review the CNA Code of Ethics (2002). What does fair treatment of individuals and groups mean to you?*

---

The family, more than anyone else, must live with the memories of their loved one and the events surrounding the death. It is a violation of the family's dignity to rush death, even though a less-involved person might say, "Why don't they turn off the machines!" This person should be ignored until all those closely involved with the client can say with acceptance and assurance, "Now is the time." Increasingly, the *person* is saying that he or she has the right to decide how long machines should maintain personal life, or that of a loved one. Family, health care providers, the ethical committee, and hospital legal counsel may all be involved in discussions about when to end life. The nurse should advocate for the patient when he or she cannot speak for self.

## Organ and Tissue Donation

Although organ transplantation is growing in Canada, shortages of needed organs still exist.[14] Molzahn, Starzomski, and McCormick claim that over a five-year period from 1996 to 2000, the waiting list grew by 62 percent, while the available transplants increased by only 22 percent. By the end of 2001, almost 4000 Canadians were waiting for organ transplants—a 15 percent increase in three years.[15] In 2001, the federal, provincial, and territorial governments established the Canadian Council for Donation and Transplantation. The council's role is to provide advice on national strategies to enhance organ and tissue donation and transportation across the country, and to improve the support afforded to donor families.[16]

The CNA Fact Sheet on Organ Donation and Tissue Transplantation claims that heading the list of single-organ transplants in Canada are kidneys (62 percent), followed by livers (22 percent) and hearts (10 percent). Eighty-six percent of transplant recipients are between 18 and 64 years of age, and men make up the majority (64 percent) of those requiring transplants, particularly heart transplants.[17]All provinces and territories have enacted legislation, which is remarkably uniform across Canada, dealing with organ donation before and after the death of the donor.[18] However, a new process has been developed to allow the residents of New Brunswick to indicate on their Medicare cards that they wish to become organ donors in the event of their death.[19]

Kidney transplantation is limited in Canada by the availability of organs—not by financial constraints. Every new client placed on a transplant list must compete with other clients for organs.[20] The reasons for the shortage of organs are varied, numerous, and complex. For example, Canada does not have a single national transplant organization with coordinated organ sharing and allocation.[21] Bowman and Richard claim that the effects of culture on attitudes toward organ donation can be overlooked by examining more pragmatic explanations for organ transplants, and by discussing either the organization of medical care or the relationship between the health care system and the public. As a result, we may significantly underestimate the effect of culture on Canadian attitudes toward organ donation.[22] For example, the practices of autopsy and organ removal are both in opposition to the belief system of the First Nations people in Canada.[23]

## CRITICAL THINKING

*What other cultural groups may not support organ donation?*

The CNA states that nurses can support organ donation and tissue transplantation in the following ways:

- Collaborate with and support other members of the transplant team, taking into account the client/family during the donation, retrieval, and transplantation phases

- Acknowledge, differentiate, and comprehend the roles of members of the health care team, volunteer agencies, and organ procurement service

- Encourage and support health care facilities to provide support programs for clients, family members, and health care providers in transplantation service

- Know about agency policies and procedures regarding organ and tissue transplantation. Formulate interdisciplinary policies and procedures to direct the team in the transplantation process

- Be aware of policies related to legal and ethical issues, such as consent and confidentiality

- Comprehend the cost–benefit aspects of organ and tissue transplantation

Many ethical issues exist around the matter of organ donation and tissue transplantation. In recent years, xenotransplantation (the adoption of animal organs for transplantation into human beings) has received renewed attention in the medical field, as well as in the media. At the same time, scientists are exploring cloning as a means of producing organs for transplants. The emerging ethical issues surrounding new discoveries are complex. It is critical that the nursing profession participate in future developments.

## CRITICAL THINKING

*What are your thoughts and feelings regarding organ donation and tissue transplantation?*

Stem cell research holds great potential to treat human disease and to prevent suffering. A stem cell can be thought of as a blank cell that has yet to become specialized. Scientists are fascinated by the ability of stem cells to become any type of cell. Stem cells have the potential to provide treatments for a host of debilitating diseases, including Parkinson's, multiple sclerosis, and Alzheimer's disease. The Canadian Institutes of Health Research (CIHR) has announced Guidelines for Human Pluripotent Stem Research. Subsequently, the guidelines were incorporated into the Tri-Council Policy Statement: Ethical Conduct for Research Involving Humans. While CIHR developed and implemented its guidelines, the federal government developed the *Act Respecting Assisted Human Reproduction and Related Research*, which became law. This Act applies to the derivation of stem cells from human embryos, but does not apply to research using human embryonic stem cell lines that have been already derived. However, the guidelines apply to both types of research.[24] With the introduction of these guidelines, Canadian researchers will be able to move forward and remain at the forefront of their field, while conducting their research according to ethical standards. In Canada, the Assisted Human Reproduction Act bans all forms of human cloning.[25]

The CNA believes that nurses have a critical role to play in advocating the availability of good information and public participation in shaping policies about assisted human reproduction, genetic testing, therapy and enhancements, the

## CONTROVERSY DEBATE

Howard is a 14-year-old boy who has been diagnosed with leukemia. He wants to donate his corneas for transplant if he should die. His parents strongly disapprove of his wish and believe it is wrong for him to do so. They have said that they will not co-sign a donor card for him. Howard has asked you to be his advocate in this matter.

1. As a health professional, how will you support Howard?
2. How will you counsel this family? What is your rationale?

human genome project and privacy concerns, and human cloning.[26] In Canada, nurses can make an invaluable contribution to these emerging fields, but they need more professional development opportunities to enable them to achieve competencies to provide the genetic services.[27]

## Euthanasia

**Euthanasia** is legally defined as *the act or practice of painlessly putting to death persons suffering from incurable or distressing diseases*. Commonly referred to as "mercy killing," it is seen as a means to finalize the suffering and pain of patients who otherwise would experience an undignified and distressed death.[28]

Although maintaining life beyond all reason is an ethical dilemma for the nurse, an equally taxing ethical dilemma occurs when the doctor deliberately hastens the client's death by increasing the dose of a narcotic analgesic such as morphine to the point of lethality. Responsible, moral caregivers, such as nurses, promote quality of life and the right to die with dignity.[29] If each human life is seen as being of infinite value, it will be worth the efforts to ease pain and help the person find meaning in the current situation.

Euthanasia is illegal throughout the world. In the Netherlands, immunity is granted to the physician who follows specific guidelines.[30] In Belgium, Verpoort and her researchers conducted a study of the view of palliative care nurses about euthanasia. Their findings indicated that a majority of nurses were not a priori for or against euthanasia, and that their views were largely dependent on the situation. What was emphasized in the study was the degree of suffering and available palliative options. Thus, depending on the situation, the researchers noted both resistance and acceptance of euthanasia. They conclude that in the light of the worldwide debate on euthanasia, it is essential to know how nurses, who are confronted with terminally ill clients every day, regard euthanasia. In addition, knowledge of these views can contribute to a realistic and qualified view on euthanasia itself, and it can further enlighten the personal views of caregivers in a diverse range of settings.[31] Apparent from this study is the need for specific support for nurses in their role in caring for clients who have made a euthanasia request.

Most Western countries consider **active euthanasia,** *deliberately hastening death*, as first-degree murder. On the other hand, court decisions have been inconsistent about **passive euthanasia**, *omission of care, or inaction, to prolong life*. Euthanasia is based on two fundamental legal premises: the right to privacy, and the right to refuse treatment when informed. The competent client may choose to decline treatment on the basis of religious reasons, fear of pain or suffering, exhaustion of finances, and the unlikelihood of recovery. The incompetent client is not allowed the right to refuse in similar situations due to fear of an irrational choice. Medical practice then defers to the wishes of the family. Nurses and other health care workers must explore their personal beliefs in and stances on active euthanasia, passive euthanasia, and physician-assisted death. Deep personal consideration is called for regarding the use of health care workers with those patients who request euthanasia measures and the ethical principles that balance the conflicting moral claims.[32]

In Quebec, Marcoux and her researchers conducted a telephone public opinion poll about the support of respondents for euthanasia and treatment withdrawal. It is interesting to note that the researchers included a previously used question on euthanasia (from Gallup) that had been criticized for methodological problems. The results indicated that 11 percent more people supported euthanasia with the Gallup question than was shown on the question developed for the current study. The researchers found a significant relationship between opinions about the acceptability of euthanasia and inaccurate knowledge of the nature of euthanasia. They concluded that the education of the population concerning euthanasia, and other end-of-life decisions, is probably a notable prerequisite to engage in public debate concerning the legalization of euthanasia.[33]

In any discussion of euthanasia, it is important to recognize the benefits and problems surrounding the practice. One such benefit is that if euthanasia were permitted, it would be possible to respect the self-determination of competent clients who want it but currently cannot have it because of its illegality. One negated consequence of euthanasia is that the practice of permitting physicians to perform euthanasia would be incompatible with their professional and moral commitment as healers to care for clients and to protect life.[34] As a society, we are obligated to think carefully about all aspects of the matter. Ultimately, health professionals are expected to ensure that people can live well until they die. When the time of death approaches, the health professional's main responsibility is to determine the way in which the patient can achieve a good death. This is a critical discussion, and we are all involved.

## Right-to-Die Movement, the Compassionate Healthcare Network, and Advance Directives

An increasingly publicized facet, with moral and ethical aspects, is the right-to-die movement, which began in England, Holland, and the Scandinavian countries, and which has gained considerable momentum in the United States.

Originally, the Right-to-Die Society and the movement insisted that people should have the last word about their own lives, either to maintain or to discontinue treatment when they are ill or dying. In 1991, the Right to Die (Society) of Canada was developed for the purpose of allowing Canadians a practical means of changing the law to permit choice-in-dying. In 1998, the Society was restructured to become an "umbrella organization" known as the Right to Die Network Canada. The network's basic field of operation is in Ottawa, so they can work more easily with federal politicians to change certain laws.[35] It has a 24-hour toll-free line with a bilingual operator.

It is noteworthy to mention that the Compassionate Healthcare Network (CHN) was founded in 1991 by President Cheryl M. Eckstein, who is an anti-euthanasia activist. The organization's work includes providing informational material on euthanasia, assisted suicide, suicide, and palliative care to health professionals, government officials, students, disability rights advocates, lawyers, and the public at large on a national and international basis (www.chninternational.com).[36]

**Advance Directives** Advance directives are written instructions provided by patients to identify their future health care preferences in the event that they become incompetent to make such decisions.[37] All provinces, except New Brunswick, have legislation in place that recognizes the directives expressed in living wills. Living wills exist in several formats depending on the province or territory in which one resides.[38]

The Canadian Association of Critical Nurses identifies the first of two major groups/forms of advance directives as instructional—commonly referred to as the living will. A living will allows individuals to identify life-sustaining treatments they would like, or not like, in given situations. The second group is the proxy directive—a document that allows individuals to specify who is to make health care decisions in the event that they become incompetent.[39] *Proxy* is a legal term used to designate a substitute decision-maker. Such a designation is frequently referred to as a power of attorney for personal care. Many health care institutions have policies in place regarding the use of advance directives. According to Martin and his associates, advance directives should contain both instruction and proxy directives.[40] Advance directives can be generic or disease-specific. Studies show that a substantial percentage of people living with HIV or cancer prefer the HIV- and cancer-specific forms.[41]

Even though advance directives are promoted widely in our society, health professionals should be aware of a few of their advantages and limitations. One of the primary advantages of advance directives is to support individuals in making decisions on their own behalf, promoting the principle of self-determination. They provide directives in advance for the fair treatment of incompetent individuals by providing a mechanism whereby prior wishes regarding life-sustaining treatment can be communicated. Advance directives are intended to decrease the intensity of the dilemmas faced by families and loved ones regarding an individual in a life-threatening situation. One of the main arguments against advance directives is that the written documentation can be somewhat vague, or challenging to apply, in a specific clinical situation. Advance directives can sometimes lead to inappropriate treatment decisions if situations arise that an individual could not foresee or consider at the time of writing the directive. Patients might change their mind regarding the type of treatment they wish to receive, but inadvertently forget to change their advance directives.

The role of the nurse is important in implementing advance directives. The Canadian Association of Critical Care Nurses (CACCN) states that the nurse should have adequate knowledge to provide patients and family members with sufficient information about the goals, advantages, and limitations of advance directives.[42] Values taken from The CNA Code of Ethics for Registered Nurses (2002) are important for end-of-life decision making, and for advance directives. These values include health and well being, choice, and dignity.[43] In addition, CNA argues that the first step in supporting clients who are considering end-of-life decisions must be for nurses to reflect on their values and beliefs associated with these issues, and to become comfortable with those values and beliefs. Another important end-of-life step is for the nurse to enter into dialogues with clients to assist them to clarify their beliefs, values, and awareness of themselves in the context of their current situation. It is imperative that: (1) individuals make their own decisions autonomously about advance directives, and (2) they are not coerced by any family member or health professional. The nurse's role is to ensure the effective communication to other members of the health care team regarding the client's treatment wishes as written in the advance directive.

Beliefs held by Canadian nurses that influence their intention to respect an advance directive document were measured by a questionnaire. The researchers found that nurses carry a strong intention to comply with advance directives written by clients.[44]

In summary, the nursing profession as a whole views and supports advance directives as an effective tool that enhances the quality of nursing care being delivered. However, the nurse must be mindful of the legal and ethical implications of advance directives.

## Assisted Suicide

In Canada, the assisted suicide debate received considerable attention during the early part of the 1990s. Keatings and Smith define assisted suicide as an act whereby an individual who is lacking the means of completing the act of taking one's own life requires the assistance of another to complete the act.[45] Under Section 241 of the Criminal Code, it is an offence to counsel, aide, or support anyone to commit suicide.[46] The CNA Code of Ethics does not address the issue of assisted suicide. Meanwhile, the much publicized case of Sue Rodriguez in British Columbia has made it clear that it is the responsibility of every nurse to become prepared for the moral challenges involved in the debate over assisted suicide.[47]

The nursing profession and all health care providers have a great deal at stake. It is important that nurses be aware of their own beliefs and personal feelings regarding assisted suicide while recognizing the acceptable ethical and legal implications within the scope of their practice.

CRITICAL THINKING

*Reflect for a moment and determine what your opinion of assisted suicide really is.*

**Physician-assisted suicide (PAS)** is *the prescription of medication or counselling of an ill patient so that he or she may use a drug overdose to end his or her own life*. Dr. Jack Kevorkian, well-known for PAS, has attended numerous deaths by suicide. He is responsible for developing the "suicide machine" to inject lethal drugs into those seeking his help in dying. Boehnlein, a physician, discusses ethical, social, and economic opposition to PAS. He maintains that it is not a compassionate act and that dignified death does not come from the inappropriate use of medical technology and expertise.[48]

This issue encompasses the autonomy and individual rights of the patient, the role of the nurse and/or the physician, and society's stake. Each perspective is a complicated issue. We need to establish safeguards so that the true wishes of the patient can be expressed and legally accounted for. Many people know that they can write living will directives, but they do not do so.

Our society suggests that we still hope for a quick fix with technology, but the aging population reminds us otherwise. We are looking at the Netherlands' experience, referred to as the "slippery slope," where, in 1990, there were 8100 intentional opiate overdoses, 1000 lethal injections *without request*, and physician-assisted suicides of which only 41 percent met regulatory requirements. A study conducted by Wilson and his researchers regarding the attitudes of terminally ill patients toward euthanasia and PAS revealed that many patients with advanced cancer favour policies that would allow them access to both euthanasia and PAS in the event that pain and physical symptoms became intolerable. However, the results also indicated that for patients who would actually make the requests for PAS, the psychological considerations may be at least as prominent as the physical symptoms.[49]

It is important for nurses to struggle with the values and issues of death—accidental death, long-term dying, active or passive euthanasia, and right-to-die choices—and consequently the issues and values of life. You will often be asked about your thoughts and beliefs. It is impossible to be value-free, but you can be non-judgmental and accepting of another's values. How you proceed with nursing care of the chronically ill or dying person will be influenced by your own personal beliefs. *Certainly, do all that is possible so that the person does not face dying and death alone.*

## CONCEPTS OF DEATH ACROSS THE LIFESPAN

As you work with people of all ages, both well and ill, you will need to understand how people perceive death. A review is given here of how the child, adolescent, and adult perceives death. The concept of death is understood differently by persons in the different life eras because of general maturity, experience, ability to form ideas, and understanding of cause and effect. Culture, religious beliefs, and the historical era also influence the concept of death, ideas about how to grieve, and customs for handling the dead person and the mourners.

## Children's Concepts of Death

Most children under age seven see death as reversible, a temporary departure like sleep or a trip, being less alive, or a decrease in life functions that result in a person being very still or unable to move.[50] Children think that grown people will not die, that nothing can happen to them. There is much curiosity about what happens to the person after death. The child connects death with external events: what is eaten at funerals, cemeteries, and absence. He or she thinks that dead persons are still capable of growth, that they can breathe and eat and feel, and that they know what is happening on earth. Death is disturbing to children because it separates people from each other and because life in the grave seems dull and unpleasant.

Around age seven (at the concrete operations stage), most children begin to think of death as final, irreversible, and universal. During this period, the concepts of causation become more sophisticated.[51] Children can be helped to understand death if they are introduced to the concept at an early age and are encouraged to share their thoughts and feelings.[52] Children need reassurance that they will continue to receive care from loving parents.

However, the child's ideas and anxiety about separation and death, and the ability to handle loss, are influenced by many factors:

1. Experiences with rejecting or punitive parents
2. Strong sibling rivalry
3. Domestic or social violence
4. Loss, illness, or death in the family
5. Reactions to, and the teachings of adults regarding, separation and death
6. Ability to conceptualize and assimilate the experience[53]

Children who live in a war-torn area have a more complete concept of death than do children who grew up in a peaceful environment. Terrorist attacks, acts of war, and sudden violent attacks are upsetting for children, even if they only view them on television or, conversely, observe the impact on the adults they care about. One of the most important things that parents or significant caregivers can do is to reassure children that they are safe and that they will be protected from danger.[54] (See the box entitled "Dos and Don'ts for Discussing Death with Children.")

## CRITICAL THINKING

*What important losses did you experience in your own childhood? How did you cope with them?*

## Adolescents' Concepts of Death

The adolescent understands the finality of death better than children do.[55] However, it is not something they think about much unless faced with it. Usually, the subject of death will be glossed over, kidded about, or avoided. Adolescents tend to develop abstract conceptions of death more than children do.[56]

Adolescents ponder the meaning of life. They are concerned about their bodies and a personal future. They are relatively realistic in thinking, but because of dependency–independency conflicts with parents and efforts to establish individuality, there is a low tolerance for accepting death. The healthy young person perceives self as invincible and will sometimes engage in risky behaviour.[57] He or she seldom thinks about death, particularly as something

## Dos and Don'ts for Discussing Death with Children

| Do | Don't |
|---|---|
| ■ Ask the child what he or she is feeling. Bring up the subject of death naturally in the context of a dead pet, a book character, television show, movie, or news item. | ■ Admonish the child not to cry; it is a universal way to show grief and anxiety. |
| ■ Help the child have a funeral for a dead pet. | ■ Tell a mystical story about the loss of the person; it could cause confusion and anxiety. |
| ■ Help the child realize that he or she is not responsible for the death. | ■ Give long, exclusively detailed explanations beyond the level of understanding. |
| ■ Tell the child what has happened on his or her level (but not in morbid detail). | ■ Associate death with sleep, which could result in chronic sleep disturbances. |
| ■ Explain the funeral service briefly beforehand; attendance depends on the child's age and wishes. | ■ Force the child to attend funerals, nor ignore signs of grieving visible in the child. |
| ■ Answer questions honestly, with responses geared to the child's age. | |
| ■ Remember that expressions of pain, anger, loneliness, or aloneness do not constitute symptoms of an illness, but they are part of a natural process of grieving. | |
| ■ Help the child to realize that the adults are also grieving and feel upset, anger, despair, and guilt. | |

that will happen to them, despite the fact that media reports of school violence have probably influenced his or her thoughts. He or she fears the prospect of a lingering death, and usually views death in religious or philosophic terms. He or she believes that death means a lack of fulfillment for them and that there is too much to lose with death.[58]

Because of inexperience in coping with crisis and the viewpoints of death, and of wanting to appear in control, the adolescent may not cry at the death of a loved one or parent. Instead, he or she may continue to play games, listen to records, engage in antisocial behaviour, withdraw into seclusion or vigorous study, or go about usual activities. If the young person cannot talk, such activities provide a catharsis. Adolescents are more interested in world events than are children. Adolescents may be affected strongly by stressful events such as terrorist attacks, acts of war, and other violent events such as the disasters of floods and blizzards. Even though most adolescents can cope with stressful events, parents and significant caregivers can help by being present to them, listening, and supporting them as necessary.[59]

## Adults' Concepts of Death

The adult's attitudes toward, and concepts about, dying and death are influenced by cultural and religious backgrounds. A number of references provide insightful information.[60] The adult's reactions to death are influenced by the experience of death of loved ones, or of others, and whether the death event is sudden or has been anticipated. A life-threatening illness can threaten the goals and plans for the future of young adults in many areas, such as getting married, having children, and pursuing either educational or vocational aspirations. As the adult progresses in the life cycle, one learns from one's own life experiences, and encounters a newly personalized sense of mortality.[61] The implications of death play a prominent role in the re-evaluation of life and self that characterizes middle adulthood. In middle and late adulthood, the understanding of death goes well beyond the simple understanding of finality. A death changes the relationships and roles of everyone in the family. For example, for a middle-aged adult, the death of a parent can be particularly unsettling, especially if the adult has not yet taken the necessary time to consider taking on the elder role. The older adult thinks and talks about death more than people do at any other age. Interestingly, such behaviours lead to less anxiety.[62]

**Meaning of Death** To the adult facing death because of illness, particularly the elderly, death can have many meanings. Death can convey certain positive meanings: a teacher of transcendental truths not comprehended during life; an adventure; a friend who brings an end to pain and suffering; or an escape from an unbearable situation into a new life without the present difficulties.

The spiritual search for meaning in one's life is often intensified by the reality of death. Individuals who are dying often seek to identify, recognize, or formulate meaning for their lives.[63] Religious and spiritual believers tend to seek to enrich and deepen their connections with a God, or some force of energy. For example, Jewish scriptures, the Muslim Quran, and the Christian Bible contain many stories that convey the idea that death comes when one's purpose in life has been fulfilled.[64] In reading these stories, individuals focus on the contributions that the dying person has made during their life, rather than on the losses that will be experienced at their deaths.

### CRITICAL THINKING

*What sorts of death-related losses do you think are most frequently experienced among middle-aged adults?*

## Near-Death Experiences

Moody coined the term *near-death experience*, and he has recorded and analyzed many reports of near-death experiences.[65] Atwater, who has distinguished herself as one of the best researchers in the field of near-death experiences, argues that health care providers are at a loss in how to recognize a near-death experience in one of their patients. This particular inability also holds true for the general public.[66]

Several reports are available about men and women of wide ranges of age, education, backgrounds, religious and non-religious beliefs, and temperament who came close to death or had a near-death experience. Some have reported an **out-of-body experience (OBE)**, *a feeling that one's consciousness or centre of awareness is at a different location than one's body.* Such reports often occur in relation to being resuscitated.

Regarding near-death experiences, there appears to be a need for careful study and analysis. At times, individuals who are not near to death have had similar experiences to those who claim to have had near-death experiences.[67]

## Nearing-Death Awareness

**Nearing-death awareness (NDA)** differs from near-death experiences. It is *an extraordinary awareness of how death will unfold, and what the person will need to die well.* This awareness is often communicated symbolically, or in obscure messages by people who are dying slowly. The person may speak of a reunion or a wonderful place, describe heaven or a Higher Power, talk about having a dream, or talk about a certain day being sad (and then die on that day). The person may call to someone, seeking reconciliation and forgiveness. A spiritual care provider should be called.[68] Keep in mind that dying patients in any setting—intensive care unit, emergency department, home, or hospice—may

express nearing-death awareness. If we listen with care to our dying patients, we will often be able to comprehend their special awareness and help their loved ones to share in it—to receive the parting gifts the dying want to give. We, too, can benefit. We have much to learn about dying, and our patients are the best possible teachers.[69]

### CRITICAL THINKING

*What is your assessment of what near-death experiences can tell us about life after death?*

# BEHAVIOUR AND FEELINGS OF THE PERSON FACING DEATH

When death comes accidentally and swiftly, there is no time to prepare for death. However, death is a normal, expected event to the old, and most old people anticipate death with equanimity and without fear. The crisis is not death itself, but where and how the person will die.

## Awareness of Dying

When the person approaches death gradually by virtue of many years lived, or from a terminal illness, he or she will go through a predictable sequence of feelings and behaviour.

Glaser and Strauss[70] describe the *stages of awareness* that the terminally ill or dying person will most likely experience, depending on the behaviour of the health team and family.

**Closed awareness** *occurs when the person is dying but has neither been informed nor made the discovery.* He or she may not be knowledgeable about the signs of terminal illness, and the health team and family may not want the person to know for fear that "he will go to pieces." Maintaining closed awareness is less likely to occur if the dying person is at home.

**Suspicious awareness** *develops for the reasons previously described. The person may or may not voice suspicions to others, and they are likely to deny his or her verbal suspicions.* The client watches more closely for signs from others to confirm suspicions.

**Mutual pretence** *occurs when staff and family become aware that the client knows he or she is dying but all continue to pretend otherwise.* There is no conversation about impending death unless the client initiates it, although sometimes staff members purposely drop cues because they believe the client has a right to know.

**Open awareness** *exists when the person and family are fully aware of the terminal condition, although neither realizes the nearness of death, nor all the complications of the condition and the mode of death.*

With the certainty of death established, the person can plan to end life in accord with personal ideas about proper dying, finish important work, and make appropriate plans for farewells with the family. He or she and the family can talk frankly, make plans, share grief, and support each other.

**Health Team** The health team in the hospital and community usually has thoughts, although not always verbalized, about how the person ought to die, morally and stylistically. The wishes of the client and the family should always have priority, particularly when they ask that no heroic measures be taken to prolong life. Wright, Watson, and Bell, in their book *Beliefs: The Heart of Healing in Families and Illness*, outline clearly in table form the death and dying issues related to religious beliefs.[71]

## Sequence of Reactions to Approaching Death

When the person becomes aware of the diagnosis and prognosis, whether he or she is told directly or learns by advancing through the stages of awareness discussed previously, he or she and the family usually go through a predictable sequence of reactions described by Kübler-Ross.[72] It is interesting to note that the only systematic approach to the dying process to which health professionals-in-training are exposed is the Kübler-Ross model.[73] Her ideas and terminology are still widely used. In your practice, assessment and intervention must be individualized. Do not assume that everyone is experiencing each stage as the research results describe.

**Denial and Isolation** **Denial** and **isolation** are *the initial and natural reactions when the person learns of terminal illness:* "It can't be true. I don't believe it's me." The person will often go through a number of rituals to support this denial, even to the point of finding another doctor. He or she needs time to mobilize resources. Denial serves as a necessary buffer against overwhelming anxiety. Recognize the client's need. Respond to this behaviour, and let him or her set the pace in conversation. Later, the person will gradually consider the possibility of the prognosis. Anxiety will lessen, and the need to deny will diminish.

If the client continues to deny for a prolonged time, despite advancing symptoms, he or she will need much warmth, compassion, and support as death comes closer. Your contacts with the client may consist of sitting in silence, using touch communication, giving meticulous physical care, conveying acceptance and security, and looking in on him or her frequently. If denial is extensive, he or she cannot grieve or face the inevitable separation. Yet, Kübler-Ross found that few persons maintain denial to the end of life.

**Anger** The second reaction, **anger**, *occurs with an acknowledgment of the reality of the prognosis.* It is necessary for an eventual acceptance of approaching death. As denial and isolation decrease, anger, envy, and resentment of the living are felt. Often, the direct expression of anger is unacceptable, so this stage is difficult for the client and others. Anger is displaced onto things or people: "The doctor is no good," "The food is no good," "The hospital is no good," "The nurses are neglectful," and "People don't care." The family also bears the brunt of the anger.

Do not take the anger personally. The dying person, whose life will soon end, needs empathy. The person who is respected, understood, and given time and attention will soon lower the angry voice and decrease his or her demands. The person will realize that he or she is considered a valuable person who will be cared for and yet allowed to function at maximum potential for as long as possible. Your calm approach will lower anxiety and defensive anger.

**Bargaining** The third reaction, **bargaining**, *occurs when the person tries to enter into some kind of agreement that may postpone death.* He or she may try to be on best behaviour. He or she knows the bargaining procedure and hopes to be granted the special wish—an extension of life, preferably without pain.

The individual continues to hope for life, to express faith in God's willingness to let him or her live, and to engage actively in positive, health promoting practices. The belief may be expressed by the person that his or her body defences will be enhanced by mental or emotional processes yet unknown. Hope, which is involved in bargaining and which you can support, gives each person a chance for more effective treatment and care as new discoveries are made.

**Depression** **Depression** is the fourth reaction, and it *occurs when the person gets weaker, needs increasing treatment, and worries about self, family, and necessities.* Role reversal and related problems add to the strain. Depression arises about past losses and the present condition. Feelings of shame about the illness arise, sometimes interpreted as punishment for past deeds, and hopelessness can enshroud the person and extend to the loved ones.

Depression is normal. The family and staff need to encourage the person by giving realistic praise and recognition. The person should be allowed to express feelings of guilt, work through earlier losses, finish mourning, and build self-esteem. He or she should stay involved with the family for as long as possible.

**Acceptance** The final reaction, **acceptance** or *a kind of resolution,* comes if the person is afforded sufficient time and does not experience a sudden or unexpected death. It helps, too, if that person is given some help in working through previous reactions. He or she will no longer be angry or depressed about his or her fate, and will no longer be envious or resentful of the living. Acceptance is difficult, and it takes time. It depends in part on the client's awareness of the prognosis of illness so that he or she can plan ahead—religiously, philosophically, financially, socially, and emotionally. This last stage is almost devoid of feeling.

Priorities change. Family and close friends become of most importance. Gradually, the person becomes able to plan for the not-too-far future. The person must adjust to fatigue, changes in body function or structure, effects of chemotherapy or radiation, the continuing treatment appointments, and the loss of control.

Whereas Kübler-Ross looks at the dying person with the family implied, Corr states that Walsh and McGoldrick have argued that two major tasks confront family members and family units.[74] The first task is to share acknowledgment of the reality of death and to share the experience of loss. The second task is to reorganize the family system and to reinvest in other relationships and life pursuits. Reorganizing the family system calls for the family members to reconstruct their understanding of what the family means to them, and to clarify their sense of identity as a family. In addition, family members must abandon roles and activities previously assigned to the deceased. Reinvestment involves restructuring or transforming the relationship with the deceased so as to allow family members to maintain a sense of connection with that person and with their past, even as they move toward the future. Open, honest, and supportive interaction within the family system is essential to each of these tasks.[75]

Kübler-Ross's model of the sequence of reactions has been criticized, mainly on the issues of stages.[76] Many clinicians and researchers who have attempted to study the

process systematically have discovered that not all dying clients exhibit these five reactions, let alone in a specific order. Since the publication of Kübler-Ross's book in 1969, there has been no independent confirmation of the validity and reliability of her model. In fact, many clinicians who have worked with the model have found it to be inadequate, misleading, and superficial. Perhaps it would be better just to speak of a broad range of responses to the experience of dying.[77] On the other hand, Herz Brown states that one of the major contributions of Kübler-Ross's work lies partly in defining the stages of dying, but mainly in making death "a subject" that it is acceptable to talk about.[78]

---

## CRITICAL THINKING

*Think about a loved one in your family who was gravely ill or dying. How did you respond initially to the seriousness of the situation?*

---

## Anniversary Reaction

**Anniversary reaction** refers to *feelings of grief and sadness, or to a reliving of the mourning process, that occur about a year following the death of the loved one. The grief and mourning response, including physical symptoms, may be more intense at the person's birth date, or at one of several of the major holidays* throughout the year.

Some individuals, despite impending death, maintain hope and endurance, apparently refuse to die, and live for some time beyond the time of their expected death. A person can program, through unconscious or conscious will, the onset of illness, recovery from severe illness, or time of death. A strong will to live is often associated with the person's being highly interested, involved, or active in life, or the person may have near them a loved one, spouse, or dependant whom he or she desires to be with, or for whom he or she feels responsible. For some, the death month is related to the birth month in that some people postpone death to witness their birthdays or another important holiday. The person with an excessive fear of death may be unable to die until he or she is able to express and work through conscious fears or phobias.

## Planning for Death

While the person is still healthy and capable of making the many decisions needed in relation to death, he or she can do much to relieve his or her own worries and the burden of those decisions from others. You will be in a position to provide professional information to others. In working with the family, you can inform them that in 2003, the Government of Canada announced a new type of employment insurance

---

### NARRATIVE VIGNETTE
## Using Compassionate Care Benefits

You are the only health care professional, an occupational nurse, in a gold mine in a small rural community. You have been on the job for three months. One of your own family members has become gravely ill. You need to stay with your loved one for a few weeks until your sister comes from New Brunswick to stay with your relative. You have heard about Compassionate Care Benefits.

#### Questions

1. How do you apply for this benefit in your province/territory?
2. What assistance can you expect to receive?

---

benefit called the Compassionate Care Benefit. This benefit allows a person to leave his or her place of employment temporarily to care for a dying family member—and receive support from the federal employment insurance program.[79]

Representatives from nursing and funeral homes and cemeteries are educating people to maintain a folder, revised periodically, containing all information that will be used by those making arrangements at the time of death. Such a folder may include the names of advisers, such as attorney, banker, life insurance broker, and accountant. Personal and vital information should be included, such as birth certificate, marriage licence, military discharge papers, and copies of wills, including the willing of body parts to various organizations. Financial records (or a copy of those held in a safety deposit box), estimated assets and liabilities, and insurance and social insurance information should be there. Personal requests and wishes, listing who is to receive which items, should be written out and kept along with funeral arrangements and cemetery deeds.

These are intellectual preparations. They cannot ease the sense of loss in the living, but they can foster peace of mind, realizing that the wishes of the deceased were carried out.

---

## CRITICAL THINKING

*With which aspects of emotional preparation might you be able to assist family members as the death of a loved one nears?*

---

# HEALTH PROMOTION IN NURSING PRACTICE

Death is an intensely poignant event. It is an event that causes deep anguish, but it is one you may encounter frequently in client and family care.

## Self-Assessment

Personal assessment, being aware of and coping with your personal feelings about death, is essential to assess accurately or intervene helpfully with the client, family, or other health care providers. How can you protect yourself from the anxiety and despair that will undoubtedly result from repeated exposure to personal sufferings? The defences of isolation, denial, and "professional" behaviour are common in making attempts to cope with feelings of helplessness, guilt, frustration, and ambivalence regarding the client's not getting well, or the secret wish that the client would just die. It takes courage and maturity to undergo the experience of death with clients and families, and at the same time remain an open, compassionate human being. You are a product of the culture, just as the client and the family are. Hence, you will experience many of the same kinds of

reactions. Spiritual, religious, philosophic, educational, and all of the other family experiences and their general maturity will affect your ability to cope with feelings related to death.

The dying client may seek an identification or partnership with someone. Often, this person is the nurse. If you are that nurse, think of this as a positive experience—it may be a privilege to share with someone the last hours or days of his or her life.

Dying in the hospital has become so organized, and care is sometimes so fragmented, that you are not necessarily vulnerable to personal involvement in the client's death. However, you are more likely to be personally affected by, and feel a sense of loss from, the client's death if an attachment has been formed to the client and family because of prolonged hospitalization or hospice care or if the death is actually unexpected. If you perform nursing measures that you even remotely believe may have contributed to the client's death, if you have worked hard to save a life, or if the client's social or personal characteristics are similar to your own, you will feel the loss rather strongly.

Glaser and Strauss describe how health care workers first judge a client's value according to social status and then respond accordingly. The client's death is considered less of a social loss (and is therefore less mourned by the nursing staff) if he or she is elderly, comatose, or confused, of a lower socioeconomic class or a minority group, poorly educated, not famous, unattractive, or is considered "responsible" for having the disease. The dying client in these categories is likely to receive less care or only routine care. The client with high social value, whose death is mourned and who receives optimum care by the nursing staff, is often the person who is young, alert, and likable, has prominent family status, has a high-status occupation or profession, is from the middle or upper socioeconomic class, or is considered talented or pretty.

If the client's death is very painful or disfiguring, you will possibly tend to avoid the client because of feelings of guilt or helplessness. In addition, you may be aware of the varied attitudes held by health team members, or of the decision of the family and doctor about prolonging life with heroic measures, or not prolonging life. These situations can provoke intense negative reactions, especially if you disapprove of the approaches of other members of the health team.

You must attempt to deal with the various potential pitfalls of working with the dying. These include the following:

1. Withdrawal from the client

2. Isolation of emotions

3. Failure to perceive one's own feelings, or the feelings of the client and family

4. Displacing one's own feelings onto other team members

5. "Burning out" from intense emotional involvement

6. Fearing illness and death

## Support for Nurses

A support system should be available. Specific times should be set aside for staff members to share emotional needs related to a specific dying client, or to learn the specifics of the dying process. Often, nurses can help each other, but there should also be another health professional available who can be called on for spontaneous sessions.

Some administrations encourage and sponsor nurses in taking certification courses so they can gain in-depth perspectives. Health care professionals should join interdisciplinary organizations in which they share problems and solutions and gain support. Staff may change departments, either temporarily or permanently, to feel the accomplishment of working with those who recover. If you work with cancer clients exclusively, you may need special assistance from time to time. If you can think of death as the last stage of life and as fulfillment, you can mature and learn from the client as he or she comes to terms with personal illness. With time and experience, you will come to view the role of the comforter as being as important as that of promoting care. Then, the client who is dying will be less of a personal threat.

Some *guidelines for the nurse working with dying clients*:

- Individual staff members should be encouraged to gain personal insight and acknowledge their own limits. Extra support or time off may be necessary when staff members are under a high degree of stress.

- A healthy balance must be maintained between work and an outside life. This type of work demands considerable personal involvement. There must be times when each staff member is left totally off call so they can pursue personally affirming activities.

- The individual must be careful when the "need to be needed" becomes too great and he or she attempts to be everything to everyone. This work is probably best accomplished by an interdisciplinary team.

- The individual must maintain a support system at work and outside the work setting. In addition, individuals should be encouraged to seek relationships outside the work setting for additional support and enjoyment.

- For those working in isolation, it is wise to consider ongoing sessions with an outside consultant or therapist who can offer guidance and provide support.

Dean claims that humour can function as a coping mechanism to deal with the potential vulnerability that accompanies constant exposure to loss and death.[80] At times, of course, humour is inappropriate in a hospice/palliative care setting. Experienced health professionals will recognize, however, the importance of sensitivity and intuition as indicators of when and how humour may be introduced.

---

### CRITICAL THINKING

*What guidelines for the use of humour by a nurse do you think should be followed?*

---

## Assessment of Client and Family

The assessment of the client and family is carried out according to the standard methods of assessment. The total person (physical, intellectual, emotional, social, including spiritual needs and status) must be assessed to plan effective care. In planning for a consistent approach, learn what the client and family know about the client's condition, and know what the doctor has told them. It is also pertinent to assess the strengths of the client, as well as those of the family, and then plan care accordingly.

Recognize also that people differ in the way they express their feelings about dying and death. Mourning can be private or public. Listen to the topics of conversation the dying person discusses, observe for rituals in behaviour, and learn of typical health-related behaviours from him or her, or from the family, to get clues about what is important. Observe family members for pathologic responses—physical or emotional—because grief after loss from death increases the risk of mortality for the survivor, especially for the male spouse or relative who is in late middle age or older.

## Intervention with the Family

The family will be comforted as they see *compassionate care being given to their loved one*. Your attitude is important. Both family members and clients are highly perceptive about your real feelings, whether you are interested and available, affirming false reassurance, or just going about a job. Family members often judge your personal relationship with their loved one as even more important than your technical skill. In order to provide sensitive, quality care, note the cultural differences and structure of each family. For example, the structure of the First Nations family is not based on the nuclear family, but on the extended family. It is extremely common to find multi-generational households in First Nations communities. As a result, when a health crisis arises within the family, it is not unusual for a large extended family to gather around. This gathering demonstrates respect for the ill or dying individual and indicates support for those family members most affected by the crisis.

Try to *help the relatives compensate for their feelings of helplessness, frustration, or guilt.* Their participation in assisting the client with feeding, grooming, or other time-consuming but non-technical aspects of care can be most helpful to them, the client, and the nursing staff. The family may seem to be acting toward, or caring for, the client in a way that seems strange or even non-therapeutic to the nursing staff. Yet, these measures or the approaches may be quite acceptable to the client because of family patterns or rituals. In turn, be alert to recognize when family members are fatigued or anxious, and relieve them of responsibility at that point. Encourage the family to take time to rest and to meet their own needs adequately. A lounge or other suitable place where the family can alternately rest and yet be near the client is helpful.

*Show acceptance of grief.* By helping the family members express their grief and by giving them support, you are helping them, in turn, to support the client.

*Prepare the family for sudden, worsening changes in the client's condition or appearance.* Doing so will help to avoid shock and feelings of being overwhelmed.

The crisis of the death of a loved one often results in a *life crisis for the surviving family members.* The problems with changes in daily routines of living, living arrangements, leisure-time activities, role reversal and assuming additional responsibilities, communicating with other family members, or meeting financial obligations can seem overwhelming. You can help by being an attentive listener, exploring with the family ways in which they might cope with their problems. You might make referrals or encourage them to seek other persons or agencies for help. Often your willingness to accept and share their feelings of loss and other concerns can be enough to help the family mobilize their strengths and energies to cope with current and outstanding problems. It is important to be sensitive to their cultural beliefs and practices around death.

The most heartbreaking time for the family occurs *when the client is disengaging from life,* and from them. The *family will need help to understand this process* and to accept it as normal behaviour. The dying person has found peace. His or her circle of interests has narrowed, and he or she wishes to be left primarily alone and not disturbed by any news of the outside world. The dying person's behaviour with others can be so withdrawn that he or she seems unreachable and unco-operative. The family needs help in realizing that their silent presence can be a most satisfying comfort, and that it shows that he or she is loved and not forgotten.

This could be the time when some family members insist on additional life-sustaining or heroic measures, although doing so will only prolong suffering. The nurse can listen to their desire to prolong life, explain the needs and what is happening to the patient, act as a mediator when various family members make contradictory statements, calm angry tempers, and start a rational discussion about what's best for the patient. Having a meeting that includes family, nurse, pastoral care, the physician, members of an ethics committee, and other health care workers or significant others is useful. For example, research to date has produced good qualitative descriptions of the decision-making process that occurs when families confront the possibility of life-sustaining therapy (LST).[81]

*News of impending or actual death is best communicated to a family unit or group, rather than to a lone individual.* Doing so will allow the people involved to give mutual support to each other. This should be done in privacy so they can express grief without the restraints imposed by public observation. Stay and comfort the person facing death, at least until a religious leader or close friends can come.

Requests by an individual or family to view the deceased should *not* be denied on the grounds that it would be too upsetting.

Sometimes the survivor of an accident will ask about people who were with him or her at the time of the accident. The interdisciplinary health team should confer on when and how to answer these questions. *Well-timed honesty is the healthiest approach.* Otherwise, the person will have unnecessary difficulty in adapting to the reality of the accidental death. The person's initial response of shock, denial, and tears or later grief will neither surprise nor upset the interdisciplinary team who understand the normal steps in resolving crisis and loss.

Parents who are in the process of grieving for their dying or fatally injured child must be respected. They must be given the opportunity to minister to the child when they wish, and they need to be relieved of responsibilities at times. Encourage the parents to share their feelings. Nurses usually work to complement, rather than compete with, the parents in caring for the child. Also, remember that grandparents, siblings, peers, and sometimes the babysitter will need special understanding in their grieving. The timing and type of support provided after the accidental death of a child are extremely important.

Gudmundsdottir and Chesla conducted a study to describe and understand significant habits and practices developed by families recently bereaved by the sudden and unexpected loss of their children. They concluded that the practices and rituals revealed in the family narratives were of utmost significance to the family healing. All healing practices honoured the memory of the dead child, and they constituted a continuing connection between the surviving family members and the child. Some of the healing practices were extensions of everyday practices, such as cooking. Others, it turned out, were highly individual and unique practices, such as smelling the child's clothes.[82]

# Factors which Influence Coping: Home-based Family Caregiving of Persons with Advanced Cancer

In a qualitative study, 15 family caregivers were interviewed following the death of their particular family member, for whom they had provided care. Coping emerged as a category needing further analysis. Factors were identified that either facilitated or interfered with caregiving coping. The caregivers in the study ranged in age from 37 to 81 years. Of the 11 women in the study, 6 were wives, 3 were daughters, 1 a daughter-in-law, and 1 a sister. Of the four men, three were husbands and one a son. The length of time in the primary caregiving role ranged from 1 to 11 months. The first of two interviews occurred from 1 to 12 months following the death of the family member.

## Results

A. Three main categories that *facilitated* their coping included the characteristics of the caregivers themselves, the contributions made by the dying person, and supportive networks, both formal and informal, that were available to the caregivers.

B. Interfering factors, evident to a lesser extent in the data, related to their experiences with the informal and formal systems. For example, caregivers identified the less-than-adequate coordination and scheduling of health services coming into the home.

## Practice Implications

1. Clinicians are challenged to recognize the centrality of the reciprocal caring partnership between caregivers and the dying person.

2. Service providers, external to the intimate duality, must seek to support both of its members in order to facilitate the coping capacity and emotional tenacity of both.

3. The dying person must be recognized as not just the passive recipient of care, but an active and participating member in the care giving process.

4. Clinicians must recognize the emotional intensity of home-based palliative caregiving and be sensitive to the tremendous responsibility carried by family caregivers. They must work with family caregivers, the dying persons, and with each other as true and equal partners in the caregiving process.

5. Clinicians must make themselves available to families for support and guidance through the maze of caregiving.

6. Clinicians must recognize the effects that their attitudes and values have on the care they deliver.

7. Health care providers must continually engage with caregivers in anticipatory guidance, interpretation, and monitoring of the inevitable decline and dying process of the ill person, so that the caregivers can feel secure and supported in their emotionally exhausting work.

Source: Strang, V.R., and P.M. Koop, Factors which Influence Coping: Home-based Family Caregiving of Persons with Advanced Cancer, *Journal of Palliative Care*, 19(2)(2003), 107–114. Used with permission.

Accident, suicide, and homicide are the leading causes of death before age 40. Consequently, survivors often include children and adolescents. The grief and mourning that surrounds each of these death events differ from those related to an anticipated death. The suddenness of each causes shock, confusion, helplessness, emptiness, and intense sadness. With suicide comes guilt and shame, a sense of being responsible, as well as anger at the person who committed the suicide. With homicide there is almost always intense feelings of anger, rage, and revenge. And the sadness is always intensified by the imagery related to brutality and what the person suffered in their last moments alive. With each of these types of death, the family longs to undo certain acts, and to be able to say goodbye in a loving way. Long-term therapy is often needed.

## CRITICAL THINKING

*What role (if any) do you believe serious accidents play in one's encounters with death?*

## Other Grief Responses

As you care for the family of the dying person, or interact with the family after death, you will sometimes perceive that they are not grieving in what you consider the usual or normal way. You will assess their grief and mourning, both in anticipation of and at the time of death as absent or delayed, as complicated, pathologic, neurotic, or dysfunctional. You may wish to classify it as a clinical depression.[83]

**Delayed grief response** may be identified when *there is no anticipatory grieving, or no expression of grief at death.*

Later, there could be manifestations of not having grieved the loss:

- Continuing to act as if the person still lives, or looking for them
- Various physical symptoms, such as insomnia, loss of appetite and loss of weight, pain, and actual malfunction of the body
- Expressions of frustration or anger that are out of context or excessive, or personality changes
- Complaints of excessive stress at work or home
- Increased smoking and use of alcohol or other drugs
- Difficulty in interpersonal and family relationships
- Nightmares, illusions of seeing the person and then realizing he or she was someone else, or hallucinations of the person
- Statements about "shutting down at the time of death"

**Complicated grief responses** may occur *when the person is experiencing unresolved grief associated with the past.* It is manifested in several ways:

- Multiple physical complaints, often with no significant findings or physical examination (often the symptoms mimic those of the deceased)
- Suicidal ideas or attempts, wanting to join the dead person
- Intense grief when speaking of the deceased; inappropriate, angry affect; or the mechanism of emotional isolation (e.g., smiling while talking about the dead person)
- Withdrawal from others, failure to participate in the usual family or social activities, radical life changes
- Inability to talk about the deceased without intense grief expressions
- Intense grief reactions triggered by minor events
- Repeated verbalization of themes of loss
- Extreme sadness at certain times of the year (e.g., anniversary dates or special holidays)

Through counselling, the person may remember past losses or rejections and grieve these as well as the current loss.

**Dysfunctional grief response** may occur when: (1) *the person had a very dependent or ambivalent relationship with the deceased;* (2) *the circumstances surrounding death were uncertain, sudden, or overwhelming,* such as homicide, *or complicated with assault,* such as rape or violent attack; or (3) *a loss is socially unspeakable or socially negated,* such as capital punishment, or death or the murder of someone who had been a gang member or a child molester or who had a criminal history. If there has been a history of mental illness or suicide, or if the person has minimal support systems, another loss will be even more difficult to handle.

**Pathologic grief response** is an *intensification of grief to the point that the person is overwhelmed, demonstrates prolonged maladaptive behaviour, manifests excessive symptoms and extensive interruptions in healing,* and does not progress to the point of integrating the loss.

## Intervention for the Dying Person

The care of the dying client falls primarily on the nurse. You have had sustained contact with the client and you understand dying and the many needs of the dying person. You know the value of compassionate service of mind and hands. You can protect the vulnerable person, and you understand at least some of the distress felt by the client and family. You have an opportunity to help the client bring life to a satisfactory close, truly to live until he or she dies, and to promote comfort. The client needs your unqualified interest and response to help decrease loneliness and make the pain and physical care or treatment more bearable.

To assist you and other health care professionals, a publication called *A Guide to the End of Life Care for Seniors* has been developed as a manual of national guidelines.[84] This guide is intended to support end-of-life care for seniors in Canada. In addition, it provides health care information for other groups, such as family caregivers and social service providers. Ethical issues concerning end of life and how to deliver end-of-life care are considered. Spirituality and cultural issues are presented, with a significant focus on the diverse needs of Canada's Aboriginal peoples.

While providing care to the dying person, you will experience many frustrations. One of the earliest experiences is the challenge of talking with or listening to the client. Will he or she talk about death? Pain may be constant and difficult to relieve, causing you to feel incompetent. The family may visit so often and for so long that they interfere with necessary care of the client. Subtle, or not so subtle, accusations from the client or family about neglect may occur, or be feared. As you rework personal feelings about crisis, dying, and death, and as you become more comfortable with your own personal negative feelings and emotional upset, you will be able to serve more spontaneously and openly in situations previously avoided. *Physical care* of the dying person includes providing for nutrition, hygiene, rest, elimination, relief of pain or other symptoms, care of the mouth, nose, eyes, skin, and peripheral circulation, positioning, and environmental considerations. Analgesics and comfort measures to promote rest can be used along with crisis therapy. Spend sufficient time with the client to establish a supportive relationship. Provide continuity of care. Try to exchange information realistically within the whole interdisciplinary team, including client and family, to reduce uncertainty and feelings of neglect. Clients can withstand great pain and much distress as long as they feel wanted and believe that their life has meaning.

Thorough and meticulous physical care is essential to promote physical well-being, but it also helps to *prevent emotional distress*. During the periods of prolonged and close contact that giving physical care provides, you can listen, counsel, and teach, using principles of effective communication. But let the client sleep often, without sedation if possible.

Let the client make some decisions about what he or she is going to do within safe limits. Modify care procedures as necessary for comfort. Through the consistent and comprehensive care you provide, you assure the client that you are available and that you will do everything possible for their continued well-being.

During care, conversation should be directed to the client. Explain nursing procedures, even though the client is comatose, because hearing is the last sense lost. Responses to questions should be simple, encouraging, and as honest as possible. Offer the person opportunities to talk about self and feelings through open-ended questions. When the client indicates a desire to talk about death, listen. Recognize when the client is unable to express feelings verbally, and help him or her to reduce tension and depression through other means—physical activity, crying, or sublimate activities.

If the client has an intense desire to live, and is denying or fearful of death, be accepting but help him or her to maintain a sense of balance. Follow the conversational lead. If the topics are concerned with life, respond accordingly.

*Encourage communication* among the interdisciplinary team. Encourage the client to ask questions and state their own needs and feelings instead of doing it for him or her, but be an advocate if the person cannot speak for self.

*Explore with family members* the ways they can communicate with and support the client. Explain to the family that because the comatose client can probably understand what is being said, they should talk in ways that promote security and should avoid whispering, which can increase the person's fears and suspicions.

*Psychological care* includes showing genuine concern, acceptance, and understanding. It involves promoting a sense of trust and dignity and a realistic body image and self-concept. Being an attentive listener and providing for privacy, optimum sensory stimulation, independence, and participation in self-care and decision making are helpful. You will provide nonverbally a feeling of security and

trust by frequently looking in on the client and using touch communication.

*Spiritual needs* of the dying person, regardless of the spiritual beliefs, can be categorized as follows:

- Search for meaning and purpose in life and in suffering. Try to make dying and death less fearful by affirming the value of life.

- Sense of forgiveness in the face of guilt about unfulfilled expectations for self, accepting non-fulfillment or incompleteness and making the most of remaining life, acts of omission or acts of commission toward others, resolving human differences.

- Need for love through others' words and acts of kindness and silent, compassionate presence. If family and friends are not present, the nurse may be the primary source of love.

- Need for hope, which connotes the possibility of future good. Hope may be expressed as the belief about afterlife, reunion with deceased loved ones, and union with God, a superior alternative to present existence. If there is no belief in the afterlife, hope may be expressed as belief about transfer of physical energy from the deceased body, belief about contributing to another's life through an organ donation, or belief in leaving a legacy in his or her children or community or organizational contributions.

You can assist with meeting the person's spiritual needs if requested, and if you feel comfortable in doing so. Certainly, you should know whom to contact if you feel inadequate. The religious adviser is a member of the health team.

*Consider the social needs* of the client until he or she is comatose or wishes to be left alone. Visitors, family, or friends can contribute significantly to the client's welfare when visiting hours are flexible. If possible, help the client to dress appropriately and groom them to receive visitors, to go out of the room to a lounge, to meet and socialize with other clients, or to eat in a client's dining room or on the unit.

Community health nurses have found two distinct attitudes in families of dying clients. The first attitude is, "If he is going to die soon, let's get him to the hospital!" For these families the thought of watching the actual death is probably abhorrent. They feel personally unable to handle the situation and feel comforted by the thought of their loved one dying in a place where qualified professionals can manage all of the details. If possible, these families should have their wishes met.

The second attitude is, "I want her to die at home. This is the place she loved. I can do everything that the hospital personnel can do." This attitude, too, can be supported by the visiting nurse. The visiting nurse can usually coordinate community resources so that a home health aide, home-maker services, the proper drug and nutrition supplies, and all necessary equipment can be made available in the home.

Clients and family members often select the *home as the place of care in the terminal stages of disease, and as the place to die*. Being with family and friends and living in their own home are often high priorities for clients. Home represents their life's work and being there helps to maintain a sense of dignity, identity, and control over dying.[85] The family wants the client at home because it is his or her wish, and because they believe they would desire to be at home if they were dying. Clients and families who choose the hospital as the place of death believe that clients will receive better care there. Clients do not want to burden their families. Families are concerned about their loved one's comfort.[86]

## CRITICAL THINKING

*Suppose that someone in your family has died. What activities or rituals would you like to have carried out at the funeral or memorial service?*

Findings from a research study conducted by Dr. Harvey Max Chochinov, head of the Psychosocial Oncology Department at Cancer Care Manitoba and a member of the Department of Psychiatry, University of Manitoba, resulted in a dignity-conserving care model complete with practical tools for palliative care providers.[87] Dr. Chochinov explains that dignity has a unique meaning for each patient and family, and that meaning must be discovered by health care providers in order for them to be able to provide comprehensive, empathetic care.

**Hospice and Palliative Care** The first hospice palliative care programs in Canada were developed in the 1970s to respond to the needs of the dying. Initially, these programs were largely grassroots initiatives that gradually evolved into a single movement that now aims to relieve suffering and to advance the quality of life for those who are living with, or dying from, an illness.[88] In a consensus-building process led by the Standards Committee of the Canadian Hospice Palliative Care Association, caregivers, organizations, and consumers joined to share their experiences and to formulate a clear vision for hospice palliative care that everyone could use. This resulted in a national model for hospice and palliative care based on nationally accepted principles and norms of practice. All are encouraged to use the model to guide activities related to it. The new Model to Guide Hospice Palliative Care is now available free online at www.chpca.net.

The Canadian Hospice Palliative Care Association consensus-building process regarding standards (norms) of practice has directed the development of hospice palliative care nursing standards. The purpose of those nursing standards is fourfold:

- To establish knowledge for the nursing care of individuals and families with advanced illness

- To support an ongoing development of hospice palliative care nursing

- To promote hospice palliative care nursing as a specialty

- To serve as a base for the development of certification in hospice palliative care nursing.[89]

The focus of the hospice palliative care nurse is to bring comprehensive, coordinated, and compassionate care to all individuals and families living with advanced illness.

In Canada, the Quality End-of-Life Care Coalition (QELCC) was formed in 2000 with a group of 24 national stakeholders who met in Toronto. At that time, the Blueprint for Action was created to achieve the goal of quality end-of-life care for all Canadians. Since then, the QELCC has developed an annual working plan to provide a framework for education and advocacy activities aimed at advancing the end-of-life care agenda across Canada, at both the national and the provincial levels.[90] The primary mandate of the coalition is to act as an advocate for quality end-of-life care for all Canadians.[91]

It is important to commend the work of Senator Sharon Carstairs. During her appointment as Minister with Special Responsibilities for Palliative Care (March 2001 to December 2003), she raised the profile of palliative care with her federal colleagues. As advocate and champion for the best quality of care for all Canadians who are dying, her efforts provided profound support to the palliative care community in its works to advance the relevant issues.[92]

## Evaluation

Throughout intervention with the dying client, or his or her family, you must continually consider whether your intervention is appropriate and effective, based on their needs rather than yours. Observation alone of their condition or behaviour will not provide adequate evaluation. Ask yourself and others how you could be more effective, whether a certain measure was comforting and skilfully administered, and how the client and family perceived your approach and attitude. Through careful and objective evaluation you can learn how to be even more skilful at intervention in similar situations in the future.

# SUMMARY

The concept of, and reaction to, dying and death depend on such matters as the person's cultural background and developmental level, the kind of death, the extent of support from significant others, and the quality of care given by nurses and other health care providers. Nurses and other health care workers must work through their own feelings as they face ethical and moral dilemmas related to the use of technology, and either prolonging or shortening life deliberately. There is much to learn from people who have a nearing-of-death awareness, a near-death experience, and premonitions about death, or other kinds of dying experiences. The dying process and the afterlife are indeed the last stage of development.

## Interesting Websites

### Canadian Hospice Palliative Care Association (CHPCA)
www.acsp.net
The CHPCA is the national association that provides leadership in hospice palliative care within Canada. It offers leadership in the pursuit of excellence in care for persons approaching death so that the burdens of suffering, loneliness, and grief are lessened.

### Canadian Virtual Hospice
www.virtualhospice.ca
The Canadian Virtual Hospice (CVH) facilitates mutual support, the exchange of information, and easier and more efficient communication and collaboration between and among health care professionals, palliative care researchers, the terminally ill, and their families. The website offers information and resources that may help people better understand the physical, emotional, and spiritual aspects of their experiences.

### World Health Organization (WHO)
www.who.int/about/en
The World Health Organization, the United Nations' specialized agency for health, was established on April 7, 1948. WHO's objective, as set out in its constitution, is the attainment by all peoples of the highest possible level of health. Health is defined in WHO's constitution as a state of complete physical, mental, and social well-being and not merely the absence of disease or infirmity.

### Living Wills Registry Canada
www.sentex.net/~lwr
The Living Wills Registry Canada is unique to this country. The registry was established by Dr. David Williams, a Stratford family physician, and his wife, Maureen, in 1992. Its mandate is to assist people in directing their own medical treatment in the event of incapacitating illnesses or injuries. The website contains information about living wills, the organization, ordering a living will, and links.

## Key Terms

acceptance (625)

active euthanasia (619)

anger (625)

anniversary reaction (626)

bargaining (625)

closed awareness (624)

coma (616)

complicated grief response (631)

death (616)

delayed grief response (630)

denial (625)

depression (625)

dysfunctional grief response (631)

euthanasia (619)

isolation (625)

mutual pretence (624)

nearing-death awareness (NDA) (624)

open awareness (624)

out-of-body experience (OBE) (624)

passive euthanasia (619)

pathologic grief response (631)

physician-assisted suicide (PAS) (621)

suspicious awareness (624)

# Endnotes

## Chapter 1

1. Kikuchi, J.F., Cultural Theories of Nursing Responsive to Human Needs and Values, *Journal of Nursing Scholarship, 37*(4) (2005), 302–307.
2. Priest, A., A Champion of Diversity, *Canadian Nurse, 103*(2) (2007), 18–19.
3. Kikuchi, Cultural Theories of Nursing Responsive to Human Needs and Values.
4. Srivastava, R., Understanding Cultural Competence in Health Care. In R. Srivastava (ed.), *The Healthcare Professional's Guide to Clinical Cultural Competence* (pp. 3, 14). Toronto: Elsevier, 2007.
5. Canadian Nurses Association. *Position Statement: Promoting Culturally Competent Care.* Website: http://www.cna-nurses.ca/ (accessed May 2007); Dreher, M., and N. MacNaughton, Cultural Competence in Nursing: Foundation or Fallacy? *Nursing Outlook, 50* (2002), 181–186.
6. Klessig, J., The Effects of Values and Culture on Life Support Decisions. In F. Baylis, J. Downie, B. Hoffmaster, and S. Sherwin (eds.), *Health Care Ethics in Canada*, 2nd ed. (pp. 41–78). Toronto: Thomson Nelson, 2004.
7. Srivastava, R., Culture Care Framework I: Overview and Cultural Sensitivity. In R. Srivastava (ed.), *The Healthcare Professional's Guide to Clinical Cultural Competence* (pp. 53, 59). Toronto: Elsevier, 2007.
8. Spector, R.E., *Cultural Diversity in Health & Illness*, 6th ed. Upper Saddle River, NJ: Pearson Prentice Hall, 2004.
9. Statistics Canada. *Portrait of the Canadian Population in 2006, 2006 Census: Population and Dwelling Counts, 2006 Census* (Catalogue no. 97-550-XIE). Ottawa: Statistics Canada, 2007.
10. Canada. *Royal Commission on Aboriginal Peoples: Report of the Royal Commission on Aboriginal Peoples, Vol. 2: Looking Forward, Looking Back.* Ottawa: Minister of Supply and Services Canada, 1996.
11. Statistics Canada, *Portrait of the Canadian Population in 2006.*
12. Statistics Canada, *Portrait of the Canadian Population in 2006.*
13. Canadian Heritage. *History of Bilingualism in Canada.* Ottawa: Statistics Canada, 2007. Website: http://www.pch.gc.ca/progs/lo-ol/biling/hist_e.cfm (accessed June 2007).
14. Office of the Commissioner of Official Languages. *Official Languages Act.* Ottawa: Author, 2003. Website: http://www.ocol-do.gc.ca/legislation/olo_llo.asp (accessed June 2007).
15. Mackay, B., News: Changing Face of Canada Is Changing the Face of Medicine, *Canadian Medical Association Journal, 168*(5) (2003).
16. James, C.E. *Seeing Ourselves: Exploring Ethnicity, Race and Culture*, 3rd ed. Toronto: Thompson Educational Publishing, 2003.
17. Andrews, M., and J. Boyle. *Transcultural Concepts in Nursing Care*, 2nd ed. Philadelphia: J.B. Lippincott, 1999; Seifert, K., R. Hoffnung, and M. Hoffnung. *Lifespan Development.* Boston: Houghton Mifflin, 1997.
18. Statistics Canada, *Portrait of the Canadian Population in 2006.*
19. Statistics Canada. *2001 Census Handbook: Reference.* Ottawa: Minister of Industry, 2003.
20. Statistics Canada, *Portrait of the Canadian Population in 2006.*
21. Ryan-Nicholls, K.D., F.E. Racher, and J.R. Robinson, Providers' Perceptions of How Rural Consumers Access and Use Mental Health Services, *Journal of Psychosocial Nursing, 41*(6) (2003), 34–43.
22. Srivastava, Culture Care Framework I: Overview and Cultural Sensitivity.
23. Macionis, J., and L. Gerber. *Sociology*, 6th Canadian ed. Toronto: Pearson Prentice Hall, 2008.
24. Macionis and Gerber, *Sociology.*
25. Kendall, D., R. Linden, and J. Lothian Murray. *Sociology in Our Times: The Essentials*, 2nd Canadian ed. Scarborough, ON: Nelson Thomson Learning, 2001.
26. CHASS Inuktitut. Website: http://www.chass.utoronto.ca/~ajohns/Inuktitut.html (accessed May 2007).
27. Andrews and Boyle, *Transcultural Concepts in Nursing Care.*
28. Kendall et al., *Sociology in Our Times: The Essentials.*
29. Macionis and Gerber, *Sociology.*
30. Foster, C.H., What Nurses Should Know When Working in Aboriginal Communities, *Canadian Nurse, 102*(4) (2006), 28–31.
31. Macionis and Gerber, *Sociology.*
32. Srivastava, Culture Care Framework I: Overview and Cultural Sensitivity.
33. Zbilut, J., Contradictions of Nursing in a Post-modern World, *IMAGE: Journal of Nursing Scholarship, 28*(3) (1996), 188–189.
34. Srivastava, Culture Care Framework I: Overview and Cultural Sensitivity; Zbilut, Contradictions of Nursing in a Post-modern World; James, *Seeing Ourselves: Exploring Ethnicity, Race and Culture.*
35. Stewart, M.J. *Community Nursing: Promoting Canadians' Health*, 2nd ed. Toronto: W.B. Saunders, 2000.
36. Canadian Heritage. *Multiculturalism.* Ottawa: Minister of Public Works and Government Services, 2008.
37. Canadian Heritage, *Multiculturalism.*
38. Leininger, M., and M. McFarland. *Transcultural Nursing: Concepts, Theories, Research, and Practice*, 3rd ed. New York: McGraw-Hill, 2002.
39. Leininger and McFarland, *Transcultural Nursing: Concepts, Theories, Research, and Practice.*
40. Andrews, M.M., J.S. Boyle, and T.J. Carr, Transcultural Nursing Assessment Guide, Appendix A. In M.M. Andrews, J.S. Boyle, and T.J. Carr (eds.), *Transcultural Concepts in Nursing Care*, 4th ed. (pp. 533–539). Philadelphia: Lippincott Wilkins & Williams, 2003.
41. Culley, L. A Critique of Multiculturalism in Health Care: The Challenge of Nursing Education, *Journal of Advanced Nursing, 23*(3) (1996), 546–570.
42. Rattansi, A. Changing the subject? Racism, culture and education. In J. Donald & A. Rattansi (eds.), "Race," *Culture and Difference*, (1992), 11–48.
43. Betancourt, J.R., A.R. Green, J.E. Carrillo, and O. Ananeh-Firempong, Defining Cultural Competence: A Practical Framework for Addressing Racial/Ethnic Disparities in Health and Health Care. *Public Health Reports, 118* (2003), 293–302.
44. Betancourt et al., Defining Cultural Competence: A Practical Framework for Addressing Racial/Ethnic Disparities in Health and Health Care.
45. Smye, V., and A.J. Browne, "Cultural Safety" and the Analysis of Health Policy Affecting Aboriginal People. *Nurse Researcher, 9*(3), (2002), 42–56.
46. Macionis and Gerber, *Sociology.*
47. Chevannes, M. Issues in Educating Health Professionals to Meet the Diverse Needs of Patients and Other Service Users, *Journal of Advanced Nursing, 39*(3) (2002), 290–298.
48. Statistics Canada, *Portrait of the Canadian Population in 2006.*
49. Statistics Canada. *Aboriginal Peoples of Canada: A Demographic Profile, 2001 Census: Analysis Series* (Catalogue no. 96F0030XIE2001

007). Ottawa: Minister Responsible for Statistics Canada, 2003; Tjepkema, M., The Health of the Off-Reserve Aboriginal Population, *Health Reports* (Catalogue no. 82-003), 13, Supplement (2002), 73–88.

50. Statistics Canada, *Aboriginal Peoples Survey 2001—Initial Findings: Well-being of the Non-Reserve Aboriginal Population* (Catalogue no. 89-589-XIE). Ottawa: Minister of Industry, 2003.

51. Canada. *Royal Commission on Aboriginal Peoples: Report of the Royal Commission on Aboriginal Peoples*.

52. Kirmayer, L.J., G.M. Brass, and C.L. Tait, Review: The Mental Health of Aboriginal Peoples: Transformations of Identity and Community, *Canadian Journal of Psychiatry*, 45(7) (2000), 607–616.

53. Statistics Canada. *2001 Census—Release 5, Jan. 21, 2003: Ethnocultural Portrait of Canada*. Ottawa: Statistics Canada, 2001. Website: http://www12.statcan.ca/english/census01/release/release5.cfm (accessed June 2007).

54. Health Canada. *Diseases & Conditions: Diabetes*. Ottawa: Author, 2006. Website: http://www.hc-sc.gc.ca/ (accessed June 2007); Iwasaki, Y., J. Bartlett, and J. O'Neil, Coping with Stress among Aboriginal Women and Men with Diabetes in Winnipeg, Canada, *Social Science & Medicine*, 60 (2005), 977–988.

55. McShane, K.E., J.K. Smylie, P.D. Hastings, C.M. Martin, and Tungasuvvingat Inuit Family Resource Centre, Guiding Health Promotion Efforts with Urban Inuit: A Community-Specific Perspective on Health Information Sources and Dissemination Strategies, *Canadian Journal of Public Health*, 97(4) (2006), 296–299.

56. Young, T.K., Review of Research on Aboriginal Populations in Canada: Relevance to Their Health Needs, *British Medical Journal*, 327(23) (August 2002), 419–422.

57. Statistics Canada, *Aboriginal Peoples Survey 2001—Initial Findings*.

58. Health Canada. *Diabetes among Aboriginal (First Nations, Inuit and Métis) People in Canada: The Evidence*. Ottawa: Health Canada, 2000.

59. Statistics Canada, *Aboriginal Peoples Survey 2001—Initial Findings*.

60. Tester, F.J., and P. McNicoll, Isumagijaksaq: Mindful of the State: Social Constructions of Inuit Suicide, *Social Science & Medicine*, 58 (2004), 2625–2636.

61. Young, Review of Research on Aboriginal Populations in Canada.

62. Jenkins, A.L., T.W. Gyrokos, K.N. Culman, B.J. Ward, G.S. Pekeles, and E.L. Mills, An Overview of Factors Influencing the Health of Canadian Inuit Infants, *International Journal of Circumpolar Health*, 62(1) (2003), 17–39.

63. Health Canada, *Diabetes among Aboriginal (First Nations, Inuit and Métis) People in Canada: The Evidence*.

64. Reading, J., and E. Nowgesic, Improving the Health of Future Generations: The Canadian Institutes of Health, Research Institute of Aboriginal Peoples' Health, *American Journal of Public Health*, 92(9) (2002), 1396–1401.

65. Tester and McNicoll, Isumagijaksaq: Mindful of the State: Social Constructions of Inuit Suicide.

66. Reading and Nowgesic, Improving the Health of Future Generations.

67. Ponting, J.R., *First Nations in Canada: Perspectives on Opportunity, Empowerment, and Self-Determination*. Toronto: McGraw-Hill Ryerson, 1997.

68. Clarke, H.F., R. Joseph, M. Deschamps, T.G. Hislop, P.R. Band, and R. Atleo, Reducing Cervical Cancer among First Nations Women, *The Canadian Nurse*, 94(3) (1998), 36–41.

69. Statistics Canada. *Portrait of the Canadian Population in 2006*.

70. Statistics Canada. *Portrait of the Canadian Population in 2006*.

71. Statistics Canada. *Population Projections of Visible Minority Groups, Canada, Provinces and Regions, 2001–2017* (Catalogue no. 91-541-XIE). Ottawa: Statistics Canada, 2005.

72. McDonald, J.T. *The Health Behaviours of Immigrants and Native-Born People in Canada*: Working Paper No. 01-06. Halifax: Atlantic Metropolis Centre—Working Paper Series, 2006.

73. Bottorff, J.L., L.G. Balneaves, L. Sent, S. Grewal, and A.J. Browne, An Explanation of Women-centred Care in the Context of Cervical Cancer Screening in Ethnocultural Groups, *Research Bulletin: Centres of Excellence for Women's Health*, 1(2), 8–9; C.E. Perez, Health Status and Health Behaviour among Immigrants, *Supplement to Health Reports* (Catalogue no. 82–003), 13 (2002). Statistics Canada; Dunn, J.R., and I. Dyck, Social Determinants of Health in Canada's Immigrant Population: Results from the National Population Health Survey. *Social Science & Medicine*, 51(11) (2000), 1573–1593.

74. Dunn and Dyck, Social Determinants of Health in Canada's Immigrant Population.

75. Adams, M. *Book Summary: Sex in the Snow—Canadian Social Values at the End of the Millennium*. Toronto: Viking, 1997.

76. Kendall et al., *Sociology in Our Times: The Essentials*.

77. Kostash, M. *The Next Canada: In Search of Our Future Nation*. Toronto: McClelland and Stewart, 2000.

78. Mangold, K., Educating a New Generation: Teaching Baby Boomer Faculty about Millennial Students, *Nurse Educator*, 32(1) (2007), 21–23.

79. Adams, M. *Clouds Over Canada: The New Social Climate*. Toronto: Environics Research Group Ltd., 1999.

80. Canadian Paediatrics Society. *Impact of Media use on Children and Youth*. Ottawa: Author, 2003. Website: http://www.cps.ca/english/statements/PP/pp03-01.htm (accessed June 2007).

81. Statistics Canada. *Television Viewing, by Age, Sex, by Province*. Ottawa: Statistics Canada, 2006. Website: http://www40.statcan.ca/l01/cst01/arts23.htm (accessed June 2007).

82. Johnson, J.G., P. Cohen, E.M. Smailes, S. Kasen, and J.S. Brook, Television Viewing and Aggressive Behaviour During Adolescence and Adulthood, *Science*, 295 (2002), 2468–2471.

83. Canadian Broadcasting Corporation. *Pinky Dinky Doo*. Toronto: Author, 2007. Website: http://www.cbc.ca/ (accessed May 2007).

84. Public Health Agency of Canada. *Canada's Physical Activity Guides for Children and Youth*. Ottawa: Author, 2002. Website: http://www.phac-aspc.gc.ca/ (accessed May 2007).

85. Ozmert, E., M. Yoyran, and K. Yurdakok, Behavioral Correlates of Television Viewing in Primary School Children Evaluated by the Child Behavior Checklist, *Archives of Pediatrics and Adolescent Medicine*, 156(9) (2002), 910–914.

86. Canadian Paediatrics Society, *Impact of Media use on Children and Youth*.

87. Canadian Paediatrics Society, *Impact of Media use on Children and Youth*.

88. Canadian Paediatrics Society, Healthy Active Living for Children and Youth. *Paediatrics and Child Health*, 7 (2002), 339–345.

89. Vail, S. *Canadians' Values and Attitudes on Canada's Health Care System: A Synthesis of Survey Results*. Ottawa: The Conference Board of Canada, 2001.

90. Mendelsohn, M. *Canadians' Thoughts on Their Health Care System: Preserving the Canadian Model Through Innovation*. Ottawa: Commission on the Future of Health Care in Canada, 2002. Website: http://www.arts.uwaterloo.ca/~gboychuk/psci491/mendelsohn.doc (accessed June 2007).

91. Soroka, S.N. *Canadian Perceptions of the Health Care System: A Report to the Health Council of Canada*. Toronto: Health Council of Canada, 2007.

92. Commission on the Future of Health Care in Canada. *Report on Citizens' Dialogue on the Future of Health Care in Canada*. Ottawa: Author, 2002.

93. Shah, C.P. *Public Health and Preventative Medicine in Canada*, 5th ed. Toronto: Elsevier Canada, 2003.

94. Raphael, D., T. Bryant, and A. Curry-Stevens, Toronto Charter Outlines Future Health Policy Directions for Canada and Elsewhere, *Health Promotion International, 19*(2) (2004), 269–273.

95. Macionis and Gerber, *Sociology*.

96. Campaign 2000. *Oh Canada! Too Many Children in Poverty for Too Long … 2006 Report Card on Child and Family Poverty in Canada.* Toronto: Author, 2006.

97. Curtis, L.J., and M. Pennock, Social Assistance, Lone Parents and Health: What Do We Know, Where Do We Go? *Canadian Journal of Public Health, 97*, Supplement 3 (2006), S4–S10.

98. Raphael, *Social Justice Is Good for Our Hearts*.

99. Macionis and Gerber, *Sociology*.

100. Campaign 2000, *Oh Canada! Too Many Children in Poverty for Too Long.*

101. Campaign 2000, *Oh Canada! Too Many Children in Poverty for Too Long.*

102. National Advisory Council on Aging. *Seniors in Canada: 2006 Report Card.* Ottawa: Minister of Public Works and Governmental Services Canada, 2006.

103. Statistics Canada. *A Portrait of Seniors in Canada.* (Catalogue no. 89-519-XIE). Ottawa: Minister of Industry, 2007.

104. National Advisory Council on Aging, *Seniors in Canada: 2006 Report Card.*

105. National Advisory Council on Aging, *Seniors in Canada: 2006 Report Card.*

106. Podymow, T., J. Turnbull, V. Tadic, and W, Muckle, Shelter-based Convalescence for Homeless Adults, *Canadian Journal of Public Health, 97*(5) (2006), 379–383.

107. Campaign 2000, *Oh Canada! Too Many Children in Poverty for Too Long.*

108. Boyle, Culture, Family, and Community.

109. Segall, A., and N. Chappell. *Health and Health Care in Canada.* Toronto: Prentice Hall, 2000.

110. Ship, S., and L. Norton, HIV/AIDS and Aboriginal Women in Canada, *Canadian Woman Studies, 21*(2) (2001), 25–31.

111. Public Health Agency of Canada. *Population Health, Towards a Canadian Understanding: Clarifying the Core Concepts of Population Health.* Ottawa: Author, 2002. Website: http://www.phac-aspc.gc.ca/ (accessed June 2007).

112. Gilmore, J., and B. Wannell, Life Expectancy, *Health Reports,* (Catalogue no. 82-003), *11*(3) (1999), 9–24.

113. Roos, N.P., and C.A. Mustard, Variation in Health and Health Care Use by Socioeconomic Status in Winnipeg, Canada: Does the System Work Well? Yes and No. *Milbank Quarterly, 75*(1) (1997), 89–111.

114. Kosteniuk, J.G., and H.D. Dickinson, Tracing the Social Gradient in the Health of Canadians: Primary and Secondary Determinants. *Social Science & Medicine, 57*(2) (2003), 263–276.

115. Seguin, L., Q. Xu, L. Potvin, M. Zunzunegui, and K.L. Frohlick, Effects of Low Income on Infant Health, *Canadian Medical Association Journal, 168*(12) (2003), 1533–1538.

116. Dooley, M.D., L. Curtis, E.L. Lipman, and D.H. Feeny, Child Health and Family Socioeconomic Status, *Policy Options* (September 1998), 13–18.

117. Ing, J.D., and L. Reutter, Socioeconomic Status, Sense of Coherence, and Health in Canadian Women, *Canadian Journal of Public Health, 94*(3) (2003), 224–228.

118. AMO/ROMA. *Rural Poverty.* Toronto: Association of Municipalities of Ontario/Rural Ontario Municipal Association, 2007. Website: www.amo.on.ca/ (accessed June 2007).

119. RDI. *Reflections on Rural and Northern Poverty: Presentation to the Standing Senate Committee on Agriculture and Forestry.* Brandon, MB: Rural Development Institute, Brandon University, 2007. Website: www.brandonu.ca/rdi (accessed June 2007).

120. Lee, K.K. *Urban Poverty in Canada: A Statistical Profile.* Ottawa: Canadian Council on Social Development, 2000.

121. Pender, N.J., C.L. Murdaugh, and M.A. Parsons, *Health Promotion in Nursing Practice,* 5th ed. New Jersey: Pearson Prentice Hall, 2006.

122. Public Health Agency of Canada, *Population Health, Towards a Canadian Understanding.*

123. Labonte, R. *Health Promotion and Empowerment: Practice and Framework.* Toronto: University of Toronto, 1993.

124. Canadian Nurses Association. *Nursing Now: Primary Health Care—The Time Has Come.* Ottawa: Author, 2003.

125. Vollman, A.R. The Canadian Health Care Delivery System. In P.A. Potter, A.G. Perry, J.C. Ross-Kerr, and M.J. Wood (eds.), *Canadian Fundamentals of Nursing,* 3rd ed. (pp. 18–33). Toronto: Elsevier Canada, 2006.

126. Health Council of Canada. *Population Health, Health Care Renewal in Canada: Clearing the Road to Quality.* Toronto: Author, 2006.

127. Intersectorial Healthy Living Network. *The Integrated Pan-Canadian Healthy Living Strategy.* Ottawa: Author, 2005.

128. Health Canada. *Healthy Canadians: A Federal Report on Comparable Health Indicators 2006.* Ottawa: Author, 2006.

129. Katzmarzyk, P.T., and C. Mason, Prevalence of Class I, II and III Obesity in Canada, *Canadian Medical Association Journal, 174*(2) (2006), 156–157.

130. Intersectorial Healthy Living Network, *The Integrated Pan-Canadian Healthy Living Strategy.*

131. Soroka, S.N. *Canadian Perceptions of the Health Care System: A Report to the Health Council of Canada.*

132. Intersectorial Healthy Living Network, *The Integrated Pan-Canadian Healthy Living Strategy.*

133. Canadian Nurses Association, *Nursing Now: Primary Health Care—The Time Has Come.*

134. Plotnikoff, R.C., J.C. Spence, L.S. Tavares, L.S. Rovniak, A. Bauman, S.A. Lear, and L. McCargar, Characteristics of Participants Visiting the Canada on the Move Website. *Canadian Journal of Public Health, 97*, Supplement 1 (2006), S28–S35.

135. Dietz, W.H., Canada on the Move: A Novel Effort to Increase Physical Activity among Canadians, *Canadian Journal of Public Health, 97*, Supplement 1 (2006), S3–S4.

136. Plotnikoff et al., Characteristics of Participants Visiting the Canada on the Move Website.

137. Leininger, M. *Care: The Essence of Nursing and Health.* Detroit: Wayne State University, 1988.

138. Kilty, H.L. *Nursing Leadership Development in Canada—A Descriptive Status Report and Analysis of Leadership Programs, Approaches and Strategies: Domains and Competencies; Knowledge Skills; Gaps and Opportunities.* Ottawa: Canadian Nurses Association, 2003.

139. Raphael, *Social Justice Is Good for Our Hearts*

140. Canadian Nurses Association. *CNA Backgrounder: Primary Health Care: A Summary of the Issues.* Ottawa: Author, 2005.

141. Canadian Nurses Association, Cultural Diversity—Changes and Challenges, *Nursing Now: Issues and Trends in Canadian Nursing, 7* (February 2000).

142. Green-Hernandez, C., S. Denman-Vitale, and T. Judge-Ellis, Making Nursing Care Culturally Competent, *The Nurse Practitioner, 29*(6) (2004), 49–55.

143. *Public Health Agency of Canada. Ottawa Charter for Health Promotion.* Ottawa: Author, 2004. Website: http://www.phac-aspc.gc.ca/ (accessed June 2007).

144. Kikuchi, Cultural Theories of Nursing Responsive to Human Needs and Values.

145. Hrycak, N., and S.L. Jakubec, Cultural Awareness: Listening to Different Voices, *Canadian Nurse, 102*(6), 24–28.

146. Lynam, M.J., B. Gurm, and R. Dhari, Exploring Perinatal Health in Indo-Canadian Women, *The Canadian Nurse, 96*(4) (2000), 18–24.

147. Health Council of Canada. *Primary Health Care 2006 Annual Report.* Ottawa: Author, 2007.

148. Manitoba Telehealth. *Telesante Manitoba.* Winnipeg: Telehealth News, 2007. Website: http://www.mbtelehealth.ca/ (accessed June 2007).

149. Sibbald, B., A Telehealth Pioneer, *Canadian Nurse,* 99(3) (2003), 52.

150. National Initiative for Telehealth Guidelines. *National Initiative for Telehealth (NIFTE) Framework of Guidelines.* Ottawa: NIFTE, 2003.

151. Ross-Kerr, J.C., and M.J. Wood. *Canadian Nursing: Issues and Perspectives,* 4th ed. Toronto: Elsevier Science Canada, 2003.

152. Hannah, K.J., The State of Nursing Informatics in Canada, *Canadian Nurse,* 103(5) (2007), 18–22.

153. Hilton, B.A., R. Thompson, L. Moore-Dempsey, and R.G. Janzen, Harm Reduction Theories and Strategies for Control of Human Immunodeficiency Virus: A Review of the Literature, *Journal of Advanced Nursing,* 33(3) (2001), 357–370.

154. Hilton et al., Harm Reduction Theories and Strategies for Control of Human Immunodeficiency Virus.

155. Wood, E., T. Kerr, E. Lloyd-Smith, C. Buchner, D.C. Marsh, J. Montaner, and M.W. Tyndall, Methodology for Evaluating Insite: Canada's First Medically Supervised Safer Injection Facility for Injection Drug Users, *Harm Reduction Journal I* (2004), 9.

156. Dienemann, J. (ed.). *Cultural Diversity in Nursing: Issues, Strategies, and Outcomes.* Waldorf, MD: American Nurses Association, 1997; Dossey, B., and L. Dossey, Body-Mind-Spirit: Attending to Holistic Care, *American Journal of Nursing,* 98(8) (1998), 35–38.

157. Canadian Nurses Association, Complementary Therapies: Finding the Right Balance, *Nursing Now: Issues and Trends in Canadian Nursing,* 6 (1999).

158. ALS Society of Canada. *Fact Sheet #11: Making Sense of Complimentary or Alternative Medicines.* Toronto: Author, 2005. Website: http://www.als.ca/ (accessed June 2007).

159. Health Canada. *Drugs & Health Products: Natural Health Products.* Ottawa: Health Canada, 2006. Website: http://www.hc-sc.gc.ca/ (accessed June 2007).

160. Montbriand, M., Alternative Therapies: Health Professionals' Attitudes, *The Canadian Nurse,* 96(3) (2000), 22–26.

161. Mulkins, A., J.M. Morse, and A. Best, Complementary Therapy Use in HIV/AIDS, *Canadian Journal of Public Health,* 93(4) (2002), 308–312.

162. Thorne, S., B. Paterson, C. Russell, and A. Schultz, Complementary/Alternative Medicine in Chronic Illness as Informed Self-Care Decision Making. *International Journal of Nursing Studies,* 39(7) (2002), 671–683.

163. Canadian Nurses Association. *Position Statement: Clinical Nurse Specialist.* Ottawa: Author, 2003.

164. Canadian Nurses Association. *The Canadian Nurse Practitioner Initiative.* Ottawa: Author, 2007.

165. Canadian Nurses Association. *Certification Bulletin: Certification Statistics for 2005.* Ottawa: Author, 2006.

## Chapter 2

1. Thomlinson, E., Environmental Health and Nursing. In M. McIntyre and E. Thomlinson (eds.), *Realities of Canadian Nursing: Professional, Practice, and Power Issues.* Philadelphia: Lippincott Williams & Wilkins, 2003.

2. Furgal, C., and P. Gosselin, Challenges and Directions for Environmental Public Health Indicators and Surveillance, *Canadian Journal of Public Health,* 93, Supplement 1 (2003), s5–s8.

3. Furgal and Gosselin, Challenges and Directions for Environmental Public Health Indicators and Surveillance.

4. Shah, C.P. *Public Health and Preventative Medicine in Canada* (5th ed.). Toronto: Elsevier Canada, 2003.

5. Health Canada, *Environment & Workplace Health, Environmental Health Assessment.* Website: http://www.hc-sc.gc.ca/ (accessed August 2007).

6. Western Economic Diversification Canada, *Canadian Environmental Assessment Act.* Website: http://www.wd.gc.ca/ (accessed August 2007).

7. Health Canada, *Environmental & Workplace Health, Reports & Publications, Environmental Health Assessment, Environmental Assessment and Human Health.* Website: http://www.hc-sc.gc.ca/ (accessed August 2007).

8. Western Economic Diversification Canada, *Canadian Environmental Assessment Act.*

9. Canadian Environmental Assessment Agency. Website: http://www.ceaa.gc.ca/ (accessed March 2008).

10. Western Economic Diversification Canada, *Canadian Environmental Assessment Act.*

11. Brundtland Report, 1987. Website: http://www.are.admin.ch/ (accessed August 2007).

12. Health Canada, *Environmental & Workplace Health, Reports & Publications, Environmental Health Assessment, Environmental Assessment and Human Health.*

13. Furgal and Gosselin, Challenges and Directions for Environmental Public Health Indicators and Surveillance.

14. National Round Table on the Environment and Economy, *Environment and Sustainable Development Indicators for Canada.* Website: http://ww.nrtee-trnee.ca/eng/media/media-releases/20030508-ESDI-eng.htm (accessed August 2007).

15. Government of Canada. *Canadian Environmental Sustainability Indicators.* Ottawa: Author, 2006. Catalogue no. 16-251-XIE.

16. Government of Canada. *Canadian Environmental Sustainability Indicators.*

17. The Canadian Environmental Network, *CEPA.* Website: http://www.cen-rce.org/eng/cepa/phase2/index.html (accessed August 2007).

18. Bill C-32: *The Canadian Environmental Protection Act,* 1999. Website: http://www.ec.gc.ca/CEPARegistry/the_act/ (accessed August 2007).

19. Environment Canada, *Informing Canadians on Pollution 2002.* Highlights of the 2000 National Pollutant Release Inventory (NPRI).

20. Environment Canada, *Informing Canadians on Pollution 2002.*

21. Environment Canada, *National Pollutant Release Inventory (NPRI),* Website: http://www.ec.gc.ca/pdb/npri/npri_home_e.cfm/ (accessed August 2007).

22. Environment Canada, *Informing Canadians on Pollution 2002.*

23. Dickinson, G., M. Liepner, S. Talos, and D. Buckingham. *Understanding the Law* (2nd ed.). Toronto: McGraw-Hill Ryerson Ltd., 1996.

24. Shah, *Public Health and Preventative Medicine in Canada.*

25. Quebec City Consensus Conference on Environmental Health Indicators, Selected Papers, *Canadian Journal of Public Health,* 93, Supplement 1 (2002), s1–s70.

26. Shah, *Public Health and Preventative Medicine in Canada.*

27. Health Canada, *Environment & Workplace Health, Environmental Health Assessment.*

28. Maller, C., M. Townsend, A. Pryor, P. Brown, and L. St. Leger, Healthy Nature Healthy People: 'Contact with Nature' as an Upstream Health Promotion Intervention for Populations, *Health Promotion International,* 21(1) (2005), 45–54.

29. Environment Canada. *Informing Environmental Decisions: First Steps Towards a Canadian Information System for the Environment.* The Interim Report of the Task Force on a Canadian Information System for the Environment to the Minister of the Environment. Ottawa: Minister of Public Works and Governmental Services, 2001.

30. Government of Canada, *Canadian Environmental Sustainability Indicators.*

31. Boyd, D.R. *The Air We Breathe: An International Comparison of Air Quality Standards and Guidelines.* Vancouver: David Suzuki Foundation, 2006.

32. Shah, *Public Health and Preventative Medicine in Canada*.
33. Edwards, P., Climate Change: Air Pollution and Your Health, *Canadian Journal of Public Health, 92*(3) (2001), I1–I12.
34. Edwards, Climate Change: Air Pollution and Your Health.
35. Manfreda, J., M.R. Becklake, M.R. Sears, M. Chan-Yeung, H. Dimich-Ward, H.C. Siersted, P. Ernst, et al., Prevalence of Asthma Symptoms among Adults Aged 20–40 Years in Canada, *Canadian Medical Association Journal, 164*(7) (2001), 995–1001.
36. Boulet, L-P, A. Becker, D. Berube, R. Beveridge, and P. Ernst, Summary of Recommendations from the Canadian Asthma Consensus Report, 1999, *Canadian Medical Association Journal, 161*(11) (1999), Supplement 2.
37. Boulet et al. Summary of Recommendations from the Canadian Asthma Consensus Report, 1999.
38. Manfreda et al., Prevalence of Asthma Symptoms among Adults Aged 20–40 Years in Canada.
39. Boulet et al. Summary of Recommendations from the Canadian Asthma Consensus Report, 1999.
40. Svavarsdottir, E.K., M.A. McCubbin, and J.H. Kane, Well-Being of Parents of Young Children with Asthma, *Research in Nursing & Health, 23* (2000), 346–358.
41. Health Care Without Harm. *Risks to Asthma Posed by Indoor Health Care Environments: A Guide to Identifying and Reducing Problematic Exposures.* Lowell, MA: Author, 2006.
42. McCarthy, M.J., J. Hansen, R. Herbert, D. Wong, M. Brimacombe, and M. Zelman, Empowering Parents through Asthma Education, *Pediatric Nursing, 28*(5) (2002), 65–73.
43. Government of Canada, *Canadian Environmental Sustainability Indicators*.
44. Government of Canada, *Canadian Environmental Sustainability Indicators*.
45. Frank, J., CIHR Research: Catching Your Breath: Research Efforts to Analyze the Negative Effects of Air Pollution on Human Health, *Healthcare Quarterly, 9*(4) (2006), 18–20.
46. Schwartz, J., Air Pollution and Children's Health, *Pediatrics, 113*(4) (2004), 1037–1043.
47. Boyd, *The Air We Breathe: An International Comparison of Air Quality Standards and Guidelines*.
48. Government of Canada, *Canadian Environmental Sustainability Indicators*.
49. Government of Canada, *Canadian Environmental Sustainability Indicators*.
50. Environment Canada, *Canada–United States Air Quality Agreement—Progress Report 2006*. Website: http://www.ec.gc.ca/ (accessed August 2007).
51. Health Canada, *Environment Canada. National Ambient Air Quality Objectives for Ground-Level Ozone, Part 1*. A report by the Federal-Provincial Working Group on Air Quality Objectives and Guidelines. Ottawa: Authors, 1999.
52. Health Canada, *Environment Canada, National Ambient Air Quality Objectives for Ground-Level Ozone*.
53. Environment Canada, *Air Quality Index (AQI) and Smog Alert Program*. Website: http://www.ene.gov.on.ca/envision/techdocs/4226e_f.pdf (accessed August 2007).
54. Ontario Ministry of the Environment, *Air Quality Ontario*. Website: http://www.airqualityontario.com (accessed August 2007).
55. Environment Canada, *Canada–United States Air Quality Agreement—Progress Report 2006*.
56. Transport Canada, *Green Travel Tips—What You Can Do*. Website: http://www.tc.gc.ca/ (accessed August 2007).
57. Environment Canada, *Clean Air Online: Clean Air in Canada 2003 Progress Report*. Website: http://www.ec.gc.ca/cleanair-airpur/CAOL/air?PM_resp_03/s1_e.html (accessed August 2007).
58. Government of Canada, *Canadian Environmental Sustainability Indicators*.
59. Transport Canada, *Green Travel Tips—What You Can Do*.
60. Mehdi, B. (ed.). *Adapting to Climate Change: An Introduction for Canadian Municipalities*. Ottawa: Canadian Climate Impacts and Adaptation Network (C-CIARN), 2006.
61. Government of Canada, *Canadian Environmental Sustainability Indicators*.
62. Lemmen, D.S., and F.J. Warren. *Climate Change Impacts and Adaptation: A Canadian Perspective*. Ottawa: Natural Resources Canada, 2004.
63. Lemmen and Warren, *Climate Change Impacts and Adaptation: A Canadian Perspective*.
64. Redlich, C., J. Sparer, and M. Callen, Sick Building Syndrome, *Lancet, 349*(9059) (1997), 1013–1016.
65. Sabo, B. Indoor Air Quality in Canadian Schools, *Canadian Nurse, 97*(2) (2001), 28–31.
66. de Groh, M., and H.I. Morrison, Environmental Tobacco Smoke and Deaths from Coronary Heart Disease in Canada, *Chronic Diseases in Canada, 23*(1) (2002), 13–16.
67. Labour Environmental Alliance Society, *Toxins in Household Products*. Website: http://leas.ca/Toxins-in-Household-Products.html (accessed August 2007).
68. Van Dongen, C., Environmental Health Risks, *American Journal of Nursing, 98*(9) (1998), 16B, 16D–16E.
69. Government of Canada, *Canadian Environmental Sustainability Indicators*.
70. Davies, J-M., and A. Mazumder, Health and Environmental Policy Issues in Canada: The Role of Watershed Management in Sustaining Clean Drinking Water Quality at Surface Sources. *Journal of Environmental Management, 68*(3) (2003), 273–286.
71. McQuigge, M., Water: A Clear and Present Danger, *Canadian Journal of Public Health, 93*(1) (2002), 10–11.
72. Raina, P., F. Pollari, G. Teare, M. Goss, D. Barry, and J. Wilson, The Relationship between E. coli Indicator Bacteria in Well-Water and Gastrointestinal Illnesses in Rural Families, *Canadian Journal of Public Health, 90*(3) (1999), 172–175.
73. Davies and Mazumder, Health and Environmental Policy Issues in Canada: The Role of Watershed Management in Sustaining Clean Drinking Water Quality at Surface Sources.
74. Government of Canada, *Canadian Environmental Sustainability Indicators*.
75. Health Canada, *Environment & Workplace Health, Water Quality, Drinking Water, Drinking Water Guidelines*. Website: http://www.hc-sc.gc.ca/ (accessed August 2007).
76. Health Canada, *Environment & Workplace Health, Water Quality, Drinking Water, Drinking Water Guidelines*.
77. Pip, E., Survey of Bottled Drinking Water Available in Manitoba, Canada, *Environmental Health Perspectives, 108*(9) (2000), 863–866.
78. Woo, D.M., and K.J. Vincente, Sociotechnical Systems, Risk Management, and Public Health: Comparing the North Battleford and Walkerton Outbreaks, *Reliability Engineering & System Safety, 80*(3) (2003), 253–269.
79. Petersen, K., The High Cost of Lousy Water: Water Crisis in Indigenous 'Canadian' Communities, *The Dominion*, November 22, 2006. Website: http://www.dominionpaper.ca/ (accessed September 2007).
80. Christensen, R., *Waterproof 2: Canada's Drinking Water Report Card*. Vancouver: Sierra Legal Defence Fund, 2006.
81. Lukovich, J.V. *Saving Lake Winnipeg: Report of the 2006 Lake Winnipeg Environment Forum*. Winnipeg: Lake Winnipeg Environment Forum, 2006.
82. Environment Canada, *Environmental Emergencies*. Website: http://manitobawildlands.org/water_act.htm (accessed September 2007).
83. Pike-MacDonald, S., D.G. Best, C. Twomey, L. Bennett, and J. Blakeley, Promoting Safe Drinking Water, *Canadian Nurse, 103*(1) (2007), 15–19.
84. Pike-MacDonald et al., *Promoting Safe Drinking Water*.
85. Shah, *Public Health and Preventative Medicine in Canada*.

86. Shah, *Public Health and Preventative Medicine in Canada*.
87. Canadian Chlorine Chemistry Council, *Dioxins*. Website: http://www.cfour.org/cms/index.php?id=18 (accessed September 2007).
88. Gaudry, J., and K. Skiehar, Promoting Environmentally Responsible Health Care, *Canadian Nurse*, 103(1) (2007), 23–26.
89. Weinhold, B., Making Health Care Healthier: A Prescription for Change, *Environmental Health Perspectives*, 109(8) (2001), A370–A377.
90. Gilmore Hall, A., Nurses: Taking Precautionary Action on a Pediatric Environmental Exposure: DEHP, *Pediatric Nursing*, 32(1) (2006), 91–93.
91. Health Canada, *Information for Parents and Caregivers of Very Young Children*. Website: http://www.hc-sc.gc.ca/ (accessed September 2007).
92. *Dioxin Pollution in Northern Canada*. Website: http://inuitcircumpolar.com/index.php?ID=132&Lang=En (accessed September 2007).
93. *Dioxin Pollution in Northern Canada*
94. Gaudry and Skiehar, Promoting Environmentally Responsible Health Care.
95. Health Canada, *Food and Nutrition*. Website: http://www.hc-sc.gc.ca/ (accessed September 2007).
96. Health Canada, *Food and Nutrition*.
97. Government of Canada. *Voluntary Labelling and Advertising of Foods That Are Not Products of Genetic Engineering*. Ottawa: Canadian General Standards Board, 2004.
98. Weir, E., Botulism in Canada, *Canadian Medical Association Journal*, 164(4) (2001), 538–541.
99. Weir, Botulism in Canada.
100. Health Canada, *Emergencies & Disasters, Emergency Response, Annex 2 Foodborne Illness Outbreak Response Protocol*. Website: http://www.hc-sc.gc.ca/ (accessed September 2007).
101. Health Canada, *Emergencies & Disasters, Emergency Response, Annex 2 Foodborne Illness Outbreak Response Protocol*.
102. Canadian Cancer Society, *Food Additives and Cancer*. Website: http://www.cancer.ca/css (accessed September 2007).
103. Canadian Cancer Society, *Food Additives and Cancer*.
104. Canadian Nurses Association, *Position Statement: Food Safety and Security Are Determinants of Health*. Website: http://www.cna-nurses.ca (accessed August 2007).
105. Canadian Nurses Association, *Position Statement: Food Safety and Security Are Determinants of Health*.
106. Health Canada, *Food & Nutrition: Food Labelling, Nutrition Labelling*. Website: http://www.hc-sc.gc.ca/ (accessed September 2007).
107. Inuit Tapiriit Kanatemi, *Northern Environmental Contaminants*. Website: http://www.itk.ca/ (accessed August 2007).
108. Inuit Tapiriit Kanatemi, *Northern Environmental Contaminants*.
109. Ontario Agriculture, *Reduced-Risk Pesticides and Biopesticides*. Website: http://www.omafra.gov.on.ca/english/crops/hort/news/vegnews/2005/vg1105a5.htm (accessed August 2007).
110. Ontario Agriculture, *Reduced-Risk Pesticides and Biopesticides*.
111. Manitoba Agriculture, *Pest Control Safety*. Website: http://www.gov.mb.ca/ (accessed August 2007).
112. Health Canada, *Environmental & Workplace Health, Noise*. Website: http://www.hc-sc.gc.ca/ (accessed September 2007).
113. Shah, *Public Health and Preventative Medicine in Canada*.
114. Health Canada, *Food and Nutrition: Food Labelling, Nutrition Labelling*.
115. Health Canada, *Environmental & Workplace Health, Noise*.
116. Shah, *Public Health and Preventative Medicine in Canada*.
117. Shah, *Public Health and Preventative Medicine in Canada*.
118. Weir, E., Hospitals and the Environment, *Canadian Medical Association Journal*, 166(3) (2002), 354.
119. Shah, *Public Health and Preventative Medicine in Canada*.
120. Environment Canada, *The 4Rs: Reduce, Reuse, Recycle, Recover*. Website: http://www.atl.ec.gc.ca/udo/reuse.html (accessed August 2007).

121. Environment Canada, *The 4Rs: Reduce, Reuse, Recycle, Recover*.
122. *Waste Reduction Week—Canada*. Website: http://www.wrwcanada.com/ (accessed August 2007).
123. Shah, *Public Health and Preventative Medicine in Canada*.
124. Government of Canada, *Hazardous Waste Management: Canadian Directions*. Ottawa: Depository Services Program, 2006. Website: http://dsp-psd.pwgsc.gc.ca/ (accessed September 2007).
125. Government of Canada, *Hazardous Waste Management: Canadian Directions*.
126. Government of Canada, *Voluntary Labelling and Advertising of Foods That Are Not Products of Genetic Engineering*.
127. Ratoff, I., and D.E. Thomsen, Chernobyl May Be Worst Nuclear Accident, *Science News*, 129 (1986), 276.
128. Weir, *Hospitals and the Environment*.
129. Escaf, M., and R.N. Shurtleff, A Program for Reducing Biomedical Waste: The Wellesley Hospital Experience, *Canadian Journal of Infection Control*, 11 (1996), 7–11.
130. International Council of Nurses, *Position Statement: Medical Waste: Role of Nurses and Nursing*. Geneva: Author, 2004. Website: http://www.icn.ch/ (accessed September 2007).
131. International Council of Nurses, *Position Statement: Medical Waste: Role of Nurses and Nursing*.
132. International Council of Nurses, *Position Statement: Medical Waste: Role of Nurses and Nursing*.
133. Sanborn, M.D., A. Abelsohn, M. Campbell, and E. Weir, Identifying and Managing Adverse Environmental Health Effects: 3. Lead Exposure, *Canadian Medical Association Journal*, 166(10) (2002), 1287.
134. Escaf and Shurtleff, A Program for Reducing Biomedical Waste: The Wellesley Hospital Experience.
135. Escaf and Shurtleff, A Program for Reducing Biomedical Waste: The Wellesley Hospital Experience.
136. Wigle, D. *Child Health and the Environment*. New York: Oxford University Press, 2003.
137. Environment Canada, *Informing Canadians on Pollution 2002*.
138. Rogers, B., Is Health Care a Risky Business? *American Nurse*, 31(5) (1997), 5.
139. Shah, *Public Health and Preventative Medicine in Canada*.
140. Shah, *Public Health and Preventative Medicine in Canada*.
141. Welsh, M.S., M. Lamesse, and E. Karpinski, The Verification of Hazardous Ingredients: Disclosures in Selected Material Safety Data Sheets, *Applied Occupational and Environmental Hygiene*, 15(5) (2000), 409–420.
142. Health Canada, *Environment & Workplace Health, Occupational Health & Safety, Workplace Hazardous Materials Information System*. Website: http://www.hc-sc.gc.ca/ (accessed August 2007).
143. Shah, *Public Health and Preventative Medicine in Canada*.
144. Welsh et al., The Verification of Hazardous Ingredients: Disclosures in Selected Material Safety Data Sheets.
145. Shah, *Public Health and Preventative Medicine in Canada*.
146. Canadian Centre for Occupational Health and Safety, *Background*. Website: http://www.ccohs.ca/ccohs.html (accessed August 2007).
147. Canadian Standards Association, *Standards*. Website: http://www.csa.ca (accessed August 2007).
148. Canadian Heritage, *Human Rights Program*. Website: http://www.pch.gc.ca (accessed August 2007).
149. Johns, G., and A.M. Saks, *Organizational Behaviour* (6th ed.). Toronto: Addison Wesley Longman, 2008.
150. Baumann, A., L. O'Brien-Pallas, B.J. Armstrong-Strassen, R. Bourbonnais, S. Cameron, D. Doran, M. Kerr, et al. *Commitment and Care: The Benefits of Health Workplaces for Nurses, Their Patients and the System, a Policy Synthesis*. Ottawa: Canadian Health Research Foundation, 2001.
151. Canadian Nurses Association, *Position Statement, Quality Professional Practice Environments for Registered Nurses*. Website: http://www.cna-nurses.ca/CNA/ (accessed August 2007).

152. Aiden, L., D. Sloans, and J. Klocinski, Hospital Nurses' Occupational Exposure to Blood: Prospective, Retrospective, and Institutional Reports, *American Journal of Public Health*, 87(1) (1997), 103–107; Bruser, S., Workplace Violence: Getting Hospitals Focused on Prevention, *American Nurse*, 32(3) (1998), 11; Trossman, S., RN Explores Agent Orange's Lasting Effects on Women Vets, *American Nurse*, 31(3) (1999), 24.

153. Del Gaudio, D., and D. Menonna-Quinn, Chemotherapy: Potential Occupational Hazards, *American Journal of Nursing*, 98(11) (1998), 59–65; Health and Safety on the Job, *American Nurse*, September–October 1997, 1, 12; Wigle, *Child Health and the Environment;* Topf, M., Theoretical Considerations for Research on Environmental Stress and Health, *IMAGE: Journal of Nursing Scholarship*, 26 (1994), 289–294; Trossman, RN Explores Agent Orange's Lasting Effects on Women Vets.

154. WHO Reports on New, Re-emerging Diseases Threatening World Health, *The Nation's Health*, 25(10) (1995), 24.

155. Topf, Theoretical Considerations for Research on Environmental Stress and Health.

156. Hynes-Gay, P., J. Bennett, A. Sarjoo-Devries, H. Jones, and A. McGeer, Severe Acute Respiratory Syndrome: The Mount Sinai Experience, *Canadian Nurse*, 99(5) (2003), 17–19.

157. Nickell, L.A., E.J. Crighton, C.S. Tracy, H. Al-Enazy, Y. Bolaji, S. Hanjrah, et al., Psychosocial Effects of SARS on Hospital Staff: Survey of a Large Tertiary Care Institution, *Canadian Medical Association Journal*, 170(5) (2004), 793–798.

158. Loutfy, M.R., T. Wallington, T. Rutledge, B. Mederski, K. Rose, S. Kwolek, et al., Hospital Preparedness and SARS, *Emerging Infectious Diseases*, 10(5) (2004), 771–776.

159. Baumann, A., J.M. Blythe, and J.M. Underwood, Surge Capacity and Casualization: Human Resource Issues in the Post-SARS Health System, *Canadian Journal of Public Health*, 97(3) (2006), 230–232.

160. Canadian Medical Association, West Nile Virus, *Canadian Medical Association Journal*, 168(11) (2003), 1443–1444.

161. Nickell et al., Psychosocial Effects of SARS on Hospital Staff: Survey of a Large Tertiary Care Institution.

162. Sayao, A-L., O. Suchowersky, A. Al-Khathaami, B. Klassen, N.R. Katz, R. Sevick, et al., Calgary Experience with West Nile Virus Neurological Syndrome During the Late Summer of 2003, *Canadian Journal of Neurological Science*, 31(2) (2004), 194–203.

163. Canadian Medical Association, West Nile Virus.

164. Schellenberg, T.L., M.F. Anderson, M.A. Drebot, M T.R. Vooght, A.R. Findlater, P.S. Curry, et al., Seroprevalence of West Nile Virus in Saskatchewan's Five Hills Health Region, 2003, *Canadian Journal of Public Health*, 97(5) (2006), 369–373.

165. Canadian Food Inspection Agency, *Bovine Spongiform Encephalopathy (BSE)*. Website: http://www.inspection.gc.ca/ (accessed August 2007).

166. Sayao et al., Calgary Experience with West Nile Virus Neurological Syndrome During the Late Summer of 2003.

167. Mount Sinai Hospital, *Department of Microbiology, FAQ: Norwalk and Noroviruses*. Website: http://microbiology.mtsinai.on.ca/faq/norwalkfaq.shtml (accessed September 2007).

168. Sheff, B., Avian Influenza: Are You Ready for a Pandemic? *Nursing 2005*, 35(9) (2005), 26–27.

169. Canadian Nurses Association, *Position Statement: Global Health Equity*, Ottawa: Author, 2003.

170. Greenpeace Canada, *About Greenpeace*. Website: http://www.greenpeace.org/canada/ca (accessed August 2007).

171. Canadian Nurses Association, *Policy Statement, Joint CNA/CMA Position Statement on Environmentally Responsible Activity in the Health Sector*. Website: http://www.cna-nurses.ca/CNA/ (accessed August 2007).

172. Greenpeace Canada, *About Greenpeace*.

173. Health Canada, *Environment & Workplace Health, Reports & Publications, Environmental Health Assessment, Canadian Handbook on Health Impact Assessment*. Website: http://www.hc-sc.gc.ca/ (accessed August 2007).

174. Canadian Nurses Association, *Policy Statement, Joint CNA/CMA Position Statement on Environmentally Responsible Activity in the Health Sector*.

175. Fraser, G., Environmental Health and Nursing, *Canadian Nurse*, 100(1) (2004), 17–19.

176. Canadian Nurses Association, *Position Statement, The Environment Is a Determinant of Health*. Website: http://www.cna-nurses.ca (accessed September 2007).

177. Fraser, Environmental Health and Nursing.

178. RNs Facing New Dangers at Works, *American Journal of Nursing*, 95(10) (1995), 78, 81; Wigle, *Child Health and the Environment;* Bruser, S., Workplace Violence: Getting Hospitals Focused on Prevention; Trossman, RN Explores Agent Orange's Lasting Effects on Women Vets.

179. Borland, R., H.H. Young, M. Siahpush, A. Hyland, S. Campbell, G. Hastings, et al., Support and Reported Compliance with Smoke-free Restaurants and Bars by Smokers in Four Countries: Findings from the International Tobacco Control (ITC) Four Country Survey, *Tobacco Control, Supplement* 3(iii) (2006), 34–41.

180. Parle, D., S. Parker, and D. Steeves, Making Canadian Healthcare Facilities 100 Percent Smoke-Free: A National Trend Emerges. *Healthcare Quarterly*, 8(4) (2005), 53–57.

181. Petruk, J., Sharp Injuries: Time to Change Our Equipment and Our Attitudes, *Canadian Nurse*, 99(9) (2003), 19–22.

182. Canadian Nurses Association, *Policy Statement, Joint CNA/CMA Position Statement on Environmentally Responsible Activity in the Health Sector*.

183. Canadian Centre for Occupational Health and Safety, *OSH Answers: Diseases, Disorders & Injuries, SARS*. Website: http://www.ccohs.ca/ (accessed September 2007).

184. College of Registered Nurses of Manitoba, *Welcome to our Hand Washing Resource Page*. Website: http://www.crnm.mb.ca/ (accessed September 2007).

185. College of Registered Nurses of Manitoba, *Welcome to our Hand Washing Resource Page*.

## Chapter 3

1. Macrae, J., Nightingale's Spiritual Philosophy and Its Significance for Modern Nursing, *IMAGE: Journal of Nursing Scholarship*, 27(1) (1995), 8–14.

2. Canadian Nurses Association. *Code of Ethics for Registered Nurses*. Ottawa: Author, 2002; Wright, L.M., *Spirituality, Suffering, and Illness: Ideas for Healing*, Philadelphia: F.A. Davis Company, 2005.

3. Rubin, M., The Healing Power of Prayer, *Journal of Christian Nursing*, 16(3) (1999), 4–7; Craig, C., C. Weinert, J. Walton, and B. Derwinski-Robinson, Spirituality, Chronic Illness, and Rural Life, *Journal of Holistic Nursing*, 24(1) (2006), 27–35.

4. Pangman, V.C., Canadian Perspectives: A Canadian Context of Spirituality. In Perri J. Bomar (ed.), *Promoting Health in Families: Applying Family Research and Theory in Nursing Practice*, 3rd ed. (pp. 208–209). Philadelphia: Saunders Publishing, 2004.

5. Can Religion Be Good Medicine? *The Johns Hopkins Medical Letter*, 10(9) (1998), 3.

6. Mackenzie, E.T., D.E. Rajagopal, M. Meilbohm, and R. Lavizzo-Mourey, Spiritual Support and Psychological Wellbeing: Older Adults' Perceptions of Religion and Health Connection, *Alternative Therapies in Health and Medicine*, 6(6) (2000), 37–45.

7. Chilton, B., Recognizing Spirituality, *IMAGE: Journal of Nursing Scholarship*, 30(4) (1998), 400–401; O'Neill, D., and E. Kenny, Spirituality and Chronic Illness, *IMAGE: Journal of Nursing Scholarship*, 30(3) (1998), 275–280.

8. Lindsey, E., Health within Illness: Experiences of Chronically Ill/Disabled People, *Journal of Advanced Nursing*, 24 (1996), 465–472.

9. Lindsey, Health within Illness: Experiences of Chronically Ill/Disabled People.

10. Baetz, M., D.B. Larson, G. Marcoux, R. Bowen, and R. Griffin, Canadian Psychiatric Inpatient Religious Commitment: An Association with Mental Health, *Canadian Journal of Psychiatry*, 47(2) (2002), 159–166.

11. Easton, K., and J. Andrews, Nursing the Soul: A Team Approach, *Journal of Christian Nursing*, 16(3) (1999), 26–29; Plante, P., Formula for a Miracle, *Journal of Christian Nursing*, 16(3) (1999), 34–35.

12. Johnston Taylor, E., Prayers, Clinical Issues and Implications, *Holistic Nursing Practice*, 17(4) (2003), 179–188; Cavendish, R., B. Kraynyak, L. Konecny, and M. Lanza, Nurses Enhance Performance through Prayer, *Holistic Nursing Practice*, 18(1) (2004), 26–31.

13. Childe, G., Spiritual Healing, *Nursing Standard*, 16(44) (2002), 27–32; Friedmann, M.L., J. Mouch, and T. Racey, Nursing the Spirit: The Framework of Systemic Organization, *Journal of Advanced Nursing*, 39(4) (2002), 325–332; McSherry, W. *Making Sense of Spirituality in Nursing and Health Care Practice: An Interactive Approach*, 2nd ed. Philadelphia: Jessica Kingsley Publishers, 2006.

14. Chilton, Recognizing Spirituality.

15. Bopp, J., M. Bopp, L. Brown, and P. Lane, Jr. *The Sacred Tree*. Lethbridge, AB: Four Worlds International Institute for Human and Community Development, 1984.

16. Bopp et al., *The Sacred Tree*; Mullin, J., L. Lee, S. Hertwig, G. Silverthorn, Final Journey: A Native Smudging Ceremony, *Canadian Nurse*, 97(9) (2001), 20–22.

17. Murray, R.B., J.P. Zentner, V. Pangman, and C. Pangman, *Health Promotion Strategies through the Lifespan*, Canadian ed. Toronto: Pearson Education Canada, 2006.

18. Statistics Canada, *2001 Census: Analysis Series, Religions in Canada*. Website: http://www.12.statcan.ca/English/census01/Proucts/Analytic/companion/rel/pdf/96F0030XIE2001015.pdf (accessed May 2007).

19. Pottinger, A., A. Perivolaris, and D. Howes, The End of Life. In R.H. Srivastava (ed.), *The Health Professional's Guide to Clinical Cultural Competence* (pp. 227–235). Toronto: Elsevier Canada, 2007.

20. Interview: Desai, A.D., Boulder, CO, November 26, 1998. Interview: Desai, B., Boulder, CO, May 5, 1997.

21. Interview: Desai, D., and A. Desai, Wedding at Boulder, Colorado, May 17, 1997.

22. Pottinger et al., The End of Life.

23. Bibby, R.W. *Restless Gods: The Renaissance of Religion in Canada*. Toronto: Stoddart, 2002.

24. Andrews, M.M., and P.A. Hanson, Religion, Culture, and Nursing. In M.M. Andrews and J.S. Boyle (eds.), *Transcultural Concepts in Nursing Care*, 4th ed. (pp. 432–469). Philadelphia, Lippincott, 2003.

25. Choquette, R., *Canada's Religions*. Ottawa: University of Ottawa Press, 2004.

26. Choquette, *Canada's Religions*.

27. Mauk, K.L., and N.A. Schmidt. *Spiritual Care in Nursing Practice*. Philadelphia: Lippincott Williams and Wilkins, 2004.

28. Muramoto, O., Jehovah's Witnesses and Artificial Blood. *Canadian Medical Association Journal* 164(7) (2001), 969.

29. Andrews and Hanson, Religion, Culture, and Nursing.

30. Andrews and Hanson, Religion, Culture, and Nursing.

31. Kulig, J.C., and C. McCaslin, Health Care for the Mexican Mennonites in Canada, *Canadian Nurse*, 94(6) (1998), 34–39.

32. Wenger, A.F., and M.R. Wenger, The Amish. In L.D. Purnell and B.J. Paulanka (eds.), *Transcultural Health Care: A Culturally Competent Approach*, 2nd ed. (pp. 54–67). Philadelphia, F.A. Davis Company, 2003.

33. Choquette, *Canada's Religions*.

34. Correctional Services Canada. *Chaplaincy Services*. Website: http://www.csc-scc.gc.ca/text/prgm/chap_e.shtml (accessed May 2007).

35. Hajela, R., A Working Guide to Illness Beliefs and Paths of Healing. In R.H. Srivastava (ed.), *The Health Professional's Guide to Clinical Cultural Competence* (pp. 172–183). Toronto: Elsevier Canada, 2007.

36. Correctional Services Canada, *Chaplaincy Services*.

37. Hunter, L.M., J. Logan, J-G. Goulet, and S. Barton, Aboriginal Healing: Regaining Balance and Culture, *Journal of Transcultural Nursing*, 17(1) (2006), 13–22.

38. Hunter et al., Aboriginal Healing: Regaining Balance and Culture.

39. Correctional Services Canada, *Chaplaincy Services*.

40. Choquette, *Canada's Religions*.

41. Andrews and Hanson, Religion, Culture, and Nursing.

42. Choquette, *Canada's Religions*.

43. Choquette, *Canada's Religions*.

44. Bibby, *Restless Gods: The Renaissance of Religion in Canada*.

45. Choquette, *Canada's Religions*.

46. Choquette, *Canada's Religions*.

47. Ontario Consultants on Religious Tolerance. *New Age Spirituality*. Website: http://www.religioustolerence.org/ (accessed May 2007).

48. Choquette, *Canada's Religions*.

49. Wright, K., Professional, Ethical, and Legal Implications for Spiritual Care in Nursing, *IMAGE: Journal of Nursing Scholarship*, 30(1) (1998), 81–83.

50. Stafford, T., The Hidden Gospel of the 12 Steps, *Christianity Today*, 35(8) (1991), 14–19.

51. Statistics Canada, *2001 Census: Analysis Series, Religions in Canada*.

52. Choquette, *Canada's Religions*; Bibby, R.W. *Fragmented Gods: The Poverty and Potential of Religion in Canada*. Toronto: Stoddart, 1987; Bibby, R.W. *Unknown Gods: The Ongoing Story of Religions in Canada*. Toronto: Stoddart, 1993; Bibby, *Restless Gods: The Renaissance of Religion in Canada*; Fay, T.J. *A History of Canadian Catholics*. Montreal: McGill-Queen's University Press, 2002; Stackhouse, J.G., Jr. *Canadian Evangelicalism in the Twentieth Century: An Introduction to Its Character*. Toronto: University of Toronto Press, 1993.

53. Choquette, *Canada's Religions*.

54. Bibby, *Fragmented Gods: The Poverty and Potential of Religion in Canada*; Bibby, *Unknown Gods: The Ongoing Story of Religions in Canada*.

55. Bibby, *Restless Gods: The Renaissance of Religion in Canada*.

56. Fay, *A History of Canadian Catholics*.

57. Clark, W., and G. Schellenberg, Who's Religious? *Canadian Social Trends*, 81(Summer) (2006), 2–9.

58. Macionis, J.J., and L.M. Gerber, *Sociology*, 6th Canadian ed. Toronto: Pearson Education Canada, 2008.

59. Macionis and Gerber, *Sociology*.

60. Choquette, *Canada's Religions*.

61. Potter, P.A., and S. Grypma, Spiritual Health. In P.A. Potter, A.G. Perry, J.C. Ross-Kerr, and M.J. Wood (eds.), *Canadian Fundamentals of Nursing*, 3rd ed. Toronto: Elsevier Canada, 2006.

62. Taylor, E.J. *Spiritual Care: Nursing Theory, Research, and Practice*. Upper Saddle River, NJ: Prentice Hall, 2002.

63. Mauk, K.L., and N.K. Schmidt. *Spiritual Care in Nursing Practice*. Philadelphia: Lippincott Williams & Wilkins, 2004.

64. Potter and Grypma, *Spiritual Health*.

65. Sandor, M.K., and R.D. Froman, Exploring the Effects of Walking the Labyrinth, *Journal of Holistic Nursing*, 24(2) (2006), 103–110.

66. Potter and Grypma, *Spiritual Health*.

67. Olson, J.K., P. Paul, L. Douglass, M.B. Clark, J. Simington, and N. Goddard, Addressing the Spiritual Dimension in Canadian

Undergraduate Nursing Education, *Canadian Journal of Nursing Research*, 35(3) (2003), 94–107.

68. Kirsh, B.D., S. Antolikova, and L. Reynolds, Developing Awareness of Spirituality in Occupational Therapy Students: Are Our Curricula Up to the Task? *Occupational Therapy International*, 8(2) (2001), 119–125.

69. Grabovac, A., and S. Ganesan, Spirituality and Religion in Canadian Psychiatric Residency Training, *Canadian Journal of Psychiatry*, 48(3) (2003), 171–175.

70. Petersen, B., The Mind–Body Connection, *The Canadian Nurse*, 92(1) (1996), 29–31; Canadian Nurses Association, Association Promotes Holistic Nursing Practice, *Canadian Nurse*, 103(1) (2007), 10.

71. Canadian Holistic Nurses Association. *Philosophy and Objectives*. Website: http://mypage.direct.ca/h/hutchings/chna.html (accessed May 2007).

72. CNA, Association Promotes Holistic Nursing Practice.

73. Wright, Professional, Ethical, and Legal Implications for Spiritual Care in Nursing.

74. Meyerhoff, H., L. van Hofwegen, C. Hoe Harwood, M. Drury, and J. Emblen, Emotional Rescue: Spiritual Nursing Interventions, *Canadian Nurse*, 98(3) (2002), 21–24.

75. Wright, Spirituality, Suffering, and Illness: Ideas for Healing.

76. Pesut, B., The Development of Nursing Students' Spirituality and Spiritual Care-Giving, *Nurse Educator Today*, 22 (2002), 128–135.

77. Chilton, Recognizing Spirituality; Plante, Formula for a Miracle; Rubin, The Healing Power of Prayer.

78. Hurley, J., Breaking the Spiritual Care Barrier, *Journal of Christian Nursing*, 16(3) (1999), 8–13.

79. Wallace, N., My Name Is Jim? Do You Know Me? *Journal of Christian Nursing*, 16(3) (1999), 36–37.

80. Wright, L.M., Suffering and Spirituality: The Soul of Clinical Work with Families, *Journal of Family Nursing*, 3(1) (1997), 3–14.

81. Buijs, R., and J. Olson, Parish Nurses Influencing Determinants of Health, *Journal of Community Health Nursing*, 92(1) (2001), 13–23.

82. Martin, L.B., Parish Nursing: Keeping Body and Soul Together, *The Canadian Nurse*, 92(1) (1996), 25–28.

83. Canadian Association for Parish Nursing Ministry. *Historical Perspective of Parish Nursing in Canada*. Website: http://www.capnm.ca/historical_overview.htm (accessed May 2007).

84. Clark, M., and J. Olson. *Nursing within a Faith Community: Promoting Health in Time of Transition*. Thousand Oaks, CA: Sage, 2000.

85. Simington, J., J. Olson, and L. Douglass, Promoting Well-Being within a Parish, *The Canadian Nurse*, 92(1) (1996), 20–34.

86. Fredland, N., Promoting Healthy Partnerships with Faith Communities. In A.R. Vollman, E.T. Anderson, and J. McFarlane (eds.), *Canadian Community as Partner: Theory and Practice in Nursing*. Philadelphia: Lippincott Williams & Wilkins, 2004.

87. Simington et al. Promoting Well-Being within a Parish; Canadian Association for Parish Nursing Ministry. *Guide for Parish Nursing Core Competencies*. Website: http://www.capnm.ca/core_competencies_standards_print.doc (accessed May 2007).

88. Meyerhoff et al., Emotional Rescue: Spiritual Nursing Interventions.

89. Koenig, H.G., Religion, Spirituality, and Medicine: Research Findings and Implications for Clinical Practice, *Southern Medical Journal*, 97(12) (2004), 1194–1200.

90. O'Mathuna, D., Prayer Research: What Are We Measuring? *Journal of Christian Nursing*, 16(3) (1999), 17–21.

91. Hudson, T., Measuring the Results of Faith, *Hospitals and Health Networks*, September 20, 1996, 23–28.

92. Chiu, L., J.D. Emblen, L. Van Hofwegen, R. Sawatzky, and H. Meyerhoff, An Integrative Review of the Concept of Spirituality in the Health Sciences, *Western Journal of Nursing Research*, 26(4) (2004), 405–428.

93. Stranahan, S., Spiritual Perception, Attitudes about Spiritual Care, and Spiritual Care Practices among Nurse Practitioners, *Western Journal of Nursing*, 23(1) (2001), 90.

94. Rankin, E.A., and M.B. DeLashmutt, Finding Spirituality and Nursing Presence: The Student's Challenge, *Journal of Holistic Nursing*, 24(4) (2006), 282–288.

95. Potter and Grypma, Spiritual Health.

96. Donley, Sr., R., Spiritual Dimensions of Health Care: Nursing's Mission, *Nursing and Health Care*, 12(4) (1991), 178–183.

## Chapter 4

1. Seifert, K., R. Hoffnung, and M. Hoffnung. *Lifespan Development*. Boston: Houghton Mifflin, 1997.

2. Ambert, A-M. *Changing Families: Relationships in Context*, Canadian ed. Toronto: Pearson Education Canada, 2005.

3. Baker, M., Definitions, Cultural Variations, and Demographic Trends. In M. Baker (ed.), *Families: Changing Trends in Canada*, 4th ed. (pp. 3, 4). Toronto: McGraw-Hill Ryerson, 2001.

4. Canadian Health Network. *Canadian Families*. Website: http://www.canadian-health-network.ca/ (accessed July 2007).

5. Canadian Health Network, *Canadian Families*.

6. Hanson, S.M., V. Gedaly-Duff, and J.R. Kaakinen. *Family Health Care Nursing: Theory, Practice, and Research*, 3rd ed. Philadelphia: F.A. Davis, 2005.

7. Doane, G.H., and C. Varcoe. *Family Nursing as Relational Inquiry: Developing Health-Promoting Practice*. Philadelphia: Lippincott Williams & Wilkins, 2005.

8. Wright, L.M., M. Leahey, and A.G. Perry, Family Nursing. In P.A. Potter, A.G. Perry, J.C. Ross-Kerr, and M.J. Wood (eds.), *Canadian Fundamentals of Nursing* (pp. 295, 299). Toronto: Elsevier, 2006.

9. Vanier Institute of the Family. *Contemporary Family Trends, Aboriginal Family Trends*. Website: http://www.vifamily.ca/library/cft/aboriginal.html/ (accessed July 2007).

10. Dion Stout, M., with C.R. Bruyere, Stopping Family Violence: Aboriginal Communities Enspirited. In J.R. Ponting (ed.), *First Nations in Canada: Perspectives on Opportunity, Empowerment, and Self-Determination* (pp. 273–288). Toronto: McGraw-Hill Ryerson, 1997.

11. Vanier Institute of the Family, *Contemporary Family Trends, Aboriginal Family Trends*.

12. Vanier Institute of the Family, *Contemporary Family Trends, Aboriginal Family Trends*.

13. Friedman, M., V. Bowden, and E. Jones. *Family Nursing: Research, Theory and Family Practice*, 5th ed. Upper Saddle River, NJ: Prentice Hall, 2003.

14. Papalia, D., S. Olds, and R. Feldman. *Human Development*, 9th ed. Boston: McGraw-Hill, 2004. Arnup, K., Lesbian and Gay Parents. In N. Mandell and A. Duffy (eds.), *Canadian Families: Diversity, Conflict and Change*, 3rd ed. (p. 176). Toronto: Harcourt Canada, 2005.

15. Alderson, K.G., A Phenomenological Investigation of Same-Sex Marriage, *The Canadian Journal of Human Sexuality*, 13(2) (2004), 107–123.

16. Vanier Institute of the Family. *Contemporary Family Trends: Same-Sex Couples and Same-Sex-Parent Families: Relationships, Parenting, and Issues of Marriage*. Website: http://www.vifamily.ca/ (accessed July 2007).

17. Brotman, S., B. Ryan, Y. Jalbert, and B. Rowe, The Impact of Coming Out on Health and Health Care Access: The Experience of Gay, Lesbian, Bisexual and Two-Spirit People, *Journal of Health & Social Policy*, 15(1) (2002), 1–29.

18. Panetta, A. *Canada Approves Same-Sex Marriage*. Website: http://www.canada.com/ (accessed July 2007).
19. Conservative Party of Canada. *Federal Election Platform 2006*. Ottawa: Author, 2006.
20. Canadian Broadcasting Corporation. *MPs Defeat Bid to Reopen Same-Sex Marriage Debate*, Thursday, Dec. 7, 2006. Website: http://www.cbc.ca/ (accessed July 2007).
21. Canadian Health Network, *Canadian Families*.
22. Canadian Health Network, *Canadian Families*.
23. Friedman et al. *Family Nursing: Research, Theory and Family Practice*.
24. Vanier Institute of the Family. *It Keeps Getting Faster: Changing Patterns of Time in Families*. Website: http://www.vifamily.ca/ (accessed July 2007).
25. Vanier Institute of the Family, *It Keeps Getting Faster: Changing Patterns of Time in Families*.
26. Vanier Institute of the Family, *It Keeps Getting Faster: Changing Patterns of Time in Families*.
27. Vanier Institute of the Family, *It Keeps Getting Faster: Changing Patterns of Time in Families*.
28. Frederick, J.A. *As Time Goes By ... Time Use by Canadians*. Ottawa: Ministry of Supply and Services and Statistics Canada, 1995.
29. Vanier Institute of the Family. *Contemporary Family Trends: The Effects of the Changing Age Structure on Households and Families to 2026*. Website: http://www.vifamily.ca/ (accessed July 2007).
30. Hall, W.A., and P. Callery, Balancing Personal and Family Trajectories: An International Study of Dual-Earner Couples with Pre-school Children, *International Journal of Nursing Studies*, 40(4) (2003), 401–412.
31. Hall, W.A., and P. Callery, Balancing Personal and Family Trajectories: An International Study of Dual-Earner Couples with Pre-school Children, *International Journal of Nursing Studies*, 40(4) (2003), 401–412.
32. Friedman et al. *Family Nursing: Research, Theory and Family Practice*.
33. Papalia et al. *Human Development*.
34. Papalia et al. *Human Development*.
35. Jones, E., Deaf and Hearing Parents' Perceptions of Family Functioning, *Nursing Research*, 44(2) (1995), 102–105.
36. White, J.M., L.E. Larson, J.W. Goltz, and B.E. Munro. *Families in Canada: Social Contexts, Continuities, and Changes*, 3rd ed. Toronto: Pearson Prentice Hall, 2005.
37. Rutter, M., Nature, Nurture, and Development: From Evangelism through Science toward Policy and Practice, *Child Development*, 73 (2002), 1–21.
38. Friedman et al. *Family Nursing: Research, Theory, & Practice*.
39. Friedman et al. *Family Nursing: Research, Theory, & Practice*.
40. Dion Stout & Bruyere, Stopping Family Violence: Aboriginal Communities Enspirited.
41. Dion Stout & Bruyere, Stopping Family Violence: Aboriginal Communities Enspirited.
42. Canada. *Report of the Royal Commission on Aboriginal Peoples*, Vol. 3: Gathering Strength. Ottawa: Minister of Supply and Services, 1996.
43. Friedman et al. *Family Nursing: Research, Theory, & Practice*.
44. Friedman et al. *Family Nursing: Research, Theory, & Practice*.
45. Bee, H., D. Boyd, and P. Johnson. *Lifespan Development*, 2nd Canadian ed. Toronto: Pearson Education Canada, 2006; Friedman et al. *Family Nursing: Research, Theory, & Practice*; Papalia et al., *Human Development*; Wright, L., and M. Leahey. *Nurses and Families: A Guide to Family Assessment and Intervention*, 4th ed. Philadelphia: F.A. Davis, 2005.
46. Carter, B., and M. McGoldrick, Overview: The Expanded Family Life Cycle: Individual, Family, and Social Perspectives. In B. Carter and M. McGoldrick (eds.), *The Expanded Family Life Cycle: Individual, Family, and Social Perspectives*, 3rd ed. (pp. 1–26). Boston: Allyn & Bacon, 1999.
47. Wright and Leahey, *Nurses and Families: A Guide to Family Assessment and Intervention*, 4th ed.
48. McGoldrick, M., and B. Carter, The Family Circle. In F. Walsh (ed.), *Normal Family Processes: Growing Diversity and Complexity*, 3rd ed. (pp. 375–392). New York: The Guilford Press, 2003.
49. McGoldrick and Carter, The Family Circle.
50. Wright and Leahey. *Nurses and Families: A Guide to Family Assessment and Intervention*, 4th ed.; McGoldrick and Carter, The Family Circle.
51. Wright and Leahey, *Nurses and Families: A Guide to Family Assessment and Intervention*, 4th ed.
52. McGoldrick and Carter, The Family Circle.
53. Wright and Leahey, *Nurses and Families: A Guide to Family Assessment and Intervention*, 4th ed.
54. Vanier Institute of the Family. *Contemporary Family Trends–Divorce: Facts, Causes, and Consequences*. Ottawa: Author, 2005.
55. Kelly, J.B., and E. Emery, Children's Adjustment Following Divorce: Risk and Resilience Perspectives, *Family Relations*, 52 (2003), 352–362.
56. Vanier Institute of the Family, Canada's Stepfamilies, *Transition Magazine*, 33(4) (Winter 2003–2004). Website: http://www.vifamily.ca/library/transition/334/334.html (accessed July 2007).
57. Wright and Leahey, *Nurses and Families: A Guide to Family Assessment and Intervention*, 4th ed.
58. Fulmer, R.H. Lower-Income and Professional Families: A Comparison of Structure and Life Cycle Processes. In B. Carter and M. McGoldrick (eds.), *The Expanded Family Life Cycle: Individual Family and Social Perspectives*, 3rd ed. (pp. 545–578). Boston: Allyn & Bacon, 1999.
59. Fulmer, Lower-Income and Professional Families: A Comparison of Structure and Life Cycle Processes.
60. Wright and Leahey, *Nurses and Families: A Guide to Family Assessment and Intervention*, 4th ed.
61. Papalia et al., *Human Development*.
62. Johnson, T.W., and P. Colucci, Lesbians, Gay Men, and the Family Life Cycle. In B. Carter and M. McGoldrick (eds.), *The Expanded Family Life Cycle: Individual Family and Social Perspectives*, 3rd ed. (pp. 346–361). Boston: Allyn & Bacon, 1999.
63. Roberts, S.J., Health Care Recommendations for Lesbian Women, *Journal of Obstetric, Gynecologic, & Neonatal Nursing*, 35(5) (2006), 583–591.
64. Papalia et al., *Human Development*; Wright and Leahey, *Nurses and Families: A Guide to Family Assessment and Intervention*, 4th ed.
65. Vanier Institute of the Family. *Contemporary Family Trends, Portraits of Fathers*. Website: http://www.vifamily.ca/ (accessed July 2007).
66. Steinberg, S., L. Kruckman, and S. Steinberg, Reinventing Fatherhood in Japan and Canada, *Social Science & Medicine*, 50(9) (2000), 1257–1272.
67. Steinberg et al., Reinventing Fatherhood in Japan and Canada.
68. Leininger, M., Japanese Americans and Culture Care. In M. Leininger and M.R. McFarland (eds.), *Transcultural Nursing: Concepts, Theories, Research & Practice*, 3rd ed. (pp. 453–463). New York: McGraw-Hill, 2002.
69. Steinberg et al., Reinventing Fatherhood in Japan and Canada.
70. Leininger, Japanese Americans and Culture Care.
71. Crawford, J.A. and M.A. Tarko, Family Communication. In P.J. Bomar (ed.), *Promoting Health in Families*, 3rd ed. (pp. 162–186). Philadelphia: Saunders Press, 2004.
72. Smalley, G., *Advice You Can Bank On, Focus on the Family*, February 1997, 2–4.
73. Bee et al., *Lifespan Development*.
74. Kahana, E., D. Biegel, and M. Wykle. *Family Caregiving across the Lifespan*. Thousand Oaks, CA: Sage, 1994.
75. Wright and Leahey. *Nurses and Families: A Guide to Family Assessment and Intervention*, 4th ed.

76. Papalia et al., *Human Development*; Wright and Leahey. *Nurses and Families: A Guide to Family Assessment and Intervention*, 4th ed.
77. Ambert, *Changing Families: Relationships in Context*.
78. Ricci, S.S., Infant. In C.L. Edelman and C.L. Mandle (eds.), *Health Promotion throughout the Life-Span*, 6th ed. (pp. 376–415). St. Louis: Mosby, 2006.
79. Bee et al., *Lifespan Development*.
80. Sulloway, F., Birth Order and Personality, *Harvard Mental Health Letter*, *14*(3) (1997), 5–7.
81. Sulloway, *Birth Order and Personality*.
82. Baker, M., The Future of Family Life. In M. Baker (ed.), *Families: Changing Trends in Canada*, 4th ed. (pp. 285–302). Toronto: McGraw-Hill Ryerson, 2001.
83. Wen, S.W., Multiple Birth Rate in Health Canada. *In Health Canada, Canadian Perinatal Health Report*. Ottawa: Minister of Public Works and Government Services Canada, 2003.
84. Canadian Council on Social Development. *A Profile of Canadian Families*. Ottawa: Author, 2004.
85. Multiple Births Canada. Website: http://www.multiplebirthscanada.org/ (accessed July 2007).
86. Mom2many: Parents of Multiples across Canada. Website: http://www.mom2many.com/ (accessed July 2007).
87. Papalia et al., *Human Development*.
88. Damato, E., Prenatal Attachment and Other Correlates of Postnatal Maternal Attachment to Twins, *Advance Neonatal Care*, *4*(5) (2004), 274–291.
89. Bee et al., *Lifespan Development*.
90. Smit, E., Unique Issues of the Adopted Child, *Journal of Psychosocial Nursing*, *34*(7) (1996), 29–36.
91. International Adoption—Canada. Website: http://www.canada.com/ (accessed July 2007).
92. Canada Adopts. Website: http://www.canadaadopts.com/ (accessed July 2007).
93. Baker, M. *Families: Changing Trends in Canada*, 4th ed. Toronto: McGraw-Hill Ryerson, 2001.
94. Ward, M. *The Family Dynamic: A Canadian Perspective*, 3rd ed. Toronto: Nelson Thomson Learning, 2002.
95. Canada Adopts. Website: http://www.canadaadopts.com/ (accessed July 2007).
96. Schaffer, J., and C. Londstrum, *How to Raise an Adopted Child*. New York: Crown, 1989.
97. Bird, G. W., R. Peterson, and S.H. Miller, Factors Associated with Distress among Support-seeking Adoptive Families, *Family Relations*, *51* (2002), 215–220.
98. Barth, R.P., and J.M. Miller, Building Effective Post Adoption Services: What is the Empirical Foundation? *Family Relations*, *49* (2000), 447–455.
99. Ritchie, C., Adoption: An Option Often Overlooked, *American Journal of Nursing*, *89*(9) (1989), 1156–1157; Schaffer and Londstrum, *How to Raise an Adopted Child*.
100. Carriere, J. Connectedness and Health for First Nations Adoptees, *Paediatric Child Health*, *10*(9) (2005), 545–548.
101. Carleton GLBTQ Centre for Sexual and Gender Diversity. *Education, Advocacy and Support*. Ottawa: Carleton University Students' Association. Website: http://www.carlton.ca/ (accessed July 2007).
102. Erich, S., P. Leung, P. Kindle, and S. Carter, Gay and Lesbian Adoptive Families: An Exploratory Study of family Functioning, Adoptive Child's Behaviour, and Familial Support Networks, *Journal of Family Social Work*, *9*(1) (2005), 17–28.
103. Lansford, J.E., Does Family Structure Matter? A Comparison of Adoptive, Two-Parent Biological, Single-Mother, Stepfather, and Stepmother Households, *Journal of Marriage and Family*, *63* (2001), 840–851.
104. Schaffer and Londstrum, *How to Raise an Adopted Child*.
105. Bee et al., *Lifespan Development*; Webster, P., and A. Herzog, Effects of Parental Divorce and Memories of Family Problems in Relationships between Adult Children and Their Parents, *Journal of Gerontology: Social Sciences*, *50B*(1) (1995), 823–834.
106. Vanier Institute of the Family. *Contemporary Family Trends: The Changing Culture of Parenting*. Website: http://www.vifamily.ca/ (accessed July 2007).
107. Lynn, M.M., Single-Parent Families. In M.M. Lynn (ed.), *Voices: Essays on Canadian Families*, 2nd ed. (pp. 32–33). Toronto: Thomson Nelson, 2003.
108. Lynn, Single-Parent Families.
109. Ford-Gilboe, M., Family Strengths, Motivation, and Resources as Predictors of Health Promotion Behavior in Single-parent and Two-parent Families, *Research in Nursing*, *20*(3) (1997), 205–217; McLanahan, S., and G. Sandefur. *Growing up With a Single Parent*. Cambridge, MA: Harvard University Press, 1994.
110. Ambert, *Changing Families: Relationships in Context*.
111. Ford-Gilboe, M., Dispelling Myths and Creating Opportunity: A Comparison of the Strengths of Single-Parent and Two-Parent Families, *Advances in Nursing Science*, *23*(1) (2000), 41–58.
112. Ford-Gilboe, Dispelling Myths and Creating Opportunity: A Comparison of the Strengths of Single-Parent and Two-Parent Families.
113. Church, E., Kinship and Stepfamilies. In M. Lynn (ed.), *Voices: Essays on Canadian Families*, 2nd ed. (pp. 32–33). Toronto: Thomson Nelson, 2003.
114. Statistics Canada, Census Operations Division. *2001 Census Handbook*. Ottawa: Minister of Industry, 2003.
115. Church, Kinship and Stepfamilies.
116. McDaniel, S.A., and L. Tepperman. *Close Relations: An Introduction to the Sociology of Families*, brief ed. Toronto: Prentice Hall, 2002.
117. Church, Kinship and Stepfamilies.
118. Mikan, A., and A. Peters, Couples Living Apart, *Canadian Social Trends*, Summer 2003. Statistics Canada Catalogue no. 11-008.
119. Mikan and Peters, Couples Living Apart.
120. Bee et al., *Lifespan Development*; Papalia et al., *Human Development*.
121. Santrock, J.W., A. MacKenzie-Rivers, K.H. Leung, and T. Malcomson. *Life-Span Development*, 1st Canadian ed. Toronto: McGraw-Hill Ryerson, 2003.
122. Riedmann, A., M.A. Lamanna, and A. Nelson. *Marriages and Families*, 1st Canadian ed. Toronto: Nelson Thomson Learning, 2003.
123. Vanier Institute of the Family, *Contemporary Family Trends, Grandparenthood in Canada*; Inwood, S. Family Ties: Grandparents Raising Grandchildren, *Canadian Nurse*, *98*(4) (2002), 21–25; Cangrands, Website: http://www.cangrands.com/ (accessed July 2007).
124. Canadian Health Network, *Canadian Families*.
125. Canadian Health Network, *Canadian Families*.
126. Statistics Canada. *2006 Census: Profile of Marital Status, Common-Law Status, Families, Dwellings and Households*. Website: http://www.statcan.ca/ (accessed July 2007).
127. Dicicco-Bloom, B., and D. Cohen, Home Nurses: A Study of the Occurrences of Culturally Competent Care, *Journal of Transcultural Nursing*, *14*(1) (2003), 25–31.
128. Bee et al., *Lifespan Development*.
129. Greenberg, P., Stay-Home Moms Need Support, Not Bad Mouthing, *American Family Association Journal*, May, 1998, 20.
130. Cheal, D., The One and the Many: Modernity and Post-Modernity. In C.J. Richardson (ed.), *Family Life: Patterns and Perspectives* (pp. 52–53). New York: McGraw-Hill, 1996.
131. Wright, L.M. and M. Leahey. *Nurses and Families: A Guide to Family Assessment and Intervention*, 3rd ed. Philadelphia: F.A. Davis Company, 2000.
132. Chan, E., Child Care: A Holistic and Family-Centred Approach, *Transition*, *31*(4) (2002), 6–9.

133. Papalia et al., *Human Development*.
134. Ward, *The Family Dynamic: A Canadian Perspective*.
135. Das Gupta, T., Families of Native People, Immigrants, and People of Colour. In N. Mandell and A. Duffy (eds.), *Canadian Families: Diversity, Conflict, and Change*, 2nd ed. (pp. 146–147). Toronto: Harcourt Brace Canada, 2000.
136. Canadian Institutes of Health Research. *Institute of Aboriginal Peoples' Health*. Website: http://www.cihr-irsc.gc.ca/ (accessed July 2007).
137. Vanier Institute of the Family. *Contemporary Family Trends, Strengths in Families: Accentuating the Positive*. Website: http://www.vifamily.ca/ (accessed July 2007).
138. Segarid, C.A. and W.A. Hall, The Family Theory-Practice Gap: A Matter of Clarity? *Nursing Inquiry, 12*(3) (2005), 210–218.
139. Wright, L.M. and J.M. Bell, Retrospective—Nurses, Families, and Illness: A New Combination, *Journal of Family Nursing, 10*(1) (2004), 3–11.
140. Rentfro, A.R., Health Promotion and the Family. In C.L. Edelman and C.L. Mandle (eds.), *Health Promotion throughout the Life-Span*, 6th ed. (pp. 152–177). St. Louis: Mosby, 2006; Wright and Leahey, *Nurses and Families: A Guide to Family Assessment and Intervention*, 4th ed.
141. Haugh, E.B., and B.L. Mildon, Practice Settings, Roles, and Functions. In L.L. Stamler and L. Yiu (eds.), *Community Health Nursing: A Canadian Perspective* (pp. 55–71). Toronto: Pearson, 2005.
142. Crawford and Tarko, Family Communication.
143. Crawford and Tarko, Family Communication.
144. Deering, C., and J. Frederick, Therapeutic Relationships and Communication. In W.K. Mohr (ed.), *Johnson's Psychiatric-Mental Health Nursing*, 5th ed. (pp. 53–75). Philadelphia: Lippincott, 2003.
145. Faulkner, A. *Effective Interaction with Patients*, 2nd ed. New York: Churchill Livingstone, 1998.
146. Fountaine, K.L. *Mental Health Nursing*, 5th ed. Upper Saddle River, NJ: Prentice Hall, 2003.
147. Wright, and Leahey, *Nurses and Families: A Guide to Family Assessment and Intervention*, 4th ed.
148. Stolte, K.M. Wellness: *Nursing Diagnosis for Health Promotion*. Philadelphia: Lippincott, 1996.
149. Stolte, Wellness: *Nursing Diagnosis for Health Promotion*.
150. Crawford, J.A., and M.A. Tarko, Family Communication. In P.J. Bomar (ed.), *Promoting Health in Families: Applying Family Research and Theory to Nursing Practice*, 3rd ed. (pp. 162–174). Philadelphia: Saunders, 2004.
151. Wright et al., Family Nursing.
152. Gottlieb, L.N., and B. Gottlieb, The Developmental/Health Framework within the McGill Model of Nursing "Laws of Nature" Guiding Whole Person Care, *Advances in Nursing Science, 30*(1) (2007), E43–E57.
153. Papalia et al., *Human Development*.
154. Papalia et al., *Human Development*.
155. Papalia et al., *Human Development*.
156. Papalia et al., *Human Development*.
157. Wright et al., Family Nursing.
158. Papalia et al., *Human Development*.
159. McNeill, T., Fathers' Experience of Parenting a Child with Juvenile Rheumatoid Arthritis, *Qualitative Health Research, 14*(4) (2004), 526–545.
160. Bee et al., *Lifespan Development*.
161. Papalia et al., *Human Development*.

**Chapter 5**

1. Nutbeam, D., and E. Harris. *Theory in a Nutshell*, 2nd ed. Toronto: McGraw-Hill, 2004.
2. Bee, H., D. Boyd, and P. Johnson. *Lifespan Development*, 2nd Canadian ed. Toronto: Pearson Education, 2006.
3. Fellous, J-M, and J.E. Ledoux, Toward Basic Principles for Emotional Processing: What the Fearful Brain Tells the Robot. In J-M. Fellous and M.A. Arbib (eds.), *Who Needs Emotions? The Brain Meets the Robot* (pp. 79, 83). New York: Oxford University Press, 2005.
4. Papalia, D., S. Olds, and R. Feldman. *Human Development*, 9th ed. Toronto: McGraw-Hill, 2004.
5. Collins, F., E. Green, A. Guttmacher, and M. Guyer, A Vision for the Future of Genomics Research, *Nature, 422* (2003), 835–847.
6. Bottorff, J.L., M. McCullum, L.G. Balneaves, M.J. Esplen, J. Carroll, M. Kelly, and S. Kieffer, Canadian Nursing in the Genomic Era: A Call for Leadership, *Nursing Research, 18* (2005), 56–72; Loescher, L. J., and C.J. Merkle, The Interface of Genomic Technologies and Nursing, *Journal of Nursing Scholarship*, 2nd Quarter (2005), 111–119.
7. Papalia et al., *Human Development*.
8. Thibodeau, G.A., and K.T. Patton, *Anatomy & Physiology*, 6th ed. St. Louis, MO: Mosby Elsevier, 2007.
9. Thibodeau and Patton, *Anatomy & Physiology*; Talon, J., Brain Study Finds Depression Clue: A Severe Depletion of Key Support Cells, *NAMI Advocate*, January–February 1998, 20.
10. Papalia et al., *Human Development*.
11. Jang, K.L., P.A. Vernon, W.J. Livesley, M.B. Stein, and H. Wolf, Intra- and Extra-Familial Influences on Alcohol and Drug Misuse: A Twin Study of Gene-Environment Correlation, *Addiction, 96* (2001) 1307–1318.
12. Katzmarzyk, P.T., R.M. Malina, L. Perusse, T. Rice, M.A. Province, D.C. Rao, and C. Bouchard, Familial Resemblance in Fatness and Fat Distribution, *American Journal of Human Biology, 12*(3) (2000), 395–404.
13. Simonen, R.L., L. Perusse, T. Rankinen, T. Rice, D.C. Rao, and C. Bouchard, Familial Aggregation of Physical Activity Levels in the Quebec Family Study, *Medicine and Science in Sports and Exercise, 34* (2002), 1137–1142.
14. Thibodeau and Patton, *Anatomy & Physiology*.
15. Papalia et al., *Human Development*.
16. Collins et al., A Vision for the Future of Genomics Research.
17. Bee et al. *Lifespan Development*; O'Connor, C., Are We More Than the Sum of Our Genes? *Washington University Outlook*, Fall 1997, 10–15; Papalia et al., *Human Development*.
18. Rutter, M. Gene-Environment Interdependence. *Developmental Science, 10*(1) (2007), 12–18.
19. Lewin, B., *Genes VII*, Upper Saddle River, NJ: Pearson Prentice Hall, 2004.
20. Peedicayil, J., Epigenetic Therapy—A New Development in Pharmacology, *Indian Journal of Medical Research, 123*(1) (2006), 17–24.
21. Hegele, R.A., Environmental Modulation of Atherosclerosis End Points in Familial Hypercholesterolemia, *Atherosclerosis Supplements, 2*(3) (2002), 5–7.
22. Public Health Agency of Canada, *The Healthy Heart Kit: Controlling Your Blood Cholesterol*. Website: www.healthyheartkit.com (accessed April 2007).
23. Public Health Agency of Canada, *The Healthy Heart Kit: Controlling Your Blood Cholesterol*.
24. Hegle, R.A., H. Cao, A.J.G. Hanley, B. Zinman, S.B. Harris, and C.M. Anderson, Clinical Utility of HNF1A Genotyping for Diabetes in Aboriginal Canadians, *Diabetes Care, 23*(6) (2002) 775–778.
25. Hegle et al., Clinical Utility of HNF1A Genotyping for Diabetes in Aboriginal Canadians.
26. Young, T.K., J. Reading, B. Elias, and J.D. O'Neil, Type 2 Diabetes Mellitus in Canada's First Nations: Status of an Epidemic in Progress, *Canadian Medical Association Journal, 163*(5) (2000), 561–566.
27. Hegle et al., Clinical Utility of HNF1A Genotyping for Diabetes in Aboriginal Canadians.

28. Pranke, P., Fetal Development. In M.A. Hogan and R.S. Glazebrook (eds.), *Maternal-Newborn Nursing* (pp. 77–80). Upper Saddle River, NJ: Prentice-Hall, 2003; Shah, C.P., *Public Health and Preventative Medicine in Canada*, 5th ed. Toronto: Elsevier Canada, 2003.

29. Collins, F., and V. McKusick, Implications of the Human Genome Project for Medical Science, *Journal of the American Medical Association*, 285(19) (2001), 2447–2448.

30. Ontario Report to Premiers, *Genetics and Gene Patenting: Charting New Territory in Healthcare*. Website: www.health.gov.on.ca/english/public/pub/ministry_reports/geneticsrep02/report_e.pdf (accessed April 2007).

31. Shah, C.P., *Public Health and Preventative Medicine in Canada*.

32. Guttman, M., S.J. Kish, and Y. Furukawa, Current Concepts in the Diagnosis and Management of Parkinson's Disease, *Canadian Medical Association Journal*, 168(3) (2003), 293–301.

33. Genome Canada, *About Genome Canada*. Website: http://www.genomecanada.ca (accessed April 2007).

34. Genome Canada, *Media*. Website: http://www.genomecanada.ca (accessed April 2007).

35. Ontario Genomics Institute, *About OGI*. Website: http://www.ontariogenomics.ca/ (accessed April 2007).

36. Ontario Genomics Institute, *Annual Report 2005–2006: The Future Is in Our Genes*. Toronto: Author. Website: http://www.ontariogenomics.ca/ogi/docs/OGI_AnnualReport_2006.pdf (accessed April 2007).

37. Hockenberry, M.J., D. Wilson, M.L. Winkelstein, and N.E. Kline. *Wong's Nursing Care of Infants and Children*, 7th ed. St. Louis, MO: Mosby, 2003.

38. Wilson, R.D., G. Davies, V. Desilets, G.J. Reid, D. Shaw, A. Summers, P. Wyatt et al., Cystic Fibrosis Carrier Testing in Pregnancy in Canada, *Journal of Obstetrics and Gynaecology Canada*, 24(8) (2002), 644–651.

39. Allen, V.M., R.D. Wilson, and A. Cheung, Pregnancy Outcomes after Assisted Reproductive Technology, *Journal of Obstetrics and Gynaecology of Canada*, 28(3) (2006), 220–250.

40. Canadian Nurses Association, *Position Statement: The Role of the Nurse in Reproductive and Genetic Technologies*. Website: http://www.cna-nurses.ca/ (accessed April 2007).

41. Cox, S.M., Human Genetics, Ethics, and Disability. In J.L. Storch, P. Rodney, and R. Starzomski (eds.), *Toward a Moral Horizon: Nursing Ethics for Leadership and Practice* (pp. 378–379). Toronto: Pearson Education Canada, 2004.

42. Loescher and Merkle, The Interface of Genomic Technologies and Nursing.

43. Bottorff et al., Canadian Nursing in the Genomic Era: A Call for Leadership.

44. Bottorff, J.L., M. McCullum, L. Balneaves, M. Esplen, J. Carroll, M. Kelly, and S. Kieffer, Nursing and Genetics, *Canadian Nurse*, 100(8) (2004), 24–28.

45. Thibodeau and Patton, *Anatomy & Physiology*.

46. Day, R.A., P. Paul, B. Williams, S.C. Smeltzer, and B.G. Bare, *Brunner & Suddarth's Textbook of Medical-Surgical Nursing*, 1st Canadian ed. Philadelphia: Lippincott Williams & Wilkins, 2007.

47. Liu, S., R. Semenciw, A-M Ugnat, and Y. Mao, Increasing Thyroid Cancer Incidence in Canada, 1970–1996: Time Trends and Age-Period-Cohort Effects. *British Journal of Cancer*, 85(9) (2001), 1335–1339.

48. Kail, R.V., J.C. Cavanaugh, and C.A. Ateah, *Human Development: A Life-Span View*, 1st Canadian ed. Toronto: Thomson Nelson, 2006.

49. Thibodeau and Patton, *Anatomy & Physiology*.

50. Thibodeau and Patton, *Anatomy & Physiology*.

51. Bee et al. *Lifespan Development*.

52. Thibodeau and Patton, *Anatomy & Physiology*.

53. Talon, Brain Study Finds Depression Clue: A Severe Depletion of Key Support Cells.

54. Young Johnson, J. *Handbook for Brunner and Suddarth's Textbook of Medical Surgical Nursing*, 10th ed. Philadelphia: Lippincott Williams & Wilkins, 2004.

55. Peschken, C.A., and J.M. Esdaile, Systematic Lupus Erythematosus in North American Indians: A Population Based Study, *Journal of Rheumatology*, 27(8) (2000), 1884–1891.

56. Hockenberry et al., *Wong's Nursing Care of Infants and Children*.

57. Public Health Agency of Canada, *Canada's Report on HIV/AIDS*. Website: http://www.phac-aspc.gc.ca/ (accessed April 2007).

58. Seifert, K., R. Hoffnung, and M. Hoffnung. *Lifespan Development*. Boston: Houghton Mifflin, 1997.

59. Ward, M. *The Family Dynamic: A Canadian Perspective*, 3rd Canadian ed. Scarborough, ON: Nelson Thomson Learning, 2002.

60. Harman, L.D., Family Poverty and Economic Struggles. In N. Mandell and A. Duffy (eds.), *Canadian Families* (pp. 241, 260). Toronto: Harcourt Brace, 2005.

61. Seifert et al., Lifespan Development.

62. Zhang, J., and M.J. Verhoef, Illness Management Strategies among Chinese Immigrants Living with Arthritis, *Social Science & Medicine*, 55(10) (2002), 1795–1802.

63. Ward, *The Family Dynamic: A Canadian Perspective*.

64. DeWit, D.J., Frequent Childhood Geographical Relocation: Its Impact on Drug Use Initiation and the Development of Alcohol and Other Drug-Related Problems among Adolescents and Young Adults, *Addictive Behaviors*, 23(5) (1998), 623–634.

65. DeWit, Frequent Childhood Geographical Relocation: Its Impact on Drug Use Initiation and the Development of Alcohol and Other Drug-Related Problems among Adolescents and Young Adults.

66. Ward, *The Family Dynamic: A Canadian Perspective*.

67. Von Bertalanffy, L., *General System Theory*. New York: George Braziller, 1968.

68. Wright, L.M., and M. Leahey, *Nurses and Families: A Guide to Family Assessment and Intervention*, 4th ed. Philadelphia: F.A. Davis, 2005; Friedman, M.M., V.R. Bowden, and E.G. Jones, *Family Nursing: Research, Theory, & Practice*, 5th ed. Upper Saddle River, NJ: Pearson Education, 2003.

69. Von Bertalanffy, L., The History and Status of General Systems Theory. In G. Klir (ed.), *Trends in General Systems Theory*. New York: Wiley, 1972; Von Bertalanffy, *General System Theory*.

70. Wright and Leahey, *Nurses and Families: A Guide to Family Assessment and Intervention*. Friedman et al. *Family Nursing: Research, Theory, & Practice*.

71. Wright and Leahey, *Nurses and Families: A Guide to Family Assessment and Intervention*; Friedman et al. *Family Nursing: Research, Theory, & Practice*; Von Bertalanffy, *The History and Status of General Systems Theory*; Von Bertalanffy, *General System Theory*; Sierchio, G.P., A Multidisciplinary Approach for Improving Outcomes, *Journal of Infusion Nursing*, 26(1) (2003), 34–43.

72. Friedman et al. *Family Nursing: Research, Theory, & Practice*.

73. Friedman et al. *Family Nursing: Research, Theory, & Practice*.

74. Wright and Leahey, *Nurses and Families: A Guide to Family Assessment and Intervention*.

75. Best, A., D. Stokols, L.W. Green, S. Leischow, B. Holmes, and K. Bucholz, An Integrative Framework for Community Partnering to Translate Theory into Effective Health Promotion Strategy, *The Science of Health Promotion*, 18(2) (2003), 168–176.

76. Wright and Leahey, *Nurses and Families: A Guide to Family Assessment and Intervention*.

77. Bee et al., *Lifespan Development*.

78. Sierchio, A Multidisciplinary Approach for Improving Outcomes.

79. Bronfenbrenner, U., The Ecology of Cognitive Development: Research Models and Fugitive Findings. In R. Wozniak and K. Fischer (eds.), *Development in Context: Acting and Thinking in*

*Specific Environments* (pp. 56, 83). Hillsdale, NJ: Lawrence Erlbaum Associates, 1993; Schaffer, D.R., E. Wood, and T. Willoughby, *Developmental Psychology: Childhood and Adolescence*, 1st Canadian ed. Scarborough, ON: Thomson Nelson, 2002.

80. Schaffer et al., *Developmental Psychology: Childhood and Adolescence*.

81. Patterson, C., and C. Watkins, *Theories of Psychotherapy*, 5th ed. New York: HarperCollins, 1996.

82. Patterson and Watkins, *Theories of Psychotherapy*.

83. Wade, C., C. Tavris, D. Saucier, and L. Elias, *Psychology*, 2nd Canadian ed. Toronto: Pearson Education Canada, 2007.

84. Wade et al. *Psychology*; Bee et al. *Lifespan Development*.

85. Patterson and Watkins, *Theories of Psychotherapy*.

86. Skinner, B.F., *Walden Two*. New York: Macmillan, 1948; Skinner, B.F., *Cumulative Record*, 3rd ed. New York: Appleton-Century-Crofts, 1972; Wade et al. *Psychology*.

87. Wade et al., *Psychology*; Santrock, J.W., A. MacKenzie-Rivers, K.H. Leung, and T. Malcomson, *Life-Span Development*, 2nd Canadian ed. Toronto: McGraw-Hill Ryerson, 2005.

88. Wade et al., *Psychology*.

89. Wade et al., *Psychology*; Bee et al., *Lifespan Development*.

90. Wade et al., *Psychology*; Bee et al., *Lifespan Development*.

91. Wade et al., *Psychology*.

92. Martin, G., and J. Pear. *Behavior Modification: What It Is and How to Do It*, 7th ed. Englewood Cliffs, NJ: Prentice-Hall, 2003.

93. Wade et al., *Psychology*.

94. Wade et al., *Psychology*.

95. Patterson and Watkins, *Theories of Psychotherapy*.

96. Patterson and Watkins, *Theories of Psychotherapy*.

97. Wade et al., *Psychology*.

98. Wade et al., *Psychology*; Frisch, N.C., and L.E. Frisch, *Psychiatric Mental Health Nursing*, 3rd ed. Scarborough, ON: Thomson Delmar Learning, 2006.

99. Frisch and Frisch, *Psychiatric Mental Health Nursing*.

100. Frisch and Frisch, *Psychiatric Mental Health Nursing*.

101. Papalia and Feldman, *Human Development*.

102. Sullivan, H.S. *The Interpersonal Theory of Psychiatry*. New York: W.W. Norton, 1953.

103. Sullivan, *The Interpersonal Theory of Psychiatry*.

104. Townsend, M.C. *Psychiatric Mental Health Nursing: Concepts of Care in Evidence-Based Practice*, 5th ed. Philadelphia: F.A. Davis, 2006.

105. Townsend, *Psychiatric Mental Health Nursing: Concepts of Care in Evidence-Based Practice*.

106. Erikson, E. *Childhood and Society*, 2nd ed. New York: W.W. Norton, 1963.

107. Bee et al., *Lifespan Development*.

108. Erikson, *Childhood and Society*.

109. Bee et al., *Lifespan Development*; Santrock et al., *Life-Span Development*.

110. Patterson and Watkins, *Theories of Psychotherapy*.

111. Townsend, *Psychiatric Mental Health Nursing: Concepts of Care in Evidence-Based Practice*.

112. Townsend, *Psychiatric Mental Health Nursing: Concepts of Care in Evidence-Based Practice*; Patterson, and Watkins, *Theories of Psychotherapy*.

113. Wade et al., *Psychology*.

114. Wade et al., *Psychology*.

115. Bandura, A., Regulation of Cognitive Processes through Perceived Self-efficacy, *Developmental Psychology*, 25 (1989), 729–735; Bandura, A., Social Cognitive Theory. In R. Vasta (ed.), *Annals of Child Development: Six Theories of Child Development: Revised Formulations and Current Issues* (pp. 1–60). Greenwich, CT: Jai Press, 1989; Bandura, A., Social Cognitive Theory of Self-Regulation, *Organizational Behavior and Human Decision Processes*, 50 (1991), 248–287.

116. Schaffer et al., *Developmental Psychology: Childhood and Adolescence*; Papalia and Feldman, *Human Development*.

117. Wade et al., *Psychology*.

118. Bee et al., *Lifespan Development*.

119. Bandura, A. *Social Foundations of Thought and Action: A Social Cognitive Theory*. Englewood Cliffs, NJ: Prentice-Hall, 1986.

120. Wade et al., *Psychology*.

121. Bee et al., *Lifespan Development*.

122. Patterson, and Watkins, *Theories of Psychotherapy*.

123. Piaget, J. *The Child's Conception of Physical Causality*. London: Kegan Paul, 1930; Piaget, J. *The Moral Judgment of the Child*. New York: Free Press of Glencoe, 1948; Piaget, J., *Play, Dreams, and Imitation in Childhood*. New York: W.W. Norton, 1951; Piaget, J. *The Child's Conception of the World*. London: Routledge and Kegan Paul, 1951; Piaget, J. *Judgment and Reasoning in the Child*. London: Routledge and Kegan Paul, 1951; Piaget, J. *The Origins of Intelligence in Children*. New York: W. W. Norton, 1963; Piaget, J. *Six Psychological Studies*. New York: Random House, 1967; Piaget, J. *Biology and Knowledge*. Chicago: University of Chicago Press, 1971; Piaget, J. *Psychology and Epistemology*. New York: Orion Press, 1971; Piaget, J. *Understanding Causality*. New York: W.W. Norton, 1974; Piaget, J. *The Grasp of Consciousness*. Cambridge, MA: Harvard University Press, 1976.

124. Schaffer et al., *Developmental Psychology: Childhood and Adolescence*.

125. Wadsworth, B. *Piaget's Theory of Cognitive and Affective Development*, 5th ed. New York: Longman, 1996; Bee et al., *Lifespan Development*.

126. Schaffer et al., *Developmental Psychology: Childhood and Adolescence*.

127. Wadsworth, *Piaget's Theory of Cognitive and Affective Development*.

128. Bee et al., *Lifespan Development*; Papalia and Feldman, *Human Development*.

129. Seifert et al., *Lifespan Development*.

130. Kohlberg, L. (ed.). *Collected Papers on Moral Development and Moral Education*. Cambridge, MA: Moral Educational Research Foundation, 1973; Kohlberg, L., Moral Stages and Moralization: The Cognitive Developmental Approach. In T. Lickona (ed.), *Moral Development and Behavior* (pp. 31–53). New York: Holt, Rinehart, & Winston, 1976; Kohlberg, L. *Recent Research in Moral Development*. New York: Holt, Rinehart, & Winston, 1977; Kohlberg, L., The Cognitive-Developmental Approach to Moral Education. In P. Scharf (ed.), *Readings in Moral Education* (pp. 36–51). Minneapolis: Winston Press, 1978.

131. Wade et al., *Psychology*; Rest, J., The Legacy of Lawrence Kohlberg, *Counseling and Values*, 32(3) (1988), 156–162.

132. Schaffer et al., *Developmental Psychology: Childhood and Adolescence*.

133. Bee et al., *Lifespan Development*.

134. Bee et al., *Lifespan Development*.

135. Wade et al., *Psychology*; Papalia and Feldman, *Human Development*.

136. Rest, The Legacy of Lawrence Kohlberg.

137. Gilligan, C., In a Different Voice: Women's Conceptualization of Self and of Mortality, *Harvard Educational Review*, 47(4) (1977), 481–517; Gilligan, C. *In a Different Voice: Psychological Theory and Women's Development*. Cambridge, MA: Harvard University Press, 1982; Gilligan, C., and D. Attanucci, Two Moral Orientations: Gender Differences and Similarities, *Merrill-Palmer Quarterly*, 34(3) (1988), 332–333.

138. Wade et al., *Psychology*.

139. Friedman et al. *Family Nursing: Research, Theory, & Practice*.

140. Frankl, V., *Man's Search for Meaning*. New York: Washington Square Press, 1967; Frankl, V. *The Unheard Cry for Meaning*. New York: Washington Square Press, 1978; Travelbee, J., *Interpersonal Aspects of Nursing*. Philadelphia: F.A. Davis, 1971.

141. Maslow, A. *Motivation and Personality*, 2nd ed. New York: Harper & Row, 1970; May, R. *Psychology and the Human Dilemma*. New York: D. Van Nostrand, 1967.

142. Maslow, A. *The Farther Reaches of Human Nature*. New York: Viking Press, 1971.

143. Bee et al., *Lifespan Development*; Kail et al., *Human Development: A Life-Span View*; Maslow, A. *Towards a Psychology of Being*, 2nd ed. New York: D. Van Nostrand, 1968.

144. Maslow, *The Farther Reaches of Human Nature*.

145. Wade et al., *Psychology*.

146. Rogers, C. *Client-Centered Therapy*. Boston: Houghton-Mifflin, 1951; Rogers, C. *On Becoming a Person*. Boston: Houghton-Mifflin, 1961; Rogers, C. *Freedom to Learn*. Columbus, OH: Charles E. Merrill, 1969; Rogers, C. *On Encounter Groups*. New York: Harper & Row, 1970; Rogers, C., A Theory of Personality. In T. Millan (ed.), *Theories of Psychopathology*. Philadelphia: W.B. Saunders, 1973; Rogers, C. *Way of Being*. Boston: Houghton Mifflin, 1980.

147. Rogers, *Client-Centered Therapy*.

148. Wade et al., *Psychology*.

149. Osachuk, T.A.G., and S.L. Cairns, Relationship Issues. In D.G. Martin and A.D. Moore (eds.), *First Steps in the Art of Intervention* (pp. 19, 21). Pacific Grove, CA: Brooks/Cole, 1995.

150. Maslow, *Towards a Psychology of Being*; Maslow, *The Farther Reaches of Human Nature*.

151. Santrock et al., *Life-Span Development*.

152. Rogers, *Client-Centered Therapy*; Rogers, *On Becoming a Person*; Rogers, *Freedom to Learn*; Rogers, *A Theory of Personality*; Rogers, *Way of Being*.

153. Townsend, *Psychiatric Mental Health Nursing: Concepts of Care in Evidence-Based Practice*.

154. Santrock et al., *Life-Span Development*.

155. Parke, R., The Society for Research in Child Development at 70: Progress and Promise, *Child Development*, 75(1) (2004), 1–24.

156. Selye, H., Stress Syndrome, *American Journal of Nursing*, 65(3) (1965), 97–99; Selye, H. *Stress without Distress*. Philadelphia: J.B. Lippincott, 1974; Selye, H., Implications of Stress Concept, *New York State Journal of Medicine*, October 1975, 2139–2145; Selye, H., Forty Years of Stress Research: Principal Remaining Problems and Misconceptions, *Canadian Medical Association Journal*, 115 (July 3, 1976), 53–56; Selye, H. *The Stress of Life*, revised ed. New York: McGraw-Hill, 1976; Selye, H., Stress and the Reduction of Distress, *Primary Cardiology*, 5(8) (1979), 22–30; Selye, H., The Stress Concept Today. In I.C. Kutash and L.B. Schlesinger (eds.), *Handbook on Stress and Anxiety* (pp. 127–144). New York: Jossey-Bass, 1980.

157. Frisch and Frisch, *Psychiatric Mental Health Nursing*.

158. Townsend, *Psychiatric Mental Health Nursing: Concepts of Care in Evidence-Based Practice*.

159. Selye, *Stress without Distress*; Selye, Stress and the Reduction of Distress.

160. Selye, Stress Syndrome; Selye, The Stress Concept Today.

161. Wade et al., *Psychology*.

162. Thibodeau and Patton, *Anatomy & Physiology*.

163. Lazarus, R., *Psychological Stress and the Coping Process*. New York: McGraw-Hill, 1966; Townsend, *Psychiatric Mental Health Nursing: Concepts of Care in Evidence-Based Practice*.

164. Thibodeau and Patton, *Anatomy & Physiology*; Wade et al., *Psychology*.

165. Townsend, *Psychiatric Mental Health Nursing: Concepts of Care in Evidence-Based Practice*.

166. Thibodeau and Patton, *Anatomy & Physiology*.

167. McEwen, B.S., Allostasis and Allostasis Load: Implications for Neuropsychopharmacology, *Neuropsychopharmacology*, 22 (2000), 108–124.

168. Thibodeau and Patton, *Anatomy & Physiology*; Wade et al., *Psychology*.

169. Wade et al., *Psychology*.

170. Townsend, *Psychiatric Mental Health Nursing: Concepts of Care in Evidence-Based Practice*.

171. Cox, B.J., P.S.R. MacPherson, M.W. Enns, and L.A. McWilliams, Neuroticism and Self-Criticism Associated with Posttraumatic Stress Disorder in a Nationally Representative Sample, *Behaviour Research and Therapy*, 42(1) (2003), 105–114.

172. Iwasaki, Y., J. Bartlett, and J. O'Neil, Coping with Stress among Aboriginal Women and Men with Diabetes in Winnipeg, Canada, *Social Science & Medicine*, 60 (2005), 977–988.

173. Townsend, *Psychiatric Mental Health Nursing: Concepts of Care in Evidence-Based Practice*.

174. Caplan, G. *Principles of Preventive Psychiatry*. New York: Basic Books, 1964.

175. Frisch and Frisch, *Psychiatric Mental Health Nursing*.

176. Townsend, *Psychiatric Mental Health Nursing: Concepts of Care in Evidence-Based Practice*.

177. Townsend, *Psychiatric Mental Health Nursing: Concepts of Care in Evidence-Based Practice*.

178. Schumacher, K., and A. Meleis, Transitions: A Central Concept in Nursing, *IMAGE: Journal of Nursing Scholarship*, 26(2) (1994), 119–127.

179. Hoff, L.A. *People in Crisis: Understanding and Helping*, 3rd ed. Redwood City, CA: Addison-Wesley, 1987.

180. Townsend, *Psychiatric Mental Health Nursing: Concepts of Care in Evidence-Based Practice*.

181. Hoff, *People in Crisis: Understanding and Helping*.

182. Hoff, *People in Crisis: Understanding and Helping*.

183. Townsend, *Psychiatric Mental Health Nursing: Concepts of Care in Evidence-Based Practice*.

184. Aguilera, D.C. *Crisis Intervention: Theory and Methodology*, 8th ed. St. Louis, MO: C.V. Mosby, 1998.

185. Hoff, *People in Crisis: Understanding and Helping*.

186. Friedman et al., *Family Nursing: Research, Theory, & Practice*.

187. Hoff, *People in Crisis: Understanding and Helping*.

188. Hoff, *People in Crisis: Understanding and Helping*.

189. Connell, C., Storm, *International Educator*, 15(5) (2006), 32–41.

190. Hoff, *People in Crisis: Understanding and Helping*; Weeks, S., Disaster Mental Health Services: A Personal Perspective, *Journal of Psychosocial Nursing*, 37(2) (1999), 14–18.

191. Public Health Agency of Canada, *Emergency Preparedness: Bioterrorism and Emergency Preparedness*. Website: http://www.phac-aspc.gc.ca/ (accessed April 2007).

## Chapter 6

1. Papalia, D., S. Olds, and R. Feldman, *Human Development*, 9th ed. Boston: McGraw-Hill, 2004.

2. Papalia et al., *Human Development*.

3. Papalia et al., *Human Development*.

4. Papalia et al., *Human Development*.

5. Papalia et al., *Human Development*.

6. Bee, H., D. Boyd, and P. Johnson, *Lifespan Development*, 2nd Canadian ed. Toronto: Pearson Education, 2006; Gormly, A., *Lifespan Human Development*, 6th ed. Fort Worth, TX: Harcourt Brace, 1997; Papalia et al., *Human Development*; Seifert, K., R. Hoffnung, and M. Hoffnung, *Lifespan Development*. Boston: Houghton Mifflin, 1997.

7. Gormly, *Lifespan Human Development*.

8. Guyton, A. *A Textbook of Medical Physiology*, 9th ed. Philadelphia: W.B. Saunders, 1996.

9. Guyton, *A Textbook of Medical Physiology*.

10. Seifert et al., *Lifespan Development*.

11. Bee et al., *Lifespan Development*.

12. Papalia et al., *Human Development*.

13. Gormly, *Lifespan Human Development*.

14. Gormly, *Lifespan Human Development*.

15. London, M.L., P. Wieland Ladewig, J.W. Ball, and R.C. McGillis Bindler, *Maternal-Newborn & Child Nursing: Family Centered Care*. Upper Saddle River, NJ: Pearson Education. 2003.

16. Papalia et al., *Human Development*; Guyton, *A Textbook of Medical Physiology*.

17. Guyton, *A Textbook of Medical Physiology*; Wong, D.L., M.J. Hochenberry, S.E. Perry, D.L. Lowdermilk, and D. Wilson, *Maternal Child Nursing Care*, 3rd ed. Philadelphia: Mosby Elsevier, 2006.

18. Wong et al., *Maternal Child Nursing Care*; Sherwen, L., M. Scoleveno, and C. Weingarten, *Nursing Care of the Childbearing Family*, 3rd ed. Norwalk, CT: Appleton & Lange, 1999.

19. Wong et al., *Maternal Child Nursing Care*; Sherwen et al., *Nursing Care of the Childbearing Family*.

20. Bee et al., *Lifespan Development*.

21. Bee et al., *Lifespan Development*. Gormly, *Lifespan Human Development*.

22. Wong et al., *Maternal Child Nursing Care*.

23. Gormly, *Lifespan Human Development*.

24. Guyton, *A Textbook of Medical Physiology*.

25. Guyton, *A Textbook of Medical Physiology*.

26. Wong et al., *Maternal Child Nursing Care*; Sherwen et al., *Nursing Care of the Childbearing Family*.

27. Wong et al., *Maternal Child Nursing Care*; Sherwen et al., *Nursing Care of the Childbearing Family*.

28. Guyton, *A Textbook of Medical Physiology*.

29. Wong et al., *Maternal Child Nursing Care*; Sherwen et al., *Nursing Care of the Childbearing Family*; Thibodeau, G.A., and K.T. Patton, *Anatomy and Physiology*, 6th ed. St. Louis, MO: Mosby Elsevier, 2007.

30. Baltes, P.B., U.M. Staudinger, and U. Lindenberger, Lifespan Psychology: Theory and Application to Intellectual Functioning, *Annual Review of Psychology*, 50 (1999), 471–507l; Lindenberger, U., and P.B. Baltes, Life Span Psychology Theory, *American Psychological Association: Encyclopedia of Psychology*, 5 (2000), 52–57; Lindenberger, U., Lifespan Theories of Cognitive Development, *International Encyclopedia of the Social and Behavioral Sciences*, 13 (2001), 884–885.

31. Lindenberger, Lifespan Theories of Cognitive Development.

32. Lindenberger and Baltes. Life Span Psychology Theory.

33. Thibodeau and Patton, *Anatomy and Physiology*; Papalia et al., *Human Development*; Sherwen et al., *Nursing Care of the Childbearing Family*; Wong et al., *Maternal Child Nursing Care*.

34. Thibodeau and Patton, *Anatomy and Physiology*; Papalia et al., *Human Development*.

35. Sherwen et al., *Nursing Care of the Childbearing Family*; Wong et al., *Maternal Child Nursing Care*.

36. Thibodeau and Patton, *Anatomy and Physiology*; Papalia et al., *Human Development*.

37. Thibodeau and Patton, *Anatomy and Physiology*; Papalia et al., *Human Development*.

38. Guyton, *A Textbook of Medical Physiology*; Papalia et al., *Human Development*.

39. London et al., *Maternal-Newborn & Child Nursing: Family Centered Care*.

40. Thibodeau and Patton, *Anatomy and Physiology*; Papalia et al., *Human Development*.

41. London et al., *Maternal-Newborn & Child Nursing: Family Centered Care*.

42. Mariano, C., and R. Hickey, Multiple Pregnancy, Multiple Needs, *The Canadian Nurse*, 94(9) (1998), 26–30.

43. Blondel, B., and M. Kaminski, Trends in the Occurrence, Determinants, and Consequences of Multiple Births, *Seminars in Perinatology*, 26 (2002), 239–249.

44. Mariano and Hickey, Multiple Pregnancy, Multiple Needs.

45. Multiple Births Canada. *Multiple Births Canada 2006 Annual Report*. Wasaga Beach, ON: Author, n.d. Website: http://www.multiplebirthscanada.org/english/documents/2006AnnualReport-web.pdf (accessed March 2007).

46. Health Canada. *Assisted Human Reproduction Legislation Becomes Law*. Website: http://www.hc-sc.gc.ca/ (accessed February 2007).

47. Treasury Board of Canada Secretariat. *2006–2007 Reports on Plans and Priorities: Assisted Human Reproduction Agency of Canada*. Ottawa: Government of Canada. Website: http://www.tbs-sct.gc.ca/rpp/0607/AHRAC-ACCPA/ahrac-accpa01_easp (accessed March 2007).

48. London et al., *Maternal-Newborn & Child Nursing: Family Centered Care*; Thibodeau and Patton, *Anatomy and Physiology*.

49. London et al., *Maternal-Newborn & Child Nursing: Family Centered Care*; Thibodeau and Patton, *Anatomy and Physiology*; Sherwen et al., *Nursing Care of the Childbearing Family*; Wong et al., *Maternal Child Nursing Care*; Seifert et al., *Lifespan Development*.

50. London et al., *Maternal-Newborn & Child Nursing: Family Centered Care*; Papalia et al., *Human Development*; Sherwen et al., *Nursing Care of the Childbearing Family*; Wong et al., *Maternal Child Nursing Care*; Seifert et al., *Lifespan Development*.

51. London et al., *Maternal-Newborn & Child Nursing: Family Centered Care*; Papalia et al., *Human Development*.

52. Health Canada. *Congenital Anomalies in Canada: A Perinatal Health Report, 2002*. Ottawa: Minister of Public Works and Government Services Canada, 2002.

53. Wong et al., *Maternal Child Nursing Care*.

54. Bee et al., *Lifespan Development*.

55. Health Canada, *Congenital Anomalies in Canada: A Perinatal Health Report*.

56. London et al., *Maternal-Newborn & Child Nursing: Family Centered Care*; Papalia et al., *Human Development*.

57. Bee et al., *Lifespan Development*; Papalia et al., *Human Development*.

58. London et al., *Maternal-Newborn & Child Nursing: Family Centered Care*; Sherwen et al., *Nursing Care of the Childbearing Family*; Wong et al., *Maternal Child Nursing Care*; Seifert et al., *Lifespan Development*.

59. The Society of Obstetricians and Gynaecologists of Canada. *Facts and Statistics: Sexual Health and Canadian Youth*. Ottawa: Author. Website: http://www.sogc.org/ (accessed February 2007).

60. London et al., *Maternal-Newborn & Child Nursing: Family Centered Care*; Sherwen et al., *Nursing Care of the Childbearing Family*; Wong et al., *Maternal Child Nursing Care*; Seifert et al., *Lifespan Development*; Papalia et al., *Human Development*.

61. Sherwen et al., *Nursing Care of the Childbearing Family*; Wong et al., *Maternal Child Nursing Care*.

62. Prysak, M., R.P. Lorenz, and A. Kisly, Pregnancy Outcome in Nulliparous Women 35 Years and Older, *Obstetrics and Gynecology*, 85 (1995), 65–70.

63. Health Canada, *Congenital Anomalies in Canada: A Perinatal Health Report*.

64. Prysak et al., Pregnancy Outcome in Nulliparous Women 35 Years and Older.

65. London et al., *Maternal-Newborn & Child Nursing: Family Centered Care*; Sherwen et al., *Nursing Care of the Childbearing Family*; Wong et al., *Maternal Child Nursing Care*.

66. London et al., *Maternal-Newborn & Child Nursing: Family Centered Care*.

67. London et al., *Maternal-Newborn & Child Nursing: Family Centered Care*; Sherwen et al., *Nursing Care of the Childbearing Family*; Wong et al., *Maternal Child Nursing Care*; Thibodeau and Patton, *Anatomy and Physiology*; Papalia et al., *Human Development*.

68. Bee et al., *Lifespan Development*.

69. London et al., *Maternal-Newborn & Child Nursing: Family Centered Care*.

70. Thibodeau and Patton, *Anatomy and Physiology*.

71. London et al., *Maternal-Newborn & Child Nursing: Family Centered Care*; Guyton, *A Textbook of Medical Physiology*.

72. Fraser Askin, D., Acquired Problems of the Newborn. In D.L. Lowdermilk and S.E. Perry (eds.), *Maternity & Women's Health Care*, 8th ed. (pp. 1051, 1056). St Louis, MO: Mosby, 2004.

73. Health Canada. *Nutrition for a Healthy Pregnancy: National Guidelines for the Childbearing Years*. Ottawa: Minister of Public Works and Government Services Canada, 2002.

74. Health Canada. *Food & Nutrition, Canada's Food Guide, Background on the Food Guide, The Evidence Base*. Website: http://www.hc-sc.gc.ca/ (accessed February 2007).

75. Health Canada, *Nutrition for a Healthy Pregnancy: National Guidelines for the Childbearing Years*.

76. Health Canada, *Food & Nutrition, Canada's Food Guide, Background on the Food Guide, The Evidence Base*.

77. Health Canada, *Food & Nutrition, Canada's Food Guide, Background on the Food Guide, The Evidence Base*.

78. Health Canada. *Food & Nutrition, Nutrition & Healthy Eating, Dietary Reference Intakes, Using the Dietary Intakes*. Website: http://www.hc-sc.gc.ca/ (accessed February 2007).

79. Health Canada. *Food & Nutrition, Nutrition & Healthy Eating, Healthy Weights, Canadian Guidelines for Body Weight Classification in Adults*. Website: http://www.hc-sc.gc.ca/ (accessed February 2007).

80. Health Canada, *Nutrition for a Healthy Pregnancy: National Guidelines for the Childbearing Years*.

81. Dudek, S.G. *Nutrition Essentials for Nursing Practice*, 5th ed., revised reprint. Philadelphia: Lippincott Williams & Wilkins, 2007.

82. Human Resource Development Canada and Health Canada, *The Well-Being of Canada's Young Children*. Ottawa: Government of Canada, 2003.

83. Health Canada, *Nutrition for a Healthy Pregnancy: National Guidelines for the Childbearing Years*.

84. Health Canada, *Nutrition for a Healthy Pregnancy: National Guidelines for the Childbearing Years*.

85. London et al., *Maternal-Newborn & Child Nursing: Family Centered Care*.

86. Health Canada, *Nutrition for a Healthy Pregnancy: National Guidelines for the Childbearing Years*.

87. Health Canada. *Preconception Health and Folic Acid, Primary Prevention of Neural Tube Defects with Folic Acid*. Website: http://www.phac-aspc.gc.ca/fa-af/report/index.html (accessed March 2007).

88. Dudek, *Nutrition Essentials for Nursing Practice*.

89. Health Canada, *Nutrition for a Healthy Pregnancy: National Guidelines for the Childbearing Years*.

90. Health Canada, *Nutrition for a Healthy Pregnancy: National Guidelines for the Childbearing Years*.

91. Dudek, *Nutrition Essentials for Nursing Practice*.

92. Health Canada, *Food & Nutrition, Canada's Food Guide, Background on the Food Guide, The Evidence Base*.

93. Rodwell Williams, S., and E.D. Schlenker. *Essentials of Nutrition and Diet Therapy*, 8th ed. St Louis, MO: Mosby, 2003.

94. Health Canada, *Food & Nutrition, Canada's Food Guide, Background on the Food Guide, The Evidence Base*.

95. Health Canada, *Preconception Health and Folic Acid, Primary Prevention of Neural Tube Defects with Folic Acid*.

96. London et al., *Maternal-Newborn & Child Nursing: Family Centered Care*.

97. House, J.D., S.B. March, S. Ratnam, M. Crowley, and J.K. Friel, Improvements in the Status of Folate and Cobalamin in Pregnant Newfoundland Women are Consistent with Observed Reductions in the Incidence of Neural Tube Defects, *Canadian Journal of Public Health*, 97(2) (2006), 132–135.

98. Health Canada, *Preconception Health and Folic Acid, Primary Prevention of Neural Tube Defects with Folic Acid*.

99. Health Canada, *Nutrition for a Healthy Pregnancy: National Guidelines for the Childbearing Years*.

100. Dudek, S.G., *Nutrition Essentials for Nursing Practice*; Sherwen et al., *Nursing Care of the Childbearing Family*; Wong et al., *Maternal Child Nursing* Care.

101. Health Canada, *Nutrition for a Healthy Pregnancy: National Guidelines for the Childbearing Years*.

102. Health Canada. *First Nations and Inuit Health Branch, Clinical Practice Guidelines for Nurses in Primary Care*. Ottawa: Minister of Public Works and Government Services Canada, 2000.

103. Dudek, *Nutrition Essentials for Nursing Practice*.

104. Willows, N.D., J. Morel, and K. Gray-Donald, Prevalence of Anemia Among James Bay Cree Infants of Northern Quebec, *Canadian Medical Association Journal*, 162(3) (2000), 323–326.

105. Willows, N.D., E. Dewally, and K. Gray-Donald, Anemia and Iron Status in Inuit Infants from Northern Quebec, *Canadian Journal of Public Health*, 91(6) (2000), 407–410.

106. London et al., *Maternal-Newborn & Child Nursing: Family Centered Care*; Sherwen et al., *Nursing Care of the Childbearing Family*; Wong et al., *Maternal Child Nursing* Care.

107. Dudek, *Nutrition Essentials for Nursing Practice*; Sherwen et al., *Nursing Care of the Childbearing Family*.

108. Health Canada, *Nutrition for a Healthy Pregnancy: National Guidelines for the Childbearing Years*.

109. Gormly, *Lifespan Human Development*; Papalia et al., *Human Development*.

110. London et al., *Maternal-Newborn & Child Nursing: Family Centered Care*.

111. London et al., *Maternal-Newborn & Child Nursing: Family Centered Care*; Sherwen et al., *Nursing Care of the Childbearing Family*; Papalia et al., *Human Development*; Guyton, *A Textbook of Medical Physiology*.

112. Papalia et al., *Human Development*.

113. London et al., *Maternal-Newborn & Child Nursing: Family Centered Care*; Sherwen et al., *Nursing Care of the Childbearing Family*; Wong et al., *Maternal Child Nursing Care*.

114. London et al., *Maternal-Newborn & Child Nursing: Family Centered Care*; Bee et al., *Lifespan Development*.

115. Van Dongen, C., Environmental Health Risks, *American Journal of Nursing*, 98(9) (1998), 16B–16E.

116. Van Dongen, C., Environmental Health Risks; Papalia et al., *Human Development*.

117. Allender, J.A., and B. Walton Spradley. *Community Health Nursing: Promoting and Protecting the Public's Health*, 8th ed. Philadelphia: Lippincott Williams & Wilkins, 2005; Chadwick, S.L., and B. Doyle, Environmental and Occupational Health. In L. Leeseberg Stamler and L. Yiu (eds.), *Community Health Nursing: A Canadian Perspective* (pp. 173, 175). Toronto: Pearson Education Canada, 2005.

118. Santrock, J.W., A. MacKenzie-Rivers, K.H. Leung and T. Malcomson. *Life-span Development*, 2nd Canadian ed. Toronto: McGraw-Hill Ryerson, 2005.

119. Markowitz, M., Lead Poisoning, *Pediatrics in Review*, 21(10) (2000), 327–335.

120. Public Health Agency of Canada. *Family-Centred Maternity and Newborn Care: National Guidelines*. Website: http://www.phac-aspc.gc.ca/dca-dea/publications/maternity_paper_e.html (accessed March 2007).

121. Ayotte, P., G. Muckle, J.L. Jacobson, S.W. Jacobson, and E. Dewailly, Assessment of Pre- and Postnatal Exposure to Polychlorinated Biphenyls: Lessons from the Inuit Cohort Study, *Environmental Health Perspectives*, 111(9) (2003), 1253–1258.

122. Van Dongen, Environmental Health Risks.

123. Health Canada. *Healthy Living, Tobacco, About Tobacco Control, Role of Governments, Federal, Federal Tobacco Control Strategy*. Website: http://www.hc-sc.gc.ca/ (accessed March 2007).

124. London et al., *Maternal-Newborn & Child Nursing: Family Centered Care*; Wong et al., *Maternal Child Nursing Care*.

125. Papalia et al., *Human Development*.

126. Papalia et al., *Human Development*; Bee et al., *Lifespan Development*.

127. Wong et al., *Maternal Child Nursing Care*; Sherwen et al., *Nursing Care of the Childbearing Family*.

128. Wong et al., *Maternal Child Nursing Care*; Sherwen et al., *Nursing Care of the Childbearing Family*; Papalia et al., *Human Development*.

129. *Drugs in Pregnancy*. Website: http://www.theberries.ns.ca/ Archives/drugs_pregnancy.html (accessed March 2007).

130. Johnson, J.L., P.A. Ratner, J.L. Bottorff, W. Hall, and S. Dahinten, Qualitative Study: Preventing Smoking Relapse in Postpartum Women, *Nursing Research*, 49(1) (2000), 44–52.

131. Canadian Nurses Association. *Position Statement, Tobacco: The Role of Health Professionals in Smoking Cessation, Joint Statement*. Website: http://www.cna-nurses.ca (accessed June 2004).

132. Meeker, J.D., S.A. Missmer, D.W. Cramer, and R. Hauser, Maternal Exposure to Second-Hand Tobacco Smoke and Pregnancy Outcome among Couples Undergoing Assisted Reproduction, *Human Reproduction*, 22(2) (2007), 337–345.

133. *Drugs in Pregnancy*.

134. The Society of Obstetricians and Gynaecologists of Canada, *Facts and Statistics: Sexual Health and Canadian Youth*.

135. Motherisk. Website: http://www.motherisk.org (accessed March 2007).

136. Wong et al., *Maternal Child Nursing Care*.

137. Papalia et al., *Human Development*; Bee et al., *Lifespan Development*; London et al., *Maternal-Newborn & Child Nursing: Family Centered Care*; Sherwen et al., *Nursing Care of the Childbearing Family*.

138. Public Health Agency of Canada, Family-Centred Maternity and Newborn Care: National Guidelines.

139. Fried, P.A., and A.M. Smith, A Literature Review of the Consequences of Prenatal Marijuana Exposure: An Emerging Theme of a Deficiency in Aspects of Executive Function, *Neurotoxicology and Teratology*, 23 (2001), 1–11.

140. Hurd, Y.L., X. Wong, V. Anderson, O. Beck, H. Minkoff, and D. Dow-Edwards, Marijuana Impairs Growth in Mid-Gestation Fetuses, *Neurotoxicology and Teratology*, 27 (2005), 221–229.

141. Porath, A.J., and P.A. Fried, Effects of Prenatal Cigarette and Marijuana Exposure on Drug Use among Offspring, *Neurotoxicology and Teratology*, 27 (2005), 267–277.

142. Fraser Askin, D., and B. Diehl-Jones, Cocaine: Effects of In Utero Exposure on the Fetus and Neonate, *Journal of Perinatal and Neonatal Nursing*, 14(4) (2001), 83–102.

143. Fraser Askin, Acquired Problems of the Newborn.

144. Fraser Askin and Diehl-Jones, Cocaine: Effects of In Utero Exposure on the Fetus and Neonate.

145. Chiriboga, C.A., L. Kuhn, and G.A. Wasserman. Prenatal Cocaine Exposures and Dose-Related Cocaine Effects on Infant Tone and Behavior, *Neurotoxicology and Teratology*, 29(3) (2007), 323–330.

146. Fraser Askin and Diehl-Jones, Cocaine: Effects of In Utero Exposure on the Fetus and Neonate.

147. Miller-Loncar, C., B. Lester, R. Seifer, L. Lagasse, C. Bauer, S. Shankaran, et al., Predictors of Motor Development in Children Prenatally Exposed to Cocaine, *Neurotoxicology and Teratology*, 27 (2005), 213–220.

148. Motherisk, *Cocaine Use by Pregnant Women in Toronto*. Website: http://www.motherisk.org/updates/index.php?id=106 (accessed March 2007).

149. Ho, E., L. Karimi-Tabesh, and G. Koren, Characteristics of Pregnant Women Who Use Ecstasy (3,4-methylene-dioxymethamphetamine), *Neurotoxicology and Teratology*, 23 (2001), 561–567.

150. Wong et al., *Maternal Child Nursing Care*; Papalia et al., *Human Development*; Bee et al., *Lifespan Development*.

151. Wong et al., *Maternal Child Nursing Care*; Sherwen et al., *Nursing Care of the Childbearing Family*.

152. Wong et al., *Maternal Child Nursing Care*.

153. Sherwen et al., *Nursing Care of the Childbearing Family*; Papalia et al., *Human Development*; Seifert et al., *Lifespan Development*.

154. Wong et al., *Maternal Child Nursing Care*.

155. Fraser Askin, Acquired Problems of the Newborn.

156. Canadian Institute of Child Health. *The Health of Canada's Children: A CICH Profile*, 3rd ed. Ottawa: Author, 2000.

157. Wong et al., *Maternal Child Nursing Care*.

158. Fraser Askin, Acquired Problems of the Newborn; Motherisk. *Fetal Alcohol Syndrome: Role of the Family Physician*. Website: http://www.motherisk.org/updates/index.php?id=299 (accessed March 2007).

159. Canadian Institute of Child Health, *The Health of Canada's Children: A CICH Profile*; London et al., *Maternal-Newborn & Child Nursing: Family Centered Care*.

160. Motherisk, Fetal Alcohol Syndrome: Role of the Family Physician.

161. Koren, G. *The Children of Neverland: The Silent Human Disaster*. Toronto: The Kids in Us Ltd., 1997.

162. Dudek, *Nutrition Essentials for Nursing Practice*.

163. Fraser Askin, Acquired Problems of the Newborn.

164. Koren, *The Children of Neverland: The Silent Human Disaster*.

165. Health Canada. *Fetal Alcohol Spectrum Disorder (FASD)*. Website: http://www.hc-sc.gc.ca/ (accessed March 2007).

166. Public Health Agency of Canada. *Fetal Alcohol Spectrum Disorder (FASD): A Framework for Action*. Website: http://www.phac-aspc.gc.ca/ (accessed March 2007).

167. London et al., *Maternal-Newborn & Child Nursing: Family Centered Care*.

168. The Society of Obstetricians and Gynaecologists of Canada, *Facts and Statistics: Sexual Health and Canadian Youth*.

169. Sherwen et al., *Nursing Care of the Childbearing Family*; Seifert et al., *Lifespan Development*; Wong et al., *Maternal Child Nursing Care*.

170. The Society of Obstetricians and Gynaecologists of Canada, *Facts and Statistics: Sexual Health and Canadian Youth*.

171. Public Health Agency of Canada. *Fetal Alcohol Spectrum Disorder (FASD): A Framework for Action*.

172. Sherwen et al., *Nursing Care of the Childbearing Family*; London et al., *Maternal-Newborn & Child Nursing: Family Centered Care*; Wong et al., *Maternal Child Nursing Care*.

173. The Society of Obstetricians and Gynaecologists of Canada, *Facts and Statistics: Sexual Health and Canadian Youth*.

174. Health Canada. Healthy Living: *Children & Adolescents*. Website: http://www.hc-sc.gc.ca/ (accessed March 2007).

175. The Society of Obstetricians and Gynaecologists of Canada, *Facts and Statistics: Sexual Health and Canadian Youth*.

176. Katz, A., The Evolving Art of Caring For Pregnant Women with HIV Infection, *Journal of Obstetrics, Gynecologic, and Neonatal Nursing*, 32(1) (2003), 102–108.

177. Health Canada, *Healthy Living: Children & Adolescents*.

178. The Society of Obstetricians and Gynaecologists of Canada, *Facts and Statistics: Sexual Health and Canadian Youth*.

179. Wong et al., *Maternal Child Nursing Care*.

180. Sherwen et al., *Nursing Care of the Childbearing Family*; Wong et al., *Maternal Child Nursing Care*.

181. London et al., *Maternal-Newborn & Child Nursing: Family Centered Care*.

182. The Society of Obstetricians and Gynaecologists of Canada, *Facts and Statistics: Sexual Health and Canadian Youth*.

183. The Society of Obstetricians and Gynaecologists of Canada, *Facts and Statistics: Sexual Health and Canadian Youth*.

184. London et al., *Maternal-Newborn & Child Nursing: Family Centered Care*; Wong et al., *Maternal Child Nursing Care*.

185. The Society of Obstetricians and Gynaecologists of Canada, *Facts and Statistics: Sexual Health and Canadian Youth*.

186. The Society of Obstetricians and Gynaecologists of Canada, *Facts and Statistics: Sexual Health and Canadian Youth*.

187. The Society of Obstetricians and Gynaecologists of Canada and Canadian Paediatric Society, National Consensus Statement on the Prevention of Early-Onset Group B Streptococcal Infections in the Newborn, *Journal of the SOGC*, *19*(7) (1997), 751–758.

188. London et al., *Maternal-Newborn & Child Nursing: Family Centered Care*.

189. The Society of Obstetricians and Gynaecologists of Canada and Canadian Paediatric Society, National Consensus Statement on the Prevention of Early-Onset Group B Streptococcal Infections in the Newborn.

190. Logsdon, M.C., K.L. Wisner, and M.D. Pinto-Foltz, The Impact of Postpartum Depression on Mothering, *Journal of Obstetric, Gynecologic, & Neonatal Nursing*, *35*(5) (2006), 652–658.

191. Koniak-Grifffin, D., C. Logsdon, V. Hines-Martin, and C. Turner, Contemporary Mothering in a Diverse Society, *Journal of Obstetric, Gynecologic, & Neonatal Nursing*, *35*(5) (2006), 671–678.

192. Stewart, D.E., Incidence of Postpartum Abuse in Women with a History of Abuse during Pregnancy, *Canadian Medical Association Journal*, *151*(11) (1994), 1601–1604; Seifert et al., *Lifespan Development*.

193. Stewart, Incidence of Postpartum Abuse in Women with a History of Abuse during Pregnancy.

194. Wong et al., *Maternal Child Nursing Care*.

195. Stewart, Incidence of Postpartum Abuse in Women with a History of Abuse during Pregnancy.

196. London et al., *Maternal-Newborn & Child Nursing: Family Centered Care*; Papalia et al., *Human Development*.

197. London et al., *Maternal-Newborn & Child Nursing: Family Centered Care*; Wong et al., *Maternal Child Nursing Care*; Sherwen et al., *Nursing Care of the Childbearing Family*.

198. Papalia et al., *Human Development*.

199. London et al., *Maternal-Newborn & Child Nursing: Family Centered Care*; Wong et al., *Maternal Child Nursing Care*; Sherwen et al., *Nursing Care of the Childbearing Family*.

200. Wong et al., *Maternal Child Nursing Care*; Sherwen et al., *Nursing Care of the Childbearing Family*.

201. London et al., *Maternal-Newborn & Child Nursing: Family Centered Care*.

202. Bee et al., *Lifespan Development*.

203. Gormly, *Lifespan Human Development*.

204. Lindenberger, Lifespan Theories of Cognitive Development; Gormly, *Lifespan Human Development*; Wong et al., *Maternal Child Nursing Care*; Sherwen et al., *Nursing Care of the Childbearing Family*; Dudek, *Nutrition Essentials for Nursing Practice*; Health Canada, *Nutrition for a Healthy Pregnancy: National Guidelines for the Childbearing Years*.

205. Papalia et al., *Human Development*.

206. Heaman, M.I., A.E. Sprague, and P.J. Stewart, Reducing the Preterm Birth Rate: A Population Health Strategy, *Journal of Obstetric, Gynecologic, and Neonatal Nursing*, *30*(1) (2001), 20–29.

207. Papalia et al., *Human Development*; London et al., *Maternal-Newborn & Child Nursing: Family Centered Care*; Seifert et al., *Lifespan Development*.

208. Dudek, *Nutrition Essentials for Nursing Practice*.

209. Veugelers, P.J., and A.L. Fitzgerald, Prevalence of and Risk Factors for Childhood Overweight and Obesity, *Canadian Medical Association Journal*, *173*(6) (2005), 607–613.

210. White, J.M., L.E. Larsun, J.W. Goltz, and B.E. Munro. *Families in Canada: Social Contexts, Continuities, and Changes*, 3rd ed. Toronto: Pearson Prentice Hall, 2005.

211. Wong et al., *Maternal Child Nursing Care*; Sherwen et al., *Nursing Care of the Childbearing Family*; Dudek, *Nutrition Essentials for Nursing Practice*; London et al., *Maternal-Newborn & Child Nursing: Family Centered Care*.

212. Wong et al., *Maternal Child Nursing Care*; Sherwen et al., *Nursing Care of the Childbearing Family*; London et al., *Maternal-Newborn & Child Nursing: Family Centered Care*.

213. Guyton, *A Textbook of Medical Physiology*.

214. Guyton, *A Textbook of Medical Physiology*.

215. Sin, D.D., H.M. Sharpe, R.L. Cowie, and S.F. Man, Spirometric Findings among School-Aged First Nations Children on a Reserve: A Pilot Study, *Canadian Respiratory Journal*, *11*(1) (2004), 45–48.

216. Williams, R., Social Ties and Health, *The Harvard Mental Health Letter*, *15*(19) (1999), 4–5.

217. Dumanoski, D., Child's Plague, *Sierra*, November/December 1997, 47–51, 80; Van Dongen, Environmental Health Risks.

218. Parish, N., Lack of Good Housing Hurts Children's Health, Study Says, *St. Louis Post-Dispatch*, April 8, 1999, B1, B3; Wong et al., *Maternal Child Nursing Care*.

219. White, J.M., L.E. Larsun, J.W. Goltz, and B.E. Munro. *Families in Canada: Social Contexts, Continuities, and Changes*, 3rd ed. Toronto: Pearson Prentice Hall, 2005.

220. Ford-Gilboe, M., Family Strengths, Motivation and Resources as Predictors of Health Promotion Behavior in Single-Parent and Two-Parent Families, *Research in Nursing and Health*, *20*(3) (1997), 205–217.

221. Papalia et al., *Human Development*; Werner, E., Risk and Resilience in Individuals with Learning Disabilities: Lessons Learned from the Kauai Longitudinal Study, *Learning Disabilities: Research and Practice*, *8*, 28–34.

222. Ford-Gilboe, M., Family Strengths, Motivation and Resources as Predictors of Health Promotion Behavior in Single-Parent and Two-Parent Families; Bee et al., *Lifespan Development* (2nd Canadian ed.). Papalia et al., *Human Development* (9th ed.).

223. Papalia et al., *Human Development* (9th ed.). Ford-Gilboe, M., Family Strengths, Motivation and Resources as Predictors of Health Promotion Behavior in Single-Parent and Two-Parent Families.

224. Centre of Excellence for Child Welfare. *2003 Canadian Incidence Study of Reported Child Abuse and Neglect* (CIS-2003). Website: http://www.cecw-cepb.ca/Pubs?PubsCIS2003.shtml (accessed March 2007).

225. Wong et al., *Maternal Child Nursing Care*; Sherwen et al., *Nursing Care of the Childbearing Family*.

226. Centre of Excellence for Child Welfare, *2003 Canadian Incidence Study of Reported Child Abuse and Neglect* (CIS-2003).

227. Sherwen et al., *Nursing Care of the Childbearing Family*; Wong et al., *Maternal Child Nursing Care*; Sin et al., Spirometric Findings Among School-Aged First Nations Children on a Reserve: A Pilot Study; Stewart, Incidence of Postpartum Abuse in Women with a History of Abuse during Pregnancy.

228. Sherwen et al., *Nursing Care of the Childbearing Family*; Wong et al., *Maternal Child Nursing Care*; Papalia et al., *Human Development*; Bee et al., *Lifespan Development*; Gormly, *Lifespan Human Development*; Seifert et al., *Lifespan Development*.

229. Sherwen et al., *Nursing Care of the Childbearing Family*; Wong et al., *Maternal Child Nursing Care*.

## Chapter 7

1. Andrews, M., and J. Boyle. *Transcultural Concepts in Nursing Care*, 3rd ed. Philadelphia: Lippincott, 1999.

2. Hoff, L. *People in Crisis: Understanding and Helping*, 4th ed. Stamford, CT: Appleton-Lange, 1995.

3. Public Health Agency of Canada. *Family Centred Maternity and Newborn Care: National Guidelines*, 4th ed. Website: www.phac-aspc.gc.ca/dca-dea/publications/fcmc06_e.html (accessed August 2007).

4. *Motherisk*. Website: http://www.motherisk.org/ (accessed July 2007).

5. Canada, Royal Commission on Aboriginal Peoples. *Report, Vol. 3* (p 11). Ottawa: Author, 1996.

6. Social Union. *Young Aboriginal Children in Canada: An Overview.* Website: http://www.socialunion.ca/ecd/2002/b-4.htm (accessed July 2007).
7. Kioke, S.J. *Revisiting the Past: Discovering Traditional Care and the Cultural Meaning of Pregnancy and Birth in a Cree Community* (master's thesis, p. 92). Kingston, ON: Queen's University, 1999.
8. Aboriginal Children's Circle of Early Learning. *Children are a Gift to Us: Aboriginal-specific Early Childhood Programs and Services in Canada.* Website: http://www.accel-capea.ca/pdf/FinalGreenwood.pdf (accessed July 2007).
9. Hammersmith, B., and L. Sawatsky. *The Beat of a Different Drum: An Aboriginal Cross-Cultural Handbook for Child-Care Workers.* Saanichton, BC: Association of Aboriginal Friendship Centres, 2000.
10. London, M.L., P.W. Ladewig, J.W. Ball, and R.C. Bindler. *Maternal-Newborn & Child Nursing: Family-Centered Care.* Upper Saddle River, NJ: Pearson Education, Inc., 2003.
11. Hoff, *People in Crisis: Understanding and Helping*; Maloni, J., and M. Ponder, Father's Experience of Their Partner's Antepartum Bed Rest, *IMAGE: Journal of Nursing Scholarship, 29*(2) (1997), 183–187.
12. Strass, P., Postpartum Depression Support, *Canadian Nurse, 98*(3) (2002), 25–28.
13. Barrett, H., Parents and Children: Facts and Fallacies about Attachment Theory, *Journal of Family Healthcare, 16*(1) (2006), 3–4.
14. Bowlby, J. *Attachment and Loss, Vol. 1.* New York: Basic Books, 1969.
15. Chess, S., and A. Thomas, Infant Bonding: Mystique and Reality, *American Journal of Orthopsychiatry, 52* (1982), 421–425.
16. Bowlby, J., Disruption of Affectional Bonds and Its Effect on Behaviour, *Canada's Mental Health Supplement, 59* (January–February 1969), 2–12.
17. Bee, H., D. Boyd, and P. Johnson, *Lifespan Development*, 2nd Canadian ed. Toronto: Pearson, 2006.
18. *Motherisk.* Website: http://www.motherisk.org/ (accessed July 2007).
19. Hammersmith and Sawatsky, *The Beat of a Different Drum: An Aboriginal Cross-Cultural Handbook for Child-Care Workers.*
20. Bee et al., *Lifespan Development.*
21. Saxon, T., J. Colombo, E. Robinson, and J. Frick, Dyadic Interaction Profiles in Infancy and Preschool Intelligence, *Journal of School Psychology, 38* (2000), 9–25.
22. Letch, D., Mother–Infant Interaction: Achieving Synchrony, *Nursing Research, 48*(1) (1999), 55–57.
23. Byrd, M., Questioning the Quality of Maternal Caregiving during Home Visiting, *IMAGE: Journal of Nursing Scholarship, 31*(1) (1999), 27–32.
24. Bee et al., *Lifespan Development.*
25. Hart, S., N. Jones, T. Field, and B. Lundy, One Year Old Infants of Intrusive and Withdrawn Depressed Mothers, *Child Psychiatry and Human Development, 30* (1999), 111–120.
26. Wong, D.L., S.E. Perry, M-J. Hockenberry, D.L. Lowdermilk, and D. Wilson. *Maternal Child Nursing Care*, 3rd ed. St. Louis, MO: Mosby Elsevier, 2006.
27. Vanier Institute of the Family. *Portraits of Fathers.* Website: http://www.vifamily.ca (accessed July 2007).
28. Ferketich, S., and R. Mercer, Predictors of Role Competence for Experienced and Inexperienced Fathers, *Nursing Research, 44* (1995), 89–95.
29. Jones, M., What Is the Influence of Self-Image and Perceived Parenting Role Expectations on Adolescent Fathers' Perceived Role Performance? *Journal of Pediatric and Adolescent Gynecology, 13*(2) (2000), 99.
30. Wong et al., *Maternal Child Nursing Care.*
31. Bee et al., *Lifespan Development.*
32. Vanier Institute of the Family. *Grandparenthood in Canada.* Website: http://www.vifamily.ca (accessed July 2007).
33. Inwood, S., Grandparents Raising Grandchildren, *The Canadian Nurse, 98*(4) (2002), 21.
34. Public Health Agency of Canada. *Canadian Incidence Study of Reported Child Abuse and Neglect.* Website: www.phac-aspc.gc.ca/ (accessed July 2007).
35. Public Health Agency of Canada, *Canadian Incidence Study of Reported Child Abuse and Neglect.*
36. Public Health Agency of Canada, *Canadian Incidence Study of Reported Child Abuse and Neglect.*
37. Public Health Agency of Canada, *Canadian Incidence Study of Reported Child Abuse and Neglect*; Trocome, N., B. MacLaurin, B. Fallon, J. Daciuk, M. Tourny, and D. Billingsley, Canadian Incidence Study of Reported Neglect: Methodology, *Canadian Journal of Public Health, 92*(4) (2001), 259–263.
38. Public Health Agency of Canada, *Canadian Incidence Study of Reported Child Abuse and Neglect.*
39. Trocome, N., B. Fallon, B. MacLaurin, J. Daciuk, C. Felstiner, T. Black, et al. *Canadian Incidence Study of Reported Child Abuse and Neglect 2003: Major Findings.* Ottawa: Minister of Public Works and Government Services Canada, 2005.
40. Trocome et al., *Canadian Incidence Study of Reported Child Abuse and Neglect 2003: Major Findings.*
41. Loo, S., N. Bala, M. Clarke, and J. Hornick. *Child Abuse: Reporting and Classification in Health Care Settings.* Ottawa: National Clearinghouse on Family Violence, Family Violence Prevention Division, Health Canada, 1998.
42. Papalia, D., S. Olds, and R. Feldman, *Human Development*, 9th ed. Boston: McGraw-Hill, 2004.
43. MacMillan, H., Child Maltreatment: What We Know in the Year 2000, *Canadian Journal of Psychiatry, 45*(8) (2000), 702–709.
44. Papalia et al., *Human Development.*
45. Tonmyr, L., H. MacMillan, E. Jamieson, and K. Kelly, The Population Health Perspective as a Framework for Studying Child Maltreatment Outcomes, *Chronic Diseases in Canada, 23*(4) (2002), 123–129.
46. Papalia et al., *Human Development.*
47. Aboriginal Peoples Collection, Solicitor General of Canada. *A Cost-Benefit Analysis of Hollow Water's Community Holistic Circle Healing Process.* Ottawa: Solicitor General of Canada, 2001.
48. Baker, M. *Changing Trends in Canada*, 4th ed. Toronto: McGraw-Hill Ryerson, 2001.
49. MacMillan, Child Maltreatment: What We Know in the Year 2000.
50. Baker, *Changing Trends in Canada.*
51. Tonmyr et al., The Population Health Perspective as a Framework for Studying Child Maltreatment Outcomes.
52. Public Health Agency of Canada. *Joint Statement on Shaken Baby Syndrome.* Website: http://www.phac-aspc.gc.ca/dca-dea/publications/jointstatement_web_e.html (accessed August 2007).
53. Public Health Agency of Canada, *Joint Statement on Shaken Baby Syndrome.*
54. Bee et al., *Lifespan Development*; Papalia et al., *Human Development*; Seifert, K., R. Hoffnung, and M. Hoffnung. *Lifespan Development.* Boston: Houghton Mifflin, 1997; Wong et al., *Maternal Child Nursing Care.*
55. Bee et al., *Lifespan Development.*
56. Wong, D.L., and M.J. Hockenberry, *Wong's Nursing Care of Infants and Children*, 7th ed. St. Louis, MO: Mosby, 2003.
57. Ballard, J.L., J.C. Khoury, K. Wedig, L. Wang, B.L. Eilers-Walsman, and R. Lipp, New Ballard Score, Expanded to Include Extremely Premature Infants, *The Journal of Pediatrics, 119*(3) (1991), 417–423.
58. Wong et al., *Maternal Child Nursing Care.*
59. Dore, S., D. Buchan, S. Coulas, L. Hamber, M. Stewart, D. Cowan, and L. Jamieson, Alcohol Versus Natural Drying for Newborn Cord Care, *Journal of Obstetric, Gynecologic and Neonatal Nursing, 27*(6) (1998), 621–627.

60. Evens, K., J. George, D. Angst, and L. Schweig, Does Umbilical Cord Care in Preterm Infants Influence Cord Bacterial Colonization or Detachment? *Journal of Perinatology, 24*(2) (2004), 100–104.

61. Janssen, P.A., B.L. Selwood, S.R. Dobson, D. Peacock, and P.N. Thiessen, To Dye or Not to Dye: A Randomized Clinical Trial of a Triple Dye/Alcohol Regime versus Dry Cord Care, *Pediatrics, 111*(1) (2003), 15–20.

62. Dore et al., Alcohol versus Natural Drying for Newborn Cord Care.

63. Public Health Agency of Canada. *Family Centred Maternity and Newborn Care,* Chapter 6: Early Postpartum Care of the Mother and Infant and Transition to the Community. Website: www.phac-aspc.gc.ca/dca-dea/prenatal/fcmc1_e.html (accessed July 2007).

64. Canadian Institute of Child Health. *The Health of Canada's Children,* 3rd ed. Ottawa: Canadian Institute of Child Health, 2000.

65. MacMillan, Child Maltreatment: What We Know in the Year 2000.

66. Health Canada. *Pediatric Clinical Practice Guidelines for Nurses in Primary Care,* Chapter 3: Prevention. Website: http://www.hc-sc.gc.ca/fnih-spni/pubs/nursing-infirm/2001_ped_guide/chap_03_e.html (accessed July 2007).

67. Wong et al., *Maternal Child Nursing Care.*

68. MacMillan, Child Maltreatment: What We Know in the Year 2000.

69. MacMillan, Child Maltreatment: What We Know in the Year 2000.

70. Manitoba Centre for Health Policy and Evaluation. *Assessing the Health of Children in Manitoba: A Population-Based Study.* Winnipeg: Manitoba Centre for Health Policy and Evaluation, 2001.

71. Public Health Agency of Canada. *Toward a Healthy Future: Second Report on the Health of Canadians.* Website: http://www.phac-aspc.gc.ca/ph-sp/phdd/report/toward/ (accessed August 2007).

72. MacMillan, Child Maltreatment: What We Know in the Year 2000.

73. Baker, *Changing Trends in Canada.*

74. Wong et al., *Maternal Child Nursing Care.*

75. Baker, *Changing Trends in Canada.*

76. Wong et al., *Maternal Child Nursing Care.*

77. Wong et al., *Maternal Child Nursing Care.*

78. Papalia et al., *Human Development.*

79. Wong et al., *Maternal Child Nursing Care.*

80. Wong et al., *Maternal Child Nursing Care.*

81. Papalia et al., *Human Development.*

82. Wong et al., *Maternal Child Nursing Care.*

83. Wong et al., *Maternal Child Nursing Care.*

84. Wong et al., *Maternal Child Nursing Care.*

85. Canadian Medical Association. *Complete Book of Mother and Baby Care: A Parent's Practical Handbook from Conception to Three Years,* 3rd ed. Toronto: Tourmaline Editions Inc, 2001.

86. Berk, L.E., and E.A. Levin, *Child Development,* Canadian ed. Toronto: Pearson Education Canada, 2003.

87. Wong et al., *Maternal Child Nursing Care.*

88. Berk and Levin, *Child Development.*

89. Berk and Levin, *Child Development.*

90. Bergson, T., and S. Trehub, Mothers' Singing to Infants and Preschool Children, *Infant Behavior and Development, 22* (1999), 53–64.

91. Papalia et al., *Human Development.*

92. Wong et al., *Maternal Child Nursing Care.*

93. Wong et al., *Maternal Child Nursing Care.*

94. Bergson and Trehub, Mothers' Singing to Infants and Preschool Children.

95. Papalia et al., *Human Development.*

96. Papalia et al., *Human Development.*

97. Papalia et al., *Human Development.*

98. Santrock, J.W., A. MacKenzie-Rivers, K.H. Leung, and T. Malcomson. *Life-span Development,* 2nd Canadian ed. Toronto: McGraw-Hill Ryerson, 2005.

99. Andrews and Boyle, *Transcultural Concepts in Nursing Care.*

100. Wong et al., *Maternal Child Nursing Care.*

101. Edelman, C., and C. Mandle. *Health Promotion Throughout The Life Span,* 4th ed. St. Louis, MO: Mosby, 1998; Papalia et al., *Human Development.*

102. Wong et al., *Maternal Child Nursing Care.*

103. Wong et al., *Maternal Child Nursing Care.*

104. Seifert et al., *Lifespan Development.* Papalia et al., *Human Development.* Wong et al., *Maternal Child Nursing Care.*

105. Papalia et al., *Human Development.* Trocome et al., *Canadian Incidence Study of Reported Child Abuse and Neglect 2003: Major Findings.*

106. Papalia et al., *Human Development.*

107. Papalia et al., *Human Development.*

108. Kail, R.V., J.C. Cavanaugh, and C.A. Ateah, *Human Development: A Life-Span View,* 1st Canadian ed. Toronto: Thomson Nelson, 2006.

109. Kail et al., *Human Development: A Life-Span View.*

110. Kellman, P. J., and M.S. Banks, Infant Visual Perception. In W. Damon (ed.), *Handbook of Child Psychology,* Vol. 2. New York: Wiley, 1998.

111. Bee et al., *Lifespan Development.*

112. Papalia et al., *Human Development.*

113. Bergson and Trehub, Mothers' Singing to Infants and Preschool Children.

114. Wong et al., *Maternal Child Nursing Care.*

115. Bee et al., *Lifespan Development.*

116. Wong et al., *Maternal Child Nursing Care.*

117. Canadian Medical Association, *Complete Book of Mother and Baby Care: A Parent's Practical Handbook from Conception to Three Years.*

118. Health Canada. *Pediatric Clinical Practice: Guidelines for Nurses in Primary Care,* Chapter 7: Nutrition. Website: http://www.hc-sc.gc.ca/ (accessed August 2007).

119. Wong et al., *Maternal Child Nursing Care.*

120. Bee et al., *Lifespan Development.* Toronto Public Health, *Growing Healthy Together: Birth to Two Years,* Toronto: Author, 1998.

121. Wong et al., *Maternal Child Nursing Care.*

122. Bee et al., *Lifespan Development.*

123. Wong et al., *Maternal Child Nursing Care.*

124. Wong et al., *Maternal Child Nursing Care.*

125. Wong et al., *Maternal Child Nursing Care.*

126. Wong et al., *Maternal Child Nursing Care.*

127. Public Health Agency of Canada. *Health Promotion: Childhood and Adolescence: Prenatal–6 years: Infant Nutrition.* Website: http://www.phac-aspc.gc.ca/ (accessed August 2007).

128. Health Canada, *Nutrition for a Healthy Pregnancy: National Guidelines for the Childbearing Years.* Ottawa: Minister of Public Works and Government Services, 1999.

129. Health Canada. *Exclusive Breastfeeding Duration: 2004 Health Canada Recommendation.* Website: http://www.hc-sc.gc.ca/ (accessed August 2007).

130. Sheehan, D., S. Watt, P. Krueger, and W. Sword, The Impact of a New Universal Postpartum Program on Breastfeeding Outcomes, *Journal of Human Lactation, 22*(4) (2006), 398–408; Palda, V.A., J-M. Guise, C.N. Wathen, Interventions to Promote Breast-Feeding: Applying the Evidence in Clinical Practice, *Canadian Medical Association Journal, 170*(6) (2004), 976–978.

131. Clifford, T.J., K. Campbell, K.N. Speechley, and F. Gorodzinsky, Factors Influencing Full Breastfeeding in a Southwestern Ontario Community: Assessments at 1 Week and at 6 Months Postpartum, *Journal of Human Lactation, 22*(3) (2006), 292–304.

132. Dennis, C.L., Breastfeeding Initiation and Duration: A 1990–2000 Literature Review, *Journal of Obstetrics Gynecology and Neonatal Nursing, 31* (2002), 12–32.

133. Knaak, S.J., The Problem with Breastfeeding Discourse, *Canadian Journal of Public Health*, 97(5) (2006), 412–415.

134. Registered Nurses Association of Ontario. *Breastfeeding Best Practice Guidelines for Nurses*. Toronto: Author, 2003.

135. Health Canada, *Nutrition for a Healthy Pregnancy: National Guidelines for the Childbearing Years*.

136. Registered Nurses Association of Ontario, *Breastfeeding Best Practice Guidelines for Nurses*.

137. Health Canada, Food & Nutrition. *Canada's Food Guide: Eating Well with Canada's Food Guide: First Nations, Inuit and Métis*. Website: http://www.hc-sc.gc.ca/ (accessed August 2007).

138. Williams, S.R., *Nutrition and Diet Therapy*, 11th ed. St. Louis, MO: Times Mirror/Mosby, 2001.

139. Kail et al., *Human Development: A Life-Span View*.

140. Wong et al., *Maternal Child Nursing Care*.

141. MacMillan, Child Maltreatment: What We Know in the Year 2000.

142. Papalia et al., *Human Development*.

143. Wong et al., *Maternal Child Nursing Care*.

144. Public Health Agency of Canada, Health Promotion. *Childhood and Adolescence, Programs: Canada Prenatal Nutrition Program (CPNP)*. Website: http://www.phac-aspc.gc.ca/ (accessed August 2007).

145. Public Health Agency of Canada, Health Promotion. *Childhood and Adolescence, Programs: Canada Prenatal Nutrition Program (CPNP)*. Website: http://www.phac-aspc.gc.ca/ (accessed August 2007).

146. Wong et al., *Maternal Child Nursing Care*.

147. Wong et al., *Maternal Child Nursing Care*.

148. Canadian Medical Association, *Complete Book of Mother and Baby Care: A Parent's Practical Handbook from Conception to Three Years*.

149. Tatone-Tokuda, F., L. Dubois, and M. Girard, Psychosocial Determinants of the Early Introduction of Complementary Foods. *Health Education & Behavior OnlineFirst*, July 9, 2007, 1–19.

150. Fiocchi, A., A. Assa'ad, and S. Bahna, Food Allergy and the Introduction of Solid Foods to Infants: A Consensus Document, *Annals of Allergy, Asthma, & Immunology*, 97 (2006), 10–21.

151. Papalia et al., *Human Development*.

152. Health Canada. *Alternate Milks*. Website: http://www.hc-sc.gc.ca/ (accessed August 2007).

153. Toronto Public Health, *Growing Healthy Together: Birth to Two Years*.

154. Health Canada, *Alternate Milks*.

155. Health Canada, *Alternate Milks*.

156. Wong et al., *Maternal Child Nursing Care*.

157. Caring for Kids. Cow's Milk. Website: http://www.caringforkids.cps.ca/ babies/CowMilk.htm (accessed August 2004).

158. BC Women's Hospital & Health Centre. *Breastfeeding: BC Women's Milk Bank*. Website: http://www.bcwomens.ca/ (accessed August 2007).

159. Health Canada, *Family Centred Maternity and Newborn Care: National Guidelines*.

160. Health Canada, *Family Centred Maternity and Newborn Care: National Guidelines*.

161. Wong et al., *Maternal Child Nursing Care*.

162. Health Canada. *Food & Nutrition: Food Safety, Water Quality, Bottled Water*. Website: www.hc-sc.gc.ca/ (accessed July 2007).

163. Wong et al., *Maternal Child Nursing Care*.

164. Tatone-Tokuda et al., Psychosocial Determinants of the Early Introduction of Complementary Foods.

165. Kail et al., *Human Development: A Life-Span View*.

166. Knaak, The Problem with Breastfeeding Discourse.

167. MacMillan, Child Maltreatment: What We Know in the Year 2000.

168. MacMillan, Child Maltreatment: What We Know in the Year 2000.

169. Bee et al., *Lifespan Development*.

170. Wong et al., *Maternal Child Nursing Care*.

171. Health Canada. Crib Safety. Website: http://www.hc-sc.gc.ca/ (accessed July 2007).

172. Canadian Child Care Federation. *Back to Sleep*. Website: http://www.qualiteservicesdegardecanada.ca/practice/health percent20watch/sleep_en.html (accessed August 2007).

173. Health Canada. *SIDS*. Website: http://www.hc-sc.gc.ca/ (accessed August 2007).

174. Wadsworth, B. *Piaget's Theory of Cognitive and Affective Development Foundations of Constructivism*, 5th ed. New York: Longman, 1996.

175. Canadian Toy Testing Council (CTTC). Website: http://www.toy-testing.org/ (accessed August 2007).

176. Hammersmith and Sawatsky, *The Beat of a Different Drum: An Aboriginal Cross-Cultural Handbook for Child-Care Workers*.

177. Wong et al., *Maternal Child Nursing Care*.

178. Wong et al., *Maternal Child Nursing Care*.

179. Health Council of Canada. *Health Care Renewal in Canada: Measuring Up? Annual Report to Canadians 2006*. Toronto: Author, 2007.

180. Canadian Paediatric Society. *PID Note: Routine Immunization Schedule*. Website: http://www.cps.ca/ (accessed August 2007).

181. Public Health Agency of Canada. *Immunization & Vaccines: Immunization Schedules*. Website: http://www.phac-aspc.gc.ca/ (accessed August 2007).

182. Public Health Agency of Canada. *Canadian Immunization Guide*, 7th ed. Ottawa: Public Works and Government Services Canada, 2006.

183. Manitoba Centre for Health Policy. *The Health and Health Care Use of Registered First Nations People Living in Manitoba: A Population-Based Study*. Winnipeg: Author, 2002.

184. Health Canada. *Advisories, Warnings & Recalls: Advisories & Warnings, Regulatory Initiative—Proposed Ban of Baby Walkers*. Website: http://www.hc-sc.gc.ca/ (accessed August 2007).

185. Public Health Agency of Canada. *Infant Mortality—Measuring Up: A Health Surveillance Update on Canadian Children and Youth*. Website: http://www.phac-aspc.gc.ca/publicat/meas-haut/mu_c_e.html (accessed April 2008).

186. Burgess, A., E. Dowdell, C. Hartman, C. Nakemy, and J. Rabun, Infant Abductors, *Journal of Psychosocial Nursing*, 33(9) (1995), 30–37.

187. Statistics Canada, *Child Care in Canada: Children and Youth Research Paper Series*. Ottawa: Special Surveys Division, 2006.

188. Blizzard, L., A-L. Ponsonby, T. Dwyer, A. Venn, and J.A. Cochrane, Parental Smoking and Infant Respiratory Infection: How Important Is Not Smoking in the Same Room with the Baby? *American Journal of Public Health*, 93(3) (2003), 482–488.

189. Health Canada, *Population Health Approach, Toward a Healthy Future: Second Report on the Health of Canadians*.

190. Papalia et al., *Human Development*.

191. Manitoba Centre for Health Policy and Evaluation, *Assessing the Health of Children in Manitoba: A Population-Based Study*; Health Canada, *Population Health Approach, Toward a Healthy Future: Second Report on the Health of Canadians*; Papalia et al., *Human Development*.

192. Seifert et al., *Lifespan Development*; Manitoba Centre for Health Policy and Evaluation, *Assessing the Health of Children in Manitoba: A Population-Based Study*; Health Canada, *Population Health Approach, Toward a Healthy Future: Second Report on the Health of Canadians*; Papalia et al., *Human Development*.

193. Bee et al., *Lifespan Development*.

194. Bee et al., *Lifespan Development*.

195. Bee et al., *Lifespan Development*.

196. Santrock et al., *Life-span Development*.

197. Bee et al., *Lifespan Development*.

198. Papalia et al., *Human Development*.

199. Papalia et al., *Human Development*.

200. Erikson, E., *Childhood and Society*, 2nd ed. New York: W.W. Norton, 1963; Bee et al., *Lifespan Development*.
201. Santrock et al., *Life-span Development*.
202. Bee et al., *Lifespan Development*.
203. Vanier Institute of the Family, Portraits of Fathers.
204. Bee et al., *Lifespan Development*.
205. Bee et al., *Lifespan Development*.
206. Low-Birth-Weight Infants Catch Up in Adolescence, *American Journal of Nursing*, 98(10) (1998), 9.
207. Letch, D., Mother–Infant Interaction: Achieving Synchrony, *Nursing Research*, 48(1) (1999), 55–57.
208. Health Canada, *Family Centred Maternity and Newborn Care*, Chapter 6: Early Postpartum Care of the Mother and Infant and Transition to the Community.
209. Lindahl, L., and M. Heimann, Social Proximity in Early Mother-Infant Interactions: Implications for Gender Differences? *Early Development & Parenting*, 6 (1997), 83–88.
210. Bee et al., *Lifespan Development*.
211. Papalia et al., *Human Development*.
212. Baker, *Changing Trends in Canada*.
213. Paneth, N., The Problem of Low Birth Weight, *The Future of Children: Low Birth Weight*, 5(1) (Spring 1995).
214. Bee et al., *Lifespan Development*.
215. Health Canada, *Canadian Perinatal Surveillance System. Congenital Anomalies in Canada: A Perinatal Health Report*. Ottawa: Minister of Public Works and Government Services Canada, 2002.
216. Health Canada, *Canadian Perinatal Surveillance System. Perinatal Health Indicators for Canada: A Resource Manual*. Ottawa: Minister of Public Works and Government Services Canada, 2000.
217. Health Canada, *Canadian Perinatal Surveillance System, Congenital Anomalies in Canada: A Perinatal Health Report*.
218. Health Canada, *Canadian Perinatal Surveillance System, Congenital Anomalies in Canada: A Perinatal Health Report*.
219. Schloman, P., and S. Fister, Parental Perspectives Related to Decision-making and Neonatal Death, *Pediatric Nursing*, 21 (1995), 243–248.
220. Canadian Paediatric Society. *Guidelines for Health Care Professionals Supporting Families Experiencing a Perinatal Loss*. Website: www.cps.ca/english/statements/FN/fn01-02.htm (accessed August 2007).
221. Canadian Paediatric Society, *Guidelines for Health Care Professionals Supporting Families Experiencing a Perinatal Loss*.

## Chapter 8

1. LaRossa, R., Fatherhood and Social Change, *Family Relations*, 37 (1988), 451–457; Papalia, D., S. Olds, and R. Feldman, *Human Development*, 9th ed. Boston: McGraw-Hill, 2004.
2. Dubeau, D., The Involved Father, *Transition Magazine*, 32(2) (2002), 8–14.
3. Wilson, D., Health Promotion of the Toddler and Family. In M. Hockenberry and D. Wilson (eds.), *Wong's Nursing Care of Infants and Children* (pp. 607–642). St. Louis, MO: Mosby, 2007.
4. Public Health Agency of Canada, *Canadian Health Network. Babies' Mental Health: First Connections Matter for Life*. Website: http://www.canadian-health-network.ca/ (accessed August 2007).
5. Public Health Agency of Canada, Canadian Health Network, *Babies' Mental Health: First Connections Matter for Life*.
6. Bowlby, J. *Attachment and Loss*, Vol. I: Attachment. New York: Basic Books, 1969.
7. Schneider, B.H., L. Atkinson, and C. Tardif, Child–Parent Attachment and Children's Peer Relations: A Quantitative Review, *Developmental Psychology*, 37(1) (2001), 86–100.
8. Pederson, D.R., and G. Moran, Expressions of the Attachment Relationship Outside of the Strange Situation, *Child Development*, 67 (1996), 915–927; Pederson, D.R., K.E. Gleason, G. Moran, and S. Bento, Maternal Attachment Representations, Maternal Sensitivity, and the Infant–Mother Attachment

Relationship, *Developmental Psychology*, 34(5) (1998), 925–933; Krakow, E., Lasting Comfort, *Bulletin of the Centre of Excellence for Early Childhood Development*, 5(1) (2006), 2–3; Growing Healthy Canadians. *Life Transitions: Transition to the First Year*. Website: http://www.growinghealthykids.com/ (accessed August 2007).
9. Bowlby, *Attachment and Loss*, Vol. I: Attachment.
10. Bowlby, *Attachment and Loss*, Vol. I: Attachment.
11. Bowlby, *Attachment and Loss*, Vol. I: Attachment.
12. Bowlby, *Attachment and Loss*, Vol. I: Attachment.
13. Bowlby, *Attachment and Loss*, Vol. I: Attachment.
14. Public Health Agency of Canada. *Health Promotion: Mental Health Promotion*. Website: http://www.phac-aspc.gc.ca/ (accessed July 2007).
15. Onyskiw, J.E., Health and the Use of Health Services of Children Exposed to Violence in Their Families, *Canadian Journal of Public Health*, 93(6) (2002), 416–420.
16. Seifert, K., R. Hoffnung, and M. Hoffnung. *Lifespan Development*. Boston: Houghton Mifflin, 1997.
17. Bee, H., D. Boyd, and P. Johnson, *Lifespan Development*, 2nd Canadian ed. Toronto: Pearson Education Canada, 2006; Papalia et al., *Human Development*; Wong, D., S. Perry, M. Hockenberry, D. Lowdermilk, and D. Wilson. *Maternal Child Nursing Care*, 3rd ed. St. Louis, MO: Mosby, 2006.
18. Wong et al., *Maternal Child Nursing Care*.
19. Bee et al., *Lifespan Development*; Papalia et al., *Human Development*; Seifert et al., *Lifespan Development*; Santrock, J.W., A. MacKenzie-Rivers, K.H. Leung, and T. Malcomson. *Life-Span Development*, 2nd Canadian ed. Toronto: McGraw-Hill Ryerson, 2005.
20. Indian and Inuit Health Committee, Canadian Paediatric Society, Growth Charts for Indian and Inuit Children, *Canadian Medical Association Journal*, 136(1) (1987), 118–119.
21. Bee et al., *Lifespan Development*; Canadian Child Care Federation. *Supporting Children to Learn Through Play: Resource Sheet #77*. Ottawa: CCCF, 2005; Papalia et al., *Human Development*; Seifert et al., *Lifespan Development*.
22. Papalia et al., *Human Development*; Wong et al., *Maternal Child Nursing Care*.
23. Bee et al., *Lifespan Development*; Santrock et al., *Life-Span Development*; Papalia et al., *Human Development*; Seifert et al., *Lifespan Development*.
24. Papalia et al., *Human Development*; Wong et al., *Maternal Child Nursing Care*.
25. Wong et al., *Maternal Child Nursing Care*.
26. Wong et al., *Maternal Child Nursing Care*.
27. Wong et al., *Maternal Child Nursing Care*.
28. Wong et al., *Maternal Child Nursing Care*.
29. Wong et al., *Maternal Child Nursing Care*.
30. Wong et al., *Maternal Child Nursing Care*.
31. Wong et al., *Maternal Child Nursing Care*.
32. Health Canada, First Nations and Inuit Health Branch. *Pediatric Clinical Practice Guidelines for Nurses in Primary Care*. Ottawa: Minister of Public Works and Governmental Services Canada, 2001.
33. Hoole, A., C. Pickard, R. Ouimette, J. Lohr, and W. Powell. *Patient Care Guidelines for Nurse Practitioner*, 5th ed. Philadelphia: J.B. Lippincott, 1999.
34. Hoole et al., *Patient Care Guidelines for Nurse Practitioner*.
35. Hoole et al., *Patient Care Guidelines for Nurse Practitioner*.
36. Hoole et al., *Patient Care Guidelines for Nurse Practitioner*.
37. Hoole et al., *Patient Care Guidelines for Nurse Practitioner*.
38. Hoole et al., *Patient Care Guidelines for Nurse Practitioner*.
39. Hoole et al., *Patient Care Guidelines for Nurse Practitioner*.
40. Hoole et al., *Patient Care Guidelines for Nurse Practitioner*.
41. Wong et al., *Maternal Child Nursing Care*.
42. Health Canada. *Eating Well with Canada's Food Guide*. Website: http://www.healthcanada.gc.ca/ (accessed August 2007).

43. Health Canada, *Eating Well with Canada's Food Guide*.
44. Health Canada, *Eating Well with Canada's Food Guide*.
45. Wong et al., *Maternal Child Nursing Care*.
46. Wong et al., *Maternal Child Nursing Care*.
47. Canadian Child Care Federation, *Supporting Children to Learn Through Play*.
48. Father Involvement Initiative—Ontario Network. *Daddy ... Come Play with Me*. Website: http://www.dadstoday.org/ (accessed August 2007).
49. Papalia et al., *Human Development*.
50. Seifert et al., *Lifespan Development*.
51. Seifert et al., *Lifespan Development*.
52. Public Health Agency of Canada. *Canadian Health Network. How Much Sleep Do Children Need?* Website: http://www.canadian-health-network.ca/ (accessed August 2007).
53. Public Health Agency of Canada, Canadian Health Network. *How Can I Protect My Child from Being Poisoned at Home?* Website: http://www.canadian-health-network.ca/ (accessed August 2007).
54. Parents Canada. *A Safe Environment for Your Toddler: In and Around the Home*. Website: http://www.parentscanada.com/ (accessed August 2007).
55. Public Health Agency of Canada. *Health Promotion: Childhood and Adolescence*. Website: http://www.phac-aspc.gc.ca/ (accessed August 2007).
56. Bee et al., *Lifespan Development*; Hoole et al., *Patient Care Guidelines for Nurse Practitioner*; Wong et al., *Maternal Child Nursing Care*.
57. Wilson, Health Promotion of the Toddler and Family.
58. Onyskiw, J.E., Health and the Use of Health Services of Children Exposed to Violence in Their Families, *Canadian Journal of Public Health*, 93(6) (2002), 416–420; Papalia et al., *Human Development*; Seifert et al., *Lifespan Development*.
59. Wadsworth, B. *Piaget's Theory of Cognitive and Affective Development: Foundations of Constructivism*, 5th ed. New York: Longman, 1996.
60. Wadsworth, *Piaget's Theory of Cognitive and Affective Development: Foundations of Constructivism*.
61. Wadsworth, *Piaget's Theory of Cognitive and Affective Development: Foundations of Constructivism*.
62. Wadsworth, *Piaget's Theory of Cognitive and Affective Development: Foundations of Constructivism*.
63. Papalia et al., *Human Development*; Wadsworth, *Piaget's Theory of Cognitive and Affective Development: Foundations of Constructivism*.
64. Bee et al., *Lifespan Development*.
65. Aguiar, A., and R. Baillargeon, Eight-and-a-Half-Month-Old Infants' Reasoning about Containment Events, *Child Development*, 69(3) (1998), 636–653.
66. Papalia et al., *Human Development*.
67. Santrock et al., *Life-Span Development*.
68. Lipari, J., Four Things You Need to Know about Raising Baby. In K.L. Freiberg (ed.), *Annual Editions: Human Development*, 31st ed. (pp. 34–35). Guilford, CN, McGraw-Hill/Dushkin, 2003/2004.
69. Craig, G.J., M.D. Kermis, and N.L. Digdon. *Children Today*, 2nd Canadian ed. Toronto: Prentice Hall. 2001.
70. Papalia et al., *Human Development*.
71. Papalia et al., *Human Development*.
72. Papalia et al., *Human Development*.
73. Stevens, E., J. Blake, G. Vitale, and S. MacDonald, Mother–Infant Object Involvement at 9 and 15 Months: Relation to Infant Cognition and Early Vocabulary, *First Language*, 18 (1998), 203–222.
74. Bee et al., *Lifespan Development*.
75. Santrock et al., *Life-Span Development*; Papalia et al., *Human Development*; Seifert et al., *Lifespan Development*.
76. Papalia et al., *Human Development*.
77. Bee et al., *Lifespan Development*.
78. Senechal, M., J-A. LeFevre, E. Hudson, and E.P. Lawson, Knowledge of Storybooks as a Predictor of Young Children's Vocabulary, *Journal of Educational Psychology*, 88(3) (1996), 520–536.
79. Senechal et al., Knowledge of Storybooks as a Predictor of Young Children's Vocabulary.
80. Wong et al., *Maternal Child Nursing Care*.
81. Kirkness, V.J., The Critical State of Aboriginal Languages in Canada, *Canadian Journal of Native Education*, 22(1) (1998), 93–107.
82. Kirkness, The Critical State of Aboriginal Languages in Canada.
83. Santrock et al., *Life-Span Development*.
84. Santrock et al., *Life-Span Development*.
85. Driessnack, M., Toddler. In C.L. Edelman and C.L. Mandle (eds.), *Health Promotion throughout the Life Span*, 6th ed. (pp. 416–435). St. Louis, MO: Elsevier Mosby, 2006.
86. Community Paediatrics Committee, Canadian Paediatric Society, Toilet Learning: Anticipatory Guidance with a Child-Oriented Approach, *Paediatrics and Child Health*, 5(6) (2000), 333–335.
87. Community Paediatrics Committee, Canadian Paediatric Society, Toilet Learning: Anticipatory Guidance with a Child-Oriented Approach.
88. Andrews, M., and J. Boyle, *Transcultural Concepts in Nursing Care*, 3rd ed. Philadelphia: Lippincott, 1999.
89. Community Paediatrics Committee, Canadian Paediatric Society, Toilet Learning: Anticipatory Guidance with a Child-Oriented Approach.
90. Canadian Child Care Federation. *Flexible Toilet Learning: A Child-Oriented Approach*. Website: http://www.cccf-fcsge.ca/ (accessed August 2007).
91. Canadian Child Care Federation, *Flexible Toilet Learning: A Child-Oriented Approach*.
92. Canadian Child Care Federation, *Flexible Toilet Learning: A Child-Oriented Approach*.
93. Berk, L.E., L.E. Berk, and E.A. Levin. *Child Development*, Canadian ed. Toronto: Pearson Education Canada, 2003.
94. Berk et al., *Child Development*.
95. Papalia et al., *Human Development*.
96. Papalia et al., *Human Development*.
97. Papalia et al., *Human Development*.
98. Papalia et al., *Human Development*.
99. Berk et al., *Child Development*.
100. Papalia et al., *Human Development*.
101. Driessnack, Toddler.

Chapter 9

1. Bee, H., D. Boyd, and P. Johnson. *Lifespan Development*, 2nd Canadian ed. Toronto: Pearson Education Canada Inc., 2006; Seifert, K., R. Hoffnung, and M. Hoffnung. *Lifespan Development*. Boston: Houghton Mifflin, 1997. Santrock, J., A. MacKenzie-Rivers, K.H. Leung, T. Malcomson. *Lifespan Development*, 2nd Canadian ed. Toronto: McGraw-Hill Ryerson, 2005.
2. Bee et al., *Lifespan Development*; Seifert et al., *Lifespan Development*.
3. Chen, X., P.D. Hastings, K.H. Rubim, H. Chen, G. Cen, and S.L. Stewart, Child-Rearing Attitudes and Behavioural Inhibition in Chinese and Canadian Toddlers: A Cross-Cultural Study, *Developmental Psychology*, 34(4) (1998), 677–686.
4. McGrath, M., M. Sullivan, and R. Seifer, Maternal Interaction Patterns and Preschool Competence in High Risk Children, *Nursing Research*, 47(6) (1998), 309–316.
5. Magill-Evans, J., and M.J. Harrison, Parent–Child Interactions and Development of Toddlers Born Preterm, *Western Journal of Nursing Research*, 21(3) (1999), 292–307.

6. Harrison, M.J., J. Magill-Evans, and K. Menzies, Fathers' Scores on the Nursing Child Assessment Teaching Scale: Are They Different from Those of Mothers? *Journal of Pediatric Nursing, 14*(4) (1999), 248–254.

7. Broom, B.L., Parental Differences and Changes in Marital Quality, Psychological Well-Being, and Sensitivity with First-Born Children, *Journal of Family Nursing, 4* (1998), 87–112.

8. Harrison, M.J., J. Magill-Evans, and D. Sadoway, Scores on the Nurses Child Assessment Teaching Scale for Father-Toddler Dyads, *Public Health Nursing, 18*(2) (2001), 94–100.

9. Dubeau, D., The Involved Father, *Transition Magazine, 32*(2) (2002), 8–14.

10. Bee et al., *Lifespan Development*; Santrock et al., *Lifespan Development*.

11. Moss, E., D. Rousseau, S. Parent, D. St-Laurent, and J. Saintonge, Correlates of Attachment at School Age: Maternal Reported Stress, Mother-Child Interaction, and Behaviour Problems, *Child Development, 69*(5) (1998), 1390–1405.

12. Child Trauma Academy, *Stress, Trauma and Post-traumatic Stress Disorders in Children.* Website: http://www.childtrauma.org/ctmaterials/ptsd_interdisc.asp (accessed July 2007).

13. Teicher, M.H., Scars That Won't Heal: The Neurobiology of Child Abuse, *Scientific American, 286*(3), (2002), 68–75.

14. Arnup, K., Lesbian and Gay Parents. In N. Mandell and A. Duffy (eds.), *Canadian Families*, 3rd ed. (pp. 176–177). Toronto: Thomson Nelson, 2005.

15. Arnup, Lesbian and Gay Parents.

16. Public Health Agency of Canada, *Because Life Goes On … Helping Children and Youth Live with Separation and Divorce.* Website: http://www.phac-aspc.gc.ca/publicat/mh-sm/divorce/4_e.html (accessed July 2007); Skitka, L., and M. Frazier, Ameliorating the Effects of Parental Divorce: Do Small Group Interventions Work? *Journal of Divorce and Marriage, 24* (1995), 3–4.

17. Ross, C.E., and J. Mirowsky, Parental Divorce, Life-Course Disruption, and Adult Depression, *Journal of Marriage and the Family, 61* (1999), 1034–1045.

18. Connidis, I.A., Divorce and Union Dissolution: Reverberations over Three Generations, *Canadian Journal of Aging, 22*(4) (2003), 353–368.

19. Berk, L., and E.A. Levin, *Child Development*, Canadian ed. Toronto: Pearson Education Canada, 2003.

20. Papalia, D., S. Olds, and R. Feldman, *Human Development*, 9th ed. Boston: McGraw-Hill, 2004.

21. Rentfro, A.R., Preschool Child. In C.L. Edelman and C.L. Mandle (eds.), *Health Promotion Throughout the Life Span.* St. Louis, MO: Elsevier Mosby, 2006.

22. Health Canada, *Canadian Guidelines for Sexual Health Education.* Ottawa: Minister of Health, 2003.

23. Papalia et al., *Human Development*.

24. Downey, D.B., and D.J. Condron, Playing Well with Others in Kindergarten: The Benefit of Siblings at Home, *Journal of Marriage and Family, 66*(2) (2004), 333–350.

25. Gass, K., J. Jenkins, and J. Dunn, Are Sibling Relationships Protective? A Longitudinal Study, *Journal of Child Psychology and Psychiatry, 48*(2) (2007), 167–175.

26. Berk and Levin, *Child Development* (Canadian ed.).

27. Ram, A., and H. Ross, Problem Solving, Contention and Struggle: How Siblings Resolve a Conflict of Interests. *Child Development, 72* (2001), 1710–1722.

28. Berk, and Levin, *Child Development*.

29. Vanier Institute of the Family. *Contemporary Family Trends—Grandparenthood in Canada.* Website: http://www.vifamily.ca/ (accessed August 2007).

30. Vanier Institute of the Family, *Contemporary Family Trends—Grandparenthood in Canada.*

31. Strom, R., and S. Strom, Building a Theory of Grandparent Development, *International Journal of Aging and Human Development, 45*(4) (1997), 255–286.

32. Inwood, S., Grandparents Raising Grandchildren, *Canadian Nurse, 98*(4) (2002), 21–25.

33. Bee et al., *Lifespan Development*.

34. Vanier Institute of the Family, *Contemporary Family Trends—Grandparenthood in Canada.*

35. Lidz, *op cit.*

36. B.C. Children's Hospital. *Safety for Children and Pets.* Website: http://www.bcchildrens.ca/KidsTeensFam/ChildSafety/SafeStart/SafetyTips/Safetyforchildrenandpets.htm (accessed August 2007).

37. Bushnik, T. *Child Care in Canada.* Ottawa: Minister of Industry, 2006.

38. Canadian Child Care Federation. Website: http://www.cccf-fcsge.ca/ (accessed August 2007).

39. Canadian Child Care Federation.

40. Canadian Child Care Federation.

41. Child and Family Canada. *Choosing a Child Care, Types of Child Care*, Chapter 2. Website: http://www.cfc-efc.ca/ (accessed August 2007).

42. Child and Family Canada, *Choosing a Child Care, Types of Child Care*, Chapter 2.

43. Canadian Child Care Federation. *Code of Ethics.* Website: http://www.cccf-fcsge.ca/ (accessed August 2007).

44. Canadian Child Care Federation, *Code of Ethics.*

45. Bee et al., *Lifespan Development*.

46. Santrock et al., *Lifespan Development*.

47. Papalia et al., *Human Development*.

48. Santrock et al., *Lifespan Development*.

49. Papalia et al., *Human Development*.

50. Pence, A., and M. McCallum, Developing Cross-Cultural Partnerships: Implications for Child Care Quality Research and Practice. In P. Moss and A. Pence (eds.), *Valuing Quality in Early Childhood Services: New Approaches to Defining Quality* (pp. 108–116). New York: Teachers College Press, Columbia University, 1994

51. Pence and McCallum, Developing Cross-Cultural Partnerships: Implications for Child Care Quality Research and Practice.

52. Papalia et al., *Human Development*.

53. Bee et al., *Lifespan Development*; Papalia et al., *Human Development*.

54. Bee et al., *Lifespan Development*; Papalia et al., *Human Development*; Seifert et al., *Lifespan Development*.

55. Monroe, A. R., Health Promotion of the Preschooler and Family, in M. Hockenberry and D. Wilson, eds., *Wong's Nursing Care of Infants and Children* (643–662). St. Louis, Mosby, 2007.

56. Papalia et al., *Human Development* (9th ed.); Seifert et al., *Lifespan Development*; Monroe, Health Promotion of the Preschooler and Family.

57. Monroe, Health Promotion of the Preschooler and Family.

58. Frankenburg, W., and J.B. Dobbs. *Denver II—Revision and Restandardization of the Denver Developmental Screening Test.* Denver, CO: Denver Developmental Materials, 1990.

59. Monroe, Health Promotion of the Preschooler and Family; Frankenburg and Dobbs, *Denver II—Revision and Restandardization of the Denver Developmental Screening Test.*

60. Monroe, Health Promotion of the Preschooler and Family.

61. Papalia et al., *Human Development*; Seifert et al., *Lifespan Development*.

62. Monroe, Health Promotion of the Preschooler and Family.

63. Monroe, Health Promotion of the Preschooler and Family.

64. Health Canada. *Eating Well with Canada's Food Guide.* Website: http://www.healthcanada.gc.ca/ (accessed August 2007).

65. Potter, P.A., A. Griffin Perry, J.C. Ross-Kerr, and M.J. Wood. *Canadian Fundamentals of Nursing*, 2nd ed. Toronto: Mosby, 2001.

66. Canadian Child Care Federation.

67. Potter et al., *Canadian Fundamentals of Nursing.*

68. Broughton, M.A., P.S. Janssen, C. Hertzman, S.M. Innis, and C.J. Frankish, Predictors and Outcomes of Household Food Insecurity among Inner City Families with Preschool Children in Vancouver, *Canadian Journal of Public Health, 97*(3) (2006), 214–216.

69. Lawrence, H., M. Romanetz, L. Rutherford, L. Cappel, D. Binguis, and J.B. Rogers, Oral Health of Aboriginal Preschool Children in Northern Ontario, *Probe, 38*(4) (2004), 172–188.

70. Health Canada, *Eating Well with Canada's Food Guide.*

71. Potter et al., *Canadian Fundamentals of Nursing.*

72. Monroe, Health Promotion of the Preschooler and Family.

73. Public Health Agency of Canada, *Canada's Physical Activity Guides for Children and Youth.* Website: http://www.phac-aspc.gc.ca/pau-uap/paguide/child_youth/index.html (accessed August 2007).

74. Monroe, Health Promotion of the Preschooler and Family.

75. Public Health Agency of Canada. *Canadian Immunization Guide,* 7th ed. Ottawa: Public Works and Government Services Canada, 2006.

76. Swan, E., Dietary Fluoride Supplement Protocol for the New Millennium, *Journal of the Canadian Dental Association, 66* (2000), 362–363.

77. Morrongiello, B.A., T.I. MacIssac, and N. Klemencic, Older Siblings as Supervisors: Does this Influence Young Children's Risk of Unintentional Injury? *Social Science and Medicine, 64* (2007), 807–817.

78. Monroe, Health Promotion of the Preschooler and Family.

79. Bruce, B.S., J.P. Lake, V.A. Eden, and J.C. Denny, Children at Risk of Injury, *Journal of Pediatric Nursing, 19*(2) (2004), 121–127.

80. Bruce et al., Children at Risk of Injury.

81. Brison, R.J., W. Pickett, R.L. Berg, J. Linneman, J. Zentner, and B. Marlenga, Fatal Agricultural Injuries in Preschool Children: Risks, Injury Patterns and Strategies for Prevention, *Canadian Medical Association Journal, 174*(12) (2006), 1723–1726.

82. Monroe, Health Promotion of the Preschooler and Family.

83. Safe Kids Canada. *Safe Kids Canada Position Statement on Bicycle Helmet Legislation.* Website: http://www.safekids.ca (accessed August 2007).

84. Canada Safety Council. *Helmets: Attitudes and Actions.* Website: http://www.safety-council.org (accessed August 2007).

85. Monroe, Health Promotion of the Preschooler and Family.

86. Monroe, Health Promotion of the Preschooler and Family.

87. Monroe, Health Promotion of the Preschooler and Family.

88. Monroe, Health Promotion of the Preschooler and Family.

89. Monroe, Health Promotion of the Preschooler and Family.

90. Haslam, R.H.A., Lead Poisoning, *Paediatrics and Child Health, 8*(8) (2003), 489–490.

91. Bailey, B., Lead Poisoning in Children, *Canadian Medical Association Journal, 171*(5) (2004), 430.

92. Monroe, Health Promotion of the Preschooler and Family; Rentfro, Preschool Child.

93. Public Health Agency of Canada. *Canadian Incidence Study of Reported Child Abuse and Neglect.* Website: http://www.phac-aspc.gc.ca/ (accessed July 2007); Trocmé, N., B. MacLaurin, B. Fallon, J. Daciuk, M. Tourigny, and D. Billingsley, Canadian Incidence Study of Reported Neglect: Methodology, *Canadian Journal of Public Health, 92*(4) (2001), 259–263; Trocome, N., B. Fallon, B. MacLaurin, J. Daciuk, C. Felstiner, T. Black, et al. *Canadian Incidence Study of Reported Child Abuse and Neglect 2003: Major Findings.* Ottawa: Minister of Public Works and Government Services Canada, 2005.

94. Ateah, C.A., J.E. Durrant, and J. Mirwaldt, Physical Punishment and Physical Abuse of Children: Strategies for Prevention. In C. Ateah and J. Mirwaldt (eds.), *Within Our Reach: Preventative Abuse across the Lifespan* (pp. 11–25). Winnipeg: Fernwood, 2004.

95. Ateah et al., Physical Punishment and Physical Abuse of Children: Strategies for Prevention.

96. Barnett, O., C.L. Miller-Perrin, and R.D. Perrin. *Family Violence Across the Lifespan: An Introduction,* 2nd ed. Thousand Oaks, CA: Sage, 2005.

97. Youngblut, J., and D. Brooten, Alternate Child Care, History of Hospitalization, and Preschool Behavior, *Nursing Research, 48*(1) (1999), 29–34.

98. Monroe, Health Promotion of the Preschooler and Family.

99. Pacquiao, D.F., People of Filipino Heritage. In L.D. Purnell and B.J. Paulanka (eds.), *Transcultural Health Care: A Culturally Competent Approach,* 2nd ed. (pp. 138, 145). Philadelphia: F.A. Davis, 2003.

100 Wadsworth, B. *Piaget's Theory of Cognitive and Affective Development: Foundations of Constructivism,* 5th ed. New York: Longman, 1996.

101. Papalia et al., *Human Development;* Wadsworth, *Piaget's Theory of Cognitive and Affective Development: Foundations of Constructivism.*

102. Papalia et al., *Human Development;* Wadsworth, *Piaget's Theory of Cognitive and Affective Development: Foundations of Constructivism;* Piaget, J. *The Equilibration of Cognitive Structures: The Central Problem of Intellectual Development* (trans. by T. Brown and K.J. Thampy). Chicago: University of Chicago Press, 1985.

103. Wadsworth, *Piaget's Theory of Cognitive and Affective Development: Foundations of Constructivism.*

104. Wadsworth, *Piaget's Theory of Cognitive and Affective Development: Foundations of Constructivism.*

105. Papalia et al., *Human Development;* Wadsworth, *Piaget's Theory of Cognitive and Affective Development: Foundations of Constructivism.*

106. Piaget, J., *The Equilibration of Cognitive Structures: The Central Problem of Intellectual Development;* Wadsworth, *Piaget's Theory of Cognitive and Affective Development: Foundations of Constructivism.*

107. Wadsworth, *Piaget's Theory of Cognitive and Affective Development: Foundations of Constructivism.*

108. Klein, J.S., and J. Bisanz, Preschoolers Doing Arithmetic: The Concepts Are Willing but the Working Memory Is Weak, *Canadian Journal of Experimental Psychology, 54*(1) (2000), 105–115.

109. Wadsworth, *Piaget's Theory of Cognitive and Affective Development: Foundations of Constructivism.*

110. Wadsworth, *Piaget's Theory of Cognitive and Affective Development: Foundations of Constructivism.*

111. Wadsworth, *Piaget's Theory of Cognitive and Affective Development: Foundations of Constructivism.*

112. Kail, R.V., J.C. Cavanaugh, and C.A. Ateah. *Human Development: A Life-span View,* 1st Canadian ed. Toronto: Thomson Nelson, 2006.

113. Bodrova, E., and D. Leong. *Tools of the Mind: The Vygotskian Approach to Early Childhood Education.* Englewood Cliffs, NJ: Prentice-Hall, 1996.

114. Bodrova and Leong, *Tools of the Mind: The Vygotskian Approach to Early Childhood Education.*

115. Seifert et al., *Lifespan Development;* Wadsworth, *Piaget's Theory of Cognitive and Affective Development: Foundations of Constructivism.*

116. Bodrova and Leong, *Tools of the Mind: The Vygotskian Approach to Early Childhood Education;* Monroe, Health Promotion of the Preschooler and Family.

117. Bodrova and Leong, *Tools of the Mind: The Vygotskian Approach to Early Childhood Education.*

118. Berk and Levin, *Child Development.*

119. Eisenberg, N., I.K. Guthrie, B.C. Murphy, S.A. Shepard, A. Cumberland, and G. Carlo, Consistency and Development of Prosocial Dispositions: A Longitudinal Study, *Child Development, 70*(6) (1999), 1360–1372.

120. Roberts, W., and J. Strayer, Empathy, Emotional Expressiveness, and Prosocial Behavior, *Child Development, 67* (1996), 449–470.

121. Thompson, C., J. Barresi, and C. Moore, The Development of Future-Oriented Prudence and Altruism in Preschoolers, *Cognitive Development, 12* (1997), 199–212.
122. Thompson et al., The Development of Future-Oriented Prudence and Altruism in Preschoolers.
123. Canadian Paediatrics Society. *Impact of Media Use on Children and Youth*. Ottawa: Author, 2003. Website: http://www.cps.ca/english/statements/PP/pp03-01.htm (accessed August 2007).
124. LeFrançois, G.R., *Of Children: An Introduction to Child and Adolescent Development*, 9th ed. Toronto: Wadsworth/Thomson Learning, 2001.
125. Santrock et al., *Lifespan Development*.
126. Johnson, M.O., Television Violence and Its Effect on Children, *Journal of Pediatric Nursing, 11*(2) (1996), 94–99.
127. Bodrova and Leong, *Tools of the Mind: The Vygotskian Approach to Early Childhood Education*.
128. Bodrova and Leong, *Tools of the Mind: The Vygotskian Approach to Early Childhood Education*.
129. Santrock et al., *Lifespan Development*.
130. Gaines, B.R., Screening for Childhood Speech-Language Problems, *Canadian Nurse, 98*(5) (2002), 15–16.
131. Gaines, Screening for Childhood Speech-Language Problems.
132. Piaget, *The Equilibration of Cognitive Structures: The Central Problem of Intellectual Development*; Berk and Levin, *Child Development*.
133. Erikson, E.H. *Childhood and Society*, 2nd ed. New York: W.W. Norton, 1963.
134. Bee et al., *Lifespan Development*.
135. Papalia et al., *Human Development*.
136. Papalia et al., *Human Development*; Seifert et al., *Lifespan Development*; Monroe, Health Promotion of the Preschooler and Family.
137. Bee et al., *Lifespan Development*; Monroe, Health Promotion of the Preschooler and Family.
138. Bee et al., *Lifespan Development*; Monroe, Health Promotion of the Preschooler and Family.
139. Papalia et al., *Human Development*.
140. Dubeau, The Involved Father.
141. Papalia et al., *Human Development*; Seifert et al., *Lifespan Development*.
142. Ateah et al., Physical Punishment and Physical Abuse of Children: Strategies for Prevention.
143. Waschbusch, D.A., H.L. Kipp, and W.E. Pelham, Jr., Generalization of Behavioural and Psychostimulant Treatment of Attention-Deficit/Hyperactivity Disorder (ADHD): Discussion and Examples, *Behaviour Research and Therapy, 36*(7–8) (1998), 675–694.
144. Bee et al., *Lifespan Development*.
145. Canadian Paediatrics Society, Effective Discipline for Children, *Paediatrics & Child Health, 9*(1) (2004), 37-41; Durrant, J., Distinguishing Physical Punishment from Physical Abuse: Implications for Professionals, *Ontario Association of Children's Aid Societies Journal, 48*(2) (2004), 15–20.
146. Santrock et al., *Lifespan Development*.
147. Erikson, Childhood and Society.
148. Erikson, Childhood and Society.
149. Monroe, Health Promotion of the Preschooler and Family.
150. Monroe, Health Promotion of the Preschooler and Family.
151. Perlman, M., and H.S. Ross, The Benefits of Parent Intervention in Children's Disputes: An Examination of Current Changes in Children's Fighting Styles, *Child Development, 64*(4) (1997), 690–700.
152. Perlman and Ross, The Benefits of Parent Intervention in Children's Disputes: An Examination of Current Changes in Children's Fighting Styles.
153. Santrock et al., *Lifespan Development*.
154. Monroe, Health Promotion of the Preschooler and Family.

155. Burgess, A., C. Hartman, and T. Baker, Memory Presentations of Childhood Sexual Abuse, *Journal of Psychosocial Nursing, 33*(9) (1995), 9–16.
156. Monroe, Health Promotion of the Preschooler and Family.
157. Monroe, Health Promotion of the Preschooler and Family.
158. Monroe, Health Promotion of the Preschooler and Family.
159. Rentfro, Preschool Child.
160. Monroe, Health Promotion of the Preschooler and Family.

**Chapter 10**

1. Novick, M. *Summoned to Stewardship: Making Poverty Reduction a Collective Legacy, Campaign 2000 Policy Perspectives*. Toronto: Campaign 2000, 2007.
2. Novick, *Summoned to Stewardship: Making Poverty Reduction a Collective Legacy, Campaign 2000 Policy Perspectives*.
3. Canadian Institute of Child Health, *The Health of Canada's Children*, 3rd ed. Ottawa: CICH, 2000.
4. Canadian Institute of Child Health, *The Health of Canada's Children*.
5. Séguin, L., Q. Xu, L. Potvin, M-V. Zunzunegui, and K.L. Frohlich, Effects of Low Income on Infant Health, *Canadian Medical Association Journal, 168*(12) (2003), 1523–1538.
6. Martin-Matthews, A., Aging and Families: Ties over Time and across Generations. In N. Mandell and A. Duffy (eds.), *Canadian Families: Diversity, Conflict and Change* (pp. 311–337). Toronto: Thomson Nelson, 2005.
7. Newman, B., and P. Newman, *Development Through Life: A Psychosocial Approach*, 7th ed. Belmont, CA: Brooks/Cole, 1999; Papalia, D., S. Olds, and R. Feldman, *Human Development*, 9th ed. Boston: McGraw-Hill, 2004.
8. Bee, H., D. Boyd, & P. Johnson. *Lifespan Development*, 2nd Canadian ed. Toronto: Pearson Education Canada, 2006; Papalia et al., *Human Development*; Sigelman, C., *Life-Span Human Development*, 3rd ed. Pacific Grove, CA: Brooks/Cole, 1999.
9. Cloutier, R., and G. Alain, Family Transitions Related to Parental Separation, *Canadian Journal of Community Mental Health, Special Supplement*, no. 4 (2002), 5–11.
10. Cloutier and Alain, Family Transitions Related to Parental Separation.
11. Statistics Canada. *Census: Families and Households Profile*. Website: http://www12.statcan.ca/ (accessed August 2007).
12. Canadian Council on Social Development. *Aboriginal Children in Poverty in Urban Communities*. Website: http://www.ccsd.ca/ (accessed August 2007).
13. Child & Family Canada. *Canada's Kids: Thriving? Or Just Surviving?* Website: http://www.cfc-efc.ca/docs/vinif/00000899.htm (accessed August 2007).
14. Child & Family Canada, *Canada's Kids: Thriving? Or Just Surviving?*
15. Public Health Agency of Canada. *Because Life Goes On ... Helping Children and Youth Live with Separation and Divorce: A Guide for Parents*. Website: http://www.phac-aspc.gc.ca/publicat/mh-sm/divorce/index.html (accessed August 2007).
16. Public Health Agency of Canada, *Because Life Goes On ... Helping Children and Youth Live with Separation and Divorce: A Guide for Parents*.
17. Public Health Agency of Canada, *Because Life Goes On ... Helping Children and Youth Live with Separation and Divorce: A Guide for Parents*.
18. Public Health Agency of Canada, *Because Life Goes On ... Helping Children and Youth Live with Separation and Divorce: A Guide for Parents*.
19. Canada Safety Council. *Children Home Alone*. Website: http://www.safety-council.org/info/child/alone.html (accessed August 2007).
20. Canada Safety Council, *Children Home Alone*.

21. Canada Safety Council, *Children Home Alone*.
22. Berk, L.E., and E.A. Levin, *Child Development*, Canadian ed. Toronto: Pearson Education Canada, 2003.
23. Ram, A., and H. Ross, Problem Solving, Contention and Struggle: How Siblings Resolve a Conflict of Interests. *Child Development, 72* (2001), 1710–1722.
24. Child & Family Canada. Adoption: So Many Issues, So Little Understanding. Website: http://www.cfc-efc.ca/docs/vanif/0000 0063.htm (accessed August 2007).
25. Schneider, B.H., A Multi-method Exploration of the Friendships of Children Considered Socially Withdrawn by School Peers, *Journal of Abnormal Child Psychology, 27*(2) (1999), 115–119.
26. Bee et al., *Lifespan Development*; Papalia et al., *Human Development*; Seifert, K., R. Hoffnung, and M. Hoffnung. *Lifespan Development*. Boston: Houghton Mifflin, 1997. Rodgers, C., Health Promotion of the School-Aged Child and Family. In M. Hockenberry and D. Wilson (eds.), *Wong's Nursing Care of Infants and Children* (pp. 712–751). St. Louis, MO: Mosby, 2007.
27. Rodgers, Health Promotion of the School-Aged Child and Family.
28. Bee et al., *Lifespan Development*; Papalia et al., *Human Development*; Seifert et al., *Lifespan Development*; Rodgers, Health Promotion of the School-Aged Child and Family.
29. Bee et al., *Lifespan Development*.
30. Bee et al., *Lifespan Development*; Papalia et al., *Human Development*; Seifert et al., *Lifespan Development*; Rodgers, Health Promotion of the School-Aged Child and Family.
31. Bee et al., *Lifespan Development*; Papalia et al., *Human Development*; Seifert et al., *Lifespan Development*; Rodgers, Health Promotion of the School-Aged Child and Family.
32. Bee et al., *Lifespan Development*; Papalia et al., *Human Development*; Seifert et al., *Lifespan Development*.
33. Seifert et al. *Lifespan Development*; Rodgers, Health Promotion of the School-Aged Child and Family.
34. Health Canada, *It's Your Health*. Website: http://www.hc-sc.gc.ca/iyh-vsv/index_e.html (accessed August 2007).
35. Canadian Paediatric Society, The Use of Fluoride in Infants and Children, *Paediatrics & Child Health, 7*(8) (2002), 569–572. Reaffirmed February 2006 as a position statement.
36. Health Canada, *It's Your Health*.
37. Papalia et al., *Human Development*.
38. Papalia et al., *Human Development*; Rodgers, Health Promotion of the School-Aged Child and Family.
39. Papalia et al., *Human Development*; Rodgers, Health Promotion of the School-Aged Child and Family.
40. Rodgers, Health Promotion of the School-Aged Child and Family.
41. Seifert et al., *Lifespan Development*; Rodgers, Health Promotion of the School-Aged Child and Family.
42. Hoole, A., C. Pickard, R. Ouimette, J. Lohr, and W. Powell. *Patient Care Guidelines for Nurse Practitioners*, 5th ed. Philadelphia: J.B. Lippincott, 1999.
43. Hoole et al., *Patient Care Guidelines for Nurse Practitioners*.
44. Hoole et al., *Patient Care Guidelines for Nurse Practitioners*. Rodgers, Health Promotion of the School-Aged Child and Family.
45. Hoole et al., *Patient Care Guidelines for Nurse Practitioners*. Rodgers, Health Promotion of the School-Aged Child and Family.
46. Peckenpaugh, N.J. *Nutrition Essentials and Diet Therapy*, 9th ed. St. Louis, MO: Saunders, 2003.
47. Stockmyer, C., Remember When Mom Wanted You Home for Dinner? *Nutrition Reviews, 59*(2) (2001), 57–61.
48. Health Canada. *Eating Well with Canada's Food Guide*. Website: http://www.healthcanada.gc.ca/ (accessed August 2007).
49. Health Canada, *Eating Well with Canada's Food Guide*.
50. Health Canada, *Eating Well with Canada's Food Guide*.
51. Health Canada, *Eating Well with Canada's Food Guide*.
52. Andrews, M., and J. Boyle. *Transcultural Concepts in Nursing Care*, 3rd ed. Philadelphia: Lippincott, 1999.
53. Birch, L., J.S. Savage, and A. Ventura, Influences on the Development of Children's Eating Behaviours: From Infancy to Adolescence, *Canadian Journal of Dietetic Practice and Research, 68*(1) (2007), S1–S5.
54. Taylor, J.P., S. Evers, and M. McKenna, Determinants of Healthy Eating in Children and Youth, *Canadian Journal of Public Health, 96*(3) (2005), S20–S27.
55. Health Canada, *Eating Well with Canada's Food Guide*.
56. McIntyre, L., S.K. Connor, and J. Warren, Child Hunger in Canada: Results of the 1994 National Longitudinal Survey of Children and Youth, *Canadian Medical Association Journal, 163* (2000), 1429–1433.
57. McIntyre et al., Child Hunger in Canada: Results of the 1994 National Longitudinal Survey of Children and Youth.
58. Lefrançois, G.R. *Of Children: An Introduction to Child and Adolescent Development*, 9th ed. Toronto: Nelson Thomson Learning, 2001; Tremblay, M.S., and J.D. Willms, Secular Trends in the Body Mass Index of Canadian Children, *Canadian Medical Association Journal, 163* (2000), 1429–1433.
59. Taylor et al., Determinants of Healthy Eating in Children and Youth.
60. Canadian Institute for Health Information. *Overweight and Obesity in Canada: A Population Health Perspective*. Ottawa: Author, 2004. Website: http://secure.cihi.ca/ (accessed September 2007).
61. Rodgers, Health Promotion of the School-Aged Child and Family.
62. Ball, G.D.C., and L.J. McCargar, Childhood Obesity in Canada: A Review of Prevalence Estimates and Risk Factors for Cardiovascular Diseases and Type 2 Diabetes, *Canadian Journal of Applied Physiology, 28*(1) (2003), 117–140.
63. Berry, D., R. Sheehan, R. Heschel, K. Knafl, G. Melkus, and M. Grey, Family-Based Interventions for Childhood Obesity: A Review, *Journal of Family Nursing, 10*(4) (2004), 429–449.
64. Society for Nutrition Education, Guidelines for Childhood Obesity Prevention Programs: Promoting Healthy Weight in Children, *Journal of Nutrition Education and Behavior, 35*(1) (2003), 1–4.
65. Andrews and Boyle, *Transcultural Concepts in Nursing Care*.
66. Rodgers, Health Promotion of the School-Aged Child and Family.
67. Taylor et al., Determinants of Healthy Eating in Children and Youth.
68. Public Health Agency of Canada. *Canada's Physical Activity Guide for Children and Youth*. Website: http://www.phac-aspc.gc.ca/ (accessed August 2007).
69. Public Health Agency of Canada, *Canada's Physical Activity Guide for Children and Youth*.
70. Public Health Agency of Canada, *Canada's Physical Activity Guide for Children and Youth*.
71. Public Health Agency of Canada, *Canada's Physical Activity Guide for Children and Youth*.
72. Heurter, H., K. Breen-Reid, L. Aronson, D. Manning, and E.L. Ford-Jones, Childhood Immunization: How Knowledgeable Are We? *Canadian Nurse, 99*(4) (2003), 27–31.
73. Public Health Agency of Canada. *Immunization & Vaccines: Immunization Schedules*. Website: http://www.phac-aspc.gc.ca/ (accessed September 2007).
74. Bigham, M., and M. Hoefer, Comparing Benefits and Risks of Immunization, *Canadian Journal of Public Health, 92*(3) (2001), 173–177.
75. Heurter et al., Childhood Immunization: How Knowledgeable Are We?
76. Bigham and Hoefer, Comparing Benefits and Risks of Immunization.

77. Halperin, S.A., How to Manage Parents Unsure about Immunization, *The Canadian Journal of Continuing Medical Education*, *1* (2000), 62–75.

78. Public Health Agency of Canada, *Immunization & Vaccines: Immunization Schedules*.

79. Canadian Nurses Association, Nurses and Immunization—What You Need to Know, *Nursing Now, 12* (November 2001), 1–4.

80. Birken, C.S., P.C. Parkin, T. To, and C. MacArthur, Trends in Rates of Death from Unintentional Injury among Canadian Children in Urban Areas: Influence of Sociocultural Status, *Canadian Medical Association Journal*, *175*(8) (2006), 867–868.

81. Bolaria, B.S., and R. Bolaria, Inequality, Family, and Child Health. In B.S. Bolaria and H.D. Dickinson, (eds.), *Health, Illness, and Health Care in Canada*, 3rd ed. (pp. 247–253). Toronto: Nelson Thomson Learning, 2002.

82. LeBlanc, J.C., T.L. Beattie, and C. Culligan, Effect of Legislation on the Use of Bicycle Helmets, *Canadian Medical Association Journal*, *166*(5) (2002), 592–595.

83. LeBlanc et al., Effect of Legislation on the Use of Bicycle Helmets.

84. Howard, A.W., Injury in Children: A Vexingly Simple Problem, *Canadian Medical Association Journal*, *175*(8) (2006), 899–900.

85. Howard, A., Automobile Restraints for Children: A Review for Clinicians, *Canadian Medical Association Journal*, *167*(7) (2002), 769–773.

86. Lapner, P.C., M. McKay, A. Howard, B. Gardner, A. German, and M. Letts, Children in Crashes: Mechanisms of Injury and Restraint Systems, *Canadian Journal of Surgery*, *44*(6) (2001), 445–449.

87. MacPherson, A., L. Rothman, and A. Howard, Body-Checking Rules and Childhood Injuries in Ice Hockey, *Pediatrics*, *117*(2) (2006), e143–e147.

88. Drkulec, J.A., and M. Letts, Snowboarding Injuries in Children, *Canadian Journal of Surgery*, *44*(6) (2001), 435–439.

89. Drkulec and Letts, Snowboarding Injuries in Children.

90. Manitoba Association of School Trustees. *Planning Ski and Snowboarding Education Programs: A Reference Guide for Schools*. Winnipeg: MAST, 2007. Website: http://www.mast.mb.ca/ (accessed September 2007).

91. Wesner, M., An Evaluation of Think First Saskatchewan: A Head and Spinal Cord Injury Prevention Program, *Canadian Journal of Public Health*, *94*(2) (2003), 115–120.

92. Canadian Institute of Child Health, *The Health of Canada's Children: A CICH Profile*, 3rd ed. Ottawa: CICH, 2000.

93. Bristow, K.M., J.B. Carson, L. Warda, and R. Wartman, Childhood Drowning in Manitoba: A 10-Year Review of Provincial Paediatric Death Review Committee Data, *Paediatric Child Health*, *7*(9) (2002), 637–641.

94. MacMillan, H., C. Walsh, and E. Jamieson. *Children's Health*. Ottawa: First Nations and Inuit Regional Health Survey National Steering Committee, 1999.

95. Rodgers, Health Promotion of the School-Aged Child and Family.

96. Rodgers, Health Promotion of the School-Aged Child and Family.

97. Bolaria and Bolaria, Inequality, Family, and Child Health.

98. Seifert et al., *Lifespan Development*.

99. Hoole et al., *Patient Care Guidelines for Nurse Practitioners*.

100. Becker, A., C. Lemiere, D. Berube, L-P. Boulet, F. M. Ducharme, M. FitzGerald, et al., Summary of Recommendations from the Canadian Asthma Consensus Guidelines, 2003, *Canadian Medical Association Journal*, *173* (6suppl) (2005), S1–S11.

101. Hoole et al., *Patient Care Guidelines for Nurse Practitioners*; Hockenberry, M., and P. Barrera, Health Problems of Early Childhood. In M. Hockenberry and D. Wilson (eds.), *Wong's Nursing Care of Infants and Children* (pp. 663–711). St. Louis, MO, Mosby, 2007.

102. Hoole et al., *Patient Care Guidelines for Nurse Practitioners*.

103. Hoole et al., *Patient Care Guidelines for Nurse Practitioners*; Ball, J., and R. Bindler. *Pediatric Nursing, Caring for Children*, 4th ed. Upper Saddle River, NJ: Pearson Education, 2008.

104. Hoole et al., *Patient Care Guidelines for Nurse Practitioners*.

105. Hockenberry and Barrera, Health Problems of Early Childhood.

106. Boynton, R., E. Dunn and G. Stephens, *Manual of Ambulatory Pediatrics* (3rd ed.) Philadelphia: J.B. Lippincott, 1994.

107. Public Health Agency of Canada. *Population Health Approach: What Determines Health?* Website: http://www.phac-aspc.gc.ca/ (accessed September 2007).

108. Wadsworth, B. *Piaget's Theory of Cognitive and Affective Development: Foundations of Constructivism*, 5th ed. New York: Longman, 1996.

109. Berk and Levin, *Child Development*.

110. Piaget, J., and B. Inhelder. *The Psychology of the Child*. New York: Basic Books, 1969; Piaget, J., and B. Inhelder, *Memory and Intelligence*. New York: Basic Books, 1973; Piaget, J. *The Equilibration of Cognitive Structures: The Central Problem of Intellectual Development* (trans. by T. Brown and K.J. Thampy). Chicago: University of Chicago Press, 1985.

111. Newman and Newman, *Development Through Life: A Psychosocial Approach*.

112. Wadsworth, *Piaget's Theory of Cognitive and Affective Development: Foundations of Constructivism*.

113. Santrock, J.W., A. MacKenzie-Rivers, K.H. Leung, and T. Malcomson, *Life-Span Development*, 2nd Canadian ed. Toronto: McGraw-Hill Ryerson, 2005.

114. Santrock et al., *Life-Span Development*.

115. Kail, R.V., J.C. Cavanaugh, and C.A. Ateah, *Human Development: A Life-Span View*, 1st Canadian ed. Toronto: Thomson Nelson, 2006.

116. Santrock et al., *Life-Span Development*.

117. Bee et al., *Lifespan Development*.

118. Santrock et al., *Life-Span Development*.

119. Santrock et al., *Life-Span Development*.

120. Pressley, M., Literacy and Literacy Instruction. In I.B. Weiner (ed.), *Handbook of Psychology*, Vol. 7. New York: Wiley, 2003.

121. Public Health Agency of Canada. *Helping Children Cope: Responding to Stressful Events*. Website: http://www.phac-aspc.gc.ca/ (accessed September 2007).

122. Piaget and Inhelder, *The Psychology of the Child*; Piaget and Inhelder, *Memory and Intelligence*; Piaget, *The Equilibration of Cognitive Structures: The Central Problem of Intellectual Development*.

123. Seifert et al. *Lifespan Development*; Wadsworth, *Piaget's Theory of Cognitive and Affective Development: Foundations of Constructivism*.

124. Wadsworth, *Piaget's Theory of Cognitive and Affective Development: Foundations of Constructivism*.

125. Wadsworth, *Piaget's Theory of Cognitive and Affective Development: Foundations of Constructivism*.

126. Berk and Levin, *Child Development*.

127. Seifert et al. *Lifespan Development*; Sternberg, R., *Thinking and Problem Solving*. San Diego: Academic Press, 1994; Sternberg, R., and R. Wagner (eds.). *Mind in Context: Interactionist Perspectives in Human Intelligence*. New York: Cambridge University Press, 1994.

128. Berk and Levin, *Child Development*.

129. Gardner, H. *Frames of Mind: The Theory of Multiple Intelligences*, 2nd ed. New York: Basic Books, 1993; Gardner, H. *Multiple Intelligence: Theory in Practice*. New York: Basic Books, 1993.

130. Berk and Levin, *Child Development*.

131. Glenwright, M.H., and P.M. Pexman, Children's Perceptions of the Social Functions of Verbal Irony. In R.W. Gibbs, Jr. and H.L. Colston (eds.), *Irony in Language and Thought: A Cognitive Science Reader* (pp. 447–466). New York: Lawrence Erlbaun Associates, Taylor & Francis Group, 2007.

132. Pexman, P.M., and M. Glenwright, How Do Typically Developing Children Grasp the Meaning of Verbal Irony? *Journal of Neurolinguistics*, *20* (2007), 178–196.

133. Pexman and Glenwright, How Do Typically Developing Children Grasp the Meaning of Verbal Irony?
134. Pexman and Glenwright, How Do Typically Developing Children Grasp the Meaning of Verbal Irony?
135. Pexman, P.M., M. Glenwright, S. Hala, S.L. Kowbel, and S. Jungen, Children's Use of Trait Information in Understanding Verbal Irony, *Metaphor and Symbol*, 21(1) (2006), 39–60.
136. Pexman and Glenwright, How Do Typically Developing Children Grasp the Meaning of Verbal Irony?
137. Pexman and Glenwright, How Do Typically Developing Children Grasp the Meaning of Verbal Irony?
138. Andrews and Boyle, *Transcultural Concepts in Nursing Care*.
139. Canadian Council on Social Development. *The Progress of Canada's Children and Youth: 2006*. Ottawa: The Canadian Council on Social Development, 2006.
140. Canadian Council on Social Development, *The Progress of Canada's Children and Youth: 2006*; Hanvey, L. *Issues Affecting the Well-Being of Canadian Children in the Middle Years—6 to 12: A Discussion Paper*. Ottawa: National Children's Alliance, n.d.
141. Statistics Canada. *Portrait of the Canadian Population in 2006, by Age and Sex, 2006 Census*. Ottawa: Author, 2006.
142. Debs-Ivall, S., Caring for Diverse Families. In R.H. Srivastava (ed.), *The Healthcare Professional's Guide to Clinical Cultural Competence* (pp. 144–171). Toronto: Elsevier Canada, 2007.
143. Papalia et al., *Human Development*; Rodgers, Health Promotion of the School-Aged Child and Family.
144. Child & Family Canada. *Middle Childhood (6–12 Years Old)*. Website: http://www.cfc-efc.ca/ (accessed September 2007).
145. Bee et al., *Lifespan Development*.
146. Canadian Institute of Child Health, *The Health of Canada's Children: A CICH Profile*.
147. Hamilton, D., Preparing for the People to Come: Secwepemc Activism in British Columbia, *Journal of Living*, 26 (2002), 28–37.
148. Seifert et al., *Lifespan Development*.
149. Bee et al., *Lifespan Development*.
150. Goleman, D. *Working with Emotional Intelligence*. New York: Bantam Books, 1998.
151. Snow, J.L., Looking beyond Nursing for Clues to Effective Leadership, *Journal of Nursing Administration*, 31(9) (2001), 440–443.
152. Bee et al., *Lifespan Development*.
153. Snow, Looking beyond Nursing for Clues to Effective Leadership.
154. Seifert et al., *Lifespan Development*.
155. Seifert et al., *Lifespan Development*.
156. Papalia et al., *Human Development*.
157. Ray, L.D., Parenting and Childhood Chronicity: Making Visible the Invisible Work, *Journal of Pediatric Nursing*, 17(6) (2002), 424–438.
158. Ray, Parenting and Childhood Chronicity: Making Visible the Invisible Work.
159. Wilkins, K., Sibling Adaptation to the Family Crisis of Childhood Cancer, *Canadian Oncology Nursing Journal*, 13(1) (2003), 46–48.
160. Woodgate, R.L., Children's Cancer Symptom Experiences: Keeping the Spirit Alive in Children and Their Families, *Canadian Oncology Nursing Journal*, 13(3) (2003), 142–150.
161. Fernandes, E., and B.W. McCrindle, Diagnosis and Treatment of Hypertension in Children and Adolescents, *Canadian Journal of Cardiology*, 44 (September 2000), 1869–1877.
162. Debs-Ivall, Caring for Diverse Families.
163. Health Canada. *First Nations & Inuit Health: Family Health, Healthy Pregnancy & Babies, Fetal Alcohol Syndrome/Fetal Alcohol Effects*. Website: http://www.hc-sc.gc.ca/ (accessed September 2007).
164. Health Canada. *First Nations & Inuit Health: Family Health, Healthy Pregnancy & Babies, Early Childhood Development Strategy for Aboriginal Children*. Website: http://www.hc-sc.gc.ca/ (accessed September 2007).
165. Harris, S.B., R. Glazier, K. Eng, and L. McMurray, Disease Patterns among Canadian Aboriginal Children, *Canadian Family Physician*, 44 (September 1998), 1869–1877.
166. Ball, G.D.C., and L.J. McCargar, Childhood Obesity in Canada: A Review of Prevalence Estimates and Risk Factors for Cardiovascular Diseases and Type 2 Diabetes, *Canadian Journal of Applied Physiology*, 28(1) (2003), 117–140.
167. Abidi, S.S.R., A. Finley, E. Milos, M. Shepherd, and D. Zitner. *Knowledge Management in Pediatric Pain: Mapping On-Line Expert Discussions to Medical Literature*. Website: users@cs.dal.ca/ (accessed September 2007).
168. Hospital for Sick Children. *10 Ways to Ease Pain in Children*. Website: http://www.sickkids.ca/ (accessed September 2007).
169. Papalia et al., *Human Development*.
170. Bee et al., *Lifespan Development*.
171. Papalia et al., *Human Development*.
172. Papalia et al., *Human Development*.
173. Berk and Levin, *Child Development*.
174. Office of the Commissioner of Official Languages. *A Look at Bilingualism*. Website: http://www.ocol-clo.gc.ca/ (accessed September 2007).
175. Bialystok, E., and J. Herman, Does Bilingualism Matter for Early Literacy? *Language and Cognition*, 2 (1999), 35–44.
176. Berk and Levin, *Child Development*.
177. Vanier Institute of the Family. *Did You Know*. Website: http://www.vifamily.ca/ (accessed September 2007).
178. Canadian Paediatric Society, Healthy Active Living for Children and Youth, *Paediatrics and Child Health*, 7(5) (2002), 339–345.
179. Swift, C., and A. Taylor, The Digital Divide—A New Generation Gap: Parental Knowledge of the Children's Internet Use, *Paediatric Child Health*, 8(5) (2003), 275–278.
180. Piaget, *The Equilibration of Cognitive Structures: The Central Problem of Intellectual Development*.
181. Bee et al., *Lifespan Development*; Lego, S., Children Killing Children, *Perspectives in Psychiatric Care*, 34(3) (1998), 3–4; Newman and Newman, *Development Through Life: A Psychosocial Approach*; Papalia et al., *Human Development*; Seifert et al., *Lifespan Development*.
182. Newman and Newman, *Development Through Life: A Psychosocial Approach*.
183. Newman and Newman, *Development Through Life: A Psychosocial Approach*.
184. Newman and Newman, *Development Through Life: A Psychosocial Approach*.
185. Newman and Newman, *Development Through Life: A Psychosocial Approach*; Seifert et al., *Lifespan Development*.
186. Newman and Newman, *Development Through Life: A Psychosocial Approach*.
187. Papalia et al., *Human Development*; Seifert et al., *Lifespan Development*.
188. Human Resources and Social Development Canada. *Bullying and Victimization among Canadian School Children*. Website: http://www.hrsd.gc.ca/ (accessed August 2007).
189. Marini, Z., L. Fairbain, and R. Zuber, Peer Harassment in Individuals with Developmental Disabilities: Towards the Development of a Multidimensional Bullying Identification Model, *Aggressive Behavior*, 32 (2006), 1–19.
190. Janssen, I., W.M. Craig, W.F. Boyce, and W. Pickett, Associations Between Overweight and Obesity with Bullying Behaviors in School-Aged Children, *Pediatrics*, 113(5) (2004), 1187–1194.
191. Bosacki, S.L., Z.A. Marini, and A.V. Dane, Voices from the Classroom: Pictorial and Narrative Representations of Children's Bullying Experiences, *Journal of Moral Education*, 35(2) (2006), 231–245.

192. Public Safety Canada. *Keeping Canadians Safe: First Steps to Stop Bullying.* Website: http://www.publicsafety.gc.ca/ (accessed September 2007).

193. Hanvey, *Issues Affecting the Well-Being of Canadian Children in the Middle Years—6 to 12: A Discussion Paper.*

194. Newman and Newman, *Development Through Life: A Psychosocial Approach;* Papalia et al., *Human Development.*

195. Andrews and Boyle, *Transcultural Concepts in Nursing Care;* Newman and Newman, *Development Through Life: A Psychosocial Approach;* Seifert et al., *Lifespan Development.*

196. Erikson, E. *Childhood and Society,* 2nd ed. New York: W.W. Norton, 1963.

197. Erikson, *Childhood and Society.*

198. Bee et al., *Lifespan Development;* Papalia et al., *Human Development.*

199. Bee et al., *Lifespan Development;* Papalia et al., *Human Development.*

200. Bee et al., *Lifespan Development.*

201. Papalia et al., *Human Development.*

202. Bee et al., *Lifespan Development;* Papalia et al., *Human Development.*

203. Newman and Newman, *Development Through Life: A Psychosocial Approach.*

204. Newman and Newman, *Development Through Life: A Psychosocial Approach;* Rodgers, Health Promotion of the School-Aged Child and Family.

205. Public Health Agency of Canada. Canadian Guidelines for Sexual Health Education. Website: http://www.phac-aspc.gc.ca/ (accessed August 2007).

206. Public Health Agency of Canada, Canadian Guidelines for Sexual Health Education.

207. Wackett, J., and L. Evans, An Evaluation of the Choices and Changes Student Program: A Grade Four to Seven Sexual Health Education Program Based on the Canadian Guidelines for Sexual Health Education, *The Canadian Journal of Human Sexuality,* 9(4) (2000), 265–273.

208. Wackett and Evans, An Evaluation of the Choices and Changes Student Program: A Grade Four to Seven Sexual Health Education Program Based on the Canadian Guidelines for Sexual Health Education.

209. Kohlberg, L., Development of Moral Character and Moral Ideology. In M.L. Hoffman (ed.), *Review of Child Development Research,* Vol. 1 (pp. 383–432). New York: Russell Sage, 1964; Kohlberg, L., Stages of Moral Development as a Basis for Moral Education. In C.M. Beck, B.S. Crittenden, and E.V. Sullivan (eds.), *Moral Education: Interdisciplinary Approaches* (pp. 23ff). New York: Paulist Press, 1972.

210. Kohlberg, Development of Moral Character and Moral Ideology; Kohlberg, Stages of Moral Development as a Basis for Moral Education.

## Chapter 11

1. Santrock, J.W., A. MacKenzie-Rivers, K.H. Leung, and T. Malcomson. *Life-span Development,* 2nd Canadian ed. Toronto: McGraw-Hill Ryerson, 2005.

2. Kail, R.V., J.C. Cavanaugh, C.A. Ateah. *Human Development: A Life-Span View,* 1st Canadian ed. Toronto: Thomson Nelson, 2006.

3. Kail et al., *Human Development: A Life-Span View;* Papalia, D., S. Olds, and R. Feldman. *Human Development,* 9th ed. Boston: McGraw Hill, 2004.

4. Santrock et al., *Life-span Development.*

5. Kail et al., *Human Development: A Life-Span View.*

6. Bee, H., D. Boyd, and P. Johnson. *Lifespan Development,* 2nd ed. Toronto: Pearson Education Canada, Inc., 2006.

7. Kail et al., *Human Development: A Life-Span View.*

8. Santrock et al., *Life-span Development.*

9. Carter, B., and M. McGoldrick, Overview: *The Expanded Family Life Cycle: Individual, Family, and Social Perspectives.* In B. Carter and M. McGoldrick (eds.), *The Expanded Family Life Cycle: Individual, Family, and Social Perspectives,* 3rd ed. (pp. 1–26). Toronto: Allyn & Bacon, 2005.

10. Kail et al., *Human Development: A Life-Span View.*

11. Sigelman, C. *Lifespan Human Development,* 3rd ed. Pacific Groves, CA: Brooks/Cole, 1999.

12. Kail et al., *Human Development: A Life-Span View.*

13. Saewyc, E.M., Health Promotion of the Adolescent. In M.J. Hockenberry and D. Wilson (eds.), *Wong's Nursing Care of Infants and Children,* 7th ed. (pp. 811–848). St. Louis, MO: Mosby Elsevier, 2007.

14. Saewyc, Health Promotion of the Adolescent.

15. Grant, C., Teens, Sex, and the Media: Is There a Connection? *Paediatric Child Health,* 8(5) (2003), 285–286.

16. Ryan, C., D. Futterman, and K. Stine, Helping Our Hidden Youth, *American Journal of Nursing,* 98(12) (1998), 37–41.

17. Saewyc, Health Promotion of the Adolescent.

18. Mahon, N.E., A. Yarcheski, and T.J. Yarcheski, Anger, Anxiety, and Depression in Early Adolescence from Intact and Divorced Families, *Journal of Pediatric Nursing,* 18(4) (2003), 267–273.

19. Ball, J.W., and R.C. Bindler. *Wong's Nursing Care of Infants and Children.* Upper Saddle River, NJ: Pearson Education, 2006.

20. Berman, H., Stories of Growing Up Amid Violence by Refugee Children of War and Children of Battered Women Living in Canada, *IMAGE: Journal of Nursing Scholarship,* 31(1) (1999), 52–63.

21. Bee et al., *Lifespan Development.*

22. Fenstermacher, K., and B. Hudson. *Practice Guidelines for Family Nurse Practitioners.* Philadelphia: Saunders, 1997.

23. Bee et al., *Lifespan Development.*

24. Polan, E.U., and S. Solberg, Conception Through Adolescence. In P.A. Potter, A. Griffin Perry, J.C. Ross-Kerr, and M.J. Wood (eds.), *Canadian Fundamentals of Nursing,* 3rd ed. (pp. 356–396). Toronto: Elsevier Canada, 2006.

25. Saewyc, Health Promotion of the Adolescent.

26. Papalia et al., *Human Development* (9th ed.).

27. Saewyc, Health Promotion of the Adolescent.

28. Papalia et al., *Human Development.*

29. Bee et al., *Lifespan Development;* Papalia et al., *Human Development;* Seifert, K., R. Hoffnung, and M. Hoffnung. *Lifespan Development.* Boston: Houghton Mifflin, 1997.

30. Bee et al., *Lifespan Development.*

31. Saewyc, Health Promotion of the Adolescent.

32. Seifert et al., *Lifespan Development;* Saewyc, Health Promotion of the Adolescent.

33. Saewyc, Health Promotion of the Adolescent.

34. Papalia et al. *Human Development.*

35. Saewyc, Health Promotion of the Adolescent; Papalia et al., *Human Development;* Seifert et al., *Lifespan Development.*

36. Saewyc, Health Promotion of the Adolescent.

37. Thibodeau, G.A., and K.T. Patton. *Anatomy & Physiology,* 6th ed. Philadelphia: Mosby Elsevier, 2007.

38. Ingram Fogel, C., Reproductive System Concerns. In D.L. Lowdermilk and S.E. Perry (eds.), *Maternity & Women's Health Care,* 8th ed. (pp. 155–183). St. Louis, MO: Mosby, 2004.

39. Blackburn, S. *Maternal, Fetal, & Neonatal Physiology: A Clinical Perspective,* 3rd ed. Philadelphia: Saunders, 2003.

40. Ingram Fogel, Reproductive System Concerns.

41. Thibodeau and Patton, *Anatomy & Physiology.*

42. Thibodeau and Patton, *Anatomy & Physiology.*

43. Ingram Fogel, Reproductive System Concerns.

44. Kollar, L.M., Physical Health Problems of Adolescence. In M.J. Hockenberry and D. Wilson (eds.), *Wong's Nursing Care of Infants and Children,* 7th ed. (pp. 849–879), St. Louis, MO: Mosby Elsevier, 2007.

45. Ingram Fogel, Reproductive System Concerns.

46. Kollar, Physical Health Problems of Adolescence.

47. Thibodeau and Patton, *Anatomy & Physiology.*

48. Thibodeau and Patton, *Anatomy & Physiology*.
49. Papalia et al., *Human Development*. Seifert et al., *Lifespan Development*.
50. Papalia et al., *Human Development*.
51. Saewyc, Health Promotion of the Adolescent.
52. Saewyc, Health Promotion of the Adolescent.
53. Saewyc, Health Promotion of the Adolescent.
54. Health Canada. *Canadian Guidelines for Sexual Health Education*. Ottawa: Minister of Public Works and Government Services Canada, 2003.
55. Muscari, M., The First Gynecologic Exam, *American Journal of Nursing*, 99(1) (1999), 68–69; Muscari, M., Rebels with a Cause: When Adolescents Won't Follow Medical Advice, *American Journal of Nursing*, 98(12) (1998), 28–35; Sharts-Hopko, N., STDs in Women: What You Need to Know, *American Journal of Nursing and Special Women's Health Issue*, 97(4) (1997), 5–7.
56. Hockenberry, M.J., and P. Barrera, Communication and Physical and Developmental Assessment of the Child. In M.J. Hockenberry and D. Wilson (eds.), *Wong's Nursing Care of Infants and Children*, 7th ed. (pp. 141–204). St. Louis, MO: Mosby Elsevier, 2007.
57. Hockenberry and Barrera, Communication and Physical and Developmental Assessment of the Child.
58. Hospital for Sick Children. *AboutKidsHealth News: Was that a Pap smear or not?* Website: http://www.aboutkidshealth.ca/ (accessed December 2007); Blake, D.R., B.M. Weber, and K.E. Fletcher, Adolescent and Young Adult Women's Misunderstanding of the Term Pap Smear, *Archives of Pediatric and Adolescent Medicine*, 158(10) (2004), 966–970.
59. Gillis, A., Teens for Healthy Living, *The Canadian Nurse*, 92(6) (1996), 26–30.
60. Gillis, Teens for Healthy Living.
61. Vingilis, E.R., T.J. Wade, and J.S. Seeley, Predictors of Adolescent Self-Rated Health, *Canadian Journal of Public Health*, 93(3) (2002), 193–197.
62. Health Canada. *Nutrition for a Healthy Pregnancy: National Guidelines for the Childbearing Years*. Ottawa: Minister of Public Works and Government Services, 1999.
63. McVey, G., S. Tweed, and E. Blackmore, Dieting among Preadolescent and Young Adolescent Females, *Canadian Medical Association Journal*, 170(10) (2004), 1559–1561
64. Rodwell Williams, S., and E.D. Schlenker, *Essentials of Nutrition & Diet Therapy*, 8th ed. St. Louis, MO: Mosby, 2003.
65. Health Canada. *Canada's Food Guide: Educators and Communicators*. Website: http://www.hc-sc.gc.ca/ (accessed December 2007).
66. Health Canada, *Canada's Food Guide: Educators and Communicators*.
67. Health Canada, *Nutrition for a Healthy Pregnancy: National Guidelines for the Childbearing Years*.
68. Rodwell Williams and Schlenker, Essentials of Nutrition & Diet Therapy.
69. Taylor, J.P., S. Evers, and M. McKenna, Determinants of Healthy Eating in Children and Youth, *Canadian Journal of Public Health*, 96(S.3) (2005), S20–S26.
70. Philips, S., L. Jacobs Starkey, and K. Gray-Donald, Food Habits of Canadians: Food Sources of Nutrients for the Adolescent Sample, *Canadian Journal of Dietetic Practice and Research*, 65(2) (2004), 81–84.
71. Philips et al., Food Habits of Canadians: Food Sources of Nutrients for the Adolescent Sample.
72. McVey et al., Dieting among Preadolescent and Young Adolescent Females.
73. Daigneau, C.V., and E.M. Saewyc, Behavioral Health Problems of Adolescence. In M.J. Hockenberry and D. Wilson (eds.), *Wong's Nursing Care of Infants and Children*, 7th ed. (pp. 880–920). St. Louis, MO: Mosby Elsevier, 2007.
74. Jones, J.M., S. Bennett, M.P. Olmstead, M.L. Lawson, and G. Rodin, Disordered Eating Attitudes and Behaviours in Teenaged Girls: A School-Based Study, *Canadian Medical Association Journal*, 165(5) (2001), 547–558.
75. Kirsh, G., G. McVey, S. Tweed, and D.K. Katzman, Psychosocial Profiles of Young Adolescent Females Seeking Treatment for an Eating Disorder, *Journal of Adolescent Health*, 40 (2007), 351–356.
76. Tierney, L., S. McPhee, and M. Papadakis, *Current Medical Diagnosis & Treatment, 1999*, 38th ed. Stamford, CT: Appleton & Lange, 1999; Daigneau and Saewyc, Behavioral Health Problems of Adolescence.
77. Turrell, S.L., R. Davis, H. Graham, and I. Weiss, Adolescents with Anorexia Nervosa: Multiple Perspectives of Discharge Readiness, *Journal of Child and Adolescent Psychiatric Nursing*, 18(3) (2005), 116–126.
78. Tierney et al., *Current Medical Diagnosis & Treatment, 1999*.
79. Tierney et al., *Current Medical Diagnosis & Treatment, 1999*.
80. Daigneau and Saewyc, Behavioral Health Problems of Adolescence; Tierney et al., *Current Medical Diagnosis & Treatment, 1999*.
81. Daigneau and Saewyc, Behavioral Health Problems of Adolescence; Tierney et al., *Current Medical Diagnosis & Treatment, 1999*.
82. Daigneau and Saewyc, Behavioral Health Problems of Adolescence; Tierney et al., Current Medical Diagnosis & Treatment, *1999*.
83. Decker, S.D., The Client with an Eating Disorder. In W.K. Mohr (ed.), *Johnson's Psychiatric-Mental Health Nursing*, 5th ed. (pp. 455–474). Philadelphia: Lippincott Williams & Wilkins, 2003.
84. Canadian Population Health Initiative. *Overweight and Obesity in Canada: A Population Health Perspective*. Ottawa: CPHI-CIHI, 2004.
85. Anonymous, The Continuing Challenge of Obesity, *Canadian Journal of Public Health*, 97(6) (2006), 428.
86. Janssen, I., W.F. Boyce, K. Simpson, and W. Pickett, Influence of Individual- and Area-Level Measures of Socioeconomic Status on Obesity, Unhealthy Eating, and Physical Inactivity in Canadian Adolescents, *American Journal of Clinical Nutrition*, 83 (2006), 139–145.
87. Canadian Institute for Health Information. *Improving the Health of Canadians*. Ottawa: Canadian Institute for Health Information, 2004.
88. Fernandes, E., and B.W. McCrindle, Diagnosis and Treatment of Hypertension in Children and Adolescents, *Canadian Journal of Cardiology*, 16(6) (2000), 801–811.
89. Katzmarzyk, P.T., The Canadian Obesity Epidemic, 1985–1998, *Canadian Medical Association Journal*, 166(8) (2002), 1039–1040.
90. Hanley, A.J.G., S.B. Harris, J. Gittelsohn, T.M.S. Wolever, B. Saksvig, and B. Zinman, Overweight among Children and Adolescents in a Native Canadian Community: Prevalence and Associated Factors, *The American Journal of Clinical Nutrition*, 71(3) (2000), 693–700.
91. Janssen, I., P.T. Katzmarzyk, W.T. Boyce, M.A. King, and W. Pickett, Overweight and Obesity in Canadian Adolescents and Their Associations with Dietary Habits and Physical Activity Patterns, *Journal of Adolescent Health*, 35 (2004), 360–367.
92. Shields, M., Overweight and Obesity among Children and Youth, *Health Reports*, 17(3) (2006), 27–43.
93. Shields, Overweight and Obesity among Children and Youth.
94. Raine, K.D. *Overweight and Obesity in Canada: A Population Health Perspective*. Ottawa: Canadian Institute for Health Information, 2004.
95. Raine, *Overweight and Obesity in Canada: A Population Health Perspective*.
96. Health Canada. The Vitality Approach: A Guide for Leaders. Ottawa: Health Canada, 2000.

97. Daigneau and Saewyc, Behavioral Health Problems of Adolescence.
98. Stanhope, M., J. Lancaster, H. Jessup-Falcioni, and G.A. Viverais-Dresler, *Community Health Nursing in Canada*, 1st Canadian ed. Toronto: Elsevier Canada, 2008.
99. Plotnikoff, R.C., K. Bercovitz, and C.A. Loucaides, Physical Activity, Smoking, and Obesity among Canadian School Youth: Comparison between Urban and Rural Schools, *Canadian Journal of Public Health, 95*(6) (2004), 413–418.
100. Public Health Agency of Canada. *Canada's Physical Activity Guide for Youth*. Website: http://www.phac-aspc.gc.ca/ (accessed December 2007).
101. Public Health Agency of Canada. *Canada's Physical Activity Guide for Youth: Teacher's Guide*. Website: http://www.phac-aspc.gc.ca/ (accessed December 2007).
102. Public Health Agency of Canada. *Canada's Physical Activity Guide to Healthy Active Living: "Let's Get Active" Interactive Magazine for Youth*. Website: http://www.phac-aspc.gc.ca/ (accessed December 2007).
103. Public Health Agency of Canada. *Canada's Physical Activity Guide to Healthy Active Living: Teacher's Guide, Physical Inactivity and Youth*. Website: http://www.phac-aspc.gc.ca/ (accessed December 2007).
104. Saewyc, Health Promotion of the Adolescent.
105. Santrock et al., *Life-span Development*.
106. Saewyc, Health Promotion of the Adolescent.
107. Wadsworth, B. *Piaget's Theory of Cognitive and Affective Development: Foundations of Constructivism*, 5th ed. New York: Longman, 1996.
108. Papalia et al., *Human Development*.
109. Dill-Schreiber, V. *A Peaceable School: Cultivating a Culture of Non-violence*. Bloomington, IN: Phi Delta Kappa, 1997.
110. Papalia et al., *Human Development*.
111. Tutty, L.M., and C. Bradshaw, Violence against Children and Youth: Do School-based Prevention Programs Work? In C.A. Ateah and J. Mirwaldt (eds.), *Within Our Reach: Preventing Abuse across the Lifespan* (pp. 47–53). Winnipeg: Fernwood, 2004.
112. Donnon, T., and W. Hammond, Understanding the Relationship between Resiliency and Bullying in Adolescence: An Assessment of Youth Resiliency from Five Urban Junior High Schools, *Child and Adolescent Psychiatric Clinics of North America, 16* (2007), 449–471.
113. Canadian Adolescents at Risk Research Network. *Fact Sheet: Adolescent Bullying*. Website: http://www.educ.queensu.ca/~caarrn (accessed August 2007).
114. Canadian Adolescents at Risk Research Network, *Fact Sheet: Adolescent Bullying*.
115. Volk, A., W. Craig, W. Boyce, and M. King, Adolescent Risk Correlates of Bullying and Different Types of Victimization, *International Journal of Adolescent Medicine and Health, 18*(4) (2006), 375–386.
116. Public Safety Canada, *First Steps to Stop Bullying and Harassment: Adults Helping Youth Aged 12 to 17*. Website: http://www.publicsafety.gc.ca/ (accessed December 2007).
117. Canadian Adolescents at Risk Research Network, *Fact Sheet: Adolescent Bullying*.
118. Public Safety Canada. *Bullying Prevention in Schools*. Website: http://www.publicsafety.gc.ca/ (accessed December 2007).
119. Santrock et al., *Life-span Development*.
120. Papalia et al., *Human Development*; Seifert et al., *Lifespan Development*.
121. Banister, E.M., S.L. Jakubec, and J.A. Stein, "Like, What Am I Supposed to Do?": Adolescent Girls' Health Concerns in Their Dating Relationships, *Canadian Journal of Nursing Research, 35*(2) (2003), 17–33.
122. Banister et al., "Like, What Am I Supposed to Do?": Adolescent Girls' Health Concerns in Their Dating Relationships.
123. Larson, R.W., Toward a Psychology of Positive Youth Development, *American Psychologist, 55* (2000), 170–183.
124. Coatsworth, J.D., E.H. Sharp, L-A., Palen, N. Darling, P. Cumsille, and E. Marta, Exploring Adolescent Self-Defining Leisure Activities and Identity Experiences across Three Countries, *International Journal of Behavioral Development, 29* (2005), 361–370.
125. Campbell, J. Adolescent Identity Development: The Relationship with Leisure Lifestyle and Motivation. Waterloo, ON: University of Waterloo, Graduate Student Leisure Research Symposium, Oral Presentation, 2007.
126. Public Health Agency of Canada. *Publications: Trends in the Health of Canadian Youth: Health Behaviours in School-Aged Children, Chapter 8: Exercise and Leisure Activities*. Website: http://www.phac-aspc.gc.ca/ (accessed December 2007).
127. Papalia et al., *Human Development*; Seifert et al., *Lifespan Development*; Bee et al., *Lifespan Development*.
128. Alfons, A., M. Crijnen, J. Ackenbach, and F. Verhulst, Comparisons of Problems Reported by Parents of Children in 12 Cultures: Total Problems, Externalizing, and Internalizing, *Journal of the American Academy of Psychiatry, 36*(9) (1997), 1269–1277.
129. Santrock et al., *Life-span Development*.
130. Bee et al., *Lifespan Development*.
131. Bee et al., *Lifespan Development*.
132. Bee et al., *Lifespan Development*.
133. Park, J., Adolescent Self-Concept and Health into Adulthood, *Health Reports, 14*(suppl.) (2003).
134. Muscari, M., When to Worry About Adolescent Angst, *American Journal of Nursing, 98*(3) (1998), 22.
135. Public Health Agency of Canada. *Publications: Trends in the Health of Canadian Youth: Summary*. Website: http://www.phac-aspc.gc.ca/ (accessed December 2007).
136. Bee et al., *Lifespan Development*.
137. Saewyc, Health Promotion of the Adolescent.
138. Garriguet, D., Early Sexual Intercourse, *Health Reports, 16*(3) (2005), 9–18.
139. Saewyc, Health Promotion of the Adolescent.
140. Evans, S.J., B.L. Wright, L. Goodbrand, J.P. Kilbreath, and J. Young, Teen Sexuality: Reaching Out in the Malls, *Canadian Journal of Public Health, 93*(1) (2002), 47–51.
141. Health Canada. *Canadian Guidelines for Sexual Health Education*. Ottawa: Minister of Public Works and Government Services Canada, 2003.
142. Kohlberg, L., Moral Stages and Moralization: The Cognitive Development Approach. In T. Lickera (ed.), *Moral Development and Behavior*. New York: Holt Rinehart & Winston, 1976.
143. Muuss, R., Carol Gilligan's Theory of Sex Differences in the Development of Moral Reasoning during Adolescence, *Adolescence, 23*(89) (1988), 229–243.
144. Shepherd, B., When Moms Pray, *Focus on the Family*, August 1999, 3–5.
145. Code, M., and K. Bernes. *Adolescents' Perceptions of Career Concern*. The National Consultation on Career Development (NATCON).
146. Saewyc, Health Promotion of the Adolescent.
147. Hoole, A., C. Pickard, R. Ouimette, J. Lohr, and W. Powell, *Patient Care Guidelines for Nurse Practitioners*, 5th ed. Philadelphia: J.B. Lippincott, 1999; Hockenberry, M.J., and D. Wilson (eds.), *Wong's Nursing Care of Infants and Children*, 7th ed. St. Louis, MO: Mosby Elsevier, 2007.
148. Stanhope et al., *Community Health Nursing in Canada*.
149. Canadian Population Health Initiative (CPHI). *Improving the Health of Canadians*. Ottawa: CPHI, 2004.

150. Stolte, K.M. *Wellness: Nursing Diagnosis for Health Promotion.* Philadelphia: Lippincott, 1996.
151. Canadian Population Health Initiative (CPHI), *Improving the Health of Canadians.*
152. Canadian Population Health Initiative (CPHI), *Improving the Health of Canadians.*
153. Canadian Adolescents at Risk Research Network, *Fact Sheet: Adolescent Injuries.*
154. Canadian Nurses Association, CNA Backgrounder, *The Built Environment, Injury Prevention and Nursing: A Summary of the Issues.* Ottawa: Author, 2005.
155. Bee et al., *Lifespan Development*; Papalia et al., *Human Development*; Saewyc, Health Promotion of the Adolescent.
156. Health Canada. *The Health Behaviour of School-Aged Children (HBSC) Study, Young People in Canada: Their Health and Well-Being.* Ottawa: Author, n.d.
157. Health Canada, *The Health Behaviour of School-Aged Children (HBSC) Study.*
158. Hoole et al., *Patient Care Guidelines for Nurse Practitioners.*
159. Saewyc, Health Promotion of the Adolescent.
160. Papalia et al., *op. cit.*
161. Canadian Nurses Association, CNA Backgrounder, *The Built Environment, Injury Prevention and Nursing.*
162. Canadian Injury Prevention Strategy. *Developing an Integrated Canadian Injury Prevention Strategy.* Website: http://www.injurypreventionstrategy.ca/ (accessed December 2007).
163. Stanhope et al., *Community Health Nursing in Canada.*
164. Muscari, M., Preventing Sports Injuries, *American Journal of Nursing, 98*(7) (1998), 58–59.
165. Hoole et al., *Patient Care Guidelines for Nurse Practitioners.*
166. Hoole et al., *Patient Care Guidelines for Nurse Practitioners.*
167. Hoole et al., *Patient Care Guidelines for Nurse Practitioners.*
168. Hockenberry, M.J., and P. Barrera, Communication and Physical and Developmental Assessment of the Child. In M.J. Hockenberry and D. Wilson (eds.), *Wong's Nursing Care of Infants and Children*, 7th ed. (pp. 141–204). St. Louis, MO: Mosby Elsevier, 2007; Health Canada. First Nations & Inuit Health: *Pediatric Clinical Practice Guidelines for Nurses in Primary Care.* Ottawa: Author, 2001.
169. Kollar, Physical Health Problems of Adolescence; Hoole et al., *Patient Care Guidelines for Nurse Practitioners*; Ball and Bindler, *Wong's Nursing Care of Infants and Children.*
170. Feinberg, S.L., The Child with Cancer. In M.J. Hockenberry, and D. Wilson (eds.), *Wong's Nursing Care of Infants and Children*, 7th ed. (pp. 1558–1611). St. Louis, MO: Mosby Elsevier, 2007.
171. Public Health Agency of Canada. *Human Papillomavirus (HPV) Prevention and HPV Vaccine: Questions and Answers.* Website: http://www.phac-aspc.gc.ca/ (accessed December 2007).
172. Bryant, R., Family-Centered Care of the Child with Chronic Illness or Disability. In M.J. Hockenberry and D. Wilson (eds.), *Wong's Nursing Care of Infants and Children*, 7th ed. (pp. 921–956). St. Louis, MO: Mosby Elsevier, 2007.
173. Woodgate, R., Adolescents' Perspectives of Chronic Illness: "It's Hard," *Journal of Pediatric Nursing, 13*(4) (1998), 210–223.
174. Ball and Bindler, *Wong's Nursing Care of Infants and Children.*
175. Ball and Bindler, *Wong's Nursing Care of Infants and Children.*
176. Canadian Mental Health Association. Youth and Suicide. Website: http://www.cmha.ca/ (accessed December 2007).
177. Papalia et al., *Human Development.*
178. Canadian Population Health Initiative (CPHI), Improving the Health of Canadians.
179. Boothroyd, L.J., L.J. Kirmayer, S. Spreng, M. Malus, and S. Hodgins, Completed Suicides among the Inuit of Northern Quebec, 1982–1996: A Case-Control Study, *Canadian Medical Association Journal, 165*(6) (2001), 749–755.
180. Boothroyd et al., Completed Suicides among the Inuit of Northern Quebec, 1982–1996.

181. Chandler, M., and T. Proulx, Changing Selves in Changing Worlds: Youth Suicide on the Fault-Lines of Colliding Cultures, *Archives of Suicide Research, 10*(2) (2006), 125–140.
182. Pinhas, L., H. Weaver, P. Bryden, N. Ghabbour, and B. Toner, Gender-Role Conflict and Suicidal Behaviour in Adolescent Girls, *Canadian Journal of Psychiatry, 47*(5) (2002), 473–476.
183. Daigneau and Saewyc, Behavioral Health Problems of Adolescence; Ball and Bindler, *Wong's Nursing Care of Infants and Children.*
184. Daigneau and Saewyc, Behavioral Health Problems of Adolescence; Ball and Bindler, *Wong's Nursing Care of Infants and Children.*
185. Daigneau and Saewyc, Behavioral Health Problems of Adolescence.
186. Daigneau and Saewyc, Behavioral Health Problems of Adolescence; Ball and Bindler, *Wong's Nursing Care of Infants and Children.*
187. Kidd, S., C.C. Henrich, K.A. Brookmeyer, L. Davidson, R.A. King, and G. Shahar, The Social Context of Adolescent Suicide Attempts: Interactive Effects of Parent, Peer, and School Social Relations, *Suicide and Life-Threatening Behavior, 36*(4) (2006), 386–395.
188. Kidd et al., The Social Context of Adolescent Suicide Attempts.
189. Hotton, T., and D. Haans, Alcohol and Drug Use in Early Adolescence, *Health Reports, 15*(3) (2004), 9–19.
190. Boyle, M.H., M. Sanford, P. Szatmarie, K. Merikangas, and D.R. Offord, Familial Influences on Substance Use by Adolescents and Young Adults, *Canadian Journal of Public Health, 92*(3) (2001), 206–209.
191. Williams, R.J., and S.Y. Chang, A Comprehensive and Comparative Review of Adolescent Substance Abuse Treatment Outcome, *Clinical Psychology: Science and Practice, 7*(2) (2000), 138–166.
192. Rehm, J., R. Room, K. Graham, M. Monteiro, G. Gmel, and C.T. Sempos, The Relationship of Average Volume of Alcohol Consumption and Patterns of Drinking to Burden of Disease—An Overview, *Addiction, 98* (2003), 1209–1228; Klingemann, H., and G. Gmel. *Mapping Social Consequences of Alcohol Consumption.* Boston: Kluwer, 2001.
193. Babor, T.F., J.C. Higgins-Biddle, J.B. Saunders, and M.G. Monteiro. *The Alcohol Use Disorders Identification Test: Guidelines for Use in Primary Care*, 2nd ed. Geneva, Switzerland: World Health Organization, 2001.
194. Rehm, J., N. Monga, E. Adlaf, B. Taylor, S.J. Bondy, and J-S. Fallu, School Matters: Drinking Dimensions and Their Effects on Alcohol-Related Problems among Ontario Secondary School Students, *Alcohol & Alcoholism, 40*(6) (2005), 569–574.
195. Maes, L., and J. Lievens, Can the School Make a Difference? A Multilevel Analysis of Adolescent Risk and Health Behaviour, *Social Science and Medicine, 3* (2003), 125–133.
196. National Alcohol Strategy Working Group. *Reducing Alcohol-Related Harm in Canada: Toward a Culture of Moderation.* Ottawa: Author, 2007.
197. National Alcohol Strategy Working Group, *Reducing Alcohol-Related Harm in Canada: Toward a Culture of Moderation.*
198. Daigneau and Saewyc, Behavioral Health Problems of Adolescence.
199. Schissel, B., The Pathology of Powerlessness: Adolescent Health in Canada. In B.S. Bolaria and H.D. Dickinson (eds.), *Health, Illness, and Health Care in Canada*, 3rd ed. (pp. 265–273). Toronto: Nelson Thomson Learning, 2002.
200. Adlaf, E.M., A. Demers, and L. Gliksman (eds.). *Canadian Campus Survey 2004.* Toronto: Centre for Addiction and Mental Health, 2005.
201. Cox, B.J., N. Yu, T.O. Afifi, and R. Ladouceur, A National Survey of Gambling Problems in Canada, *Canadian Journal of Psychiatry, 50*(4) (2005), 213–217.
202. Ball and Bindler, *Child Health Nursing: Partnering with Children & Family.*
203. American Psychiatric Association. *Diagnostic and Statistical Manual of Mental Disorders*, 4th ed., text revision. Washington, DC: American Psychiatric Association, 2000.

204. Seifert et al., *Lifespan Development*.
205. Health Canada. *Preventing Substance Abuse Problems among Young People: A Compendium of Best Practices*. Ottawa: Minister of Public Works and Government Services Canada, 2001.
206. Health Canada, *Preventing Substance Abuse Problems among Young People*.
207. Council of Ministers of Education, Canada. Canadian Youth, Sexual Health and HIV/AIDS Study. Toronto: Author, 2003.
208. Rotermann, M., Sex, Condoms and STDs among Young People, *Health Reports*, 16(3) (2005), 39–45.
209. Bee et al., *Lifespan Development*; Papalia et al., *Human Development*; Seifert et al., *Lifespan Development*.
210. Public Health Agency of Canada, Canadian Sexually Transmitted Infections Surveillance Report, *Canada Communicable Disease Report*, 33(S1) (2007), 1–69.
211. Public Health Agency of Canada, *Canadian Sexually Transmitted Infections Surveillance Report*.
212. Public Health Agency of Canada, *Canadian Sexually Transmitted Infections Surveillance Report*.
213. Public Health Agency of Canada, *2002 Canadian Sexually Transmitted Infections Surveillance Report*. Canada Communicable Disease Report (2005).
214. Steenbeek, A., Empowering Health Promotion: A Holistic Approach in Preventing Sexually Transmitted Infections among First Nations and Inuit Adolescents in Canada, *Journal of Holistic Nursing*, 22(3) (2004), 254–266.
215. Steenbeek, Empowering Health Promotion: A Holistic Approach in Preventing Sexually Transmitted Infections among First Nations and Inuit Adolescents in Canada.
216. Steenbeek, A., M. Tyndall, R. Rothenberg, and S. Sheps, Determinants of Sexually Transmitted Infections among Canadian Inuit Adolescent Populations, *Public Health Nursing*, 23(6) (2006), 531–534.
217. Steenbeek et al., Determinants of Sexually Transmitted Infections among Canadian Inuit Adolescent Populations.
218. Society of Obstetricians and Gynaecologists of Canada. *Sex Sense: Canadian Contraception Guide*, 2nd, revised ed. Ottawa: Author, 2005.
219. Fisher, W.A., R. Boroditsky, and B. Morris, The 2002 Canadian Contraception Study: Part 1, *Journal of Obstetrics and Gynaecology of Canada*, 26 (2004), 580–590; Fisher, W.A., R. Boroditsky, and B. Morris, The 2002 Canadian Contraception Study: Part 2, *Journal of Obstetrics and Gynaecology of Canada*, 26 (2004), 646–656.
220. Society of Obstetricians and Gynaecologists of Canada, Sex Sense: Canadian Contraception Guide; Fisher, W.A., and A. Black, Contraception in Canada: A Review of Method Choices, Characteristics, Adherence and Approaches to Counselling, *Canadian Medical Association Journal*, 176(7) (2007), 953–961; McKay, A., Adolescent Sexual and Reproductive Health in Canada: A Report Card in 2004, *The Canadian Journal of Human Sexuality*, 13(2) (2004), 67–81.
221. Fisher and Black, Contraception in Canada: A Review of Method Choices, Characteristics, Adherence and Approaches to Counselling.
222. McKay, Adolescent Sexual and Reproductive Health in Canada.
223. McKay, Adolescent Sexual and Reproductive Health in Canada.
224. Council of Ministers of Education, Canada, Canadian Youth, Sexual Health and HIV/AIDS Study.
225. Maticka-Tyndale, E., M. Barrett, and A. McKay, Adolescent Sexual and Reproductive Health in Canada: A Review of National Data Sources and Their Limitations, *The Canadian Journal of Human Sexuality*, 9 (2000), 41–65.
226. Wackett, J., Factors Affecting Yukon Teen Pregnancy Decline in the Mid and Late 1990s, *Journal of Obstetrics and Gynaecology in Canada*, 24(11) (2002), 889–893.
227. Kollar, Physical Health Problems of Adolescence.
228. Kollar, Physical Health Problems of Adolescence.
229. Kollar, Physical Health Problems of Adolescence; Mannion, C., Adolescent Sexual Health and Pregnancy. In L. Leeseberg Stamler and L. Yiu (eds.), *Community Health Nursing: A Canadian Perspective*, 2nd ed. (pp. 360–367). Toronto: Pearson Education Canada, 2008.
230. Langille, D.B., Teenage Pregnancy: Trends, Contributing Factors and the Physician's Role, *Canadian Medical Association Journal*, 176(11) (2007), 1601–1615.
231. Peterson, W., W. Sword, C. Charles, and A. DiCenso, Adolescents' Perceptions of Inpatient Postpartum Nursing Care, *Qualitative Health Research*, 17(2) (2007), 201–212.
232. McKay, Adolescent Sexual and Reproductive Health in Canada.
233. Rentschler, D.D., Pregnant Adolescents' Perspectives of Pregnancy, *MCN American Journal of Maternal/Child Nursing*, 28(6) (2003), 377–383; Stiles, A.S., Parenting Needs, Goals, & Strategies of Adolescent Mothers, *MCN American Journal of Maternal/Child Nursing*, 30(5) (2005), 327–333; Herrman, J.W., The Voices of Teen Mothers: The Experience of Repeat Pregnancy, *MCN American Journal of Maternal/Child Nursing*, 31(4) (2006), 243–249.
234. Dryburgh, H., Teenage Pregnancy, *Health Reports*, 12(1) (2000), 9–20.
235. McKay, Adolescent Sexual and Reproductive Health in Canada.
236. McKay, Adolescent Sexual and Reproductive Health in Canada.

## Chapter 12

1. Swearingen, S., and A. Liberman, Nursing Generations: An Expanded Look at the Emergence of Conflict and its Resolution, *The Health Care Manager*, 23(1) (2004), 54–64.
2. Weston, M., Coaching Generations in the Workplace, *Nursing Administration Quarterly*, 25(2) (2001), 11–21.
3. Papalia, D., S. Olds, and R. Feldman, *Human Development*, 9th ed. Boston: McGraw Hill, 2004.
4. Santrock, J.W., A. MacKenzie-Rivers, K.H. Leung, and T. Malcomson, *Life-span Development*, 2nd Canadian ed. Toronto: McGraw-Hill Ryerson, 2005.
5. Boyd, D., H. Bee, and P. Johnson, *Lifespan Development*, 3rd Canadian ed. Toronto: Pearson Education Canada Inc., 2009.
6. Boyd et al., *Lifespan Development*.
7. Kudzma, E.C., Young Adult. In C.L. Edelman and C.L. Mandel (eds.), *Health Promotion through the Lifespan*, 5th ed. (pp. 649–680). Toronto: Mosby, 2002.
8. Ateah, C.A., R.V. Kail, and J.C. Cavanaugh. *Human Development: A Life-Span View*, 2nd Canadian ed. Toronto: Nelson Education, 2009.
9. Boyd et al., *Lifespan Development*.
10. Kudzma, Young Adult.
11. Health Canada. Food and Nutrition, *Canadian Guidelines for Body Weight Classification in Adults*. Website: http://www.hc-sc.gc.ca/ (accessed March 2008).
12. Health Canada, Food and Nutrition, *Canadian Guidelines for Body Weight Classification in Adults*.
13. Brien, S.E., P.T. Katzmarzyk, C.L. Craig, and L. Gauvin, Physical Activity, Cardiorespiratory Fitness and Body Mass Index as Predictors of Substantial Weight Gain and Obesity: The Canadian Physical Activity Longitudinal Study, *Canadian Journal of Public Health*, 98(2) (2007), 121–124.
14. Brien et al., Physical Activity, Cardiorespiratory Fitness and Body Mass Index as Predictors of Substantial Weight Gain and Obesity.
15. Chen, Y., and Y. Mao, Obesity and Leisure Time Physical Activity among Canadians, *Preventive Medicine*, 42 (2006), 261–265.
16. Chen and Mao, Obesity and Leisure Time Physical Activity among Canadians.
17. Health Canada, Food and Nutrition, *Canadian Guidelines for Body Weight Classification in Adults*.
18. Phillips, W.T., R.M. Kierman, and A.C. King, The Effects of Physical Activity on Physical and Psychological Health. In

A. Baum, T.A. Revenson, and J.E. Singer (eds.), *Handbook of Health Psychology*. Mahwah, NJ: Erlbaum, 2001.

19. Boyd et al., *Lifespan Development*.
20. Santrock et al., *Life-span Development*.
21. Santrock et al., *Life-span Development*.
22. Newman, B., and P. Newman. *Development Through Life: A Psychosocial Approach*, 7th ed. Belmont, CA: Brooks/Cole, 1999.
23. Stanhope, M., J. Lancaster, H. Jessup-Falcioni, and G.A. Viverais-Dresler, *Community Health Nursing in Canada* (pp. 291–325). Toronto: Elsevier Canada, 2008.
24. Davidson, M.R., M.L. London, and P.A. Ladewig, *Olds' Maternal-Newborn Nursing & Women's Health across the Lifespan*, 8th ed. Upper Saddle River, NJ: Pearson Education, Inc., 2008.
25. Davidson et al., *Olds' Maternal-Newborn Nursing & Women's Health across the Lifespan*.
26. Erlick Robinson, G., The Problem with Premenstrual Syndrome, *Canadian Family Physician*, 48 (2002), 1753–1755.
27. Davidson et al., *Olds' Maternal-Newborn Nursing & Women's Health across the Lifespan*.
28. Davidson et al., *Olds' Maternal-Newborn Nursing & Women's Health across the Lifespan*.
29. Erlick Robinson, The Problem with Premenstrual Syndrome.
30. Fogel, C.I., Reproductive System Concerns. In D.L. Lowdermilk and S.E. Perry (eds.), *Maternity & Women's Health Care*, 8th ed. (pp. 155–184). St. Louis, MO: Mosby, 2004.
31. Davidson et al., *Olds' Maternal-Newborn Nursing & Women's Health across the Lifespan*.
32. Davidson et al., *Olds' Maternal-Newborn Nursing & Women's Health across the Lifespan*.
33. Thibodeau, G.A., and K.T. Patton. *Anatomy & Physiology*, 6th ed. St. Louis, MO: Mosby Elsevier, 2007.
34. Thibodeau and Patton, *Anatomy & Physiology*.
35. Thibodeau and Patton, *Anatomy & Physiology*.
36. Stanhope et al., *Community Health Nursing in Canada*.
37. Pangman, V.C., and M. Sequire, Sexuality and the Chronically Ill Older Adult: A Social Justice Issue, *Sexuality and Disability*, 18(1) (2000), 49–59.
38. Klingman, L., Assessing the Female Reproductive System, *American Journal of Nursing*, 99(8) (1999), 37–43
39. Klingman, Assessing the Female Reproductive System.
40. Klingman, L., Assessing the Male Genitalia, *American Journal of Nursing*, 99(7) (1999), 47–50.
41. Ambert, A-M. *Contemporary Family Trends, Same-Sex Couples and Same-Sex Parent Families: Relationships, Parenting and Issues of Marriage*. Ottawa: Vanier Institute of the Family, 2005. Website: http://www.vifamily.ca/ (accessed March 2008).
42. Ambert, *Contemporary Family Trends, Same-Sex Couples and Same-Sex Parent Families*.
43. Epstein, R., Lesbian Families. In M. Lynn (ed.), *Voices: Essays on Canadian Families*, 2nd ed. (pp. 76–102). Scarborough, ON: Thomson Nelson, 2003.
44. Ambert, *Contemporary Family Trends, Same-Sex Couples and Same-Sex Parent Families*.
45. Canadian Bar Association, British Columbia. *Gay & Lesbian Relationships*. Website: http://www.cba.org/BC/public_media/family/163.aspx (accessed February 2008).
46. Ward, M. *The Family Dynamic: A Canadian Perspective*, 3rd ed. Scarborough, ON: Nelson Thomson Learning, 2002.
47. Vanier Institute of the Family. *Marriage and Legal Recognition of Same-Sex Unions: A Discussion Paper Submission to the House of Commons Committee on Justice and Human Rights*. Ottawa: Author, 2007. Website: http://www.vifamily.ca/ (accessed February 2008).
48. Vanier Institute of the Family, *Marriage and Legal Recognition of Same-Sex Unions*.
49. Vanier Institute of the Family, *Marriage and Legal Recognition of Same-Sex Unions*.
50. Papalia et al., *Human Development*.
51. Blum, D., "What Made Troy Gay?" *Health*, April 1998, 82–86.
52. Katz, A., "Mom, I Have Something to Tell You"—Disclosing HIV Infection, *Journal of Advanced Nursing*, 25 (1997), 139–143.
53. Brotman, S., B. Ryan, Y. Jalbert, and B. Rowe, The Impact of Coming Out on Health and Health Care Access: The Experiences of Gay, Lesbian, Bisexual and Two-Spirit People, *Journal of Health & Social Policy*, 15(1) (2002), 1–29.
54. Davis, V., Social and Sexual Issues Committee Members, Lesbian Health Guidelines, *Journal of Society of Gynaecologists and Obstetricians in Canada*, 22(3) (2000), 202–205.
55. Davis, V., Social and Sexual Issues Committee Members, Lesbian Health Guidelines.
56. Canadian Federation for Sexual Health, *Sexual Health in Canada: Baseline 2007*. Ottawa: Author, 2007.
57. Canadian Federation for Sexual Health, *Sexual Health in Canada*.
58. O'Byrne, P., and D. Holmes, Re-Evaluating Current Public Health Policy: Alternative Public Health Nursing Approaches to Sexually Transmitted Infection Testing for Teens and Males who Have Sex with Males, *Public Health Nursing*, 22(6) (2005), 523–528.
59. Budinski, R.A., and F. Trovato, The Effect of Premarital Cohabitation on Marital Stability over the Duration of Marriage, *Canadian Studies in Population*, 32(1) (2005), 69–95.
60. Mandell, N., and A. Duffy, Explaining Family Lives. In N. Mandell and A. Duffy (eds.), *Canadian Families: Diversity, Conflict, and Change*, 3rd ed. (pp. 3–16). Toronto: Thomson Nelson, 2005.
61. Statistics Canada. *Profile of Canadian Families and Households: Diversification Continues*. Ottawa: Author, 2002.
62. Mandell and Duffy, Explaining Family Lives.
63. Papalia et al., *Human Development*.
64. Pangman and Sequire, Sexuality and the Chronically Ill Older Adult.
65. Kralik, D., T. Koch, and K. Telford, Constructions of Sexuality for Midlife Women Living with Chronic Illness, *Journal of Advanced Nursing*, 35(2) (2001), 180–187.
66. Canadian Fitness and Lifestyle Research Institute (CFLRI). *Physical Activity Levels among Canadian Adults: Canadian Community Health Survey 2004/05*. Ottawa: Canadian Fitness and Lifestyle Research Institute, 2005.
67. Butler, G., H.M. Orpana, and A.J. Wiens, By Your Own Two Feet: Factors Associated with Active Transportation in Canada, *Canadian Journal of Public Health*, 98(4) (2007), 259–264.
68. Public Health Agency of Canada. *Handbook for Canada's Physical Activity Guide to Healthy Active Living*. Ottawa: Author, n.d.
69. Public Health Agency of Canada, *Handbook for Canada's Physical Activity Guide to Healthy Active Living*.
70. Taylor, B.V., G.Y. Oudit, and M.F. Evans, Walking or Vigorous Exercise? Which Best Helps Prevent Coronary Heart Disease in Women? *Canadian Family Physician*, 46 (2000), 316–318.
71. Taylor et al., Walking or Vigorous Exercise?
72. Papalia et al., *Human Development*. Taylor et al., Walking or Vigorous Exercise?
73. Taylor et al., Walking or Vigorous Exercise?
74. Public Health Agency of Canada. *Aging and Seniors: Foot Care Info-sheet for Seniors*. Ottawa: Author, 2005.
75. Health Canada. *Eating Well with Canada's Food Guide*. Website: http://www.healthcanada.gc.ca/ (accessed March 2008).
76. Health Canada. *Eating Well with Canada's Food Guide: A Resource for Educators and Communicators*. Website: http://www.hc-sc.gc.ca/ (accessed March 2008).
77. Health Canada, *Eating Well with Canada's Food Guide: A Resource for Educators and Communicators*.
78. Dudek, S.G. *Nutrition Essentials for Nursing Practice*, 5th ed., revised reprint. Philadelphia: Lippincott Williams & Wilkins, 2007.

79. Dudek, *Nutrition Essentials for Nursing Practice.*
80. Strychar, I., Fighting Obesity: A Call to Arms, *Canadian Journal of Public Health*, 95(1) (2004), 12–14.
81. Dudek, *Nutrition Essentials for Nursing Practice.*
82. Health Canada. *Nutrition for a Healthy Pregnancy: National Guidelines for the Childbearing Years*. Ottawa: Minister of Public Works and Government Services Canada, 1999.
83. Health Canada, *Nutrition for a Healthy Pregnancy.*
84. Dudek, *Nutrition Essentials for Nursing Practice*; Health Canada, Nutrition for a Healthy Pregnancy.
85. Health Canada, Nutrition for a Healthy Pregnancy.
86. Boyle, J.S., Culture, Family, and Community. In M.M. Andrews and J.S. Boyle (eds.), *Transcultural Concepts in Nursing Care*, 5th ed. (pp. 261–296). Philadelphia: Wolters Kluwer Health/ Lippincott Williams & Wilkins, 2008.
87. Boyle, Culture, Family, and Community.
88. Boyle, Culture, Family, and Community.
89. Health Canada. *Eating Well with Canada's Food Guide: First Nations, Inuit and Métis*. Website: http://www.healthcanada. gc.ca/ (accessed March 2008).
90. Health Canada. *Eating Well with Canada's Food Guide: My Food Guide*. Website: http://www.healthcanada.gc.ca/ (accessed March 2008).
91. Purnell, L.D., and B.J. Paulanka. *Transcultural Health Care: A Culturally Competent Approach*, 2nd ed. Philadelphia: F.A. Davis Company, 2003.
92. Health Canada, *Eating Well with Canada's Food Guide.*
93. Wade, C., C. Tavris, D. Saucier, and L. Elias. *Psychology*, 2nd Canadian ed. Toronto: Pearson Prentice Hall, 2006.
94. Fontaine, K.L. *Mental Health Nursing*, 5th ed. Upper Saddle River, NJ: Pearson Education, Inc., 2003.
95. Fontaine, *Mental Health Nursing.*
96. Stockert, P.A., Sleep. In P.A. Potter, A.G. Perry, J.C. Ross-Kerr, and M.J. Wood (eds.), *Canadian Fundamentals of Nursing*, 3rd ed. (pp. 1209–1234). Toronto: Elsevier Canada, 2006.
97. Wade et al., *Psychology.*
98. Thibodeau, G.A., and K.T. Patton. *Anatomy & Physiology*, 6th ed. St. Louis, MO: Mosby Elsevier, 2007.
99. Kozier, B., G. Erb, A.J. Berman, K. Burke, D.S.R. Bouchal, and S.P. Hirst. *Fundamentals of Nursing: The Nature of Nursing Practice in Canada*, 1st Canadian ed. Toronto: Pearson Education Canada Inc., 2004.
100. Archer, S., D. Robilliard, D. Skene, M. Smits, A. Williams, J. Arendt, and M. von Schantz, A Length Polymorphism in the Circadian Clock Gene Per 3 is Linked to Delayed Sleep Phase Syndrome and Extreme Diurnal Preference, *Sleep, 26* (2003), 413–415.
101. Stockert, Sleep.
102. Boivin, D., and E.W. Lamont. *Human Circadian Rhythms*. Montreal: Canadian Sleep Society, 2006.
103. Boivin and Lamont, *Human Circadian Rhythms.*
104. Boivin and Lamont, *Human Circadian Rhythms.*
105. Wade et al., *Psychology.*
106. Marcus, P., C.R. Kneisl, E. Trigoboff, Psychobiology. In C.R. Kneisl, H.S. Wilson, and E. Trigoboff (eds.), *Contemporary Psychiatric-Mental Health Nursing*, Upper Saddle River, NJ: Pearson Education, Inc., 2004.
107. Thurston, N.E., S.M. Tanguay, and K.L. Fraser, Sleep and Shift Work I, *The Canadian Nurse*, 96(9) (2000), 35–38.
108. Kozier et al., *Fundamentals of Nursing.*
109. Wade et al., *Psychology.*
110. McCance, K.L., and S.E. Huether. *Pathophysiology: The Biologic Basis for Disease in Adults and Children*, 4th ed. St. Louis, MO: Mosby, 2002.
111. Stockert, Sleep.
112. Wilkinson, J.M., and K. van Leuven. *Fundamentals of Nursing: Theory, Concepts & Applications*, Volume 1. Philadelphia: F.A. Davis Company, 2007.
113. Wilkinson and van Leuven, *Fundamentals of Nursing.*
114. Wade et al., *Psychology.*
115. Wade et al., *Psychology.*
116. Wade et al., *Psychology.*
117. Wilkinson and van Leuven, *Fundamentals of Nursing.*
118. Kozier et al., *Fundamentals of Nursing.*
119. Kozier et al., *Fundamentals of Nursing.*
120. Wilkinson and van Leuven, *Fundamentals of Nursing.*
121. Kozier et al., *Fundamentals of Nursing.*
122. Stockert, Sleep.
123. Stockert, Sleep; Sigurdson, K., and N.T. Ayas, The Public Health and Safety Consequences of Sleep Disorders, *Canadian Journal of Physiology and Pharmacology*, 85 (2007), 179–183.
124. Sigurdson and Ayas, The Public Health and Safety Consequences of Sleep Disorders.
125. Kozier et al., *Fundamentals of Nursing.*
126. Papalia et al., *Human Development.*
127. Boyd et al., *Lifespan Development*; Santrock et al., *Life-span Development.*
128. Wadsworth, B. *Piaget's Theory of Cognitive and Affective Development: Foundations of Constructivism*, 5th ed. New York: Longman, 1996.
129. Arlin, P., Cognitive Development in Adulthood: A Fifth Stage? *Developmental Psychology, 11*(5) (1975), 602–606.
130. King, V., and K.S. Kitchener, Reflective Judgement: Theory and Research on the Development of Epistemic Assumptions through Adulthood, *Educational Psychologist, 39* (2004), 5–18.
131. Ateah et al., *Human Development.*
132. King and Kitchener, Reflective Judgement.
133. Ateah et al., *Human Development.*
134. Sternberg, R. *Beyond IQ: A Triarchic Theory of Human Intelligence*. New York: Cambridge University Press, 1985.
135. Schuster, P.M. *Communication: The Key to the Therapeutic Relationship*. Philadelphia: F.A. Davis, 2000.
136. Rankin, S.H., K.D. Stallings, and F. London. *Patient Education: Principles & Practice*, 5th ed. Philadelphia: Lippincott Williams & Wilkins, 2005.
137. Schuster, *Communication: The Key to the Therapeutic Relationship.*
138. Nunnery, R.K., Teaching-Learning Process. In R.K. Nunnery (ed.), *Advancing Your Career: Concepts of Professional Nursing*, 3rd ed. Philadelphia: F.A. Davis, 2005.
139. Boyd et al., *Lifespan Development.*
140. Cooke-Reynolds, M., and N. Zukewich, The Feminization of Work, *Canadian Social Trends, 72* (Spring 2004), 24–29.
141. Boyd et al., *Lifespan Development.*
142. Santrock et al., *Life-span Development.*
143. Shannon, H.S., S.A. Ibrahim, L.S. Robson, and F. Zarinpoush, Changes in Job Stressors in Canadian Working Population, *Canadian Journal of Public Health*, 97(3) (2006), 225–229.
144. Manteler, J., A. Matejicek, K. Matheson, and H. Anisman, Coping with Employment Uncertainty: A Comparison of Employed and Unemployed Workers, *Journal of Occupational Health Psychology, 10* (2005), 200–209.
145. Manteler et al., Coping with Employment Uncertainty.
146. Vanier Institute of the Family. *Tracking the Links between Jobs and Family: Job, Family and Stress among Husbands, Wives and Lone-Parents 15–64 from 1990 to 2000*. Ottawa: Contemporary Family Trends, Connections, Author, 2002.
147. Santrock et al., *Life-span Development.*
148. Canada WorkinfoNet. Website: www.workinfonet.ca/ (accessed March 2008).
149. Papalia et al., *Human Development.*
150. Blumenthal, T., Harassment in the Workplace, *In Brief, 4* (April 1999), 1–2.
151. Macdonald, S., R. Csiernik, P. Durand, M. Rylett, and T.C. Wild, Prevalence and Factors Related to Canadian Workplace Health Programs, *Canadian Journal of Public Health*, 97(2) (2006), 121–125.

152. Papalia et al., *Human Development*. Seifert, K., R. Hoffnung, and M. Hoffnung. *Lifespan Development*. Boston: Houghton Mifflin, 1997.

153. Papalia et al., *Human Development*.

154. Strickland, D., Emotional Intelligence: The Most Potent Factor in the Success Equation, *Journal of Nursing Administration*, 30(3) (2000), 112–117.

155. Herbert, R., and L. Edgar, Emotional Intelligence: A Primal Dimension of Nursing Leadership? *Nursing Leadership*, 17(4) (2004), 56–63.

156. Levinson, D. *The Seasons of a Man's Life*. New York: Ballantine Books, 1978; Levinson, D., et al., Periods in the Adult Development of Men: Ages 18 to 45, *Counseling Psychologist*, 6(1) (1976), 21–25; Levinson, D., A Conception of Adult Development, *American Psychologist*, 41 (1986), 3–13.

157. Boyd et al., *Lifespan Development*.

158. Santrock et al., *Life-span Development*.

159. Santrock et al., *Life-span Development*.

160. Santrock et al., *Life-span Development*.

161. Papalia et al., *Human Development*.

162. Macionis, J.J., and L.M. Gerber. *Sociology*, 6th Canadian ed. Toronto: Pearson Education Canada, 2008.

163. Papalia et al., *Human Development*.

164. Gottman, J.M., and N. Silver. *The Seven Principles of Making Marriages Work*. New York: Crown, 1999; Gottman, J.M., and C.I. Notarious, Decade Review: Observing Marital Interaction, *Journal of Marriage and the Family*, 62 (2000), 927–947.

165. Santrock et al., *Life-span Development*.

166. Kohlberg, L. *Recent Research in Moral Development*. New York: Holt, Rinehart & Winston, 1971.

167. Seifert et al., *Lifespan Development*.

168. Papalia et al., *Human Development*; Seifert et al., *Lifespan Development*.

169. Seifert et al., *Lifespan Development*.

170. Seifert et al., *Lifespan Development*.

171. Biordi, D.L., A.M. Warner, and G.P. Knapik, Body Image. In I.M. Lubkin and P.D. Larsen (eds.), *Chronic Illness: Impact and Interventions*, 6th ed. (pp. 181–197). Toronto: Jones and Bartlett Publishers, 2006.

172. Gorman, L.M., M.L. Raines, and D.F. Sultan. *Psychosocial Nursing for General Patient Care*, 2nd ed. Philadelphia: F.A. Davis Company, 2002.

173. Price, B., Assessing Altered Body Image, *Journal of Psychiatric and Mental Health Nursing*, 2 (1995), 169–175; Townsend, M.C. *Psychiatric Mental Health Nursing: Concepts of Care in Evidence-Based Practice*, 5th ed. Philadelphia: F.A. Davis Company, 2006.

174. Biordi et al., Body Image.

175. Townsend, *Psychiatric Mental Health Nursing*.

176. Papalia et al., *Human Development*; Seifert et al., *Lifespan Development*.

177. Compton, S., Always a Bridesmaid: People Who Don't Expect to Marry, *Canadian Social Trends*, 77 (Summer 2005), 2–8.

178. Davies, L., Singlehood: Transitions within a Gendered World, *Canadian Journal on Aging*, 22(4) (2003), 343–352.

179. Boyd et al., *Lifespan Development*.

180. Smith-Battle, L., Change and Continuity in Family Caregiving Practices with Young Mothers and Their Children, *IMAGE: Journal of Nursing Scholarship*, 29(2) (1997), 145–149.

181. Maloni, J., and M. Ponder, Fathers' Experience of Their Partner's Antepartum Bed Rest, *IMAGE: Journal of Nursing Scholarship*, 29(2) (1997), 183–188.

182. Andrews, M., and S. Boyle. *Transcultural Concepts in Nursing Care*, 5th ed. Philadelphia: Lippincott Williams & Wilkins, 2008.

183. Public Health Agency of Canada. *Canadian Perinatal Surveillance System: Physical Abuse during Pregnancy*. Ottawa: Her Majesty the Queen in Right of Canada, 2004.

184. Health Canada. *Perinatal Health Indicators for Canada: A Resource Manual*. Ottawa: Minister of Public Works and Government Services Canada, 2000.

185. Cokkinides, V.E., A.L. Coker, M. Sanderson, C. Addy, and L. Bethea, Physical Violence during Pregnancy: Maternal Complications and Birth Outcomes, *Obstetrics and Gynaecology*, 93(5) (1999), 661–666.

186. Boyd et al., *Lifespan Development*.

187. Public Health Agency of Canada. *Canadian Immunization Guide*, 7th ed. Ottawa: Minister of Public Works and Government Services Canada, 2006.

188. Public Health Agency of Canada, *Canadian Immunization Guide*.

189. Public Health Agency of Canada, *Canadian Immunization Guide*.

190. Public Health Agency of Canada, *Canadian Immunization Guide*.

191. Whitney, L., S. Marchant-Short, and L. Yiu, Communicable Diseases. In L.L. Stamler and L. Yiu (eds.), *Community Health Nursing: A Canadian Perspective*, 2nd ed. (pp 142–161). Toronto: Pearson Education Canada, 2008.

192. Drebot, M.A., and H. Artsob, West Nile Virus: A Pathogen of Concern for Older Adults, *Geriatrics and Aging*, 9(7) (2006), 465–471.

193. Public Health Agency of Canada, *Canadian Immunization Guide*.

194. Hoole, A., R.G. Pickard, R. Ouimette, J. Lohr, and W. Powell. *Patient Care Guidelines for Nurse Practitioners*, 5th ed. Philadelphia: Lippincott Williams & Wilkins, 1999.

195. Tierney, L., S. McPhee, and M. Papadakis. *Current Medical Diagnosis and Treatment, 1999*, 38th ed. Stamford, CT: Appleton-Lange, 1999.

196. Shah, C.P. *Public Health and Preventive Medicine in Canada*, 5th ed. Toronto: Elsevier Saunders, 2003.

197. Public Health Agency of Canada. *Ministerial Council on HIV/AIDS Annual Report April 1, 2004–March 31, 2005*. Website: http://www.phac-aspc.gc.ca/ (accessed March 2008).

198. Public Health Agency of Canada, *Ministerial Council on HIV/AIDS Annual Report April 1, 2004–March 31, 2005*.

199. Health Canada. *Diseases & Conditions, HIV and AIDS*. Website: http://www.hc-sc.gc.ca/ (accessed March 2008).

200. Shah, *Public Health and Preventive Medicine in Canada*.

201. Shah, *Public Health and Preventive Medicine in Canada*.

202. Strychar, I., Fighting Obesity: A Call to Arms, *Canadian Journal of Public Health*, 95(1) (2004), 12–14; Gray, J., The Difficulties of Women Living with HIV Infection, *Journal of Psychosocial Nursing*, 37(5) (1999), 39, 43.

203. Papalia et al., *Human Development*.

204. Gray, The Difficulties of Women Living with HIV Infection.

205. Croft, J., and J. Mill (adaptors), Management of Patients with HIV Infection and AIDS. In R.A. Day, P. Paul, B. Williams, S.C. Smeltzer, and B.G. Bare (eds.), *Brunner & Suddarth's Textbook of Medical-Surgical Nursing*, 1st Canadian ed. (pp 1553–1587). Philadelphia: Lippincott Williams & Wilkins, 2007.

206. Croft and Mill, Management of Patients with HIV Infection and AIDS.

207. Sherman, D., HIV/AIDS Update, *Nursing Clinics of North America*, 34(1) (1999), 1–233.

208. Croft and Mill, Management of Patients with HIV Infection and AIDS.

209. MayoClinic.com. *HIV/AIDS*. Website: http://www.mayoclinic.com/health/hiv-aids/DS00005 (accessed March 2008).

210. MayoClinic.com, *HIV/AIDS*.

211. Croft and Mill, Management of Patients with HIV Infection and AIDS.

212. Canadian Association of Nurses in AIDS Care. Website: http://www.canac.org/ (accessed March 2008).

213. CATIE. Website: http://www.catie.ca/ (accessed March 2008).

214. Canadian Nurses Association. *Position Statement: Blood-Borne Pathogens*. Website: http://www.cna-nurses.ca/ (accessed March 2008).

215. Health Canada. *Activities & Responsibilities, Strategies & Initiatives, HIV/AIDS*. Website: http://www.hc-sc.gc.ca/ (accessed March 2008).
216. Whitney et al., Communicable Diseases.
217. Public Health Agency of Canada. *Tuberculosis in Canada 2006 Pre-Release*. Ottawa: Author, 2007.
218. Canada's Role in Fighting Tuberculosis. *Prevention of Tuberculosis*. Website: http://www.lung.ca/tb/ (accessed March 2008).
219. Canadian Centre for Occupational Health & Safety. *Inquiry Rates & Statistics*. Website: http://www.ccohs.ca/oshlinks (accessed March 2008).
220. Canadian Centre for Occupational Health & Safety, *Inquiry Rates & Statistics*.
221. Canadian Cancer Society. *General Cancer Stats for 2007*. Website: http://www.cancer.ca/ (accessed March 2008).
222. Public Health Agency of Canada. *Cancer in Young Adults in Canada*. Website: http://www/phac-aspc.gc.ca/ (accessed March 2008).
223. Public Health Agency of Canada, *Cancer in Young Adults in Canada*.
224. Public Health Agency of Canada, *Cancer in Young Adults in Canada*.
225. Public Health Agency of Canada, *Cancer in Young Adults in Canada*.
226. Demers, A.A., D. Turner, D. Mo, and E.V. Kliewer, Breast Cancer Trends in Manitoba: 40 Years of Follow-Up, *Chronic Diseases in Canada, 26*(1) (2005), 13–19.
227. Canadian Cancer Society. *Breast Cancer Stats*. Website: http://129.33.170.32/ccs/internet/standard/0,3172_14435_langld-en,00.html (accessed March 2008).
228. Public Health Agency of Canada, *Cancer in Young Adults in Canada*.
229. Demers et al., *Breast Cancer Trends in Manitoba*.
230. Boon, H.S., F. Olatunde, and S.M. Zick, Trends in Complementary/Alternative Medicine Use by Breast Cancer Survivors: Comparing Survey Data from 1998 and 2005, *BioMed Central Women's Health, 7*(4) (2007). Available: http://www.bimedcentral.com/1472-6874-7-4 (accessed March 2008).
231. Canadian Cancer Society, *Breast Cancer Stats*.
232. Canadian Cancer Society. *Knowing Your Breasts*. Website: www.cancer.ca (accessed March 2008).
233. Wadden, N., Breast Cancer Screening in Canada: A Review, *Canadian Association of Radiologists Journal, 56*(5) (2005), 271–275.
234. Boon et al., Trends in Complementary/Alternative Medicine use by Breast Cancer Survivors.
235. Jermal, A., T. Murray, E. Ward, A Samuels, R. Tiwari, A. Ghafoor, E. Feuer, and M. Thun, Cancer Statistics 2005, *CA Cancer Journal for Clinicians, 55*(1) (2005), 10–30.
236. Canadian Cancer Society. *Early Detection of Testicular Cancer*. Website: http://www.cancer.ca/ccs/internet/standard/0,3182,3172_10175_74554325_langId_en,00.html (accessed March 2008).
237. Cheung, W.Y., A. Demers, D. Hossain, T. Owen, S. Ahmed, and P.M. Czaykowski, Appropriateness of Testicular Cancer Management: A Population-Based Cohort Study, *The Canadian Journal of Urology, 14*(3) (2007), 3542–3549.
238. Health Canada. *Preventing Skin Cancer*. Website: http://www.hc-sc.gc.ca/ (accessed March 2008).
239. Public Health Agency of Canada, Cancer in Young Adults in Canada.
240. International Agency for Research on Cancer. *Sunscreens* (IARC Handbooks of Cancer Prevention, Volume 5). Lyon, France: Author, 2001.
241. Public Health Agency of Canada, *Cancer in Young Adults in Canada*.
242. Health Canada, *Preventing Skin Cancer*.
243. Health Canada, *Preventing Skin Cancer*.
244. Marrett, L.D., J. Frood, D. Nishri, A-M. Ugnat, and the Cancer in Young Adults in Canada (CYAC) Working Group, Cancer Incidence in Young Adults in Canada: Preliminary Results of a Cancer Surveillance Project, *Chronic Diseases in Canada, 23*(2) (2002), 58–64.
245. Health Canada. *Special Report on Youth Piercing, Tattooing, and Hepatitis C: Trends and Findings*. Ottawa: Population and Public Health Branch, 2001.
246. Public Health Agency of Canada. *Hepatitis C*. Website: http://www.phac-aspc.gc.ca/hepc/ (accessed March 2008).
247. Zou, S., M. Tepper, and A. Giulivi, Current Status of Hepatitis C in Canada, *Canadian Journal of Public Health, 91S1* (2000), S10–S15.
248. Cote, P., J. Baril, M. Hebert, M. Klein, R. Lalonde, M. Poliquin, D. Rouleau, et al., Management and Treatment of Hepatitis C Virus in Patients with HIV and Hepatitis C Virus Co-infection: A Practical Guide for Health Care Professionals, *The Canadian Journal of Infectious Diseases & Medical Microbiology, 18*(5) (2007), 293–303.
249. Andrews, M., and J. Boyle. *Transcultural Concepts in Nursing Care*, 3rd ed. Philadelphia: Lippincott, 1999; Hoole et al., Patient Care Guidelines for Nurse Practitioners.
250. Postpartum Disorders, *The Harvard Mental Health Letter, 14*(2) (1997), 1–4.
251. Bolaria, B.S., and R. Bolaria, Women's Lives, Women's Health. In B.S. Bolaria and H.D. Dickinson (eds.), *Health, Illness, and Health Care in Canada*, 3rd ed. (pp. 169–173). Toronto: Nelson Thomson Learning, 2002.
252. Turecki, G., Suicidal Behavior: Is There a Genetic Predisposition? *Bipolar Disorder, 3* (2001), 335–349; Kelly, T.M., J.R. Cornelius, and D.R. Clark, Psychiatric Disorders and Attempted Suicide among Adolescents with Substance Use Disorders, *Drug & Alcohol Dependence, 73* (2004), 87–97.
253. Brezo, J., J. Paris, R. Tremblay, F. Vitaro, M. Zoccolillo, M. Hebert, and G. Turecki, Personality Traits as Correlates of Suicide Attempts and Suicidal Ideation in Young Adults, *Psychological Medicine, 36* (2006), 191–202.
254. McGirr, A., M. Sequin, J. Renaud, C. Benkelfat, M. Alda, and G. Turecki, Gender and Risk Factors for Suicide: Evidence for Heterogeneity in Predisposing Mechanisms in a Psychological Autopsy Study, *Journal of Clinical Psychiatry, 67*(10) (2006), 1612–1617.
255. World Health Organization. *The World Health Report 2001—Mental Health: New Understanding, New Hope*. Geneva: Author, 2001.
256. Stanhope et al., *Community Health Nursing in Canada*.
257. Public Health Agency of Canada. *A Report on Mental Illnesses in Canada*. Website: http://www.phac-aspc.gc.ca/ (accessed March 2008).
258. Public Health Agency of Canada, *A Report on Mental Illnesses in Canada*.
259. Canadian Psychiatric Association, Canadian Clinical Practice Guidelines for the Treatment of Depressive Disorders, *Canadian Journal of Psychiatry, 46*(Supplement 1) (2001).
260. Alcohol Policy Network. *Statistical Overview of Alcohol Use*. Website: http://www.apolnet.ca/ (accessed March 2008).
261. Health Canada. *Canadian Addiction Survey (CAS)*. Website: http://www.statcan.ca/ (accessed March 2008).
262. Ateah et al., *Human Development*.
263. Statistics Canada. *Canadian Community Health Survey: Mental Health and Well-being*. Website: http://www.statcan.ca/ (accessed March 2008).
264. Ateah et al., *Human Development*.
265. Wilkinson, H.P., Substance Abuse. In L.L. Stamler and L. Yiu (eds.), *Community Health Nursing: A Canadian Perspective*, 2nd ed. (pp. 385–394). Toronto: Pearson Education Canada, 2008.
266. Addictions Foundation of Manitoba. *Overview*. Website: http://www.afm.mb.ca/ (accessed March 2008).
267. Wilkinson, Substance Abuse.
268. Health Canada, *Canadian Addiction Survey (CAS)*.
269. Addictions Foundation of Manitoba, *Overview*.

270. Wilkinson, Substance Abuse.
271. Cox, B., N. Yu, T. Afifi, and R. Ladouceur, A National Survey of Gambling Problems in Canada, *Canadian Journal of Psychiatry*, 50(4) (2005), 213–217.
272. Cox et al., A National Survey of Gambling Problems in Canada.
273. Wilkinson, Substance Abuse.
274. *The Daily*. Canadian Community Health Survey 2003. Website: http://www.statcan.ca/ (accessed March 2008).
275. Stanhope et al., *Community Health Nursing in Canada*.
276. Public Health Agency of Canada. *Respiratory Disease in Canada*. Website: http://www.phac-aspc.gc.ca/ (accessed March 2008).
277. Public Health Agency of Canada, *Cancer in Young Adults in Canada*.
278. Canadian Lung Association. *Smoking & Tobacco*. Website: http://www.lung.ca/ (accessed March 2008).
279. Canadian Lung Association, *Smoking & Tobacco*.
280. Stanhope et al., *Community Health Nursing in Canada*.
281. Statistics Canada. *Family Violence in Canada: A Statistical Profile 2006*. Ottawa: Public Health Agency of Canada, 2006.
282. Statistics Canada, *Family Violence in Canada*.
283. Boyd et al., *Lifespan Development*.
284. Buchbinder, E., and Z. Eisikovits, Battered Women's Entrapment in Shame: A Phenomenological Study, *American Journal of Orthopsychiatry*, 73 (2003), 355–366.
285. Wuest, J., M. Merritt-Gray, and M. Ford-Gilboe, Regenerating Family: Strengthening the Emotional Health of Mothers and Children in the Context of Intimate Partner Violence, *Advances in Nursing Science*, 27(4) (2004), 257–274.
286. Stanhope et al., *Community Health Nursing in Canada*.
287. Draucker, C., Impact of Violence in the Lives of Women: Restriction and Resolve, *Issues in Mental Health*, 18 (1997), 59–80; Krane, J., and L. Davies, Mothering under Difficult Circumstances: Challenges to Working with Battered Women, *Journal of Women and Social Work*, 22(1) (2007), 23–38.
288. Burgess, A., W. Fehder, and C. Hartman, Delayed Reporting of the Rape Victim, *Journal of Psychosocial Nursing*, 33(9) (1995), 21–29; O'Campo, P., A. Grelen, R. Faden, N. Xine, N. Kass, and N. Wang, Violence by Male Partners against Women during the Childbearing Years: A Contextual Analysis, *American Journal of Public*, 85 (1995), 1092–1097.
289. Canadian Nurses Association. *Position Statement: Violence*. Website: http://www.cna-aiic.ca/ (accessed March 2008).
290. Canadian Nurses Association, *Position Statement: Violence*.
291. Campbell, J., If I Can't Have You, No One Can: Murder Linked to Battery During Pregnancy, *Reflections*, Third Quarter 1999, 6–12; Draucker, Impact of Violence in the Lives of Women.
292. Stanhope et al., *Community Health Nursing in Canada*.
293. Hall, L., B. Sachs, and M. Rayens, Mothers' Potential for Child Abuse: The Roles of Childhood Abuse and Social Resources, *Nursing Research*, 47(2) (1998), 87–95; Sachs, B., L. Holly, M. Lutenbacher, and M. Rayens, Potential for Abusive Parenting by Rural Mothers with Low-Birth-Weight Children, *IMAGE: Journal of Nursing Scholarship*, 31(1) (1999), 21–25.
294. Wright, L., and M. Leahey, *Nursing Families: A Guide to Family Assessment and Intervention*, 2nd ed. Philadelphia: F.A. Davis, 1994.
295. Papalia et al., *Human Development*; Seifert et al., *Lifespan Development*.
296. Ambert, A. *Divorce: Facts, Causes, and Consequences*. Ottawa: Vanier Institute of the Family, 2005.
297. Macionis and Gerber, *Sociology*.
298. Macionis and Gerber, *Sociology*.

## Chapter 13

1. Heckhausen, J., Adaption and Resilience in Midlife. In M.E. Lachman (ed.), *Handbook of Midlife Development* (pp. 345–94). New York: Wiley, 2001.
2. Papalia, D., and S. Olds. *Human Development*, 9th ed. Boston: McGraw Hill, 2004.
3. Santrock, J.W., A. MacKenzie-Rivers, K.H. Leung, and T. Malcomson. *Life Span Development*, 2nd Canadian ed. Toronto: McGraw-Hill Ryerson, 2005.
4. Santrock, J., *Life Span Development* (6th ed.). Chicago: Brown & Benchmark, 1997.
5. Bee, H., D. Boyd, and P. Johnson. *Lifespan Development*, 2nd Canadian ed. Toronto: Pearson Education Canada, 2006.
6. Papalia and Olds, *Human Development*; Santrock et al., *Life Span Development*.
7. Hoff, L. *People in Crisis: Understanding and Helping*, 4th ed. Redwood City, CA: Addison-Wesley, 1995.
8. Santrock et al., *Life Span Development*.
9. Bee et al., *Lifespan Development*.
10. Papalia and Olds, *Human Development*; Seifert, K., R. Hoffnung, and M. Hoffnung. *Lifespan Development*. Boston: Houghton Mifflin, 1997.
11. Bee et al., *Lifespan Development*.
12. Neugarten, Adaptation and the Lifecycle, *The Counseling Psychologist*, 6, no.1 (1976), 16–20; Papalia D., and S.Olds, *Human Development* (3rd ed.) Boston: McGraw Hill, 1998; Santrock, J., *Life Span Development* (6th ed.). Chicago: Brown & Benchmark, 1997; Sigelman, C., *Life-span Human Development* (3rd ed.) Pacific Grove, CA: Brooks/Cole, 1998.
13. Martin-Matthew, A., Aging and Families: Ties over Time and across Generations. In N. Mandell and A. Duffy (eds.), *Canadian Families: Diversity, Conflict, and Change*, 3rd ed. (pp. 311–331). Toronto: Thomson Nelson, 2005.
14. McPherson, B.D. *Aging as a Social Process*, 3rd ed. Toronto: Harcourt Brace, 1998.
15. Barrette, G., Grandparenting Today, Expression: *National Advisory Council on Aging*, 18(3) (2005), 1–8.
16. Barrette, Grandparenting Today; Waldrop, D.P., and J.A. Weber, From Grandparent to Caregiver: The Stress and Satisfaction of Raising Grandchildren, *Families in Society*, 82 (2001), 461–472.
17. Martin-Matthew, Aging and Families.
18. Barrette, Grandparenting Today.
19. Milan, A., and B. Hamm, Across the Generations: Grandparents and Grandchildren, *Canadian Social Trends*, 71 (2003), 2–7.
20. Waldrop and Weber, From Grandparent to Caregiver: The Stress and Satisfaction of Raising Grandchildren.
21. Barrette, Grandparenting Today.
22. Inwood, S., Grandparents Raising Grandchildren, *Canadian Nurse*, 98(4) (2002), 21–25.
23. Inwood, Grandparents Raising Grandchildren.
24. Fuller-Thomson, E., Canadian First Nations Grandparents Raising Grandchildren: A Portrait in Resilience, *International Journal of Aging and Human Development*, 60(4) (2005), 331–342.
25. Inwood, Grandparents Raising Grandchildren.
26. Santrock et al., *Life Span Development*.
27. Bee et al., *Lifespan Development*.
28. Barrette, Grandparenting Today.
29. Chappell, N., E. Gee, L. McDonald, and M. Stone. *Aging in Contemporary Canada*. Toronto: Pearson Education Canada, 2003.
30. Mitchell, B.A., and E.M. Gee, Young Adults Returning Home: Implications for Social Policy. In B. Galaway and J. Hudson (eds.), *Youth in Transition to Adulthood: Research and Policy Implications* (pp. 61–65). Toronto, Thomson Educational Publishing, 1996.
31. Mitchell and Gee, Young Adults Returning Home: Implications for Social Policy.
32. Santrock et al., *Life Span Development*.
33. Papalia and Olds, *Human Development*; Santrock et al., *Life Span Development*; Seifert et al., *Lifespan Development*.
34. Papalia and Olds, *Human Development*.
35. Ruchala, P.L., and M. Clauson, Young to Middle Adult. In P.A. Potter, A.G. Perry, J.C. Ross-Kerr, and M.J. Wood (eds.), *Canadian Fundamentals of Nursing*, 3rd ed. (pp 397–412). Toronto: Elsevier Canada, 2006.

36. Corr, C. A., C. M. Nabe, and D. M. Corr, *Death and Dying, Life and Living* (3rd ed.) Scarborough, ON: Nelson Thomson Learning, 2000.
37. Papalia and Olds, *Human Development*.
38. Hoff, People in Crisis; Lund, D.C., and M.S. Caserta, Older Men Coping with Widowhood, *Geriatrics & Aging, 7*(6) (2004), 29–33.
39. Caserta, M.S., D.A. Lund, and S.J. Rice, Pathfinders: A Self-Care and Health Education Program for Older Widows and Widowers, *Gerontologist, 39* (1999), 615–620.
40. Caserta et al., Pathfinders.
41. Martin-Matthew, Aging and Families.
42. Campbell, L.D., and A. Martin-Matthews, Primary and Proximate: Implications of Distance and Relationship in Men's Caring Roles, *Journal of Family Issues, 21*(8) (2000), 1007–1031.
43. Clemens-Stone, S., D.G. Eigsti, and S. McGuire. *Comprehensive Community Health Nursing: Family, Aggregate, and Community Practice*, 4th ed. St. Louis, MO: C.V. Mosby, 1995; Papalia and Olds, *Human Development*.
44. Martin-Matthew, Aging and Families.
45. Houde, S.C., Men Providing Care to Older Adults in the Home, *Journal of Gerontological Nursing, 27*(8) (2001), 13–19.
46. Turcotte, M., and G. Schellenberg. *A Portrait of Seniors in Canada*, 2006. Ottawa: Statistics Canada, 2007.
47. Turcotte, and Schellenberg, *A Portrait of Seniors in Canada*, 2006.
48. Ward-Griffin, C., and V.W. Marshall, Reconceptualising the Relationship between "Public" and "Private" Eldercare, *Journal of Aging Studies, 17* (2003), 189–208.
49. Hawranik, P.G., and L.A. Strain, Giving Voice to Informal Caregivers of Older Adults, *Canadian Journal of Nursing Research, 39*(1) (2007), 156–172.
50. Hawranik and Strain, Giving Voice to Informal Caregivers of Older Adults.
51. Gahagan, J., C. Loppie, L. Rehman, M. MacLellan, and K. Side, "Far as I Get is the Clothesline": The Impact of Leisure on Women's Health and Unpaid Caregiving Experiences in Nova Scotia, Canada, *Health Care for Women International, 28* (2007), 47–68.
52. Gahagan et al., "Far as I Get is the Clothesline."
53. Brody, E.M., S.J. Litvin, C. Hoffman, and M.H. Kleban, Marital Status of Caregiving Daughters and Co-residence with Dependent Parents, *The Gerontologist, 35*(1) (1995), 75–84; Houde, Men Providing Care to Older Adults in the Home; Dunbrack, J. *The Information Needs of Informal Caregivers Involved in Providing Support to a Critically Ill Loved One*. Ottawa: Health Canada, 2005; Fink, S.V., The Influence of Family Resources and Family Demands on the Strains and Well-being of Caregiving Families, *Nursing Research, 44*(3) (1995), 139–146; Franks, M.M., and M.A.P. Stephens, Social Support in the Context of Caregiving: Husband's Provision of Support to Wives Involved in Parent Care, *Journal of Gerontology, 51B*(1) (1996), P43–P52.
54. Brody et al., Marital Status of Caregiving Daughters and Co-residence with Dependent Parents; Fink, The Influence of Family Resources and Family Demands on the Strains and Well-being of Caregiving Families; Mui, A.C., Caring for Frail Elderly Parents: A Comparison of Adult Sons and Daughters, *The Gerontologist, 35*(1) (1995), 86–93; Papalia and Olds, *Human Development*.
55. Schumacher, K.L., B.J. Stewart, P.G. Archbold, M.J. Dodd, and S.L. Dibble, Family Caregiving Skill: Development of the Concept, *Research in Nursing & Health, 23* (2000), 191–203.
56. Prince, M.J., *Respecting Family Caregivers: What's Been Happening Recently?* Remarks to the Family Caregiver Network Society Annual General Meeting, Victoria Health Unit, Victoria, BC. September 23, 2003. Available: http://web.uvic.ca/spp/documents/respfamilycaregivers.pdf (accessed October 2007).
57. Fast, J.E., and N.C. Keating. *Informal Caregivers in Canada: A Snapshot*. Ottawa: Health Canada, 2001.
58. Taylor, S., and M.H. Kopot, The Breakfast Club: Providing Support for Male Caregivers of Persons with Alzheimer Disease or Related Dementia, *Geriatrics Today: Journal of the Canadian Geriatric Society, 4*(3) (2001), 136–140.
59. Taylor and Kopot, The Breakfast Club.
60. Zarit, S.H., P.A. Todd, and J.M. Zarit, Subjective Burden of Husbands and Wives as Caregivers: A Longitudinal Study, *The Gerontologist, 26* (1986), 260–266.
61. Perry, J., Wives Giving Care to Husbands with Alzheimer's Disease: A Process of Interpretive Caring, *Research in Nursing & Health, 25* (2002), 307–316.
62. Bar-David, G., Three Phase Development of Caring Capacity in Primary Caregivers for Relatives with Alzheimer Disease, *Journal of Aging Studies, 13*(2) (1999), 177–197.
63. Bar-David, Three Phase Development of Caring Capacity in Primary Caregivers for Relatives with Alzheimer Disease.
64. Eakes, G., M. Burke, and M. Hainsworth, Middle-Range Theory of Chronic Sorrow, *IMAGE: Journal of Nursing Scholarship, 30*(2) (1998), 179–184.
65. Martin-Matthew, Aging and Families.
66. Andrews, M., and J. Boyle. *Transcultural Concepts in Nursing Care*, 3rd ed. Philadelphia: Lippincott, 1999.
67. Bee et al., *Lifespan Development*; Papalia and Olds, *Human Development*; Santrock et al., *Life Span Development*; Seifert et al., *Lifespan Development*.
68. Bee et al., *Lifespan Development*; Papalia and Olds, *Human Development*; Santrock et al., *Life Span Development*; Seifert et al., *Lifespan Development*.
69. Santrock et al., *Life Span Development*; Wasaha, S., What Every Woman Should Know about Menopause, *American Journal of Nursing, 96*(1) (1996), 24–32.
70. Santrock et al., *Life Span Development*.
71. Santrock et al., *Life Span Development*.
72. Kail, R.V., J.C. Cavanaugh, and C.A. Ateah. *Human Development: A Life-Span View*, 1st Canadian ed. Toronto: Thomson Nelson, 2006.
73. Santrock et al., *Life Span Development*.
74. Health Canada. *Health Canada Endorsed Important Safety Information on Cialis, Levitra and Viagra*. Ottawa: Author, 2006. Website: http://www.hc-sc.gc.ca/ (accessed October 2007).
75. Santrock et al., *Life Span Development*.
76. Santrock et al., *Life Span Development*.
77. Thibodeau, G.A., and K.T. Patton. *Anatomy & Physiology*, 6th ed. Philadelphia: Mosby Elsevier, 2007.
78. Wasaha, What Every Woman Should Know about Menopause.
79. Hoff, People in Crisis.
80. Health Canada. *It's Your Health: Benefits and Risks of Hormone Replacement Therapy*. Website: http://www.hc-sc.gc.ca/ (accessed August 2007).
81. Health Canada, *It's Your Health: Benefits and Risks of Hormone Replacement Therapy*.
82. Health Canada, *It's Your Health: Benefits and Risks of Hormone Replacement Therapy*.
83. Blake, J.M., J.A. Collins, R.L. Reid, D.M. Fedorkow, and A.B. Lalonde, The SOGC Statement on the WHI Report on Estrogen and Progestin Use in Postmenopausal Women, *Journal of Obstetrics and Gynaecology Canada, 24*(10) (2002), 783–787.
84. Blake et al., The SOGC Statement on the WHI Report on Estrogen and Progestin Use in Postmenopausal Women.
85. Women's Health Initiative Steering Committee, Effects of Conjugated Equine Estrogen in Postmenopausal Women with Hysterectomy. *Journal of the American Medical Association, 291*(14) (2004), 1701–1712.
86. Wathen, C.N., D.S. Feig, J.W. Feightner, B.L. Abramson, A.M. Cheung, and the Canadian Task Force on Preventive Health Care, Hormone Replacement Therapy for the Primary Prevention of Chronic Disease: Recommendation Statement from the Canadian Task Force on Preventive Health Care, *Canadian Medical Association Journal, 288*(3) (2002), 321–333.

87. MacLennan, A., S. Lester, and V. Moore, Oral Estrogen Replacement Therapy versus Placebo for Hot Flushes: A Systematic Review, *Climacteric*, 4(1) (2001), 58–74; Cheung, A.M., D. Feig, M. Kapral, N. Diaz-Granados, S. Dodin, and the Canadian Task Force on Preventive Health Care, Prevention of Osteoporoses and Osteoporotic Fractures in Postmenopausal Women: Recommendation Statement from the Canadian Task Force on Preventive Health Care, *Canadian Medical Association Journal*, 170(11) (2004), 1665–1667.

88. Guay, M-P., A. Dragomir, D. Pilon, Y. Moride, and S. Perreault, Changes in Pattern of Use, Clinical Characteristics and Persistence Rate of Hormone Replacement Therapy among Postmenopausal Women after WHI Publication, *Pharmacoepidemiology and Drug Safety*, 16 (2007), 17–27.

89. Wathen, C.N., Health Information Seeking in Context: How Women Make Decisions Regarding Hormone Replacement Therapy, *Journal of Health Communication*, 11 (2006), 477–493.

90. Humphries, K., and S. Gill, Risks and Benefits of Hormone Replacement Therapy: The Evidence Speaks, *Canadian Medical Association Journal*, 168(8) (2003), 1001–1010.

91. Santrock et al., *Life Span Development*; Papalia and Olds, *Human Development*.

92. Papalia and Olds, *Human Development*; The Phytoestrogen Question, *The New England Journal of Medicine Health News*, 3(15) (1999), 1, 4.

93. Health Canada. *Eating Well with Canada's Food Guide*. Website: http://www.healthcanada.gc.ca/ (accessed October 2007).

94. Health Canada, *Eating Well with Canada's Food Guide*.

95. Health Canada, *Eating Well with Canada's Food Guide*.

96. Health Canada. *Canadian Guidelines for Body Weight Classification in Adults*. Website: http://www/hc-sc.gc.ca/ (accessed October 2007).

97. Spanier, P.A., S.J. Marshall, and G.E. Faulkner, Tackling the Obesity Pandemic: A Call for Sedentary Behaviour Research, *Canadian Journal of Public Health*, 97(3) (2006), 255–257.

98. Brien, S.E., P.T. Katzmarzyk, C.L. Craig, and L. Gauvin, Physical Activity, Cardiorespiratory Fitness and Body Mass Index as Predictors of Substantial Weight Gain and Obesity, *Canadian Journal of Public Health*, 98(2) (2007), 121–124.

99. Dudek, S.G. *Nutrition Essentials for Nursing Practice*, 5th ed., revised reprint. Philadelphia: Lippincott Williams & Wilkins, 2007.

100. Dudek, *Nutrition Essentials for Nursing Practice*.

101. Raine, K.D., Determinants of Healthy Eating in Canada: An Overview and Synthesis, *Canadian Journal of Public Health*, 96(S3) (2005), S8–S14.

102. Public Health Agency of Canada. *Canada's Physical Activity Guide to Healthy Active Living for Older Adults*. Website: http://www.phac-aspc.gc.ca/ (accessed October 2007); Fenstermacher, K., and B. Hudson. *Practice Guidelines for Family Nurse Practitioners*. Philadelphia: Saunders, 1997.

103. Public Health Agency of Canada, *Canada's Physical Activity Guide to Healthy Active Living for Older Adults*.

104. Tannenbaum, C., and B. Shatenstein, Exercise and Nutrition in Older Canadian Women: Opportunities for Community Intervention, *Canadian Journal of Public Health*, 98(3) (2007), 187–193.

105. Edelman, C., and C. Mandel. *Health Promotion throughout the Lifespan*, 6th ed. St. Louis, MO: C.V. Mosby, 2006.

106. Getting Relief: Your Aching Feet, *Harvard Health Letter*, 24(5) (1999), 1–3.

107. Getting Relief: Your Aching Feet.

108. Wolkove, N., O. Elkholy, M. Baltzan, and M. Palayew, Sleep and Aging: 1. Sleep Disorders Commonly Found in Older People, *Canadian Medical Association Journal*, 176(9) (2007), 1299–1304.

109. Trouble Sleeping? *Mount Sinai School of Medicine Focus on Healthy Aging*, 2(2) (1999), 2.

110. Mayo Clinic. *Sleep Apnea*. Mayo Foundation for Medical Education and Research, 2006. Website: http://www.mayoclinic.com/ (accessed October 2007).

111. Mayo Clinic, *Sleep Apnea*.

112. Wolkove et al., Sleep and Aging.

113. Shamsuzzaman, A.S., B.J. Gersh, and V.K. Somers, Obstructive Sleep Apnea: Implications for Cardiac and Vascular Disease, *Journal of the American Medical Association*, 290 (2003), 1906–1914.

114. Wolkove et al., Sleep and Aging.

115. Health Canada. *Canadian Immunization Guide*, 7th ed. Ottawa: Minister of Public Works and Government Services Canada, 2006.

116. Bee et al., *Lifespan Development*; Edelman and Mandel, *Health Promotion throughout the Lifespan*.

117. Bee et al., *Lifespan Development*; Fenstermacher and Hudson, *Practice Guidelines for Family Nurse Practitioners*.

118. Health Canada. *The Health Effects of Second-Hand Smoke*. Website: http://www.hc-sc.gc.ca/ (accessed October 2007).

119. Health Canada, *Canadian Guidelines for Body Weight Classification in Adults*.

120. Health Canada, *Canadian Guidelines for Body Weight Classification in Adults*.

121. Hoole, A., G. Pickard, R. Ouimete, J. Lohr, and W. Powell. *Patient Care Guidelines for Nurse Practitioners*, 5th ed. Philadelphia: J.B. Lippincott, 1999; Bee et al., *Lifespan Development*; Public Health Agency of Canada. *Centre for Chronic Prevention and Control Cervical Cancer*. Website: http://www.phac-aspc.gc.ca/ccdpc-cpcmc/cc-ccu/index_e.html (accessed August 2007).

122. Cole, D.E.C., New Genetic Technologies: Clinical Application and Ethical Issues in Familial Ovarian Cancer, *Clinical and Investigative Medicine*, 27(1) (2004), 16–18.

123. Fenstermacher and Hudson, *Practice Guidelines for Family Nurse Practitioners*; Spencer-Cisek, P., Overview of Cancer Prevention, Screening, and Detection, *Nurse Practitioner Forum*, 9(3) (1998), 134–146.

124. Public Health Agency of Canada, *Centre for Chronic Prevention and Control Cervical Cancer*; Sibbald, B., Cervical Cancer Vaccine May Come Soon to Canada, *Canadian Medical Association Journal*, 175(3) (2006), 235.

125. Health Canada. *Notice of Decision for Gardasil*. Website: http://www.hc-sc.gc.ca/ (accessed October 2007).

126. Kwon, J.S., M.S. Carey, E.F. Cook, F. Qiu, and L. Paszat, Patterns of Practice and Outcomes in Intermediate- and High-Risk Stage I and II Endometrial Cancer: A Population-Based Study, *International Journal of Gynecological Cancer*, 17 (2007), 433–440.

127. Fenstermacher and Hudson, *Practice Guidelines for Family Nurse Practitioners*.

128. Canadian Cancer Society. *What Is Colorectal Cancer?* Website: http://www.cancer.ca/ (accessed October 2007).

129. Canadian Cancer Society, *What Is Colorectal Cancer?*

130. Spencer-Cisek, Overview of Cancer Prevention, Screening, and Detection.

131. Pickles, T., Current Status of PSA Screening, *Canadian Family Physician*, 50(1) (2004), 57–63.

132. Svendsen, A., The Current Status of Cardiovascular Disease in Canada—A Call to Action, *Canadian Journal of Cardiovascular Nursing*, 14(1) (2004), 5–7.

133. Svendsen, The Current Status of Cardiovascular Disease in Canada—A Call to Action.

134. Tanuseputro, P., D.G. Manuel, M. Leung, K. Nguyen, and H. Johansen, Risk Factors for Cardiovascular Disease in Canada, *Canadian Journal of Cardiology*, 19(11) (2003), 1249–1259.

135. Fenstermacher and Hudson, *Practice Guidelines for Family Nurse Practitioners*; Thyroid Testing for Women Over 50, *Mount Sinai School of Medicine Focus on Healthy Aging*, 2(2) (1999), 2.

136. Schaefer, K., Women Living in Paradox: Loss and Discovery in Chronic Illness, *Holistic Nursing Practice, 9*(3) (1995), 63–74.
137. Schaefer, Women Living in Paradox.
138. Eakes et al., Middle-Range Theory of Chronic Sorrow.
139. Dowd, R., and J. Cavalieri, Help Your Patient Live with Osteoporosis, *American Journal of Nursing, 99*(4) (1999), 56–60.
140. Jacobs, P., J.F. Blanchard, R.C. James, and N. Depen, Excess Costs of Diabetes in the Aboriginal Population of Manitoba, Canada, *Canadian Journal of Public Health, 91*(4) (2000), 298–301.
141. Papalia and Olds, *Human Development.*
142. Papalia and Olds, *Human Development.*
143. Wadsworth, B. *Piaget's Theory of Cognitive and Affective Development: Foundations of Constructivism,* 5th ed. New York: Longman, 1996.
144. Papalia and Olds, *Human Development;* Seifert et al., *Lifespan Development.*
145. Papalia and Olds, *Human Development;* Seifert et al., *Lifespan Development;* Santrock et al., *Life Span Development.*
146. Santrock et al., *Life Span Development.*
147. Papalia and Olds, *Human Development.*
148. Papalia and Olds, *Human Development;* Santrock et al., *Life Span Development;* Seifert et al., *Lifespan Development;* Wadsworth, *Piaget's Theory of Cognitive and Affective Development.*
149. Papalia and Olds, *Human Development;* Santrock et al., *Life Span Development;* Seifert et al., *Lifespan Development;* Wadsworth, *Piaget's Theory of Cognitive and Affective Development.*
150. Wadsworth, *Piaget's Theory of Cognitive and Affective Development.*
151. Papalia and Olds, *Human Development;* Santrock et al., *Life Span Development;* Seifert et al., *Lifespan Development.*
152. Simonton, D., Creativity: Cognitive, Personal, Developmental, and Social Aspects. *American Psychologist, 55* (2000), 151–158.
153. Streufert, S., R. Pogash, M. Piasecki, and G.M. Post, Age and Management Team Performance, *Psychology and Aging, 5* (1990), 551–559.
154. Bee et al., *Lifespan Development.*
155. Bee et al., *Lifespan Development;* Papalia and Olds, *Human Development;* Seifert et al., *Lifespan Development.*
156. Parton, D., Out of Work: One Family's Journey, *Focus on the Family,* January 1994, 2–4.
157. Hunter, M., Work, Work, *Modern Maturity,* May–June 1999, 36–49.
158. Papalia and Olds, *Human Development.*
159. Schellenberg, G., M. Turcotte, and B. Ram, Preparing for Retirement, *Canadian Social Trends, 78* (Fall 2005).
160. Moen, P., J. Kim, and H. Hofmeister, Couples' Work/Retirement Transitions, Gender, and Marital Quality, *Social Psychology Quarterly, 64*(1) (2001), 55–71.
161. Bee et al., *Lifespan Development.*
162. Duchesne, D., Seniors at Work, *Perspectives on Labor and Income, 14*(2) (2002), 33–44.
163. Dosman, D., J. Fast, S.A. Chapman, and N. Keating, Retirement and Productive Activity in Later Life, *Journal of Family and Economic Issues, 27* (2006), 401–419.
164. Bee et al., *Lifespan Development.*
165. Seifert et al., *Lifespan Development.*
166. Erikson, E. *Childhood and Society,* 2nd ed. New York: W.W. Norton, 1963.
167. Vance, C., and R. Olson. *The Mentoring Connection in Nursing.* New York: Springhill, 1998.
168. Erikson, *Childhood and Society.*
169. Goleman, D., R. Boyatzis, and A. McKee. *Primal Leadership: Realizing the Power of Emotional Intelligence.* Boston: Harvard Business School Press, 2002.
170. Bee et al., *Lifespan Development;* Papalia and Olds, *Human Development;* Seifert et al., *Lifespan Development.*
171. Seifert et al., *Lifespan Development.*
172. Bee et al., *Lifespan Development;* Papalia and Olds, *Human Development.*
173. Kohlberg, L. *Recent Research in Moral Development.* New York: Holt, Rinehart & Winston, 1977.
174. Kohlberg, *Recent Research in Moral Development.*
175. Gilligan, C., In a Different Voice: Women's Conceptions of Self and of Mortality, *Harvard Educational Review, 47*(4) (1977), 481–517; Gilligan, C., N. Lyons, and T. Hammer (eds.). *Making Connections.* Cambridge, MA: Harvard University Press, 1990.
176. Stolte, K.M. *Wellness: Nursing Diagnosis for Health Promotion.* Philadelphia: Lippincott, 1996.

## Chapter 14

1. Andrews, M., and J. Boyle. *Transcultural Concepts in Nursing Care,* 5th ed. Philadelphia: Lippincott, 2008; Boyd, D., H. Bee, and P. Johnson. *Lifespan Development,* 3rd Canadian ed. Toronto: Pearson Education Canada, 2009.
2. Andrews and Boyle, *Transcultural Concepts in Nursing Care;* Boyd et al., *Lifespan Development.*
3. Ebersole, P., P. Hess, T. Touhy, and K. Jett. *Gerontological Nursing & Healthy Aging,* 2nd ed. Philadelphia: Mosby, 2005; Papalia, D., S. Olds, and R. Feldman. *Human Development,* 9th ed. Boston: McGraw Hill, 2004; Seifert, K., R. Hoffnung, and M. Hoffnung. *Lifespan Development.* Boston: Houghton Mifflin, 1997.
4. Boyd et al., *Lifespan Development;* Lookinland, S., and K. Anson, Perpetuation of Ageism Attitudes among Present and Future Health Care Personnel: Implications for Elder Care, *Journal of Advanced Nursing, 21*(1) (1995), 47–56; Seifert et al., *Lifespan Development.*
5. Elsner, R., M. Quinn, S. Fanning, S. Cueldner, and L. Poon, Ethical and Policy Considerations for Centenarians: The Oldest Old, *Journal of Nursing Scholarship, 31*(3) (1999), 263–267.
6. Boyd et al., *Lifespan Development;* Seifert et al., *Lifespan Development.*
7. Kaufert, P.A., and M. Lock, Medicalization of Women's Third Age, *Journal of Psychosomatic Obstetrics and Gynaecology, 18* (1997), 81–86.
8. Macionis, J., and L. Gerber. *Sociology,* 6th Canadian ed. Toronto: Pearson Education Canada, 2008.
9. Novak, M., and L. Campbell. *Aging and Society: A Canadian Perspective,* 5th ed. Toronto: Nelson, 2006.
10. Grant, M.J., A.S. Ross, C.M. Button, T.E. Hannah, and R. Hoskins, Attitudes and Stereotypes about Attitudes across the Lifespan, *Social Behavior and Personality, 29*(8) (2001), 749–762.
11. Ebersole et al., *Gerontological Nursing & Healthy Aging;* Papalia et al., *Human Development;* Seifert et al., *Lifespan Development.*
12. Ebersole et al., *Gerontological Nursing & Healthy Aging.*
13. National Advisory Council on Aging. *Seniors in Canada 2006 Report Card.* Ottawa: Minister of Public Works and Government Services Canada, 2006.
14. Edelman, C., and C. Mandle. *Health Promotion throughout the Lifespan,* 3rd ed. St. Louis, MO: C.V. Mosby, 1994.
15. Ebersole et al., *Gerontological Nursing & Healthy Aging.*
16. Prull, M.W., J.D.E. Gabrieli, and S.A. Bunge, Age-Related Changes in Memory: A Cognitive Neuroscience Perspective. In F.I.M. Craik and T.A. Salthouse (eds.), *The Handbook of Aging and Cognition,* 2nd ed. (pp. 91, 103). Hillsdale, NJ: Lawrence Erlbaum Associates, 2000.
17. Novak and Campbell. *Aging and Society.*
18. Ebersole et al., *Gerontological Nursing & Healthy Aging.*
19. National Advisory Council on Aging, *Seniors in Canada 2006 Report Card.*
20. National Advisory Council on Aging, *Seniors in Canada 2006 Report Card;* Ebersole et al., *Gerontological Nursing & Healthy Aging.*
21. Kemp, C., The Social and Demographic Contours of Contemporary Grandparenthood: Mapping Patterns in Canada and the

United States, *Journal of Comparative Family Studies*, 34(2) (2003), 187–212.

22. Milan, A.M., and B. Hamm, Across the Generations: Grandparents and Grandchildren, *Canadian Social Trends, 71* (Winter 2003), 2–7.

23. Waldrop, D.P., and J.A. Weber, From Grandparent to Caregiver: The Stress and Satisfaction of Raising Grandchildren, *Families in Society, 82*(5) (2001), 361–472.

24. Novak and Campbell. *Aging and Society.*

25. Novak and Campbell. *Aging and Society.*

26. Clark, W., Time Alone, *Canadian Social Trends,* 66 (2002), 2–7.

27. Novak and Campbell. *Aging and Society.*

28. Ebersole et al., *Gerontological Nursing & Healthy Aging.*

29. Ebersole et al., *Gerontological Nursing & Healthy Aging.*

30. Bowling, A., and E. Grundy, Activities of Daily Living: Changes in Functional Ability in Three Samples of Elderly and Very Elderly People, *Age and Aging, 26* (1997), 107–114; Papalia et al., *Human Development.*

31. Beattie, E., Long-Term Care for the Elderly in Australia, *Journal of Nursing Scholarship, 31*(2) (1999), 134–135; Pascucci, M.A., and G.L. Loving, Ingredients of an Old and Healthy Life: A Centenarian Perspective, *Journal of Holistic Nursing, 15*(2) (1997), 199–213; Rowe, J.W., and R.L. Kahn, Successful Aging, *The Gerontologist, 37* (1997), 433–440; Ruffing-Rahal, M., Individuation and Varieties of Well-Being Experience among Older Women, *Advances in Nursing Science, 20*(3) (1998), 13–20.

32. Andrews and Boyle, *Transcultural Concepts in Nursing Care.*

33. Barusch, A.S., Self-Concepts of Low-Income Older Women: Not Old or Poor, but Fortunate and Blessed, *International Journal of Aging and Human Development, 44*(4) (1997), 269–282; Fenstermacher, K., and B. Hudson. *Practice Guidelines for Family Nurse Practitioners.* Philadelphia: Saunders, 1997; Heidrich, S.M., Older Women's Lives through Time, *Advances in Nursing Science, 20*(3) (1998), 65–75.

34. Stanhope, M., J. Lancaster, H. Jessup-Falcioni, and G.A. Viverais-Dresler. *Community Health Nursing in Canada.* Toronto: Elsevier Canada, 2008.

35. Boyd et al., *Lifespan Development*; Papalia et al., *Human Development*; Seifert et al., *Lifespan Development.*

36. Miller, C.A. *Nursing for Wellness in Older Adults: Theory and Practice,* 4th ed. Philadelphia: Lippincott Williams & Wilkins, 2004.

37. Miller, *Nursing for Wellness in Older Adults.*

38. Meiner, S.E., Theories of Aging. In S. Meiner and A.G. Lueckenotte (eds.). *Gerontologic Nursing,* 3rd ed. (pp. 19–32). Philadelphia: Mosby Inc., 2006.

39. Boyd et al., *Lifespan Development*; Papalia et al., *Human Development*; Seifert et al., *Lifespan Development*; Edelman and Mandle, *Health Promotion throughout the Lifespan*; Miller, *Nursing for Wellness in Older Adults*; Meiner, Theories of Aging.

40. Meiner, Theories of Aging.

41. Ebersole et al., *Gerontological Nursing & Healthy Aging*; Papalia et al., *Human Development*; Meiner, Theories of Aging.

42. Miller, *Nursing for Wellness in Older Adults.*

43. Russell, R., In Sickness and in Health: A Qualitative Study of Elderly Men Who Care for Wives with Dementia, *Journal of Aging Studies, 15*(4) (2001), 351–367.

44. Erikson, E. *Adulthood.* New York: W.W. Norton, 1978.

45. Peck, R.C., Psychological Development in the Second Half of Life. In B. Neugarten (ed.), *Middle Age and Aging.* Chicago: University of Chicago Press, 1968.

46. Miller, *Nursing for Wellness in Older Adults.*

47. Meiner, Theories of Aging.

48. Boyd et al., *Lifespan Development*; Johansson, B., S. Hofer, J. Allaire, M. Maldonado-Molina, A. Piccinin, S. Berg, N. Pederson, and G. McClearn, Change in Cognitive Capabilities in the Oldest Old: The Effects of Proximity to Death in Genetically Related Individuals over a 6-Year Period, *Psychology & Aging, 19*(1) (2004), 145–156.

49. Boyd et al., *Lifespan Development*; Papalia et al., *Human Development*; Seifert et al., *Lifespan Development.*

50. Meiner, Theories of Aging.

51. Meiner, Theories of Aging.

52. Russell, In Sickness and in Health.

53. Novak and Campbell, *Aging and Society.*

54. Ducharme, F., L. Levesque, S.H. Zarit, L. Lachance, and F. Giroux, Changes in Health Outcomes among Older Husband Caregivers: A One-Year Longitudinal Study, *International Journal of Aging and Human Development, 65*(1) (2007), 73–96.

55. Novak and Campbell., *Aging and Society.*

56. Townsend-Batten, B., Staying in Touch: Contact between Adults and their Parents, *Canadian Social Trends,* 64 (Spring 2002), 9–12.

57. Novak and Campbell., *Aging and Society.*

58. Smale, B., and S.L. Dupuis. *In Their Own Voices: Guiding Principles & Strategies for Change Identified by and for Caregivers in Ontario, Stage 3: Working Focus Group.* Waterloo, ON: Murray Alzheimer Research and Education Program (MAREP), University of Waterloo, 2004.

59. Keefe, J.M., and P.J. Fancey, Work and Eldercare: Reciprocity between Older Mothers and Their Employed Daughters, *Canadian Journal of Aging, 21*(2) (2002), 229–241.

60. Papalia et al., *Human Development*; Seifert et al., *Lifespan Development.*

61. Boyd et al., *Lifespan Development*; Papalia et al., *Human Development.*

62. Novak and Campbell., *Aging and Society.*

63. Boyd et al., *Lifespan Development*; Papalia et al., *Human Development*; Edelman and Mandle, *Health Promotion throughout the Lifespan*; Seifert et al., *Lifespan Development.*

64. Solomon, J., and J. Marx, "To Grandmother's House We Go": Health and School Adjustment of Children Raised Solely by Grandparents, *The Gerontologist, 35*(3) (1995), 386–394.

65. Cooney, T., and L. Smith, Young Adults' Relations with Grandparents Following Recent Parental Divorce, *Journal of Gerontology: Social Sciences, 51B*(2) (1996), S91–S95.

66. Kemp, C.L., Dimensions of Grandparent–Adult Grandchild Relationships: From Family Ties to Intergenerational Friendships, *Canadian Journal on Aging, 24*(20) (2005), 161–178.

67. Boyd et al., *Lifespan Development*; Papalia et al., *Human Development*; Seifert et al., *Lifespan Development.*

68. Collins, C.E., F.R. Butler, S.H. Gueldner, and M.H. Palmer, Models for Community-Based Long-Term Care for the Elderly in a Changing Health System, *Nursing Outlook, 45*(2) (1997), 59–63.

69. Boyd et al., *Lifespan Development*; Papalia et al., *Human Development*; Seifert et al., *Lifespan Development*; Thompson, E., A. Futterman, D. Gallagher-Thompson, J. Rose, and S. Lovett, Social Support and Caregiving Burden in Family Caregivers of Frail Elders, *Journal of Gerontology: Social Sciences, 48*(5) (1995), S245–S254.

70. Boyd et al., *Lifespan Development*; Papalia et al., *Human Development.*

71. Jackson, S.A., and M.B. Mittelmark, Unmet Needs for Formal Home and Community Services among African-American and White Older Adults: The Forsyth County Aging Study, *The Journal of Applied Gerontology, 16*(3) (1997), 298–316.

72. Boyd et al., *Lifespan Development*; Papalia et al., *Human Development.*

73. Boyd et al., *Lifespan Development*; Papalia et al., *Human Development*; Seifert et al., *Lifespan Development.*

74. Boyd et al., *Lifespan Development*; Papalia et al., *Human Development*; Seifert et al., *Lifespan Development.*

75. Roberts, J., G. Browne, C. Milne, L. Spooner, A. Gafni, M. Drummond-Young, J. LeGris, et al., Problem-Solving Counseling for Caregivers of the Cognitively Impaired: Effective for

Whom? *Nursing Research, 48*(3) (1999), 162–172; Szabo, V., and V. Shang, Experiencing Control in Caregiving, *Journal of Nursing Scholarship, 31*(1) (1999), 71–75.

76. Burton, L., Age Norms, the Timing of Family Role Transitions, and Intergenerational Caregiving among Aging African-American Women, *The Gerontologist, 36*(2) (1996), 199–208.

77. Seifert et al., *Lifespan Development.*

78. Szabo and Shang, Experiencing Control in Caregiving.

79. Chang, B., Cognitive-Behavioral Interventions with Home-bound Caregivers of Persons with Dementia, *Nursing Research, 48*(3) (1999), 173–182; Ebersole et al., *Gerontological Nursing & Healthy Aging*; Szabo and Shang, Experiencing Control in Caregiving.

80. Liddy, C., J.J. Dusseault, S. Dahrouge, W. Hogg, J. Lemlin, and J. Humbert, Telehomecare for Patients with Multiple Chronic Illnesses: Pilot Study, *Canadian Family Physician, 54* (2008), 58–65.

81. Miller, *Nursing for Wellness in Older Adults.*

82. Hegge, M., and C. Fischer, Grief Responses of Seniors and Elders: Practice Implications, *Journal of Gerontological Nursing, 26*(2) (2000), 35–43.

83. Boyd et al., *Lifespan Development*; Papalia et al., *Human Development*; Seifert et al., *Lifespan Development.*

84. Chipperfield, J.G., and B. Havens, Gender Differences in the Relationship between Marital Status Transitions in Later Life, *Journals of Gerontology Series B, 56*(30) (2001), 176–186.

85. Moire, E., M.W. Rosenberg, and D. McGuiness. *Growing Old in Canada: Demographic and Geographic Perspectives.* Toronto: ITP Nelson and Statistics Canada, 1997.

86. Novak and Campbell, *Aging and Society.*

87. Novak and Campbell, *Aging and Society.*

88. Novak and Campbell, *Aging and Society.*

89. Novak and Campbell, *Aging and Society.*

90. Katz, S. Pet Therapy: *Soothing Troubled Seniors.* Website: http://www.en.50plus.com/ (accessed April 2008).

91. Public Health Agency of Canada. *Community Awareness and Response: Abuse and Neglect of Older Adults, 2006.* Website: http://www.phac-aspc.gc.ca/ (accessed April 2008).

92. Hawranik, P., and E. McKean, The Abuse of Older Adults: Issues and Prevention Strategies. In C. Ateah and J. Mirwaldt (eds.), *Within Our Reach: Preventing Abuse across the Lifespan* (pp. 90, 91). Winnipeg: Fernwood Publishing, 2004.

93. Novak and Campbell, *Aging and Society.*

94. Public Health Agency of Canada, *Community Awareness and Response.*

95. Boyd et al., *Lifespan Development*; Papalia et al., *Human Development*; Seifert et al., *Lifespan Development*; Edelman and Mandle, *Health Promotion throughout the Lifespan.*

96. Boyd et al., *Lifespan Development.*

97. Public Health Agency of Canada, *Community Awareness and Response.*

98. Government of Canada. *Directory of Services and Programs Addressing the Needs of Older Adult Victims of Violence in Canada.* Ottawa: Minister of Health, 2002.

99. Public Health Agency of Canada, *Community Awareness and Response.*

100. Manitoba Government. *Manitoba Seniors' Guide, 2007/2008.* Winnipeg: Minister Responsible for Seniors, n.d.

101. Department of Justice Canada. *Abuse of Older Adults: A Fact Sheet from the Department of Justice Canada.* Website: http://www.canada.justice.gc.ca/en/ps/fm/adultsfs.html (accessed April 2008).

102. Baker, M., and M.M. Heitkemper, The Roles of Nurses on Interprofessional Teams to Combat Elder Mistreatment, *Nursing Outlook, 53*(5) (2005), 253–259.

103. Ebersole et al., *Gerontological Nursing & Healthy Aging.*

104. Kiecolt-Glaser, J.K., and R. Glaser, Stress and Immunity: Age Enhances the Risks, *Current Directions in Psychological Science, 10* (2001), 18–21.

105. Papalia et al., *Human Development.*

106. Ebersole et al., *Gerontological Nursing & Healthy Aging.*

107. Olivieri, R., The Integument. In P.A. Tabloski (ed.), *Gerontological Nursing* (pp. 328, 335). Upper Saddle River, NJ: Pearson Education, Inc., 2006.

108. Olivieri, The Integument.

109. Ebersole et al., *Gerontological Nursing & Healthy Aging.*

110. Ebersole et al., *Gerontological Nursing & Healthy Aging*; Papalia et al., *Human Development.*

111. Burke, J., and G. Kamen, Changes in Spinal Reflexes Preceding a Voluntary Movement in Young and Old Adults, *Journal of Gerontology: Medical Sciences, 51A*(1) (1996), M17–M22; Ebersole et al., *Gerontological Nursing & Healthy Aging*; Edelman and Mandle, *Health Promotion throughout the Lifespan*; Papalia et al., *Human Development*; Seifert et al., *Lifespan Development.*

112. Ebersole et al., *Gerontological Nursing & Healthy Aging*; Edelman and Mandle, *Health Promotion throughout the Lifespan*; Papalia et al., *Human Development.*

113. Papalia et al., *Human Development.*

114. Boyd et al., *Lifespan Development.*

115. Galli, R.L., B. Shukitt-Hale, K.A. Youdim, and J.A. Joseph, Fruit Polyphenolics and Brain Aging: Nutritional Interventions Targeting Age-Related Neuronal and Behavioral Deficits, *Annals of the New York Academy of Science, 959*(1) (2002), 128–132.

116. Papalia et al., *Human Development*; Seifert et al., *Lifespan Development*; Boyd et al., *Lifespan Development.*

117. Maclaughlin Warnat, B., and P.A. Tabloski, Sensation: Hearing, Vision, Taste, Touch, and Smell. In P.A. Tabloski (ed.), *Gerontological Nursing* (pp. 383–420). Upper Saddle River, NJ: Pearson Education, Inc., 2006.

118. Papalia et al., *Human Development.*

119. Boyd et al., *Lifespan Development.*

120. Ebersole et al., *Gerontological Nursing & Healthy Aging*; Edelman and Mandle, *Health Promotion throughout the Lifespan.*

121. Edelman and Mandle, *Health Promotion throughout the Lifespan*; Papalia et al., *Human Development*; Boyd et al., *Lifespan Development.*

122. Edelman and Mandle, *Health Promotion throughout the Lifespan*; Papalia et al., *Human Development*; Ebersole et al., *Gerontological Nursing & Healthy Aging.*

123. Papalia et al., *Human Development*; Ebersole et al., *Gerontological Nursing & Healthy Aging.*

124. Ebersole et al., *Gerontological Nursing & Healthy Aging.*

125. Maclaughlin Warnat and Tabloski, Sensation: Hearing, Vision, Taste, Touch, and Smell.

126. Ebersole et al., *Gerontological Nursing & Healthy Aging*; Maclaughlin Warnat and Tabloski, Sensation: Hearing, Vision, Taste, Touch, and Smell.

127. Edelman and Mandle, *Health Promotion throughout the Lifespan*; Papalia et al., *Human Development*; Boyd et al., *Lifespan Development*; Ebersole et al., *Gerontological Nursing & Healthy Aging*; Chase, S.K., The Cardiovascular System. In P.A. Tabloski (ed.), *Gerontological Nursing* (pp. 422–431, 453–454). Upper Saddle River, NJ: Pearson Education, Inc., 2006.

128. Ebersole et al., *Gerontological Nursing & Healthy Aging*; Edelman and Mandle, *Health Promotion throughout the Lifespan*; Tabloski, P.A. (ed.). *Gerontological Nursing* (pp. 459–516). Upper Saddle River, NJ: Pearson Education, Inc., 2006.

129. Papalia et al., *Human Development*; Boyd et al., *Lifespan Development*; Olivieri, R., The Musculoskeletal System. In P.A. Tabloski (ed.), *Gerontological Nursing* (pp. 551–599). Upper Saddle River, NJ: Pearson Education, Inc., 2006; Eliopoulos, C. *Gerontological Nursing*, 6th ed. Philadelphia: Lippincott Williams & Wilkins, 2005.

130. Papalia et al., *Human Development.*

131. Foldvari, M., M. Clark, L.C. Laviolette, M.A. Bernstein, D. Kaliton, C. Castaneda, C.T. Pu, J.M. Hausdorff, R.A. Fielding,

and M.A. Singh, Association of Muscle Power with Functional Status in Community-Dwelling Elderly Women, *Journal of Gerontology: Biological and Medical Sciences*, 55 (2000), M192–199.

132. Ham, R.J., P.D. Sloane, and G.A. Warshaw. *Primary Care Geriatrics*, 4th ed. St. Louis, MO: Mosby, 2002.

133. Ebersole et al., *Gerontological Nursing & Healthy Aging*; Edelman and Mandle, *Health Promotion throughout the Lifespan*; Miller, *Nursing for Wellness in Older Adults*.

134. Miller, *Nursing for Wellness in Older Adults*.

135. Tabloski, P.A. (ed.). *Gerontological Nursing* (pp. 366–382). Upper Saddle River, NJ: Pearson Education, Inc., 2006.

136. Ebersole et al., *Gerontological Nursing & Healthy Aging*; Edelman and Mandle, *Health Promotion throughout the Lifespan*.

137. Tabloski, *Gerontological Nursing*.

138. Zurakowski, T.L., The Genitourinary and Renal Systems. In P.A. Tabloski (ed.), *Gerontological Nursing* (pp. 517–550). Upper Saddle River, NJ: Pearson Education, Inc., 2006.

139. Zurakowski, The Genitourinary and Renal Systems.

140. Zurakowski, The Genitourinary and Renal Systems.

141. Zurakowski, The Genitourinary and Renal Systems; Ebersole et al., *Gerontological Nursing & Healthy Aging*; Edelman and Mandle, *Health Promotion throughout the Lifespan*.

142. Papalia et al., *Human Development*; Roach, S.S. *Introductory Gerontological Nursing*. Philadelphia: Lippincott Williams & Wilkins, 2001.

143. Ebersole et al., *Gerontological Nursing & Healthy Aging*; Roach, *Introductory Gerontological Nursing*.

144. Tabloski, P.A. (ed.). *Gerontological Nursing* (pp. 642–683). Upper Saddle River, NJ: Pearson Education, Inc., 2006.

145. Papalia et al., *Human Development*; Tabloski, *Gerontological Nursing* (pp. 642–683).

146. Ebersole et al., *Gerontological Nursing & Healthy Aging*; Tabloski, *Gerontological Nursing* (pp. 642–683).

147. McCance, K., and S. Huether. *Pathophysiology: The Biologic Basis for Disease in Adults and Children*. St. Louis, MO: Mosby, 2001.

148. Roach, *Introductory Gerontological Nursing*; Tabloski, P.A. (ed.). *Gerontological Nursing* (pp. 600–641). Upper Saddle River, NJ: Pearson Education, Inc., 2006.

149. Ebersole et al., *Gerontological Nursing & Healthy Aging*.

150. Hoole, J., C. Pickard, R. Ouimette, J. Lohr, and W. Powell. *Patient Care Guidelines for Nurse Practitioners*, 5th ed. Philadelphia: J.B. Lippincott, 1999.

151. McCance and Huether, *Pathophysiology*.

152. Tabloski, *Gerontological Nursing* (pp. 600–641).

153. Harkness, G.A., The Immune System. In P.A. Tabloski (ed.), *Gerontological Nursing* (pp. 754–786). Upper Saddle River, NJ: Pearson Education, Inc., 2006.

154. Harkness, The Immune System.

155. Ebersole et al., *Gerontological Nursing & Healthy Aging*; Harkness, The Immune System.

156. Tabloski, P.A. (ed.). *Gerontological Nursing* (pp. 684–710). Upper Saddle River, NJ: Pearson Education, Inc., 2006.

157. Roach, *Introductory Gerontological Nursing*.

158. Pangman, V.C., and M. Seguire, Sexuality and the Chronically Ill Older Adult: A Social Justice Issue, *Sexuality and Disability*, 18(1) (2000), 49–59.

159. Hajjar, R.R., and H.K. Kamel, Sexuality in the Nursing Home, Part 1: Attitudes and Barriers to Sexual Expression, *Journal of the American Medical Directors Association*, 5(2) (2004), S43–S47.

160. Steinke, E.E., Intimacy Needs and Chronic Illness: Strategies for Sexual Counseling and Self-Management, *Journal of Gerontological Nursing*, 31(5) (2005), 40–50.

161. Wallace, M., Sexuality, *Try This: Best Practices in Nursing Care to Older Adults*, 10 (2007).

162. Wallace, Sexuality.

163. Health Canada. *Eating Well with Canada's Food Guide*. Website: http://www.healthcanada.gc.ca/ (accessed April 2008).

164. Health Canada, *Eating Well with Canada's Food Guide*.

165. Ebersole et al., *Gerontological Nursing & Healthy Aging*; Morrison, S., Feeding the Elderly Population, *Nursing Clinics of North America*, 32(4) (1997), 791–801; Dudek, S.G. *Nutrition Essentials for Nursing Practice*, 5th ed, revised reprint. Philadelphia: Lippincott Williams & Wilkins, 2007.

166. Payette, H., and B. Shatenstein, Determinants of Healthy Eating in Community-dwelling Elderly People, *Canadian Journal of Public Health*, 96(Supplement 3) (2005), S27–S31.

167. Health Canada, *Eating Well with Canada's Food Guide*.

168. Keller, H., and J.D. McKenzie, Nutritional Risk in Vulnerable Community-Living Seniors, *Canadian Journal of Dietetic Practice and Research*, 64(4) (2003), 195–201.

169. Keller and McKenzie, Nutritional Risk in Vulnerable Community-Living Seniors.

170. Werner, K., D. Christoph, J. Born, and H. Fehm, Changes in Cortisol and Growth Hormone Secretion during Nocturnal Sleep in the Course of Aging, *Journal of Gerontology: Medical Sciences*, 51A(1) (1996), M3–M9.

171. Public Health Agency of Canada. *Healthy Living Unit: Physical Activity Guide for Older Adults*. Website: http://www.phac-aspc.gc.ca/ (accessed April 2008).

172. Public Health Agency of Canada, *Healthy Living Unit: Physical Activity Guide for Older Adults*.

173. Ebersole et al., *Gerontological Nursing & Healthy Aging*; Edelman and Mandle, *Health Promotion throughout the Lifespan*; Miller, *Nursing for Wellness in Older Adults*.

174. Stanley, M., K.A. Blair, and P.G. Beare. *Gerontological Nursing: Promoting Successful Aging with Older Adults*, 3rd ed. (pp. 215–224, 313–318). Philadelphia: F.A. Davis Company, 2005.

175. Clark, C., Wellness Self-Care by Healthy Older Adults, *Journal of Nursing Scholarship*, 30(4) (1998), 351–355; Edelman and Mandle, *Health Promotion throughout the Lifespan*.

176. Miller, *Nursing for Wellness in Older Adults*.

177. Edelman and Mandle, *Health Promotion throughout the Lifespan*.

178. Miller, *Nursing for Wellness in Older Adults*.

179. Carter, N., K.M. Khan, H. McKay, M. Petit, C. Waterman, A. Heinonen, P. Janssen, et al., Community-Based Exercise Program Reduces Risk Factors for Falls in 65- to 75-Year-Old Women with Osteoporosis: Randomized Controlled Trial, *Canadian Medical Association Journal*, 167(9) (2002), 997–1004.

180. Government of Canada. *Go for It! A Guide to Choosing and Using Assistance Devices*. Ottawa: Minister of Public Works and Government Services Canada, 2002.

181. Edelman and Mandle, *Health Promotion throughout the Lifespan*.

182. Clark, Wellness Self-Care by Healthy Older Adults.

183. Boult, C., M. Altmann, D. Gilbertson, C. Yu, and R. Kane, Decreasing Disability in the 21st Century: The Future Effects of Controlling Six Fatal and Nonfatal Conditions, *American Journal of Public Health*, 86(10) (1996), 1388–1393.

184. Menec, V., J. Chipperfield, and R. Perry, Self Perceptions of Health: A Prospective Analysis of Mortality, Control, and Health, *Journal of Gerontology: Psychological Sciences*, 54B(2) (1999), 85–93.

185. Papalia et al., *Human Development*; Boyd et al., *Lifespan Development*.

186. Papalia et al., *Human Development*; Boyd et al., *Lifespan Development*; Ebersole et al., *Gerontological Nursing & Healthy Aging*; Fenstermacher, K., and B. Hudson. *Practice Guidelines for Family Nurse Practitioners*. Philadelphia: Saunders, 1997.

187. Health Canada. *Canadian Immunization Guide*, 7th ed. Ottawa: Her Majesty the Queen in Right of Canada, 2006.

188. Whitney, L., S. Marchant-Short, and L. Yiu, Communicable Diseases. In L. Leeseberg Stamler and L. Yiu (eds.), *Community Health Nursing: A Canadian Perspective*, 2nd ed. (pp. 142, 144). Toronto: Pearson Education Canada, 2008.

189. Meiner, S.E., Safety. In S.E. Meiner and A.G. Lueckenotte (eds.), *Gerontologic Nursing*, 3rd ed. (pp. 245–261). St. Louis, MO: Mosby Elsevier, 2006.
190. Public Health Agency of Canada. *Aging and Seniors: Enhancing Safety and Security for Canadian Seniors*, Chapter 5: Crimes against Seniors. Website: http://www.hc-sc.gc.ca/seniors-aines/pubs/enhancing/chap5_e.htm (accessed April 2008).
191. Ebersole et al., *Gerontological Nursing & Healthy Aging*.
192. Ebersole et al., *Gerontological Nursing & Healthy Aging*; Miller, *Nursing for Wellness in Older Adults*.
193. Batscha, C., Heat Stroke: Keeping Your Clients Cool in the Summer, *Journal of Psychosocial Nursing*, 35(7) (1997), 12–17.
194. Ebersole et al., *Gerontological Nursing & Healthy Aging*.
195. Batscha, Heat Stroke.
196. Batscha, Heat Stroke; Ebersole et al., *Gerontological Nursing & Healthy Aging*.
197. Schneider, J., Chronic Pain Management in Older Adults: With Coxibs under Fire, What Now? *Geriatrics*, 60(5) (2005), 26–31.
198. Schneider, Chronic Pain Management in Older Adults.
199. Springhouse, Lippincott, and Springhouse (eds.). *ElderCare Strategies: Expert Care Plans for Older Adults* (pp. 1–25). Springhouse, PA: Lippincott Williams & Wilkins, 2003.
200. Springhouse, Lippincott, and Springhouse (eds.), *ElderCare Strategies*.
201. Ebersole et al., *Gerontological Nursing & Healthy Aging*; Fenstermacher and Hudson, *Practice Guidelines for Family Nurse Practitioners*; Tierney, L., S. McPhee, and M. Papadakis. *Current Medical Diagnosis and Treatment, 1999*, 38th ed. Stamford, CT: Appleton-Lange, 1999.
202. Ebersole et al., *Gerontological Nursing & Healthy Aging*; Fenstermacher and Hudson, *Practice Guidelines for Family Nurse Practitioners*; Tierney et al., *Current Medical Diagnosis and Treatment, 1999*.
203. Stanley et al., *Gerontological Nursing*.
204. Miller, *Nursing for Wellness in Older Adults*.
205. Miller, *Nursing for Wellness in Older Adults*.
206. Gibbons, L.W., and S.M. Clark, Exercise in the Reduction of Cardiovascular Events: Lessons for Epidemiologic Trails, *Cardiology Clinics*, 19(3) (2001), 347–355.
207. Roach, *Introductory Gerontological Nursing*.
208. Canadian Cancer Society. *General Cancer Stats for 2007*. Website: http://www.cancer.ca/ (accessed April 2008).
209. Canadian Cancer Society. *Progress in Cancer Prevention: Modifiable Risk Factors*. Website: http://www.cancer.ca/ (accessed April 2008).
210. Tierney et al., *Current Medical Diagnosis and Treatment, 1999*.
211. Leenaars, A.A., Can a Theory of Suicide Predict All "Suicides" in the Elderly? *Crisis*, 24(1) (2003), 7–16.
212. Havens, B., M. Hall, G. Sylvestre, and T. Jivan, Social Isolation and Loneliness: Differences between Older Rural and Urban Manitobans, *Canadian Journal of Aging*, 23(2) (2004), 129–140.
213. Adams, M.P., L.N. Holland, and P. Manuel Bostwick. *Pharmacology for Nurses: A Pathophysiologic Approach*, 2nd ed. (pp. 85, 86). Upper Saddle River, NJ: Pearson Education, Inc., 2008.
214. Stanley et al., *Gerontological Nursing*.
215. Adams et al., *Pharmacology for Nurses*.
216. Adams et al., *Pharmacology for Nurses*.
217. Miller, *Nursing for Wellness in Older Adults*.
218. Dudek, Nutrition Essentials for Nursing Practice.
219. Gill, S., B. Misiaszek, and C. Brymer, Improving Prescribing in the Elderly: A Study in the Long Term Care Setting, *Canadian Journal of Clinical Pharmacology*, 8(2) (2001), 78–83.
220. Gill et al., Improving Prescribing in the Elderly.
221. Public Health Agency of Canada. *How You Can Help Seniors Use Medication Safely*. Website: http://www.phac-aspc.gc.ca/seniors-aines/pubs/med_matters/intro_e.htm (accessed April 2008).
222. Spencer, C. *Alcohol and Seniors*. Website: www.agingincanada.ca/ (accessed April 2008).
223. D'Agostino, C.S., K.L. Barry, F.C. Blow, and C. Podgorski, Community Interventions for Older Adults with Comorbid Substance Abuse: The Geriatric Addictions Program (GAP), *Journal of Dual Diagnosis* 2(3) (2006), 31–45.
224. Canadian Network of Substance Abuse and Allied Professionals. *Seniors*. Website: http://www.cnsaap.ca/ (accessed April 2008).
225. Miller, *Nursing for Wellness in Older Adults*.
226. Levenson, M.R., and C.M. Aldwin. *A Generation at Risk ... Applying Prevention Concepts to the Elderly: Prevention Tactics*. Folsom, CA: Evaluation Management Training (EMT) Group, Inc., 2001.
227. Spencer, *Alcohol and Seniors*.
228. Centre for Addiction and Mental Health (CAMH). *Responding to Older Adults with Substance Use, Mental Health and Gambling Challenges: A Guide for Workers and Volunteers*. Toronto: CAMH, 2006.
229. Papalia et al., *Human Development*.
230. Papalia et al., *Human Development*.
231. Tabloski, P.A. (ed.). *Gerontological Nursing* (pp. 189–194). Upper Saddle River, NJ: Pearson Education, Inc., 2006.
232. Papalia et al., *Human Development*.
233. Miller, *Nursing for Wellness in Older Adults*; Boyd et al., *Lifespan Development*.
234. Papalia et al., *Human Development*; Boyd et al., *Lifespan Development*; Edelman and Mandle, *Health Promotion throughout the Lifespan*; Seifert et al., *Lifespan Development*.
235. Papalia et al., *Human Development*; Boyd et al., *Lifespan Development*; Edelman and Mandle, *Health Promotion throughout the Lifespan*; Seifert et al., *Lifespan Development*; Miller, *Nursing for Wellness in Older Adults*.
236. Papalia et al., *Human Development*; Boyd et al., *Lifespan Development*; Tabloski, *Gerontological Nursing* (pp. 189–194).
237. Boyd et al., *Lifespan Development*.
238. Stanhope et al., *Community Health Nursing in Canada*.
239. Miller, *Nursing for Wellness in Older Adults*.
240. Tierney, L.M., S.J. McPhee, and M.A. Papadakis. *Current Medical Diagnosis and Treatment*, 41st ed. East Norwalk, CT: Appleton & Lange, 2002; Gillis, A.J., and B. MacDonald, Gerontology: Unmasking Delirium, *Canadian Nurse*, 102(9) (2006), 19–24.
241. Ebersole et al., *Gerontological Nursing & Healthy Aging*.
242. Miller, *Nursing for Wellness in Older Adults*.
243. Miller, *Nursing for Wellness in Older Adults*.
244. Santrock, J.W., A. MacKenzie-Rivers, K.H. Leung, and T. Malcomson. *Life-Span Development*, 2nd Canadian ed. Toronto: McGraw-Hill Ryerson Limited, 2005.
245. Boyd et al., *Lifespan Development*; Miller, *Nursing for Wellness in Older Adults*.
246. Santrock et al., *Life-Span Development*.
247. Erikson, E. *Childhood and Society*, 2nd ed. New York: W.W. Norton, 1963.
248. Erikson, *Childhood and Society*.
249. Boyd et al., *Lifespan Development*.
250. Boyd et al., *Lifespan Development*.
251. Boyd et al., *Lifespan Development*; Santrock et al., *Life-Span Development*.
252. Miller, *Nursing for Wellness in Older Adults*.
253. Kolanowski, A., and A. Whall, Life-Span Perspective of Personality of Dementia, *Journal of Nursing Scholarship*, 28(4) (1996), 315–320; Light, J., J. Grigsby, and M. Bligh, Aging and Heterogeneity: Genetics, Social Structure, and Personality, *The Gerontologist*, 36(2) (1996), 147–156.
254. Krause, N., Social Support. In R.H. Binstock and L.K. George (eds.), *Handbook of Aging and the Social Sciences*, 5th ed. (pp. 272–294). San Diego: Academic Press, 2001.
255. Ryff, C.D., C.M. Kwan, and B.H. Singer, Personality and Aging: Flourishing Agendas and Future Challenges. In J.E. Birren, and

K.W. Schaie (eds.), *Handbook of the Psychology of Aging*, 5th ed. (pp. 477–499). San Diego: Academic Press, 2001.

256. Tabloski, *Gerontological Nursing*.
257. Krause, N., Stress and the Devaluation of Highly Salient Roles in Late Life, *Journal of Gerontology: Social Sciences, 54B*(2) (1999), S99–S108.
258. Miller, *Nursing for Wellness in Older Adults*.
259. Peck, Psychological Development in the Second Half of Life.
260. Krause, Stress and the Devaluation of Highly Salient Roles in Late Life.
261. Krause, Stress and the Devaluation of Highly Salient Roles in Late Life.
262. Boyd et al., *Lifespan Development*.
263. Rowe, J., and R. Kahn, Successful Aging, *Gerontologist, 37*(4) (1997), 433–440; Rowe, J., and R. Kahn. *Successful Aging.* New York: Pantheon, 1998.
264. Papalia et al., *Human Development*; Boyd et al., *Lifespan Development*; Seifert et al., *Lifespan Development*; Novak and Campbell, *Aging and Society*.
265. Maclaughlin Warnat and Tabloski, Sensation: Hearing, Vision, Taste, Touch, and Smell; Miller, *Nursing for Wellness in Older Adults*.
266. Maclaughlin Warnat and Tabloski, Sensation: Hearing, Vision, Taste, Touch, and Smell.
267. Maclaughlin Warnat and Tabloski, Sensation: Hearing, Vision, Taste, Touch, and Smell; Miller, *Nursing for Wellness in Older Adults*.
268. Ebersole et al., *Gerontological Nursing & Healthy Aging*.
269. Miller, *Nursing for Wellness in Older Adults*.
270. Isaia, D., V. Parker, and E. Murrow, Spiritual Well-Being Among Older Adults, *Journal of Gerontological Nursing, 25*(8) (1999), 16–21.
271. Andrews and Boyle, *Transcultural Concepts in Nursing Care*.
272. Erikson, *Adulthood*.
273. Stanley et al., *Gerontological Nursing*.
274. Andrews and Boyle.,*Transcultural Concepts in Nursing Care*; Calasanti, T., Gender and Life Satisfaction in Retirement: An Assessment of the Male Model, *Journal of Gerontology: Social Science, 51B*(1) (1996), S18–S29.
275. Boyd et al., *Lifespan Development*.
276. Papalia et al., *Human Development*; Boyd et al., *Lifespan Development*; Seifert et al., *Lifespan Development*; Turcotte, M., and G. Schellenberg. *A Portrait of Seniors in Canada 2006*. Ottawa: Statistics Canada, 2007.
277. Santrock et al., *Life-Span Development*.
278. Papalia et al., *Human Development*.
279. Turcotte and Schellenberg. A Portrait of Seniors in Canada 2006.
280. Rathje, K., Retirement Trends in Canada, *The Expert Witness Newsletter, 8*(1) (2003), 26–32.
281. Rathje, Retirement Trends in Canada.
282. Wilson, D.M., and P. Palha, A Systematic Review of Published Research Articles on Health Promotion at Retirement, *Journal of Nursing Scholarship, 39*(4) (2007), 330–337.
283. Novak and Campbell, *Aging and Society*.
284. Tompa, E. Transitions to Retirement: *Determinants of Age of Social Security Take up, Social and Economic Dimensions of an Aging Society Research Program*, (SEDAP) Research Paper no. 6. Hamilton, ON: McMaster University, 1999.
285. Andrews and Boyle, *Transcultural Concepts in Nursing Care*.
286. Papalia et al., *Human Development*; Seifert et al., *Lifespan Development*.
287. Iwasaki, Y., J. Zuzanck, and R. Mandell, The Effects of Physically Active Leisure on Stress-Health Relationships, *Canadian Journal of Public Health, 92*(3) (2001), 214–218.
288. Wilson and Palha, A Systematic Review of Published Research Articles on Health Promotion at Retirement.
289. Wilson and Palha, A Systematic Review of Published Research Articles on Health Promotion at Retirement; McDonald, L. *Retiring to Caregive, 2005–2008*. Toronto: Institute for Life Course and Aging, University of Toronto, 2008.
290. Government of Canada. *Liberal Task Force Report*, February, 2000. Ottawa: Liberal Task Force on Seniors, 2004.
291. McDonald, *Retiring to Caregive, 2005–2008*.
292. McDonald, *Retiring to Caregive, 2005–2008*.
293. National Advisory Council on Aging, *Seniors in Canada: 2006 Report Card*. Ottawa: Author, 2006.
294. National Advisory Council on Aging, *Seniors in Canada*.
295. Elsner, R., M. Quinn, S. Fanning, S. Cueldner, and L. Poon, Ethical and Policy Considerations for Centenarians: The Oldest Old, *Journal of Nursing Scholarship, 31*(3) (1999), 263–267.
296. King, T., Status and Standards of Care for Older Adults, *Canadian Nurse, 100*(5) (2004), 23–26.
297. Stanhope et al., *Community Health Nursing in Canada*.
298. Cranswick, K. *General Social Survey Cycle 16: Caring for an Aging Society*. Ottawa: Statistics Canada, 2003.
299. Government of Canada. *Seniors Canada*. Website: http://www.seniors.gc.ca/home.jsp?lang=en (accessed April 2008).
300. Edelman and Mandle, *Health Promotion throughout the Lifespan*.
301. Community Legal Education Ontario (CLEO). *Every Resident: Bill of Rights for People Who Live in Ontario Long Term Care Homes. Advocacy Centre for the Elderly (ACE) and CLEO*, 2005. Website: http://www.cleonet.ca/instance.php?instance_id=275 (accessed April 2008).
302. Papalia et al., *Human Development*; Seifert et al., *Lifespan Development*.
303. Life Lease Associates of Canada. *What Is Life Lease?* Website: http://www.life-lease.com/whatis.htm (accessed April 2008).
304. Bailey, L., and R. Hanssen, Psychological Obstacles to Job or Career Change in Late Life, *Journal of Gerontology: Psychological Sciences, 50B* (1995), P280–P288; Novak and Campbell. *Aging and Society: A Canadian Perspective*; Boyd et al., *Lifespan Development*.
305. Edelman and Mandle, *Health Promotion throughout the Lifespan*; Ebersole et al., *Gerontological Nursing & Healthy Aging*.

## Chapter 15

1. Santrock, J.W., A. MacKenzie-Rivers, K.H. Leung, and T. Malcomson. *Life-span Development*, 2nd Canadian ed. Toronto: McGraw-Hill Ryerson, 2005.
2. Canadian Hospice Palliative Care Association. *The Pan-Canadian Gold Standard for Palliative Home Care: Towards Equitable Access to High Quality Hospice Palliative and End-of-Life Care at Home*. Ottawa: Canadian Hospice Palliative Care Association, 2006.
3. Wilson, D., S. Smith, M. Anderson, H. Northcott, R. Fainsinger, M. Stingl, and C. Truman, Twentieth-Century Social and Health Care Influences on Location of Death in Canada, *Canadian Journal of Nursing Research, 34*(3) (2002), 141–161.
4. Stajduhar, K.I., Examining the Perspectives of Family Members Involved in the Delivery of Palliative Care at Home, *Journal of Palliative Care, 19*(1) (2003), 27–35.
5. Canadian Hospice Palliative Care Association, *The Pan-Canadian Gold Standard for Palliative Home Care*.
6. Tierney, L., S. McPhee, and M. Papadakis. *Current Medical Diagnosis & Treatment, 1999*, 38th ed. Stamford, CT: Appleton & Lange, 1999; Lazar, N.M., S. Shemie, G.C. Webster, and B.M. Dickens, Bioethics for Clinicians: 24. Brain Death, *Canadian Medical Association Journal, 164*(6) (2001), 833–836.
7. Schemie, S.D., C. Doig, and P. Belitsky, Advancing Toward a Modern Death: The Path from Severe Brain Injury to Neurological Determination of Death, *Canadian Medical Association Journal, 168*(8) (2003), 993–997.
8. Wijdicks, E.F.M., Brain Death Worldwide, *Neurology, 58*(1) (2002), 20–25.

9. Canadian Congress Committee on Brain Death, Death and Brain Death: A New Formulation for Canadian Medicine, *Canadian Medical Association Journal*, 138(5) (1988), 405–406; Canadian Neurological Care Group, Guidelines for the Diagnosis of Brain Death, *Canadian Journal of Neurological Science*, 26(1) (1999), 64–66.

10. Lazar et al., Bioethics for Clinicians: 24. Brain Death.

11. Canadian Association of Critical Care Nurses. *Withholding and Withdrawing of Life Support*. Website: http://caccn.ca/ new/index.php?fuseaction=view.content&item=55 (accessed September 2007).

12. Canadian Nurses Association. *Joint Statement on Resuscitative Interventions*. Website: http://www.cna-nurses.ca (accessed September 2007).

13. Canadian Nurses Association. *Code of Ethics for Registered Nurses, 2002*. Ottawa: Author, 2002.

14. Shemie, S.D., C. Doig, G. Rocker, and P. Belitsky, How to Improve Organ Donation Rates, *Canadian Medical Association Journal*, 170(3) (2004), 318–320.

15. Molzahn, A.E., R. Starzomski, and J. McCormick, The Supply of Organs for Transplantation: Issues and Challenges, *Nephrology Nursing Journal*, 30(1) (2003), 17–26.

16. Gillham-Eisen, L.A., and E. Holmgren, The Ottawa Hospital Organ and Tissue Donation Program, *Canadian Nurse*, 98(8) (2002), 18–24.

17. Canadian Nurses Association. *Fact Sheet: Organ Donation and Tissue Transplantation*. Website: http://www.cna-nurses.ca/CNA/ (accessed September 2007).

18. Keatings, M., and O. Smith, *Ethical & Legal Issues in Canadian Nursing*, 2nd ed. Toronto: W.B. Saunders Canada, 2000.

19. Nursing News, Organ Donor Preference Now Indicated on NB Medicare Cards, *Nursing Leadership*, 20(2) (2007), 14.

20. Zaltzman, J.S., Kidney Transplantation in Canada: Unequal Access, *Canadian Medical Association Journal*, 175(5) (2006), 489–490.

21. Zaltzman, Kidney Transplantation in Canada.

22. Bowman, K.W., and S.A. Richardson, Cultural Considerations for Canadians in the Diagnosis of Brain Death, *Canadian Journal of Anesthesia*, 51(3) (2004), 273–280.

23. Canadian Nurses Association. *Everyday Ethics: Putting the Code into Practice*. Ottawa: Author, n.d.

24. Canadian Institutes of Health Research, *Updated Guidelines for Human Pluripotent Stem Cell Research, June 2007*. Website: http://cihr-irsc.gc.ca/e/34460.html (accessed September 2007).

25. Caulfield, T., Human Cloning a Decade after Dolly, *Canadian Medical Association Journal*, 176(5) (2007), 613.

26. Canadian Nurses Association. *Position Statement: The Role of the Nurse in Reproductive and Genetic Technologies*. Ottawa: Author, 2002.

27. Canadian Association of Nurses, Nursing and Genetics: Are You Ready? *Nursing Now*, May 1, 2005, 20.

28. Santrock et al., *Life-span Development*.

29. Canadian Nurses Association. *Position Statement: Code of Ethics for Registered Nurses*. Ottawa: Author, 2002.

30. Gordon, C., Euthanasia: It's No Dutch Treat, *Focus on the Family*, June 1997, 10–11; Papalia, D., S. Olds, and R.D. Feldman. *Human Development*, 9th ed. Boston: McGraw Hill, 2004; Seifert, K., R. Hoffnung, and M. Hoffnung. *Lifespan Development*. Boston: Houghton Mifflin, 1997.

31. Verpoort, C., C. Gastmans, and B. Dierckx de Casterlé, Palliative Care Nurses' Views on Euthanasia. *Journal of Advanced Nursing*, 47(6) (2004), 592–600.

32. Roy, D.J., Palliative Care and Euthanasia: A Continuing Need to Think Again, *Journal of Palliative Care*, 18(1) (2002), 3–5.

33. Marcoux, I., B.L. Mishara, and C. Durand, Confusion between Euthanasia and Other End-of-Life Decisions: Influences on Public Opinion Poll Results, *Canadian Journal of Public Health*, 98(3) (2007), 235–239.

34. Brock, D., Voluntary Active Euthanasia. In F. Baylis, J. Downie, B. Hoffmaster, and S. Sherwin (eds.), *Health Care Ethics in Canada*, 2nd ed. (pp. 468–483). Toronto: Thomson Nelson, 2004.

35. Right to Die Society of Canada. Website: http://www.righttodie.ca/ (accessed September 2007).

36. Compassionate Healthcare Network. Website: http://www.chninternational.com/ (accessed October 2007).

37. Canadian Association of Critical Care Nurses. *Advanced Directives*. Website: http://www.caccn.ca/ (accessed October 2007).

38. Bee, H., D. Boyd, and P. Johnson. *Lifespan Development*, 2nd Canadian ed. Toronto: Pearson Education Canada, Inc., 2006.

39. Canadian Association of Critical Care Nurses, *Advanced Directives*.

40. Martin, D.K., L.L. Emanuel, and A. Singer, Planning for the End of Life, *The Lancet*, 356(9242) (2000), 1672–1676.

41. Singer, P.A., E.C. Thiel, I. Salit, and W. Flanagan, The HIV-Specific Advance Directive, *Journal of General Internal Medicine*, 12(12) (1997), 729–735; Berry, S.R., and P.A. Singer, The Cancer Specific Advance Directive, *Cancer*, 82(8) (1998), 1570–1577.

42. Canadian Association of Critical Care Nurses, *Advanced Directives*.

43. Canadian Nurses Association, *Position Statement: Code of Ethics for Registered Nurses*.

44. Blondeau, D., M. Lavoie, P. Valois, E.W. Keyserlingk, M. Hebert, and I. Martineau, The Attitude of Canadian Nurses Toward Advance Directives, *Nursing Ethics*, 7(5) (2000), 399–411.

45. Keatings, M., and O.B. Smith. *Ethical & Legal Issues in Canadian Nursing*, 2nd ed. Toronto: W.B. Saunders Canada, 2000.

46. Galbraith, K.M., and K. Dobson, The Role of the Psychologist in Determining Competence for Assisted Suicide/Euthanasia in the Terminally Ill, *Canadian Psychology*, 41(3) (2000), 174–183.

47. Van Weel, H., Euthanasia: Mercy, Morals and Medicine, *Canadian Nurse*, 91(8) (1995), 35–40; Shapiro, C., R. Dean, and M. Seguire, Assisted Suicide: A Challenge for Today's Nurses, *Canadian Nurse*, 98(1) (2002), 24–26.

48. Boehnlein, J., The Case against Physician-Assisted Suicide, *Community Mental Health Journal*, 35(1) (1999), 5–24.

49. Wilson, K.G., J.F. Scott, I.D. Graham, J. Kozak, S. Chater, R. Viola, et al., Attitudes of Terminally Ill Patients toward Euthanasia and Physician-Assisted Suicide, *Archives of Internal Medicine*, 160 (2000), 2454–2460.

50. Santrock et al., *Life-span Development*.

51. Papalia et al., *Human Development*.

52. Bee et al., *Lifespan Development*.

53. Papalia et al., *Human Development*.

54. Health Canada. *Helping Your Child Cope—Responding to the Stress of Terrorism and Armed Conflicts, 2002*. Website: http://www.hc-sc.gc.ca/pphb-dgspsp/emergency-urgence/index_e.html (accessed September 2007).

55. Papalia et al., *Human Development*.

56. Santrock et al., *Life-span Development*.

57. Kail, R.V., J.C. Cavanaugh, and C. Ateah. *Human Development: A Life-Span View*, 1st Canadian ed. Toronto: Thomson Nelson, 2006.

58. Noppe, I., and L. Noppe, Evolving Meanings of Death during Early, Middle, and Later Adolescence, *Death Studies*, 21 (1997), 253–275.

59. Public Health Agency of Canada. *Stressful Events: Helping Teens Cope*. Website: http://www.phac-aspc.gc.ca/ (accessed September 2007).

60. Kennard, M., A Visit from an Angel, *American Journal of Nursing*, 98(3) (1998), 48–51; Kübler-Ross, E. (ed.). *On Death and Dying*. New York: Collier-Macmillan, 1969; Kübler-Ross, E. *Death, the Final Stage of Growth*. Englewood Cliffs, NJ: Prentice-Hall, 1975; Kübler-Ross, E. (ed.). *Living with Dying*.

New York: Macmillan, 1981; Wylie, N., T.A. Mast, and J. Kennerly. *Sharing the Final Journey: Walking with the Dying.* Hantsport, NS: Robert Pope Foundation, 1996; Ufema, J. *Insights on Death & Dying.* Philadelphia: Lippincott, Williams & Wilkins, 2007; Albom, M. *Tuesdays with Morrie: An Old Man, a Young Man, and Life's Greatest Lesson.* Toronto: Doubleday, 1998.

61. Corr, C.A., C.M. Nabe, and D.M. Corr. *Death and Dying, Life and Living,* 3rd ed. Scarborough, ON: Wadsworth Thomson Learning, 2000.
62. Santrock et al., *Life-span Development.*
63. Corr et al., *Death and Dying, Life and Living.*
64. Bee et al., *Lifespan Development.*
65. Moody, R.A. *Life after Life.* New York: Bantam Books, 1975.
66. Atwater, P.M.H. *In Search of a Common Criteria for Identifying Near-Death States.* Website: http://www.cinemind.com/atwater/criter.html (accessed September 2007).
67. Corr et al., *Death and Dying, Life and Living.*
68. Boltz, L., A Time to Every Purpose, *American Journal of Nursing,* 98(11) (1998), 47.
69. Ufema, *Insights on Death & Dying.*
70. Glaser, B., and A. Strauss. *Awareness of Dying.* Chicago: Aldine, 1965; Glaser, B., and A. Strauss. *Time for Dying.* Chicago: Aldine, 1968.
71. Wright, L., W.L. Watson, and J.M. Bell. *Beliefs: The Heart of Healing in Families and Illness.* New York: Basic Books, 1996.
72. Kübler-Ross (ed.), *On Death and Dying.*
73. Downe-Wamboldt, B., and D. Tamblyn, An International Survey of Death Education Trends in Faculties of Nursing and Medicine, *Death Studies,* 21 (1997), 177–188.
74. Corr et al., *Death and Dying, Life and Living.*
75. Corr et al., *Death and Dying, Life and Living.*
76. Bee et al., *Lifespan Development.*
77. Corr et al., *Death and Dying, Life and Living.*
78. Brown, F.H., The Impact of Death and Serious Illness on the Family Life Cycle. In B. Carter and M. McGoldrick (eds.), *The Changing Family Life Cycle: A Framework for Family Therapy,* 2nd ed. (pp. 457–475). Needham Heights, MA: Allyn and Bacon, 1989.
79. Canadian Hospice Palliative Care Association. *A History.* Website: http://www.chpca.net/ (accessed September 2007).

80. Dean, R., Death, Humor, and Spirituality: Strange Bedfellows. In G.R. Cox, R.A. Bendiksen, and R.G. Stevenson (eds.), *Making Sense of Death* (pp. 73, 75). Amityville, NY: Baywood Publishing Co. Inc., 2003.
81. Wiegand, D.L., Families and Withdrawal of Life-Sustaining Therapy: State of the Science, *Journal of Family Nursing,* 12(2) (2006), 165–184.
82. Gudmundsdottir, M., and C.A. Chesla, Building a New World: Habits and Practices of Healing Following the Death of a Child, *Journal of Family Nursing,* 12(2) (2006), 143–164.
83. Levin, B., Grief Counselling, *American Journal of Nursing,* 98(5) (1998), 69–71.
84. Health Canada. *A Guide to End-of-Life Care for Seniors.* Toronto and Ottawa: Faculty of Medicine, University of Toronto and University of Ottawa, 2000.
85. Canadian Hospice Palliative Care Association, *The Pan-Canadian Gold Standard for Palliative Home Care.*
86. Zerwekh, J., Do Dying Patients Really Need IV Fluids? *American Journal of Nursing,* 97(3) (1997), 26–30.
87. Chochinov, H.M., Dignity-Conserving Care—A New Model for Palliative Care, *Journal of American Medical Association,* 287(17) (2002), 2253–2260.
88. Canadian Hospice Palliative Care Association. *A History: A Model to Guide Hospice Palliative Care.* Website: http://www.chpca.net (accessed September 2007).
89. Canadian Hospice Palliative Care Association. *Interest Groups, Nurses, Hospice Palliative Care Nursing Standards of Practice.* Website: http://www.chpca.net/ (accessed September 2007).
90. Quality End-of-Life Care Coalition. *Dying for Care: Status Report June 2004.* Ottawa: Canadian Hospice Palliative Care Association, 2004; Quality End-of-Life Care Coalition. *2006 Workplan.* Ottawa: Secretariat, Canadian Hospice Palliative Care Association, 2006.
91. Canadian Hospice Palliative Care Association. *A History: Quality End-of-Life Care Coalition.* Website: http://www.chpca.net/ (accessed September 2007).
92. Health Canada. Canadian Strategy on Palliative and End-of-Life Care: Progress Report of the Coordinating Committee, December 2002 to March 2004. Ottawa: Authority of the Minister of Health, 2005.

# Photo Credits

**Chapter 1** p. 21, Image 100
**Chapter 7** p. 235, Kathleen Finlay/Masterfile; p. 248, Marc Vaughn/Masterfile; p. 267, George Dodson/Lightworks Studio
**Chapter 8** p. 293, Jennie Woodcock, Reflections Photolibrary/ CORBIS
**Chapter 9** p. 314, Masterfile
**Chapter 10** p. 375, J. Hardie/Masterfile; p. 379, dk & dennie cody/Masterfile

**Chapter 11** p. 449, Will Hart/Photo Edit
**Chapter 12** p. 483, Miep van Damm/Masterfile
**Chapter 13** p. 530, Peter Griffith/Masterfile
**Chapter 14** p. 552, Peter Griffith/Masterfile; p. 559, Rick Gomez/Masterfile; p. 579, Berger, K. J. and M. B. Williams, *Fundamentals of Nursing: Collaborating for Optimal Health.* Stamford, CT: Appleton & Lange, 1992, p. 1317; p. 607, Health Canada website and media photo gallery, Health Canada, *www.hc-sc.gc.ca.*

# Index

## A

abandonment, 224
able elderly, 610–611
Aboriginal children
    adolescent pregnancies, 450
    adoption of, 11
    disease patterns, 379
    Early Childhood Caries (ECC), 324
    FAS/FAE rates, 379
    growth charts, and regional variations, 282–283
    immunization rates, 267
    poverty and, 15
Aboriginal peoples
    attachment, 235
    average age of, 351
    children. See Aboriginal children
    Chlamydia, 444
    chronic conditions, 10
    cultural groups, 3
    cultural population, 10–11
    cultural revival, 11
    diabetes, 181, 206
    family, 96, 232
    family healer, 103
    gonorrhea, 444
    Government of Canada categories, 3
    healing practices, 61–62, 103
    and health inequalities, 18
    health status, 10–11, 11t
    high birth weight, 244
    Hollow Water First Nations Holistic Healing Circle (CHCH), 239
    and injuries, 364–365, 420, 495
    language, 4, 5–6, 301
    life expectancy, 606
    low birth weight, 244
    Medicine Wheel, 61
    mental health and, 9
    Native American Church, 79
    parenting practices, 120
    pollution and food contaminants, 38
    poverty, 15
    preterm birth, 220
    skipped-generation households, 512
    spirituality, 79
    suicide, 425–426, 500
    three groups, 10
    transmission of culture, 5
    Two-spirit people, 97
    type 2 diabetes, 10
    women of child-bearing age, 206
Aboriginal Peoples Survey (2001), 10

abortion
    and adolescence, 449–450
    spontaneous abortion, 201t
absolute poverty, 15
absorption, 577t
abstract reasoning, 594t
abstract space, 333
abuse
    battered women, myths and realities, 505–506
    child maltreatment. See child maltreatment
    domestic violence, 217
    elder abuse and neglect, 562–564
    family violence, 503–507
    identification of partner abuse, 504
    physical abuse, 238
    of pregnant women, 217
    sexual abuse, 224, 238, 346, 353t
academic performance, 595t
acceptance, 625–626
accession, 183
accidents. See injury and injury control
accommodation, 169
accommodative esophoria, 367t
achievement tests, 377
acid, 430t
acid rain, 28
acknowledgment of reality, 185t
acne, 403
acne vulgaris, 422t
acrocyanosis, 242
action, 335–336
action groups, 610
action space, 333
active euthanasia, 619
activity theory, 556, 557
acute cervical adenitis, 329t
acute nonspecific gastroenteritis, 295t
acute pyelonephritis, 492t
Adam, 430t
Adams, Michael, 13
adaptation, 169
adaptive mechanisms
    adolescence, 418
    infants, 273
    later adulthood, 600–601
    middle age, 545
    positive adaptive mechanisms, 181
    preschool years, 344
    school-aged years, 392–393
    toddler stage, 304
    young adults, 485

adaptive responses in the family, 103
Addiction Centre Adolescent Research Group, 427
Addictions Foundation of Manitoba, 214
adequacy, 175
adolescence
    abortion, 449–450
    abuse, neglect and maltreatment, 400
    adaptive mechanisms, 418
    alcohol, 427–428
    anorexia nervosa, 405–406
    body image, 416–417
    brain development, 403
    bulimia, 406–407
    bullying, 411
    cardiovascular system, 403
    career selection, 419
    chronic illness, 424–425
    cognitive development, 410–411
    common health problems, 422–424, 422t–423t
    communication, 399
    conflict, 511
    contraceptive practices, 444–447
    counselling, 452
    cultural differences in physical development, 403
    dating patterns, 412
    death, concepts of, 622–623
    defined, 398
    developmental crisis, 414–416
    early adolescence, 398
    emotional characteristics, 413–414
    emotional development, 413–416, 414t
    family life cycle, 398
    family relationships, 398–400
    formal operations period, 410–411
    gambling, 428–429
    gender differences in growth, 401
    grief, 630
    growth, 401
    health promotion, 419–443, 451–452
    identity diffusion, 414, 415, 416
    identity formation, 414–415
    identity statuses, 415–416
    immunization, 420
    injury and injury control, 420, 421–422
    late adolescence, 398–399, 418–419

gay men (*continued*)
    gay family life cycle, 107
    LAT arrangements, 118
    parents, 312
gender
    constancy, 312
    and infants, 273
    primary identification, 305
gender differences
    anorexia nervosa, 406
    cardiovascular disease, 585
    cognitive development, 478
    growth, during adolescence, 401
    hypothyroidism, 575
    jobs, 479
    longevity, 580–581
    malnutrition, effects of, 288
    moral reasoning, 418
    physical exercise, 468
    playing with children, 340
    relationship concerns, 482
    sexual behaviour, 514
    size, during school-aged years, 355
    smoking, 502
    vision, 358
    wages, 479
gender identity, 273, 305, 312–313
gender-role conflicts, 426
general adaptation syndrome, 179–181
General Injury Prevention Guidelines, 365
general knowledge, 595t
General Social Survey (GSS), 81
general systems theory, 188t
generalization, 159t
generation, 457
generation gap, 511
generativity, 542–544
genes, 145–146, 198, 203
genetic counselling, 56
genetic defects, 204
genetic gene theory, 556t
genetic influences, 145
genetic linkage, 115
genetic predisposition, 147
genetic technologies, 147–148
genetic traits, 144–147
genetically modified foods, 37
genital stage, 164t
genitourinary diseases, 587t
genogram, 126, 128f
Genome Canada, 148
genuineness, 124
geographic moves, 152, 393–394
geriatrics, 552
German measles, 215
germinal stage, 200, 200t–201t
gerontology, 552
gestational age assessment, 241–242
gestational diabetes, 206
gestational weight gain, 207, 207t
gestures, 271

gifted child, 378
Gilligan, Carol, 172–174, 175t, 189t, 418, 548
gingivitis, 422t
"Gita is a way of life" (Desai), 64f
glaucoma, 567
global responsibility and the environment, 44–51
global warming, 28
globalists, 540
globalization of food supply, 37
globesity, 362, 407
glutaraldehyde, 34
*Go for It: A Guide for Choosing and Using Assistive Devices,* 580
goal achievement, 153
goals, 154t
Golden Rule, 62, 63f
Goleman, Daniel, 377, 481
gonadotropin, 206, 400
gonorrhea, 216, 444, 445t
Good Friday, 71
gout, 534t
government, 7t
Government of Canada, 187, 317, 607
grandparenthood, 559
grandparents
    divorce of children, 316
    expansion of intrafamily relationships, 238
    and infants, 238
    maternal grandmother, 238
    and preschoolers, 315–316
    role, 512
    skipped-generation households, 512
    spiritual sustenance, 315
    stepgeneration family, 119
    tips for, 513
grass, 438t–441t
Grave's disease, 534t
great-grandparents, 559
great-great-grandparents, 559
Greek Eastern Orthodox faith, 72, 76t, 80
Green Plan, 40
greenhouse gas emissions, 29, 30, 32–33
Greenpeace, 51
gridlock, 483
grief, 630–631
gross motor coordination, 283
ground-level ozone, 32
group action, 610
group in crisis, 183–186
group teaching, 21
growing pains, 365
growth
    adolescence, 401
    asynchronous growth, 197
    cultural comparisons, 355
    defined, 195
    incremental growth, 195
    infants, 250–251

    of parents, 232–233
    physical growth, in adolescence, 400–401
    principles of growth, 197–198, 355
    replacement growth, 195
    secular growth trends, 398
growth hormone deficiency, 322
growth hormone (GH), 221, 283, 400
growth hormone-releasing factor (GHF), 221
growth rate
    discontinuity of, 197
    in toddlers, 282–283
grunting, 271
Guaranteed Income Supplement (GIS), 15, 606
guidance
    preschoolers, 342–343
    school-aged years, 386–387
    toddlers, 305
*Guide to the End of Life Care for Seniors,* 631
guided participation, 336
*Guidelines for Canadian Drinking Water Quality,* 357
guilt, 343
gynecologic cancers, 533

# H

Hadith, 67
hair, 522t, 565t, 566
hallucinogens, 430t–433t
hand-foot-and-mouth disease, 368t
handedness, 283
handwriting, 381
happy marriage, 513–514
Hare Krishna, 79
harm reduction approach, 23
hatha yoga, 65
Hayward, Pat, 214
hazard exposure, 42
*Hazardous Materials Information Review Act,* 42
*Hazardous Products Act,* 42, 43, 267
hazardous waste disposal, 40–42
HDL cholesterol, 146
head
    circumference, of infants, 244
    injuries, 327, 364
    of school-aged children, 357
head lice, 368t
health
    defined, 19
    human health and global ecosystems, 30
    importance of, 22
    key definitions, 19
    nature, role of, 30
    and religion, link between, 61
    and stress, 150
Health Behaviour in School Aged Children (HBSC), 420–421

interpersonal communication studies, 377
interpersonal problem solving, 125–126
interpersonal security, 165
interpersonal skill, 374
interpersonal theory of psychiatry, 165, 188t
interpreter, 19–20, 20t
interventions
    adoptive families, 116
    biological rhythms, 474
    body image, 486–487
    Calgary Family Intervention Model
      (CFIM), 132
    child maltreatment, 346–347
    child maltreatment, preventive
      interventions for, 240
    children of abused women, 505–507
    circular questions, 132–133, 133t
    for the dying person, 631–633
    faith communities, 86
    family care, 132–134, 135t
    family crisis intervention, 134
    family of dying clients, 628–630
    later adulthood, 611–612
    life review, 612
    linear questions, 132–133
    McGill Model of Nursing, 133–134
    recall, 597
    reminiscence, 612
    resuscitative interventions, 617
    sleep, 476–477
    spiritual care, 85–88
    substance abuse, 442t
    suicide, 426–427
intimacy, 482
intracytoplasmic sperm injection (ICSI), 148
intrapersonal skill, 374
intrauterine growth restrictions
  (IUGRs), 209
intrauterine system (IUS), 446t
introjection, 163t
intuitive phase, 334
Inuit, 3, 10, 38
    *see also* Aboriginal peoples
IQ tests, 377
iron deficiency anemia, 269t, 491t
iron-fortified infant cereal, 260
ironic compliments, 374–375
ironic criticism, 374–375
irony, 374–375
Islam, 67–68, 74t
isolation, 393, 484, 625
Izaak Walton Killam (IWK) Telehealth
  Program, 22

## J

Jainism, 65–66
James Bay, 36
jaundice, 242
Jehovah's Witnesses, 77t, 78, 88
Jen, 67
jet lag, 473

jogging, 467
joint, 438t–441t
*Journal of Christian Nursing,* 81
Judaism, 69–70, 74t
jumping to conclusions, 167t
Jung, Carl, 193
juvenile diabetes, 368t
juvenile hypertension, 329t
juvenile period, 350, 355
juvenile rheumatoid arthritis, 380

## K

karma yoga, 64
Katz, Anne, 464
Kellogg Canada, 18
ketoacidosis, 206
Kevorkian, Jack, 621
Keys to Care Giving program, 235
kidney transplants, 618
kidneys, 358, 573, 588
Kids Help Line, 240
*Kids Talk About Divorce,* 352
kindergarten, 318
kinesthetic skill, 374
knee jerk reflex, 247t
knowledge, 8t, 177t, 443
Kohlberg, Lawrence, 172, 189t, 418, 547
kosher, 69
Kübler-Ross, E., 625, 626

## L

La Leche League Canada, 258, 259
labelling, 167t
labour, 136–137
labyrinth, 82
lacto-ovo-vegetarians, 73
lactose intolerance, 492t
lalling, 271
Lamaze, 156
Lamaze, Fernand, 218–219
Landau reflex, 247t
language
    Aboriginal peoples, 4, 5–6, 301
    acquisition theories, 298
    assessment of development, 300
    contraction, 299
    culture, stabilizing aspect of, 5–6
    development, 301, 338t
    dialect, 6
    expansion, 299
    Indo-European languages, 5–6
    interactionist theory, 298
    interpreter, 19–20, 20t
    learning, 336
    meeting ground between cultures, 6
    pragmatics, 381
    school-aged years, 381
    skill, 374
    toddler stage, 298–301
    uses of, 336
lanugo, 202t

Lao-tzu, 67
large families, 112
large sport utility vehicles, 32
last-born child, 112
latchkey child, 353
late adolescence, 398–399, 418–419
late childhood, 350
latency stage, 164t
later adulthood
    *see also* aging
    able elderly, 610–611
    adaptive mechanisms, 600–601
    adverse drug reactions, 589–590
    alcohol, 590, 591
    assessment, 611
    assisted living, 609
    assistive devices, 580
    beginning of, 552
    body image, 601–602
    the brain, 566
    cardiovascular disease, 571
    cardiovascular system, 571t–572t
    caregiver role, 560
    children, relationships with, 558
    cognitive development, 591–598,
      592t–595t
    common health problems, 585–591
    community planning, 606–611
    community services, 606–607
    creativity, 596, 598
    crystallized intelligence, 591–592
    death, concepts of, 623–624
    definitions, 552–553
    despair, 599
    divorce, 561
    economic status, 15
    ego integrity, 598
    elder abuse and neglect, 562–564
    emotional development, 598–599
    endocrine system, 575
    extended-care facility, 608–609
    family development and
      relationships, 557–564
    farming hazards, 44
    federal planning for the aged in
      Canada, 606
    fluid intelligence, 592
    foot care, 468
    gastrointestinal system, 575
    general appearance, 564–566
    grandparenthood and great-
      grandparenthood, 559
    group action, 610
    hair, 566
    health prevention, 580–584
    health promotion, 580–584,
      611–612
    hearing, 568–569
    hematologic system, 576
    immune system, 576
    immunization, 581

maturation, 195
maturational factors, 150–151, 169
mature baptism, 73
maturity, 544
matzo, 70
McGill Model of Nursing, 133–134
MDMA, 213, 430t
Meadow Lake Tribal Council, 319
measles, 329t, 490
mechanical hazard exposure, 42
meconium, 245
media
    *see also* Internet; television
    Child Behavior Checklist (CBCL),
        13–14
    psychosocial development of
        children, 13–14, 335
    roles of, 335
    and school-aged years, 381–384
    violence, 14
Media Awareness Network (MNet), 381
*Medical Waste: Role of Nurses and Nursing*
    (ICN), 41
*Medication Matters*, 590
Medicine Wheel, 61
meditation, 81, 82
Meichenbaum, Donald, 167–168
meiosis, 199
memory
    declarative (episodic) memory, 593t
    forgetfulness, 596
    information theory, 172
    interventions, 597
    life review, 598, 612
    long-term memory, 536–537, 593t
    in middle age, 536–537
    and modelling, 168
    recall, 597
    reminiscence, 597–598, 612
    sensory memory, 536, 592t
    short-term memory, 172, 536, 593t
men
    *see also* fathers; gender differences;
        men's health
    caregiver role for spouse, 558
    male climacteric, 524–525
    male reproductive cycle, 198–199
    nocturnal emissions, 401
    spermarche, 401
    toxic agents, exposure to, 211
menarche, 401, 417
Mendelian Law of Inheritance, 144–145
Mennonites, 77t, 78
menopause, 513, 524, 525, 526, 527
menorah, 69
men's health
    *see also* men
    generally, 463
    information site, 463
    physical changes and characteristics,
        520t–524t

prostate cancer, 533, 575
    sexual dysfunctions, 463–464
    testicular cancer, 422, 497–499
Men's Health Canada, 463
menstrual cycle, 402
menstrual patterns, 402
menstrual period, 402
menstruation, 398, 401
mental filter, 167t
Mental Health Plan, 9
mentor, 543
mercury, 211
mesoderm, 201t
mesosystems, 153
metabolic function, 206
metabolism, 577t
metacognition, 172, 372
Methodist, 77t
methylene chloride, 34
Métis, 3, 10
    *see also* Aboriginal peoples
microbial pesticides, 38
microsystems, 153, 239
mid-life crisis, 545–547
mid-life transition, 545–547
mid-old, 552
middle age
    adaptive mechanisms, 545
    aging parents, relationship with,
        515–519
    body image, 544–545
    cancer, 533
    cardiovascular disease, 535
    caregiver role, 516–519
    children, relationship with, 511–513
    chronic illness, 535–536
    cognitive ability, 536
    cognitive development, 536–539
    common health problems, 533–536,
        534t–535t
    continued learning, 537–539
    creativity, 537
    death, concepts of, 623–624
    death of parents, 519
    defined, 511
    developmental crisis, 542–544
    early dementia, 538
    elderly relatives, responsibility for,
        515–516
    emotional changes related to
        physical changes, 527
    emotional development, 542–544
    family life cycle, 511
    female climacteric, 524
    foot balance, 531
    foot care, 531
    foot problems, 531
    formal operations stage, 537
    generativity, 542–544
    health care role, 519
    health prevention, 532–536

    health promotion, 532–533,
        548–549
    hormonal changes, 524–527
    hormone replacement therapy,
        526–527
    hypothyroidism, 535
    illness prevention, 532–533
    immunization, 532
    injury and accidents, 532
    leadership role, 541–542
    leisure, 542
    male climacteric, 524–525
    maturity, 544
    menopause, 513, 526
    mid-life crisis, 545–547
    mid-life transition, 545–547
    moral-spiritual development,
        547–548
    nutritional needs, 528–530
    obesity, 533
    physical activity, 530–531
    physical changes, 520, 520t–524t
    physical characteristics, 520–527
    physiological development, 520–532
    psychosocial development, 536–548
    respiratory conditions, 535
    retirement, 541
    sandwich generation, 515
    sexual dysfunction, 525–526
    sleep, 531–532
    spouse or partner, relationship with,
        513–514
    work, 539–541
middle childhood, 350, 355
middle-class North American family life
    cycle, 104–107
migraine headache, 493t
mikvah, 69
milia, 242
miliaria rubra, 296t
military families, 140
milk malabsorption syndrome, 492t
mind-body relationship, 181
mind reading, 167t
Mini-Mental State Exam (MMSE), 596
minimization, 167t
minister, 73
minor ankle sprain, 421–422
minor lacerations, 327
minor strains and sprains, 421
miscarriage, 201t
mislabelling, 167t
mitosis, 203–204
mitral value prolapse, 491t
mitzvah, 70
mobility devices, 580
modelling, 168
*Modernization of Benefits and Obligations*
    *Act*, 464
Moffitt, P., 2
money concept, 373

play (continued)
    symbolic play, 340
    toddler stage, 288–290,
        290t–291t, 298
pleasure principle, 160t
PLISSIT model, 576
point sources of pollution, 34
poisoning
    lead poisoning, 41–42, 327
    preschool years, 327
    prevention, 297
pollution
    air pollution, 30–32, 31f, 222
    chemical pollution, 55
    early childhood, effect on,
        221–222
    noise pollution, 38–40
    paradigm shift, 29f
    soil pollution, 36–37
    surface pollution, 40–42
    water pollution, 34–36
poly-chlorinated biphenyls (PCBs), 38
polygenic inheritance, 146
polypharmacy, 588, 589–590, 591
polyvinyl chloride (PVC), 37
population
    density, 5
    growth rate, in Canada, 11–12
    size, 5
    visible minority population, 12
Population Health Perspective (PHP), 240
positive adaptive mechanisms, 181
positive coping strategies, 181
positive reinforcement, 156, 158t
possessiveness, 304
post-formal thought, 478
post-industrialism, 6
post-traumatic stress disorder (PTSD),
    16, 181
postconventional morality, 172, 173t–174t
posterior fontanel, 241
postindustrial society, 6
postmenstrual phase, 402
postmodern family, 95
postmodern society, 6
postpartum period, 137–138, 233
postural problems, 329t
posture, 566
pot, 438t–441t
poverty
    Aboriginal children, 15
    absolute poverty, 15
    in Canada, 15–16
    child poverty rates, 15
    children and, 350
    and infant mortality, 15
    location of, 17
    municipal governments, 17
    reduction of, 350
    relative poverty, 15
    rural poverty, 17

urban poverty, 17
    vulnerable populations, 15
Poverty Reduction Strategy, 15
practical intelligence, 478
pragmatics, 381
praying, 81
pre-religious stage, 306
preadolescence, 350, 358
preconceptual phase, 333
preconscious, 161t
preconventional morality, 172, 173t
pregnancy
    see also prenatal development
    childbirth, 218–220
    dietary problems, 470
    domestic violence, 217
    major physiological changes,
        203t–204t
    maternal diabetes, 206
    occupational hazards and fetal
        damage, 44
    well-baby care, 134–138
prejudice, 9–10
premarital sexual activity, 417
prematurity, 219–220, 274–275
premenstrual dysphoric disorder (PMDD),
    461–462
premenstrual phase, 402
premenstrual syndrome (PMS), 460–462
prenatal care, 135–136
prenatal development
    the beginning, 198–200
    critical periods, 210f
    embryonic stage, 200, 201t–202t
    environmental hazards. See prenatal
        environmental hazards
    fetal stage, 200, 202t–203t
    germinal stage, 200, 200t–201t
    heredity, 203–205
    maternal nutrition, 206–209
    and parental age, 205
    prenatal endocrine and metabolic
        functions, 206
    stages of, 200–203, 200t–203t
prenatal environmental hazards
    alcohol, 214
    cocaine, 212–213, 213f
    drug hazards, 212–214
    Ecstasy, 213
    external environmental factors,
        210–211
    fathers and, 218
    fetal infection, 217
    immunologic factors, 217
    industrial wastes, 211
    marijuana, 212
    maternal emotions, 217
    maternal infections, 215–216
    mercury, 211
    narcotics, 213–214
    occupational hazards, 211

radiation, 211
    smoking tobacco, 211–212
    substance abuse and addiction, 212
    teratogens, 209–210
preoperational period, 170t–171t, 297
preoperational stage, 333–334
prepubertal sexual development, 358
prepuberty, 358
prepubescence, 350
presbycusis, 569
presbyopia, 567
preschool years
    adaptive mechanisms, 344
    attachment, 311–313
    body image, 343–344
    causality concepts, 333
    cerebral cortex, 320
    child care, 272–273, 316–320
    child maltreatment, 328–330,
        346–347
    common health problems, 328–330,
        328t–329t
    communication, 335–336, 337t
    concept formation, 331
    defined, 310
    dental care, 325
    developmental assessment, 320–322
    developmental crisis, 343
    discipline, 342–343
    emotional development, 343
    exercise, 324–325
    eye-hand coordination, 320
    family, role of, 335
    family life cycle, 310–311
    gender identity, 312–313
    grandparents, 315–316
    guidance, 342–343
    health prevention, 325–328
    health promotion, 325–328,
        345–347
    hospitalization, 330
    illness, reaction to, 330
    immunization, 325
    injury control, 325–328
    intervention, 346–347
    intuitive phase, 334
    mental development, assessment
        of, 332t
    moral-spiritual development,
        344–345
    motor control, 321t
    motor nerves, 320
    new baby, arrival of, 314–315
    nutritional needs, 322–324
    older siblings, 315
    other adults and non-family
        members, influence of, 316–320
    parents, relationships with, 311–313
    physical characteristics, 320–322
    play, 337–340, 341t
    preconceptual phase, 333

preoperational stage, 333–334
problem-solving abilities, 335
prosocial behaviour, 335
psychosocial development, 330–345
  quantitative concepts, 333
  relationships, concepts of, 331
  safety, 325–328
  self-concept, 343–344
  sex education, 313
  sexuality development, 343–344
  siblings, 313–315
  single-parent families, 312
  sleep, 325
  sociocultural perspective, 334
  spatial concepts, 333
  stepfamilies, 312
  time concept, 331
  transductive logic, 334
  vital signs, 320
pressure, 247
preterm birth, 219
prevention. *See* health prevention
Preventive Interventions for Child
  Maltreatment, 240
prickly heat, 296t
primary circular reactions, 269–270
primary dysmenorrhea, 402
primary health care (PHC), 17
primary identification, 304, 305
primary prevention, 19
primary process thinking, 160t
primary sleep disorders, 476
Principle of Asynchronous Growth, 197
principle of communal existence, 165
Principle of Development toward Self-
  Knowledge and Autonomy, 196–197
Principle of Differentiation, 197
Principle of Discontinuity of Growth
  Rate, 197
principle of functional activity, 165
principle of organization, 165
Principle of Readiness, 197
principles of development, 195–197, 401
principles of growth, 197–198
private pension plans, 15
private speech, 336
problem-finding stage, 478
problem solving, 125–126, 335, 410,
  537, 594t
professional family life cycle, 104–107
professional responsibility and the
  environment, 51–52
progesterone, 199, 402
progestin-only pill, 446t
programmed learning, 21
progressive differentiation, 196
Project Canada 2000, 80–81
projection, 163t, 304, 393
prolactin, 259
prolonged separation, 224
property, forms of, 7t

prosocial behaviour, 335
prostate cancer, 533, 575
prostatitis, acute, 534t
prostatitis, chronic, 535t
protective clothing, 55
protective factors, 180
protest, 280
Protestant bodies, 73
Protestantism, 72–73, 76t, 80
Proximodistal Principle, 197
proxy, 620
prudent behaviour, 335
psilocybin, 432t
psychic determination, 160t, 161t
psychic structures of the personality, 160t
psychoanalytical theory
  described, 159
  education, view of, 160
  health implications of, 188t
  the human, view of, 160
  neo-analytic theory, 165–166
  overview, 160
  psychodynamic perspective,
    160–164
  reality, 160
  therapy, view of, 160
psychodynamic perspective, 160–164
psychological age, 195, 511, 552
psychological theories
  behavioural theory, 155–157
  interpersonal theory of
    psychiatry, 165
  neo-analytic theory, 165–166
  overview, 155
  psychoanalytical theory, 159–164
  psychosocial theory of personality
    development, 165–166
psychologically extended family, 97
psychology, 142
psychoneuroimmunology, 150
psychosexual crisis. *See* psychosexual
  development
psychosexual development
  adolescence, 414–415
  middle age, 541–542
  school-aged years, 387–388
  stages of, 164, 164t
  toddlers, 301
  young adults, 482
psychosocial development
  adolescence, 410–419
  described, 268
  infants, 268–273
  later adulthood, 591–602
  middle age, 536–548
  preschool years, 330–345
  school-aged years, 369–394
  toddler stage, 293–306
  young adults, 477–490
psychosocial hazard exposure, 42
psychosocial theories of aging, 556–557

psychosocial theory of personality
  development, 165–166
puberty
  *see also* adolescence
  defined, 398
  menarche, 401
  nocturnal emissions, 401
  physical characteristics, 401
  primary dysmenorrhea, 402
  secondary sex characteristics,
    401–402
  sex hormones, 402
  spermarche, 401
  spermatogenesis, 398, 401
  timing of, 398
  variation in, 398
Public Health Agency of Canada (PHAC),
  256, 366, 409, 468, 495, 500, 530, 607
pulse rate, 320, 355
punishment, 156, 158t
pupillary response reflex, 246t

### Q

Quakers, 77t
Quality-End-of-Life Care Coalition, 633
quantitative concepts, 333
Quebec City Consensus Conference on
  Environmental Health Indicators, 29
Quebec Family Study, 145
Quebec Pension Plan (QPP), 606
quickening, 202t
quiet play, 340
Quran, 67–68

### R

rabies, 327, 366
radiation, 56, 211
Raine, Kim, 408
raja yoga, 64
Ramadan, 68
Ramakrishna, 62
rational thought, 418
rationalization, 163t, 393
reaching reflex, 246t
reaction formation, 163t, 304, 393
reaction range, 205
reaction time, 536, 594t
Read, Grantly Dick, 218
readiness, principle of, 197
reading, 380
real identity, 415
reality, 160, 176
reality principle, 161t
realms of cognition, 373–374
reasoned action, theory of, 143
recall, 597
reciprocal determinism, 168f
recognition, 593t
recreation, 8t
red measles, 215
reefer, 438t–441t

referral guidelines, 22t
reflex stage, 269
reflexes, 245, 246t–247t
reflexive learning, 593t
Reform Jews, 69
refugees, 16, 22
refusal of medical treatment, 88
regional culture, 4–5
Registered Nurses Association of Ontario
    (RNAO), 258
regression, 163t, 393
regulation, 221
reinforcement, 156
reinforcement schedule, 156, 157
relationship concepts, 331
relative poverty, 15
religion
        see also spiritual care
        agnosticism, 80
        atheism, 80
        defined, 61
        and health, link between, 61
        health care implications, 74t
        and health promotion, 81–90
        "no religion," 80
        refusal of medical treatment, 88
        religious education, 344
        special religious groups, 73–80
        world religions. See world religions
religiosity, 81
religious culture, 4
REM sleep, 475, 476
remarriage
        remarried family life cycle, 104, 107t
        stepchild, 117
        stepfamily, 96t, 118
reminiscence, 597–598, 612
replacement growth, 195
Report Card on Child and Family Poverty
    (2006), 15, 350
Report Card on Seniors in Canada, 606
Report of the Royal Commission on
    Aboriginal Peoples, 10
Report on Reflections on Rural and Northern
    Poverty, 17
repression, 163t, 304
reproductive cycles, 198–199
reproductive screening, 148
reproductive system, 520t–521t, 576
reproductive technology. See assisted
    reproductive technology
rescue marriage, 483
resilient children, 223, 389–390
resistance stage, 180
resolution adaptation, 185t
respect, 123
respiratory conditions, 365, 535
respiratory diseases, 586t
respiratory efforts at birth, 244–245
respiratory infections, 34
respiratory muscles, 572t

respiratory rate, 320, 355
respiratory system
        adolescence, 403
        infants, 254–255
        later adulthood, 571–572, 572t–573t
        middle age, 524t
        toddler stage, 283
        young adults, 458
respondent conditioning, 158t
rest, 291–292, 363, 409–410, 474–477, 578
        see also sleep
resuscitative interventions, 617
reticular activating system (RAS), 475
retirement, 541, 602–604
retirement communities, 610, 611
retirement planning, 604–605
retreads, 540
reversibility, 371
rewards, 160
Rh factor, 217
rib cage, 572t
RICE, 421
right brain processing, 144t
right-to-die movement, 619–620
Right to Die Network Canada, 620
Rio Earth Summit, 1992, 28
risk, 19
risk factors
        cardiovascular disease, 585
        coronary heart disease, 365
        defined, 19
        depression, 500
        obesity as risk factor, 379, 459
        overweight as risk factor, 459
        spontaneous preterm birth (SPB), 220
        tobacco use, 502
risk reduction behaviours, 23
ritual, 4, 387
ritualistic behaviour, 302, 393
Robinson, Erlick, 460
Rocky Mountain spotted fever, 423t
Rodriguez, Sue, 621
Rogers, Carl, 178, 190t
Rohypnol®, 434t
role complementarity, 99t
role conflict, 99t
role models, 354
role overload, 100t
role reciprocity, 99t
role strain, 99t
role theory, 99t
roles, 5, 101–102
Roman Catholic Church, 71–72, 75t, 80, 81
romantic marriage, 483
roofies, 434t
rooting reflex, 246t
rope, 434t
Rosh Hashanah, 70
rubella, 215, 296t
rubeola, 215
runaways, 419

rural area, 5
Rural Ontario Municipal Association
    (ROMA), 17
rural poverty, 17
ruralness, 5
Russian Orthodox, 76t, 80

S
Sabbath, 69
Sacraments, 71
Safe Kids Canada, 293, 327
safer injecting facility (SIF), 23
safety
        adolescence, 420–421
        food safety, 37–38
        infants, 267–268
        later adulthood, 582–584
        needs, 177t
        and play, 290
        preschool years, 325–328
        school-aged years, 364–365
        toddler stage, 292–293
same-sex couples, 351
same-sex/homosexual family, 96t
same-sex marriage, 96–97
sample menus
        middle age, 469f, 529f
        school-aged years, 361f
        toddler stage, 287t
        young adult vegetarian, 471f
sanctification, 73
sandwich generation, 515
satiation, 159t
satisfaction of needs, 165
scabies, 491t
scaffolding, 298
scams, 582–583
schema, 169
school-aged years
        adaptive mechanisms, 392–393
        adoptive parents, 354, 354t
        body image, 390, 391, 392t
        bullying, 385–386
        cardiovascular system, 355
        changing behavioural
            characteristics, 387t–388t
        child in transition, 393–394
        chronic illness, 365
        cognitive characteristics, 369t–370t
        cognitive development, 369–379
        common health problems, 365–369,
            367t–368t
        communication patterns, 379–384
        concepts, 372–373
        concrete operations period, 369–371
        developmental crisis, 387–390
        discipline, 386–387
        eating patterns, 360–362
        emotional development, 387–390
        family life cycle, 350–351
        gastrointestinal system, 358

trans-theoretical (stages of change) model, 143
transcultural nursing, 8–9
transdermal contraceptive patch, 446t
transductive logic, 334
transfer, 156
transference, 161t
transformation, 371
transformation of wastes, 40
transgendered family life cycle, 107
transition, 182, 196, 393–394
translocation syndrome, 609–610
transportation, 7t, 267
*Transportation of Dangerous Goods Act*, 40
travel, 7t
treyfe, 69
triadic question, 133t
Triarchic Theory of Intelligence, 373–374, 478
trunk incurvation reflex, 247t
trust *versus* mistrust, 272, 403
tuberculosis, 495, 588t
12-step programs, 80
twin study method, 145
twins, 112, 145
two-egg twins. *See* fraternal twins
Two-spirit people, 97
type 1 diabetes, 368t
type 2 diabetes, 10, 534t

## U

Ukrainian Orthodox, 80
ultradian rhythms, 472
umbilical cord, 201t, 242
unconscious, 161t
Unction of the Sick, 72
understanding, 177t
underweight, 405–407
undoing, 163t, 393
unemployment, 539
Unitarian/Universalist, 77t
United Nations, 507
*United Nations Declaration on the Rights of the Child*, 317
universal focus, 174t
unlicensed child care, 317
unstable marital relationship, 514
unwed parents, 136
Upanishads, 62
upper respiratory infection, 491t
urban area, 4–5
urban poverty, 17
*Urban Poverty in Canada: A Statistical Profile*, 17
urbanization, 152
urinary infection, 365
urinary system
    infants, 255
    later adulthood, 573–575
    middle age, 524t

school-aged years, 358
toddler stage, 255
urinary tract infection, 329t
urticaria, 491t
U.S. National Ambulatory Health and Nutrition Survey, 283
U.S. National Institutes of Health, 526

## V

vaccine-associated adverse events (VAAEs), 363–364
vaccines, 222, 265
    *see also* immunization
value system, 9
Vanier Institute of the Family, 381
varicella, 295t
vascularization, 468
Vedas, 62
vegetarian families, 324
vegetarianism, 470–471
verbal expression, 336
vernix caseosa, 242
very-low-birth-weight (VLBW), 219
victimization, 411
videotapes, 21
violence
    *see also* abuse
    CNA position statement, 504
    domestic violence, 503–507
    family violence, 503–507
    sexual assault, 504–505
    in television, 14, 383
    on television, 14
viral croup, 296t
Vishnu, 62
visible minority population, 12
vision
    age-related macular degeneration (AMD), 567
    blind persons, 568
    cataracts, 567
    gender differences, 358
    glaucoma, 567
    infants, 254
    later adulthood, 567
    middle age, 523t
    neurological changes in the eye, 567t–568t
    newborns, 247–249
    presbyopia, 567
    school-aged years, 358, 365, 366
    toddler stage, 283
vital signs
    infants, 254
    newborns, 244–245
    preschool years, 320
    school-aged years, 355–357
Vitality program, 408
vitamin D, 528
vitamin K, 265
voice, 523t

volunteer work, 481, 605
vulnerable children, 223, 389, 390
Vygotsky, Lev, 334, 336

## W

waist circumference (WC), 458
wake, 71
Walkerton, Ontario, 36
walking exercise, 580
walking reflex, 246t
warmth, 123
warning, 180
warts, 368t
waste management, 40
Waste Management Branch, Environment Canada, 40
Waste Reduction Week, 40
water
    and breastfeeding babies, 260
    fluid intake, 578
    fluoridation of, 357
    fresh water quality. *See* fresh water quality
    purification issues, 36
water pollution. *See* fresh water quality
*Water Protection Act*, 36
Watson, John B., 156
weaning, 261
wear and tear theory, 555t
weed, 438t–441t
weight
    newborns, 243–244
    school-aged years, 355
    young adults, 458–459
weight concepts, 331
Weight Realities Division, Society for Nutrition Education, 362
well-baby care
    childbirth. *See* childbirth
    childbirth education classes, 136
    delivery, 136–137, 219
    labour, 136–137
    nurse, role of, 134–138
    postpartum period, 137–138
    prenatal care, 135–136
    prenatal development. *See* prenatal development
well elderly, 610–611
well water, 35
wellness, 19
wellness programs, 23
Wen, 67
West Nile virus (WNV), 50
White, Ellen G., 78
whole-being approach, 78
widow, 515, 561
widower, 515
widowhood, 560–561
wisdom, 595t, 599
wisdom teeth, 357
withdrawing reflex, 246t

withdrawn child, 354
women
  see also gender differences; mothers;
    women's health
  battered women, myths and realities,
    505–506
  caregiver role, 560
  and caregiver role, 517
  childbearing age, 468
  depression, 500
  emotional changes related to
    physical changes, 527
  family violence, 503–507
  female climacteric, 524
  female reproductive cycle, 198
  Gilligan's theory of moral
    development, 172–174
  gynecologic cancers, 533
  homemaker, 120
  menarche, 401, 417
  menopause, 513, 524, 525, 526, 527
  menstruation, 402
  moral development, 548, 548t
  perimenopausal years, 524
  sexual harassment, 480–481
  vascularization, 468
  work-life balance, 480
  working, in middle age, 540
women's health
  see also women
  breast cancer, 497
  cervical cancer, 533
  dysmenorrhea, 461
  endometrial cancer, 533
  hormone replacement therapy,
    526–527
  information site, 460
  natural family planning, 462–463
  ovarian cancer, 533
  physical changes and characteristics,
    520t–524t
  premenstrual dysphoric disorder
    (PMDD), 461–462
  premenstrual phenomena, 460–462
  premenstrual syndrome (PMS),
    460–462
  sexual dysfunctions, 463–464
Women's Health Initiative (WHI),
  526–527
Word of Wisdom, 78
work, in middle age, 539–541
work-life balance, 480
work options and attitudes, 479–481
work schedules, 474
Workers' Compensation Act, 43
Workers' Compensation Board, 43
working mothers, 272, 353
workload, 97
Workplace Hazardous Materials
  Information System (WHMIS), 42
workplace health programs, 481

World Commission on Environment and
  Development (WCED), 29
World Health Organization (WHO), 17,
  50, 58, 267, 357, 362, 407, 427–428,
  459, 500, 552
world religions
  see also religion
  Buddhism, 65, 74t
  Christianity, 70–73, 75t
  Confucianism, 66–67
  Golden Rule, 62, 63f
  Hinduism, 62–65, 74t
  Islam, 67–68, 74t
  Jainism, 65–66
  Judaism, 69–70, 74t
  profile of changing world religions
    in Canada, 80–81
  Shintoism, 65, 66
  Sikhism, 65
  similarities, 62
  Taoism, 66–67
Wright, Lorraine, 85
writing skill, 380
Wuest, J., 2

## X

X, 430t
XTC, 430t

## Y

yang, 66
yarmulke, 69
yin, 66
yin-yang symbol, 66
yoga, 64–65, 79
Yom Kippur, 70
young adults
  adaptive mechanisms, 485
  AIDS (acquired immunodeficiency
    syndrome), 490–495
  alcohol, 501
  biological rhythms, 472–473
  body image, 485–487
  cancer, 495–499, 496t
  cardiovascular system, 458
  childbearing age, 468
  cognitive development, 477–479
  cohabitation, 465
  common health problems, 490–508,
    491t–493t
  continuing health promotion, 507
  death, concepts of, 623–624
  developmental crisis, 482
  divorce, 507
  emotional development, 481–484
  emotional health problems, 500–501
  family life cycle, 457
  family planning, 487–490
  family relationships, 457–458
  family violence, 503–507
  formal operations period, 477–478

gambling, 501–502
health prevention, 490–507
health promotion, 490–507
hepatitis C, 499–500
immune system, 458
immunization, 490
injuries, 495
intellectual development, 477
intimacy, 482
leisure, 481
lifestyle and physical illness, 500
lifestyle options, 487
love, 482–483
marriage, 483–484
men's health, 463
moral-spiritual development,
  484–485
musculoskeletal system, 458
nursing goals, 458
nutrition, 468–472
nutrition assessment, 470
obesity, 459, 470
overview, 457
physical development and age,
  458–459
physical fitness and exercise,
  466–468
physical problems, 490–507
psychosocial development,
  477–490
respiratory system, 458
returning home, 512, 513–514
self-concept, 485–487
sexual behaviour variations,
  464–465
sexual dysfunctions, 463–464
sexual-reproductive maturity,
  459–460
sexuality and sexual development,
  459–460
sleep, 474–477
smoking, 502–504
social health problems, 507
stress, 500–501
substance abuse and addiction,
  501, 502
suicide, 500–501
teaching the adult, 479
tuberculosis, 495
values of, 511
weight, 458–459
women's health, 460–463
work options and attitudes,
  479–481
young-old, 552

## Z

Zen sect, 66, 74t
Zentner, J., 3
Zoroastrianism, 67
zygote, 199